LABS ON CHIP

Principles, Design, and Technology

Devices, Circuits, and Systems

Series Editor
Krzysztof Iniewski
CMOS Emerging Technologies Research Inc.,
Vancouver, British Columbia, Canada

PUBLISHED TITLES:

PUBLISHED TITLES:

PUBLISHED TITLES:

Radiation Effects in Semiconductors
Krzysztof Iniewski

Semiconductor Radiation Detection Systems
Krzysztof Iniewski

Smart Grids: Clouds, Communications, Open Source, and Automation
David Bakken

Smart Sensors for Industrial Applications
Krzysztof Iniewski

Technologies for Smart Sensors and Sensor Fusion
Kevin Yallup and Krzysztof Iniewski

Telecommunication Networks
Eugenio Iannone

Testing for Small-Delay Defects in Nanoscale CMOS Integrated Circuits
Sandeep K. Goel and Krishnendu Chakrabarty

VLSI: Circuits for Emerging Applications
Tomasz Wojcicki

Wireless Technologies: Circuits, Systems, and Devices
Krzysztof Iniewski

FORTHCOMING TITLES:

Analog Electronics for Radiation Detection
Renato Turchetta

**Cell and Material Interface: Advances in Tissue Engineering,
Biosensor, Implant, and Imaging Technologies**
Nihal Engin Vrana

Circuits and Systems for Security and Privacy
Farhana Sheikh and Leonel Sousa

CMOS: Front-End Electronics for Radiation Sensors
Angelo Rivetti

CMOS Time-Mode Circuits and Systems: Fundamentals and Applications
Fei Yuan

**Electrostatic Discharge Protection of Semiconductor Devices
and Integrated Circuits**
Juin J. Liou

Gallium Nitride (GaN): Physics, Devices, and Technology
Farid Medjdoub and Krzysztof Iniewski

Implantable Wireless Medical Devices: Design and Applications
Pietro Salvo

FORTHCOMING TITLES:

Laser-Based Optical Detection of Explosives
Paul M. Pellegrino, Ellen L. Holthoff, and Mikella E. Farrell

Mixed-Signal Circuits
Thomas Noulis and Mani Soma

Magnetic Sensors: Technologies and Applications
Simone Gambini and Kirill Poletkin

MRI: Physics, Image Reconstruction, and Analysis
Angshul Majumdar and Rabab Ward

Multisensor Data Fusion: From Algorithm and Architecture Design to Applications
Hassen Fourati

Nanoelectronics: Devices, Circuits, and Systems
Nikos Konofaos

Nanomaterials: A Guide to Fabrication and Applications
Gordon Harling, Krzysztof Iniewski, and Sivashankar Krishnamoorthy

Optical Fiber Sensors: Advanced Techniques and Applications
Ginu Rajan

Optical Imaging and Sensing: Technology, Devices, and Applications
Dongsoo Kim and Ajit Khosla

Physical Design for 3D Integrated Circuits
Aida Todri-Sanial and Chuan Seng Tan

Power Management Integrated Circuits and Technologies
Mona M. Hella and Patrick Mercier

Radiation Detectors for Medical Imaging
Jan S. Iwanczyk and Polad M. Shikhaliev

Radio Frequency Integrated Circuit Design
Sebastian Magierowski

Reconfigurable Logic: Architecture, Tools, and Applications
Pierre-Emmanuel Gaillardon

Soft Errors: From Particles to Circuits
Jean-Luc Autran and Daniela Munteanu

Solid-State Radiation Detectors: Technology and Applications
Salah Awadalla

Wireless Transceiver Circuits: System Perspectives and Design Aspects
Woogeun Rhee

LABS ON CHIP

Principles, Design, and Technology

Eugenio Iannone

Dianax s.r.l. CEO and Founder, Milano, Italy

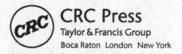

CRC Press
Taylor & Francis Group
Boca Raton London New York

CRC Press is an imprint of the
Taylor & Francis Group, an **informa** business

CRC Press
Taylor & Francis Group
6000 Broken Sound Parkway NW, Suite 300
Boca Raton, FL 33487-2742

First issued in paperback 2017

© 2015 by Taylor & Francis Group, LLC
CRC Press is an imprint of Taylor & Francis Group, an Informa business

No claim to original U.S. Government works

ISBN-13: 978-1-4665-6072-7 (hbk)
ISBN-13: 978-1-138-07628-0 (pbk)

Library of Congress Cataloging-in-Publication Data

Labs on chip : principles, design, and technology / author, Eugenio Iannone.
    pages cm. -- (Devices, circuits, and systems)
  Includes bibliographical references and index.
    ISBN 978-1-4665-6072-7 (hardcover : alk. paper) 1. Labs on a chip. I. Iannone, Eugenio.

QD54.L33L33 2015
542'.284--dc23
    2014015404

Visit the Taylor & Francis Web site at
http://www.taylorandfrancis.com

and the CRC Press Web site at
http://www.crcpress.com

Printed and bound by CPI Group (UK) Ltd, Croydon, CR0 4YY

This book is dedicated to my wife, Flavia, and to my children, Emanuele, Maria Grazia, and Gabriele. I simply would not be who I am without my family, and this book would not have been possible without their continuous encouragement and support.

Contents

SECTION II   Lab on Chip Technology

Preface

I discovered the impressive potentiality of miniaturization and integration very early in my career. In 1984, when I concluded my university studies, IBM on one side and Olivetti on the other side were struggling to reduce computer dimensions. The dream was to shrink into a tabletop machine a system occupying several great closets.

That dream now seems quite old: we hold in our hands electronic devices much more powerful, easier to use, and functionally richer than 1984 computers. Integrated electronics has radically changed our way of living: neither the Internet nor mobile communications would have been possible without it.

Miniaturization has been applied to many fields since the first revolutionary successes: miniaturized optical components, mechanical, chemical and optical sensors, and micro-actuators are present in huge numbers in our homes, in our cars, and even on our person.

Currently, a new revolution seems near the edge, with the potential to change the lifestyle itself all over the world—miniaturized biochemical analysis performed via small, electronic-like chips, called lab on chip.

A lab-on-chip device, also known as a micro-total-analysis system (µTAS), is a device that can integrate miniaturized laboratory functions on a single microprocessor-like chip, such as separation and analysis of components of a mixture. It uses extremely small fluid volumes, nanoliters or even picoliters, thus eliminating the need for large samples.

Integration also promises huge cost reduction, strong resilience, and ease of use, up to conceiving systems that can be used with no training whatsoever.

From the beginning, the first application predicted for this technology was monitoring of human health, even if huge application opportunities also exist in the fields of environmental control, food industry, security, and more.

Extended and inexpensive prevention and screening could be introduced using labs on chip while reducing the need for centralized structures. In-field diagnosis in emergencies can dramatically change the possibility of a correct intervention and save a huge number of human lives. Home monitoring of chronic patients can improve their quality of life while increasing their general health.

In advanced countries, a lab on chip could give a substantial contribution to the required decrease of healthcare expenses while improving the quality of the service. In developing countries, labs on chip can be key in allowing an effective, in-field prevention strategy without the need for expensive structures. An effective prevention and an early solution to small problems can be a way to reduce the number of critical patients in developing countries, allowing the development of a sustainable healthcare system.

The huge potential of the lab-on-chip idea fascinated me ever since I started working in this field several years ago. A huge research effort was made in the past two decades to discover and refine microfluidic systems, biochemistry miniaturization, and new technology processes. Nevertheless, about 20 years were required to arrive at the edge of a widespread introduction of a lab on chip, and a huge scientific, industrial, and engineering research study is still required.

The mere nature of a lab on chip as the synthesis of microfluidic systems, biochemical sensors, and miniaturized technologies is one of the causes of this long struggle. It is practically impossible to collect specific competencies and experiences in all these fields in a single person, and integration between researchers and engineers with different attitudes and skills is a key to succeed in this field. Such an integration is frequently difficult in universities and industries due to the strongly specialized education of technical people and the sectorial structure of many organizations.

This book is meant to be an instrument for such an integration, presenting a global view of the lab-on-chip field. The treatment of each specific subject is intended to provide a path starting with a recap of basic elements and progressing toward advanced concepts typical of a labs-on-chip study. This structure allows the different parts of the book to be useful both for specialists of the sector and for professionals coming from different specializations.

I hope this will be a small but useful contribution to the way of labs-on-chip diffusion causing a widespread, low-cost availability of effective diagnostic and prevention systems to all humankind.

Acknowledgment

I would like to acknowledge Dr. Maurizio Moroni, R&D director of Dianax s.r.l. His experience and passion were invaluable in organizing, refining, and reviewing the biochemical part of this book. I would also like to thank Dr. Giusy Nocca for his help in reviewing selected parts of Chapters 2 and 3.

Finally, I thank the whole Dianax R&D team for the continuous discussions and support.

Author

Eugenio Iannone earned the Italian Laurea degree in engineering (classical version) from Rome University "La Sapienza," Rome, Italy, in 1984.

He was a researcher in Fondazione Ugo Bordoni until 1997, and was engaged in developing new fields in optical communications to which he made relevant contributions. From 1997 to 2009 he joined Pirelli and subsequently worked at Cisco as a research leader in optical communications and as a product management leader.

Since 2009, his main interest has been in the field of industrial research, especially labs on chip. In 2011 he founded the Dianax Study Group, an independent research group active in the lab-on-chip field. Since the end of 2013, he has been the CEO of Dianax s.r.l., a start-up company operating in the same field.

Dr. Iannone is the author of three books on optical communication, among them *Telecommunication Networks* (CRC Press), which was published in 2011. He is also an author of more than 100 papers in peer-reviewcd journals. Dr. Iannone is a member of IEEE-Engineering in Medicine and Biology Society and the American Chemical Society.

Introduction

Miniaturization is one of the key technology elements that have changed human life over the past 60 years, enabling a large number of functions to be packed into a very compact space at a cost that is orders of magnitude less than that of macroscopic equipment performing the same functions.

The most astounding example of miniaturization is microelectronics, but integrated optics also has a wide role especially in sensors and telecommunications. This is demonstrated by the plot in Figure I.1, where the dimension of the channel of CMOS transistors is shown for different generations of microelectronic circuits. In the figure, each step in reducing the CMOS channel width is called a technology node, following the nomenclature used by ITRS (www.itrs.net), the international industry roadmap for semiconductor technology evolution. Miniaturization not only enables huge numbers of chips to be fabricated at a reduced cost, but also permits several different functions to be integrated in the same element, obtaining functionally rich subsystems.

Besides miniaturization, advances in biochemistry and medical chemistry have been a key factor driving progress in the past half century. The discovery of new drugs and capillary diffused medical prevention has cooperated in decreasing dramatically the impact of diseases and dysfunctions in advanced countries, and pervasive environmental control is considered a key point in fighting pollution and other environmental problems caused by human activity. Moreover, the effort to reduce cost and increase the effectiveness of medical resources is promising in that it extends their pervasive penetration to the whole world, creating a unique opportunity to transform human life.

The success of biochemistry and medical chemistry applications is strongly related to miniaturization. The design of advanced analytical systems, analysis of complex organic reactions, and study of biomolecules would all be impossible without the power of microelectronics. However, the idea of miniaturizing the chemical structure itself, that is, to fabricate miniaturized chips implementing analytical biochemical functions, is relatively recent. Different from electronics and optics, where a flow of elementary particles such as photons and electrons is processed, biochemistry deals with large and complex molecules, if not with cells. Frequently, the analysis of samples containing such components requires operations such as purification, pumping, and chemical filtering that are not easy to implement in a chip environment.

There is a large consensus on the fact that the first lab-on-chip prototype to be realized was presented in 1979 [1]: it was a complete gas chromatograph fabricated on a 2 in. (51 mm) silicon wafer. The system was able to separate hydrocarbons from a gas flux in less than 10 s, a quite shorter time period with respect to macroscopic gas chromatography. The main advantages of lab on chip, miniaturization, fast operation, and potential low cost were all present in this early prototype. Nevertheless, the lab-on-chip field was quite a niche in research up to the early 1990s, when researchers and industries worldwide started to realize that this technology could transform completely the way in which chemical and biochemical analysis is performed [2]. It was at that time that the term micro-total analysis systems, with its acronym μ-TAS, was introduced with essentially the same meaning as lab on chip.

In biochemical laboratories, the sample under test is moved from one analysis stage to the other in several different ways. In research, lab sample management is frequently made by hand although, when a high throughput is required, automatized robots are frequently used. Both these methods are not applicable if the whole analysis lab is comprised in a chip. A viable technique to move the sample among different sections of the chip is to adopt fluid dynamic systems that exploit the liquid nature of the sample. Moreover, fluid dynamic structures also allow several functions to be realized with mechanical means, such as filtering, flow rate regulation, mixing and so on.

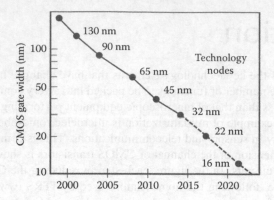

FIGURE I.1 Channel width of different generations (technology nodes) of microelectronic CMOS transistors as defined by International Technology Roadmap for Semiconductors (ITRS).

Fluid dynamic systems can be realized on chip in very small dimensions using the so-called micro-electro-mechanical (MEM) technology. This silicon-based technology was developed to implement a large variety of miniaturized mechanical elements, like membranes for sensor application, moving shutters for miniaturized cameras, suspended cantilevers for accelerometers, and so on. MEM technology is adopted in a large variety of fields such as automotive, portable electronic devices, and electrical appliances, so that billions of MEM chips are produced every year.

As a consequence, earlier research in the field of lab on chip was concentrated on microfluidic functions, with the realization of mixers and valves, micropumps and micro-separation systems. These microfluidic elements have subsequently found application in many other fields too, like fluid-cooled microsystems. In parallel, an intense technology research has been carried out, both for the adaptation of the traditional microelectronic technology to the needs of lab on chip and to introduce other materials like specialized polymers, with suitable microfabrication techniques.

Very encouraging results in the microfluidic field have hastened research toward both miniaturization of the traditional bioanalytical technique and discovery of new techniques optimized for on-chip operation.

Today, complex lab-on-chip prototypes have been presented in the technical literature and the research activity in the field has grown to an impressive volume. This is demonstrated by the plot reported in Figure I.2, where the number of articles published in peer-reviewed journals covering microfluidics and detection systems for application in analytical chemistry and biochemistry is compared with the number of similar articles in the field of microelectronics. After about 20 years

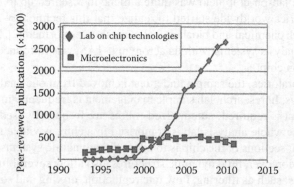

FIGURE I.2 Number of papers published in peer-reviewed scientific and technical journals covering microfluidics and detection systems for application in analytical chemistry and biochemistry compared with the number of peer-reviewed papers in the field of microelectronics.

of research, the time seems to be ripe for marketing a wide variety of industrial products based on the lab on chip concept.

I.1 WHAT IS A LAB ON CHIP?

The most general definition of a lab on chip is a chemical or a biochemical laboratory specifically conceived for a specific chemical process and completely comprised within a single chip. This definition is so wide that some restriction is needed in order to perform a specific analysis of the lab on chip technology, design, and applications. Thus, in this book, we limit our definition of lab on chip by adopting a certain number of assumptions.

First, we limit our attention to biochemical and medical applications: it is not impossible to imagine a lab on chip for application in the field of nonbiological analytical chemistry; as a matter of fact, labs on chip for artificial polymer characterization have been reported in the literature [3–5]. In any case, biological and medical applications dominate both research and industry efforts.

We also assume that a liquid sample is introduced in the lab on chip. This sample is either a natural or an artificial solution containing the analytes to be examined besides several other chemical elements. We thus exclude systems that are designed for gas and environmental analysis [6,7], which in the technical literature are generally called chemical sensors instead of labs on chip.

We will mainly concentrate on systems for molecular analysis, only occasionally considering the analysis of cells and tissues. Large amounts of literature have been produced dealing with labs on chip both for cell counting and activity monitoring [8–10] and for tissue analysis [11,12], producing several promising results. Many differences both in the required tests and in the adopted technology create a clear distinction between labs on chip for molecule processing and for cell processing. Elements of cell processing technologies will in any case be introduced to also provide inside elements in this important field.

The generic functional scheme of a lab on chip, as it is defined here, is presented in Figure 1.3. The chip has a sample input section, performing sample insertion into the system and preparation for subsequent processing. Blood anticoagulation is an example of such a preparation. After the input section, the sample is purified, generally through a cascade of purification stages, each of which eliminates a specific class of unwanted components. After purification, a detection section is present, where the assay is carried out. The assay's results are processed by a processing algorithm that is carried out generally in the external equipment hosting the lab on chip and the results are then presented to the user.

An exception to the general structure of Figure I.3 is labs on chips for selected genetic operations like amplification of nucleic acids by polymerase chain reaction or DNA sequencing (see Chapters 3 and 12). In these cases, the macromolecules to be analyzed are nucleic acids that have

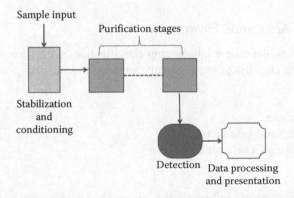

FIGURE I.3 Functional block scheme of a generic lab on chip.

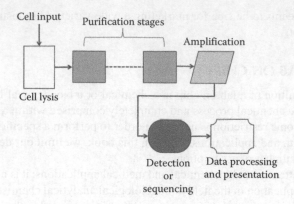

FIGURE I.4 Functional block scheme of a lab on chip for genetic analysis.

to be extracted from cells. Thus, quite frequently, the input sample is constituted by a cell population that is inserted in the input section of the chip where cells are broken and the target macromolecule is isolated to be processed in the following circuit. To allow successive processing, the nucleic acids have to be multiplied by an amplification process generally executed through the reaction, that is known as polymerase chain reaction (see Chapter 2). Once extracted and amplified, the targets can be processed by purification stages and identification tests. In this case, the most complete identification test is the nucleic acid sequencing, providing the detailed molecular structure in terms of its elementary building blocks. The structure of such a lab on chip is presented in Figure I.4.

The situation is somehow similar when cell proteins have to be analyzed. These proteins are present only inside the cell, so that before purification and identification, they have to be extracted from a cell population by breaking the cells in the first stage of the chip.

I.2 LAB-ON-CHIP APPLICATIONS

Lab-on-chip applications are suitable for a wide variety of applications, essentially whenever detection and quantification of a biological molecule within a sample are required. However, lab-on-chip requirements and, consequently, the most suitable design and technology solutions heavily depend on the considered application.

For this reason, a brief analysis of the potential lab-on-chip application fields and of their specific characteristics is fundamental to fully understand the different design and technology choices.

I.2.1 Lab-on-Chip Application Environment

An important application-dependent lab-on-chip classification can be done considering the environment where a lab on chip has to work. Mainly, we have four distinct possibilities, as shown in Figure I.5:

- Research laboratories
- Analysis and industrial laboratories
- Noncontrolled internal environments
- In the field

The target application greatly influences the lab-on-chip design, due to the presence of many specific requirements. A synthesis of application-specific requirements is reported in Table I.1.

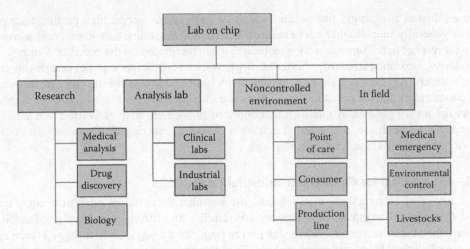

FIGURE I.5 Lab-on-chip classification on the ground of the environment where they are used.

I.2.1.1 Lab on Chip for Research Application

A lab on chip that is built to be used in research laboratories is mainly considered as a research instrument. The main advantage of using a lab on chip for research is its low cost, which takes into account both the low cost of the chip itself and the very low quantity of chemical reagents that have to be used in a lab on chip. Moreover, biochemical assays are generally much faster when operated by a lab on chip. This makes a lab on chip particularly useful when a great number of repeated measurements have to be performed or when very costly reagents are needed if a macroscopic system is used, as in the case of ELISA assays (see Section 3.7.5). In addition, a lab on chip can manage very low-quantity samples that can be a key factor for use in specific research fields.

On the one hand, since they will be used by researchers, who are highly qualified personnel, a particular design to simplify their use is not needed. Moreover, the working environment is controlled from the point of view of contamination, temperature, and mechanical stresses, up to, in a few cases, a clean room (see Section 4.3.1). This means that, in general, packaging is less critical, temperature control and strong resistance to vibrations is not required, and microfluidic interfaces can require a bit of lab work to be operated.

Selected functions can be external to the lab on chip, like detection and pumping: this allows not only a simpler lab-on-chip structure to be fabricated, but also very high sensitivity detection to be

---

TABLE I.1

Qualitative Summary of Application-Specific Requirements for a Lab on Chip

	Research	Analysis Laboratories	Noncontrolled Environments	In the Field
Cost	★★★	★★★	★★★	★★
Sensitivity	★★★	★★★	★★	★★★
Simple external equipment	★★	★	★★★	★★★
In-use resilience	★	★★	★★★	★★★
Storage resilience	★	★	★★★	★★★
Throughput	★	★★★	★	★
Ease of use	★★	★★	★★★	★★★

Note: ★★★—key factor, ★★—important, ★—nice to have.

performed. Just as an example, fluorescence spectroscopy by macroscopic high-performance equipment has generally much higher performances in terms of flexibility, sensitivity, and wavelength range with respect to the same detection technique when integrated on the board of a chip.

Sensitivity, separation efficiency, and the ability to work with different types of samples are important for a lab on chip for research use. The sensitivity has to be at least of the order of their macroscopic counterparts and the possibility to use the same chip for different kinds of assays is important.

To assure a very good assay quality, functionalized surface are frequently used in a lab on chip fabricated for research use, and external detection is also a recurring choice, to assure both high sensitivity and potential use for different assays.

I.2.1.2 Lab on Chip for Clinical and Industrial Laboratories

Besides cost- and performance-related issues, the key characteristics of analytical equipment to be used in a clinical or industrial laboratory are stability and throughput. Very good stability is required to be able to set specific references for the performed assays, such as the reference ranges in the case of clinical blood and urine analysis. Throughput is required by the very high number of repetitive assays that are performed in these cases. As an example, an average European hospital performs 700,000 blood analyses a year, that is an average of 2000 analyses per day, while a big hospital performs 1–2 million blood analyses a year [13,14].

The biggest current expense of a large analysis laboratory is biochemical reagents, so a lab on chip is quite competitive since it allows a drastic reagent quantity reduction. To guarantee suitable throughput, however, a lab on chip has to be designed as a cartridge that can be charged in a high-throughput industrial machine. This particular use influences the package and the various interfaces, which renders quite convenient the use of external detection where high sensitivity is required or when optical detection is used.

Owing to the controlled environment of a laboratory, extreme resilience is not required in this field. However, ease of use is very important due to the highly repetitive nature of operations and the need to work with standard laboratory personnel. Owing to these elements, standards for interface and dimensions are key for diffusion of the lab on chip in this application. Moreover, the use of functionalized surfaces can be the right choice in case it helps to increase sensitivity and selectivity.

I.2.1.3 Lab on Chip for the Noncontrolled Internal Environment

A lab on chip is used in a noncontrolled internal environment when it is not used in a laboratory, but in an environment where no specific care has been undertaken to control environmental conditions and to limit the presence of possible contaminants.

Three important examples of this kind of application are the use at a point of care, consumer use, and use besides an industrial line. If the lab on chip is used in a point of care or at home it has to work without any temperature control and possibly without requiring a horizontal position. If it is used near an industrial line, besides uncontrolled temperature conditions, mechanical vibrations or contaminants can be present.

The point of care and consumer applications also have a supply chain quite different from industrial applications. Operators of a point of care and consumers do not buy materials in volume and use the normal distribution system through dedicated shops such as pharmacies or small representatives of equipment vendors. This fact has a great impact on lab-on-chip design. Standard distribution means potentially a long time in warehouses, transportation through standard means, without particular care to vibrations and temperature changes, and potentially long times of exposition in shops.

Combining the characteristics of the environment where they have to be used with the nature of the distribution system selling them, exceptional resilience is required by this kind of lab on chip, both under uncontrolled environmental conditions and in the possible presence of contaminants. This requirement becomes perhaps the most important one if a lab on chip is designed to be used in an industrial environment.

The need for resilience implies several consequences on the way the system is designed. The package has to be sufficiently robust so as not to suffer vibrations and, if the internal chip does not work correctly in the environmental range of temperatures, temperature stabilization is required inside the package. Interfaces have to be robust, resilient to the contact with potential contaminants. Considering interface contamination, not only do contaminants that are present in the air have to be considered, but also other potential contamination sources, such as contact with fats and dirt that is present on the human skin if the interface is touched by the operator's hands while the lab on chip is being operated.

To obtain long storage time maintaining a wide temperature range and resistance to vibrations, many types of functionalized surfaces cannot be used for such an application. The range of usable biochemical reagents is limited by these requirements, too. The lab-on-chip substrate choice is also influenced, since polymers that tend to to change shape with prolonged temperature changes like polydimethylsiloxane (PDMS) adapt to this application with difficulty.

Labs on chip to be used in point of care, consumer houses, or factories are generally used by persons who are not specifically trained to use them. This means that ease of use and protection from usage errors are fundamental in these fields. To use a lab on chip in a consumer or point of care application, the equipment that is needed to operate the lab on chip has to be as simple as possible, the ideal being to reduce it to a simple electronic support for data elaboration and visualization like a personal computer or smartphone. This requirement strongly encourages the implementation of internal detection. In case of industrial use, the lab on chip has to probably be inserted in dedicated external equipment that can be designed suitably for the specific use.

Finally, the low cost of a lab on chip is frequently a key enabler for these applications that would be impossible in many cases with macroscopic analytic equipment.

I.2.1.4 Lab on Chip for In-Field Use

A lab on chip is designed for in-field use when it is transported to the place where some particular biochemical analysis has to be performed and operates there. Examples are a lab on chip for medical use in emergency situations or systems for monitoring environmental water, rains, and similar liquids.

A lab on chip is particularly suited for this kind of application because of their small dimension, small quantity of used reactants, simpler or no assay preparative procedure, and the possibility of integrating it with a general-purpose electronic device with the consequent possibility of direct transmission of assay data over great distances through a telecommunication network. In addition, assays performed through a lab on chip are generally much faster than corresponding assays performed with standard biochemical equipment, a key property if obtaining data in a brief time period is at a premium.

Opening this large field of possibilities, however, also requires systems with very high performance in terms of reliability, ease of use, and cost.

Not only should the lab on chip have to be resistant to long-term storage in the presence of variable environmental conditions, as happens during storage on an ambulance waiting for use, but also mechanical vibrations can be present during use, as in the case of the test of environmental water from a boat while travelling on a river. During medical emergencies, patients have to be assisted in several different ways and in complex situations, and therefore one can imagine that the most suitable position for lab-on-chip use cannot be attained, for example, if a patient is in an almost vertical position or being held with a single hand.

As far as the cost is concerned, its importance depends on the diffusion and use of such a lab on chip. In the case of environmental control, for example, a very wide diffusion can be envisioned, which can be enabled only by a very low cost. In case of a medical emergency, where using the correct and less-invasive therapy is strictly related to the knowledge of key analytical data, cost is relatively less important, as long as it is kept low.

I.2.2   ANALYTE-RELATED LAB ON CHIP CHARACTERISTICS

Another possibility for a rough classification of labs on chip is to look at the nature of the target analyte. From this point of view, we can individuate roughly four classes of systems, as shown in Figure I.6:

- Lab on chip for element and small molecule quantization
- Lab on chip for dissolved macro-molecule quantization and activity analysis
- Lab on chip for intracellular macromolecule analysis
- Lab on chip for cell analyses

The analytical and separation methods implemented in the lab on chip critically depend on the target nature and on the assay scope.

When cells are present in the sample, as in the cases of blood, milk, as and many other natural samples, they are first separated by the liquid content that is generally a water solution of molecules and ions. This operation can be done either on a chip or externally, depending on the application. On-chip cell separation is generally carried out by hydrodynamic filtering (see Section 8.5.1) or by suitable membranes (see Section 8.5). Depending on the required assay, either the cell content or the liquid residue is maintained in the chip.

I.2.2.1   Dissolved Targets

In case small molecules or ions have to be analyzed, further purification of the liquid residue could be required with very selective methods such as micro-dialysis, allowing the macromolecule content to be reduced and a suitable assay to be prepared for the desired target. If dissolved macromolecules have to be selected, ions are in general to be maintained in the solution to assure the correct pH value. Separation methods such as different types of micro-electrophoresis (see Section 8.5.2) can be used to purify the target before the assay.

The adopted detection method is usually selected on the grounds of target properties, required sensitivity, and system complexity. Electronic detection is simple to implement in the chip, even if a certain amount of data processing is required, and has the advantage of requiring neither external optical interfaces nor integration of optically active components on the board of the chip. However, electronic detection has its own weaknesses.

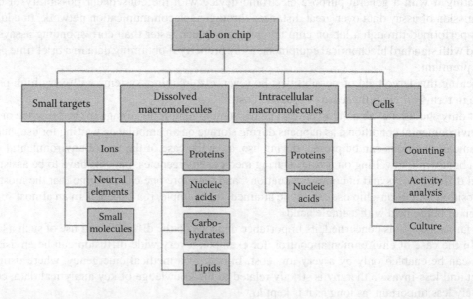

FIGURE I.6   Lab-on-chip classification by target.

Calorimeter detection is practically limited to a sufficiently exothermic process that is a rarely fulfilled condition in reactions among macromolecules. Thus, calorimetric detection use in the lab on chip is limited to particular cases. Purely mechanical detection, for example, through micro-cantilevers, is more suitable for use with macromolecules, but it requires activated surfaces and mobile parts on the chip, being not completely suitable for applications where high resilience versus temperature and mechanical vibrations is required.

Faradaic electrochemical detection requires the presence of RedOx couples, which is frequently the situation for lab-on-chip targets, and it can be performed without the need to fix the target on an activated surface as in the case of cyclic voltammetry (see Section 10.3.2). Even if electrochemical detection methods generally require a certain amount of data processing, it is in general not a problem, unless the system is meant to be used in an electromagnetic interference reach environment. Thus, in the presence of RedOx targets, electrochemical detection is a good candidate for a large set of applications.

A further advantage of electrochemical detection is the ability to provide information on the target species besides its quantization. As an example, the RedOx reaction rate can be evaluated through electrochemical detection and enzyme activity can also be detected and analyzed.

If the target does not reduce or oxidize easily, electrochemical detection is limited to non-Faradaic impedance sensing, which has limitations when complex samples are present, where the target is accompanied by several other molecules and when the sample composition is not well known.

Optical detection, either through plasma resonance or absorption and fluorescence spectroscopy, assures very good detection performances and can be adopted for almost all the target substances. The drawbacks of optical detection are the necessity of either managing external optical interfaces or integrating optically active components on the chip.

When the external optical interface is simply a transparent window on the chip package surface, coupling external sources and detectors with the assay chamber on the chip is a small problem. This configuration allows external optical systems to be coupled with the chip, fully exploiting the capabilities of tunable, high power and small linewidth lasers and high sensitivity optical systems. However, complex external equipment is required in this case, so that this solution is practically suitable only for application in laboratories.

A simpler system can be obtained by adopting an optical interface based on fiber optics (see Section 6.5.4) and integrating the optical transmitter/receiver in a small external equipment adopting semiconductor lasers and photodiodes. Semiconductor optics has been developed at an industrial level in the infrared and red regions for telecommunications and for consumer electronics so that compact equipment can be obtained at a cost in the consumer electronics range. In addition, if a fiber optics interface is adopted, on-chip interferometry can also be adopted, with the possibility of integrating all the optical circuits on the chip.

In the most frequent case, the lab on chip is a disposable element, so that it has to be hosted into a pluggable package to be inserted in the external equipment. In this case, the optical interface has to be exposed out of the package and suitably protected from the environment and from possible damages at the moment of the plug-in. Such an external optical interface system, while fully developed for other applications, has hardly a cost compatible with a disposable element that has to be used in very large volumes. Thus, this solution is suitable for premium applications, but adapts with difficulty to applications where a very low price is the key requirement, such as consumer medical use.

I.3 BOOK FOCUS AND USE

The field of a lab on chip, like an analogous field in the biotechnology area, is characterized by a strong multidisciplinary nature: a strong physical knowledge of both fluid dynamics and molecular phenomena has to be accompanied by a clear vision of the involved biological processes; sophisticated mathematical methods used for lab-on-chip design have to team with deep chemical analysis of the interactions between the different species and a solid technology experience, allowing technology potentialities and limitations to be fully taken into account.

It is practically impossible to collect all these competencies and experiences in a single person, and integration between researchers and engineers with different aptitudes and skills is a key to succeed in this field.

This book is meant to be an instrument for such an integration, presenting a global view of the lab-on-chip field. Each subject is analyzed starting from a summary of basic principles and concluding with a detailed description of the aspects that are relevant in the field of lab on chip. This structure allows the different parts of the book to be useful both for specialists in the sector and for other professionals working in the lab-on-chip sector coming from different scientific cultures.

Requisite for a full exploitation of this book's potential is the technical knowledge typical of an engineer, a molecular biologist or a biochemical expert, or a professional in applied physics. An advanced PhD student in these disciplines can find this book very useful to recover unity between the different aspects of the study of a lab on chip.

I.3.1 EXAMPLES OF POTENTIAL USERS OF THIS BOOK ARE ...

The industrial research and development leader, who can have a clear and complete idea of the field without neglecting key elements that are beyond his or her core area of competence. Owing to its strong focus on interdependence, the book offers critical guidance in the decision process and could well become a working instrument for technical and marketing managers.

The designer, who can have a global idea of new technologies so as to channel his or her work in the most suitable direction and to make design choices having a complete view of the possible alternatives.

The university professor, who can exploit the book's architecture to propose a strongly multidisciplinary approach to this field to his or her students. The book is also useful to help structure an up-to-date university course in tune with the latest trends. Finally, a university professor can also use this book to update himself or herself on aspects of microfluidics and related technology that fall out of the core area of his competencies.

The senior student, who can use this book to decide where to direct his or her activity and to acquire an organized view of the application and technical environment.

I.4   BOOK STRUCTURE

The book is divided into three parts. Section I is devoted to recalling important elements of organic chemistry and biochemistry with specific attention to standard and innovative methods of analytical biochemistry. This section is intended to assist engineers, physicists, and technology experts in becoming familiar with the biochemical elements required to work on labs on chip without dispersing in the huge technical literature that has been produced.

Special care is paid in this section to introduce gradually the specific language of molecular biology in those areas relevant for lab-on-chip applications. Properties of artificial polymers are also discussed in Chapter 1, since these materials are often used for lab-on-chip fabrication.

Section II is focused on fabrication technologies for labs on chip. The field of planar technologies and polymer microfabrication is huge and it is virtually impossible to review them all in a book section. Section II focuses on the technologies of choice for labs on chip, even if this implies neglecting important processes that are widely diffused and used sometimes also in the lab-on-chip sector. This is the case, for example, of silicon doping techniques or of technologies based on the use of III–V materials. Details of these technologies can be found in the widely reported bibliography at the end of each chapter.

Particular attention is devoted to process scalability to huge volumes, based on the assumption that labs on chip will enter the market as protagonists only if they are to be pervasively present in healthcare and biotechnology industrial processes. Thus, the cost model of silicon-based planar technology is discussed in some detail in Chapter 4 and techniques such as design for testing and test location along the process chain are evidenced in Chapters 4 and 6.

Section III, the longest section, is devoted to lab-on-chip design techniques. Whenever a working principle or a design technique is considered, the main physical and chemical principles are summarized and specific quantitative models are derived that are of help in real component design. Almost only analytical models are considered, with the aim of combining quantitative design and performance evaluation with a fundamental understanding of the trends related to a change in the value of the main design parameters. In all considered cases, the mathematical derivation of the model is kept as general as possible and the performed approximations are well evidenced so that the approach to a more accurate numerical solution of the governing equation should be easier starting from the presented analysis.

Chapters 7 and 8 are devoted completely to the discussion of microfluidic techniques related to labs on chip. The aspects rendering microfluidic phenomena so different from phenomena taking place in macroscopic fluids flow are derived in Chapter 7 from the base equations of fluid motions, and the main elements of fluid motion and solute dynamics are detailed in the same chapter in addition to a discussion on the interaction between fluid motion and static electromagnetic fields.

Microfluidic building blocks used in lab on chips such as fluid dynamic filters, microvalves and micropumps are discussed in Chapter 8.

Chapter 9 is devoted to that part of surface physics and chemistry that is relevant to lab-on-chip technology. This mainly relates to surface functionalization with molecular layers either to catalyze specific reactions in proximity of a surface or to provide selective immobilization of assay targets. At the end of the chapter, a brief exercise in the field of cell immobilization in lab-on-chip structures is also presented. A few compromises have been made while constructing this chapter. Since a huge number of different chemical species and reactions are presented, chemical and biochemical properties are frequently not presented in detail, but a bibliography allowing the interested reader to explore in depth as needed is supplied.

Attention is paid instead to the scalability characteristics of the considered processes and to their integration into the process flow of a lab on chip. In this framework, the issue of stability of functionalized surfaces is considered in some detail.

Detection techniques are considered in Chapters 10 and 11, where electronic and optical detection techniques are reviewed. An important choice was made in Chapter 11 regarding the review of electromagnetic properties of matter. A satisfactory description of the interaction of the electromagnetic radiation with matter can be carried out only within a complete quantum model, where both atomic systems and the electromagnetic fields are described using quantum mechanics. While a description of quantum mechanical properties of atomic systems in normal conditions can be carried out using classical quantum mechanics, essentially based on the Schrödinger equation, this is not true for the electromagnetic field.

Reviewing even briefly in this book the quantum field theory is simply impossible; it is quite far in general from the lab-on-chip field and even a minimal review would occupy too much space and would require a background that only theoretical physicists, in general, have. However, a classical description based on the pure phenomenological introduction of the wavelength dependence of the material electromagnetic parameter would hide almost completely the underlying physical dynamics.

Our choice was to qualitatively introduce the concept of a photon and to adopt the Einstein theory to describe absorption and fluorescence, where the fully quantized interaction between molecules and light is completely evident. Under a theoretical physics point of view, the Einstein theory is a quite old tool box, with the main defect of not taking into account correlations between the molecular populations in the different energy levels. In any case, the obtained results are valid in a sufficiently wide range of practical parameters in the case of absorption and provide a good qualitative explanation of the fluorescence dependence on the main system parameters. However, the use of the more correct optical Block equations for the density matrix has been considered beyond the scope of this book.

A whole chapter is devoted to a lab on chip for genetics at the end of Section III, since their design has many specific aspects when the genetic material is extracted from cells by an on-chip process or when sequencing is performed on the chip.

REFERENCES

1. Terry S. C., Jerman J. H., Angell J. B., Gas chromatographic air analyzer fabricated on a silicon wafer, *Transaction on Electronic Devices*, vol. 26, pp. 1880–1886, 1979.
2. Manz A., Graber N., Widmer H. M., Miniaturized total chemical analysis systems: A novel concept for chemical sensing, *Sensors and Actuators B: Chemical*, vol. 1, pp. 244–248, 1990.
3. Li W. et al., Multi-step microfluidic polymerization reactions conducted in droplets: The internal trigger approach, *Journal of American Chemical Society*, vol. 130, pp. 9935–9941, 2008.
4. Voicu D. et al., Kinetics of multicomponent polymerization reaction studied in a microfluidic format, *Macromolecules*, vol. 45, pp. 4469–4475, 2012.
5. Tonhauser C., Natalello A., Löwe H., Frey H., Microflow technology in polymer synthesis, *Macromolecules*, vol. 45, pp. 9551–9570, 2012.
6. Banica F.-G., *Chemical Sensors and Biosensors: Fundamentals and Applications*, Wiley, New York, NY; 1st edition (October 4, 2012), ISBN-13: 978-0470710678.
7. Fraden J., *Handbook of Modern Sensors: Physics, Designs, and Applications*, Springer, Berlin, Germany; 4th edition (September 29, 2010), ISBN-13: 978-1441964656.
8. El-Ali J., Sorger P. K., Jensen K. F., Cells on chip, *Nature*, vol. 442, pp. 403–411, 2006.
9. Gupta K., Kim D. H., Ellison D., Smith C., Kundu A., Tuan J., Suh K. Y., Levchenko A., Lab-on-a-chip devices as an emerging platform for stem cell biology, *Lab on a Chip*, vol. 10, pp. 2019–2031, 2010.
10. Bahnemann J. et al., A new integrated lab-on-a-chip system for fast dynamic study of mammalian cells under physiological conditions in bioreactor, *Cells*, vol. 2, pp. 349–360, 2013.
11. Hwang C. M., Khademhosseini A., Park Y., Sun K., Lee S. H., Microfluidic chip-based fabrication of plga microfiber scaffolds for tissue engineering, *Langmuir*, vol. 24, pp. 6845–6851, 2008.
12. Baker M., Tissue models: A living system on a chip, *Nature*, vol. 471, pp. 661–665, 2011.
13. Burtis C. A., Bruns D. E., *Tietz Fundamentals of Clinical Chemistry*, Saunders, Philadelphia, PA; 6th edition (November 20, 2007), ISBN-13: 978-0721638652.
14. McKenzie S. B., *Clinical Laboratory Hematology*, Prentice-Hall, Upper Saddle River, NJ; 2nd edition (2010), ISBN-13: 978-0135137321.

Section I

Biological Chemistry

1 Elements of Organic Chemistry

1.1 INTRODUCTION

As the name suggests, a lab on chip is a microscopic chemical laboratory that implements chemical reactions, generally for biological sensing applications, in a microscopic environment.

By using small amount of reagents, the nature of the chemical processes that takes place in a lab on chip is not qualitatively different from those realized in macroscopic systems, except that chemical reactions frequently do not happen in mechanical equilibrium, but are realized while the fluid containing the reagents moves [1,2].

A frequent example of this out-of-equilibrium situation is realized in a diffusion-driven micro-reactor. In this case, the microfluidic system is designed to implement the reaction between two chemical species both in diluted solution in the same solvent. The first solution is precharged into a reaction chamber, while the second is contained in a feeding duct divided by the reaction chamber by a valve. When the valve is open, no macroscopic fluid movement happens, due to the fact that the two diluted solutions are based on the same solvent.

As far as the solutes are concerned, the solute from the feeding duct diffuses into the reaction chamber and also the solute in the reaction chamber diffuses into the ducts. During diffusion of the species, they come in contact and react. Thus both reagents and the reaction product diffuse in the reaction room.

These and other similar situations can be analyzed by mixed chemical and mechanical models that join fluid dynamics elements with chemical elements.

In order to set up all the tools needed to introduce and analyze similar complex, out-of-equilibrium situations, we will start in this chapter to review a set of basic physical and chemical properties of solutions with particular attention to biological situations.

1.2 THERMODYNAMIC AND CHEMICAL PROPERTIES OF SOLUTIONS

1.2.1 THERMODYNAMIC STATE FUNCTIONS

In its general definition, a thermodynamic system [3] is described by a number of thermodynamic parameters, for example, temperature, volume, and pressure, which are not necessarily independent, but that are sufficient to completely individuate the macroscopic equilibrium state of the system.

This means that when the system is in mechanical and chemical equilibrium, that is, no motion of its parts happens and no chemical reaction is ongoing, all the macroscopic physical and chemical variables of the system can be evaluated if the state parameters are known. If we introduce a Euclidean space where the state parameters are the °coordinates, the equilibrium state of the system can be represented as a point in the state space.

The minimum number of parameters needed to describe the system is the dimension of the state space of the system (D). For example, a monatomic gas with a fixed number of particles is a simple case of a two-dimensional system (D = 2). In this example, any system is uniquely specified by two parameters, such as pressure and volume, or perhaps pressure and temperature. These choices are equivalent: they are simply different coordinate systems in the two-dimensional thermodynamic state space. An analogous statement holds for higher-dimensional spaces.

We can conceive a very slow transformation of the system so that in every moment the system is practically in an equilibrium state. This transformation is called "reversible" and it can be represented as a curve in the space state since all the intermediate states are equilibrium states with a very good approximation. It is to be observed that reversible reactions are not necessarily slow under a commonsense point of view: they can also be quite fast if considered on the typical human time scale. An important characteristic of reversible transformations is that all the thermodynamic coordinates can be univocally defined for the whole systems: for example, no relevant temperature or pressure gradient exists through the system.

For example, in a reversible transformation of a gas, we might have that pressure and volume vary with time, but in any instant, they have a single value through all the volume occupied by the gas. In this case, for example, the work operated by the gas during the transformation can be expressed as a function of the state variables as

$$W(t_1, t_0) = \int_{t_0}^{t_1} P(t) \frac{dV(t)}{dt} \, dt \tag{1.1}$$

It is clear that in order to calculate the work $W(t_1, t_0)$ in the above integral, we will have to know the functions $P(t)$ and $V(t)$ at each time t, over the entire path. A state function is a function of the parameters of the system which only depends on the parameters' values at the end points of the path. For example, suppose we wish to calculate the finite variation of the function

$$\Psi = P(t)V(t) \tag{1.2}$$

along a reversible transformation. We would have

$$\Delta\Psi(t_1, t_0) = \int_{t_0}^{t_1} \left[P(t) \frac{dV(t)}{dt} + V(t) \frac{dP(t)}{dt} \right] dt = P(t_1)V(t_1) - P(t_0)V(t_0) = \Psi(t_1) - \Psi(t_0) \tag{1.3}$$

It can be seen that the integrand can be expressed as an exact differential; therefore, it depends only on the end points of the integration path. The product PV is a state function of the system.

There are state variables that do not depend on the mass of the system: in particular, if we add mass to the system without changing the system state, these variables do not change. Examples of such state variables are the pressure against the external environment, the temperature, and, as we will see, the chemical potential. Such state variables are called intensive variables.

On the contrary, there are state variables, called extensive variables, that are simply proportional to the mass of the system. This means that if we add mass to the system, in order not to change the value of the intensive variables that somehow determine the qualitative part of the system status, extensive variables have to be scaled with the mass.

Basic thermodynamic equations associate intensive and extensive variables always at the same way.

For example, the heat is given by TdS, where the temperature is an intensive variable and the entropy is an extensive variable. In all definitions of thermodynamic function, due to the meaning of the term TdS, these variables always appear coupled, while we never find, for example, a term PdS.

As far as pressure P is concerned, it is always coupled with volume, due to the meaning of the term PdV that represents the work against the external pressure.

When a couple of variables are related in this way, the variables are called conjugated, so that the temperature is the conjugated variable of entropy, the pressure is the conjugated variable of the volume, and the number of particles is the conjugated variable of the chemical potential.

In a theoretical treatment of thermodynamics, the concept of conjugated variables can be introduced in a much more formal way in a framework similar to that used in analytical mechanics; however, here we recall certain fundamental definitions of thermodynamics that will be necessary in the development of the book, and a theoretical approach is beyond the scope of this book. The interested reader is encouraged to use the numerous theoretical books on thermodynamics for an in-depth knowledge on these aspects [4,5].

1.2.1.1 Enthalpy

The first important thermodynamic state function we want to introduce is enthalpy.

Enthalpy is a measure of the total energy of a thermodynamic system. It includes the internal energy, which is the energy required to create a system, and the amount of energy required to make room for it by displacing its environment and establishing its volume and pressure.

Enthalpy is a state function, frequently also called thermodynamic potential due to its role in stating the equilibrium states of a system, and it is an extensive quantity, that is, for a fixed system state it is proportional to the system's overall mass.

The enthalpy of a system is defined as

$$H = U + PV \qquad (1.4)$$

where H is the enthalpy, U is the internal energy, P is the pressure at the boundary of the system and its environment, and V is the volume of the system.

The expression of the enthalpy has an important physical meaning that makes it useful in a great number of practical applications.

As a matter of fact, the U term is equivalent to the energy required to create the system starting from it base components, and the term PV is equivalent to the energy that would be required to "make room" for the system if the pressure of the environment remained constant.

The meaning of this last term may be understood by the following example of an isobaric process. Consider gas changing its volume (by, e.g., a chemical reaction) in a cylinder, pushing a piston, maintaining constant pressure P.

If the piston has an area equal to A, the force exerted by the gas on the piston can be written as $F = PA$. By definition, the work W done is $W = Fd$, where d is the piston displacement. From the two expressions, we obtain that the work done by the internal chemical reaction to "make place" to the volume increase against the external pressure is exactly $W = P\Delta V$.

Including this PV term into the enthalpy expression (1.4) means that during constant pressure expansion any internal energy forfeited as work on the environment does not affect the value of enthalpy. The enthalpy change can thus be defined as

$$\Delta H = \Delta U + W = \Delta U + \Delta(PV) \qquad (1.5)$$

where ΔU is the thermal energy lost to expansion, and W the energy gained due to work done on the external environment.

Owing to the meaning we have underlined, the enthalpy is the preferred expression of system energy changes in many physical measurements, because it simplifies the description of energy transfer. This is because a change in enthalpy takes account of energy transferred to the environment through the expansion of the system under study.

In chemical reaction happening at constant pressure without change of volume, enthalpy takes a different role. As a matter of fact, if the pressure is constant and the only work done by the system performing reaction is due to change of volume, from the first principle of thermodynamics the enthalpy identifies with the heat released or absorbed during the reaction.

Thus, in this case, the change ΔH is positive in endothermic reactions, and negative in exothermic processes.

In correspondence of this chemical meaning, several standard ways are defined to measure the enthalpy variation in particular processes.

Frequently, owing to the fact that these are standard definitions, the fact that we are dealing with an enthalpy difference is dropped, simply talking about enthalpy of the process.

A few relevant standard enthalpy definitions are

- Enthalpy of reaction, defined as the enthalpy change observed when 1 mole of substance reacts completely
- Enthalpy of formation, defined as the enthalpy change observed when 1 mole of a compound is formed from its elementary antecedents
- Enthalpy of combustion, defined as the enthalpy change observed when 1 mole of a substance combusts completely with oxygen
- Enthalpy of hydrogenation, defined as the enthalpy change observed when 1 mole of an unsaturated compound reacts completely with an excess of hydrogen to form a saturated compound
- Enthalpy of atomization, defined as the enthalpy change required to atomize 1 mole of compound completely
- Enthalpy of neutralization, defined as the enthalpy change observed when 1 mole of water is produced when an acid and a base react
- Standard Enthalpy of solution, defined as the enthalpy change observed when 1 mole of a solute is dissolved completely in an excess of solvent

It is also useful to derive and expression of enthalpy as a function of the system entropy S since frequently we are in front of entropy-driven processes, that is, processes that happen spontaneously due to the fact that the overall system entropy increases.

This expression can be derived starting from the fundamental relation linking entropy with the internal energy for reversible processes, which is written as

$$dU = TdS - PdV \tag{1.6}$$

Adding VdP to both members we immediately obtain

$$dH = TdS + VdP \tag{1.7}$$

This is the required expression of the enthalpy as a function of the entropy.

1.2.1.2 Gibbs Free Energy

The Gibbs free energy, another extensive thermodynamic state function, is perhaps the most used state function in chemical applications. The free energy definition, which immediately qualifies it as a state function since it is defined as a combination of state functions, is

$$G = H - TS \tag{1.8}$$

In order to understand the importance of the Gibbs free energy, let us imagine to have a constant temperature and constant pressure transformation. These are the conditions in which more frequent chemical reactions happen. So it is very useful to consider this particular case if we mainly consider chemical reactions. In these conditions, we can write the following relations:

$$dU = dH - PdV \tag{1.9a}$$

$$dH = TdS + PdV \tag{1.9b}$$

Since T is kept constant like P, combining the above equations we get

$$dG = d(H - TS) = 0 \qquad (1.10)$$

This is an important conclusion, telling us that in constant temperature and pressure processes, the equilibrium state is characterized by a null variation of the Gibbs free energy.

Since any move from equilibrium will decrease the work below its maximum value PdV, it is immediate to evaluate that if an equilibrium state is moved out of equilibrium by an infinitesimal change of a system variable, the Gibbs free energy, that can be still defined due to the fact that we are out of equilibrium only for an infinitesimal change, tends to increase.

Thus, we can conclude that, considering all the states sufficiently near to an equilibrium so that the Gibbs free energy can be globally defined, the equilibrium state is characterized by the minimum free energy. This principle is somehow the chemical version of the general principle of classical mechanics stating that stable states correspond to a minimum of energy and it justifies the name of free energy for the state function G.

This principle has an important extension if applied to chemical reactions. Let us imagine a chemical reaction bringing the system from state S_0 to state S_1 and be able to determine not only the free energy change ΔG related to the transformation but also the free energy of all the intermediate states $S(t)$, which are all equilibrium states due to the hypothesis of reversible transformation.

We have several possible cases that are shown in Figure 1.1 and that corresponds to different types of chemical reactions:

1. $\Delta G < 0$ and $G(t)$ always decrease along the transformation; in this case the chemical reaction is spontaneous, bringing the system from the initial to the final state as soon as it assembles by joining its components.
2. $\Delta G < 0$ and $G(t)$ first increases then decreases: the reaction would bring to a decrease of free energy, but it does not happen spontaneously due to an initial potential wall to overcome; in order to obtain the reaction, a quantity of energy equal to $\Delta_i G$ has to be provided to the system, for example, via heating. In this case the heat does not increase the system temperature, but starts the reaction. However, when the reaction arrives in the spontaneous part of the transformation (where $G(t)$ is decreasing) an amount of energy equal to $\Delta G - \Delta_i G > \Delta_i G$ is released.

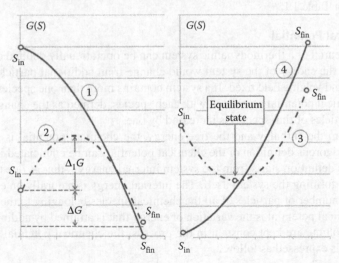

FIGURE 1.1 Different kinds of constant temperature and pressure chemical reactions depending on the value of the free energy variation along the transformation. The numbers linked to the curves relate to the different types of chemical reactions cited in the text.

TABLE 1.1
Example Values of the Free Energy of Formation for a Few Substances Both in kJ/Mole and in kcal/Mole

Substance	State (Standard Condition)	$\Delta_f G°$(kJ/Mole)	$\Delta_f G°$(kcal/Mole)
NH_3	Gas	−12.67	−3.976
H_2O	Liquid	−237.13	−56.69
H_2O	Gas	−228.6	−54.64
CO_2	Gas	−394.4	−94.26
CO	Gas	−137.2	−32.81
CH_4	Gas	−50.5	−12.14
C_2H_6	Gas	−25.05	−7.86
C_3H_8	Gas	−23.4	−5.614
C_8H_{18}	Gas	13.19	4.14
$C_{10}H_{22}$	Gas	26.23	8.23

3. $\Delta G > 0$ and $G(t)$ always increases along the transformation; the transformation is not spontaneous, in order to obtain it an amount of energy equal to ΔG has to be provided to the system.
4. $\Delta G > 0$ and $G(t)$ first decreases and then increases along the transformation; in this case the system spontaneously arrives to the equilibrium state with minimal free energy and does not spontaneously evolve beyond it.

The standard Gibbs free energy of formation of a compound is the change of Gibbs free energy that accompanies the formation of 1 mole of that substance from its component elements, at their standard states, that is, at a temperature of 25°C and at a pressure of 100 kPa. Its symbol is $\Delta_f G$.

All elements in their standard states (oxygen gas, graphite, etc.) have 0 standard Gibbs free energy of formation, as no changes are involved to obtain them from their pure molecular state.

To provide an idea of the standard Gibbs free energy of formation of a few chemical species, we report its values in Table 1.1.

1.2.1.3 Chemical Potential

The chemical potential of a thermodynamic system can be operationally defined on the basis of the amount by which the energy of the system would change if an additional particle was introduced, with the entropy and volume held fixed. If a system contains more than one species of particle, there is a separate chemical potential associated with each species, defined as the change in energy when the number of particles of that species is increased by one.

Differently from the enthalpy and the free energy, the chemical potential is an intensive state variable. A more rigorous definition of the chemical potential can be enunciated in different ways.

The most basic definition starts from the system internal energy—that is, due to the interactions from the particles forming the system itself. The internal energy is naturally an extensive variable, depending on the number of particles of all the chemical species belonging to the system.

Since the chemical potential is the variation of energy that is attained by adding a particle, if the entropy and the volume are kept constant in the process, the chemical potential of the ith species inside the system is expressed as follows:

$$\mu_i = \frac{\partial U(S,V,N_1,\ldots,N_n)}{\partial N_i}\bigg|_{S,V,N_{j\neq i}} \tag{1.11}$$

where N_1, N_2, and N_n are the numbers of molecules of the n species that are present in the system and the indices of the derivative indicate what variables have to be kept constant.

It is not so frequent in practical systems that the entropy and the volume are kept constant, thus even if the definition (1.11) has a clear physical meaning, it is not easily applicable. The conditions that are generally realized, also in reactions happening in labs on chip, are pressure and temperature constancy. In labs on chip, generally, temperature constancy is explicitly assured by a cooling system, while pressure constancy comes out from the system structure.

In this condition, we have seen that the energy of the system can be expressed through the Gibbs free energy, so that a much more operative definition of the chemical potential is

$$\mu_i = \left. \frac{\partial G(P, T, N_1, \ldots, N_n)}{\partial N_i} \right|_{P, T, N_{j \neq i}} \tag{1.12}$$

The chemical potential is particularly important when studying systems of reacting particles or systems consisting of one or more species in different states of aggregation. Consider the simplest case of two states of aggregation of one species that are in equilibrium in the sense that the mass of each of them remains constant. We can consider liquid water in equilibrium with water vapor. If the system is at equilibrium, the chemical potentials of the two species must be equal.

This is due to the fact that, for the definition of chemical potential itself, subtracting a particle to the species at higher potential generates more energy than the energy that is needed to add a particle to the species at lower potential. This implies an energy release by the system that in this way moves toward states with lower free energy; thereby realizing a spontaneous transformation as we have seen in the previous section. This transformation continues up to the moment in which the chemical potentials are kept equal or up to the moment in which one of the two states disappears; that means that in the considered conditions, the equilibrium between vapor and liquid states is not possible.

This principle enables us to understand that chemical potentials are involved in the evaluation of the equilibrium conditions of also more complex situations like a chemical reaction. This is true, but the description of the way in which this happens, that is, the so-called law of mass action is not trivial (compare Section 1.2.3); to introduce this important law for chemical equilibrium, we have to introduce the chemistry of solutions.

1.2.1.4 Quasi-Equilibrium State and Local Thermodynamic State Functions

When analyzing labs on chip, chemical reactions sometimes happens in a situation of only approximate mechanical equilibrium, for example, while slow diffusion or fluid motion happens.

In these cases, different phenomena time scales have to be compared with the time resolution of the performed observation. Phenomena that are very fast with respect to the time resolution of the measurement system are not resolved in time so that they are simply detected in their equilibrium state. This is, for example, the case of the great part of antigen–antibody neutralizations (see Section 3.7), whose dynamic is very fast with respect to the typical time resolution of labs on chip detectors. Phenomena that are very slow with respect to the integration time are well resolved, so that the percentage variation between subsequent measures is very small.

When fast and slow phenomena coexist, for example, when antibody–antigen neutralization happens while the different chemical species slowly diffuses in solution, the problem arises to define thermodynamic variables regulating the fast chemical part of the evolution. In this case, the so-called adiabatic approximation can be used, where the slow mechanical evolution can be considered not to alter a local thermodynamic equilibrium of the system, but only causing it to change in a reversible manner. In this approximation, intensive variables such as pressure and temperature are defined as fields in the volume of the system, while extensive variables are defined as densities that also depend on time and space. This is the key approximation that allows the use of thermodynamic I fluidic systems and it will be largely used in Chapters 7 through 10.

In this framework, we can define an entropy density (measured in J/K/m³), an enthalpy density (measured in J/m³), and a free energy density (measured in J/m³) so that, for example, the global entropy in a volume V and its deviation can be expressed as

$$S(t) = \int_V s(\boldsymbol{r},t)\, d^3\boldsymbol{r} \tag{1.13a}$$

$$\delta^2 S(t) = \int_V s^2(\boldsymbol{r},t)\, d^3\boldsymbol{r} - \frac{1}{V}\left[\int_V s(\boldsymbol{r},t)\, d^3\boldsymbol{r}\right]^2 \tag{1.13b}$$

Naturally, all thermodynamic relations locally hold. Thus, considering a transformation involving all the considered system at a constant temperature, we have

$$\Delta g(\boldsymbol{r}) = \Delta h(\boldsymbol{r}) - T(\boldsymbol{r})\Delta s(\boldsymbol{r}) \tag{1.14}$$

where the difference is from the initial and the final instant of the transformation.

On the contrary, standard thermodynamic equations cannot be used to relate average values of the state functions. For example, integrating Equation 1.14, we obtain

$$\Delta G = \Delta H - T\Delta S + C(T, S) \tag{1.15}$$

where the correlation function

$$C(T,S) = \int_V T(\boldsymbol{r})\Delta s(\boldsymbol{r})\, d^3\boldsymbol{r} - \int_V T(\boldsymbol{r})\, d^3\boldsymbol{r}\int_V \Delta s(\boldsymbol{r})\, d^3\boldsymbol{r} \tag{1.16}$$

is generally different from zero; this is the macroscopic effect of the dynamic nature of the situation.

In the interesting and important case of a perfect gas at constant temperature, we have that locally

$$\Delta s(\boldsymbol{r}) = \kappa c(\boldsymbol{r}) \ln\left(\frac{dV}{dV_0}\right) \tag{1.17}$$

where $c(\boldsymbol{r})$ is the gas density in terms of molecules/m³ and the term $j(\boldsymbol{r}) = (dV/dV_0) = (c(\boldsymbol{r})/c_0)$ is the local expansion of the gas due to the transformation that can be evaluated with a fluid dynamic algorithm (see Section 7.2). Introducing the expansion coefficient in the expression of the correlation function, which is the parameter describing the fact that the system is not in global equilibrium, we have

$$C(T,S) = \kappa \int_V T(\boldsymbol{r})c(\boldsymbol{r})\ln(j(\boldsymbol{r}))\, d^3\boldsymbol{r} - \kappa \int_V T(\boldsymbol{r})\, d^3\boldsymbol{r}\int_V c(\boldsymbol{r})\ln(j(\boldsymbol{r}))\, d^3\boldsymbol{r} \tag{1.18}$$

The results show that the fluid dynamic parameter $j(\boldsymbol{r})$ appears in the expression of the average free energy, as expected due to the fact that the macroscopic motion of the gas contributes besides microscopic phenomena to the gas energy.

It is interesting to evaluate the explicit expression of the average free energy for a perfect gas, which is both a simple and a very important case. Starting from the local expression (1.14) and from the local equations of the state functions for a perfect gas, we can write

$$G = \kappa \int_V c(\boldsymbol{r})T(\boldsymbol{r})\ln\left(\frac{P(\boldsymbol{r})}{\Pi}\right)d^3\boldsymbol{r} \tag{1.19}$$

where

- $c(r)$ is the gas density in molecules/m^3
- κ is the Boltzmann constant
- T is the temperature field
- P is the pressure field
- Π is a constant with the dimensions of a pressure that can be derived for low-density gases from the quantum mechanical Sackur–Tetrode equation [5]

1.2.2 Chemical Properties of Solutions

Solutions are homogeneous (single-phase) mixtures of two or more components. For convenience, we often refer to the majority component as the solvent; minority components are solutes. However, there is no fundamental distinction between them. The most common solutions, and also the solutions that almost always occur in lab on chip systems, are solutions of some substance that at environmental condition is solid, liquid, or gaseous in a liquid solvent.

The most common solvent is water, also in physiological liquids such as blood or urine, but other solvents are commonly used, such as combinations of water and some alcohol, for example.

In general chemistry, gas in gas solutions and gas or liquid in solid solutions are considered, but such solutions have no great importance in microfluidic systems and we do not consider them extensively.

1.2.2.1 Solution Concentration

Concentration is a general term that expresses the quantity of solute contained in a given amount of solution. Various ways of expressing concentration are in use; the choice is usually a matter of convenience in a particular application.

Starting from no-dimensional definitions, the concentration expressed in terms of the number of particles of solute divided by the number of particles of solution is the so-called particle concentration c_p since it is measured as a ratio between number of particles. In diluted solution, the number of moles of the solute is negligible with respect to the number of moles of the solvent and the particle concentration can also be expressed as the number of moles of the solute divided by the number of moles of the solvent.

If we refer to standard conditions (a pressure of 100 kPa and a temperature of 25°C), a mole of a given substance has an associated molar volume. Thus, we can define the concentration in terms of volumes, call it c_V as the molar volume of the solute divided by the volume of 1 mole of the solution (that in diluted solutions is quite coincident with the molar volume of the solvent).

Also, a molar weight is associated with a mole of a given substance, so that a solution concentration can also be expressed as weight concentration c_W, that is, the ratio between the molar weight of the solute divided the weight of the solvent. In any case, if the concentration is defined so as to be nondimensional, it is measured either in percentage or in parts per million (PPM) when the solution is particularly diluted.

Naturally, all the possible nondimensional ways to measure the concentration of a solution are related by the properties of the considered substances. In particular, if we call w_s and V_s the molar weight and the molar volume of the solute and w_0 and V_0 the same quantities for the solvent and indicate the standard condition molar densities for the two substances as $\rho_s = w_s/V_s$ and $\rho_0 = w_0/V_0$, we can write

$$c_V = c_p \frac{V_s}{V_0} = c_w \frac{\rho_0}{\rho_s} \qquad (1.20)$$

In biological chemistry, one observes solutions of very big molecules in a solvent with small molecules like water or some light alcohol. In this case, the values of nondimensional concentrations can be quite different depending on what expression is used.

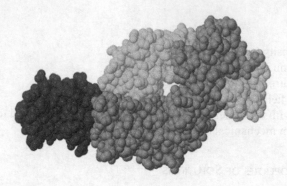

FIGURE 1.2 Molecular stereographic image of the synthetic antigen used to calculate in a practical case the different expressions of a solution concentration. The molecule is represented using the convention where each atom is a sphere approximately coincident with its external van den Waals radius (see Appendix 1).

To illustrate with an example that helps us to familiarize with data relative to biological and medical applications, let us imagine to dissolve a certain amount of the synthetic antigen in water, whose molecular structure is shown in Figure 1.2 (graphical methods to represent the structure of macromolecules are discussed in Appendix 1; in this case, the antigen is represented using the so-called volume stereographic model). The antigen has a molecular mass of 500 kDa. The unified atomic mass unit (indicated with u) or Dalton (indicated with Da) is a unit that is used for indicating mass on an atomic or molecular scale. It is defined as one-twelfth of the rest mass of an unbound neutral atom of carbon-12 in its nuclear and electronic ground state, and has a value of about 1.660×10^{-27} kg [6]. One Dalton is in a very first approximation equal to the mass of one proton or one neutron. Water molecule has a molar weight of 18 Da.

For molecules that are compact, almost spherical in shape like water and the antigen we are using in our example, the molar volume can be evaluated in a first approximation multiplying the molecular weight in Da by a fixed factor that depends on the molecular shape and is reported in tables for the most common shapes. For molecules that are compact, this factor is about 3×10^{-7} m^3/Da [7].

Let us imagine to have a very diluted solution with a molar concentration $c_p = 10^{-4}$ PPM mole, meaning that we have one antigen molecule for every 10 billion molecules of water.

The corresponding volume concentration, which in this case coincides with the weight concentration due to the almost equivalent molecules shape, is $c_V = 16$ PPM volume, due to the great difference of weight of the two molecules.

The situation is still different if we consider a water solution of an IgG immunoglobulin, a big molecule with a Y shape (see Figure 1.3). The immunoglobulin we are considering has a weight of 160 kDa, but the shape is very different from a compact shape; thus, a different factor has to be used for a first estimate of the molar volume.

The most used value for Y-shaped molecules is about 1.1×10^{-10} m^3/Da [7] whose value reflects the fact that immunoglobulins are maintained in Y shape during navigation through the solution by their rigid structure (compare Section 3.3). In this case, starting as in the previous case from a particle concentration $c_p = 10^{-4}$ PPM mole, we get a weight concentration of $c_w = 8.8$ PPM weight and a volume concentration of $c_V = 8.0810^{-3}$ PPM volume.

Nondimensional concentration definitions are very useful in problems where analytical derivations have to be done, since they reflect the nature of the concentration to express the ratio between similar quantities, but they are not traditionally the most used definitions in chemistry.

Common concentration measurements used in chemistry refers to the solution volume so that they are not nondimensional. The most used concentration definitions in chemistry are

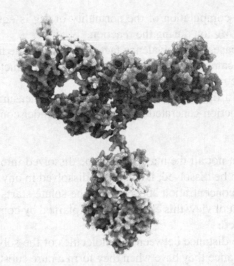

FIGURE 1.3 Stereographic image of IgG immunoglobulin used to calculate the different expressions of a solution concentration in a second practical case.

- The *molar concentration* c_m is the ratio of the solute number of moles m and the solution volume V ($c_m = m/V$); it is measured in moles/m^3, but more commonly in moles/dm^3 = moles/L (moles per liter). When measured in m/L, it is called solution molarity.
- The *mass concentration* c_M is the ratio of the solute mass M and the solution volume V.
- ($c_M = M/V$); it is measured in kg/m^3.
- The *number concentration* c_n is the ratio of the solute number of particles N and the solution volume V ($c_N = N/V$); it is measured in 1/m^3.
- The molality c_{mol} is defined as the number of moles of the solute divided by the mass of the solvent; it is measured in 1/kg; it is to underline that in the evaluation of the molality, the solvent mass also has to be considered in nondiluted solutions.

Finally, in particular types of reactions, the solution is characterized by its normality N_o. The normality of a solution is its molarity divided by an equivalent factor f_{eq} that depends on the particular reaction being considered. Thus

$$N_o = \frac{c_m}{f_{eq}} \qquad (1.21)$$

The normality should be measured in moles/L, since the equivalence factor has to be nondimensional, but it is also measured in equivalents per liter (Eq/L), since its physical meaning is generally related to the concentration in moles per liter of some substance that is produced during the considered reaction.

The normality is generally used in three particular cases, where the equivalence factor takes three different values:

Acid–base reactions: In this case, the equivalence factor is defined as the number of hydroxyl (H$^+$) or oxydril (OH$^-$) ions generated by the considered substance during the reaction. As an example, if we consider the reaction

$$Mg(OH_2)_2 + 2HCl \Rightarrow MgCl_2 + 2H_2O \qquad (1.22)$$

the equivalent factor for the computation of the normality of *Mg* is equal to 2, since two oxydril group are generated by each *Mg* ion during the reaction.

Redox reactions: In this case, the equivalence factor is equal to the number of electrons that an oxidizing or reducing agent can accept or donate. Owing to the characteristics of redox reactions, the equivalence factor can be noninteger in this case.

Precipitation reactions: In this case, the equivalence factor measures the number of ions that will precipitate in a given reaction generated by the substance under consideration.

1.2.2.2 Solvability

It is a general experience that not all the materials can be dissolved into a certain solvent and that, even if a certain material can be dissolved, it cannot be dissolved in any quantity, but there exists a maximum possible solution concentration above which the solute starts to deposit out of the solution. Under a qualitative point of view this effect can be explained by considering the steps that happens when a solution is formed.

In a first step, the average distance between the molecules of the solvent increases with respect to the average reciprocal distance they have when they form a pure substance; after that, molecules of the solvent are inserted among them forming the solute–solvent chemical bond that characterizes the solution. Since the solution does not change substantially, the molecules of the solute and of the solvent, the solute–solvent chemical bond has to be quite weak, while it can be polar or nonpolar depending on the case.

In the first phase, we can image that the greater space among molecules increase entropy, creating a more favorable situation under the entropic point of view. This is not the equilibrium situation in the stand-alone substance due to the intermolecular forces that tends to maintain the solute molecules nearer. Thus, the free energy in the first phase has to also increase. This is naturally due to the fact that energy has to be added to the solution to move from equilibrium to this new situation.

The intermolecular forces are shielded by the interposition of the solvent molecules; moreover, weak solute–solvent bonds are created. The intermolecular force shielding is surely an energy-favored process, while the creation of solvent–solute bonds can either release or absorb energy, depending on the cases.

Summarizing the overall change in free energy due to solution formation is constituted by an increase in entropy and an increase in enthalpy due to the increase in distance among solute molecules, a decrease in enthalpy due to the shielding of intermolecular forces, and an enthalpy term that can be either positive or negative due to the formation of solute–solvent bonds.

This balance can be either negative or positive depending on the case; if the balance is negative spontaneous dissolution happens.

Even if the solute can be dissolved for a certain initial concentration, further increasing the concentration of the solute, the shielding carried out by the presence of the solvent molecules greatly reduces and the situation resembles more of the stand-alone solvent, up to a moment in which the entropy increases and the other negative energy term is no longer sufficient to stabilize the solution: further, the solvent stops to be dissolved and the maximum possible concentration is reached.

The starting point for a macroscopic study of the chemical properties of solutions is the so-called Raoult law for ideal solutions. An ideal solution is a solution having zero creation enthalpy. Intuitively, this happens when enthalpy terms in the solution creation process have a zero sum.

Let us imagine a solution of n liquids that are present in the molar concentrations $c_j (j = 1,\ldots, n)$, and that the solution is contained in a container in which there was void before the introduction of the solution. If the solution does not fill the container completely, a little of every liquid present in the solution will pass in gaseous form to fill the void on top of the solution surface. A vapor pressure will be created in this way, which will be the result of the presence of n different vapors.

Since the chemical substances we are considering do not react in vapor form, we can say that the total pressure will be the sum of the pressures of every individual vapor, that is,

$$P_T = \sum_{i=1}^{n} P_i \tag{1.23}$$

The Raoult law states that individual vapor pressures are proportional to the particle concentration (moles divided by total moles) of each component of the solution multiplied by the equivalent vapor pressure of 1 mole of that components as if it was alone in the container. Thus, calling $P_{0,i}$ the molar vapor pressure of the ith component of the solution, we have

$$P_T = \sum_{i=1}^{n} c_i P_{0,i} \tag{1.24}$$

Let us now consider our solution in equilibrium with its saturated vapor and at a constant temperature.

From the general theory of gases, we know that the free energy variation ΔG_{vap} of a gas passing from pressure P_1 to pressure P_2 at a constant temperature is given by

$$\Delta G_{vap} = mRT \ln\left(\frac{P_2}{P_1}\right) \tag{1.25}$$

where m is the number of moles of the vapor.

Let us now imagine mixing two liquids (call them a and b) so as to form a solution: their vapor pressure passes from P_a^0 to P_a and from P_b^0 to P_b where, if we consider the solution ideal, the final and initial vapor pressure is related by the Raoult law.

Thus, combining Equation 1.24, written in the case of two liquids, and Equation 1.25 we can write the overall change in free energy per mole of solution ΔG_{sol} due to the mixing of the two liquids as

$$\Delta G_{sol} = m_T RT \left(c_a \ln c_a + c_b \ln c_b\right) \tag{1.26}$$

where c_a and c_b are the particle concentrations of the two liquids in the solution and m_T the solution number of moles. Since it must be by definition $c_a + c_b = 1$ we get the important result that the free energy variation for an ideal solution is always negative, meaning that in the ideal case two liquids would in any case spontaneously form a solution.

Moreover, since in our ideal case $\Delta H_{sol} = 0$, from the definition of free energy, we find

$$\Delta S_{sol} = -m_T R \left(c_a \ln c_a + c_b \ln c_b\right) > 0 \tag{1.27}$$

We have thus demonstrated the qualitative conclusion to which we arrived at the start of the section: in an ideal solution, in which the net enthalpy of formation ΔH_{sol} is zero, the disorder due to the mix of the two kinds of molecules causes an increase of entropy, making the solution state more favorable under a thermodynamic point of view with respect to the state in which the solution components are divided. We can say that the formation of an ideal solution is an entropic-driven phenomenon.

In the case of a real solution however, we generally have $\Delta H_{sol} \neq 0$, so that we have to use the general relation

$$\Delta G_{sol} = \Delta H_{sol} - T\,\Delta S_{sol} \tag{1.28}$$

Owing to the general discussion made, we have to assume that the entropy ΔS_{sol} is always positive, at least if we consider diluted solutions when one of the concentration is much greater than all the others, as it is almost always verified in biochemical cases. The solution enthalpy determines whether the solution process is spontaneous or not at a certain temperature and it is also evident from Equation 1.28 that increasing the temperature favors the spontaneous solution formation.

It is interesting to note that from Equation 1.28 it can be deduced that even if a solution absorbs heat from the environment in the process of forming, it can nevertheless form spontaneously. This is, for example, the case of KNO_3, which absorbs from the environment 8.24 kcal/mole while spontaneously dissolving in water.

The value of the solution-forming entropy depends on the concentration of the species participating in the solution. Let us refer to a diluted solution, in which the concentration of the solvent is almost one. In this case, the entropy variation will be equal to $\Delta S_{sol} = -Rc_a \ln c_a$, c_a being the molar concentration of the solute. Even if in the real case this equation could be not exact, we can try to understand what happens while increasing the solute concentration by adopting it in a very first approximation, that is valid in those cases in which the concentration of the solute is small such that both the solution entropy and the solution enthalpy are very small numbers.

Let us assume that the enthalpy is positive and that we enclose our solution into an insulating container so that no heat can be assumed from the environment. This means that the only way to form a solution absorbing energy is to decrease the solution temperature. The solution temperature decreases proportionally to the quantity of needed energy, which is conversely proportional to the solute concentration.

At the end, at least qualitatively, we have that Equation 1.28 can be written as

$$\Delta G_{sol} \approx c_a \Delta H_{sol}^0 - c_a \left(T_0 - \frac{c_a \Delta H_{sol}^0}{\beta} \right) \ln c_a = c_a (\Delta H_{sol}^0 - T_0 \ln c_a) + c_a^2 \ln c_a \tag{1.29}$$

where ΔH_{sol}^0 is the solution reference enthalpy.

The plot of Equation 1.29 with a set of reasonable parameters is presented in Figure 1.4. Even if not quantitatively accurate, Equation 1.29 reproduces the qualitative trend of the solution-free

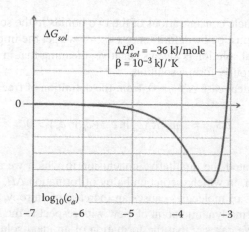

$\Delta H_{sol}^0 = -36$ kJ/mole
$\beta = 10^{-3}$ kJ/°K

FIGURE 1.4 Qualitative diagram of the solution free energy for a solution with positive solution enthalpy.

energy in the solutions that have a negative value of the molar solution enthalpy. At very small values of the concentration, the free energy is negative and varies linearly with the concentration, as foreseen for an extensive state variable. By increasing the concentration, the nonlinearity due to the presence of the enthalpy emerges up to a value of the concentration above which the free energy is no more negative, but it gets positive. This is called the saturation value of the concentration and it is the maximum value of the solute that can be put in solution at the given temperature.

A solution with concentrations greater than the saturation value is not formed spontaneously and, if more solute is added to a saturated solution, this does not pass in solution, but remains separated from the solvent, either depositing on the floor of the container if it is solid at the environment conditions or remaining in liquid phase, but completely separated from the solution.

1.2.2.3 Solution Colligative Properties

The fact that a solute is dissolved in a solvent changes the properties of the solvent, even if the concentration of the solute is quite small.

These changes, derived by lowering the vapor pressure foreseen by the Raoult law, are collectively known as solution colligative properties. While in the case of an ideal solution these properties are easily related to the Raoult law, they are also not easy to be quantitatively foreseen in solutions that have strong nonideal behavior.

It is not within the scope of this brief review of the chemical properties of solutions to study in detail the solution colligative properties, thus we limit ourselves to a simple list of the most important of them.

- *Boiling point elevation:* Liquid boils at the temperature at which its vapor pressure equals atmospheric pressure. The presence of a nonvolatile solute lowers the vapor pressure of a solution and so it is necessary to heat the solution to a higher temperature in order for it to boil.

  The amount by which the boiling point is raised is known as the boiling point elevation. In an ideal solution, due to the Raoult law, the boiling point elevation is proportional to the concentration of solute.

- *Freezing point depression:* The presence of a nonvolatile solute lowers the freezing point of a solvent. To freeze the solvent, it must be cooled to a lower temperature in order to compensate for its lower escaping tendency. The amount by which the freezing point is lowered is known as the freezing point depression.

  In an ideal solution, the freezing point depression is proportional to the concentration of solute.

- *Osmotic pressure:* When two liquids, such as a solvent and a solution, are separated by a semipermeable membrane that allows only solvent molecules to pass through, then there is a net transfer of solvent molecules from the solvent to the solution. This process is called osmosis.

  Osmosis can be stopped by applying pressure to compensate for the difference in escaping tendencies. The pressure required to stop osmosis is called osmotic pressure.

- In ideal dilute solutions, osmotic pressure is directly proportional to the molarity of the solution and its temperature in Kelvin.

1.2.3 CHEMICAL EQUILIBRIUM IN REACTIONS AMONG SOLUTES

After this review of the chemical properties of solutions, we are ready to study equilibrium of chemical reactions among reagents that come in contact with solutes in the same solvent.

1.2.3.1 Simple Reaction Equilibrium and the Law of Mass Action

In general, let us imagine n solutes R_j ($j = 1, ..., n$) dissolved in a solvent that, under the chemical point of view, does not participate to the reaction. The solutes react giving rise to h reaction products r_i ($i = 1, ..., h$).

Thus, the stoichiometry of the reaction is written as

$$\alpha_1 R_1 + \alpha_2 R_2 + \cdots + \alpha_n R_n \rightleftarrows \beta_1 r_1 + \beta_2 r_2 + \cdots + \beta_h r_h \tag{1.30}$$

where α_i and β_i are the stoichiometric coefficients of the reaction. If the reaction is at equilibrium we must have the overall variation of the free energy for each infinitesimal variation if one of the equilibrium concentrations is positive, so that the equilibrium free energy results to be the minimum possible.

The target is thus to find the minimum of the function

$$G(c_1, c_2, \ldots, c_n, c_{n+1}, \ldots, c_{n+h}) = \sum_{i=1}^{n} \alpha_i G_i - \sum_{j=1}^{h} \beta_j G_{n+j} \tag{1.31}$$

where the elements G_i indicates the free energies of formation of the equilibrium concentration of the various components appearing in the reaction and all the species has been numbered from 1 to $n+h$; the first n being the species at the first member of the reaction, the species numbered from $n+1$ to $n+h$ those at the second member.

In order to have the equilibrium concentrations, the variation of the free energy expressed by Equation 1.31 for an infinitesimal variation of the concentration, subjected to the fact that the stoichiometric equilibrium of the reaction is respected, have to be always positive. In order to respect the stoichiometric equilibrium of the reaction we have to apply to the concentrations a fluctuation equal to $dc_i = \alpha_i \, d\xi$ for the reagent on the left side of the reaction and $\delta c_j = \beta_j d\xi$ for the reagent on the right side. Substituting and dividing by $d\xi$ we get

$$\frac{dG}{d\xi} = \sum_{i=1}^{n} \alpha_i \mu_i - \sum_{j=1}^{h} \beta_j \mu_{n+j} = 0 \tag{1.32}$$

Equation 1.32 constitutes the general equilibrium condition for our reaction. In the case the solution can be approximated with an ideal solution, that is, the Raoult law can be applied with a good approximation, Equation 1.32 takes a much simpler form, which we will derive for simplicity in the case $n = 2$ and $h = 2$.

As a matter of fact, from Equation 1.25 we can write in this case

$$\mu_j = \frac{dG_{sol}}{dc_j} = RT \ln c_j + RT \tag{1.33}$$

Substituting and defining the concentration equilibrium constant K_c as

$$K_c = e^{(\beta_1 + \beta_2 - \alpha_1 - \alpha_2)} \tag{1.34}$$

we arrive to the equilibrium rule that is known as the rule of mass action

$$\frac{c_1^{\alpha_1} c_2^{\alpha_2}}{c_3^{\beta_1} c_4^{\beta_2}} = K_c \tag{1.35a}$$

Equation 1.35 can be rewritten using the Raoult law that links the concentrations of the solutes with the partial pressures, as functions of the partial pressures of the solutes as

$$\frac{p_1^{\alpha_1} \, p_2^{\alpha_2}}{p_3^{\beta_1} \, p_4^{\beta_2}} = K_p \tag{1.35b}$$

The constant K_p takes the name of pressure equilibrium constant and it is related to the concentration equilibrium constant by the equation

$$K_p = K_c \, (RT)^{(\beta_1 + \beta_2 - \alpha_1 - \alpha_2)} \tag{1.36}$$

which derives immediately from the Raoult law.

From Equation 1.37 it is possible to deduce how a reaction changes its equilibrium when the partial pressure of one of the components changes, which is a recurrent mechanism used by biological systems to regulate reaction equilibrium. The equilibrium coefficient does not depend on pressure, thus when the partial pressure of one component changes, the reaction moves the equilibrium versus the opposite side, that is, it produces more reaction products due to the abundance of one of the reaction elements.

We have obtained the law of mass action in a specific case assuming to have an ideal solution; in reality this law is much more general as it can be demonstrated with more sophisticated methods [8] and it represents the universal law of equilibrium of reactions taking place in a single phase (liquid in our case).

When the solution deviates from the ideal case or different types of phase are considered for the reaction, the expression (1.34) of the concentration equilibrium constant can be no more valid, but the relation (1.35) still holds in any case.

Deviations from the rule of mass action are observed when the concentrations of the solutes are not small. In this case, we can imagine that in a certain instant, a molecule of the jth solute may be surrounded by molecules of the same species so as to be not available for the reaction. If we consider this phenomenon under a statistical point of view intuitively, we can suppose that the effect of increasing the concentrations of the solutes beyond a critical point can be represented with the introduction of a sort of effective concentration, which has to be maintained smaller than the real concentration.

The accurate analysis of the reaction equilibrium for concentrated solutes confirms this intuition [6,8]. In particular, if we consider concentrated solutions, the mass action law (1.35) is still valid by substituting to the effective concentrations the so-called solute activity a_j, which is obtained as

$$a_j = c_j \epsilon_j \quad 0 < \epsilon_j \le 1 \tag{1.37}$$

where ϵ_j is the so-called activity coefficient of the jth solute. The value of the activity coefficient of a solute usually ranges downward from unity as the concentration is increased. For example, the mean activity coefficient of aqueous KCl decreases from 0.97 at 0.001 mol/L to 0.61 at 1.0 mol/L. Aqueous $ZnSO_4$ has a mean activity coefficient of the dissolved ions of 0.70 at 0.001 mol/L which decreases to 0.05 at 1.0 mol/L. The activity coefficient also depends on the solvent.

Finally, it is to observe that in very rare cases interaction between concentrated solutes increases the reaction probability with respect to the case of diluted solutes. This could happen, for example, in case of decay of a poorly stable molecule. Sometimes these cases are represented with an activity coefficient greater than one.

From now on we will always consider the concentrations in the analysis of equilibrium and kinetics of chemical reactions, since the case of diluted solution is by far the most common in lab on chip applications. However, if concentrated solutions have to be considered concentrations have to be substituted by activities. The activity coefficients of a large number of solutions have been experimentally measured and are tabled as a reference for chemical calculations.

1.2.3.2 Simultaneous Equilibrium of Several Reactions

If we look at practical cases occurring in biochemistry, the situation is more complex than a single reaction that goes to equilibrium. What happens is that multiple reactions occur simultaneously, in sequence, or both. This is due to the fact that molecules involved in biological processes are generally complex molecules that are able to react with a wide variety of reagents in different ways and also to the fact that biological reactions frequently involve processes more complex than a simple chemical transformation.

Let us assume that all the reagents involved either at the right or the left member of the reactions that happens in parallel during the biological process are arranged as the coordinates of a chemical species vector, call it $\mathbf{R} = (R_1, R_2, \ldots, R_n)$ and that the stoichiometry of the set of parallel reactions is characterized by a couple of reaction matrixes $\underline{A} = (\alpha_{i,j})$ and $\underline{B} = (\beta_{i,j}), i = 1, \ldots, n, j = 1, \ldots, H$, where n is the number of different substances involved in the reactions and H is the total number of parallel reactions. The substances can be either in the right member in a reaction and in the left member in another reaction, where the processes are chained so that the products of the first are reagents in the second. We can also introduce a free energy vector G whose components are the free energies of all the reactions.

In order for all the system to be in equilibrium, any reaction has to be in equilibrium, thus we can write the equilibrium condition in vector form as

$$\frac{d}{d\xi} G = (\underline{A} - \underline{B})\mu = 0 \tag{1.38}$$

where μ is the vector of the chemical potentials. If the reaction set admits an equilibrium state, this means that the system (1.38) of the chemical potential has a solution different from the null vector.

Thus, we must have

$$\det(\underline{A} - \underline{B}) = 0 \tag{1.39}$$

In this case, we have to fix arbitrarily the chemical potential of one of the species, but this is not surprising, remembering that all the classical expressions of potentials are determined with the uncertainty of an arbitrary constant. Up to now we have somehow hidden this fact only because we have assumed to set it to zero in the evaluation of the free energy.

At this point, we can substitute to the potentials the expression (1.33). Now it is even more natural that at least one of the concentrations has to be fixed: the reaction chain has to start somehow. Proceeding as in the case of a single reaction, an individual mass action law is obtained for each reaction of the set in the form

$$\prod_{j=1}^{n} c_j^{\alpha_{i,j} - \beta_{i,j}} = K_{c,i} \quad i = 1, \ldots, H \tag{1.40}$$

As an important example of this simultaneous equilibrium of more than one reaction, let us consider the transport of oxygen by hemoglobin from the lung to the body cells [9,10]. The human blood has a great capacity of transporting oxygen, about 0.01 mole per blood liter, due to the fact that hemoglobin binds oxygen chemically. As a matter of fact, pure serum dissolves in simple solution no more than 0.0001 mole of oxygen per liter, a value that is not far from the O_2 solubility in ordinary water at room conditions.

When the highly oxygenated blood passes through the capillary, the oxygen is released by the hemoglobin due to the interaction with a different oxygen binding molecule, the myoglobin that is found in the cells surrounding the capillary. The myoglobin carries out oxygen from the capillary surface to the cells where it enters into the cells metabolism.

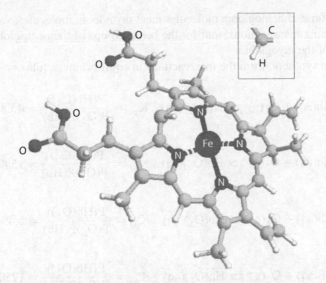

FIGURE 1.5 Molecular structure of the heme group in hemoglobin: the iron atom at the center of the molecule group is put in evidence with its coordinate bonds with nitrogen atoms.

Hemoglobin binds oxygen strongly during transit to the lungs and does not release it until encountering myoglobin, which is the end vector to bring oxygen to the cells. This dynamical behavior is the result of the characteristic of the heterogeneous equilibrium with which myoglobin and hemoglobin bind oxygen. The hemoglobin is a large protein in which four heme groups (protein parts containing an ion atom) are embedded. The molecular structure of one of the hemoglobin heme groups is graphically shown in Figure 1.5 in ball-and-stick representation (see Appendix 1).

Oxygen that is transported by hemoglobin is bound to each heme group, so that a single hemoglobin molecule can bind up to four oxygen molecules. Myoglobin, on the contrary, has only one heme group, so that a single myoglobin molecule can embed only one oxygen molecule. The plot of the whole myoglobin molecule is illustrated in Figure 1.6 using two different molecule plotting conventions.

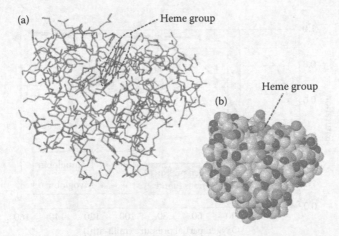

FIGURE 1.6 Molecular structure of the myoglobin reported using two different conventions. In (a), the sticks plot is reported, the same used for the heme group in Figure 1.5. In (b), the volume convention is used.

When oxygen-saturated hemoglobin molecules meet myoglobin molecules, we have a composite equilibrium comprising five reactions: four for the heme groups of the hemoglobin and one for the single heme group of the myoglobin.

We can write in a synthetic form the five reactions in equilibrium as follows:

$$Hb(aq) + O_2(g) \rightleftarrows Hb(O_2)(aq) \quad K_{p1} = \frac{P(Hb(O_2))}{P(O_2)P(Hb)} = 4.88 \tag{1.41a}$$

$$Hb(aq) + O_2(g) \rightleftarrows Hb(O_2)(aq) \quad K_{p2} = \frac{P(Hb(O_2))}{P(O_2)P(Hb)} = 15.4 \tag{1.41b}$$

$$Hb(aq) + O_2(g) \rightleftarrows Hb(O_2)(aq) \quad K_{p3} = \frac{P(Hb(O_2))}{P(O_2)P(Hb)} = 6.49 \tag{1.41c}$$

$$Hb(aq) + O_2(g) \rightleftarrows Hb(O_2)(aq) \quad K_{p4} = \frac{P(Hb(O_2))}{P(O_2)P(Hb)} = 1750 \tag{1.41d}$$

$$Mb(aq) + O_2(g) \rightleftarrows Mb(O_2)(aq) \quad K_{pM} = \frac{P(Hb(O_2))}{P(O_2)P(Hb)} = 271 \tag{1.41e}$$

Owing to the different positions of the four heme groups in the hemoglobin molecule, the pressure equilibrium coefficients are not equal; the fourth is much bigger than the other three. When the partial pressure of the oxygen changes, due to the form of the pressure equilibrium coefficients, the reactions binding oxygen to hemoglobin moves toward a greater number of saturated heme group. This is clearly viewed from the plot of Figure 1.7, where the so-called hemoglobin and myoglobin saturation curves, that is, the average number of heme groups bonded with an oxygen molecule, is represented versus the partial pressure of oxygen.

This situation occurs in the lungs, where oxygen penetrates in great quantity due to osmosis into the lung alveolus coming in contact with hemoglobin. Here a strong bond is formed between hemoglobin and oxygen that allows hemoglobin to transport oxygen effectively through the circulatory system. In arterial blood, the partial pressure of oxygen is of the order of magnitude 0.13 atm. Both

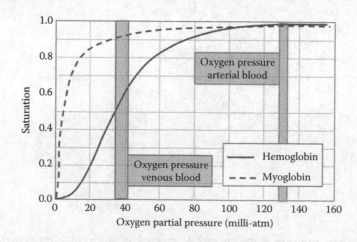

FIGURE 1.7   Hemoglobin and myoglobin saturation of oxygen as functions of the oxygen partial pressure.

hemoglobin and myoglobin are highly saturated in this condition (more than 95% both) so that oxygen transport happens effectively. In capillaries, the partial pressure of oxygen decreases greatly, the hemoglobin saturation strongly decreases so that oxygen is released to myoglobin, whose saturation remains high, and is distributed gradually to nearby cells.

In great veins, the partial oxygen pressure generally does not rise above 0.04 atm. So that hemoglobin saturation is lower than 55%, while myoglobin saturation remains of the order of 90%. At this pressure, myoglobin is still able to work as oxygen distributor to cells, but hemoglobin is quite poor and is ready to be injected in lungs again to collect other oxygen.

1.2.4 REACTION KINETICS

Up to now we have dealt with equilibrium rules, stating the characteristics of reaction stable states. However, no information has been provided on the time the reaction takes to arrive to equilibrium.

This is often a key factor, it is sufficient to note that this time changes orders of magnitude passing from one kind of reaction to another; as an example, we can consider that oxidation of a metal–organic molecule, which is a practically a unidirectional reaction, takes from 48 to 200 h to reach equilibrium while neutralization of selected antibodies by a specific IgG immunoglobulin in a lab on chip microreactor can arrive to equilibrium in a time as short as 10 μs.

In this section, we will introduce a theory of chemical kinetics, that is heuristically based on a simple molecule kinetic theory, reserving to justify it with more accurate microscopic models in the situations we are more interested in References [11,12].

The first step in this direction is to define the so-called reaction coordinate ξ that marks the microscopic time dynamics of the reaction. The physical meaning of the reaction coordinate depends essentially on the kind of reaction we are considering.

In a very simple reaction in which two ions create an ionic bond through a collision, we can describe microscopically with a good approximation what happens when the bond is constituted as the collision of two charged spheres. In this case, the reaction coordinate is simply the distance between the center of mass of the two ions. In other cases, it is not so simple to define the reaction coordinate on elementary considerations.

A general definition of the reaction coordinate is provided by the so-called transition state theory for chemical kinetics [13,14]. If we consider a system of molecules that are so far from one another to be completely isolated, they can be described with a set of N generalized spatial degrees of freedom, so that the system spatial configuration can be represented with the N generalized coordinates [15,16].

The system mechanical energy is composed of a kinetic and a potential term. In the absence of external forces, the potential term is zero for infinitely far molecules and has a finite value if the molecules are at a finite distance. If we represent the system as a point in the generalized coordinate space, we can imagine that starting from its initial position it will move always along the steepest descendent direction on the potential energy surface to reach a local minimum that is a stable equilibrium point. Once in a local minimum, the system behavior will depend on its kinetic energy and on the presence of other local minima nearby. If the kinetic energy due to temperature is high enough, the system can pass from a local minimum to another up to reaching a sufficiently deep minimum where it remains entrapped since the kinetic energy is not sufficient to overcome the surrounding potential energy barrier.

The reaction coordinate is defined as the curvilinear coordinate over the trajectory from the initial to the final reaction state. This trajectory is defined in the space of the molecular system generalized coordinates and lies over a constant potential energy surface. Average is performed with respect to the fluctuations of the thermal velocities' directions and intensities. In conditions of constant macroscopic pressure and temperature and in the absence of external forces, such as electrical fields, while the kinetic energy term is essentially due the temperature, the potential energy is proportional to the Gibbs free energy, for the definition of G itself.

Chemical reactions, as far as kinetic is concerned, can be classified into two groups: single-step and many-step reactions. Single-step reactions happen essentially through a single combination between the reagents: the molecules come in contact, they form a sort of high-energy activated complex that decays to the reaction products. This is true in both the reaction directions, as it is immediate from the reversibility of mechanical forces and the definition of reaction coordinate. In single-step reactions, the dependence of the free energy from the reaction coordinates always has the qualitative shape that is shown in Figure 1.8. The needed energy to overcome the initial potential barrier is given in a spontaneous reaction by the temperature that represents the average kinetic energy of the molecules that join in the activated composite.

We have to imagine that when the collision among the right particles happens, the reaction takes place only if the thermal energy of the colliding molecules is sufficient to overcome the activation energy. Let us call p_{RD} the probability that reaction occurs conditioned to the fact that the right collision happens. If we assume that the molecules have a Boltzmann energy distribution for all their degrees of freedom due to the equal partition principle, p_{RD} is given by [20]:

$$p_{RD} = p(E > \Delta E_+) = \frac{\vartheta}{\kappa T} \int_{\Delta E_+}^{\infty} e^{-E/\kappa T} dE = \vartheta e^{-\frac{\Delta E_+}{\kappa T}} \tag{1.42}$$

where ΔE_+ is the activation energy, ϑ is the active molecules' degrees of freedom, that is, the number of degrees of freedom that can participate in the energy exchange during the collision, and κ is the Boltzmann constant. If we apply the kinetic theory to our molecule population we can also evaluate the number of collisions of the needed type in a unit time. In the case of a simple reaction, whose equation is

$$R_1 + R_2 \rightleftarrows R_3 + R_4 \tag{1.43}$$

we need a collision between two different molecules of the correct type. From the kinetic theory, we have that in this case the collision rate per unit solution volume between the considered particles is given by

$$N_{12} = c_1 c_2 \; p_{RD} \; \Omega_{12} \tag{1.44}$$

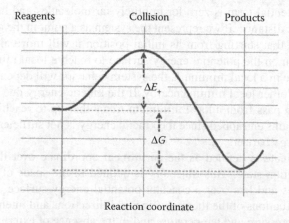

FIGURE 1.8 Qualitative diagram of the energy corresponding to the different states of the system during a collision generating a single-step reaction.

where the concentrations c_1 and c_2 are evaluated in moles/m^3 and Ω_{12} is a parameter related to the reacting molecules characteristics in solution, and finally the concentrations are expressed as moles of the solute divided by moles of the solution (compare Section 1.2.2.1).

Thus, we have to imagine that the number of effective collisions that is proportional to the concentration variation rate can be deduced by multiplying Equation 1.42 by Equation 1.43 so that the time evolution of the concentrations of the reagents in the two directions will be regulated by the following equations:

$$\frac{dc_1}{dt} = \frac{dc_2}{dt} = -v_+\, e^{-\frac{\Delta E_+}{\kappa T}}\, c_1\, c_2 + v_-\, e^{-\frac{\Delta E_-}{\kappa T}}\, c_3\, c_4 \tag{1.45a}$$

$$\frac{dc_3}{dt} = \frac{dc_4}{dt} = +v_+\, e^{-\frac{\Delta E_+}{\kappa T}}\, c_1\, c_2 - v_-\, e^{-\frac{\Delta E_-}{\kappa T}}\, c_3\, c_4 \tag{1.45b}$$

where ΔE_+ and ΔE_- are the direct and the inverse activation energies, respectively, and

$$v_+ = \vartheta\Omega_{12} \tag{1.46a}$$

$$v_- = \vartheta\Omega_{34} \tag{1.46b}$$

If the stoichiometric coefficients of reaction (1.43) are not all equal to one, a more complex activation collision is needed. Let us imagine to have the following reaction:

$$\alpha_1 R_1 + \alpha_2 R_2 \rightleftarrows \beta_3 R_3 + \beta_4 R_4 \tag{1.47}$$

In principle, from the kinetic theory it is possible to evaluate the probability of whatever collision is needed and use it besides the suitable energy probability density to evaluate the equivalent of Equation 1.38. As it is intuitive, interpreting the concentration as the probability to find a particle in a unit volume of space, is obtaining that the probability that α_1 particles will participate to the collision is proportional to $c_1^{\alpha_1}$, so that the following equations are obtained:

$$\alpha_1 \frac{dc_1}{dt} = \alpha_2 \frac{dc_2}{dt} = -v_+\, e^{-\frac{\Delta E_+}{\kappa T}}\, c_1^{\alpha_1}\, c_2^{\alpha_2} + v_-\, e^{-\frac{\Delta E_-}{\kappa T}}\, c_3^{\beta_3}\, c_4^{\beta_4} \tag{1.48a}$$

$$\beta_1 \frac{dc_1}{dt} = \beta_2 \frac{dc_2}{dt} = v_+ e^{-\frac{\Delta E_+}{\kappa T}}\, c_1^{\alpha_1}\, c_2^{\alpha_2} - v_- e^{-\frac{\Delta E_-}{\kappa T}}\, c_3^{\beta_3}\, c_4^{\beta_4} \tag{1.48a}$$

From Equation 1.45, the equilibrium concentrations can be evaluated, by starting from the fact that at equilibrium the concentration derivatives are zero. It is obtained by

$$\frac{c_{10}^{\alpha_1}\, c_{20}^{\alpha_2}}{c_{30}^{\beta_3}\, c_{40}^{\beta_4}} = \frac{v_-\, e^{\frac{\Delta E_+ - \Delta E_-}{\kappa T}}}{v_+} \tag{1.49}$$

That is nothing more than the kinetic derivation of the law of mass action.

It is now important to compare the speed of different kinds of reactions and we will start to consider a very simple decay reaction, in which an unstable chemical species forms an activated composite by joining α molecules that decays in two products that are stable at given environmental conditions. Such a reaction can be assumed almost unidirectional and be written as

$$\alpha R_1 \rightarrow R_2 + R_3 \tag{1.50}$$

We get the following evolution law for the concentrations:

$$\frac{dc_1}{dt} = -\frac{\nu_+}{\alpha} e^{-\frac{\Delta E_+}{\kappa T}} c_1^{\alpha} \tag{1.51}$$

Assuming to start with $c_1(0) = c_0$ we can easily evaluate the concentration versus time obtaining

$$c_1(t) = c_0 e^{-2\nu_+ te^{-\frac{\Delta E_+}{\kappa T}}} \quad \alpha = 1 \tag{1.52a}$$

$$c_1(t) = (\alpha - 1)^{(\alpha-1)} \sqrt{\frac{\alpha}{\nu_+} \frac{e^{\frac{\Delta E_+}{\kappa T}}}{t + A}} \quad \alpha > 1 \quad \text{and} \quad A = \left(\frac{c_0}{\alpha - 1}\right)^{(\alpha-1)} \frac{\alpha}{\nu_+} e^{\frac{\Delta E_+}{\kappa T}} \tag{1.52b}$$

The plot of the concentration time evolution is reported in Figure 1.9. It is evident that the higher the stoichiometric coefficient the slower the reaction. The reaction with the parameters we have used is completed at 90% after 0.38 s if $\alpha = 1$, after 7.85 s if $\alpha = 4$, and after 16.6 min if $\alpha = 6$.

On the one side, this is intuitive since the probability that a collision happens decreases exponentially with a number of colliding particles; on the other side, this trend would imply that no reaction with a high stoichiometric coefficient can be fast; this is clearly untrue since there are many reactions with quite high stoichiometric coefficients that are also quite fast.

The point is that practically no reaction with high stoichiometric coefficients is realized in a single step, but it has to be schematized as a reaction chain. A striking example of a kinetic mechanism in complete disagreement with the kinetic interpretation of a single-step reaction is the reaction

$$NO_2(gas) + CO(gas) \rightarrow NO(gas) + CO_2(gas) \tag{1.53}$$

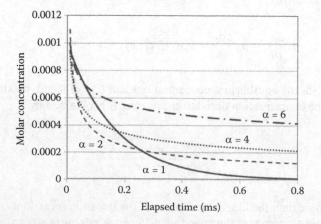

FIGURE 1.9 Decay law of the decay of multiple molecules.

Experimentally, the kinetic of this reaction is found to be second order with respect to c_{NO_2} and zero order with respect to c_{CO} so that the governing time evolution equation of this almost unidirectional oxidation of the carbon oxide that produces carbon dioxide is written as follows:

$$\frac{dc_{NO_2}}{dt} = -v_+ e^{\frac{\Delta E_+}{\kappa T}} c_{NO_2}^2 \tag{1.54}$$

There is no possible single-step mechanism that can justify this dynamics and the following multistep mechanism has been proposed:

$$\text{Step 1:} \quad 2\,NO_2(gas) \rightarrow NO_3(gas) + NO(gas)(slow) \tag{1.55a}$$

$$\text{Step 2:} \quad NO_3(gas) + CO(gas) \rightarrow NO_2(gas) + CO_2(gas)(fast) \tag{1.55b}$$

Since step 1 is the slowest step, it determines the rate of the overall reaction. Thus, the above mechanism agrees with the observed rate law.

Multistep mechanisms are the normal way in which reactions that would involve multiple particle collision happens and it is the reason why these reactions can happen at a fast pace that would be impossible with a single-step mechanism. Once a multistep mechanism is known in detail, the consequent reaction rates can be determined. As an example, we want to present the simple calculation of the reaction rate of the two-step reaction

$$2NO(gas) + O_2(gas) \rightarrow 2NO_2(gas) \tag{1.56}$$

with the following observed rate law [17]

$$\frac{dc_{NO}}{dt} = v_+ e^{-\frac{\Delta E_+}{\kappa T}} c_{NO}^2 c_{O_2} \tag{1.57}$$

The rate expression is compatible with a one-step reaction between two molecules of nitrogen oxide and a molecule of oxygen, but the observed value of v_+ is much higher than the value that would be foreseen by the kinetic theory and a great difference is not easy to justify only with the approximation of the kinetic theory in making quantitative estimations.

An alternative mechanism is provided by the following two-step process constituted by a fast equilibrium creating a population of the intermediate product N_2O_2 and a slow further oxidation of nitrogen to give NO_2. The reaction could be decomposed in

$$2\,NO(gas) \underset{v_{1-}}{\overset{v_{1+}}{\rightleftharpoons}} N_2O_2 \tag{1.58a}$$

$$N_2O_2 + O_2 \xrightarrow{v_{2+}} 2\,NO_2 \tag{1.58b}$$

where we have enclosed the Boltzmann exponential term into the terms indicating the reaction speed.

Both the steps (1.55) are bimolecular steps, much more likely to happen than a three-way collision: this naturally favors the two-step process with respect to the direct single-step process. The slow step determines the overall reaction rate, providing

$$\frac{dc_{NO_2}}{dt} = v_{2+} c_{N_2O_2} c_{O_2} \tag{1.59}$$

However, in practice this equation is not useful, implying the use of the N_2O_2 concentration that, due to the fact that it is only an intermediate component, cannot be evaluated experimentally.

Since the intermediate, dinitrogen dioxide, reacts slowly with oxygen, the reverse reaction of the first step of the decomposition (1.58) is possible. Thus, we are allowed to assume that the reaction of dinitrogen dioxide formation will reach a dynamic equilibrium that performs a reversible evolution through a series of equilibrium states. This leads to set, at every given instant: $v_{1+}c_{NO}^2 = v_{1-}c_{N_2O_2}$.

Substituting into Equation 1.59 we get

$$\frac{dc_{NO_2}}{dt} = \frac{v_{2+}v_{1+}}{v_{1-}}c_{NO}^2\,c_{O_2} \tag{1.60}$$

At this point the rates of the elementary steps can be evaluated starting from the kinetic theory and the experimental value of the overall reaction rate is obtained with a good approximation.

The mechanism of multistep reactions is the cause of the fact that, generally, when the stoichiometric coefficients of a reaction are not identical, there is almost no relation between the reaction rates and the stoichiometric coefficients themselves, and if the step decomposition of the reaction is not known, the reaction rates have to be experimentally estimated.

1.2.5 CATALYSIS

Catalysis is the change in rate of a chemical reaction due to the participation of a substance called a catalyst. Unlike other reagents that participate in the chemical reaction, a catalyst is not consumed by the reaction itself [18,19].

Catalysts that speed up the reaction are called positive catalysts while catalysts that decrease a reaction rate are called negative catalysts, even if they are quite rare in practice. Substances that slow a catalyst's effect are called inhibitors, substances that increase the activity of catalysts are called promoters, and substances that deactivate catalysts are called catalytic poisons.

Catalysis is a constant biochemical reaction with a high activation energy that is enabled and carried out at a fast pace so that the capacity of devising catalysis inhibitors or promoters is the base of many drugs whose scope is to change the reaction rate of biological reactions so as to accelerate or slow the production of particular substances inside the human body. A remarkable example of this principle is constituted by drugs based on inhibitors that lower the capability of the human body in producing immunoglobulin and immunity system cells. They are key enablers of the organs transplant procedures since they stop a possible destructive reaction of the immune system against the transplanted organ.

Catalytic reactions have a lower free energy of activation with respect to the corresponding reactions performed without catalysis, resulting in higher reaction rate at the same temperature. The free energy diagram of Figure 1.10 shows the effect of a catalyst in a hypothetical exothermic chemical reaction. The presence of the catalyst opens a different reaction pathway with a lower activation energy so as to increase the reaction rate, as shown, for example, by Equation 1.55.

Thus, catalysts have no effect on the chemical equilibrium of a reaction because the rate of both the forward and the reverse reactions are affected in the same way. The fact that a catalyst does not change the equilibrium is a consequence of the second law of thermodynamics. Suppose that a catalyst shifts a reaction equilibrium, introducing the catalyst when the reaction is at equilibrium without it causes the system to move to the new, more favorable, equilibrium, producing energy. Production of energy is a necessary result since reactions are spontaneous if and only if Gibbs free energy is produced. Removing the catalyst also causes the reaction to be out of equilibrium so that it moves to the new equilibrium state spontaneously, thereby producing energy. Both catalyst addition and removal produces energy: thus, a catalyst that could change the equilibrium would be a perpetual motion machine, a contradiction to the laws of thermodynamics.

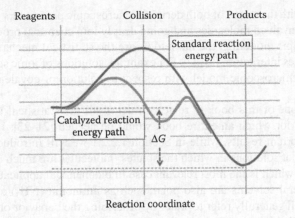

FIGURE 1.10 Alternative and favored energy path opened by the presence of a catalyst.

The basic catalysts mechanism causing the alternative and preferred reaction path to be enabled is to react with one or more reactants to form intermediate products that would not be possible without the catalyst presence. These products appear only in the middle steps of a multistep reaction, which subsequently gives the final reaction product, regenerating the catalyst in the process. The fact that standard catalysis is impossible in single-step reactions is another reason because frequently multistep reactions are preferred in the biological environment.

The following is a typical reaction scheme, where R_C represents the catalyst, R_1 and R_2 are reactants, and R_3 is the product of the reaction:

$$\text{Step 1:} \quad \alpha_1 R_1 + R_C \rightarrow R_{1\alpha_1} R_C \tag{1.61a}$$

$$\text{Step 2:} \quad \alpha_2 R_2 + R_{1\alpha_1} R_C \rightarrow R_{2\alpha_2} R_{1\alpha_1} R_C \tag{1.61b}$$

$$\text{Step 3:} \quad R_{2\alpha_2} R_{1\alpha_1} R_C \rightarrow R_{3\alpha_3} R_C \tag{1.61c}$$

$$\text{Step 4:} \quad R_{3\alpha_3} R_C \rightarrow \alpha_3 R_3 + R_C \tag{1.61d}$$

where the coefficients α_1 and α_2 are frequently equal to one and never big, so that cases in which one of them is equal to two do exist but are rare, and even rarer are cases where both are equal to two. The catalyst quantity before and after the reaction is not changed, unless the catalyst is consumed by spurious reactions or inhibited by other physical meanings such jellification of reaction products incorporating the catalyst that is physically divided by the solution in which the reaction happens. As a matter of fact, the overall reaction appears to be

$$\alpha_1 R_1 + \alpha_2 R_2 \rightarrow \alpha_3 R_3 \tag{1.62}$$

As a catalyst is regenerated in a reaction, often only small amounts are needed to increase the rate of the reaction, unless they are consumed in secondary processes.

1.2.6 SOLVABILITY IN A POLAR SOLVENT

Up to now we have analyzed the properties of solutions and of chemical reactions happening among solutes under a macroscopic point of view. Much more sophisticated microscopic model has been developed, with the scope of both deriving macroscopic parameters from the microscopic characteristics of the involved molecules and going deeply into chemical process dynamics. When dealing with microscopic modeling, the main tools are the statistical mechanics and the quantum description of molecules interaction [21,22]. For example, solutions of ionic solutes in polar solvent have a very different microscopic model with respect to solution of covalent solutes in nonpolar solvents.

It is beyond the scope of this book to review in detail all the statistical theories of the different types of solutions, for which an entire book would be needed [21–23]. Here, we qualitatively describe selected important results, while in Section 1.2.2.1 we will introduce more details about microscopic modeling of solutions in which the solutes' molecules are much bigger with respect to the solvent molecules, which is the most relevant case in biochemical applications.

Besides water, several solvents are also polar, such as ammonia (NH_3) and hydrogen cyanide (HCN) [24,25]. We will generally refer to water by describing the behavior of a solution with polar solvent, but the discussion is quite general unless it is explicitly indicated.

Liquid water consists of an extended network of H_2O molecules linked together by dipole–dipole attractions that we call hydrogen bonds, as it is shown in Figure 1.11. Because these are much weaker than ordinary chemical bonds, they are continually disrupted by thermal forces. As a result, the extended structure is highly disordered (in contrast to that of solid ice) and continually changing.

When a solute molecule is introduced into liquid water, a certain amount of energy must be expended in order to break the local hydrogen bond structure and make space for the new molecule. If the solute is itself an ion or a polar molecule, new ion–dipole or dipole–dipole attractions come into play. In favorable cases, these may release sufficient potential energy to largely compensate for the energy required to incorporate the solute into the structure.

An extreme example occurs when ammonia dissolves in water (see Figure 1.12). Each NH_3 molecule can form four hydrogen bonds, so the resulting solution is even more hydrogen-bonded than is pure water, accounting for the considerable amount of heat released in the process and the extraordinarily large solubility of ammonia in water.

When a nonpolar solute such as oxygen or hexane is introduced into a polar liquid, we might expect that the energy required to break the hydrogen bonds to make space for the new molecule is not compensated by the formation of new attractive interactions, suggesting that the process will be energetically unfavorable. We can, therefore, predict that solutes of these kinds will be only sparingly soluble in water, and this is indeed the case. Moreover, in all the cases, owing to the entropic

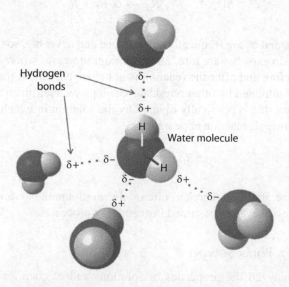

FIGURE 1.11 Hydrogen bonds formed among molecules of liquid water.

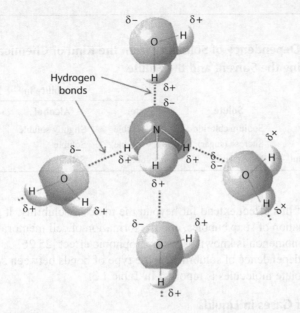

FIGURE 1.12 Scheme of hydrogen bonds forming when ammonia dissolves in water.

contribution to the solubility, we have to imagine that it increases with temperature. This is the case, as it is shown in Table 1.2.

It turns out, however, that lack of compensation for the energy needed to break solvent polar bonds accounts only partially for the small solubility of nonpolar solutes in water. As a matter of fact, H_2O molecules that surround a nonpolar intruder and find themselves unable to form energy-lowering polar interactions with it will rearrange themselves into a configuration that maximizes the hydrogen bonding between the water molecules themselves. In doing so, this creates a cage-like shell around the solute molecule. In terms of the energetics of the process, these new $H_2O–H_2O$ interactions compensate, sometimes overcompensate, for the lack of solute–H_2O interactions. But this shell of highly organized water molecules exacts its own toll on the solubility by reducing the entropy of the system. Dissolution of a solute normally increases the entropy by spreading the solute molecules (and the thermal energy they contain) through the larger volume of the solvent. But in this case, the H_2O molecules within the highly structured shell surrounding the solute molecule are themselves constrained to this location, and their number is sufficiently great to reduce the entropy more than the dissolved solute increases it. Thus, the small solubility of a nonpolar solute in water results more from the negative entropy change rather than from energetic considerations.

TABLE 1.2

Examples of Dependency of Solubility from Temperature

Compound	Type of Bonding	Solubility (g/100 mL Water)	
		At 20°C	At 100°C
Sodium chloride	Ionic	35.7	39.1
Barium sulfate	Ionic	2.3×10^{-4}	4.1×10^{-4}
Sucrose	Polar covalent	179	487
Ammonia	Polar covalent	89.9	7.4
Hydrogen chloride	Polar covalent	82.3	56.1
Oxygen	Nonpolar covalent	4.5×10^{-3}	3.3×10^{-3}

TABLE 1.3

Example of Dependency of Solubility from the Kind of Chemical Bond Characterizing the Solvent and the Solute

		Solubility In		
Kinds of Bonds	**Solute**	**Water**	**Alcohol**	**Benzene**
Ionic	Sodium chloride	Very soluble	Slightly soluble	Insoluble
Polar covalent	Sucrose (sugar)	Very soluble	Soluble	Insoluble
Nonpolar covalent	Napthalene	Insoluble	Soluble	Very soluble

The implications of this effect extend far beyond the topic of solubility. It governs the way that proteins fold, the formation of soap bubbles, and the formation of cell membranes, as we will detail in Chapter 2. This phenomenon is known as the hydrophobic effect [25,26].

A summary of the dependence of solubility on the type of bonds between solvent molecules and between solvent and solute molecules is reported in Table 1.3.

1.2.6.1 Solutions of Gases in Liquids

Gases dissolve in liquids, but usually only to a small extent. When a gas dissolves in a liquid, the ability of the gas molecules to move freely throughout the volume of the solvent is greatly restricted. If this latter volume is small, as is often the case, the gas is effectively being compressed. Both of these effects amount to a decrease in the entropy of the gas that is not usually compensated by the entropy increase due to mixing of the two kinds of molecules. Such processes greatly restrict the solubility of gases in liquids.

One important consequence of the entropy decrease when a gas dissolves in a liquid is that the solubility of a gas decreases at higher temperatures; this is in contrast to most other situations, where a rise in temperature usually leads to increased solubility. Bringing a liquid to its boiling point will completely remove a gaseous solute.

The pressure of a gas mixed in a liquid is a measure of its "escaping tendency" from the actual aggregation phase. Thus, raising the pressure of a gas in contact with a solvent will cause a larger fraction of it to pass from gaseous phase to liquid phase, increasing the solution concentration. There is a simple proportionality between gas concentration in a liquid solution with the gas external pressure that can be derived from the Raoult law, taking into account the proportionality between the concentration and the partial pressure.

As a matter of fact, equilibrium between liquid and gaseous phase is reached when the partial pressure the solution will cause when posed in a void container is exactly balanced by the external gas pressure.

1.2.6.2 Solutions of Liquids in Liquids

While all gases are more or less soluble in water, the situation is different for liquids, since there are liquids that are completely nonsoluble. A useful general rule is that liquids are completely miscible when their intermolecular forces are very similar in nature [21].

Thus, water is miscible with other liquids that can engage in hydrogen bonding, whereas a hydrocarbon liquid in which London dispersion forces are the only significant intermolecular effect will only be completely miscible with similar kinds of liquids.

Substances such as the alcohols, $CH_3(CH_2)_nOH$, which are hydrogen-bonding (and thus hydrophilic) at one end and hydrophobic at the other, tend to be at least partially miscible with both kinds of solvents. If n is large, the hydrocarbon properties dominate and the alcohol has only a limited solubility in water. Very small values of n allow the −OH group to dominate, so miscibility in water increases and becomes unlimited in ethanol ($n = 1$) and methanol ($n = 0$).

Owing to the same reason, miscibility with hydrocarbons decreases owing to the energy required to break alcohol–alcohol hydrogen bonds when a nonpolar liquid is added.

1.2.6.3 Solutions of Solids in Liquids

1.2.6.3.1 Molecular Solids

The stronger intermolecular forces in solids require more input of energy in order to disperse the molecular units into a liquid solution, but there is also a considerable increase in entropy due to the great increase of the average molecules' distance and of the much smaller order of their configuration.

As the molecular weight of the solid increases, the intermolecular forces holding the solid together also increase, and solubility tends to fall off; thus, the solid linear hydrocarbons $CH_3(CH_2)_nCH_3$ ($n > 20$) show diminishing solubility in hydrocarbon liquids.

1.2.6.3.2 Ionic Solids

Since the coulomb forces that bind ions and highly polar molecules into solids are quite strong, we might expect these solids to be insoluble in just about any solvent. Ionic solids are insoluble in most nonaqueous solvents, but the high solubility of some of them, for example, NaCl, in water suggests the need for some further explanation. The key factor here turns out to be the interaction of the ions with the solvent, as pictorially illustrated in Figure 1.13. The electrically charged ions exert a strong coulomb attraction on the end of the water molecule that has the opposite partial charge. As a consequence, ions in solution are always hydrated; that is, they are quite tightly bound to water molecules through ion–dipole interaction. The number of water molecules contained in the primary hydration shell varies with the radius and charge of the ion.

The dissolution of an ionic solid MX in water can be thought of as a sequence of two steps:

$$\text{Step 1:} \quad MX(s) \rightarrow M^+(g) + X^-(g) \quad \Delta H > 0 \quad \text{(lattice dissol.)} \tag{1.63a}$$

$$\text{Step 2:} \quad M^+(g) + X^-(g) + H_2O \rightarrow M^+(aq) + X^-(aq) \quad \Delta H < 0 \quad \text{(hydration)} \tag{1.63b}$$

The first reaction is always endothermic since it breaks up ionic bonds of the crystal lattice. The hydration step is always exothermic as H_2O molecules are attracted to the electrostatic field of the ion. The values of the enthalpy of these two steps of the solution processes are shown in

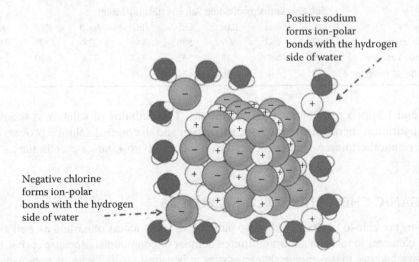

Positive sodium forms ion-polar bonds with the hydrogen side of water

Negative chlorine forms ion-polar bonds with the hydrogen side of water

FIGURE 1.13 Pictorial illustration of how water decomposes and hydrates a NaCl crystal during solvation.

TABLE 1.4

**Examples of Values of Lattice Dissociation Energies in kJ/Mole
for a Few Ionic Crystals**

	F$^-$	Cl$^-$	Br$^-$	I$^-$
	Lattice Dissociation Energies (kJ/Mole)			
Li$^+$	+1031	+848	+803	+759
Na$^+$	+918	+780	+742	+705
K$^+$	+817	+711	+679	+651
Mg^{2+}	+2957	+2526	+2440	+2327
Ca^{2+}	+2630	+2258	+2176	+2074
Sr^{2+}	+2492	+2156	+2075	+1963

TABLE 1.5

**Examples of Values of the Hydration Energy for a Few
Common Ions in kJ/Mole**

Hydration Energies (kJ/Mole)			
H$^+$(g)	−1075	F$^-$(g)	−503
Li$^+$(g)	−515	Cl$^-$(g)	−369
Na$^+$(g)	−405	Br$^-$(g)	−336
K$^+$(g)	−321	I$^-$(g)	−398
Mg^{2+}(g)	−1922	OH$^-$(g)	−460
Ca^{2+}(g)	−1592	NO$_3^-$	−328
Sr^{2+}(g)	−1445	SO$_4^{2-}$	−1145

TABLE 1.6

**Example of Calculation of the Solution Enthalpy in kJ/Mole for a Few Common
Solutions**

Substance	LiF	NaI	KBr	CsI	LiCl	NaCl	KCl	AgCl
Solution Enthalpy of Some Salt Crystals (kJ/Mole)								
Lattice energy	1021	682	669	586	846	778	707	910
Hydration energy	1017	686	649	552	884	774	690	844
Enthalpy of solution	+3	−4	+20	+34	−38	+4	+17	+66

Tables 1.4 and 1.5 for a few common ionic solutions. The enthalpy of solution is the sum of the lattice and hydration energies, and can have either sign and the overall solution process can come out as either endothermic or exothermic, and examples of both kinds are common as shown in Table 1.6.

1.3 ORGANIC CHEMISTRY BUILDING BLOCKS

Carbon atoms are able to combine with large numbers of other atoms of carbon as well as atoms of many other elements to form an almost unlimited number of compounds. Because carbon chemistry is so extensive and has many unique characteristics, it is usually called with its own name: organic chemistry.

Despite the huge number of existing and potential organic compounds, carbon chemistry can be greatly simplified once it is realized that the chemistry of organic compounds can, in large part, be reduced to the reactions that are characteristic of particular groups of atoms within the molecules. These groups of atoms are called functional groups [27,28]. The functional groups bestow most of the chemical properties on a molecule. Thus recognizing functional groups where they appear in any organic molecule is a key point to understanding the properties of the molecule.

1.3.1 Hydrocarbons: Types and Structure

The simplest organic compounds, the hydrocarbons, contain only carbon and hydrogen atoms [29,30]. They constitute the main source of our energy supply in the form of natural gas, kerosene and petroleum and are mostly derived from crude oil and natural gas.

There are several families of hydrocarbons, each distinguished by a particular functional group. Hydrocarbons may be saturated compounds in which there are no double or triple bonds between any of the carbon atoms or they may consist of unsaturated molecules containing at least one multiple bond between two carbon atoms.

The presence of a double or triple bond imparts different characteristics to unsaturated hydrocarbons compared with saturated hydrocarbons. The hydrocarbons are grouped into various families of compounds that share similar properties:

- Saturated hydrocarbons are called alkanes.
- Hydrocarbons that include at least one double bond in their molecule, that is, containing the C=C functional group, are called alkenes.
- Hydrocarbons containing at least one triple bond, that is, containing the C/C functional group, are called alkynes.

All the above classes of hydrocarbons are called aliphatic hydrocarbons and are characterized by a single, well-specified type of bond between their carbon atoms.

Hydrocarbons in which different types of bonds coexist, even in hybrid form, also exist: they are called aromatic hydrocarbons or arenes. The compound benzene is an example of an aromatic hydrocarbon.

Alkanes have so few reactions apart from combustion in oxygen that an alkane is not considered to contain a functional group. However, alkenes and alkynes are both very reactive due to the possibility of breaking the multiple bonds characterizing their functional group to bind other atoms or molecules.

1.3.1.1 Alkanes

Alkanes may contain chains of C atoms with or without branches, also called side chains. They can also form rings of C atoms in which case they are called cyclic alkanes. We can divide the alkanes into subclasses, depending on the reciprocal position of carbon atoms. The simplest class is that of the simple-chain alkanes, having the carbon atoms linked in a simple chain.

The two extreme carbon atoms have three free valences, bonding three hydrogen atoms, the carbons in the middle of the chain have the capability of linking only two hydrogen, so that the general formula for simple-chain alkanes is $C_nH_{(2n+2)}$.

The simplest alkane of this class containing only one C atom is named methane, its chemical formula is CH_4 and its structure consists of a central C atom bonded to four H atoms by single covalent bonds as shown in Figure 1.14a. Thus, the valence of the C atom (four) is saturated and the valence of each of the H atoms (one) is also saturated. The second member of the alkane family, named ethane, consists of molecules containing two C atoms joined by a single bond and each of the remaining three valences of both C atoms are used to form single bonds to H atoms (see Figure 1.14b). This gives a total of two C atoms and six H atoms, so the molecular formula of ethane is C_2H_6.

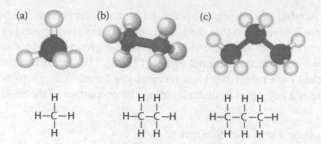

FIGURE 1.14 Chemical formulas and structural representations of methane (a), ethane (b), and propane (c). The ball-and-stick convention is used for the stereographic representation.

The third member of this family, propane, has three C atoms joined to each other in a chain and each of the two end C atoms (terminal atoms) is also bonded to three H atoms. The C atom in the middle of the chain has only two unused valences remaining, so it bonds to just two H atoms, giving a total of three C atoms and eight H atoms, thus a molecular formula of C_3H_8 and its structure is represented in Figure 1.14c.

A second class of alkanes is that of cyclic alkanes, having the carbon atoms arranged in a circular chain. The general formula for cyclic alkanes have two less H atoms than the noncyclic molecules because two of the carbon atoms in the ring use one valence each to join together in order to form the ring so it writes C_nH_{2n}. As the minimum number of C atoms that can form a ring is three, the simplest cyclic alkane would have the molecular formula C_3H_6 and is named cyclopropane.

Noncyclic alkanes that contain four carbon atoms can be bonded either as a straight chain of four C atoms or as a branched chain structure containing three C atoms with the fourth C atom bonded to the central atom of the chain as the branch as shown in Figure 1.15. Both compounds have the same chemical formula, C_4H_{10}, but are different compounds with different properties such as melting point, boiling point, and density. Compounds that have the same molecular formula but differ in some aspect of their structures are called isomers. There are several possible types of isomerism. The type of isomerism that gives rise to the two forms of the compound C_4H_{10} is called constitutional isomerism.

The formulas and names of the first alkanes are reported in Table 1.7. Also a few chemical properties of these composites are listed. Increasing the molecular weight the importance of van der Waals forces increases. As a consequence the aggregation state at standard conditions passes from gas to liquid and, beyond $n = 15$, to solid. Coherently, the boiling temperature is an increasing function of n.

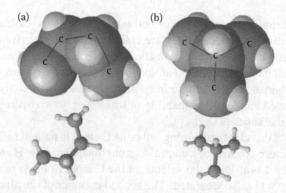

FIGURE 1.15 The isomeric forms of butane: (a) butane and (b) isobutane; molecules are represented using the volume convention and the chemical formula of the carbon chain is superimposed to the molecule graphical representation. The ball-and-stick representation is also reported.

TABLE 1.7

Chemical and Structural Formulas of the First Alkali with Isometrics Forms

n	Molecular Formula	Constitutional Formula	Name	Aggregation $T = 25°C$, $P = 1$ atm	Boiling Temperature (°C)	ΔG_{form} (kcal/Mole)
1	CH_4	CH_4	Methane	Gas	−164	−12.14
2	C_2H_6	CH_3CH_3	Ethane	Gas	−88.63	−7.86
3	C_3H_8	$CH_3CH_2CH_3$	Propane	Gas	−42.07	−5.61
4	C_4H_{10}	$CH_3CH_2CH_2CH_3CH_3(CH2)_2CH_3$	Butane	Gas	−0.5	−3.75
5	C_5H_{12}	$CH_3CH_2CH_2CH_2CH_3CH_3(CH_2)_3CH_3$	Pentane	Liquid	36.07	−1.96
6	C_6H_{14}	$CH_3CH_2CH_2CH_2CH_2CH_3CH_3(CH_2)_4CH_3$	Hexane	Liquid	68.95	+0.05
7	C_7H_{16}	$CH_3CH_2CH_2CH_2CH_2CH_2CH_3CH_3(CH_2)_5CH_3$	Heptane	Liquid	98.42	+2.09
8	C_8H_{18}	$CH_3CH_2CH_2CH_2CH_2CH_2CH_2CH_3$	Octane	Liquid	125.66	+4.14
9	C_9H_{20}	$CH_3CH_2CH_2CH_2CH_2CH_2CH_2CH_2CH_3$	Nonane	Liquid	150.80	+6.18

Also, the formation of free energy increases with n, passing from negative to positive numbers when n increases from 5 to 6. This means that the molecules become less and less stable with increasing n. On the other side, the bond energies of the C–C covalent bond and of the C–H covalent bond are 83 kcal/mole and 99 kcal/mole, respectively. These are quite high values, indicating that up to the moment in which van der Waals repulsion between nearby carbon atoms compensate partially the strong bonds, the alkanes with a small number of carbon atoms are among the most stable organic components at standard conditions.

1.3.1.2 Alkyl Groups

An alkyl compound is derived from any alkane compound by deleting one H atom from the chain and leaving a free valence on the alkyl group available to bond to some other group. This free valence is often shown as a line like a covalent bond to reinforce the fact that the alkyl group is not an independent entity. Normally, any alkyl group will be bonded to another atom in a compound and not have a free existence like a polyatomic ion.

Alkyl groups are named by removing the "ane" ending from the parent alkane and replacing it with "yl." Thus, from methane, the methyl group (represented as $CH_3\text{–}$) would be derived, from ethane, the ethyl group (represented as $C_2H_5\text{–}$), and so on. The line attached to the formula for each alkyl group represents the free valence remaining on a C atom. For convenience and because the particular alkyl group often has little effect on the functional group reactions of a compound, they are often represented simply as R– in a general structural formula.

Naming alkanes that include one or more branched chains in their molecules requires some further rules, the branches being named as alkyl groups substituting H atoms on the main chain. The longest carbon chain is named as above for compounds with an unbranched chain but any side chains are named as alkyl groups and their position on the main chain is given by a number designating the C atom to which they are bonded.

For example, the compound having the structural formula in Figure 1.16a would be named as a butane because there are four C atoms in the longest chain of carbon atoms. A methyl group, $CH_3\text{–}$, is attached to the second carbon from the end, so the name for the compound would be 2-methylbutane. Note that the C atoms in the main chain are numbered so that overall the smallest numbers are used in the name of the compound and they may not necessarily be numbered from left to right—in this example, the chain is numbered from right to left.

The next example, considering the formula reported in Figure 1.16b illustrates another rule that applies when there is more than one alkyl group attached to the main chain, namely that the groups be named in alphabetical order. This compound has seven C atoms in the longest chain so it would

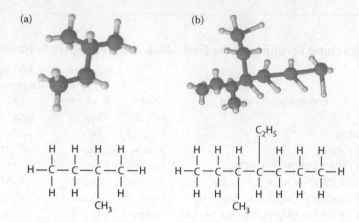

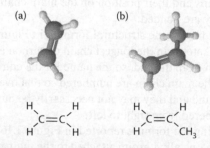

FIGURE 1.16   Structural formulas and graphical representations of 2-methylbutane (a) and 4-ethyl-3-methyl-heptane (b).

be named as a heptane with a methyl group, CH_{3-}, attached to C atom number 3 (numbering from the left this time) and an ethyl group, C_2H_{5-}, attached to C atom number 4.

This order uses the smallest numbers (3 and 4) rather than the alternative of numbering from the right, which would allocate the methyl group to C atom number 5 and the ethyl group to C atom number 4. Naming the side chains in alphabetical order, the full name for the compound is 4-ethyl-3-methylheptane.

If more than one of any given alkyl group is substituted on the main chain of an alkane, the total number of that group is indicated in the name by use of the prefixes di, tri, tetra, penta, and so on with the numbers of the C atoms to which they are bonded given first. For example, a compound with two methyl groups attached to C atoms numbers 2 and 3 would be named as 2,3-dimethyl-heptane. The prefix di- is not included in deciding the alphabetical order of the substituents in the name—ethyl still is listed ahead of dimethyl.

1.3.1.3   Alkenes

Alkenes contain the functional group consisting of a carbon/carbon double bond, represented as C=C. Naming alkenes uses the same stem as for alkanes to indicate the number of C atoms in the longest chain which includes the double bond and the ending "ene" is attached. In addition, a number is required to indicate the position of the double bond in the chain. The simplest alkene has the molecular formula C_2H_4 and has the structure shown in Figure 1.17a. It is named ethene using the systematic nomenclature. However, common names were in use long before the current system was adopted and this compound is generally named as ethylene in deference to existing practice.

FIGURE 1.17   Molecular formulas and graphical representations of ethane (a) and propene (b).

The second alkene in the series contains three C atoms and has the molecular formula C_3H_6. Its structure is represented in part (b) of Figure 1.17 and this compound is named as propene or, using the common name, propylene. The ball–stick structures are also shown for each molecule.

Inspection of these molecular formulas indicates that the alkene series of hydrocarbons has the general formula C_nH_{2n} where again n is the number of C atoms in the molecule. Neither ethene nor propene requires a number to indicate the position of the double bond as there is only one possible structure.

However, the unbranched alkene containing four carbon atoms could exist as two possible isomers, so the name must include a number to indicate the location of the double bond in the chain. The convention used is to number the C atoms in the longest chain, which includes the double bond so that the smallest number can be allocated to the first C atom of the double bond. Branched chain alkenes are named using the same procedures as for alkanes.

1.3.1.4 Alkynes

Alkynes contain the functional group consisting of a carbon/carbon triple bond which is represented as C/C. The first member of the alkyne series has the molecular formula C_2H_2 and is named as ethyne using the systematic name which incorporates the same stems used for alkanes to which is added the ending "yne." However, in practice, its trivial name, acetylene, is always used.

1.3.1.5 Stereoscopic Structure of Hydrocarbons

1.3.1.5.1 Alkanes

Up to now we have used chemical formulas as chains. These formulas, however, do not take into account spatial disposition of the atoms, which is a fundamental element to determine the properties of a certain molecule. The tetrahedral arrangement of bonds around a central atom is one common spatial disposition, the tetrahedral angle between any bonds on the atom being 109.5. In particular, this is the arrangement of the bonds around any carbon atom in a molecule where it has four single bonds such as in alkanes.

Atoms in alkanes are often referred to as being in a "chain" but this analogy is not quite accurate because any two atoms joined by a single covalent bond have the property of free rotation about the bond axis. Thus, for any C–C bond in an alkane, the two sections of the molecule joined at that bond are able to rotate relative to each other about the bond axis. A better description of an alkane would be as having a backbone of C atoms in a chain where each link is joined to the next by a swivel.

This is reproduced in the so-called ball-and-stick representation that we have used several times up to now in figures besides the molecular formula (see Appendix 1). In this representation, fixed angles are set to the correct values and the groups can rotate as permitted by the type of bond one with respect to the other.

Also, in the volume representation (also described in Appendix 1), the reciprocal position in space of the various atoms is correctly taken into account, even if the fact that atoms representing spheres superimpose to simulate electrons sharing in covalent bonds renders this property less evident. On the other hand, the volume representation gives a much better idea of the space occupied by a molecule, which is another important property of the great organic molecules.

1.3.1.5.2 Alkenes

Unlike single covalent bonds, there is no rotation possible about the C=C double bond. Instead, the two C atoms of the C=C bond plus the other four atoms joined to them remain in the same plane at all times.

For example, the unsaturated hydrocarbon ethene (ethylene) has a double bond joining the carbon atoms as shown in Figure 1.17. As a consequence, as it is represented in the stereographic molecule representation, all the atoms are constrained to be on the same plane, with bond angles of about 120.

The rigidity imposed by the nonrotation of the C=C bond leads to another type of isomerism called geometric isomerism—molecules with the same molecular and structural formulas but with different spatial arrangements.

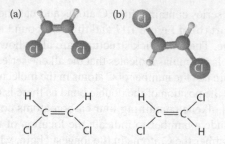

FIGURE 1.18 Geometric isomers: structure and stereographic representation of Z 1,2-dichloroethene and E 1,2-dichloroethene.

An example would be 1,2-dichloroethene (1,2- dichloroethylene), the two forms of which (called Z for "same side" and E for "opposite side" of the C=C bond) are illustrated in Figure 1.18. The two isomers have different physical and chemical properties.

1.3.1.5.3 Alkynes

When two carbon atoms are joined by a triple bond, each C atom has only one remaining valence which is, bonded to either another C atom or an H atom. In either case, both C atoms joined by the triple bond and the two other atoms to which they are bonded are all in a linear arrangement.

1.3.1.6 Aromatic Hydrocarbons

Aromatic hydrocarbons are characterized by the aromatic bond. The aromatic bond can be described with a sort of covalent bond where the shared electrons have much more distributed wave functions so as to be shared with two nearby carbon atoms. In the presence of the aromatic bond the typical hexagon shape generates with carbon atoms at the vertices. Each carbon atom shares with the nearby atoms an electron on a p orbital. This orbital is characterized by two lobes, both perpendicular to the hexagon plane, as shown in Figure 1.19a. When the molecule is formed, the minimum energy state, that is, the ground state of the molecule, is reached when the electrons completely delocalize in a molecular orbital spanning all the ring that is formed by two wide lobes, one below and one above the ring plane, as shown in Figure 1.19b. The electron sharing creates six equivalent bonds, differently from the bonds of carbon atoms in an open chain. This strongly influences the chemical properties of aromatic hydrocarbons, which results to be very resistant against reduction and oxidation and add with difficulty new functional groups to their molecule, while the most common reactions in which aromatic hydrocarbons are involved imply substitution of one carbon atom with some other atom.

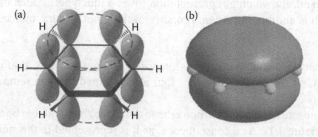

FIGURE 1.19 Principal scheme of the aromatic bond where every carbon atom shares a p electron with nearby atoms: p orbitals of the six carbon atoms forming the ring (a) and ground energy level molecular orbital of benzene (b). The molecular orbital has the needed degeneracy so that the electrons, composed of opposite spins couples, are disposed so as to satisfy Pauli principle.

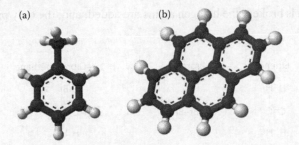

FIGURE 1.20 Stereographic structure of (a) toluene, where an aromatic ring links a methyl group, and (b) pyrene composed of four linked aromatic rings.

Different aromatic rings can combine via substitution of the hydrocarbon characteristic C–H bond with a couple of bonds between nearby aromatic rings. Examples of these structures are toluene and pyrene, whose multiring structure is shown in Figure 1.20.

Aromatic rings can also form by establishing double or even triple bonds among a few of the carbon atoms couples. In this case, the bonds are no more all equivalent and the reactivity of the composite is higher.

In every case, under a steric point of view, aromatic rings tends to be planar, while nearby aromatic rings has a limited capacity to rotate one with respect to the other. Thus, also under a spatial composition point of view, aromatic composites are rigid, thereby increasing their stability.

1.3.2 FUNCTIONAL GROUPS

Ideally, hydrocarbons constitute the backbone of all the organic molecules. Even the more complex molecules such as nucleic acids or enzymes can be built by binding several hydrocarbons and substituting to the hydrogen atoms more complex functional groups.

There are no infinite numbers of functional group, although the possibilities seem huge. Nature has selected a limited number of groups and uses them to build all the immense array of organic molecules. Here, we cannot naturally go in-depth into the role and chemical properties of each functional group when it is bonded to a particular set of hydrocarbon structures, but at least we will review the functional groups structure and main role.

1.3.2.1 Allogeneic Functional Group

The most commonly demonstrated halogenation reactions are brominations using bromine water, Br_2, which is a red-brown colored liquid in standard conditions. Under standard laboratory conditions, alkanes do not react with halogens, but they allow a substitution reaction with an allogeneic group in the presence of UV light. During this reaction, halogen atoms substitute for hydrogen atoms, one at a time, producing a haloalkane and a hydrogen halide.

An example of bromination is given by the following reaction, where we use structural formulas to clearly detect the substitution on which the reaction is based.

$$
\begin{array}{cccccccc}
\text{Ethane} & + & \text{Bromine} & \xrightarrow{\text{UV}} & \text{Bromoethane} & + & \text{Bromide} & \\[2mm]
\begin{array}{c}\text{H H}\\ |\ \ |\\ \text{H–C–C–H}\\ |\ \ |\\ \text{H H}\end{array} & + & \text{Br–Br} & \xrightarrow{\text{UV}} & \begin{array}{c}\text{H H}\\ |\ \ |\\ \text{H–C–C–Br}\\ |\ \ |\\ \text{H H}\end{array} & + & \text{H–Br} & \text{(1.64)}
\end{array}
$$

Alkenes readily react with halogens under standard laboratory conditions. In this reaction, halogen atoms are added across the double bond of the alkene. In an alkene containing only one double bond, the double bond is broken, the halogen atoms are added, and, the only product of the reaction will be a dihaloalkane.

$$
\begin{array}{ccccc}
\text{Ethene} & + & \text{Bromine} & \rightarrow & \text{1,2–Dibromoethane} \\[6pt]
\begin{array}{c} \text{H} \;\; \text{H} \\ | \;\; | \\ \text{C=C} \\ | \;\; | \\ \text{H} \;\; \text{H} \end{array} & + & \text{Br–Br} & \rightarrow & \begin{array}{c} \text{Br} \; \text{Br} \\ | \;\; | \\ \text{H–C–C–H} \\ | \;\; | \\ \text{H} \; \text{H} \end{array}
\end{array}
\tag{1.65}
$$

In a bromination reaction, if excess alkene is present, the reaction mixture will change from a red-brown color to colorless.

1.3.2.2 Alcoholic Functional Group

An alcohol is an organic compound in which the hydroxyl functional group (–OH) is bound to a carbon atom. In particular, this carbon center should be saturated, having single bonds to three other atoms [31]. An important class of alcohols is the simple acyclic alcohols that are obtained by acyclic saturated hydrocarbons, so that their general formula is $C_nH_{2n+1}OH$. Of those, ethanol (C_2H_5OH) is the type of alcohol found in alcoholic beverages, and in common speech the word "alcohol" refers specifically to ethanol.

Other alcohols are usually described with a clarifying adjective, as in isopropyl alcohol (propan-2-ol) or wood alcohol (methyl alcohol, or methanol).

In the IUPAC system, the name of the alkane chain loses the terminal "e" and adds "ol," for example, "methanol" and "ethanol" [31]. When necessary, the position of the hydroxyl group is indicated by a number between the alkane name and the "ol": propan-1-ol for $CH_3CH_2CH_2OH$ and propan-2-ol for $CH_3CH(OH)CH_3$.

Sometimes, the position number is written before the IUPAC name: 1-propanol and 2-propanol. If a higher-priority group is present (such as an aldehyde, ketone or carboxylic acid), then it is necessary to use the prefix "hydroxyl," for example, 1-hydroxy-2-propanone (CH_3COCH_2OH).

The IUPAC nomenclature is used in scientific publications and where precise identification of the substance is important. In other less formal contexts, an alcohol is often called with the name of the corresponding alkyl group followed by the word "alcohol," for example, methyl alcohol and ethyl alcohol. Propyl alcohol may be n-propyl alcohol or isopropyl alcohol, depending on whether the hydroxyl group is bonded to the first or second carbon on the propane chain.

Alcohols are classified into primary, secondary, and tertiary, based on the number of carbon atoms connected to the carbon atom that bears the hydroxyl group. The primary alcohols have general formulas RCH_2OH; secondary ones are $RR'CHOH$; and tertiary ones are $RR'R''COH$, where R, R' and R'' stand for alkyl groups.

Ethanol and n-propyl alcohol are primary alcohols; isopropyl alcohol is a secondary one. The prefixes *sec*- (or *s*-) and *tert*- (or *t*-), conventionally in italics, may be used before the alkyl group's name to distinguish secondary and tertiary alcohols, respectively, from the primary one. For example, isopropyl alcohol is occasionally called *sec*-propyl alcohol, and the tertiary alcohol ($CH_3)_3COH$, or 2-methylpropan-2-ol in IUPAC nomenclature is commonly known as *tert*-butyl alcohol or *tert*-butanol. A list of common alcohols with the common alcohol name and the IUPAC name besides the molecular formula is reported in Table 1.8.

In general, the hydroxyl group makes the alcohol molecule polar. Those groups can form hydrogen bonds to one another and to other compounds. This hydrogen bonding means that alcohols can be used as protic solvents.

The solubility of alcohols is generally influenced by two phenomena with opposite effects: the tendency of the polar OH to promote solubility in water, and the tendency of the carbon chain to resist it. Thus, methanol, ethanol, and propanol are miscible in water because the hydroxyl group

TABLE 1.8
List of Common Alcohols with the Common Alcohol Name and the IUPAC Name besides the Molecular Formula

Chemical Formula	IUPAC Name	Common Name
Monohydric Alcohols		
CH_3OH	Methanol	Wood alcohol
C_2H_5OH	Ethanol	Grain alcohol
C_3H_7OH	Isopropyl alcohol	Rubbing alcohol
C_4H_9OH	Butyl alcohol	Butanol
$C_5H_{11}OH$	Pentanol	Amyl alcohol
$C_{16}H_{33}OH$	Hexadecan-1-ol	Acetyl alcohol
Polyhydric Alcohols		
$C_2H_4(OH)_2$	Ethane-1,2-diol	Ethylene glycol
$C_3H_5(OH)_3$	Propane-1,2,3-triol	Glycerin
$C_4H_6(OH)_4$	Butane-1,2,3,4-tetraol	Erythritol
$C_5H_7(OH)_5$	Pentane-1,2,3,4,5-pentol	Xylitol
$C_6H_8(OH)_6$	Hexane-1,2,3,4,5,6-hexol	Mannitol, sorbitol
$C_7H_9(OH)_7$	Heptane-1,2,3,4,5,6,7-heptol	Volemitol
Unsaturated Aliphatic Alcohols		
C_3H_5OH	Prop-2-ene-1-ol	Allyl alcohol
$C_{10}H_{17}OH$	3,7-Dimethylocta-2,6-dien-1-ol	Geraniol
C_3H_3OH	Prop-2-in-1-ol	Propargyl alcohol
Alicyclic Alcohols		
$C_6H_6(OH)_6$	Cyclohexane-1,2,3,4,5,6-hexol	Inositol
$C_{10}H_{19}OH$	2-(2-Propyl)-5-methyl-cyclohexane-1-ol	Menthol

wins over the short carbon chain. Butanol, with a four-carbon chain, is moderately soluble because of a balance between the two trends. Alcohols of five or more carbons (pentanol and higher) are effectively insoluble in water because of the hydrocarbon chain's dominance. All simple alcohols are miscible in organic solvents.

Because of hydrogen bonding, alcohols tend to have higher boiling points than comparable hydrocarbons and ethers. The boiling point of the alcohol ethanol is 78.29°C, compared to 69°C for the hydrocarbon hexane (a common constituent of gasoline), and 34.6°C for diethyl ether.

Alcohols, like water, can show either acidic or basic properties at the –OH group. With a pK_a of around 16–19, they are, in general, slightly weaker acids than water, but they are still able to react with strong bases such as sodium hydride or reactive metals such as sodium. The salts that result are called alkoxides, with the general formula RO– M+.

Meanwhile, the oxygen atom has lone pairs of nonbonded electrons that render it weakly basic in the presence of strong acids such as sulfuric acid.

Alcohols can also undergo oxidation to give aldehydes, ketones or carboxylic acids, or they can be dehydrated to alkenes. They react to form ester compounds, and they can (if activated first) undergo substitution reactions where they work a nucleophile role. A nucleophile is a chemical species that donates an electron pair to another species (called electrophile) to form a chemical bond. All molecules or ions with a free pair of electrons or at least one pi bond can act as nucleophiles.

As one moves from primary to secondary to tertiary alcohols with the same backbone, the hydrogen bond strength, the boiling point, and the acidity typically decrease.

1.3.2.3 Ester Functional Group

Esters are chemical compounds derived by reacting an oxoacid with a hydroxyl compound such as an alcohol or phenol (see the representation of the functional group in Figure 1.21).

Esters are usually derived from an inorganic acid or organic acid in which at least one –OH (hydroxyl) group is replaced by an –O–alkyl (alkoxy) group, and most commonly from carboxylic acids and alcohols. That is, esters are formed by condensing an acid with an alcohol.

Esters are ubiquitous. Most naturally occurring fats and oils are the fatty acid esters of glycerol. Esters with low molecular weight are commonly used as fragrances and found in essential oils and pheromones. Phosphoesters form the backbone of DNA molecules. Nitrate esters, such as nitroglycerin, are known for their explosive properties, while polyesters are important plastics, with monomers linked by ester moieties.

Ester names are derived from the parent alcohol and the parent acid, where the latter may be an organic or an inorganic acid. Esters derived from the simplest carboxylic acids are commonly named according to the more traditional, so-called "trivial names," for example, as formate, acetate, propionate and butyrate, as opposed to the IUPAC nomenclature methanoate, ethanoate, propanoate, and butanoate. Esters derived from more complex carboxylic acids are, however, more frequently named using the systematic IUPAC nomenclature, based on the name for the acid followed by the suffix -oate. For example, the ester hexyl octanoate, also known under the trivial name hexyl caprylate, has the formula $CH_3(CH_2)_6CO_2(CH_2)_5CH_3$.

The chemical formulas of organic esters are typically written in the format of RCO_2R', where R and R′ are the hydrocarbon parts of the carboxylic acid and alcohol, respectively. For example, butyl acetate, derived from butanol and acetic acid, would be written as $CH_3CO_2C_4H_9$. Alternative presentations are common, including BuOAc and $CH_3COOC_4H_9$.

Cyclic esters are called lactones, regardless of whether they are derived from an organic acid or an inorganic acid. They are more polar than ethers but less polar than alcohols, participate in hydrogen bonds as hydrogen bond acceptors, but cannot act as hydrogen bond donors, unlike their parent alcohols. This ability to participate in hydrogen bonding confers some water solubility. Because of their lack of hydrogen-bond-donating ability, esters do not self-associate. Consequently, esters are more volatile than carboxylic acids of similar molecular weight.

Esters contain a carbonyl center, which gives rise to 120°C–C–O and O–C–O angles. Unlike amides, esters are structurally flexible functional groups because rotation about the C–O–C bonds has a low barrier. Their flexibility and low polarity is manifested in their physical properties; they tend to be less rigid (lower melting point) and more volatile (lower boiling point) than the corresponding amides. The pK_a of the α-hydrogens on esters is around 25.

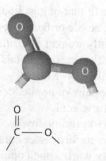

FIGURE 1.21 The ester functional group: chemical formula and graphical representation in the ball-and-stick convention.

1.3.2.4 Ether Functional Group

Ethers are a class of organic compounds that contain an ether group—an oxygen atom connected to two alkyl or aryl groups—of general formula R–O–R'. A typical example is the solvent and anesthetic diethyl ether (whose structure in the ball-and-stick and the volume representations is shown in Figure 1.22), commonly referred to simply as "ether" (CH_3CH_2–O–CH_2CH_3). Ethers are common in organic chemistry and pervasive in biochemistry, as they are common linkages in carbohydrates and lignin.

Ethers feature C–O–C linkage defined by a bond angle of about 104.5° and C–O distances of about 140 pm. The barrier to rotation about the C–O bonds is low. The bonding of oxygen in ethers, alcohols and water is similar. In the language of valence bond theory, the hybridization at oxygen is sp^3. Oxygen is more electronegative than carbon, thus the hydrogen alpha to ethers are more acidic than in simple hydrocarbons. They are far less acidic than hydrogen alpha to ketones, however.

Depending on the groups at R and R', ether is classified into two types:

- Simple ethers or symmetrical ethers
- Mixed ethers or unsymmetrical ethers

The names for simple ethers, those with none or few other functional groups, are a composite of the two substituents followed by "ether": ethyl methyl ether ($CH_3OC_2H_5$), diphenylether ($C_6H_5OC_6H_5$). IUPAC rules are often not followed for simple ethers. As for other organic compounds, very common ethers acquired names before rules for nomenclature were formalized. Diethyl ether is simply called "ether," but was once called sweet oil of vitriol. Methyl phenyl ether is anisole, because it was originally found in aniseed. The aromatic ethers include furans. Acetals (α-alkoxy ethers R–CH(–OR)–O–R) are another class of ethers with characteristic properties.

In the IUPAC nomenclature system, ethers are named using the general formula "alkoxyalkane," for example, CH_3–CH_2–O–CH_3 is methoxyethane. If the ether is part of a more complex molecule, it is described as an alkoxy substituent, so –OCH_3 would be considered a "methoxy-" group. The simpler alkyl radical is written in front, so CH_3–O–CH_2CH_3 would be given as methoxy(CH_3O) ethane(CH_2CH_3). The nomenclature of describing the two alkyl groups and appending "ether," for example, "ethyl methyl ether" in the example above, is a trivial usage.

Ether molecules cannot form hydrogen bonds with each other, resulting in a relatively low boiling point compared to those of the analogous alcohols. The difference, however, in the boiling points of the ethers and their isometric alcohols becomes lower as the carbon chains become longer, as the van der Waals interactions of the extended carbon chain dominates over the presence of hydrogen bonding.

Ethers are slightly polar. The C–O–C bond angle in the functional group is about 110°, and the C–O dipoles do not cancel out. Ethers are more polar than alkenes but not as polar as alcohols, esters, or amides of comparable structure. However, the presence of two lone pairs of electrons on the oxygen atoms makes hydrogen bonding with water molecules possible.

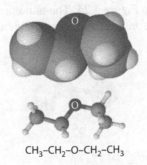

CH_3–CH_2–O–CH_2–CH_3

FIGURE 1.22 Chemical structure of diethyl ether (frequently simply called ether).

TABLE 1.9

A Few Physical Properties of Selected Ethers

	Structure	Boiling Temperature (°C)	Melting Temperature (°C)	Solubility in Water (g/L)	Dipole Moment (D)
Dimethyl ether	CH_3-O-CH_3	−138.5	−23.0	70	1.30
Diethyl ether	$CH_3CH_2-O-CH_2CH_3$	−116.3	34.4	69	1.14
Tetrahydrofuran	$O(CH_2)_4$	−108.4	66.0	Miscible	1.74
Dioxane	$O(C_2H_4)_2O$	11.8	101.3	Miscible	0.45

Cyclic ethers such as tetrahydrofuran and 1,4-dioxane are miscible in water because of the more exposed oxygen atom for hydrogen bonding as compared to aliphatic ethers. A few physical properties of selected ethers are reported in Table 1.9.

1.3.2.5 Aldehyde Functional Group

An aldehyde is an organic compound containing a formyl group. This functional group, with the structure R–CHO, consists of a carbonyl center (a carbon double bonded to oxygen) bonded to hydrogen and an R group which is, any generic alkyl or side chain, as shown in Figure 1.23.

The group without R is called the aldehyde group or formyl group. Aldehydes differ from ketones in that the carbonyl is placed at the end of a carbon skeleton rather than between two carbon atoms. Aldehydes are common in organic chemistry.

Aldehydes feature an sp²-hybridized, planar carbon center, that is connected by a double bond to oxygen and a single bond to hydrogen. The C–H bond is not acidic. Because of resonance stabilization of the conjugate base, an α-hydrogen in an aldehyde (not shown in the picture above) is far more acidic, with a pK_a near 17, than a C–H bond in a typical alkane (pK_a about 50). This acidification is attributed to

- The electron-withdrawing quality of the formyl center
- The fact that the conjugate base, an enolate anion, delocalizes its negative charge

Owing to the electron withdrawing, the aldehyde group is somewhat polar.

Aldehydes (except those without an alpha carbon, or without protons on the alpha carbon, such as formaldehyde and benzaldehyde) can exist in either the keto or the enol tautomer.

Keto-enol tautomerism refers to a particular form of isomerism between an aldehyde (or a ketone) and a corresponding alcohol. The two molecules have the same atoms in the molecule and the same molecular structure, but a different bond. The interconversion of the two forms involves the movement of a proton and the shifting of bonding electrons; this kind of isomerism involving bond changes is called tautomerism to distinguish it from purely stereographic isomerism. Tautomerism is shown through structural formulas in Figure 1.24. The tautomeric forms generally are both present in chemical equilibrium. Usually, the enol is the minority tautomer, but it is more reactive.

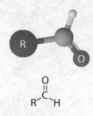

FIGURE 1.23   Structure and graphical representation of aldehydes.

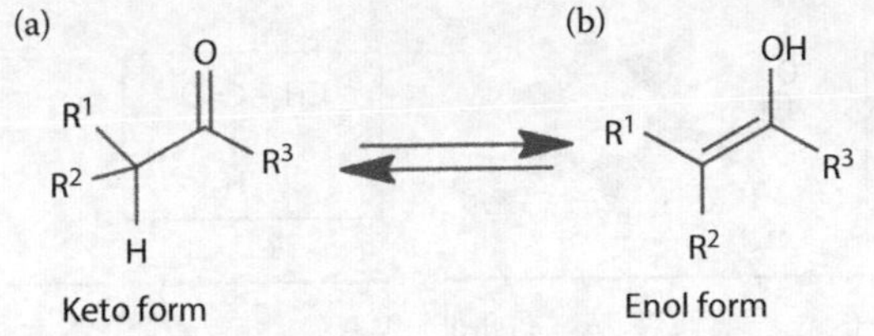

FIGURE 1.24 Keto-enol tautomerism: (a) the keto form and (b) the enol form.

IUPAC prescribes the following nomenclature for aldehydes:

1. Acyclic aliphatic aldehydes are named as derivatives of the longest carbon chain containing the aldehyde group. Thus, HCHO is named as a derivative of methane, and $CH_3CH_2CH_2CHO$ is named as a derivative of butane. The name is formed by changing the suffix -e of the parent alkane to -al, so that HCHO is named *methanal*, and $CH_3CH_2CH_2CHO$ is named *butanal*.
2. In other cases, such as when a –CHO group is attached to a ring, the suffix -*carbaldehyde* may be used. Thus, $C_6H_{11}CHO$ is known as *cyclohexanecarbaldehyde*. If the presence of another functional group demands the use of a suffix, the aldehyde group is named with the prefix *formyl-*. This prefix is preferred to *methanoyl-*.
3. If the compound is a natural product or a carboxylic acid, the prefix *oxo-* may be used to indicate which carbon atom is part of the aldehyde group; for example, $CHOCH_2COOH$ is named *3-oxopropanoic acid*.
4. If replacing the aldehyde group with a carboxyl group (–COOH) would yield a carboxylic acid with a trivial name, the aldehyde may be named by replacing the suffix -*ic acid* or -*oic acid* in this trivial name by -*aldehyde*. The pK_a of common carboxyl acids in water solution is reported in Table 1.10.

However, as usual, many aldehydes have different common names that are widely used.

Aldehydes have properties that are diverse and that depend on the remainder of the molecule. Smaller aldehydes are more soluble in water, formaldehyde and acetaldehyde completely so. The volatile aldehydes have pungent odors. Aldehydes degrade in air via the process of autoxidation.

The two aldehydes of greatest importance in industry, formaldehyde and acetaldehyde, have complicated behavior because of their tendency to oligomerize or polymerize. They also tend to hydrate, forming the geminal diol. The oligomers/polymers and the hydrates exist in equilibrium with the parent aldehyde.

TABLE 1.10

Typical pK_a in Water of Some Carboxyl Acids

Carboxylic Acid	Formula	pK_a
Formic acid	HCO_2H	3.75
Acetic acid	CH_3COOH	4.76
Chloroacetic acid	CH_2ClCO_2H	2.86
Dichloroacetic acid	$CHCl_2CO_2H$	1.29
Trichloroacetic acid	CCl_3CO_2H	0.65
Trifluoroacetic acid	CF_3CO_2H	0.5
Oxalic acid	HO_2CCO_2H	1.27
Benzoic acid	$C_6H_5CO_2H$	4.2

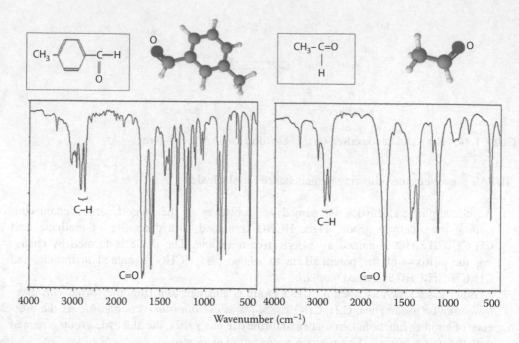

FIGURE 1.25 IR spectroscopy of acetaldehyde (on the left) and *p*-tolualdehyde (on the right). Structural formulas and graphical representations of the two composites are also reported. To correctly read the plots, the compression of the plot scale typical of wide bandwidth infrared spectroscopy is to be taken into account (compare the ordinate wavenumber scale in 1/cm).

Aldehydes are readily identified by spectroscopic methods. Using IR spectroscopy, they display a strong vCO band near 1700 cm^{-1}. In their 1H NMR spectra, the formyl hydrogen center absorbs near $\delta 9$ (i.e., the polar extreme of the ninth hydrogen atom), which is a distinctive part of the spectrum. This signal shows the characteristic coupling to any protons on the alpha carbon.

This feature is shown in Figure 1.25, where the IR spectrum of two selected aldehydes is shown evidencing the characteristic spectral features.

1.3.2.6 Ketone Functional Group

A ketone is an organic compound with the structure RC(=O)R′, where R and R′ can be a hydrocarbon radical of different kinds as shown in Figure 1.26. It features a carbonyl group (C=O) bonded to two other carbon atoms. Examples include many sugars and the industrial solvent acetone.

According to the rules of IUPAC nomenclature, ketones are named by changing the suffix -e of the parent alkane to -one. For the most important ketones, however, traditional nonsystematic names are still generally used, for example, acetone and benzophenone. These nonsystematic names are considered retained IUPAC names, although some introductory chemistry textbooks use names such as 2-propanone or propan-2-one instead of acetone, the simplest ketone (CH$_3$–CO–CH$_3$). The position of the carbonyl group is usually denoted by a number.

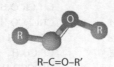

R–C=O–R′

FIGURE 1.26 Structure and graphical representation of the ketone functional group.

Although used infrequently, "oxo" is the IUPAC nomenclature for a ketone functional group. Other prefixes, however, are also used. For some common chemicals (mainly in biochemistry), "keto" or "oxo" is the term used to describe the ketone functional group.

The ketone carbon is often described as "sp^2 hybridized," terminology that describes both their electronic and molecular structure. Ketones are trigonal planar about the ketonic carbon, with C–C–O and C–C–C bond angles of approximately 120°. Ketones differ from aldehydes in that the carbonyl group (CO) is bonded to two carbons within a carbon skeleton. In aldehydes, the carbonyl is bonded to one carbon and one hydrogen and is located at the ends of carbon chains. Ketones are also distinct from other carbonyl-containing functional groups, such as carboxylic acids, esters, and amides.

The carbonyl group is polar as a consequence of the fact that the electronegativity of the oxygen center is greater than that for carbonyl carbon. Thus, ketones are nucleophilic at oxygen and electrophilic at carbon. Because the carbonyl group interacts with water by hydrogen bonding, ketones are typically more soluble in water than the related methylene compounds. Ketones are hydrogen-bond acceptors but are not usually hydrogen-bond donors and cannot hydrogen bond to itself. Because of their inability to serve both as hydrogen-bond donors and acceptors, ketones tend not to "self-associate" and are more volatile than alcohols and carboxylic acids of comparable molecular weights. These factors relate to pervasiveness of ketones in perfumery and as solvents.

Ketones, like aldehydes, give rise to keto-enol tautomerism. The reaction with a strong base gives the corresponding enolate, often by deprotonation of the enol.

Ketones are classified on the basis of their substituents. One broad classification subdivides ketones into symmetrical and unsymmetrical derivatives, depending on the equivalency of the two organic substituents attached to the carbonyl center. Acetone and benzophenone ($C_6H_5C(O)C_6H_5$) are symmetrical ketones. Acetophenone ($C_6H_5C(O)CH_3$) is an unsymmetrical ketone.

1. *Diketones:* Many kinds of diketones are known, some with unusual properties. The simplest is diacetyl ($CH_3C(O)C(O)CH_3$), once used as butter flavoring in popcorn. Acetylacetone (pentane-2,4-dione) is virtually a misnomer (inappropriate name) because this species exists mainly as the monoenol $CH_3C(O)CH=C(OH)CH_3$. Its enolate is a common ligand in coordination chemistry. Coordination chemistry is that branch of chemistry that studies coordination complexes, which consists of an atom or ion (usually metallic), and a surrounding array of bound molecules or anions, which are in turn known as ligands or complexing agents [32,33]. A simple example of coordination compound obtained using ketones as ligands (Fe(ox)$_3$) is shown in Figure 1.27.

2. *Unsaturated ketones:* Ketones containing alkene and alkyne units are often called unsaturated ketones. The most widely used member of this class of compounds is methyl vinyl ketone, $CH_3C(O)CH=CH_2$, which is useful in Robinson annulation reaction. The Robinson annulation is a chemical reaction used for the synthesis of structures formed by concatenated aromatic rings. The method uses a ketone and a methyl vinyl ketone in

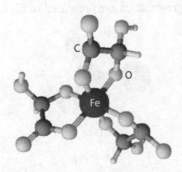

FIGURE 1.27   Example of ferrous coordination compound obtained using ketones as ligands (Fe(ox)$_3$).

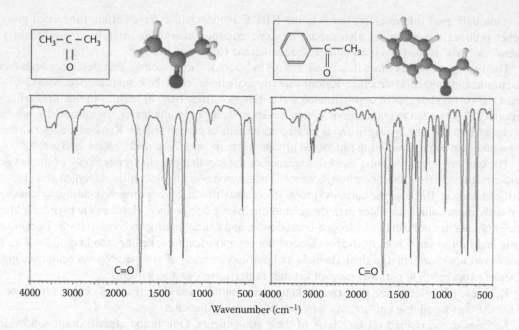

FIGURE 1.28 IR spectroscopy of acetone (on the left) and acetophenone (on the right). Structural formulas and graphical representations of the two composites are also reported. To correctly read the plots, the compression of the plot scale typical of wide bandwidth infrared spectroscopy is to be taken into account (compare the ordinate wavenumber scale in 1/cm).

its base version, while several variations exist where ketones play slightly different roles [34–36].

3. *Cyclic ketones:* Many ketones are cyclic. The simplest class has the formula $(CH_2)_nCO$, where n starts from 3 for cyclopropanone. Larger derivatives exist. Cyclohexanone, a symmetrical cyclic ketone, is an important intermediate in the production of nylon. Isophorone, derived from acetone, is an unsaturated, unsymmetrical ketone, that is the precursor to other polymers. Muscone, 3-methylpentadecanone, is an animal pheromone.

Ketones, as aldehydes, absorb strongly in infra-red spectrum near $1700\ cm^{-1}$. The exact position of the peak depends on the substituents. A typical spectroscopy trace of a solution of two ketones is reported in Figure 1.28.

1.3.2.7 Acid Functional Group

Carboxylic acids are organic acids characterized by the presence of at least one carboxyl group whose structure and graphical representation are presented in Figure 1.29.

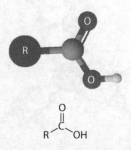

FIGURE 1.29 Structure and graphical representation of an oxylacid molecule.

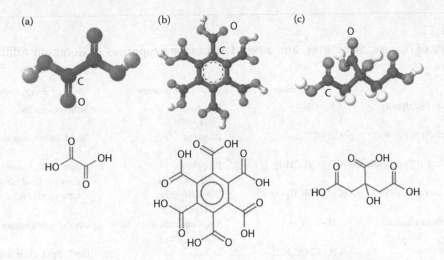

FIGURE 1.30   Different examples of organic acids: oxalic acid (a), mellitic acid (b), and citric acid (c).

The general formula of a carboxylic acid is R–COOH, where R is some monovalent functional group. A carboxyl group (or carboxy) is a functional group consisting of a carbonyl (RR′C=O) and a hydroxyl (R–O–H), which has the formula –C(=O)OH, usually written as –COOH or –CO$_2$H.

Carboxylic acids are acids (in the Brønsted–Lowry sense [6,8]) because they are proton (H$^+$) donors. They are the most common type of organic acid. Among the simplest examples are formic acid H–COOH that occurs in ants, and acetic acid CH$_3$–COOH, that gives vinegar its sour taste. Acids with two or more carboxylic groups are called dicarboxylic, tricarboxylic, and so on. The simplest dicarboxylic example is oxalic acid (COOH)$_2$, which is just two connected carboxyls. Mellitic acid is an example of a hexa-carboxylic acid. Other important natural examples are citric acid (in lemons) and tartaric acid (in tamarinds). Different examples of organic acids are provided in Figure 1.30.

Salts and esters of carboxylic acids are called carboxylates. When a carboxylic group is deprotonated, its conjugate base, a carboxylate anion, is formed. Carboxylate ions are resonance stabilized and this increased stability makes carboxylic acids more acidic than alcohols.

Carboxylic acids are polar. Because they are both hydrogen-bond acceptors (the carbonylic) and hydrogen-bond donors (the hydroxyl), they also participate in hydrogen bonding. Together, the hydroxyl and carbonylic groups form the functional group carboxyl. Carboxylic acids usually exist as dimeric pairs in nonpolar media due to their tendency to self-associate. Dimers are compounds in which two identical molecules are bonded via either a strong, covalent generally, or a weak bond [6,8]. For organic acids, the dimer is formed by hydrogen bonds, as shown in Figure 1.31, where the structure of a dimer composed by two carboxyl acids is presented.

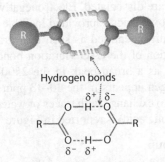

FIGURE 1.31   Structure of a dimer composed of two carboxyl acids.

TABLE 1.11

Summary of Names, Structures, and a Few Qualitative Properties of Common Addition Polymers

Name(s)	Formula	Monomer	Properties
Polyethylene low density (LDPE)	$-(CH_2-CH_2)_n-$	Ethylene $CH_2=CH_2$	Soft, waxy solid
Polyethylene high density (HDPE)	$-(CH_2-CH_2)_n-$	Ethylene $CH_2=CH_2$	Rigid, translucent solid
Polypropylene (PP) different grades	$-[CH_2-CH(CH_3)]_n-$	Propylene $CH_2=CHCH_3$	*Atactic*: soft, elastic solid *Isotactic*: hard, strong solid
Poly(vinyl chloride) (PVC)	$-(CH_2-CHCl)_n-$	Vinyl chloride $CH_2=CHCl$	Strong rigid solid
Poly(vinylidene chloride) (Saran A)	$-(CH_2-CCl_2)_n-$	Vinylidene chloride $CH_2=CCl_2$	Dense, high-melting solid
Polystyrene (PS)	$-[CH_2-CH(C_6H_5)]_n-$	Styrene $CH_2=CHC_6H_5$	Hard, rigid, clear solid soluble in organic solvents
Polyacrylonitrile (PAN, Orlon, Acrilan)	$-(CH_2-CHCN)_n-$	Acrylonitrile $CH_2=CHCN$	High-melting solid soluble in organic solvents
Polytetrafluoroethylene (PTFE, Teflon)	$-(CF_2-CF_2)_n-$	Tetrafluoroethylene $CF_2=CF_2$	Resistant, smooth solid
Poly(methyl methacrylate) (PMMA, Lucite, Plexiglas)	$-[CH_2-C(CH_3)CO_2CH_3]_n-$	Methyl methacrylate $CH_2=C(CH_3)CO_2CH_3$	Hard, transparent solid
Poly(vinyl acetate) (PVAc)	$-(CH_2-CHOCOCH_3)_n-$	Vinyl acetate $CH_2=CHOCOCH_3$	Soft, sticky solid
cis-Polyisoprene natural rubber	$-[CH_2-CH=C(CH_3) -CH_2]_n-$	Isoprene $CH_2=CH-C(CH_3)=CH_2$	Soft, sticky solid requires vulcanization for practical us
Polychloroprene (cis + trans) (Neoprene)	$-[CH_2-CH=CCl-CH_2]_n-$	Chloroprene $CH_2=CH-CCl=CH_2$	Tough, rubbery solid oil resistant

Smaller carboxylic acids (1–5 carbons) are soluble in water, whereas higher carboxylic acids are less soluble due to the increasing hydrophobic nature of the alkyl chain. These longer-chain acids tend to be rather soluble in less polar solvents such as ethers and alcohols.

Carboxylic acids tend to have higher boiling points than water, not only because of their increased surface area, but because of their tendency to form stabilized dimers so that they would tend to evaporate or to boil in dimer form. For boiling to occur, for example, either the dimer bonds must be broken or the entire dimer arrangement must be vaporized, both of which increase the enthalpy of vaporization requirements significantly.

Carboxylic acids are typically weak acids, meaning that they only partially dissociate into H^+ cations and $RCOO-$ anions in neutral aqueous solution. For example, at room temperature, only 0.4% of all acetic acid molecules are dissociated. Electronegative substituents give stronger acids. Typical pK_a in water of some carboxyl acids is provided in Table 1.11.

Carboxylic acids are most readily identified as such by infrared spectroscopy. They exhibit a sharp band associated with vibration of the C–O vibration bond between 1680 and 1725 cm^{-1}. A characteristic O–H band appears as a broad peak in the 2500–3000 cm^{-1} region. By 1H NMR spectrometry, the hydroxyl hydrogen appears in the 10–13 ppm region, although it is often either broadened or not observed owing to exchange with traces of water. The example of the IR spectrum of an organic acid (2-bromobutanolic acid) is reported in Figure 1.32.

1.3.2.8   Amino Functional Group

Amines are organic compounds and functional groups that contain a basic nitrogen atom with a electron pair. An electron pair or a Lewis pair consists of two electrons that occupy the same orbital

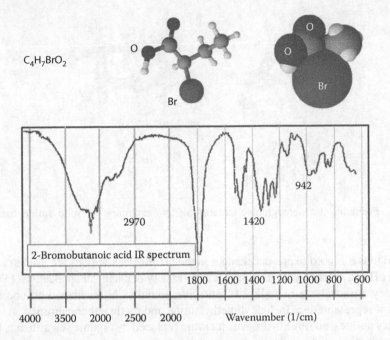

$C_4H_7BrO_2$

2970

1420

942

2-Bromobutanoic acid IR spectrum

1800 1600 1400 1200 1000 800 600

4000 3500 2000 2500 2000   Wavenumber (1/cm)

FIGURE 1.32 Structure, stereographic representations, and IR spectrum of 2-bromobutanoic acid. To correctly read the plots, the compression of the plot scale typical of wide bandwidth infrared spectroscopy is to be taken into account (compare the ordinate wavenumber scale in 1/cm).

but have opposite spins. Amines are derivatives of ammonia, wherein one or more hydrogen atoms have been replaced by a substituent such as an alkyl or aryl group. Important amines include amino acids, biogenic amines, trimethylamine, and aniline. Inorganic derivatives of ammonia are also called amines, such as chloramine ($NClH_2$).

Aliphatic amines, which do not contain aromatic rings, are classified into three groups, as shown in Figure 1.33.

- Primary amines arise when one of three hydrogen atoms in ammonia is replaced by an alkyl. Important primary alkyl amines include methylamine, ethanolamine (2-aminoethanol), and the buffering agent tris (2-amino-2-(hydroxymethyl)propane-1,3-diol). A buffer is an aqueous solution consisting of a mixture of a weak acid and its conjugate base or a weak base and its conjugate acid. Its pH changes very little when a small amount of strong acid or base is added

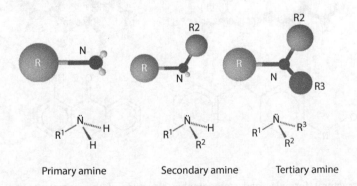

Primary amine   Secondary amine   Tertiary amine

FIGURE 1.33 Formulas and stereographic structure of the three classes of noncyclic amine.

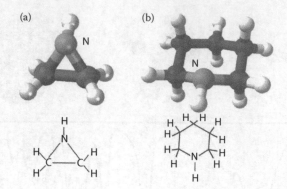

FIGURE 1.34   Formulas and stereographic structure of two examples of cyclic amine: aziridine (a) and piperidine (b).

to it, and thus it is used to prevent changes in the pH. Buffer solutions are used as a means of keeping pH at a nearly constant value in a wide variety of chemical applications [37].

- Secondary amines have two alkyl substituents bound to N together with one hydrogen. Important representatives include dimethylamine and methylethanolamine.
- In tertiary amines, all three hydrogen atoms are replaced by organic substituents. Examples include trimethylamine.
- Cyclic amines are either secondary or tertiary amines. Examples of cyclic amines include the three-member ring aziridine and the six-membered ring piperidine. N-Methylpiperidin is a cyclic tertiary amine. It is also possible to have four alkyl substituents on the nitrogen. These compounds are not amines but are called quaternary ammonium cations, have a charged nitrogen center, and necessarily come with an anion. The structural formula and stereographic representation of aziridine and piperidine are reported as an example in Figure 1.34.

Aromatic amines have the nitrogen atom connected to an aromatic ring as in anilines. The aromatic ring decreases the alkalinity of the amine, depending on its substituents. The presence of an amine group strongly increases the reactivity of the aromatic ring due to an electron-donating effect. The structure of two sample aromatic amines is shown in Figure 1.35.

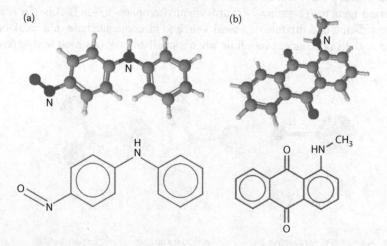

FIGURE 1.35   Structural formulas and stereographic structure of two sample aromatic cyclic amines: 4-nitrosodiphenylamine (a) and 1-(methylamino)anthraquinone (b).

Amines have various common names, depending on the origin of the molecule. Typically, the compound is given the prefix "amino-" or the suffix "-amine." The prefix "N-" shows substitution on the nitrogen atom. An organic compound with multiple amino groups is called a diamine, triamine, tetraamine, and so forth.

Hydrogen bonding significantly influences the properties of primary and secondary amines. Thus, the boiling point of amines is higher than those of the corresponding phosphines, but generally lower than those of the corresponding alcohols. For example, methylamine and ethylamine are gases under standard conditions, whereas the corresponding methyl alcohol and ethyl alcohols are liquids.

Also reflecting their ability to form hydrogen bonds, most aliphatic amines display some solubility in water. Solubility decreases with the increase in the number of carbon atoms. Aliphatic amines display significant solubility in organic solvents, especially polar organic solvents. Primary amines react with ketones such as acetone.

The aromatic amines, such as aniline, have their lone pair of electrons conjugated into the benzene ring, thus their tendency to engage in hydrogen bonding is diminished. Their boiling points are high and their solubility in water is low.

Amines of the type NHRR' and NRR'R" are chiral, that is, they are not superimposable to their mirror image: two molecules that are chiral mirror images are also called stereoisomers. The energy barrier for the inversion of the stereo-center is relatively low, ~7 kcal/mole in the case of a trialkylamine. The conversion from a stereoisomers to the other has been compared to the inversion of an open umbrella in a strong wind. Because of this low barrier, stereoisomers of amines such as NHRR' cannot be resolved optically and NRR'R" can only be resolved when the R, R', and R" groups are constrained in cyclic structures such as aziridines. Quaternary ammonium salts with four distinct groups on the nitrogen are capable of exhibiting optical activity.

Like ammonia, amines are bases. The basicity of amines depends on

1. The electronic properties of the substituents, for example, alkyl groups enhance the basicity; aryl groups diminish it.
2. Steric hindrance offered by the groups on nitrogen.
3. The degree of solvation of the protonated amine.

The nitrogen atom features a lone electron pair that can bind H^+ to form an ammonium ion R_3NH^+. The water solubility of simple amines is largely due to hydrogen bonding between protons in the water molecules and these lone electron pairs.

1.3.2.9 Amide Functional Group

The amide functional group is obtained by substitution of an acid radical group to one or more hydrogen atoms in the ammonia molecule. Thus, the generic amide has the structure reported in Figure 1.36, where the radicals can also represent simple hydrogen atoms. Depending on the number of hydrogen atoms in the ammonia that are replaced by acid radicals, the amide group can be

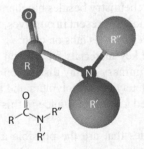

FIGURE 1.36 Structural formulas and stereographic representation of the amide functional group.

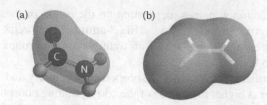

FIGURE 1.37 Representation of the delocalized π molecular orbitals of formamide (a) and equal charge surface around the formamide molecule for a charge of 1.13×10^{12} C/m^3 (b).

a primary, a secondary, or a tertiary amide. Primary amides are more common, but secondary and tertiary amides also have a role in biochemistry.

In the common nomenclature, the term "amide" is added to the stem of the parent acid's name. For instance, the amide derived from acetic acid is named acetamide (CH_3CONH_2). IUPAC recommends ethanamide, but this and related formal names are rarely encountered but in scientific literature when precise identification of similar substances is needed. When the amide is derived from a primary or secondary amine, the substituents on nitrogen are indicated first in the name. Thus, the amide formed from dimethylamine and acetic acid is N,N-dimethylacetamide $CH_3CON(CH_3)_2$. In common language, even this name is often simplified to dimethylacetamide. In the common language, cyclic amides are called lactams; they are necessarily secondary or tertiary amides.

Compared to amines, amides are very weak bases. While the conjugate acid of an amine has a pK_a of about 9.5, the conjugate acid of an amide has a pK_a around −0.5. Therefore, amides do not clearly behave as bases in water. This relative lack of basicity is explained by the electron-withdrawing nature of the carbonyl group where the lone pair of electrons on the nitrogen is delocalized by resonance [38].

As a matter of fact, amides possess a conjugated system spread over the O, C, and N atoms, consisting of molecular orbitals occupied by delocalized electrons. As an example, one of the π molecular orbitals in formamide is shown in Figure 1.37a besides the equal change surface around the molecule (at a charge density of 1.13×10^{12} C/m^3) [39]. However, amides are much stronger bases than carboxylic acids, esters, aldehydes, and ketones.

Because of the greater electronegativity of oxygen, the carbonyl (C=O) is a stronger dipole than the N–C dipole. The presence of a C=O dipole and, to a lesser extent a N–C dipole, allows amides to act as H-bond acceptors. In primary and secondary amides, the presence of N–H dipoles allows amides to function as H-bond donors as well. Thus, amides can participate in hydrogen bonding with water and other polar solvents. As a result, the water solubility of amides is greater than that of corresponding hydrocarbons.

1.4 POLYMERS

Polymer technology is perhaps the most important result of the great understanding humanity has gained in the last century of organic chemistry besides biochemical applications that we will review in Chapters 2 and 3. Polymers are uniquely present in our lives, from common everyday applications to the more sophisticated technologies such as labs on chip.

As a matter of fact, polymers are key materials for labs on chip technology, so that a review of a few key polymers qualities is preliminary to any discussion on labs on chip fabrication. A wide range of labs on chip are built completely out of polymers and technologies to fabricate small chips from polymer materials have acquired a key importance in this field. We will review the main technologies in this area in Chapter 4.

Also, in silicon-based technologies that are the possible alternative to polymers technologies for lab on chip fabrication, polymers have an important role, for example, as photoresists and also structural material, for example, in the wafer bonding technology (see Section 4.9.2).

A first factor distinguishing technologies using simple materials like Si and SiO$_2$ from technologies using polymers is the impact on technology process of the material properties.

Si and SiO$_2$ are well-known materials and while some modulation of their characteristics is possible via changing the deposition technique and introducing doping, they do not completely change the process characteristics, at least when mechanical and chemical properties are considered. Electronics and optics are other issues due to the junction and guiding effects that are completely based on doping.

On the contrary, under the family of polymers a great number of profoundly different materials are collected so that a wide range of different mechanical, chemical, and optical properties can be obtained by simply selecting a particular polymer. Thus, a correct choice of the polymer to use for a determined chip fabrication is a key success factor.

1.4.1 POLYMERIZATION AND POLYMER TYPES

Polymerization is a process of reacting monomer molecules together in a chemical reaction to form polymer chains or three-dimensional networks [40,41]. Here, we will focus on carbon-based polymers; however, it is well known that C and Si atoms have somehow similar bonding abilities, even if the C–C bond is stronger than the Si–Si bond. This property allows silicon to be used instead of carbon to construct polymeric structures, usually called polysilicate structures, like polydimethylsiloxane (PDMS) (see Table 1.12). The great part of the introductory considerations we will do regarding C-based polymers can be applied also to Si-based polymers, even if differences naturally exist, due to the different weight and bond energy of the Si atom with respect to the C atom. We cannot go in detail into the differences between C- and Si-based polymers; the interested reader is encouraged to access the huge scientific literature on polymers, starting from general works such as those reported in References [40,41].

Polymerization occurs via different reaction mechanisms that vary in complexity due to the involved functional groups and their inherent steric effects [42,43]. Steric effects arise from the fact that each atom within a molecule occupies a certain amount of space. If atoms are brought too close together, there is an associated cost in energy due to overlapping electron clouds, and this may affect the molecule's preferred shape and reactivity. An example of steric effect is the difficulty of tri-(*tert*-butyl)amine C$_3$N(CH$_3$)$_3$ to cause electrophilic reactions, like forming the tetraalkylammonium cation, even if it incorporates nitrogen atoms offering a lone electrons pair, which is generally an enabling feature for this type of reactions. This is due to the fact that the nitrogen atom is difficult to reach since it is located inside the molecule, completely surrounded by carbon atoms, as shown in Figure 1.38, where the stereographic representation of the tri-(*tert*-butyl)amine molecule is shown in both volume and ball-and-stick representations.

Different types of steric effects can occur:

- *Steric hindrance* occurs when the large size of groups within a molecule prevents chemical reactions that are observed in related molecules with smaller groups. An example is the case of tri-(*tert*-butyl)amine we have discussed earlier. Although steric hindrance is sometimes a problem, it can also be a very useful tool to change the reactivity pattern of a molecule by stopping unwanted side reactions or by leading to a preference for one reaction course among the possible once. Steric hindrance between adjacent groups can also restrict torsional bond angles.
- *Steric shielding* occurs when a charged group on a molecule is spatially shielded by less charged or oppositely charged atoms. In some cases, for an atom to interact with sterically shielded atoms, it would have to approach from a vicinity where there is less shielding, thus controlling where and from what direction a molecular interaction can take place.
- *Steric attraction* occurs when molecules have shapes or geometries that are optimized for interaction with one another. In these cases, molecules will react with each other most often in specific arrangements.

TABLE 1.12

Summary of Names, Structure, and a Few Qualitative Properties of Common Condensation Polymers

Formula	Name	Components	T_g (°C)	Notes
$\text{-[CO(CH}_2)_4\text{CO-OCH}_2\text{CH}_2\text{O]}_n^-$	Polyester	$HO_2C-(CH_2)_4-CO_2H$ $HO-CH_2CH_2-OH$	<0	
	Polyester dacron, mylar	Para $HO_2C-C_6H_4-CO_2H$ $HO-CH_2CH_2-OH$	70	
	Polyester	Meta $HO_2C-C_6H_4-CO_2H$ $HO-CH_2CH_2-OH$	50	
	Polycarbonate lexan	$(HO-C_6H_4-)_2C(CH_3)_2$ (Bisphenol A) $X_2C=O$ (X = OCH_3 or Cl)	150	Amorphous transparent glass-like rigid
$\text{-[CO(CH}_2)_4\text{CO-NH(CH}_2)_6\text{NH]}_n^-$	Polyamide nylon 66	$HO_2C-(CH_2)_4-CO_2H$ $H_2N-(CH_2)_6-NH_2$	45	
$\text{-[CO(CH}_2)_5\text{NH]}_n^-$	Polyamide nylon 6		53	
	Polyamide kevlar	Para $HO_2C-C_6H_4-CO_2H$ para $H_2N-C_6H_4-NH_2$	—	Extremely tough and resistant
	Polyamide nomex	Meta $HO_2C-C_6H_4-CO_2H$ meta $H_2N-C_6H_4-NH_2$	273	Extremely tough and resistant
	Polyurethane spandex	$HOCH_2CH_2OH$	52	
	Polymeth-acrylimide (PMI)			High tensile, compress and shear modules
	Polydimeth-ylsiloxane (PDMS)		−125	Optical transparent non-toxic, viscoelastic

- *Chain crossing* happens when a chain, a ring, or a set of rings cannot change from one conformation to another due to the fact that they are twisted in a helical-like shape of another chain passing through them. This effect is responsible for the shape of catenanes and molecular knots [44,45].
- *Steric repulsions* between different parts of molecular system were found to be of key importance to govern the direction of transition metal-mediated transformations and catalysis.

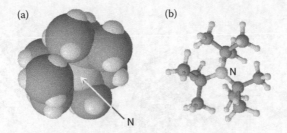

FIGURE 1.38 Stereographic representation of tri-(tert-butyl)amine in both volume (a) and ball-and-stick (b) representations.

A complete analysis of steric effects on polymerization mechanism can be attained by applying a microscopic model that describes interactions between electrons in bonding atoms. Three such models essentially exists: the molecular orbitals theory [46] that is based directly on the quantum mechanical description of the molecule, the valence electron theory that is also based on quantum mechanical behavior of electrons in the orbitals that are available for chemical bonds and is a bit simplified to be useful for big molecules [47,48], and the valence shell electron pair repulsion (VSERP) theory [49].

Molecular orbitals theory essentially relies on basic quantum mechanical analysis of the electrostates in a molecule. In simple molecules, it can be directly performed by solving the electron dynamic equation; in more complex molecules it is often carried out by studying the electron orbitals in separated atoms that are accessible to bonding and studying the effect on these orbitals implied by atoms vicinity.

The molecular orbitals theory is accurate but quite difficult, and complex molecules can be impossible to deal with even by powerful computational machines if important approximations are not carried out [46].

The premise of VSEPR is that the valence electron pairs surrounding an atom mutually repel each other, and will therefore adopt an arrangement that minimizes this repulsion, thus determining the molecular geometry. The number of electron pairs surrounding an atom, both bonding and nonbonding, is called its steric number [49]. Even if quantitative results are not easy to derive from VSEPR theory, it is almost always accurate in describing the stereographic shape of complex molecules, and much easier than the molecular orbitals theory.

In more straightforward polymerization, alkenes, which are relatively stable due to bonding between carbon atoms, form polymers through relatively simple radical reactions. A simple example of this polymerization mechanism is reported in Figure 1.39 in which each styrene monomer unit's double bond reforms as a single bond with another styrene monomer and forms polystyrene. Figure 1.39b, in which a simple polymeric chain of only 32 monomers is represented in stereographic form, is very useful.

It shows polymeric chains twisted to form complex structures: this is true even for a very simple chain of 32 monomers, while real polymeric chains are composed of thousands of monomers.

Polymers obtained simply by adding monomers from one to another are called addition polymers. The key to having an addition polymer is that no part of the original monomer is eliminated during polymerization. A summary of names, structure, and a few qualitative properties of common addition polymers are presented in Table 1.11.

Polymerization can also require more complex reactions such as those needed when bifunctional monomers react to form a long-chain polymer molecule while eliminating in the process small molecules, such as water. Such polymers are called, for this reason, condensation polymers.

An example of the formation of condensation polymer is the polyesters polymerization. In such a reaction, –OH functional group of one monomer reacts with the –COOH functional group of another monomer; water is created besides the polymer and eliminated by the reaction. This reaction is shown in Figure 1.40.

A table of composition and names of selected common condensation polymers is reported in Table 1.12.

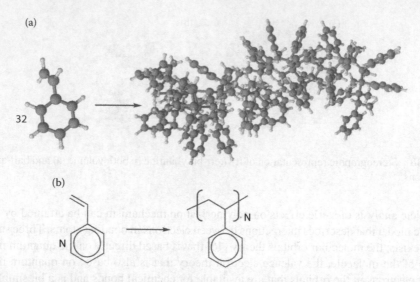

FIGURE 1.39 An example of alkene polymerization in which each styrene monomer unit's double bond reforms as a single bond with another styrene monomer and forms polystyrene. The structural formula is reported in (a) while the stereographic representation of the involved species in the case N = 32 is reported in (b).

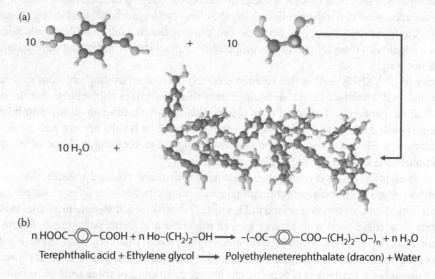

n HOOC—⟨O⟩—COOH + n Ho–$(CH_2)_2$–OH ⟶ –(–OC–⟨O⟩–COO–$(CH_2)_2$–O–)$_n$ + n H_2O

Terephthalic acid + Ethylene glycol ⟶ Polyethyleneterephthalate (dracon) + Water

FIGURE 1.40 Polyester polymerization; structure from reaction (a) and stereographic representations of the involved composites (b).

The last line of Table 1.12 deserves further comments. In this line, the structure and the characteristics of PDMS are reported. This polymer, besides having the property to be viscoelastic (see Section 7.3.6.3) and the fact that it is widely used in lab on chip technology, differentiates clearly from the other considered examples due to the fact that the main structure of the polymer chain is constructed by Si atoms instead of C atoms. It is an example of polysilicate, a silicon-based polymer.

1.4.2 POLYMERIC MATERIALS STRUCTURE

Synthetic high-density polyethylene (HDPE) macromolecules have masses ranging from 10^5 to 10^6 Da while low-density polyethylene (LDPE) molecules are more than a hundred times smaller.

Rubber and cellulose molecules have similar mass ranges, but fewer monomer units because of the monomer's larger size. The physical properties of these three polymeric substances differ from each other, and of course from their monomers [50,51]:

- HDPE is a rigid translucent solid that softens on heating above 100°C, and can be fashioned into various forms, including films. It is not as easily stretched and deformed as is LDPE. HDPE is insoluble in water and most organic solvents, although some swelling may occur on immersion in the latter. HDPE is an excellent electrical insulator.
- LDPE is a soft translucent solid that deforms badly above 75°C. Films made from LDPE stretch easily and are commonly used for wrapping. LDPE is insoluble in water, but softens and swells on exposure to hydrocarbon solvents. Both LDPE and HDPE become brittle at very low temperatures (below −80°C). Ethylene, the common monomer for these polymers, is a low-boiling (−104°C) gas.
- Natural (latex) rubber is an opaque, soft, easily deformable solid that becomes sticky when heated above 60°C, and brittle when cooled below −50°C. It swells to more than double its size in nonpolar organic solvents such as toluene, eventually dissolving, but is impermeable to water. The C_5H_8 monomer isoprene is a volatile liquid with boiling temperature of 34°C.
- Pure cellulose, in the form of cotton, is a soft flexible fiber, essentially unchanged by variations in temperature ranging from −70°C to 80°C. Cotton absorbs water readily, but is unaffected by immersion in toluene or most other organic solvents. Cellulose fibers may be bent and twisted, but do not stretch much before breaking. The monomer of cellulose is the $C_6H_{12}O_6$ aldohexose D-glucose. Glucose is a water-soluble solid melting below 150°C.

To account for the differences noted here we need to consider the nature of the aggregate macromolecular structure of each substance: the polymer morphology. Because polymer molecules are so large, they generally pack together in a nonuniform fashion, with ordered or crystalline-like regions mixed together with disordered or amorphous domains. In some cases, the entire solid may be amorphous, composed entirely of coiled and tangled macromolecular chains.

Crystal order occurs when linear polymer chains are structurally oriented in a uniform three-dimensional matrix. Increased crystal order is associated with an increase in rigidity, tensile strength, and opacity (due to light scattering). Amorphous polymers are usually less rigid, weaker, and more easily deformed. They are often transparent. Three factors that influence the degree of crystal structure are

- Chain length
- Chain branching
- Interchain bonding

The importance of the first two factors is illustrated by the differences between LDPE and HDPE. As noted earlier, HDPE is composed of very long unbranched hydrocarbon chains. These pack together easily in crystalline domains that alternate with amorphous segments, and the resulting material, while relatively strong and stiff, retains a degree of flexibility. In contrast, LDPE is composed of smaller and more highly branched chains which do not easily adopt crystalline structures. This material is therefore softer, weaker, less dense, and more easily deformed than HDPE. As a rule, mechanical properties such as ductility, tensile strength, and hardness rise and eventually level off with increasing chain length.

The nature of cellulose supports the above analysis and demonstrates the importance of the interchain bonding. Cellulose chains easily adopt a stable rod-like conformation. These molecules align themselves side by side into fibers that are stabilized by interchain hydrogen bonding between the three hydroxyl groups on each monomer unit [52]. This structure is shown in Figure 1.41, in which the molecular structure of a strand of cellulose is shown. The presence of these hydrogen

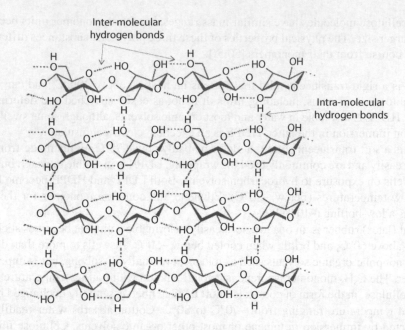

FIGURE 1.41   A strand of cellulose showing the hydrogen bonds within and between cellulose molecules as dashed lines.

bonds tends to give to the polymeric chain an ordered twist, in contrast with a more disordered twist due to the random interaction with nearby molecules and different parts of the same molecule chain, strongly favoring a crystal form.

Partial crystal states created by polymers due to hydrogen bonds are shown in Figure 1.42, in which the principal scheme of a set of local polymer crystals arranged in a random way is shown, besides the structure of one of these crystal domains. When crystal order is high, as in cellulose, the molecules do not move or slip relative to each other. The high concentration of hydroxyl groups also accounts for the facile absorption of water that is characteristic of cotton. This phenomenon also presents in biopolymers like proteins of nucleic acids and will be studied much more in detail in Chapter 2 dealing with the structure of these molecules.

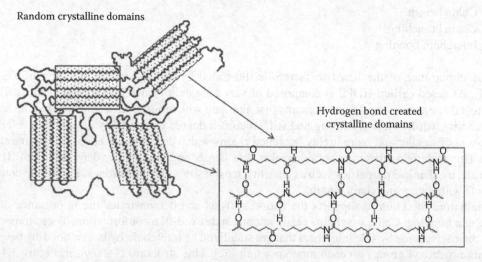

FIGURE 1.42   Example of a local crystal structure created in a polymeric material by hydrogen bonds.

Natural rubber is a completely amorphous polymer. The potentially useful properties of raw latex rubber are limited by temperature dependence. These characteristic can be completely changed by chemical processing. The double bonds in the hydrocarbon chain provide planar segments that stiffen, but do not straighten the chain. If the chains of rubber molecules are slightly cross-linked by sulfur atoms, a process called vulcanization, the desirable elastic properties of rubber are substantially improved.

At 2–3% cross-linking, a soft rubber, which no longer suffers stickiness and brittleness problems on heating and cooling, is obtained. At 25–35% cross-linking, a rigid hard rubber product is formed. Figure 1.43 shows a cross-linked section of amorphous rubber. In Figure 1.43a, the arrangement of polymeric chains in relaxed state, that is, without the application of external forces, is shown, while in Figure 1.43b, the schematic polymer structure is shown when an external traction force is applied. The more highly ordered chains in the stretched conformation have lower entropy with respect to the more disordered steady state of the chains, thus they can survive only as far as an external work is applied to the polymer. As far as the external forces cease, the polymer returns to the higher entropy initial state.

It is to be noted that proteins (see Section 2.3.1) are natural polymers: their base is a very particular form of polymer where the COOH group of a peptide reacts with the NH_2 group of the sequent peptide forming a polypeptide chain.

Contrary to biopolymers like proteins or nucleic acids, where the simple change of a radical group in a long molecule can completely change the molecule functionality, artificial polymeric material are composed generally of chains that are structurally identical (and frequently much simpler than proteins) but of different lengths so that alternation of long and shorter chains is very frequent. The HDPE molecules, for example, are all long carbon chains, but the lengths may vary by thousands of monomer units. Because of this, polymer molecular weights are usually given as averages.

Two key indicators for the polymer molecular weight distribution are generally used: the so-called number-average molecular weight, M_n, and the weight-average molecular weight, M_w. The

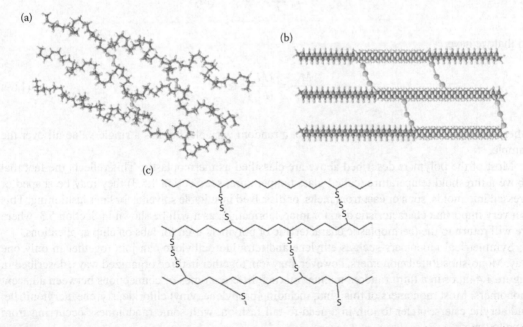

FIGURE 1.43 Sulfur cross-linked section of amorphous rubber: the arrangement of polymeric chains in relaxed state, that is, without the application of external forces, is shown in (a), while the schematic polymer structure when an external traction force is applied is shown in (b); the chain structural formula of vulcanized rubber is shown in (c).

number-average weight is calculated from the mole fraction distribution of different-sized molecules in a sample, while the weight-average weight is calculated from the weight fraction distribution of different-sized molecules.

In mathematical terms, let us call n_i the mole fraction and w_i the weight fraction of molecules with i monomers, whose molecular weight is M_i, we have

$$M_n = \sum_i n_i M_i \tag{1.66a}$$

$$M_w = \sum_i w_i M_i \tag{1.66b}$$

Since larger molecules in a sample weigh more than smaller molecules, the weight average M_w is always greater than M_n. As the weight dispersion of molecules in a sample narrows, M_w approaches M_n, and in the unlikely case that all the polymer molecules have identical weights (a pure monodisperse sample), $M_w = M_n$.

This can be analytically seen if we consider that

$$w_i = \frac{n_i M_i}{M_n} \tag{1.67}$$

Substituting in Equation 5.1b and considering that if we have a total of N molecules, $p_i = n_i/N$ is the probability that a random molecule has a molecular mass M_i, we can write

$$M_w = \frac{N}{M_n} \sum_i p_i M_i^2 = \frac{(M_i^2)}{(M_i)} \tag{1.68}$$

so that we have

$$\frac{M_w}{M_n} = \frac{(M_i^2)}{(M_i)^2} \geq 1 \tag{1.69}$$

where the equal sign indicates that M_i is not a random variable, but has a single value all over the sample.

Most of the polymers described above are classified as thermoplastic. This reflects the fact that above a threshold temperature (called glass temperature, see Section 1.5.3) they may be shaped or pressed into molds, spun or cast from melts, or dissolved in suitable solvents for later fashioning. This is a very important characteristic also for microfabrication, as it will be shown in Section 5.3, where we will return to the thermoplastic characteristic of polymers used for labs on chip applications.

Symmetrical monomers such as ethylene and tetrafluoroethylene can join together in only one way. Mono-substituted monomers, however, may join together in three organized ways, described in Figure 1.44a, or in a third random manner mixing different types of connections between adjacent monomers. Most monomers of this kind, including propylene, vinyl chloride, styrene, acrylonitrile, and acrylic esters, prefer to join in a head-to-tail fashion, with some randomness occurring from time to time.

If we then draw polymer chain using skeletal formulas (see Appendix 1), each of the substituent groups (Z) will necessarily be located above or below the plane defined by the carbon chain. Consequently, we can identify three configurational isomers of such polymers. If all the substitutes

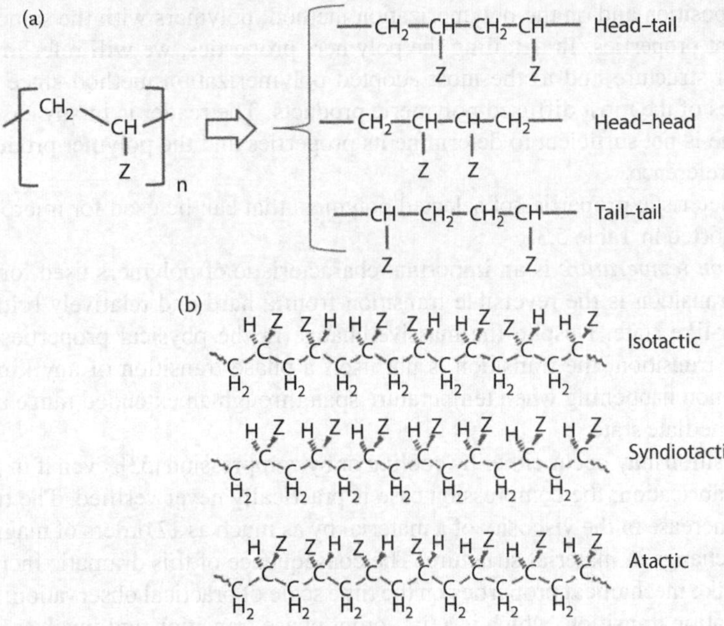

FIGURE 1.44 Polymer tacticity: definition (a) and different tactic forms (b).

lie on one side of the chain, the configuration is called isotactic. If the substitutes alternate from one side to another in a regular manner, the configuration is termed syndiotactic. Finally, a random arrangement of substituent groups is referred to as atactic. Examples of these configurations are shown in Figure 1.44b.

The properties of a given polymer will vary considerably with its tacticity. Thus, atactic polypropylene is useless as a solid construction material, and is employed mainly as a component of adhesives or as a soft matrix for composite materials. In contrast, isotactic polypropylene is generally a high-melting solid (about 170°C), which can be molded or machined into structural components. Another example of this differentiation is polypropylene, whose properties are synthetized in Table 1.11. In this case, the atactic material is soft and elastic, while the isotactic one is hard and rigid.

1.4.3 Polymers for Microfabrication Main Properties

In this section, we focus on the main polymer application we will encounter in this book, considering polymers that can be used for microfabrication processes. The particular conditions in which planar processes happen and also the requirements in terms of small critical dimension and durability of labs on chip structures differentiate the type of polymer use in this application by many polymers used to fabricate macroscopic objects. The control of the chemical and physical properties of organic polymers has been extensively investigated, allowing the fabrication of controlled microstructures with various structural and surface properties including hydrophobicity, conductivity, reflection coefficient, roughness, oxidation state, and crystal structure.

Certain functionalities (e.g., carboxyl groups) of polymers can be generated during the fabrication process, and this has attractive potential applications for the polymers used in microfluidic chips.

A last observation is important in considering properties of polymeric materials. A polymer takes its name from the main monomers chain; however, polymers with the same backbone chain can be a sensibly different one from the other both due to a different degree of cross-linking and due to the presence of lateral chains that cast the polymer particular properties. Thus, depending on the specific composition and on the polymerization method, polymers with the same generic name can have different properties. In detailing the polymers properties, we will refer in general to the simpler chemical structure and to the most adopted polymerization method since these are also the characteristics of the most diffused polymeric products. The reader is in any case advised that, the polymer name is not sufficient to determine its properties and the polymer producer data sheet is the only clear reference.

A set of characteristic properties of selected polymers that can be used for microfluidic circuits fabrication is reported in Table 5.3.

Glass transition temperature is an important characteristic of polymers used for microfabrication. The glass transition is the reversible transition from a hard and relatively brittle state into a molten or rubber-like state. Despite the massive change in the physical properties of a material through its glass transition, the transition is not itself a phase transition of any kind. It is a continuous phenomenon happening when temperature span through an extended range and implying a continuous intermediate state.

The glass transition may occur either by cooling or by compression [53], even if in practical cases regarding microfabrication, the compression case is practically never verified. The transition comprises a smooth increase in the viscosity of a material by as much as 17 orders of magnitude without any pronounced change in material structure. The consequence of this dramatic increase is a glass exhibiting solid-like mechanical properties on the time scale of practical observation. This is in contrast to crystallization transition, which is a first-order phase transition and involves discontinuities in thermodynamic and dynamic properties such as volume, energy, and viscosity.

Since glass transition is a continuous phenomenon, the individuation of a well-specified glass transition temperature is more a matter of a convention than of nature. This convention has been standardized by ISO [54]. The measurement procedure indicated in Reference [54] is qualitatively reproduced in Figure 1.45: the system from above the glass transition is cooled at 10°C/min to arrive quite below the glass transition in a zone where the heat capacity of the glass is slow varying. Starting from that point the polymer is heated at the same rate while measuring the time variation of the heat capacity. As shown in Figure 1.45, typically two flexes are individuated in the measured curve, called points 2 and 3 in the figure, while the behavior well below the transition temperature is almost linear. The transition temperature is then defined as the temperature corresponding to the intersection between the line extrapolating the low-temperature linear behavior and the tangent to the measured curve in the first flex (point 2). This point is individuated in the figure as point 1.

Different operational definitions, however, are used in the scientific community for the glass transition temperature, since due to the arbitrary nature of this polymer characteristic, often the ease

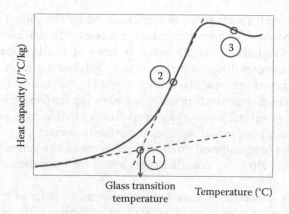

FIGURE 1.45 Typical measurement of the glass transition temperature performed measuring the specific heat versus temperature in a scanning calorimeter.

of use in the specific application is the criterion followed to select a specific definition. Different definitions yield different numeric results, generally within a few kelvins. One definition refers to the viscosity, fixing a temperature value at which viscosity is 10^{12} Pa s. As evidenced experimentally, this value is close to the annealing point of many glasses [55].

In contrast to viscosity, the thermal expansion, heat capacity, shear modulus, and many other properties of inorganic glasses show a relatively sudden change at the glass transition temperature. Any such step or kink can be used to define the glass transition temperature, and in any case, to make this definition reproducible, the cooling or heating rate must be specified.

Melting temperature is another important temperature parameter for polymers used in microfabrication. In case of polymers, the term "melting temperature" is used in a slightly different way with respect to its general meaning. As a matter of fact, the real melting point of polymers is located at the temperature at which the crystal structure of the polymer transits to the glass structure, which is more similar to a very high-viscosity liquid than a crystal solid. In practice, this correct definition of melting temperature, used frequently in scientific literature, is used besides a completely different meaning, related to a sudden change in heat capacity and viscosity that the polymer has at a temperature quite higher than the glass transition temperature, and, that is indicated as point 3 in Figure 1.45.

Above this point, the polymer becomes a much more fluid liquid, since viscosity has a sudden decrease, so that under an intuitive point of view, melting seems to happen. Although not completely correct, in case of polymers, we will reserve the term "melting temperature" to this temperature, which is higher than the glass transition temperature.

Almost all the considerations that we have done dealing with the glass transition temperature can be repeated here, and the calorimetric measure of the melting temperature is reported also in Figure 1.45 as the second flex point of the measured heat capacity versus temperature curve.

Elastic coefficients and hardness are other important mechanical characteristics of microfabrication polymers, especially when they are used with a structural role. While elastic coefficients are well-defined quantities related to the elastic behavior of a material [56,57], the definition of hardness is not so universally unified. Intuitively, hardness is the capacity of a solid to resist a force causing a localized deformation. The term can be applied to deformation from indentation, scratching, cutting, or bending. In most polymers, the considered deformation is a plastic deformation of the surface.

The lack of a fundamental definition indicates that hardness is not to be a basic property of a material, but rather a composite one with contributions from the yield strength, work hardening, true tensile strength, modulus, and others factors. Hardness measurements are in any case widely used for control of materials quality because they are quick and frequently nondestructive [58,59].

A large variety of hardness measurement methods exist, all providing different numerical values depending on the type of test. As far as polymers are concerned, largely the most used hardness measurement is performed with the so-called Shore durometer [60]. Durometer, like many other hardness tests, measures the depth of an indentation in the material created by a given force on a standardized presser foot. This depth is dependent on the hardness of the material, its viscoelastic properties, the shape of the presser foot, and the duration of the test. The basic test requires applying the force in a consistent manner, without shock, and measuring the hardness (depth of the indentation). If a timed hardness is desired, force is applied for the required time and then read. The material under test should be a minimum of 6.4 mm (0.25 inch) thick. The principal scheme of a durometer measure is reported in Figure 1.46a.

Depending on the type of tool used to cause the indentation and on the applied force there are as much as 12 different scales that can be used for durometric measures [61,62]. The two most common scales in the field of polymers characterization are type A and type D scales, both expressing hardness with a number between 0 and 100. The A scale is for softer plastics, while the D scale is for harder ones. The characteristics of the tools used for measuring scales A and D hardness are reported besides the applied load in Table 1.13 and graphically shown in Figure 1.46b. Typical ranges of Shore type A and type B scales are shown in Figure 1.47 and typical values for known types of common applications polymers in Table 1.14.

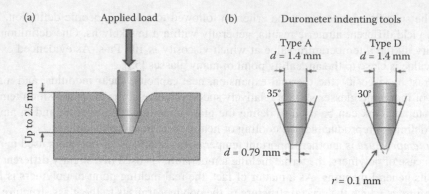

FIGURE 1.46 Principal scheme of a durometer measure (a) and indenting tools used for type A and type D scales on the durometer (b).

TABLE 1.13

Characteristics of Durometric Measures Using Type A and Type B Hardness Scales

Scale	Indenting Tool	Indenting Force (N)
Type A	1.4 mm diameter, with a truncated 35° cone, 0.79 mm diameter	8.064
Type B	1.4 mm diameter, with a 30° conical point, 0.1 mm radius tip	44.64

Several experimental attempts have been conducted to relate the Shore hardness to parameters of the elasticity theory, but it is a difficult task due to the fact that the deformation induced by the hardness measurement is complex and a theoretical elasticity analysis should produce quite involved results. Moreover, the induced deformation is not purely elastic, making the problem even more difficult.

One of the several empirical relations between the Young's modulus E measured in MPa and the hardness H (indicated as H_A or H_D depending on the scale) is presented in Reference [63] and is written as

$$\log_{10}(\varepsilon) = 0.0235(H + c) - 0.6403 \begin{cases} H = H_A & c = 0 \quad 20 < H_A < 80 \\ H = H_D & c = 50 \quad 30 < H_D < 85 \end{cases} \tag{1.70}$$

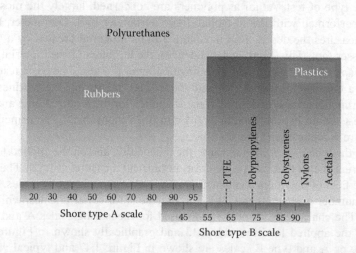

FIGURE 1.47 Common ranges of polymer hardness measured in Shore type A and type B scales.

TABLE 1.14

Values of Hardness Measured in Shore Type A and Type D Scales for Common Application Polymers

Hardness	Application
30 Shore A	Art gum erasers
35 Shore A	Rubber bands
40 Shore A	Can tester pads
50 Shore A	Rubber stamps
55 Shore A	Pencil erasers
60 Shore A	Screen wiper blades
65 Shore A	Automotive tires
70 Shore A	Shoe heels
75 Shore A	Abrasive handling pads
80 Shore A	Shoe soles
85 Shore A	Tap washers
90 Shore A	Typewriter rollers
95 Shore A	Fork lift solid tires
60 Shore D	Golf ball
80 Shore D	Paper-making rolls

For very hard polymers, it is possible that the Shore type D scale is not accurate, compressing too much high values. In this case, the Rockwell R method, which was born in the field of metallurgy, is used to measure hardness [64].

An empirical relation can be established between the type A and type D scales of the Shore method and the Rockwell method in the superposition ranges. In order to be accurate, this relation should be strictly material dependent and referred only to hardness measured by indention of flat surfaces. However, a good approximation can be performed if polymers are considered, which is reported besides experimental point in Figure 1.48.

Dielectric constant: It is often critical that a polymer substrate to be used to fabricate a microfluidics chip exhibits good electrical insulating properties, so that the electric field will drop across the fluid-filled channel and not through the substrate in microfluidic systems. Thus, a high dielectric constant is generally required. This allows, for example, effective electrophoresis to be performed in the integrated chip (see Section 8.5.2). Since frequently alternate current is used in electrohydrodynamics systems, the electric constant in alternate current is also important.

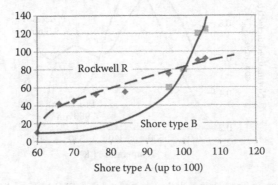

FIGURE 1.48 Approximate conversion plot between Shores type A and type B and Rockwell R hardness scales. A few experimental points measured for different polymers are also reported.

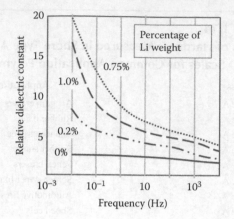

FIGURE 1.49 Dependence of the dielectric constant of a high-insulation polymer used for microfabrication of electrolyte membranes (PMMA and PMMA-LiPF$_6$). (Data from Kalyanasundaram S. et al., *Ionic Conductivity, Thermal Stability and FT-IR Studies on Plasticized PVC/PMMA Blend Polymer Electrolytes Complexed with LiAsF$_6$ and LiPF$_6$*, Ionics, vol. 7, pp. 44–52, 2001.)

The dependence of the dielectric constant of a high-insulation polymer used for microfabrication of electrolyte membranes (PMMA and PMMA-LiPF$_6$) is reported in Figure 1.49 (data from Reference [65]). It is evident from the figure how the dielectric constant depends critically on the polymer composition.

The dependence on the temperature of the dielectric constant of PMMA films [66] is reported in Figure 1.50, where it is also evident how the membrane thickness and the relative fabrication process influences the dielectric constant behavior.

Optical properties can be fundamental in polymers used as structural material in labs on chip if optical detection is used, for example, by photoluminescence or interferometry. This means that the polymer absorbance have to be low at the considered frequency. In selected case, integrated optical structures have to be built in the polymeric film to implement optical detection, so that the possibility of tuning optical properties can be important.

Interesting frequencies are in both cases in the infrared region, where many biochemical molecules show interesting fluorescence and where integrated optical sources such as semiconductor lasers preferably emit [67]. The absorption generally increases by increasing the wavelength in the

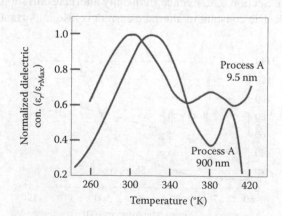

FIGURE 1.50 Dependence of the relative dielectric constant of PMMA membranes on temperature for different membrane thickness. (Data from Fukao K. et al. *Journal of Non-Crystalline Solids*, vol. 307–310, pp. 517–523, 2002.)

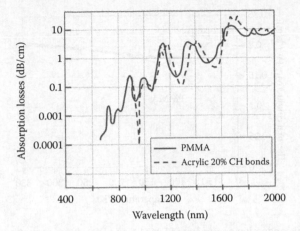

FIGURE 1.51 Absorption spectrum in the near-infrared region of PMMA and acrylic with 20% of CH bonds. (Data from Eldada L., Shacklette L. W., *IEEE Journal of Selected Topics in Quantum Electronics*, vol. 6, pp. 54–68, 2000.)

region where it is low, mainly driven by the resonances of the CH bond of the polymeric molecules [68]; however, frequent oscillations are present in the absorption curve, due to the complex interworking of the great number of absorption causes related to the great quantity of different bonds in the polymeric molecule. An example of spectral absorption in the near-infrared region of two different polymers used in integrated optics is shown in Figure 1.51 (data from Reference [68]), showing the capability of working with low losses as material for integrated optics detector systems.

Another important detection region is the UV band, where it is also possible to design polymers with suitably low absorption [69].

If polymers have to be also used with optical materials, the refraction index is also important. Generally, the refraction index of polymers that are transparent in the infrared region is comprised in the interval 1.30–1.70, but a higher refractive index is often required for specific applications. The refractive index is related to the molar refractivity, structure, and weight of the monomer. In general, high molar refractivity and low molar volumes increase the refractive index of the polymer. A great amount of data relative to polymers refraction indexes is reported in Reference [70] while an example of dependence of the refraction index on the wavelength for selected polymers is reported in Figure 1.52, showing as generally that the refraction index decreases as the wavelength increases.

Thermal conduction of structural polymers can be important in heat dissipation in labs on chip since elevated local temperatures can damage the microfluidic channels, denature more fragile

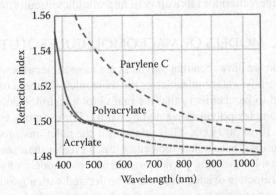

FIGURE 1.52 Refraction index of parylene C, polyacrylate, and acrylate in the near-infrared.

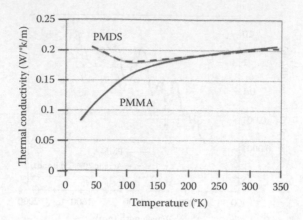

FIGURE 1.53 Thermal conduction coefficient of PMMA and PDMS versus temperature. (Data from Kline E. D., Hansen D., Thermal conductivity of polymers, from *Thermal Characterization Techniques*, Slade P. E., Jenkins L. T., editors, Dekker, 1st edition (1970), ISBN-13: 978-1114244627; Luo T. et al. *Journal of Applied Physics*, vol. 109, pp. 074321-1–074321-6, 2011.)

biological molecules, or influence the efficiency of chemical separations. Also, thermal expansion coefficient can be important when the polymer is used as a structural material in contact with other materials, such as glass or silica.

The thermal conductivity of PMMA and PDMS is shown in Figure 1.53 (data from References [70] and [71]). The behavior of the thermal conductivity versus temperature is different for various polymers, increasing or decreasing in different temperature ranges. Thermal conductivity also critically depends on tacticity, degree of polymerization, and crosslinking in the polymeric matrix [70].

Thermal expansion is also an important element, especially when a polymer is put in strict contact with some other material, for example, when a silicon wafer where labs on chip microfluidic circuits are realized is bonded with a polymer cap so as to close the fluid ducts and chambers. In this case, a very different expansion coefficient can provoke progressive weakening of the bonding due to the temperature fluctuations or prevent the adoption of processes that provoke a very high temperature increase after the bonding.

Adhesion on silicon and glass: It is quite frequent that polymers are used as caps for silicon or silica wafers containing microfabricated structures. In this case, polymer adhesion is an important factor. However, it can be better explained and discussed in the framework of a specific discussion on the specific adhesion processes, so that we will delay the discussion of this important polymer property to Chapter 4, when we will deal with silicon microfabrication. Physical and chemical characteristics of selected polymers used for fabrication of microfluidics circuits are reported in Table 1.15.

1.5 MICROSCOPIC MODELS OF MACROMOLECULE SOLUTIONS

From the previous section we have seen that polymers are huge molecules with respect of molecules of other categories, especially water molecules or the molecules of other common solvents. We will see in Chapter 2 devoted to biochemistry that the main biological molecules, such as proteins and nucleic acids, are very complex polymers created by nature. For example, typical molecular masses of proteins ranges from 10 to 300 kDa. Thus, almost all the solutions processed by labs on chip, which are biological solutions, have solute molecules much greater than solvent molecules.

This circumstance enables building particular microscopic models of biological solutions that the base macroscopic parameters of such solutions to be derived with a good approximation without the need of a detailed description of the interaction of the solvent with the solute molecules: they are called implicit solvents models [72–74].

TABLE 1.15

Physical and Chemical Selected Characteristics of Polymers Used for Fabrication of Microfluidics Circuits

	PMMA	PC	PETG	PE-LD	PDMS	SU8[a]	PI[a]
Glass transition temperature (°C)	40 (isotactic)	150	81	−35	−130	>200	>400
Melting temperature (°C)	85–105	(230)	—	130	—	30 (degradation)	Does not melt
Tensile modulus (GPa)	2.4–3.1	2.5	1.7	0.16–0.25	<0.01	4.95	0.09
Thermal expansion coefficient ($\times 10^6$ K^{-1})	50–90	68	91	100–220	10–19	30	55
Heat capacity (J/mol/K)	17–220	—	—	22–36	—	—	—
Dielectric constant	2.8	2.9	3.2	2.2	3.0–3.5	4.5 (4.2@10 GHz)	3.5
Chemical resistance (weak acids)	Good	Poor	Fair	Excellent	Fair	Excellent	Good
Chemical resistance (weak bases)	Good	Poor	Fair	Excellent	Fair	Excellent	Good
Chemical resistance (alcohols)	Fair	Poor	Fair	Excellent	—	Excellent	Excellent
Chemical resistance (ketones)	Poor	Poor	Poor	Excellent	—	Excellent	Excellent

[a] Indicates fully polymerized form after backing.

PMMA, poly(methyl methacrylate); PC, polycarbonate (high viscosity); PETG, poly(ethylene terephthalate) glycol; LDPE, polyethylene (branched); PDMS, poly(dimethyl siloxane); PI, polyimide (pyromellitic dianhydride and 4,4′ oxydianiline monomer). For SU8 definition, see Section 4.5.2.

It is beyond the scope of this book to review in detail all the possible articulation of these models, which are collectively called implicit solvent models, both for the variety of approaches to the description of the interaction among the macromolecules and the continuous medium modeling the solvent, and because a detailed analysis of such methods would require also the consideration of the numerical complexity and accuracy of the algorithms implementing them [75,76]. As a matter of fact, many implicit solvent models are developed exactly with the aim of rendering the detailed analysis of the physical and chemical property of the solution feasible using a statistical mechanical description.

We will review the principle of equilibrium implicit solvent models in the next section, leaving detailed implementation to bibliography references. Such models are intended to describe a solution in its equilibrium state via a microscopic calculation of its thermodynamic parameters, thus one of their main tasks is to evaluate the free solvation energy.

1.5.1 IMPLICIT SOLVENT MODELS FOR SOLUTION IN EQUILIBRIUM

In general, a microscopic model of a solution based on statistical mechanics has to take into account three terms when evaluating the internal energy of the solution: interaction between the solute molecules, interaction between the solvent molecules, and interaction between solvent and solute molecules.

In a complete model, generally called explicit solvent model, the molecular structure of both solute and solvent are considered generating a remarkable degree of complexity that is manageable only with a remarkable computational effort [77,78]. However, the fact that macromolecules are much bigger than solute molecules allows simplifications to be carried out.

This simplification essentially consists in considering the solvent a continuous medium in which the macromolecules are embedded so that motion in a continuous fluid can be used to model the macromolecules dynamic. This is also justified by the fact that water dynamic is much faster than the configuration change that macromolecules experiment while moving so that the water shell due to hydration that unavoidably accompany solvation moves almost unaltered around the macromolecules, shielding them and easing their motion in the mass of water.

However, the solvent results excluded from a volume internal to the folded form of the macromolecule, so that it is possible to speak of a solvent exclusion volume accompanying the solution creation [73,74].

Such a model is useful when studying a single solution, when the macroscopic parameters like the solvation free energy have to be derived from the microscopic characterization of the macromolecules, and when the dynamic of more than one solvent reacting one with the other in the same solvent has to be studied.

Several classes of continuum water models have been explored depending on the considered situation, on the target problem to be solved, and on the available calculation power [79,80]:

- Simple dielectric models characterized by a given dielectric constant (generally set equal to 80 for water)
- Dielectric models where the dielectric constant changes with distance from the considered molecule to reflect the different states of water molecules in the vicinity to a macromolecule and far from it
- Geometric models based on exposed surface area or solute volume
- Continuum dielectric models where the effect of water is taken into account by an electrostatic model; two main electrostatic models categories have been considered:
  - Poisson–Boltzmann (PB)
  - Generalized Born (GB), which has generated a great number of variations when this idea is adapted to different situations or optimized for different targets
- More complex models based on variation algorithms to evaluate the different energy terms [81]

Let us consider a biological macromolecule composed of M atoms of different species located in space in points corresponding to the position vectors r_i, where the index i run from 1 to M to indicates all the atoms.

For compactness of notation, the molecule configuration, that is, a function of all the atom's position with respect to the center of mass of the molecule, can be indicated with the matrix

$$\underline{C} = \left[r_1 - r_c, r_2 - r_c, \ldots, r_M - r_c \right] \tag{1.71}$$

where r_c is the center of mass position and the underline indicates that $\underline{C}$ is a matrix (see Appendix 2).

The effective energy function of a macromolecule, containing both intramolecular interactions and solvent–molecule coupling terms, has the form

$$E_T(r_c, \underline{C}) = H_M(r_c, \underline{C}) + \Delta G_{sol}(r_c, \underline{C}) \tag{1.72}$$

where $H_M(r_c, \underline{C})$ is the so-called configuration energy, due to the particular configuration the macromolecule is assuming and $\Delta G_{sol}(r_c, \underline{C})$ is the solvation free energy. The solvation energy ΔG_{sol} is defined as the free energy change for transferring a molecule from the gas phase to the water solvent phase without altering its conformation state.

The transfer process can be decomposed into three steps:

1. Solute molecules are extracted by the solute gaseous phase by breaking the solute-to-solute bonds and charge distribution over the surface of the macromolecules that can exist in gaseous phase, the so-called solute shell is created in this way.

2. The solute shell is transferred into aqueous solution substituting an equivalent volume of water. This requires the water–water hydrogen bonds to break.

3. The solute's van der Waals interactions and partial charges are restored; so to create effective interaction between the solute and the solvent, hydration is created in this phase.

The solvation free energy can be expressed as

$$\Delta G_{sol} = \Delta G_{el} + \Delta G_{cav} + \Delta G_{vdW} \tag{1.73}$$

where ΔG_{el} is the electrostatic contribution, which is a purely enthalpic term, while ΔG_{cav} and ΔG_{vdW} are the cavity and the van der Waals contributions that have both an enthalpic and an entropic term. The first comes from the creation of the cavity in the solvent volume where the solute shell is placed, and the second from break and, in case, restoration of van der Waals forces.

1.5.1.1 Cavity Free Solvation Energy

In order to evaluate the cavity free energy in the simple model we have introduced, it is necessary to individuate the macromolecule configuration and its volume, so as to evaluate the energy that is needed to exclude solvent molecules from that volume. In principle, it is not possible to exactly individuate the solute-occupied volume since molecule borders should be described by a spatial distribution of charge provided by molecular orbitals. Naturally, this is a very complex approach that results to be not manageable if a solution model has to be carried out. Thus, some approximation is needed. Generally, the solute molecular volume is described as a set of overlapping spheres of radius R_i centered on the atomic positions r_i, each sphere somehow representing the volume occupied by the corresponding atom.

It is not trivial to define a meaningful atomic radius and different definitions have been used in different areas of physics. In this case, the more meaningful definition of atomic radius refer to the fact that van der Waals forces are very important in establishing configuration of organic macromolecules, besides hydrogen bonds (compare Section 2.2). The origin of van der Waals forces is in the continuous fluctuations of the electron density on the molecular external orbitals. Even if the average value of the charge distribution is zero, its variance is not zero so that dipole and multipolar forces arise in time.

A typical behavior of the average van der Waals potential between two macromolecules in a selected mutual configuration is reported in Figure 1.54. The van der Waals potential exhibits an

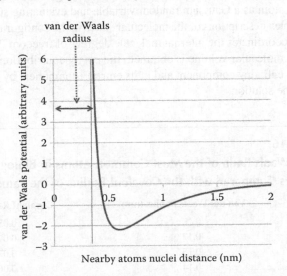

FIGURE 1.54 Typical average van der Waals potential in the interaction between two biomolecules in a given mutual configuration with the definition of van der Waals radius of the nearby atoms.

asymptote at a well-defined distance between the nuclei of the two nearer atoms. The atoms cannot be nearer than that distance owing to the strong repulsive energy due to the superposition of electronic orbitals. This suggests that, at least as far as weak intermolecular forces like van der Waals or hydrogen bonds are considered, the atom can be assumed to be a hard sphere with a radius depending on its properties, which is called van der Waals radius [82].

Van der Waals radii for different atoms may be determined with different means:

- From mechanical properties of nonideal gases by using the van der Waals state equation and fitting it with experimental data
- From the experimental measurement of the substance critical point
- Measurements of atomic spacing between pairs of unbounded atoms in crystals
- From measurements of electrical or optical properties, for example, the polarizability and the molar refractivity of crystals

These various methods give values for the van der Waals radius which are similar but not identical. Tabulated values of van der Waals radii, like those reported in Table 1.16 for the most common atoms in organic macromolecules, are obtained by taking a weighted mean of a number of different experimental values, and, for this reason, different tables will often report slightly different values. This is somehow intuitive, since there is no reason to assume that a precise value of the van der Waals radius can be defined as an absolute property of the atomic structure; this is more a relative property that assumes a precise value only when the physical and chemical environments are defined [82]. For example, it is possible to assume that the van der Waals radius of a selected atom slightly changes depending on the macromolecule where it is embedded.

Within the approximations characteristics of an implicit solvent model, the intrinsic approximation of considering an average van der Waals radius is not relevant with respect to other adopted approximations, thus this concept is very useful in this contest.

Once the van der Waals radius is associated to each atom, it is clear that the volume formally occupied by each atom is constituted by a sphere and these spheres, superimposing between nearby atoms, forms a continuous volume that constitute the molecular volume, that is, the so-called solvent exclusion volume (see Figure 1.55). Naturally, the molecule volume calculated in this way heavily depends on the molecule configuration. Different ways have been introduced to evaluate approximately an average molecular volume, from simple approximations considering the net volume that can be attributed to each individual atom as a Gaussian random variable and evaluating statistical parameters on this basis, to more complex descriptions of the molecular states in the configuration phase state, that is, in that space having as coordinates the internal molecule degrees of freedom [77,83].

Once the equivalent molecular volume is obtained, the cavity contribution to the free energy can be evaluated both in its enthalpy component and in its entropy component by analyzing in detail the ideal process to form the solution.

TABLE 1.16

Van der Waals Radii of the Most Common Atoms in Biological Molecules Compared with the Covalent Radius of the Same Atom

Atom	Van der Waals Radius (nm)	Covalent Radius (nm)
H	0.1	0.037
C	0.17	0.077
N	0.15	0.070
O	0.14	0.066
P	0.19	0.096
S	0.185	0.104

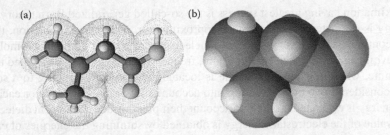

FIGURE 1.55 Stereographic representations of an organic molecule evidencing the superposition of the van der Waals spheres associated with each atom (a) and the resulting molecule volume and solvent exclusion volume (b).

The cavity free energy is composed of two terms: the first term is the energy needed to eliminate solvent molecules from the exclusion volume and the second term is the energy needed to replace them with solute molecules. During solvent elimination, both entropy is reduced, since less volume is available for the solute molecules, and positive enthalpy is expended, due to the need of imposing to the solvent molecules an ordered motion to bring them out of the exclusion volume.

During the solute molecules introduction, generally entropy increases due to the fact that the solute molecules are removed from the stable form of the solute alone and inserted into solution with a continuous solvent. This operation generally increases the number of available configurations for the solute molecules in the phase space, thereby increasing entropy.

1.5.1.2 Electromagnetic Free Solvation Energy

This is almost always the greater factor affecting the solvation free energy and it is due to the fact that water molecules are polar. The continuous model of the solvent can be thus modeled with a polar dielectric, whose dipoles are oriented by the surface charges on the solute molecule surfaces. The most correct way to take into account this effect is the so-called Poisson–Boltzmann model.

This kind of model will be analyzed in detail in Section 7.5.2. It allows the potential arising around a charged surface immersed in a continuous fluid where charges or dipoles are present to be evaluated on the ground of the Poisson equation for the electrostatic potential and the Boltzmann distribution of the thermal energy of the fluid particles. In our case the charged surface is the surface of the macromolecule, that is locally charged even if its overall charge is zero, and the fluid where the surface is immersed is the solvent.

In general, dipoles are oriented and free charges are attracted by the charged locations on the molecule surface so that a charge and oriented dipole layer is generated around the molecule surface. This is the so-called double layer (see Section 7.5.2) that in the implicit solvent model models the molecule hydration once inside the solvent. Two different forces regulate the dynamics of charges and dipoles near the charged surface: electrostatic interaction and thermal motion. Under the action of electrostatic interaction, charges adhere to the surface and dipoles are oriented in the fluid layer near the surface. While this phenomenon goes ahead, the electrostatic field is increasingly shielded up to a threshold point where it is no more sufficient to overcome completely thermal motion. This first phase generated the so-called Stern layer near the surface, which is a layer of almost still charges and dipoles completely adherent to the surface.

Out of the Stern layer, the electrostatic interaction generates an average dipole orientation and charge localization, which is continuously randomized by thermal motion, thereby generating the so-called Debye layer, where average charge and dipole is not zero, but thermal motion generates continuous random fluctuations.

While quite accurate in modeling the solvent–solute interaction once the charge distribution on the macromolecule surface is evaluated, this model is also quite complex under a computational point of view and several approximations have been introduced to render it manageable in complex situations.

The approximation having greatest success is the so-called generalized Born theory, where electrostatic energy is evaluated with a pairwise approximation. In this approximation, the solvent is considered a continuous dielectric with a fixed dielectric constant out of the macromolecules occupied volume, while a different dielectric constant, frequently equal to one, is assigned to the solvent exclusion volume, where the solute molecule is located. The atoms belonging to a solute macromolecule are considered two by two, taking into account all possible couples. For each couple, the electrostatic energy is evaluated taking into account their position and the solvent dielectric constant and the final value of the electrostatic energy is obtained by summing the energies of each different couple. A schematic representation of this pairwise approximation is reported in Figure 1.56.

In this approximation, each atom is considered like a sphere characterized by a well-defined Born radius, which is in general different from the van der Waals radius that is used to evaluate the macromolecule volume and external surface, and which is dependent on the macromolecule configuration. The Born radii and the dielectric constants of the solute and the exclusion volume are the key parameters of each Born approximation. Several different ways to assign these key parameters have been proposed [77,83] both with the scope of achieving good reproduction of experimental results and to control the numerical complexity of the obtained model. For example, either the solvent dielectric constant can be assigned simply constant outside the exclusion volume, or it can be modeled with a position depending on function so as to somehow reproduce the effect of the macromolecule hydration in changing the solvent structure in the Stern and Debye layers. Similarly, Born radii are generally assigned in strict relation to the molecule shape and to the position of the atom inside the molecule, so as to reproduce different effects.

On the ground of the structure of the Born approximation, the free solvation energy is calculated using the following equation:

$$\Delta G_{el} = \Delta G_m - \Delta G_w \tag{1.74}$$

where ΔG_m is the electrostatic energy of the molecule atoms in their real situation and ΔG_w is the energy they would have if the solvent would not be excluded by the molecule volume so that the dielectric constant would be that of water.

Equation 1.74 can be explicated with the generalized Born model approximation as (compare Figure 1.56)

$$\Delta G_{el} = -\frac{1}{2}\left(\frac{1}{\varepsilon_m} - \frac{1}{\varepsilon_w}\right)\sum_{i,j=1}^{N}\frac{q_i q_j}{\sqrt{r_{ij}^2 + B_i B_j\, e^{-r_{ij}^2/(4 B_i B_j)}}} \tag{1.75}$$

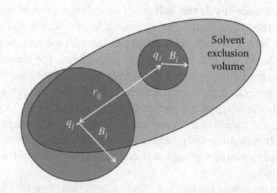

FIGURE 1.56 Schematic representation of the pairwise approximation adopted in the generalized Born model and definition of its main parameters.

where

- B_i is the Born radius of the ith atom of the solute molecule
- q_i is the electrical charge of the ith atom of the solute molecule
- r_{ij} is the distance between the ith and the jth atoms of the solute molecule
- ε_m is the dielectric constant inside the solvent exclusion volume
- ε_w is the water dielectric constant

Equation 1.68 can be rearranged by separating the double sum into one sum collecting all the terms with equal indices and one sum collecting all the terms with different indices.

The first sum represents the sum of the energies due to the position of each single atom with respect to the solvent, and can be named self-energy, ΔG_{self}, while the second term represents the contribution due to the mutual position of each atoms couple and can be named reciprocal free energy, ΔG_{rec}.

Thus, Equation 1.75 can be written as

$$\Delta G_{el} = \Delta G_{self} + \Delta G_{rec} \qquad (1.76)$$

The self-energy is largest for the atoms that are most exposed to the solvent because they are capable of inducing stronger polarization fields. This effect is captured by the generalized Born model in that atoms exposed to the solvent have smaller Born radii, whereas buried atoms tend to have larger Born radii. The pair-energy term corresponds to the dampening of electrostatic interactions in a high dielectric medium due to the screening of the solute charges.

1.5.1.3 van der Waals Free Solvation Energy

The evaluation of the van der Waals free energy term requires the introduction of a van der Waals interaction potential between the molecule accessible surface and the continuous solvent. This is generally dependent on the point of the molecule surface since different active and inert molecule sites creates van der Waals bonds with very different efficiency.

Thus, several models have been proposed to model van der Waals free energy component and this is one of the major variations among different implicit solvent models. Maintaining a pairwise approximation as in the case of generalized Born model, the interaction potential between the solvent and the solute molecules can be changed, both with the aim of better represent the real interaction and with the aim of simplifying calculation complexity of the model.

Generally, energy release is caused by establishing of van der Waals forces between the solute and the solvent, due to the fact that the van der Waals bonded molecules are more stable, that is, in a lower energy state, with respect to unbounded molecules. The negative free energy is frequently composed by a negative enthalpy term and by a lesser positive entropy term, due to the fact that establishment of van der Waals bonds reduces the number of possible configurations of water molecules around the solute molecule.

1.5.1.4 Implicit Solvent Models and Explicit Solvent Simulations

In order to evaluate the effectiveness of the different implicit solvent models it has to be observed that these methods have been applied to a variety of different applications [84–87] and in order to obtain the best results they have been carefully tuned not only in the values of the parameters, but also in the kind of applied algorithm in order to be optimized for the specific problem.

One optimized, the implicit solvent model based on the generalized Born approach gives generally good results when compared either with direct measurements or with much more cumbersome explicit solvent models. A similar comparison is carried out, for example, in Reference [88] in which a solution of the particular molecule with structural formula is shown in Figure 1.57.

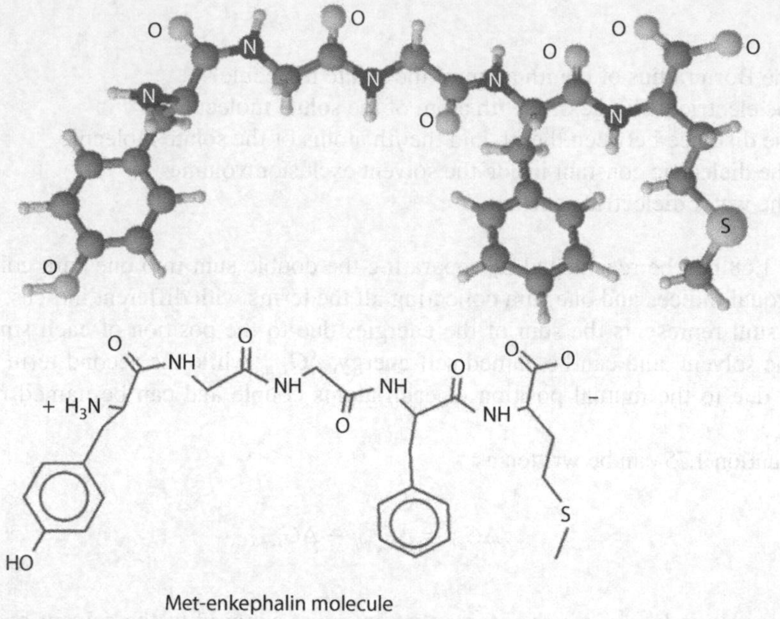

Met-enkephalin molecule

FIGURE 1.57 Structural formula of the particular molecule (Met-enkephalin) used in Reference [88] for a comparison between a generalized Born model and an explicit solvent model where the bonds between individual water molecules and the solute molecules are considered.

Owing to the two carbon rings, this molecule assumes configuration characterized by the angle between the rings planes, thus is particularly suitable to compare the two kinds of models under a structural point of view considering simple variables. Another variable that can be assumed to compare different molecule configurations is the so-called gyration radius, that, once the molecule atoms are numbered using the organic chains convention (see Section 1.4) can be defined as

$$\gamma^2 = \frac{1}{N} \sum_{i=1}^{N} \left| r_i - r_g \right|^2 \tag{1.77}$$

where r_g is the position vector of the molecule center of mass and r_i the position vector of the ith atom.

Naturally, the rotation angle and the value of γ^2 are statistical variables in a water solution of the considered molecule at equilibrium and it is very interesting to compare the distribution of these variables as estimated by different solution models. The different implicit and explicit solvents models considered in Reference [88] and their characteristics are reported in Table 1.17. In particular two different models are considered to represent nonpolar interaction between the protein surface and the water solvent, mainly constituted by van der Waals forces.

The estimate of the statistical distribution of the gyration radius produced by the different considered models is reported in Figure 1.58. From the figure, it clearly results that the consideration of a form of solvation potential, that is, the consideration of the surface energy linking the macromolecule to the water solvent, is necessary to obtain a good qualitative description of the molecular shape distribution in the equilibrium situation.

If a reasonable solvation potential is adopted, correct values for the gyration radius are obtained, but a few fine details of the distribution are in any case not correctly predicted by implicit solvent models. It is the case of the double maximum of the distribution obtained using the explicit solvent

TABLE 1.17

Acronyms and Characteristics of the Explicit and Implicit Solvent Models Used in Reference [88]

Acronym	Model Type	Model for Water Viscosity	Dielectric Constant of Water	Solvation Potential Solvent Molecule Interaction
ASPS	Implicit	Static	Experimental	Atomic solvation parameter [44]
ASPD	Implicit	Dynamic	Experimental	Atomic solvation parameter [44]
ASPE	Implicit	Static	Theoretical	Atomic solvation parameter [44]
SASA	Implicit	Static	Experimental	Solvent-accessible surface area [45,46]
NASP	Implicit	Dynamic	Experimental	No one
MD		Fully explicit atomic simulation		

simulation that represents an oscillation of the configuration between two almost stable states, as demonstrated by a fine analysis of the trajectories in the configuration space state [88]. However, reproduction of statistical distributions fine details is generally not strictly needed in determining with a good accuracy the macroscopic thermodynamic characteristics of the solution, where implicit solvent models generally performs well once optimized correctly. Other expressions of the solvation potential that has been proposed in literature are also tested in Reference [88] with quite worst results, generating completely unacceptable results, that probably also impact the macroscopic values of thermodynamic state functions.

Similar results are also obtained by comparing the statistical distribution of the molecule torsion angle. In this case, wider variations are observed, corresponding to a worst ability of implicit solvent models to catch the details of internal molecular torsion angles.

In studying the dynamic kinetic theory describing reactions of macromolecules in diluted solutions, it is very important to evaluate the thickness of the solvation water layer that surrenders the macromolecules; thus, it is useful to understand if implicit solvent models are able to evaluate this parameter with accuracy. This problem is faced, for example, in Reference [89]. Since this parameter depends on the position we consider on the theoretical protein surface, in the article, different active sites are considered and, for each site, different implicit solvent models are compared with an explicit solvent model.

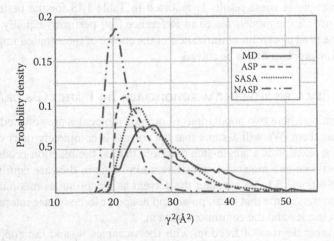

FIGURE 1.58 Probability density function of the torsion radius of a water solution at thermodynamic equilibrium as forecasted by different models: the considered models are reported in the figure and the acronym meanings in Table 1.17. (Data from Shen M., Freed K. S., *Biophysical Journal*, vol. 82, 1791–1808, 2002.)

TABLE 1.18

Example of Results from Two Explicit Solvents (ES1 and ES2) and Two Implicit Solvent (IS1 and IS2) Models When Used to Evaluate the Solvent Shell Thickness and the Solvent Accessible Area

	Solvent Shell Thickness (nm)			Surface Accessible Area (nm²)		
	Mean	Error	Error (%)	Mean	Error	Error (%)
ES1	0.245	Reference		30.64	Reference	
ES2	0.227	−0.018	−8%	31.29	0.65	2%
IS1	0.35	0.105	35%	31.43	0.79	3%
IS2	0.47	0.225	63%	32.53	1.89	6%

Source: Mashayak S. Y., Tanner D. E., *Comparing Solvent Models for Molecular Dynamics of Protein*, University of Illinois at Urbana-Champaign, Physics Department, May 12, 2011 Final Research Reports (last accessed on March 21, 2012 on http://online.physics. uiuc.edu/courses/phys466/spring11/projects/index.html).

Note: The first explicit solvent simulation is assumed as a reference.

In particular, the explicit, two full atoms simulation models (ES1 and ES2) are compared with a GB and with a coarse grain solvent model (CG) that is somehow an intermediate step where the solvent is considered as a set of coarse grains each of which is modeled as a continuum with macroscopic parameters derived from the water solvent.

In agreement with Reference [88], it is found that the two all atoms models represent accurately the shape distribution of the molecules, while this characteristic is also approximately represented by implicit solvent models. However, the average solvent concentration around the molecule in chemical equilibrium is also well represented by implicit solvent models, with errors of the order of less than 10% if we decouple it from wide bandwidth statistical errors due to the finite number of simulations. The variance of the solvent shell thickness is instead reproduced with a larger error, probably due to its greater dependence on the specific protein shape.

Another important parameter is the protein surface accessible area, which is a key steric parameter of many organic chemical reactions and that is generally well reproduced in the implicit solvent simulations. An example of these results is reported in Table 1.18 for the better implicit solvent models. However, not all the models tested in Reference [89] performs equally well, as a further demonstration of the need of careful optimization of the choice of the adopted implicit solvent algorithm when a specific problem has to be solved.

1.5.2 CHEMICAL REACTIONS BETWEEN MACROMOLECULES: THE PERFECT GAS OF MACROMOLECULES

Consider now a solution where two populations of organic molecules are solvated in order to generate a reaction among them. We will assume that the solvent is completely inert with respect to the reaction and that the reaction is a single-step reaction, that is, the reaction product is obtained by a single collision between two molecules of different kinds. As in the case equilibrium models we have discussed in Section 1.5.1, we consider the solvent as a continuous medium surrounding the macromolecules and we assume that local, polar, and nonpolar forces cause interaction between the surface of macromolecules and the continuous solvent.

Identifying the inner degrees of freedom with the variables w_j and the conjugate moments χ_j and the degrees of freedom related to rigid translation and rotation of the molecule with q_j and the associated moments with p_j, the Hamiltonian expression of the energy of a large molecule can be written as

$$H_k = \frac{1}{2} \frac{p_1^2 + p_2^2 + p_3^2}{M_k} + \frac{1}{2} \frac{p_4^2 + p_5^2 + p_6^2}{J_k} + H_{c,k}(w_j, \chi_j) + H_{s,k}(p_j, q_j, w_j, \chi_j) \qquad (1.78)$$

where the index k refers to the specific solute, $H_{c,k}(w_j, \chi_j)$ is the configurational contribution, and $H_{s,k}(p_j, q_j, w_j, \chi_j)$ is the contribution of the solvent shell that is created due to the macromolecules hydration.

Let us divide the phase space in a configuration space and a position space, where the variables of the configuration space are (w_j, χ_j). We will assume that, in a first approximation, the configuration-related energy can be divided by the molecular global translation energy, but for the fact that the molecule configuration impacts the viscous parameters that contribute to determine the motion of the whole molecule in the viscous surrounding.

If this is true, we can define a state space distribution considering only inner variables and, proceeding with standard statistical mechanics, we can arrive at the Boltzmann result for the statistical distribution of $H_{c,k}$

$$p(H_{c,k}) = \frac{1}{\kappa T} e^{-H_{c,k}/\kappa T} \qquad (1.79)$$

In this hypothesis, the distribution of large molecules always relaxes on a uniform distribution over the set of configurations having the smallest possible internal energy. This simple reasoning is confirmed by almost all equilibrium models, both implicit and explicit solvent based [72–74].

Imagining that all the molecules are in one of these stable configurations, slowly jumping among them, and that any configuration change due, for example, to a collision is rapidly recovered [72], we can assume that all the molecules have approximately the same energy related to the inner degrees of freedom $H_{c0,k}$. If this is true and we are not interested in steric properties, that is, the reaction is not essentially changed by the configuration of the molecules, we can incorporate this constant into the general constant defining energy and eliminate it.

It is worth observing that steric effects are quite important in many organic reactions. However, if the reaction is practically determined by the exposure of the molecule reaction site, generally this situation does not change considering different minimum energy configurations. This is due to the fact that in nature the reaction has to happen or not, independently of the random configuration change due to thermal motion. Thus, the model we are going to introduce in practice can also be used in many cases in which steric effects are important.

As far as the term $H_{s,k}(p_j, q_j, w_j, \chi_j)$ is concerned, this is a statistical term depending on the attraction generated between a set of bonded solvent molecules and the solute single-bonded molecule.

During motion, the effect of the hydration shell moves along with the macromolecule, thus practically increasing the macromolecule mass.

Since the surrounding solvent is not in contact with the macromolecule surface, but with the hydration shell, it is possible to assume that it sensibly reduces the viscous drag opposed to the macromolecule motion. However, this effect also renders quite difficult the change of the speed of a macromolecule if it is subject to an external force. To qualitatively understand this effect, let us imagine that the molecule starts to accelerate, the shell will be deformed remaining mainly on the rear of the macromolecule (see Figure 1.59). In this condition, the macromolecule is no more shielded on the front by a solvent shell and experiments a transient increase of the viscous resistance to motion, due to the interaction between its less-shielded surface and the solvent molecules that are encountered on its trajectory. Thus, the acceleration is thwarted and either a new equilibrium velocity is reached if the external field effect is permanent or, when the external field is switched off, the molecule will return at the original average speed. In any case, the hydration shell will return to its equilibrium configuration.

Exactly the opposite occurs if the macromolecule is decelerated, so that the shell of solvent molecules that facilitate the macromolecule motion in the solvent tends to push the macromolecules toward an equilibrium velocity.

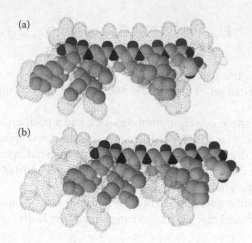

FIGURE 1.59 Scheme of a macromolecule with its hydration shell (represented by a cloud of points) in equilibrium motion (a) and during acceleration (b).

Thus, the term $H_{s,k}(p_j, q_j, w_j, \chi_j)$, as far as the quasi-equilibrium condition holds, can also be imagined as an almost constant term, having small and rapid fluctuations around its average value. A configuration dependence also exists in the rotational part of the solid motion energy, in the form of the inertia momentum tensor, but with the same principle used to eliminate the inner degrees of freedom, we can substitute it with the average value over the equilibrium configurations.

At the end, the Hamiltonian of the large molecules is, in a first approximation

$$H_k = \frac{1}{2}\frac{p_1^2 + p_2^2 + p_3^2}{M_k} + \frac{1}{2}\frac{p_4^2 + p_5^2 + p_6^2}{J_k} + H_{K0} \tag{1.80}$$

where H_{k0} is a constant. In particular, Equation 1.80 tells us that the big particles behave as a sort of ideal gas formed by rigid, nonsymmetric particles, moving in a viscous environment. These particles have, however, to be characterized by an equivalent mass and an equivalent viscous coefficient has to be introduced to take into account hydration. We can talk about a sort of macromolecule equivalent perfect gas, so explaining at least qualitatively the good success of a very simple kinetic theory in explaining the time evolution of single-step reactions. Example of parameters obtained by fitting experimental results with the molecule perfect gas theory are reported in Table 1.19. Parameters for pure waters are reported too for comparison.

1.5.3 COLLISIONS AND REACTION KINETICS

The macromolecule cross section $\sigma_k(\xi_j)$ can be evaluated by considering a configuration, characterized by a set of M configuration parameters ξ_j, in the extreme case all the elements of the configuration matric $\underline{C}$ defined in Equation 1.71. Let us imagine to define the reference system so that the macromolecule center of mass is located in the origin and to target the macromolecule with a point particle beam with a plane front (see Figure 1.60).

Let us define the following parameters:

- ϕ_0, the angle that the incident probe beam defines with the xy plane
- ψ_0 the angle that the incident probe beam defines with the xz plane
- ϕ_1, ψ_1 the angles that the generic incident particle define after deflection with the xy and the xz planes when it is so far from the macromolecule not to be influenced by it
- $\phi_{10} = \phi_1 - \phi_0$ and $\psi_{10} = \psi_1 - \psi_0$

TABLE 1.19

Approximate Values of the Average Collision Cross Section and Radii for Selected Molecules

Molecule	Notes	Cross Section (nm²)	Collision Radius (nm)
Water	Inorganic	0.25	0.28
Glucose	Almost linear sugar	0.33	0.33
Muscle troponin C (mouse)	Y shaped protein	1.24	0.63
Insulin (human)	Globular protein	78.5	5
Hemoglobin (human)	Globular Protein	113.1	6
DNA (human)	Supercoiled form	5027	40

The collision cross section of the macromolecule is defined as

$$\sigma_k(\xi_j, \phi_0, \psi_0) = \int\limits_0^{2\pi}\int\limits_0^{\pi} \delta\sigma(\xi_j, \phi_0, \psi_0, \phi_{10}, \psi_{10}) \sin(\psi_{10}) \, d\phi_{10} d\psi_{10} \tag{1.81}$$

where $\delta\sigma$ is the probability that a point particle incident with angles ϕ_0, ψ_0 is deviated due to the interaction with the macromolecule by angles ϕ_{10}, ψ_{10}.

For a given configuration of the macromolecule, the scattering cross section depends both on the potentials model assumed for the interaction of the different parts of the molecular surface in the given position and on the nature of the probe particle. For example, it completely changes in the realistic case in which active sites are present on the molecule surface that are electrically charged if the probe particle is charged or not.

Equation 1.81 can be solved analytically only in very simple cases. The simpler case is that of a sphere with an interaction potential equal to infinity if the probe particle hits the sphere, so that the probe is simply reflected in this case, and equal to zero if the particle does not hit the sphere surface. In this case, as intuitive, the cross section is independent from the incident angles and equal to

$$\sigma_k = \pi R^2 \tag{1.82}$$

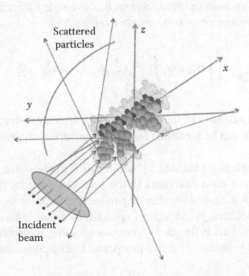

FIGURE 1.60 Geometry of the system used to evaluate the macromolecule scattering cross section.

where R is the sphere radius. In more general cases, the evaluation of the collision cross section is much more complex; depending on realistic values of the cross section, the so-called collision radius of a macromolecule is defined as

$$R(\xi_j, \phi_0, \psi_0) = \sqrt{\frac{\sigma_k(\xi_j, \phi_0, \psi_0)}{\pi}} \qquad (1.83)$$

In practical calculations what is interesting is not the cross section for the interaction with a point particle, even if in some cases it can be useful, but the mutual cross section of two macromolecules. The direct calculation using the cross section definition, due to the geometrical and interaction complexity of the two targets, is very complex and generally simplifications are used. The more frequent approximation is based on the collision radius definition.

A particular dominant interaction mechanism is identified. For example, if the collision will have a probability to create an ionic bond, the dominant interaction is electromagnetic, otherwise it can be based on dipolar repulsion or van der Waals forces. Once the dominant interaction is selected, an interaction potential model is also selected and a probe particle is fixed in such a way as to be sensible to the selected interaction mechanism. Once the point cross sections of the two macromolecules are evaluated, the mutual cross section is calculated with the equation

$$\sigma_{h,k} = \pi(R_h + R_k)^2 \qquad (1.84)$$

It is easy to demonstrate that Equation 1.84 is exact for rigid spheres, but it is a simple approximation in other cases, even if the dependence on the incident angles and on the molecular configurations is introduced in the expressions of the collision radii.

Another issue adding complexity to the statistical model we are creating is that, in general, collisions occur from a random direction, unless a particular reason exists to select a specific reciprocal position of the molecules. This reason sometimes effectively exists when the collision involves macromolecules with conjugate active sites. For example, the ionic attraction between these sites can orient the colliding molecules during their travel one toward the other so as to collide in the point where the active sites are located.

Thus, we will adopt this approximation: if a specific collision mutual position exists, the corresponding collision cross section is selected; otherwise, for example, in collisions among nonreacting molecules, we will use an average cross section. It is evaluated starting from the collision radii where the point collision average cross sections are evaluated as

$$\sigma_k = \frac{1}{2\pi^2} \int_0^{2\pi}\!\!\int_0^{\pi} d\phi_0 d\psi_0 \int .. \int \sigma_k(\xi_j, \phi_0, \psi_0) p(\xi_j)\, d\xi_1 \ldots d\xi_n \qquad (1.85)$$

where $p(\xi_j)$ is the probability density of the configuration parameters that, since we are assuming a quasi-equilibrium condition, can be identified with the equilibrium distribution of the configuration parameters.

The function $p(\xi_j)$ is generally obtained by equilibrium models, like those based on implicit solvent representation that we have described in the previous section, by representing the set of probable configurations with a limited number of parameters in order to allow Equation 1.85 to be evaluated numerically. Sometimes, $p(\xi_j)$ is simply ignored, by assuming a cross section that does not depend on the configuration. This is frequently done for globular molecules.

Let us consider a diluted solution of two solutes A and B that gives rise to a first-order reaction

$$A + B \rightleftharpoons C \qquad (1.86)$$

where C is the reaction product. Let us set the reference system so that the x axis connects the centers of the colliding molecules and one of the molecules results to be still, which results to be an inertial reference system due to the Newton's first law. In the relative system where the B molecule is still, the relative energy of the A molecule is the sum of the energies of A and B observed in the absolute system. Thus, setting

$$E_T = E_A + E_B \tag{1.87}$$

and applying the equal partition principle, we have

$$P(E_T) = \frac{1}{\kappa T} e^{-\frac{E_T}{\kappa T}} \tag{1.88}$$

Thus, for the Boltzmann energy distribution, we have, in a first approximation

$$p_{RD} = \frac{1}{\kappa T} \int_{E_+}^{\infty} e^{-\frac{E}{\kappa T}} \, dE = e^{-\frac{E_+}{\kappa T}} \tag{1.89}$$

The inverse reaction can be both due to a marginal instability of the reaction product (in this case decay is spontaneous and characterized by a given decay time τ_C) and due to the fact that the C molecule collides with another molecule with a sufficient energy to break the bound and recreate the original components. Different reactions are governed by different mechanisms, depending on the stability of the final product and on the strength of the bounds creating the reaction product starting from the reagents.

Let us consider reactions that are not only spontaneous, but also whose equilibrium favors the formation of the reaction product with respect to disjoined reagents. Almost all reactions happening in labs on chip are of this kind. In this case, it is possible to consider, among all phenomena causing the break of a C molecule in A plus B, only those depending on the concentrations at first order. All collision-related phenomena depend on the concentrations at second order or more, requiring the simultaneous participation of two different molecules. Thus, in a first approximation, they can be neglected with respect to spontaneous decay of a C molecule due to the A–B bond break by thermal energy. As a matter of fact, the probability of this phenomenon depends on the density of C molecules only at first order.

Thus, considering thermal decay of a C molecule, we obtain

$$p_{BB} = \frac{1}{\kappa T} \int_{E_-}^{\infty} e^{-\frac{E}{6\kappa T}} \, dE = e^{-\frac{E_-}{\kappa T}} \tag{1.90}$$

These results naturally coincide with those obtained in Section 1.2.4 if only one degree of freedom (the translation in the collision direction) contributes to overcome the reaction activation energy.

Now, we have to determine the collision rates. If the concentration c_k $k = (A,B,C)$ of different molecules in the considered solution is expressed in moles for total solution moles, the number of particle n_k in the unitary volume for each of the reacting species is equal to

$$n_j = c_j M_w N_{AV} \quad j = (A,B,C) \tag{1.91}$$

where N_{AV} is the Avogadro number, M_w is the solution number of moles that, in the hypothesis of highly diluted solution, can be assumed equal to the solvent number of moles. The equivalent volume spanned in a second by a molecule depends on its average velocity and on its point cross section. The square average velocity v_j^2 of a molecule in the absolute reference system can be evaluated by the Maxwell distribution and it is given by

$$v_j^2 = \frac{8\kappa T}{\pi m_j} \quad j = (A,B,C) \tag{1.92}$$

The square average velocity is reported for different temperature and different molecular masses in Figure 1.61 (data from Table 1.20) for different substances in solution and, for comparison, for molecular nitrogen in air. In order to take into account, approximately, the effect of hydration, a hydration coefficient has been introduced whose value is evaluated approximately by using an implicit solvent method where a molecular surface definition based on van der Waals sphere atomic representation is used. The case of calcium ion is naturally an exception. In this case, the approximate hydration coefficient is evaluated starting from mobility measures (compare Section 7.5.1).

The square average velocity of a particle of type j in the reference in which the square average velocity of species k is zero can be obtained by a statistical mechanics theorem by substituting in Equation 1.92 the mass m_j with the reduced mass m_{kj}, that is given by

$$m_{kj} = \frac{m_j m_k}{m_j + m_k} \tag{1.93}$$

so that the average volume $\bar{V}_j$ spanned by a particle of the type j in the reference where the particle of type k is still in average is

$$\bar{V}_j = \sqrt{\frac{8\kappa T}{\pi m_{jk}}} \, \sigma_j \tag{1.94}$$

Note that in this chapter the index summation rule (see Appendix 3) is not used.

The probability η_{kj} that a particle of type j will hit a particle of type k in the unit time and unit volume of the solution can be evaluated by considering that the collision happens if a single particle of type k is partially contained in the volume $\bar{V}_j$. This is equivalent to consider the particle of type k

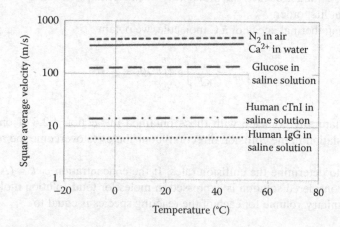

FIGURE 1.61 Thermal induced particles square average velocity for different temperature, different molecular masses, and different aggregation states. cTnI indicates human cardiac troponin I, a protein involved in heat contraction regulation; IgG indicates human immunoglobulin (see Sections 2.3.4.1 and 2.4.1). The parameters used to obtain the curves are reported in Table 1.20.

TABLE 1.20

Masses and Hydration Ratios Used in Figure 1.61

Substance	Aggregation	Molecular Mass (kg)	Hydration Ratio	Hydrated Mass (kg)
Nitrogen	Molecular in air	4.62×10^{-26}	—	—
Calcium ion	Water solution	1.99×10^{-26}	300%	7.98×10^{-26}
Glucose	Water saline solution	2.99×10^{-25}	90%	3.80×10^{-25}
cTnI	Water saline solution	3.82×10^{-23}	25%	4.40×10^{-23}
IgG	Water saline solution	2.49×10^{-22}	10%	2.71×10^{-22}

Note: cTnI indicates human cardiac troponin I, a protein involved in heat contraction regulation. IgG indicates human immunoglobulin (see Section 3.2).

as a point and to substitute in Equation 1.94 the point cross section with the reciprocal cross section, obtaining the reciprocal volume $\bar{V}_{jk}$ that can be expressed as

$$\bar{V}_{jk} = \sqrt{\frac{8\kappa T}{\pi m_{jk}}}\, \sigma_{jk} \tag{1.95}$$

Using the expression of the mutual volume we obtain

$$\eta_{kj} = c_k c_j \left(\frac{N_{AV} M_w}{V_S}\right)^2 \sqrt{\frac{8\kappa T}{\pi m_j m_k}}\, (m_j + m_k)\sigma_{kj} \tag{1.96}$$

where V_S is the solution volume. As intuitive expression (1.96) is completely symmetric in the indices j and k since no difference has to exist with the result evaluated in a reference system where the particles of species j are in average still.

Finally, the number of collisions N_{AB} for unit volume and unit time that could generate the reaction (1.86) from left to right can be written as

$$N_{AB} = c_A c_B \left(\frac{N_{AV} M_w}{V_S}\right)^2 \sqrt{\frac{8\kappa T}{\pi m_A m_B}}\, (m_A + m_B)\sigma_{AB} = \bar{c}_A \bar{c}_B \Omega_{AB} \tag{1.97}$$

where while c_A and c_B are measured in moles/moles, $\bar{c}_A$ and $\bar{c}_B$ are measured in moles/m^3. Here emerges the intuitive and fundamental property that the number of collisions between two species is essentially proportional to the product of the concentrations of the two species.

As we have seen in Section 1.2.4, this is an instrumental result in relating the kinetic theory of single-step reactions with the macroscopically observed reaction kinetic. Finally, the number N_{AB} of molecular reactions happening in the unit time and unit volume and creating the reaction product is

$$\widehat{N}_{AB} = c_A c_B \left(\frac{M_w}{V_S}\right)^2 \Omega_{AB} e^{-\frac{E_+}{\kappa T}} = \bar{c}_A \bar{c}_B\, \Omega_{AB} e^{-\frac{E_+}{\kappa T}} \tag{1.98}$$

This coincides with Equation 1.44 we used in the kinetic reaction theory to define the reaction rates.

As far as the reaction in the opposite direction is concerned, considering only thermal decay of a C molecule, we obtain

$$\widehat{N}_C = c_C \frac{M_w}{V_S} = \overline{c}_C\, e^{-\frac{E}{\kappa T}} \tag{1.99}$$

Generally, for spontaneous reactions, $E_{ib} \gg 6\kappa T$, so that Equation 1.89 provides the correct dependence of the reaction rate on the concentration of the species C.

Another important parameter that can be evaluated by the kinetic theory is the so-called average free path of a molecule. This is the average distance run by the molecule of a given species between two successive collisions. In evaluating the average free path, we have to consider that not only collisions that are potentially effective in generating a chemical reactions but also all possible collisions have to be considered.

Considering a particle of the species j, the probability p_j that in the unit time it has a collision can be evaluated, neglecting multiple collision events, as

$$p_j = \left[p_{jB}\,(1 - p_{jC} - p_{jA}) + p_{jA}\,(1 - p_{jB} - p_{jC}) + p_{jC}\,(1 - p_{jB} - p_{jA}) \right] \tag{1.100}$$

where, from Equation 1.97, we have

$$p_{jk} = c_k \frac{N_{AV} M_w}{V_S} \sqrt{\frac{8\kappa T}{\pi m_j m_k}(m_j + m_k)}\,\sigma_{jk} = \overline{c}_k\,\Omega_{jk} \tag{1.101}$$

Thus, the average number of collisions in unit time is obtained by multiplying (1.100) by $\overline{c}_j$ and the average free time τ_j is provided by

$$\tau_j = \frac{1}{\overline{c}_j \left[\overline{c}_A \Omega_{jA} + \overline{c}_B \Omega_{jB} + \overline{c}_C \Omega_{jC} \right]} \tag{1.102}$$

Since the particle has square average velocity $\overline{v} = \sqrt{v^2}$ given by Equation 1.92, the mean free path ℓ_j of the species j is given by

$$\ell_j = \sqrt{\frac{8\kappa T}{\pi m_j}} \frac{1}{\overline{c}_j \left[\overline{c}_A \Omega_{jA} + \overline{c}_B \Omega_{jB} + \overline{c}_C \Omega_{jC} \right]} \tag{1.103}$$

TABLE 1.21
Data Used for Figure 1.62

	A	B	C	AB	AC	BC
Initial concentrations (moles/m³)	0.04	0.04	0	—	—	—
Hydrated molecular mass (kDa)	0.15	1	1.15	—	—	—
Hydrated molecular mass (kg)	2.49 10⁻²⁵	1.66 10⁻²⁴	1.91 10⁻²⁴	—	—	—
Collision cross sections[a] (nm²)	20	200	400	100	100	200

[a] Mutual cross section is reported under the single-component column.

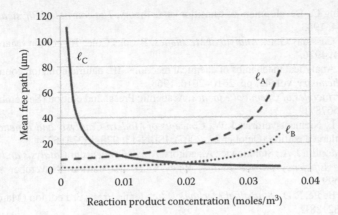

FIGURE 1.62 Mean free path of the reagents of reaction (1.82) versus the concentration of the reaction product in moles/m³. Data are reported in Table 1.21.

The mean free path decreases increasing the concentrations of the reagents and increases increasing the temperature. In the last case, the square mean velocity increases so that a longer path is run in the same mean free time.

An example of application of Equation 1.103 can be provided starting from reaction (1.86). Assuming initial concentrations of the reagents equal to 0.04 moles/m³, which are reasonable for labs biochemical reactions, and assuming the parameters of Table 1.21, where hydrated masses have to be considered, the values of the free mean path of the three chemical species involved in the reaction at 3000 K are reported in Figure 1.62 versus the concentration of the reaction product, taking into account the reaction stoichiometry that relates the concentration of the three species.

REFERENCES

1. Li P. C. H., *Fundamentals of Microfluidics and Lab on a Chip for Biological Analysis and Discovery*, CRC Press; 1st edition (February 24, 2010), ISBN-13: 978-1439818558.
2. Ghallab J. H., *Lab-on-a-Chip: Techniques, Circuits, and Biomedical Applications*, Artech House Publishers (July 2010), ISBN-13: 978-1596934184.
3. Fermi E., *Thermodynamics*, Dover Publications (June 1, 1956), ISBN-13: 978-0486603612.
4. Lavenda B. H., *A New Perspective on Thermodynamics*, Springer; 1st edition (December 3, 2009), ISBN-13: 978-1441914293.
5. Ben-Naim, A., *A Farewell to Entropy: Statistical Thermodynamics Based on Information*, World Scientific Publishing Company; 1st edition (2008), ISBN-13: 978-9812707062.
6. Timberlake K., *Chemistry: An Introduction to General, Organic, & Biological Chemistry*, Prentice-Hall; 10th edition (February 18, 2008), ISBN-13: 978-0136019701.
7. Berg J. M., Tymoczko J. L., Stryer L., *Biochemistry*, W. H. Freeman; 7th edition (December 24, 2010), ISBN-13: 978-1429229364.
8. Tro J. N., *Chemistry: A Molecular Approach*, Prentice-Hall; 2nd edition (January 15, 2010), ISBN-13: 978-0321651785.
9. Bunn F, Forger B. G., *Hemoglobin: Molecular, Genetic and Clinical Aspects*, W B Saunders Co; 2nd edition (July 1984), ISBN-13: 978-0721621814.
10. Antonini E., *Hemoglobin and Myoglobin in their Reactions with Ligands*, North-Holland Pub. Co, (1971), ISBN-13: 978-0444100962.
11. Houston P. L., *Chemical Kinetics and Reaction Dynamics*, Dover Publications (November 17, 2006), ISBN-13: 978-0486453347.
12. Connors L. A., *Chemical Kinetics: The Study of Reaction Rates in Solution*, Wiley-VCH; 1st edition (August 29, 1990), ISBN-13: 978-0471720201.
13. Truhlar D. G., Garrett B. C., Klippenstein S. J., Current status of transition-state theory, *The Journal of Physical Chemistry*, vol. 100, pp. 12771–12800, 1996.

14. Laidler K., King C., Development of transition-state theory, *The Journal of Physical Chemistry*, vol. 87, pp. 2657–2664, 1983.

15. Fowles G. R., Cassiday G. L., *Analytical Mechanics*, Brooks Cole; 7th edition (March 19, 2004), ISBN-13: 978-0534494926.

16. Marcus R. A., Analytical mechanics of chemical reactions. III. natural collision coordinates, *The Journal of Physical Chemistry*, vol. 49, pp. 2610–2616, 1968.

17. House J. E., *Principles of Chemical Kinetics*, Academic Press; 2nd edition (September 13, 2007), ISBN-13: 978-0123567871.

18. Chorkendorff I., Niemantsverdriet J. W., *Concepts of Modern Catalysis and Kinetics*, Wiley-VCH; 2nd revised and enlarged edition (October 23, 2007), ISBN-13: 978-3527316724.

19. Cybulski A., Moulijn J. A., Stankiewicz A., editors, *Novel Concepts in Catalysis and Chemical Reactors: Improving the Efficiency for the Future*, Wiley-VCH; 1st edition (November 9, 2010), ISBN-13: 978-3527324699.

20. Pathria R. K., Beale, P. D., *Statistical Mechanics*, Academic Press; 3rd edition (March 14, 2011), ISBN-13: 978-0123821881.

21. Chaikin P. M., Lubenski T. C., *Principles of Condensed Matter Physics*, Cambridge University Press; reprint edition (October 9, 2000), ISBN-13: 978-0521794503.

22. Sewel G., *Quantum Mechanics and Its Emergent Macrophysics*, Princeton University Press (July 29, 2002), ISBN-13: 978-0691058320.

23. Marcus J., *The Properties of Solvents*, Wiley; 1st edition (2 November 1998), ISBN-13: 978-0471983699.

24. Tapia O., Bertran J., *Solvent Effects and Chemical Reactivity*, Springer; 1st edition (July 31, 2003), ISBN-13: 978-1402004179.

25. Tanford C., *The Hydrophobic Effect: Formation of Micelles and Biological Membranes*, Krieger Pub Co; 2nd edition (August 1991), ISBN-13: 978-0894646218.

26. Kunz, W., *Specific Ion Effects, World Scientific Publishing Company*; 1st edition (December 17, 2009), ISBN-13: 978-9814271578.

27. Wade, L. G., *Organic Chemistry*, Prentice-Hall; 7th edition (February 1, 2009), ISBN-13: 978-0321592316.

28. Lehman J. W., *Operational Organic Chemistry*, Prentice-Hall; 4th edition (July 26, 2008), ISBN-13: 978-0136000921.

29. Hopf H., *Classics in Hydrocarbon Chemistry: Syntheses, Concepts*, Perspectives, Wiley-VCH; 1st edition (April 20, 2000), ISBN-13: 978-3527296064.

30. Olha A. G., Molnår Å., *Hydrocarbon Chemistry*, Wiley-Interscience; 2nd edition (April 17, 1995), ASIN: B001CPLFU6.

31. Dainthit J., *Oxford Dictionary of Chemistry*, Oxford University Press, USA; 6th edition (April 15, 2008), ISBN-13: 978-0199204632.

32. Gispert J. R., *Coordination Chemistry*, Wiley (May 2008), ISBN-13: 978-3527318025.

33. Laurance G. A., *Introduction to Coordination Chemistry*, Wiley; 1st edition (February 23, 2010), ISBN-13: 978-0470519318.

34. Cornelius C., Stereochemistry of the robinson anellation: Studies on the mode of formation of the intermediate hydroxy ketones, *Helvetica Chimica Acta*, vol. 73, pp. 1621–1636, 1990.

35. Scanio C. J. V., Starrett R. M., Remarkably stereoselective robinson annulation reaction, *Journal of the American Chemical Society*, vol. 93, pp. 1539–1540, 1971.

36. McMurray J. E., *Organic Chemistry*, Brooks Cole; 7th edition (January 2007), ISBN-13: 978_0495118374.

37. Scorpio R., *Fundamentals of Acids, Bases, Buffers & Their Application to Biochemical Systems*, Kendall Hunt Pub. Co. (August 2000), ISBN-13: 978-0787273743.

38. Kemnitz C. R., Loewen M. J., Amide resonance correlates with a breadth of C-N rotation barriers, *Journal of American Chemical Society*, vol. 129, pp. 2521–2528, 2007.

39. Leach A. R., *Molecular Modeling: Principles and Applications*, Prentice-Hall; 2nd edition (April 9, 2001), ISBN-13: 978-0582382107.

40. Youg R. J., Lovell P. A., *Introduction to Polymers*, CRC Press; 3rd edition (June 27, 2011), ISBN-13: 978-0849339295.

41. Hiemenz P. C., Lodge P. T., *Polymer Chemistry*, CRC Press; 2nd edition (February 15, 2007), ISBN-13: 978-1574447798.

42. Weinhold F., Chemistry. *A New Twist on Molecular Shape, Nature*, vol. 411, pp. 539–341, 2001.

43. Allinger L. N., Roger D. W., *Molecular Structure: Understanding Steric and Electronic Effects from Molecular Mechanics*, Wiley; 1st edition (August 2, 2010), ISBN-13: 978-0470195574.

44. Melaccio F., Ferré N., Olivucci M., Quantum chemical modeling of rhodopsin mutants displaying switchable colors, *Physical Chemistry Chemical Physics*, vol. 14, pp. 12485–12495, 2012.

45. Hasell T., et al., Triply interlocked covalent organic cages, *Nature Chemistry*, vol. 2, pp. 750–755, 2010.
46. Fleming I., *Molecular Orbitals and Organic Chemical Reactions: Reference Edition*, Wiley; 1st edition (May 4, 2010), ISBN-13: 978-0470746585.
47. Weinhold F., *Discovering Chemistry with Natural Bond Orbitals*, Wiley; 1st edition (July 10, 2012).
48. Shalk S. S., Hiberty P. C., *A Chemist's Guide to Valence Bond Theory*, Wiley-Interscience; 1st edition (December 4, 2007), ISBN-13: 978-0470037355.
49. Gillespie R. J., Hargittai I., *The VSEPR Model of Molecular Geometry*, Dover Publications; Reprint edition (February 15, 2012), ISBN-13: 978-0486486154.
50. Ward I. M., Sweeney J., *An Introduction to the Mechanical Properties of Solid Polymers*, Wiley; 2nd edition (May 31, 2004), ISBN-13: 978-0471496267.
51. Bicerano J., *Prediction of Polymer Properties*, CRC Press; 3rd edition (August 1, 2002), ISBN-13: 978-0824708214.
52. Dikie L. A., Labana S. S., Bauer R. S., editors, *Cross-Linked Polymers: Chemistry, Properties, and Applications*, American Chemical Society (May 5, 1988), ISBN-13: 978-0841214712.
53. Hansen J. P., McDonald I. R., *Theory of Simple Liquids*, Elsevier, 1st edition (2007), ISBN-13 978-0123705355.
54. ISO 11357-2: Plastics–Differential Scanning Calorimetry (DSC)–Part 2: Determination of Glass Transition Temperature, (1999).
55. Glass-Transition Temperature, IUPAC Compendium of Chemical Terminology, vol. 66, 1994.
56. Saada A. S., *Elasticity: Theory and Applications*, J. Ross Publishing, Inc.; 2nd edition (March 9, 2009), ISBN-13: 978-1604270198.
57. Maceri A., *Theory of Elasticity*, Springer; 1st edition (August 10, 2010), ISBN-13:978_3642113918.
58. Tweedi C. A., Van Vliet K. J., On the indentation recovery and fleeting hardness of polymers, *Journal of Material Research*, vol. 21, pp. 3029–3026, 2006.
59. Pusz A., Michalik K., Examining the hardness of the high density polyethylene with method of the cone, *Archives of Materials Science and Engineering*, vol. 28, pp. 467–470, 2007.
60. Gilman J. J., *Chemistry and Physics of Mechanical Hardness*, Wiley-Interscience; 1st edition (June 9, 2009), ISBN-13: 978-0470226520.
61. UNI ISO 7619-1:2011, Rubber, Vulcanized or Thermoplastic—Determination of Indentation Hardness—Part 1: Durometer Method (Shore Hardness).
62. UNI ISO 21509:2006, Plastics and Ebonite—Verification of Shore Durometers.
63. Qi H. J., Joyce K., Boyce M. C., Durometer hardness and the stress-strain behavior of elastomeric materials, *Rubber Chemistry and Technology*, vol. 76, 2, pp. 419–435, 2003.
64. ISO 2039-2:1987, Plastics—Determination of Hardness—Part 2: Rockwell Hardness.
65. Kalyanasundaram S. et al., Ionic conductivity, thermal stability and FT-IR studies on plasticized PVC/PMMA blend polymer electrolytes complexed with LiAsF6 and LiPF6, *Ionics*, vol. 7, pp. 44–52, 2001.
66. Fukao K., Uno S., Miyamoto Y., Hoshino A., Miyaji H., Relaxation dynamics in thin supported polymer films, *Journal of Non-Crystalline Solids*, vol. 307–310, pp. 517–523, 2002.
67. Agrawal G. P., Dutta N. K., *Semiconductor Lasers, Van Nostrand Reinhold*; 2nd edition (July 31, 1993), ISBN-13: 978-0442011024.
68. Eldada L., Shacklette L. W., Advances in polymer integrated optics, *IEEE Journal of Selected Topics in Quantum Electronics*, vol. 6, pp. 54–68, 2000.
69. Nelson N. et al., A Handheld Fluorometer for UV Excitable Fluorescence Assays, Proceedings of IEEE Biomedical Circuits and Systems Conference, BIOCAS, pp. 111–114, 2007.
70. Kline E. D., Hansen D., Thermal Conductivity of Polymers, from Thermal Characterization Techniques, Slade P. E., Jenkins L. T., editors, *Dekker*, 1st edition 1970, ISBN-13: 978-1114244627.
71. Luo T., Esfarjani K., Shiomi J., Henry A., Chen G., Molecular dynamics simulation of thermal energy transport in polydimethylsiloxane (PDMS), *Journal of Applied Physics*, vol. 109, pp. 074321-1–074321-6, 2011.
72. Cramer C. J., *Essentials of Computational Chemistry: Theories and Models*, Wiley; 2nd edition (November 22, 2004), ISBN-13: 978-0470091821.
73. *Modeling Solvent Environments: Applications to Simulations of Biomolecules*, Freight M. editor, Wiley-VCH, 1st edition (March 30, 2010), ISBN-13: 978-3527324217.
74. Chen J., Brooks III C. L., Khandogin J., Recent advances in implicit solvent-based methods for biomolecular simulations, *Current Opinion in Structural Biology*, vol. 18, pp. 140–148, 2008.
75. Backer N. A., Improving implicit solvent simulations: A poisson-centric view, *Current Opinion in Structural Biology*, vol. 15, pp. 137–143, 2005.

76. Lu B. Z., Zhou J. C., Holst M. J., McCammon J. A., Recent progress in numerical methods for the poisson boltzmann equation in biophysical applications, *Communications in Computational Physics*, vol. 3, pp. 973–1009, 2008.

77. Canuto S., *Solvation Effects on Molecules and Biomolecules: Computational Methods and Applications*, Springer; 1st edition (November 17, 2008), ISBN-13: 978-1402082696.

78. Fennel C. J., Keoe W. C., Dill K. A., Modeling aqueous solvation with semi-explicit assembly, *PNAS*, vol. 108, pp. 3234–3239, February 22, 2011.

79. Assan S. A., Mehler E., Modeling aqueous solvent effects through local properties of water, in *Modeling Solvent Environments: Applications to Simulations of Biomolecules*, Freight M. editor, Wiley-VCH; 1st edition (March 30, 2010), ISBN-13: 978-3527324217.

80. Chen J., Implicit Solvent, MMTSB/CTBP Workshop, August 4–9, 2009.

81. Cheng Li-T., Wang Z., Setny P., Dzubiella J., Bo Li, McCammon J. A., Interfaces and hydrophobic interactions in receptor-ligand systems: A level-set variational implicit solvent approach, *Journal of Chemical Physics*, vol. 131, pp. 144102, 2009.

82. Bondi A., Van der waals volumes and radii, *Journal of Physical Chemistry*, vol. 68, pp. 441–451, 1964.

83. Gallicchio E., Levy R. M., AGBNP: An analytic implicit solvent model suitable for molecular dynamics simulations and high-resolution modeling, *Wiley Journal of Computational Chemistry*, vol. 25, pp. 479–499, 2004.

84. Yu-Sum, Latour R. A., Comparison of implicit solvent models for the simulation of protein–surface interactions, *Wiley Journal of Computational Chemistry*, vol. 27, pp. 1908–1922, 2006.

85. Kessel A., Tieleman D. P., Ben-Tal N., Implicit solvent model estimates of the stability of model structures of the alamethicin channel, *European Biophysics Journal*, vol. 33, pp. 16–28, 2004.

86. Wang T., Wade C. R., Implicit solvent models for flexible protein–protein docking by molecular dynamics simulation, *Proteins: Structure, Function, and Genetics*, vol. 50, pp. 158–169, 2003.

87. Krol M., Comparison of various implicit solvent models in molecular dynamics simulations of immunoglobulin g light chain dimer, *Wiley Journal of Computational Chemistry*, vol. 24, pp. 531–546, 2003.

88. Shen M., Freed K. S., Long time dynamics of met-enkephalin: Comparison of explicit and implicit solvent models, *Biophysical Journal*, vol. 82, 1791–1808, 2002.

89. Mashayak S. Y., Tanner D. E., Comparing Solvent Models for Molecular Dynamics of Protein, University of Illinois at Urbana-Champaign, Physics Department, May 12, 2011 Final Research Reports (last accessed on March 21, 2012 on http://online.physics.uiuc.edu/courses/phys466/spring11/projects/index.html).

2 Elements of Biochemistry

2.1 INTRODUCTION

Biochemistry in its core is the chemical study of living beings, a strongly multidisciplinary study in which chemistry, biology, medicine, and abstract modeling converge in a unitary body of knowledge. Perhaps, the most important outcomes of biochemical research have been the realization that all organisms have much in common. Organisms are remarkably uniform at the molecular level. This observation is frequently referred to as the unity of biochemistry, but, in reality, it illustrates the unity of life.

This uniformity reveals that all organisms on the earth have arisen from a common ancestor. A core of essential biochemical processes appeared early in the evolution of life. The diversity of life in the modern world has been generated by evolutionary processes acting on these core processes through millions or even billions of years [1].

Only three naturally occurring elements—oxygen, hydrogen, and carbon—make up 98% of the atoms in a living organism. Moreover, the abundance of these three elements in life is vastly different from their abundance in the earth's crust, as shown in Table 2.1. One reason that oxygen and hydrogen are so common is the ubiquity of water and there is a universal consensus among biologists that water has been the life enabler on earth.

After oxygen and hydrogen, the next most common element in living organisms is carbon. Most large molecules in living systems are predominantly made up of carbon.

As a means of seeing why carbon is uniquely suited for life, let us compare it with silicon, its nearest elemental relative. Silicon is much more plentiful than carbon in the earth's crust (see Table 2.1), and, like carbon, can form four covalent bonds—a property crucial to the construction of large molecules. However, carbon–to–carbon bonds are stronger than silicon–to–silicon bonds. This difference in bond strength has three important consequences [2].

- Large molecules can be built with the use of carbon–carbon bonds as the backbone of life being structure because of the stability of these bonds;
- More energy is released when carbon–carbon bonds undergo combustion than when silicon reacts with oxygen;
- After carbon has undergone combustion, carbon dioxide is readily soluble in water and can exist as a gas; thus, it remains in biochemical circulation, to be used by other organisms. In contrast, silicon is essentially insoluble in reactions with oxygen, silicon oxide in amorphous form is glass, while in crystalline form it is quartz. After silicon has combined with oxygen, it is permanently out of circulation.

Thus, carbon-based molecules are stronger construction materials and are better fuels than silicon-based molecules.

Other elements have essential roles in living systems, for example, nitrogen, phosphorus, and sulfur. Moreover, some of the trace elements, although present in tiny amounts compared with oxygen, hydrogen, and carbon, are absolutely vital to a number of life processes, like iron and potassium.

In Section 2.2 we take a look at the whole chemical system building the base of life, from elementary metabolites to the complex cell chemistry. In Section 2.3 we will put aside the more complex structures, such as organelles and cells, and concentrate on the chemistry and functionalities of

TABLE 2.1

Abundance of Different Elements in Earth's Crust, in Sea Water, and in Human Beings

Element	Human Beings (%)	Seawater (%)	Earth's Crust (%)
Hydrogen	63	66	0.22
Oxygen	25.5	33	47
Carbon	9.5	0.0014	0.19
Nitrogen	1.4	<0.1	<0.1
Calcium	0.31	0.06	3.5
Phosphorus	0.22	<0.1	<0.1
Chloride	0.03	0.33	<0.1
Potassium	0.06	0.006	2.5
Sulfur	0.05	0.017	<0.1
Sodium	0.03	0.28	2.5
Magnesium	0.01	0.003	2.2
Silicon	<0.1	<0.1	28
Aluminum	<0.1	<0.1	7.9
Iron	<0.1	<0.1	4.5
Titanium	<0.1	<0.1	0.46

macromolecules. As a matter of fact, these are the main elements determining chemical dynamics in labs on chip even when cells are processed either to directly analyze their behavior or to extract substances from them.

2.2 STRUCTURAL ORGANIZATION OF BIOCHEMICAL MACROMOLECULES

The molecular constituents of living matter do not reflect randomly the infinite possibilities for combining C, H, O, and N atoms. Only a limited set of possibilities is exploited, sharing properties essential to the establishment and maintenance of the living state. The most prominent aspect of molecular biology is the prominent role of great molecules, called macromolecules, which are constructed from simple molecules according to a hierarchy of increasing structural complexity and by frequently using complex polymerization procedures [2]. The major precursors for the formation of biomolecules are water, carbon dioxide, and three inorganic nitrogen compounds—ammonium (NH_4), nitrate (NO_3), and dinitrogen (N_2). Metabolic processes assimilate and transform these inorganic precursors through ever more complex levels of biomolecular order [3,4].

In the first step, precursors are converted into metabolites, simple organic compounds that are intermediates in cellular energy transformation and in the biosynthesis of various sets of building blocks: amino acids, sugars, nucleotides, fatty acids, and glycerol. Through covalent linkage of these building blocks, the four classes of macromolecules are constructed:

- Proteins
- Polynucleotides (DNA and RNA)
- Polysaccharides
- Lipids

This complex and progressive construction of more complex molecules is shown schematically in Figure 2.1, while the molecular weight of biological macromolecules obtained along this path is reported in Table 2.2.

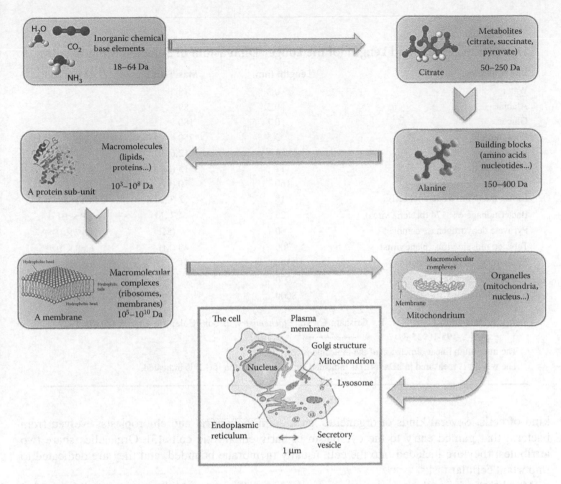

FIGURE 2.1 The hierarchy of biological structures: every successive organisation level is built by ordered composition of structures of the lower level. Examples of structures of every level and dimensions either in Da or in length are shown.

Interactions among macromolecules lead to the next level of structural organization, supra-molecular complexes. Here, various members of one or more of the classes of macromolecules come together to form specific assemblies that serve important subcellular functions. Examples of these supra-molecular assemblies are ribosomes, chromosomes, and cytoskeletal elements. For example, an eukaryotic ribosome contains four different RNA molecules and at least 70 unique proteins. The structural integrity of these supra-molecular assemblies is maintained by noncovalent forces, in contrast to the characteristic of macromolecules forming them that are largely based on covalent bonds. These noncovalent forces include hydrogen bonds, ionic attractions, and van der Waals forces. The hydrophilic and hydrophobic nature of specific molecular sites or whole macromolecules has also an important role to play at this level. Such forces maintain supra-molecular assemblies in a highly ordered functional state. Many noncovalent forces are weak, often less than 40 kJ/mol, with the remarkable exception of the ion bond that can arrive to about 800 kJ/mol in ionic crystals [5]. A large number of weak bonds, however, exists in these assemblies and thus collectively maintain the complex architecture of supra-molecular structures effectively under conditions consistent with cell life.

The next higher rung in the hierarchical ladder is occupied by the organelles, entities of considerable dimensions compared with the cell itself. Organelles are found only in eukaryotic cells, that is, the cells of "higher" organisms. The only exceptions are ribosomes that are found in all

TABLE 2.2
Dimensions in kDa and Length (of the Longer Dimension) of Selected Biomolecules

Biomolecule	Length[a] (nm)	Mass[b] (Da)	Mass (kg)
Water	0.3	18	
Alanine	0.5	89	
Glucose	0.7	180	
Phospholipid	3.5	750	
Ribonuclease	4	12.6 (k)	
Immunoglobin IgG	14	15 (k)	
Myosin	160	470 (k)	
Ribosome (from a bacterial cell)	18	2.5 (M)	4.1×10^{-21}
Bacteriophage $\phi \times 174$ (bacteria virus)	25	4.7 (M)	7.8×10^{-21}
Pyruvate dehydrogenase complex	60	7 (M)	1.17×10^{-20}
Tobacco mosaic virus (plant virus)	300	40 (M)	6.68×10^{-20}
Escherichia coli cell (bacterium)	1500		1.5×10^{-15}
Chloroplast (spinach cell)	2000		2×10^{-15}
Liver cell (human)	8000		60×10^{-15}

Source: Data from Garreth H. R., Grisham C. M., *Biochemistry*, Brooks/Cole; 4th edition (2010), ISBN-13 978-0-495-10935-8.

[a] The maximum linear dimension of the molecule is considered

[b] The weight is measured in kDa if (k) is indicated and in MegaDalton if (M) is indicated.

kind of cells. Several kinds of organelles, such as mitochondria and chloroplasts, evolved from bacteria that gained entry to the cytoplasm of early eukaryotic cells [3]. Organelles share two attributes: they are included into the cell, usually membrane bounded, and they are dedicated to important cellular tasks.

Membranes define the boundaries of cells and organelles. As such, they are not easily classified as supra-molecular assemblies or organelles, although they share the properties of both. Membranes resemble supra-molecular complexes in their construction because they are complexes of proteins and lipids maintained by noncovalent forces. Hydrophobic interactions are particularly important in maintaining membrane structure. Hydrophobic interactions arise because water molecules prefer to interact with each other rather than with nonpolar substances as underlined in Section 1.2.6, when we have described the properties of the dissolution of nonpolar solutes in polar solvents.

The presence of nonpolar molecules decreases the possible configurations of water–water interaction by forcing the water molecules into ordered arrays around the nonpolar groups; thereby decreasing the entropic contribution to the structure free energy. To decrease the free energy as much as possible in order to attain a stable equilibrium, it is needed to reduce the order in the resulting structure to increase the entropic contribution to the free energy. For this reason, nonpolar molecules redistribute from a dispersed state in water into an aggregated organic phase surrounded by water. The spontaneous assembly of membranes in the aqueous environment where life arose and exists is the natural result of the hydrophobic character of their lipids and proteins. Hydrophobic interactions are the creative means of membrane formation and the driving force that presumably established the boundary of the first cell. The membranes of organelles differ from one another, each having a characteristic protein and lipid composition tailored to the organelle's function. Furthermore, the creation of discrete volumes or compartments within cells is not only an inevitable consequence of the presence of membranes but usually an essential condition for proper organelle function.

The basic building block of life is the cell. The cell is characterized as the smallest entity capable of displaying the attributes associated uniquely with the living state: growth, metabolism, stimulus response, and replication. We will not analyze in depth the complex and fascinating cell biology, however, interested readers can refer to the bibliography [6–8].

2.2.1 General Properties of Macromolecules

If we consider what attributes of biomolecules render them so fit as components of growing, replicating systems, several biologically relevant themes of structure and organization emerge. Prominent among them is the necessity for information and energy in the maintenance of the living state [2]. Some biomolecules must have the capacity to contain the information needed for the creation of living organisms. Other biomolecules must have the capacity to translate this information so that the organized structures essential to life are synthesized. An orderly mechanism for abstracting energy from the environment must also exist in order to obtain the energy needed to drive these processes.

The first peculiar characteristics that render macromolecules and their building blocks suitable to perform these complex tasks is that they have an oriented structure, that is, their spatial structure privileges specific directions if certain types of chemical interactions are considered. The macromolecules of cells are built of units—amino acids in proteins, nucleotides in nucleic acids, and carbohydrates in polysaccharides—that have structural electrical dipole charge. Polymerization of these units to form macromolecules occurs by head-to-tail linear connections (see Section 1.4.2) forced by electromagnetic attraction. Because of this, the polymer also has a head and a tail, and hence, the macromolecule structure has polarity, as represented in Figure 2.2.

Owing to these polar characteristics, the elements of a biological macromolecule are ordered, for example, by starting from the head and arriving at the tail. They are thus capable of storing information in a sequential order of their component building blocks. As a matter of fact, when read along the length of the molecule, they appear like a word composed of symbols belonging to an alphabet. While interaction between building blocks of single macromolecules are polar and thus strong, as we have seen in the introduction, interaction between different macromolecules is driven by weak forces. These weak forces create interactions that are constantly forming and breaking at physiological temperature, unless in cases where they impart stability to the structures generated by their collective action by cumulative number.

2.2.1.1 van der Waals Forces

The origin of van der Waals forces [9,10] is due to continuous fluctuations of the electron density in the molecular external orbitals. Even if the average value of the charge distribution is zero its variance is not zero so that dipole and multipolar forces arise in time. The net effect does not vanish when averaging on long times and constitute a weak, but fundamental, source of interaction between large biomolecules. Owing to their nature, typical interaction distances are quite small, as shown in Figure 2.3, when the van der Waals average potential between two large molecules is shown.

This means that, for van der Waals forces to be effective, the atoms on interacting molecules must pack together neatly, that is, their molecular surfaces must possess a degree of structural

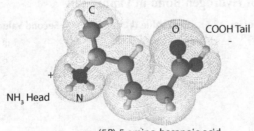

(5R)-5-amino-hesanoic-acid

FIGURE 2.2   Example of polarity of a complex organic molecule.

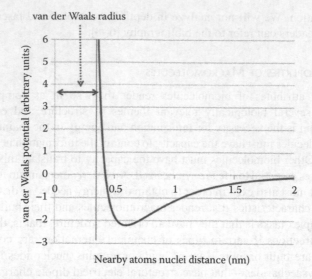

FIGURE 2.3 van der Waals average potential between two large molecules in a selected mutual configuration.

complementarity in order to allow them to stay packed without generating strong repulsion. Frequently, stability or instability of interaction between biological molecules is determined by complementarity between particular interaction sites due to their steric characteristics; this contributes to an ordered hierarchy of biological structure to emerge from the multiplicity of potential possibilities.

A single van der Waals interaction has an energy of the order of 0.1–4.0 kJ/mol. However, the sum of many such interactions between macromolecules can be substantial. Calculations indicate that the attractive van der Waals energy between the enzyme lysozyme and a sugar substrate that it binds is about 60 kJ/mol.

2.2.1.2 Hydrogen Bonds

Hydrogen bonds [11] are important in biomolecular interactions since they form a bond between two electronegative atoms, that is mediated by an hydrogen atom creating a sort of hydrogen bridge between them. Hydrogen bonds are cylindrically symmetrical and tend to be highly directional, forming straight bonds between donor, hydrogen, and acceptor atoms. Hydrogen bonds can vary in strength from very weak (1–2 kJ/mol) to extremely strong (161.5 kJ/molin the ionHF^{2-}) [12,13]. Typical enthalpies of hydrogen bond are presented in Table 2.3.

TABLE 2.3
Strength of Hydrogen Bond in Vapor State

Chemical Species	First Value (kJ/mol)	Second Value (kcal/mol)
F–H...:F	161.5	38.6
O–H...:N	29	6.9
O–H...:O	21	5.0
N–H...:N	13	3.1
N–H...:O	8	1.9

Note: Since the bond enthalpy depends on the structure of the bonded molecules, two recurring values of the bond enthalpy are reported in the table.

TABLE 2.4

Symmetry and Angle of the Hydrogen Bond in Different Substances

Acceptor...Donor	Symmetry	Angle (°)
HCN...HF	Linear	180
$H_2CO...HF$	Trigonal planar	110
$H_2O...HF$	Pyramidal	46
$H_2S...HF$	Pyramidal	89
$SO_2...HF$	Trigonal	142

Detailed quantum mechanical calculations shows that the same hydrogen bond can have quite different associated enthalpies depending on the molecules they bond. For example, the $N - H \cdots N$ hydrogen bond between guanine and cytosine is much stronger in comparison to the $N - H \cdots N$ bond between the adenine–thymine pair [14].

The length of hydrogen bonds depends on bond strength, temperature, and pressure. The typical length of a hydrogen bond in water is 1.97 Å. The ideal bond angle depends on the nature of the hydrogen bond donor. Characteristics of the hydrogen bond in different substances are presented in Table 2.4 [15].

Hydrogen bonding plays an important role in determining the three-dimensional structures adopted by proteins and nucleic bases. In these macromolecules, bonding between parts of the same macromolecule causes it to fold into a specific shape, which helps determine the molecule's physiological or biochemical role.

The double helical structure of DNA, for example, is due largely to hydrogen bonding between the base pairs, which link one complementary strand to the other and enable replication. This effect is graphically shown in Figure 2.4. Also, the protein stereographic structure largely depends on hydrogen bonds location in the protein structure. The so-called "alpha helix," is a right-handed spiral conformation. This structure occurs when every backbone N–H group is linked by an hydrogen bond to the backbone C–O group corresponding to the amino acid located four residues earlier in

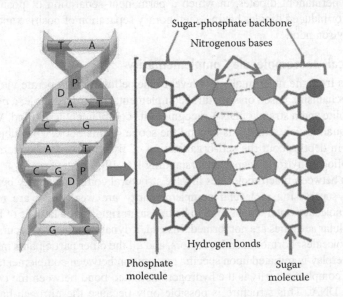

FIGURE 2.4 Graphical representation on how hydrogen bonds determine the curvature of the DNA double helix.

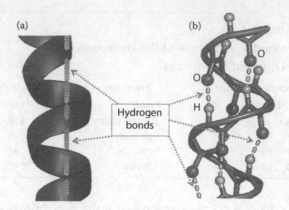

(a)   (b)

Hydrogen
bonds

FIGURE 2.5 Strip (a) and balls and sticks (b) representations of a protein α-helix segment where the hydrogen bonds generating the helix twist are evidenced.

the protein chemical chain (see Figure 2.5). As in all helicoid structures, the α-helix has an important role in the way in which the protein both diffuses in biological solutions and bonds with other molecules: as a matter of fact, helixes participate in the steric process with which the molecule twists hiding some parts and exposing other parts for interaction with the environment.

2.2.1.3 Ionic Interactions

Ionic interactions [9,10] are the result of attractive forces between oppositely charged structures, such as negative carboxyl groups and positive amino groups. These electrostatic forces average about 20 kJ/mol in aqueous solutions while are much stronger in crystals.

Typically, the electrical charge is radially distributed, so these interactions may lack the directionality of hydrogen bonds or the precise fit of van der Waals interactions. Nevertheless, because the opposite charges are restricted to spherically defined positions, ionic interactions can impart a high degree of structural specificity. The strength of electrostatic interactions is highly dependent on the nature of the interacting species and the distance between them. Electrostatic interactions may involve ions permanent dipoles, in which a permanent separation of positive and negative charge is created, or induced dipoles having a temporary separation of positive and negative charge induced by the environment.

2.2.1.4 Biological Macromolecule Complementarity

Biological systems from the macromolecular level to the cellular level operate via specific molecular recognition mechanisms based on structural complementarity, for example, a protein recognizes its specific metabolite and a strand of DNA recognizes its complementary strand. We will deal with this subject only qualitatively, since it is beyond the scope of this book. The subject is fundamental to understand in depth about the self-organization of living structures. Interested readers are directed to the bibliography for a deeper understanding [16–19].

All interactions between macromolecules involve structural complementarity between molecules. Since interactions supervising molecular complementarity are weak, they are readily reversible. Consequently, biomolecular interactions tend to be transient: rigid, static lattices of biomolecules that might paralyze cellular activities are not formed. Instead, a dynamic interplay occurs between metabolites and macromolecules, hormones and receptors, and all the other participants instrumental to life processes. This interplay is initiated upon specific recognition between complementary molecules.

An example of complementarity is the hydrogen-mediated bond between the two counter twisting helixes of the DNA. This structure is possible only because the nitrogen-based bases of the single helix are disposed along a well-defined sequence so that when the two helixes are created, they start to form hydrogen bonds and the progressive creation of bonds lowers the free energy of both the helixes up to the moment in which the bond is complete and the system is arrived at a minimum free energy state.

Complementarity is frequently constituted by the fact that two macromolecules exhibit complementary groups located in specific positions of the molecule stereographic configuration that are suitable to bond each other not only under a chemical but also under a steric point of view: these groups are generally called active sites of the macromolecule. In this way, active sites of antibodies search for and bind antigens in specific active sites called epitopes and in the same way enzymes combine with the molecules whose evolution they are catalyzing in a specific active site, complementary to the active site of the considered macromolecule.

Under a thermodynamic point of view, the ability to recognize of complementary molecules is mediated by the fact that the set of bonded molecules forms a lower free energy state with respect to the unbonded molecules so that the bonding spontaneously takes place. Since this is a process fundamentally based on the fact that macromolecules have a precise orientation and internal organization, we can somehow say that complementarity between biological macromolecules are regulated by a sort of biological grammar that states the rules with which the molecular words can be sequenced in order to obtain correct sentences in the very particular language of life. This approach has also been used with success to study in detail biological complementarity and interactions and it brings to very interesting parallels between human logical structures embedded in formal languages used in mathematics and informatics and the biological logic coded in the chemical complementarity between macromolecules. The interested reader is encouraged to start the analysis of this fascinating subject from the relevant bibliographies reported here [20–22].

This principle of structural complementarity extends to higher level interactions in the scale of biological structures. Very complex subcellular structures are actually spontaneously formed through structural complementarity.

The fact that weak forces determine, through complementarity, the assembly of biological structures restricts organisms to a narrow range of environmental conditions: macromolecules are functionally active only within a narrow range of temperature, ionic concentration, and pH; extreme conditions disrupt the forces maintaining the structure of macromolecules. The loss of structural order in these macromolecules, is called denaturation since it is accompanied by loss of function [23].

As a consequence, cells cannot tolerate reactions in which large amounts of energy are released, nor can they generate a large energy burst to drive energy-requiring processes. Instead, such transformations take place via sequential series of chemical reactions whose overall effect achieves dramatic energy changes, even though any given reaction in the series proceeds with only modest input or release of energy. These sequences of reactions are organized to provide for the release of useful energy to the cell from the breakdown of food or to take such energy and use it to drive the synthesis of biomolecules essential to the living state. Collectively, these reaction sequences constitute cellular metabolism—the ordered reaction pathways by which cellular chemistry proceeds and biological energy transformations are accomplished.

2.2.1.5 Enzymatic Catalysis

The rate at which cellular reactions proceed is a very important factor in the maintenance of the living state. The common ways chemists accelerate reactions are not available to cells; the temperature cannot be raised, acid or base cannot be added, the pressure cannot be elevated, and concentrations cannot be dramatically increased. Instead, bio-catalysts mediate cellular reactions. These catalysts, called enzymes, accelerate the reaction rates by many orders of magnitude and, by selecting the substances undergoing reaction, determine the specific reaction that takes place [24,25].

Metabolic regulation is achieved by controlling the activity of enzymes. Thousands of reactions mediated by enzymes are occurring at any given instant within the cell. Collectively, these reactions constitute cellular metabolism. The need for metabolic regulation is obvious. This metabolic regulation is achieved through controls on enzyme activity so that the rates of cellular reactions are appropriate to cellular requirements. Despite the organized pattern of metabolism and the thousands of enzymes required, cellular reactions nevertheless conform to the same thermodynamic principles that govern any chemical reaction.

Enzymes have no influence over energy changes (the thermodynamic component) in their reactions, as in all catalyzed reactions (see Section 1.2.5), enzymes only influence reaction rates. Cells are systems that take in food, release waste, and carry out complex degradation and biosynthetic reactions while operating under conditions of essentially constant temperature and pressure and maintaining a constant internal environment (homeostasis) with no outwardly apparent changes.

2.2.2 ORGANIZATION AND STRUCTURE OF THE CELL

All living cells fall into one of three broad categories—Archaea, Bacteria, and Eukarya [6–8]. Archaea and Bacteria are referred to collectively as prokaryotes. As a group, prokaryotes are single-celled organisms that lack nuclei and other organelles; the word is derived from pro meaning "prior to" and karyot meaning "nucleus." In conventional biological classification schemes, prokaryotes are grouped together as members of the kingdom Monera. The other four living kingdoms are all Eukarya—the single-celled Protists, such as amoebae, and all multicellular life forms, including the Fungi, Plant, and Animal kingdoms.

Eukaryotic cells have true nuclei and other organelles such as mitochondria, with the prefix "eu" meaning "true." For a long time, most biologists believed that eukaryotes evolved from the simpler prokaryotes in some linear progression from simple to complex over the course of geological time. However, contemporary evidence favors the view that present-day organisms are better grouped into the three classes mentioned: Eukarya, Bacteria, and Archaea. All are believed to have evolved approximately 3.5 billion years ago from an ancestral communal gene pool shared among primitive cellular entities.

Contemporary eukaryotic cells are, in reality, composite cells that harbor various bacterial contributions. Despite great diversity in form and function, cells and organisms share much biochemistry in common. This commonality and diversity has been substantiated by the results of genome study, evidencing strong commonalities between Archaea, Bacteria, and Eukarya. As an example, the genome of *Mycoplasma genitalium* consists of 523 genes, encoding 484 proteins, in just 580,074 base pairs, while number of genes around 25,000 is common for most superior animals, as reported in Table 2.5. All these genetic codes are constructed using a sequence of the same bases organized in complementary pairs.

TABLE 2.5
Number of Genes Characteristics of the DNA of Different Species

Organism	Number of Cells[a]	Number of Genes
Microbacterium genitalium (pathogenic bacterium)	1	523
Metanococcus janaschii (archaeal methanogen)	1	1800
Escherichia coli K12 (intestinal bacterium affecting human)	1	4400
Saccharomyces cereviseae (baker's yeast)	1	6000
Caenorhabditis elegans (nematode worm)	959	19,000
Drosophilia melanogaster (fruit fly)	10,000	13,500
Arabidopsis thaliana (flowering plant)	10^7	≈27,000
Fugu rubripes (pufferfish)	10^{12}	≈38,000
Homo sapiens (human)	10^{14}	≈20,500

Source: Adapted from Garreth H. R., Grisham C. M., *Biochemistry*, Brooks/Cole; 4th edition (2010), ISBN-13 978-0-495-10935-8.

Note: It is interesting to observe that, even if the pufferfish has an estimated number of genes roughly double of humans, their dimension is quite small and the overall genome of the pufferfish is about 1/8 in molecular weight of the human one.

[a] For multicellular beings, the adult form has to be considered.

This information sparks an interesting question: How many genes are needed for cellular life? Any minimum gene set must encode all the information necessary for cellular metabolism, including the vital functions essential to reproduction. The simplest cell must show at least

- Some degree of metabolism and energy production
- Genetic replication based on a template molecule that encodes information
- Formation and maintenance of a cell boundary (membrane)

Studies with the aim to discover from existing cells what the minimum gene set is, are focused on simple parasitic bacteria. This is because parasites often obtain many substances from their hosts and do not have to synthesize them from scratch; thus, they require fewer genes. However, no definitive result has been reached and no artificial cells with an artificially designed number of genes has been still built to demonstrate that there exists a well-defined minimum information amount to be stored in the cell to allow it to be called a cell.

2.2.2.1 Cell Structural Organization

Bacteria form a widely spread group. The Archaea, about which we know less, are remarkable because they can be found in unusual environments where other cells cannot survive. Archaea include the thermoacidophiles (heat- and acid-tolerant bacteria) of hot springs, the halophiles (salt-tolerant bacteria) of salt lakes and ponds, and the methanogens (bacteria that generate methane from CO_2 and H_2).

Prokaryotes are typically very small, on the order of several microns in length, and are usually surrounded by a rigid cell wall that protects the cell and gives it its shape. The characteristic structural organization of one of these cells is depicted in Figure 2.6. Prokaryotic cells have only a single membrane, the plasma membrane or cell membrane. Because they have no other membranes, prokaryotic cells contain no internal elements that are contained in a dedicated membrane. Nevertheless, they possess a distinct nuclear area where a single circular chromosome is localized, and some have an internal membranous structure called a mesosome, that is derived from and continuous with the cell membrane. Reactions of cellular respiration are localized on these membranes. In cyanobacteria, flat, sheet-like membranous structures called lamellae are formed from cell membrane infoldings. These lamellae are the sites of photosynthetic activity, but they are not contained within plastids, the organelles of photosynthesis found in higher plant cells. Prokaryotic

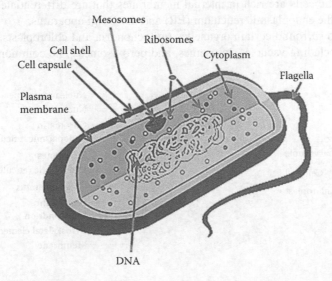

FIGURE 2.6 Graphical representation of the typical structure of a bacterium.

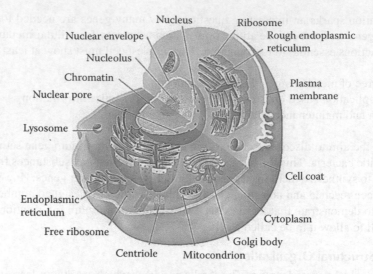

FIGURE 2.7   Graphical representation of the typical structure of an animal cell.

cells also lack a cytoskeleton; the cell wall maintains their structure. Some bacteria have flagella, single, long filaments used for motility. Prokaryotes largely reproduce by asexual division.

Structural organization of eukaryotic cells is more complex than that of prokaryotic cells; eukaryotic cells are much greater in size, typically having cell volumes 103–104 times larger and contain much more complex sub-structures. These two features require that eukaryotic cells partition their diverse metabolic processes into organized compartments, with each compartment dedicated to a particular function. A system of internal membranes accomplishes this partitioning. A typical animal cell is shown in Figure 2.7 and a typical plant cell in Figure 2.8. Eukaryotic cells possess a discrete, membrane-bounded nucleus, the repository of the cell's genetic material, which is distributed among a few or many chromosomes. During cell division, equivalent copies of this genetic material must be passed to both daughter cells through duplication and orderly partitioning of the chromosomes by the process known as mitosis.

Like prokaryotic cells, eukaryotic cells are surrounded by a plasma membrane. Unlike prokaryotic cells, eukaryotic cells are rich in internal membranes that are differentiated into specialized structures such as the endoplasmic reticulum (ER) and the Golgi apparatus.

Membranes also surround certain organelles (mitochondria and chloroplasts, for example) and various vesicles, including vacuoles, lysosomes, and peroxisomes. The common purpose of these

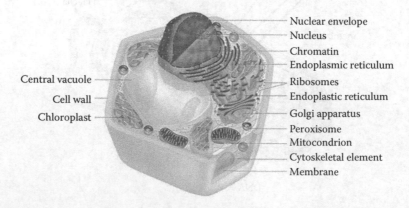

FIGURE 2.8   Graphical representation of the typical structure of a plant cell.

membranous partitioning is the creation of cellular compartments that have specific, organized metabolic functions, such as the mitochondrion's role as the principal site of cellular energy production. Eukaryotic cells also have a cytoskeleton composed of arrays of filaments that give the cell its shape and its capacity to move. Some eukaryotic cells also have long projections on their surface—cilia or flagella—which provide propulsion.

2.2.3 VIRUSES

A particular form of life is constituted by viruses [1,2]. Viruses are often not classified as cells, also no general agreement exists among biologists on this point.

A virus is completely inert, and thus incapable to duplicate, if outside a host cell. In order to duplicate, it invades a cell (infects it) and utilizes to a certain extent the host cell material to replicate itself, generally killing the host cell in the process. This is due to the fact that a virus does not contain a complete set of genetic material, but brings inside either the DNA or the RNA. A large variety of DNA and RNA structures can be found inside viruses, also quite different from the molecule structures we are accustomed to recognize in high-level life forms (see Section 2.5).

In particular, single-stranded (ss) DNA and double-strand (ds) RNA can be found in viruses and gene superposition is quite common. This large differentiation is mainly due to the need of coding the genetic viral information in a small amount of genetic material. Owing to this diversity viruses are classified in virus classes (identified by an ordeal number) on the ground of the type of genetic material they bring as

    I. dsDNA viruses
   II. ssDNA viruses
  III. dsRNA viruses
  IV. (+)ssRNA viruses
   V. (–)ssRNA viruses
  VI. ssRNA-RT viruses
 VII. dsDNA-RT viruses

From the above list it is clear that ssRNA viruses can be further classified on the basis of the sense of the RNA strands, which is an important factor since RNA duplication process inside the infected cell can directly duplicate only a strand ordered in the so-called positive sense (+). The negative sense (–) strand has to be transcribed to a positive sense strand by a suitable enzyme (RNA polymerase) before its duplication in the host cell.

Retroviruses are indicated with a code RT in the name (groups VI and VII). They use a DNA intermediate to replicate into the host cell [1,2].

When it comes into contact with a host cell, a virus can insert its genetic material into its host, literally taking over the host's functions. An infected cell produces viral proteins and genetic material instead of its usual products. Some viruses may remain dormant inside host cells for long periods, causing no obvious change in their host cells (a stage known as the lysogenic phase). When a dormant virus is stimulated, it enters the lytic phase: new viruses are formed, self-assemble, and burst out of the host cell, killing the cell and going on to infect other cells.

Viruses are the cause of many important diseases in humans and other superior living beings, but because they can transfer genetic material between different species, they are extensively used in genetic engineering. Viruses also carry out natural *genetic engineering*: a virus may incorporate some genetic material from its host as it is replicating, and transfer this genetic information to a new host, even to a host unrelated to the previous one. This is known as transduction, and in some cases it may serve as a means of evolutionary change, although it is not clear how important this evolutionary mechanism is in the overall evolution economy.

2.2.4 CLASSES OF BIOLOGICAL MACROMOLECULES

After a brief introduction to the structure and role of the cell, that is the base component of living beings, the rest of this chapter is devoted to the analysis of the main macromolecules that are the players of the cells chemistry. These biomolecules can be divided into just four classes:

- Proteins
- Nucleic acids
- Lipids
- Carbohydrates

Proteins are the most versatile of biomolecules. They are constructed from 20 building blocks, called amino acids, linked by peptide bonds to form a long polymer. This long unbranched polymer folds into a precise three-dimensional structure that facilitates a vast array of biochemical functions. Proteins serve as signal molecules and as receptors for signal molecules. As an example, human hormones that frequently work as feedback signals to regulate physiological processes, are proteins. Receptors convey to the cell that a signal has been received and initiates the cellular response. For example, insulin binds to its particular receptor, called the insulin receptor, and initiates the biological response to the presence of carbohydrates in the blood. Proteins also play structural roles, allow mobility, and provide defenses against environmental dangers. Moreover, proteins are frequently catalysts of biochemical reactions.

Nucleic acids include deoxyribonucleic acid (DNA) and ribonucleic acid (RNA). Together with proteins, nucleic acids make up the most important macromolecules; each is found in abundance in all living beings, where they function in encoding, transmitting, and expressing genetic information.

Lipids are much smaller than proteins or nucleic acids. The key characteristic of polar lipids is their dual chemical nature: part of the molecule is hydrophilic, meaning that it can dissolve in water, whereas the other part, made up of one or more hydrocarbon chains, is hydrophobic and cannot dissolve in water. This dual nature allows lipids to form barriers that delineate the cell and the cellular compartments. Lipids allow the development of "inside" and "outside" at a biochemical level. The hydrocarbon chains cannot interact with water and, instead, interact with those of other lipids to form a barrier, or membrane, whereas the water-soluble components interact with the aqueous environment on either side of the membrane.

Lipids are also an important storage form of energy: the hydrophobic component of lipids can undergo combustion to provide large amounts of cellular energy. Lipids are crucial signal molecules as well.

Carbohydrates are mainly involved in oxidation processes to provide energy to living beings. The most common carbohydrate used in this way is the simple sugar glucose. Glucose is stored in animals as glycogen, which consists of many glucose molecules linked end to end and having occasional branches. In plants, the storage form of glucose is starch, which is similar to glycogen in molecular composition. There are thousands of different carbohydrates. They can be linked together in chains, and these chains can be highly branched, much more than in glycogen or starch. Such chains of carbohydrates play important roles in helping cells to recognize one another. Many of the components of the cell exterior are patterned with various carbohydrates that can be recognized by other cells and serve as sites of cell-to-cell interactions.

2.3 PROTEIN STRUCTURE AND CHEMISTRY

2.3.1 PROTEIN CHEMICAL STRUCTURE

Proteins are essentially formed by articulated amino acids structures. We will, therefore, begin the analysis of proteins chemistry from the analysis of the main amino acids characteristics [1,2,16]. Although a very high number of amino acids can be obtained by combining all the possible radical groups with the basic amino acid structure, all the proteins that are found in high-level living forms are formed by a simple set of 20 base amino acids, whose chemical composition and selected characteristics are reported in Appendix 2.2. The 20 basic amino acids are as a sort of protein alphabets, and protein characteristics and functionalities depends on the properties of the amino acids composing the protein and on their interactions.

2.3.1.1 Acid–Base Reactions of Amino Acids

An amino acid has both a basic amine group and an acid carboxylic group as shown in Figure 2.9. This is caused by an internal transfer of a hydrogen ion from the –COOH group to the –NH_2 group to leave an ion with both a negative charge and a positive charge. The central group constituted by the nitrogen group and the carbon chain is indicated as a zwitterion.

Under an electrochemical point of view zwitterions can either act as true ions or give rise to very strong polar interactions. Increasing the pH of a zwitterion solution by adding hydroxide ions, the hydrogen ion is removed from the –NH_3+ group. In this condition, the molecule is a negative ion, with an overall negative charge.

Adding an acid to a solution of an amino acid, the –COO– part of the zwitterion picks up a hydrogen ion as in the following reaction:

$$
\begin{array}{ccc}
NH_3^+ & & NH_3^+ \\
| & \rightarrow & | \\
R - CH - COO^- + H_{(aq)}^+ & & R - CH - COOH
\end{array}
\qquad (2.1)
$$

The molecule has now a net positive charge and completely behaves as a positive ion.

Starting from a water solution obtained from the reaction (2.1) and progressively adding alkali to decrease the pH the positive charged molecule is put in the condition of losing an hydrogen ion attracted by the alkali solutes. Two hydrogen atoms showing acid behavior are present at the extremes of the molecule: one in the NH_3^+ group and one in the –COOH group. The most acid part is the one in the –COOH group such that it is removed first so that the original zwitterion is recreated. The pH at which this happens is known as the isoelectric point of the amino acid and varies from amino acid to amino acid.

The isoelectric point could be expected to be at the neutral point of the zwitterion solution, at pH = 7, but this is not true and generally it is near pH = 6, even if a dependence on the particular

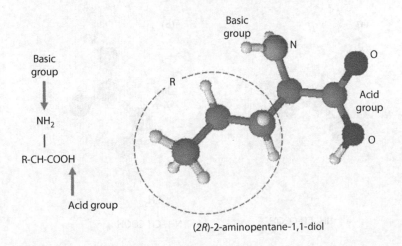

(2R)-2-aminopentane-1,1-diol

FIGURE 2.9 Acid–base structure of an amino acid.

amino acid exists. The reason relies in the interaction with the zwitterion with the solute molecules, that reflects its mixed acid–base nature.

We have two possible reactions taking place in a zwitterion aqueous solution that form a contemporary reaction set that have to reach equilibrium as detailed in Section 1.2.3. In particular, considering the zwitterion as an acid we have

$$
\begin{array}{cc}
NH_3^+ & NH_2 \\
| & | \\
R-CH-COO^- + H_2O \rightleftharpoons & R-CH-COO^- + H_3O^+
\end{array}
\tag{2.2}
$$

The NH_3^+ group is a weak acid and donates a hydrogen ion to a water molecule. Because it is only a weak acid, the reaction equilibrium is quite moved on the left side. Considering the zwitterion as a base:

$$
\begin{array}{cc}
NH_3^+ & NH_3^+ \\
| & | \\
R-CH-COO^- + H_2O \rightleftharpoons & R-CH-COOH + OH^-
\end{array}
\tag{2.3}
$$

Since the basic strength of the COOH group is weak, this reaction is also in equilibrium when it is quite moved towards the left side.

The positions of the two equilibria are not identical: they vary depending on the influence of the R group. For the simpler amino acids, the position of the first equilibrium lies a bit further to the right than the second one. This means that there will be more negative ion than the positive one in the solution. To return to a neutral solution eliminating all the electrolytes, the amount of negative ion has to be cut down so that the concentrations of the two ions are identical. This can be done adding the right amount of an acid that do not interact with the zwitterion to the solution, moving the position of the first equilibrium further to the left. Typically, the pH has to be lowered to about 6 to achieve this. The isoelectric point for all base amino acids is reported in the tables of Appendix 2.2.

2.3.1.2 Protein General Chemical Composition

Let us consider two simple amino acids, glycine and alanine, whose formulas and stereographic representations are depicted in Figure 2.10 (cf. Appendix 2.2).

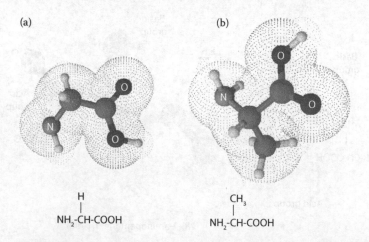

(a)   (b)

H   CH$_3$
| |
NH$_2$-CH-COOH   NH$_2$-CH-COOH

FIGURE 2.10 Structural formula and stereographic representation of glycine (a) and alanine (b).

Glycine and alanine can combine together with the elimination of a molecule of water to produce a dipeptide. This is possible in one of two different ways so you might get two different dipeptides that are produced by the following reactions (that naturally, in general, coexists if simple synthesis of the dipeptides is performed):

$$
\begin{array}{ccc}
& CH_3 & H\ H \\
& | & |\ | \\
NH_2\text{-}CH\text{-}C\text{-OH} & + & H\text{-}N\text{-}CH\text{-}COOH \\
\| & & \\
O & &
\end{array}
\longrightarrow
NH_2\text{-}CH\text{-}C\text{-}N\text{-}CH\,COOH \quad +H_2O \qquad (2.4a)
$$

$$
\begin{array}{ccc}
H & & H\ CH_3 \\
| & & |\ | \\
NH_2\text{-}CH\text{-}C\text{-OH} & + & H\text{-}N\text{-}CH\text{-}COOH \\
\| & & \\
O & &
\end{array}
\longrightarrow
NH_2\text{-}CH\text{-}C\text{-}N\text{-}CH\text{-}COOH \quad +H_2O \qquad (2.4b)
$$

The linkage between the two amino acids in the structure of the dipeptide (that is evidenced in the formulas) is known as a peptide link in biology, whereas in chemistry it is often called an amide bond.

If three amino acids are joined together with a similar bond a tripeptide is obtained and the molecule obtained by joining a chain of different amino acids, as in a protein chain, is called polypeptide. A protein chain will have somewhere in the range of 50–2000 amino acid residues, as they are called the amino acid radicals that are left after the joining reaction that cause the production of one water molecule for each peptide bond created.

By convention, when drawing peptide chains are represented, the NH_2 group which has not been converted into a peptide bond is written on the left-hand end. The unchanged COOH group is written on the right-hand end. The end of the peptide chain with the NH_2 group is known as the N-terminal, and the end with a -COOH group is the C-terminal.

A protein chain (with the N-terminal on the left) will, therefore, look like the structure that is shown below.

$$
\begin{array}{c}
R \quad\quad H\ R \quad\ O\ H\ R \quad\quad H\ R \\
| \quad\quad\ |\ |\quad\ \|\ |\ |\quad\quad\ |\ | \\
NH_2-CH-C-N-CH-C-N-CH-C-N-CH-COOH \\
\| \quad\quad\quad\quad\quad\quad \| \\
O \quad\quad\quad\quad\quad\quad\ O
\end{array}
\qquad (2.5)
$$

In Figure 2.11, a particular chain realization is shown as an example of the complexity of the peptide chain structure. An interesting particular case happens in the case where the "R" group comes from the amino acid proline, as a matter of fact in this case the general pattern is broken: the hydrogen on the nitrogen nearest the "R" group is missing, and the "R" group loops around and is attached to that nitrogen as well as to the carbon atom in the chain. This is due to the particular bonding characteristics of proline [26,27].

2.3.1.3 Protein Primary Structure

The term "primary structure" is used in two different ways when referred to a protein. At its simplest, the term is used to describe the order of the amino acids joined together to make the protein. This primary structure is usually shown using abbreviations for the amino acid residues (the complete list of abbreviations is reported in the tables of Appendix 2.2 from [27]). These abbreviations commonly consist of three letters, but an alternative list of one letter abbreviations also exists [27].

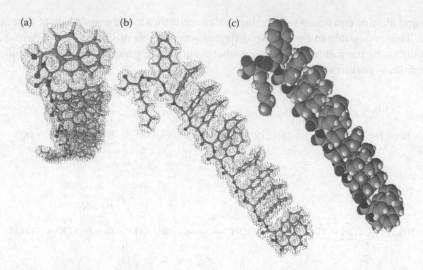

FIGURE 2.11 Different views and representations of a polypeptide chain. In part (a), the chain is represented in the balls and sticks representations in a frontal view, while the same representation is used to show a lateral view in part (b). In part (c), the lateral view is also shown in the volume representation.

Using three-letter abbreviations, a bit of a protein chain might be represented by, for example:

$$\text{Try-Gly-Lys-Lys-Ala-Pro-Val-Lys-Lys-Gly-Gly-Pro-Ala-Gly-Lys-} \ldots\ldots \tag{2.6}$$

The N protein terminal is placed on the left-hand end, while the C terminal is placed on the right-hand end of the chain. The positions of these two terminals in the chain representation are conventional and render unique the way in which the chain (or every part of it) is written as a residues sequence.

It could seem that the connection between the amino acid residue fix all the protein characteristics that are related to covalent bonds between groups, so that it is natural to define the primary protein structure as the structure derived from covalent bonds. In real proteins however, there is also another feature deriving from a covalent bond that is not represented by the residue chains.

The cysteine, whose structure formula is reported in Equation 2.7, due to the presence of a sulfur atom in its residue, bestows a particular property to chains containing it.

$$\begin{array}{c} CH_2SH \\ | \\ NH_2\text{-CH-COOH} \end{array} \tag{2.7}$$

If two cysteine side chains end up next to each other because of folding in the peptide chain, they can react to form a sulfur bridge, as shown in Figure 2.12. This is another covalent bond and so sometimes it is included in literature as a part of the primary structure of the protein while other fonts include it as a part of tertiary structure due to the fact that is one of the causes of proteins chain folding.

2.3.2 Protein Stereography: Secondary Structure

Within the long protein chains there are regions in which the chains are organized into regular structures known as helixes and pleated sheets [27]. We have already briefly introduced one of these structures, the α-helix, dealing with the important role of hydrogen bond in biological macromolecules: the group of these structures constitutes the secondary structures in proteins. The way in which hydrogen bond rises among peptide links is shown in Figure 2.13.

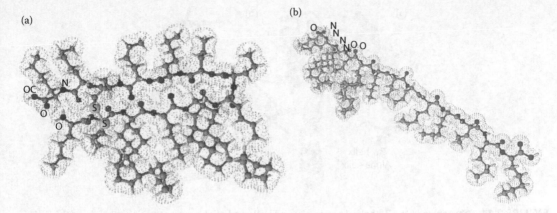

FIGURE 2.12 A peptide chain incorporating the sulfur bridge is shown in part (a), evidencing the chain folding due to the connection between the two groups containing the S atom. To further showing the effect, in part (b) the same chain with the group SH substituted by a single H atom is represented, where no folding is present in the absence of external forces causing it.

2.3.2.1 The Protein Helixes

In an α-helix, the protein chain is coiled like a loosely coiled spring, as shown in Figure 2.5. The "alpha" means that if you look down the length of the spring, the coiling is happening in a clockwise direction. The amino acids in an α helix are arranged in a right-handed helical structure where each amino acid residue corresponds to a 100° turn in the helix (i.e., the helix has 3.6 residues per turn), and a translation of 1.5 Å (0.15 nm) along the helical axis. Short pieces of left-handed helix sometimes occur with a large content of glycine amino acids, but are unfavorable for the other normal, biological L-amino acids.

The pitch of the α-helix (the vertical distance between one consecutive turn of the helix) is 5.4 Å (0.54 nm) which is the product of 1.5 and 3.6. What is most important is that the N–H group of an amino acid forms a hydrogen bond with the C–O group of the amino acid four residues earlier; this repeated hydrogen bonding is the most prominent characteristic of an α-helix. Official international

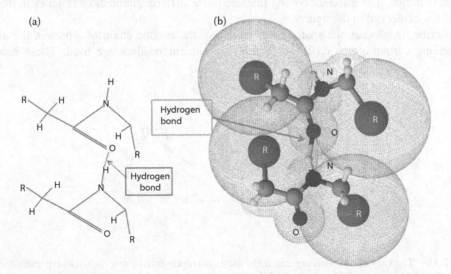

FIGURE 2.13 Structure of the hydrogen bond creating helixes and sheets in the secondary structure of proteins. Both structural formula (a) and stereographical representation in balls and sticks convention (b) are shown.

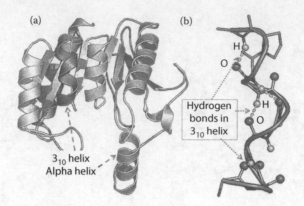

FIGURE 2.14 Structure of the 3_{10} helix in strips (a) and balls and sticks representations (b) where the hydrogen bonds and the twisted side chains structure are evidenced.

nomenclature [28] specifies two ways of defining α-helices, rule 6.2 in terms of repeating φ, ψ torsion angles and rule 6.3 in terms of the combined pattern of pitch and hydrogen bonding. The α-helix is the most common, but not the only helicoid structure recurring in proteins. Similar structures include the 3_{10} and the π-helix, both based as the α-helix on hydrogen bonds.

All the helixes constructed by hydrogen bonds can be described using an analytical language, like the 3_{10} helix. In particular, a protein helix can be indicated with the symbol X_Y, where X represents the number of chain residue that are present per turn, that can be a noninteger number as in the case of a helix, and the index Y represents the number of atoms, including hydrogen, that are present in the closed loop between two consecutive hydrogen bonds.

In the case of the 3_{10} helix, every helix turn is composed by three residues and a total of 10 atoms comprises between two adjacent hydrogen bonds. Using the same type of nomenclature, a helix should be called a 3.6_{13} helix, and a π helix has to be called a 4.1_{13} helix. An example of a 3_{10} helix structure is reported in Figure 2.14 both in strips representation and in balls and sticks representations, where the hydrogen bonds are evidenced. The α helix and the 3_{10} helix are also compared in Figure 2.15, where the top view of the two helicoid structures is shown representing them in sticks only representation. The different coiling rate due to the different number of residues in the single helix twist is evidenced in the figure.

To describe, in general, the spatial arrangement of the residue chain of a protein the dihedral angles among carbon atoms on the C termini subsequent residues are used. These atoms are

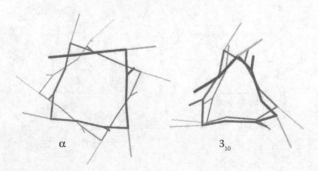

FIGURE 2.15 Top view of an α helix (a) and a 310° helix (b) represented using the sticks representation. This representation evidences the difference in the helices rounding rate due to the different number of residues in a single helix twist. (Reproduced under open CC license granted by the owner, Jane Shelby Richardson, James B. Duke Professor of Biochemistry at Duke University in Durham NC, USA.)

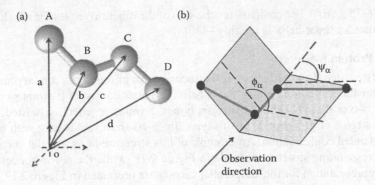

FIGURE 2.16 Definition of the dihedral angles of a protein chain: vectors associated to four consecutive α carbons in a protein chain (a), planes and dihedral angles associated to the considered chain (b).

generally called α-atoms and identified with numbers on the protein chain in its conventional orientation. Once the position of these atoms is known through the dihedral angles, all the other atoms can be easily positioned on the ground of the fixed angles formed by the bonds in the considered residue [28]. Once an observation point is selected as origin of an orthonormal reference system, four α- atoms along the chain are individuated with the four vectors joining the observation point to the atoms centers, as shown in Figure 2.16a. The four vectors, when considered in the order dictated by the protein chain, individuate two planes in space, as shown in Figure 2.14b, whose geometrical dihedral angles (also represented in Figure 2.16b) are the dihedral angles associated to the selected segment of the protein chain.

To evidence the differences among different helix structures the so-called Ramachandran plot is used (also called ϕ, ψ plot due to the representation in polar coordinates). It is a way to visualize backbone dihedral angles ψ against ϕ of amino acid residues in protein structure. Examples of general Ramachandran plot and a Ramachandran plot for glycine are reported in Figure 2.17. Because dihedral angle values are circular and 0° is the same as 360°, the edges of the Ramachandran plot "wrap" right to left and bottom to top. For instance, the small strip of allowed values along the lower-left edge of the plot are a continuation of the large, extended-chain region at upper left.

Ramachandran plot with data points for α-helical residues form a dense diagonal cluster below and left of center, around the global energy minimum for backbone conformation [29]. Residues in α-helices typically adopt backbone (ϕ, ψ) dihedral angles around (–60°, –45°), as shown in Figure 2.17. In more general terms, they adopt dihedral angles such that the ψ dihedral angle of one residue and the ϕ dihedral angle of the next residue sum to roughly –105°. As a consequence, α-helical dihedral angles, in general, fall on a diagonal stripe on the Ramachandran diagram, ranging from

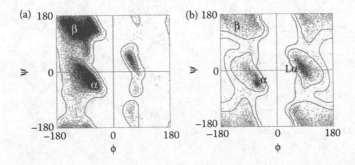

FIGURE 2.17 Generic Ramachandran plot (a) and Ramachandran plot for glycine (b). (Reproduced under open CC license granted by the owner, Jane Shelby Richardson at Duke University.)

$(-90°, -15°)$ to $(-35°, -70°)$. For comparison, the sum of the dihedral angles for a 3_{10} helix is roughly $-75°$, whereas that for the π-helix is roughly $-130°$.

2.3.2.2 The Protein β-Sheets

The β-sheet, also called β-pleated sheet, is the second form of regular secondary structure in proteins, only somewhat less common than the α-helix. β-Sheets consist of β-strands connected laterally by at least two or three backbone hydrogen bonds, forming a generally twisted, pleated sheet. A β strand is a stretch of polypeptide chains typically 3–10 amino acids long with backbone in an almost fully extended conformation. An example of this structure in its parallel version is reported besides the corresponding structure formula in Figure 2.18, while the correspondent formula and stereographic representation for the antiparallel version are presented in Figure 2.19.

The majority of β strands are arranged adjacent to other strands and form an extensive hydrogen bond network with their neighbors in which the N–H groups in the backbone of one strand establish hydrogen bonds with the C=O groups in the backbone of the adjacent strands.

In the fully extended β strand, successive side chains point straight up, then straight down, then straight up, and so forth. Adjacent β strands in a β sheet are aligned so that their α C atoms are adjacent and their side chains point in the same direction. The "pleated" appearance of β strands arises from tetrahedral chemical bonding at the α C atom. The pleating causes the distance between C_i^α and C_{i+1}^α to be approximately 6 Å, rather than the 7.6 Å (2×3.8 Å) expected from two fully extended

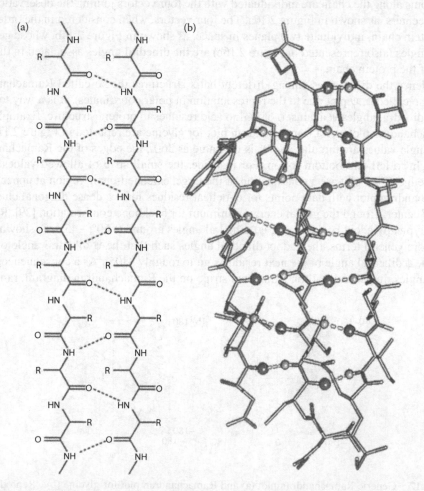

FIGURE 2.18 Structure formula (a) and stereographic representation (b) of a parallel β-sheet.

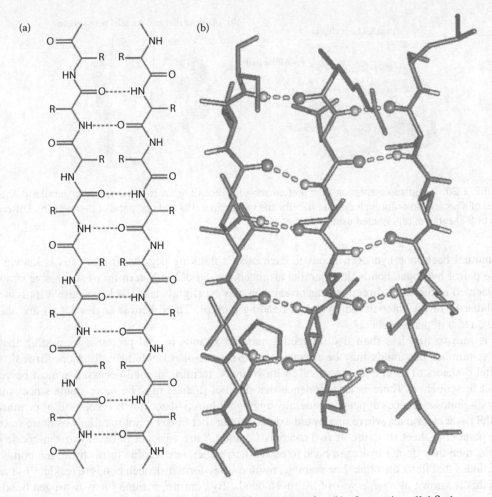

FIGURE 2.19 Structure formula (a) and stereographic representation (b) of an antiparallel β-sheet.

transpeptide virtual bonds. The sideways distance between adjacent C^α atoms in hydrogen-bonded β strands is roughly 5 Å.

However, β strands are rarely perfectly extended; rather, they exhibit a twist due to the chirality of their component amino acids. The energetically preferred dihedral angles near $(\phi, \psi) = (-135°, 135°)$, broadly, the upper left region of the Ramachandran plot, see Figure 2.17, diverge significantly from the fully extended conformation $(\phi, \psi) = (-180°, 180°)$. The twist is often associated with alternating fluctuations in the dihedral angles to prevent the individual β strands in a larger sheet from splaying apart. The side chains point outwards from the folds of the pleats, roughly perpendicular to the plane of the sheet; successive residues point outwards on alternating faces of the sheet.

Because peptide chains have a directionality conferred by their N-terminus and C-terminus, β strands too can be said to be directional. They are usually represented in protein topology diagrams by an arrow pointing toward the C-terminus. Adjacent β strands can form hydrogen bonds in antiparallel, parallel, or mixed arrangements. In an antiparallel arrangement, the successive β strands alternate directions so that the N-terminus of one strand is adjacent to the C-terminus of the next. This is the arrangement that produces the strongest inter-strand stability because it allows the inter-strand hydrogen bonds between carbonyls and amines to be planar, which is their preferred orientation. The peptide backbone dihedral angles (ϕ, ψ) are about $(-140°, 135°)$ in antiparallel sheets. In this case, if two atoms C_i^α and C_j^α are adjacent in two hydrogen-bonded β strands, then they form

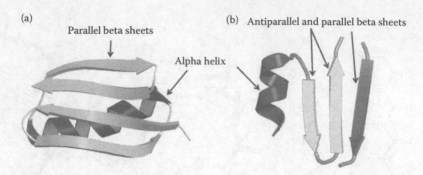

FIGURE 2.20 Strip representation of a protein sub-unit including an α-helix and four parallel β-sheets (a) and of a protein sub-unit including an α-helix and two antiparallel and one parallel β-sheets (b). Different types of β-sheets are represented using different colors.

two mutual backbone hydrogen bonds to each other's flanking peptide groups; this is known as aclose pairof hydrogen bonds. In a parallel arrangement, all of the N-termini of successive strands are oriented in the same direction; this orientation may be slightly less stable because it introduces nonplanarity in the inter-strand hydrogen bonding pattern. The dihedral angles (ϕ, ψ) are about ($-120°$, $115°$) in parallel sheets.

It is rare to find less than five interacting parallel strands in real proteins, suggesting that a smaller number of strands may be unstable, however it is also fundamentally more difficult for parallel β-sheets to form because strands with N and C termini aligned necessarily must be very distant in sequence. There is also evidence that parallel β-sheet may be more stable since small amyloid-genic sequences appear to generally aggregate into β-sheet fibrils composed of primarily parallel β-sheet strands, where one would expect antiparallel fibrils if antiparallel was more stable.

In parallel β-sheet structure, if two α-atoms C_i^α and C_j^α are adjacent in two hydrogen-bonded β strands, then they do not hydrogen bond to each other; rather, one residue forms hydrogen bonds to the residues that flank the other. For example, residue i may form hydrogen bonds to residues $j-1$ and $j+1$; this is known as a *wide pair* of hydrogen bonds. By contrast, residue j may hydrogen bond to different residues altogether, or to none at all. The hydrogen bonding of β strands need not be perfect, but can exhibit localized disruptions known as β bulges. In any case, it lies roughly in the plane of the sheet, with the peptide carbonyl groups pointing in alternating directions with successive residues.

An example of strip representation of parallel and antiparallel b sheets embedded in a protein structure is reported in Figure 2.20: both sheets are represented with flat sheets with a terminal arrow representing the sheet conventional direction, which is the direction of the chains in parallel sheets and the direction of the right-handed twist right always present in antiparallel sheets due to the chirality of their component amino acids. If parallel and antiparallel sheets have to be distinguished they can be evidenced with different colors or gray scales.

2.3.3 PROTEIN STEREOGRAPHY: TERTIARY STRUCTURE

The tertiary structure of a protein is a description of the way the whole chain (including the secondary structures) folds itself into its final three-dimensional shape. This is often simplified into strips models, where the chains and the sheets are represented as twisted and plain strips, respectively [27]. This incorporates all the atomic bonds in a continuous structure and allows the effective tertiary structure to be evidenced as shown in more detail in Appendix 1.

Also, the tertiary structure is caused by the weak forces we have discussed in Section 2.2, van der Waals forces, hydrogen bonds, ion bonds, besides the sulfur bridge: all these forces create secondary bonds between faraway parts of the protein chain, causing it to fold and twist. An example of ionic bond between residues in protein chains is presented in Figure 2.21, the effective exploitation

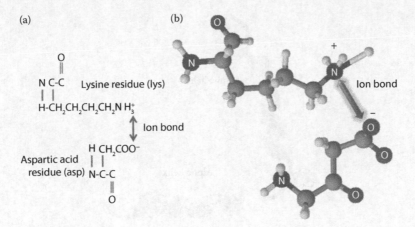

FIGURE 2.21 Example of an ion bond between residue in different positions in a protein chain that can cause the chain folding determining the tertiary protein structure; the structural formula is reported in part (a) while the stereographic representation is reported in part (b).

of the mixed acid–base nature of zwitterions residues is evident: one of the extremes is engaged in the main chain bonds and the other is free to form ionic bonds. A similar example of weak force that caused chain folding exploiting a hydrogen bond is reported in Figure 2.22.

Structural motifs are configurations involving several sheets and helixes and that are sufficiently recurrent in the tertiary architecture of real proteins to be considered typical configurations. These motifs can be substantially involved in the way in which the protein individuates the complementary molecules and it is individuated by them. As a matter of fact, there are motifs that mainly determine the protein steric characteristics, stable twists and turns tends to hide particular parts of the protein rendering it difficult to reach for interacting molecules and expose other parts that becomes the most reactive parts of the protein [17,19]. The presence of determined motifs has been supposed to be the enabler of the disabler of specific chemical behaviors of selected proteins and the same molecule with completely different tertiary structure can exhibit different chemical behavior.

Several motifs have been individuated and we cannot detail the characteristics of them all. We will limit ourselves to illustrate rapidly the simpler and more diffused, leaving a complete analysis to specialized texts [30–32].

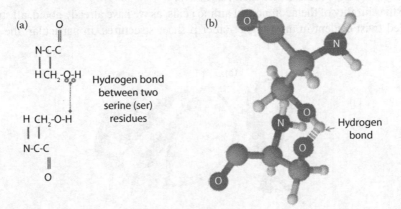

FIGURE 2.22 Example of an hydrogen bond between residues in different positions in a protein chain that can cause the chain folding determining the tertiary protein structure; the structural formula is reported in part (a) while the stereographic representation is reported in part (b).

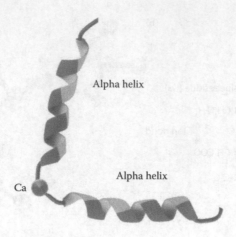

FIGURE 2.23   Example of helix-turn-helix motif.

The simplest motif based on the α helix is the very common α–α motif that consists of two α helixes linked by a short chain of residues. When the two α helixes are linked by a calcium-based radical they tend to assume orthogonal positions, as shown in Figure 2.23 and the motif is generally called *helix-turn-helix motif.* A very simple structural motif involving β sheets is the β hairpin, in which two antiparallel strands are linked by a short loop of two to five residues, of which one is frequently a glycineor a proline, that can assume the unusual dihedral-angle conformations required for a tight turn. Individual strands can also be linked in more elaborate ways with long loops that may contain α-helixes or even entire protein domains. Two examples of β hairpins are reported in Figure 2.24, the first simply formed by two β sheets and a short interconnection chain, the second much more complex, formed by a sequence of two β hairpins, one simple and the second incorporating an α helix between the two β sheets.

The Greek key motif consists of three antiparallel β sheets connected by hairpins, while the fourth is adjacent to the first and linked to the third by a longer loop. This type of structure forms easily during the protein folding process [33]. The scheme of the Greek key motif and an example of the motif embedded in a real protein structure are shown in Figure 2.25. The Greek key motif tends to form a sort of barrel shape in the protein folding regularly as shown in Figure 2.26. These structures are exceptionally hard with respect to other structures found in proteins and are commonly used, among other reasons, for their resistance.

Owing to the chirality of their component amino acids, as we have already noted, all strands exhibit a right-handed twist evident in most higher-order β sheet structures. In particular, the linking loop

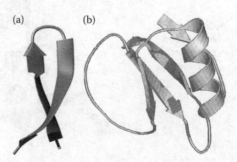

FIGURE 2.24   Two examples of β hairpins, the first part (a) simply formed by two β sheets and a short inter-connection chain, the second part (b) much more complex, formed by a sequence of two β hairpins, one simple and the second incorporating an α helix between the two β sheets.

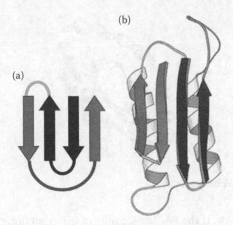

FIGURE 2.25   Schematic representation (a) and positioning inside a real protein (b) of a Greek key motif composed by four interconnected β sheets.

between two parallel strands almost always has a right-handed crossover chirality, which is strongly favored by the inherent twist of the sheet. This linking loop frequently contains a helical region, in which case it is called a β-α-β motif. A closely related motif called a β-α-β-α motif forms the basic component of the most commonly observed protein tertiary structure, the TIM barrel. An example of such structure is reported in Figure 2.27. This fold consists of eight parallel strands connected by right-handed helical crossovers and is one of the most common folds found in enzymes. The TIM barrel typically contains approximately 200 amino acid residues. Contrary to the appearance of the strip drawing, the interior of the barrel is closely packed by the side chains protruding from the strands. The strands are inclined at an angle of approximately 30° to barrel axis, which is necessary to allow efficient packing of the interior. The necessity to form a closely packed interior explains why these barrels are almost always formed from eight strands.

In a traditional approach to proteins stereographic structure, a quaternary protein structure is also introduced. Many proteins are composed of more than one polypeptide chain that are linked by different kinds of weak forces, like ion bridges or ionic bonds, so as to form a single element

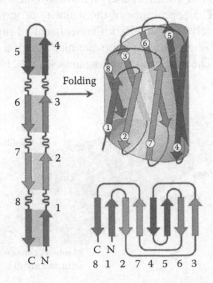

FIGURE 2.26   Composition of a barrel structure starting from the straight form of a Greek key motif.

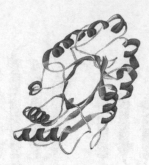

FIGURE 2.27   Example of TIM barrel motif.

under a functional point of view. If the whole assembly of different polypeptide chains is referred as a protein, individual chains are called protein sub-units and the arrangement of different sub-units is considered as the quaternary protein structure.

Recently, this approach is frequently substituted by a more rigorous approach in which a protein is a single polypeptide chain and an arrangement of different polypeptide chains is considered to be a protein complex, regulated by protein–protein interactions. This approach allows intra- and inter-protein bonds to be treated separately, seems to be more functional to the study of protein complexes functionalities and chemical characteristics. In this context, the quaternary protein structures no more exist, substituted by the stereographic properties of protein complexes.

2.3.4   Role of Proteins in Biochemistry

Proteins are the most diffused macromolecules and those having more varied structures [24,27,30]. It is thus not surprising that they perform a variety of roles in the biochemistry of living organisms. A different structure corresponds to each function, that is optimized for its application. In the following, we will review the main role of specialized proteins.

2.3.4.1   Contractile Proteins

Contractile proteins are involved in muscle contraction and movement [27]. In evolved animals, the response of the transduction of chemical energy into movement of body parts are performed by structures called muscles. The appearance of the majority of muscles is characterized by the presence of a number of relatively light and dark filaments called myofibrils that collect bundles of smaller fibers called muscle fibers. Muscle fibers are made up of a number of different proteins arranged in a specific manner. The relationship among muscle cells, fibers, and myofibrils is shown in Figure 2.28.

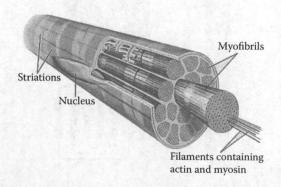

FIGURE 2.28   Striated muscle structure evidencing the particular role of muscle parts.

The protein component can be divided into three categories:

- Myofibrillar or salt-soluble proteins
- Sarcoplasmic or soluble proteins
- Stroma or insoluble proteins

Myofibrillar proteins make up about 50–55% of the total and are responsible for the actual contraction of the muscle. Sarcoplasmic proteins that make up about 25–35% of the total are almost all enzymes; the glycolytic enzymes are the major proteins of this fraction. The remainder of the protein fraction is the insoluble or stroma fraction. It contains membrane proteins, connective tissue proteins, and some large specialized structural proteins. The main muscle proteins are listed with a few of their characteristics in Table 2.6 in which the proteins are indicated in connection to the type of muscle where they have been observed and to their molecular weight.

The contraction of muscle requires coordination of the thick and thin filaments, ATP and calcium. Structure of muscle thick and thin filaments with the associated proteins is represented in Figure 2.29, whereas in Figure 2.30 the transversal structure of the thin filament is shown when in

TABLE 2.6
Main Muscle Contractive Proteins Associated to the Muscle Where They Have Been Observed and to Their Molecular Weight in Da

Protein	Muscle Type	Molecular Wt. (Da)
Thin Filament		
Actin	Rabbit	42,000
β-Actinin		
BI	Chicken fast twitch	35,000
BII		31,000
Tropomyosin		
α Tropomyosin	Chicken fast twitch	33,000
β-Tropomyosin	Chicken fast twitch	36,000
Troponin		
C	Chicken fast twitch	18,000
I	Rabbit	20,900
T	Chicken fast twitch	30,500
Thick Filament		
Myosin		
Heavy chain	Chicken fast twitch	220,000
Alkali light chain		16,000–22,000
DTNB light chain		18,000
C-Protein	Human fast twitch	128,000
H-Protein	Rabbit	69,000
X-Protein	Rabbit	152,000
Sarcomere Structure		
α-Actinin	Rabbit fast twitch	100,000
Desmin		55,000
Nebulin	Rabbit	700,000–900,000
Titin	Rabbit	1,000,000
Myomesin		170,000
I-Protein	Chicken fast twitch	50,000

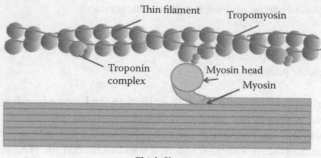

FIGURE 2.29 Schematics of the details of muscles thin and thick fibers.

contact with the mobile head of myosin in two thick filaments above and below. In the figure the thin filament proteins are evidenced, with particular attention to the Troponin complex, formed by Troponin I (TnI), Troponin T (TnT), and Troponin C (TnC), carrying the Ca bonding sites.

A nerve impulse changes the polarity of the membrane surrounding the muscle cell. This change is transmitted through the cell to the sarcoplasmic reticulum and calcium is released from the membrane. The concentration of calcium in the cell increases by a factor of about 100.

The calcium binds to the calcium-binding site of TnC. This binding causes a change in the inhibitory site of TnI which causes a change in the position of tropomyosin. The entire troponin–tropomyosin complex moves into the groove created by the twisting of the two actin chains. This removes the portion of tropomyosin that was blocking the myosin binding site. The binding of one calcium moves a complex covering seven actins. These actins are now capable of interacting with the head portion of the myosin molecule.

The release of myosin heads with actin requires ATP. An ATP molecule will bind to a myosin head and cause it to release from one of its actin binding sites. It will still be bound weakly to another site. The myosin head will hydrolyze the ATP to ADP and phosphate, which will remain bound to the myosin head. If the troponin–tropomyosin complex is in the actin groove, that is if calcium is present, then myosin will bind to actin. The energy from the hydrolysis will be used to change the myosin conformation and contraction will occur, accompanied by the release of ADP and phosphate. Thus, the cycle will be repeated as long as calcium and ATP are present. The change in structure of the myosin head is thought to cause a swivel-like motion that slides the thin filament past the thick filament in what is known as the sliding filament model. This can be compared to the action of an oar in a boat.

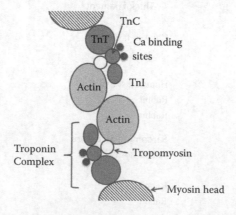

FIGURE 2.30 Transversal section of a thin muscle fiber in contact with two thick fibers (one below and one on top of it) through the mobile myosin head. The position of different thin filament proteins is evidenced.

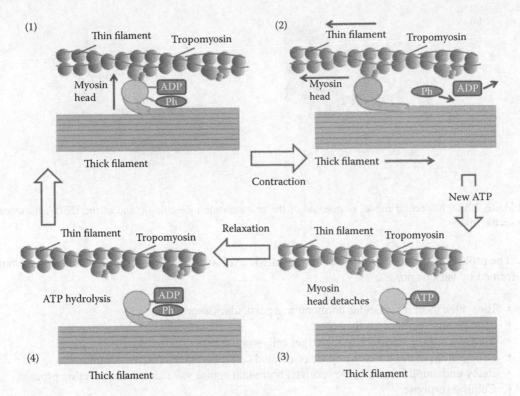

FIGURE 2.31 Schematic representation of the main phases of the muscle contraction driven by muscle proteins: Myosin head attaches to the actin filament (thin filament) (1), the myosin head pivots and bends while pushing the thin filament to slide with respect to the thick one: this is the strike phase of muscle contraction (2), as a new ATP attaches to the myosin head the myosin–actin bridges break and the myosin head detaches from the thin filament (3), the ATP is hydrolyzed in ADP and phosphates (Ph) so preparing the myosin head to attach again to the actin for the next muscle contraction (4).

When the calcium concentration falls as a consequence of a nerve impulse for relaxation, ATP will bind to myosin and cause it to release from actin. It will not be able to reattach because of the change in position of the troponin–tropomyosin complex and the filaments will slide back to their original position. This complex process is schematically shown in its main steps in Figure 2.31.

2.3.4.2 Enzymatic Proteins

Enzymes are proteins that facilitate biochemical reactions via catalysis. Examples include the enzymes lactase and pepsin. Lactase breaks down the sugar lactose found in milk; pepsin is a digestive enzyme that works in the stomach to break down proteins in food. For its importance in biological assays performed both in macroscopical systems and in labs on chip a detailed analysis of enzymatic catalysis is carried out in Section 2.4.

2.3.4.3 Hormones

Hormonal proteins are messenger proteins which help to coordinate certain bodily activities [34,35]. Examples include insulin, oxytocin, and somatotropin. Insulin regulates glucose metabolism by controlling the blood–sugar concentration, oxytocin stimulates contractions in females during childbirth, somatotropin is a growth hormone that stimulates protein production in muscle cells. Examples of the chemical structure of hormones are given in Figure 2.32.

(a)   (b)

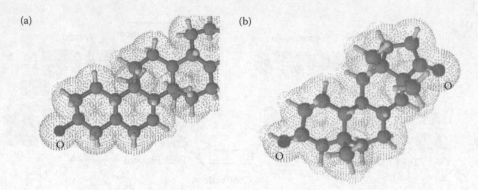

FIGURE 2.32   Molecular model of one end of the progesterone molecule (a) and of the DEHA hormone molecule (b).

The process that implies information transmission through hormones is a complex process that is formed by various phases:

• Biosynthesis of a particular hormone in a particular tissue
• Storage and secretion of the hormone
• Transport of the hormone to the target cell or cells
• Recognition of the hormone by an associated cell membrane receptor protein
• Relay and amplification of the received hormonal signal via a signal transduction process
• Cellular response
• Degradation of the hormone

The reaction of the target cells may then be recognized by the original hormone-producing cells, leading to a downregulation in hormone production. This is an example of a homeostatic negative feedback loop.

Hormone cells are typically of a specialized cell type, residing within a particular endocrine gland, such as thyroid gland, ovaries, and testes. Hormones exit their cell of origin via transport through cell membrane.

Different tissue types may respond contemporarily and differently to the same hormonal signal. Moreover, a single cell type may have several different receptors that recognize the same hormone and activates different signal transduction pathway or a cell type may have several different receptors that recognize different hormones and activate the same biochemical pathway. Because of this, hormonal signaling is elaborate and hard to dissect.

For many hormones, the receptor is membrane associated and embedded in the plasma membrane at the surface of the cell. The interaction of hormone and receptor typically triggers a cascade of secondary effects within the cytoplasm of the cell, often involving phosphorylation or dephosphorylation of various other cytoplasmic proteins, changes in ion channel permeability, or increased concentrations of intracellular molecules that may act as secondary messengers.

Receptors of other hormones such as steroid or thyroid hormones, are located within the cytoplasm of their target cell so that these hormones may cross the cell membrane. This is possible due to lipid solubility of such hormones. The combined hormone–receptor complex then moves across the nuclear membrane into the nucleus of the cell, where it binds to specific DNA sequences, effectively amplifying or suppressing the action of certain genes, and affecting protein synthesis [36,37]. However, it has been shown that not all steroid receptors are located in intracellular positions. Some are associated with the plasma membrane [38].

The rate of hormone biosynthesis and secretion is often regulated by a homeostatic negative feedback control mechanism. Such a mechanism depends on factors that influence the metabolism and excretion of hormones. Thus, higher hormone concentration alone cannot trigger the negative feedback mechanism. Negative feedback must be triggered by overproduction of an *effect* of the hormone.

Hormone secretion can be stimulated and inhibited by

- Other hormones (stimulating- or releasing hormones)
- Plasma concentrations of ions or nutrients, as well as binding globulins
- Neurons and mental activity
- Environmental changes, as light intensity or temperature

One special group of hormones is the tropic hormones that stimulate the hormone production of other endocrine glands. For example, thyroid-stimulating hormone (TSH) causes growth and increased activity of another endocrine gland, the thyroid, which increases output of thyroid hormones.

An example of how hormones regulates through mutual interaction with receptors and among themselves the biological cycles that establish homeostasis and allow life is the human reproductive cycle [39]. The concentrations of the three hormones regulating the female fertility cycle oscillate in blood in a characteristic way as represented in Figure 2.33.

Stimulated by gradually increasing amounts of estrogen in the follicular phase, discharges of blood ending the previous cycle, called menses slow down and stop, and the lining of the uterus thickens. Follicles in the ovary begin developing under the influence of a complex interplay of hormones, and after several days one or occasionally two become dominant while nondominant follicles atrophy and die. Approximately mid-cycle, 24–36 h after the luteinizing hormone (LH) surges, the dominant follicle releases an ovum in an event called ovulation. After ovulation, the egg only lives for 24 h or less without fertilization, while the remains of the dominant follicle in the ovary become a corpus luteum; this body has a primary function of producing large amounts of progesterone.

Under the influence of progesterone, the endometrium, also called uterine lining, changes to prepare for potential implantation of an embryo to establish a pregnancy. If implantation does not occur within approximately two weeks, the corpus luteum will involute, causing sharp drops in levels of both progesterone and estrogen. These hormone drops cause the uterus to shed its lining and the egg in a process termed menstruation. In the menstrual cycle, changes occur in the female reproductive system as well as other systems, which frequently lead to breast tenderness, for example.

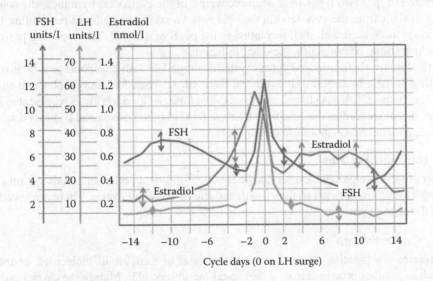

FIGURE 2.33 Hormones behavior in the human reproductive cycle: arrows indicate statistical limits of 99% on the healthy women population. (From Sadava, D. et al. *Life, The Science of Biology*, Macmillan Publishers; 9th edition (2009). ISBN-10 1429219629.)

2.3.4.4 Structural Proteins

The structural proteins are the basic building material of all the many structures constituting our body [27,30]. Proteins may have the form of long spiraling fibers such as hair, connective tissue, or muscle thick fibers. They form the semipermeable cell wall and the wall of the different vesicular or tubular structures in the cell.

In some cases some mineral is accumulated in the cell, such as in bone, or large amounts of fat or other substances are deposited in the cell. These processes are all regulated by the proteins and proteins lay out the matrix and constitute the forming material of these structures. Examples include keratin, collagen, and elastin. Keratins strengthen protective coverings such as hair, quills, feathers, horns, and beaks. Collagens and elastin provide support for connective tissues such as tendons and ligaments.

2.3.4.5 Storage Proteins

Storage proteins are proteins that are used by living organisms to store materials [27,30]. Usually, storage proteins are in reality protein complexes constituted by several polypeptide chains arranged in a quaternary structure suitable to store the target element or composite.

An important group of storage proteins comprises proteins generated mainly during seed production and stored in the seed that serve as nitrogen sources for the developing embryo during germination. The average protein content of cereal grains is 10–15% of their dry weight that of Leguminosae seeds 20–25, while it is only 3–5% in normal leaves. Besides seeds, storage proteins can also be found in root and shoot tubers, such as in potatoes.

Another important category of storage proteins are used inside the human body to store metals and other materials. The most important of these proteins is ferritin, storing mainly iron, but also aluminum and zinc, for use principally in the synthesis of other proteins. Iron, for example, is a key element for the synthesis of hemoglobin and myoglobin (cf. Section 1.2.3.2). Ferritin is a protein complex with a mass of 450 kDa consisting of 24 subunits that is present in every cell type [40]. In vertebrates, these subunits are both the light (L) and the heavy (H) type with an apparent molecular weight of 19 or 21 kDA, respectively; their sequences are about 50% homologous.

Ferritin is present in all the animals and plants species that share the need of storing iron atoms; ferritin from different species is different, even if strong similarities do exist. Amphibians have an additional ("M") type of ferritin [41]; the single ferritin of plants and bacteria most closely resemble the vertebrate H-type. Two types have been recovered in the gastropod Lymnaea, the somatic ferritin being distinct from the yolk ferritin (see below). An additional subunit resembling Lymnaea soma ferritin is associated with shell formation in the pearl oyster [42]. Two types are present in the parasite Schistosoma, one in males, the other in females.

Inside the ferritin shell, iron ions form crystallites together with phosphate and hydroxide ions. The resulting particle is similar to the mineral ferrihydrite. Each ferritin complex can store about 4500 iron (Fe^{3+}) ions [39,41]. A stereographic model of human blood ferritin is represented in Figure 2.34, where it is evidenced as the complex structure formed by α helixes and β sheets retains inside the molecule a metallic iron molecule to transport it.

2.3.4.6 Transport Proteins

A transport protein is a protein that serves the function of moving other materials within an organism. Transport proteins are vital to the growth and life of all living things. There are several different kinds of transport proteins.

2.3.4.6.1 Carrier Proteins

Carrier proteins are proteins involved in the movement of ions, small molecules, or macromolecules, such as another protein, across a biological membrane [43]. Membrane carrier proteins are membrane proteins, that is, they exist within and span the membrane across which they transport substances. Each carrier protein is designed to recognize only one substance or one group of very similar substances [44].

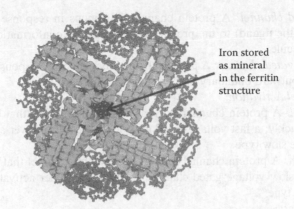

Iron stored as mineral in the ferritin structure

FIGURE 2.34 Molecular structure of the ferritin complex trapping iron in metallic form. The protein helices form a sort of cage surrounding the metallic atom and bind it with coordinate bonds without breaking the iron mineral molecules.

Generally, membrane carrier proteins, also called channel are tightly twisted around a central opening full of water thereby allowing small hydrophilic molecules to enter the cell as it is schematically shown in Figure 2.35. Sometimes the channel is even longer than the membrane, accompanying the molecules well inside the cell body. Some types of channels are always opened, other types only open as a response to a precise type of stimulus.

The main types of channels individuated in human cells are classified differently, depending on the type of channel characteristics used for classification:

- *Opening/closing stimulus*
  - *Voltage-gated channel:* A protein channel that can be opened or closed in response to changes in the electric potential across a cell membrane. See also ligand-gated channel.

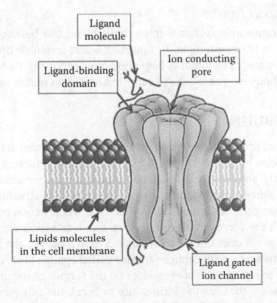

Ligand molecule

Ion conducting pore

Ligand-binding domain

Lipids molecules in the cell membrane

Ligand gated ion channel

FIGURE 2.35 Graphical representation of the role and working of channel proteins. In the example a ligand-activated channel protein is shown and, besides the channel penetrating into the cell membrane, the ligand point with the activating molecule is also evidenced.

- *Ligand-gated channel:* A protein channel that opens in response to the binding of a molecule (the ligand) to the protein, which causes a conformational change in the protein molecule.
- *Mechanical gated channel:* A protein channel that opens in response to pressure operated on the outward boundary of the channel protein.
- *Speed of Channel Activation:*
  - *Fast channel:* A protein channel, such as a sodium channel, that becomes activated relatively quickly; a fast voltage-gated channel has a much lower activation potential than does the slow type.
  - *Slow channel:* A protein channel such as the calcium channel that is slow to become activated; a slow voltage-gated channel has a much higher activation potential than does the fast type.
- *Channel Selectivity:*
  - *Calcium channel, frequently called calcium–sodium channel:* A slow voltage-gated channel very permeable to calcium ions and slightly permeable to sodium ions, existing in three subtypes designated L, M, and N and located throughout the body; calcium channels are the main way calcium ions traverse the muscle cell membrane to activate muscle contraction and the N channels regulate neurotransmitter release.
  - *Potassium channel:* A slow voltage-gated channel selective for the passage of potassium ions, found on the surface of a wide variety of cells, including nerve, muscle, and secretory cells; its functions include regulation of cell membrane excitability, regulation of repetitive low frequency firing in some neurons, and recovery of the nerve fiber membrane at the end of the action potential.
  - *Sodium channel:* A type of fast channel selective for the passage of sodium ions. Voltage-gated sodium channels are the main causes of depolarization and repolarization of nerve membranes during the action potential.
  - *Water channel:* A channel in a cell membrane that permits passage of water molecules; chemical substances such as vasopressin cause the opening of new channels and increase permeability.

2.3.4.6.2 Blood Transport Proteins

These are the proteins transporting material through the blood flux between far parts of the living organism. Serum albumin is one example. It transports water-insoluble lipids in the bloodstream. The most known blood transport protein is hemoglobin, transporting molecular oxygen from the lungs to all parts of the body to enable cells to carry out oxidation reactions.

2.4　IMMUNOGLOBULIN

Antibodies are specialized proteins involved in defending the body from antigens, the general name under which the active sites of all the dangerous external elements entering the living structure are named [45,46]. Commonly, antigens are extraneous proteins or polysaccharides, polypeptides, lipids, nucleic acids, and many other materials, belonging to most complex structures, such as viruses and bacteria, or simply infecting the organism from outside. The whole action of the antibodies is based on complementarity with the corresponding antigen so that it is a highly specific action. When an antibody attacks an antigen it does not try to bond on a casual part of the antigen molecule, but it searches for a specific attack site on the antigen surface called epitope [46]. This is usually one to six monosaccharides or five to eight amino acid residues on the surface of the antigen.

Examples of antigens are the sites the viruses use to break the cell membrane and inject their own nucleic acids infecting the cell. In this case, generally, antibodies combine with these active sites neutralizing them and so rendering the virus inactive, operation that is often called virus coating. A schematic example of this process is shown in Figure 2.36. In other cases, especially if a

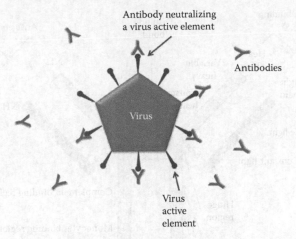

FIGURE 2.36   Schematic representation of the process of virus neutralization by antibodies.

bacterium has to be fought, antibodies attach to the surface of the bacterium and constitute a binding site for the immune system cells that are deputed to attack and eliminate the bacterium [45].

Immune response by antibodies may also be generated against smaller substances, called haptens, when they appear in large quantity inside the blood. A variety of molecules such as drugs, simple sugars, amino acids, small peptides, phospholipids, or triglycerides may function as haptens. Thus, given enough time, just about any foreign substance will be identified by the immune system and evoke specific antibody production.

Because antigen molecules exist in space, the epitope recognized by an antibody may be dependent upon the presence of a specific three-dimensional antigenic conformation, for example, a unique site formed by the interaction of two native protein loops or subunits, or the epitope may correspond to a simple primary sequence region. Such epitopes are described as conformational and linear, respectively. The range of possible binding sites is enormous, with each potential binding site having its own structural properties derived from covalent bonds, ionic bonds, and hydrophilic and hydrophobic interactions.

In the following, we will refer to the structure of human immunoglobulin. Several immunoglobulin of nonhuman origin are used in biotechnology, both for macroscopic and for lab on chip assays. They can differ from human immunoglobulin for a different molecular weight and naturally for different chemicals structure of the binding sites, but the immunoglobulin structure is the same in all evolved animals. Thus, reference to the human case, which is in any case of great importance, will not limit the generality of the discussion.

In spite of the large variety of immunoglobulin existing in the human body, they all share a common structure, based as in all proteins on polypeptides. Moreover, immunoglobulins bind at their polypeptides glycol residues, thereby being glycoproteins [47].

2.4.1   Immunoglobulin G Structure

Immunoglobulin G is the predominant Ig in the serum; it makes up about 80% of the total antibody found in a person at any given time, being 75% of the total serum antibody. It can diffuse out of the blood stream into the extravascular spaces and it is the most common Ig found there [45,47]. Its concentration in tissue fluids is increased during inflammation. It is particularly effective at the neutralization of bacterial exotoxins and viruses. IgG crosses the placental barrier, and thereby provides passive immunity to the fetus and infant for the first six months of life. The structure of IgGs is also the base of the structure of all the other immunoglobulins that are found in the immune system of human and other animals.

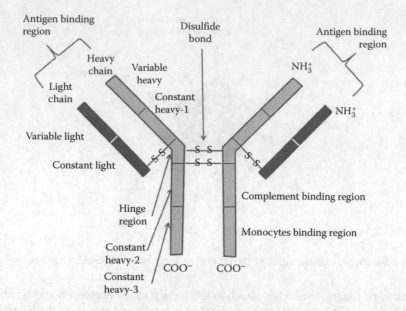

FIGURE 2.37 Y-shaped diagram of an immunoglobulin (IgG) structure where all the molecule important elements are identified.

The basic IgG, a molecule with a weight of about 150 kDa, is formed by four polypeptides, two with approximately the same weight of 50 kDa, called heavy chains, and two of a weight of approximately 25 kDa, called light chains.

Heavy and light chains are bonded by disulfide bonds (see Sections 2.3.1 and 2.3.3) and several chains exist, linked to form a longer sequence as shown in Figure 2.37. Even if multiple heavy chains (H-chains or simply H) exist in an IgG, they are all of the same type, and the same is true for the light chains (L-chains or simply L). Each L chain is connected to a H chain and the two H-chains are connected to one another by disulfide bridges. All the structural elements of an IgG are evidenced in the Y-shaped diagram reported in Figure 2.38, a conventional diagram that is frequently used for this kind of proteins.

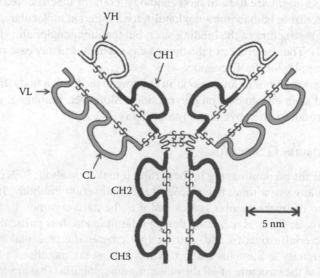

FIGURE 2.38 Schematic diagram putting in evidence domains in the IgG structure.

The stem of the Y is called the Fc region and it consists mainly of two halves of the identical H chains. Each of the arms of the Y contains one complete L-chain and half of one of the H-chains. The Y stem stands on the carboxyl termini of the H chains; the tips of the arms contain the amino termini of the H- and L-chains. Each arm is sometimes referred to as the Fab region of the molecule.

The Fab region is the antigen binding fragment of the antibody molecule, terminating with the body epitope, which is the segment of the molecule that is complimentary to the epitope of the antigen to which the IgG has to react. A specific region of the antigen will react with the antigen epitope region at the amino terminus of each Fab. Hence, the IgG molecule, which has two antigen binding fragments is said to be divalent, which means that it can bind to two antigen epitopes of the same antigen.

The polypeptide composition of the Fc region of all IgG1 antibody molecules is relatively constant regardless of antibody specificity; however, the Fab regions always differ in their exact amino acid sequences depending upon their antigenic specificity. Even though the antigen does not react with the Fc region of the IgG molecule, this should not be taken to mean that the Fc region has no importance or biological activity. On the contrary, specific amino acid regions of the Fc portion of the molecule are recognized by receptors on phagocytes and certain other cells [45], and the Fc domain contains a peptide region that will bind to and activate complement, which is often required for the manifestation of auto-immune complementary reactions. This is the region at which the arms of the antibody molecule forms a Y called the hinge region because there is some flexibility in the molecule at this point.

Even if, generally, the molecule IgG is drawn to resemble an Y, IgGs are not found in this extended configuration. The first element that determines a more complex shape is the formation of the so-called IgG domains. IgG molecule is folded into globular regions each of which contains an intra-chain disulfide bond as shown in Figure 2.39: these regions are called domains. Domains have the same structure in all the IgGs, independently from the specific antigen they are designed to attack and they can be classified as follows:

1. Light chain
    1.1. Variable light (VL—110 amino acids)
    1.2. Constant light (CL—110 amino acids)
2. Heavy chain
    2.1. Variable heavy (VH—110 amino acids)
    2.2. Constant heavy 1 (CH1—330–440 amino acids)
    2.3. Constant heavy 2 (CH2—330–440 amino acids)
    2.4. Constant heavy 3 (CH3—330–440 amino acids)

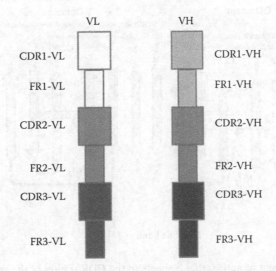

FIGURE 2.39   Sub-region alteration in the variable light chain of an IgG.

Constant domains lie in carboxyl or terminal portion of the molecule and show an unvarying amino acid sequence that is typical of all IgGs. This amino acid residue sequence is responsible for IgG biological functions that do not depend on the specific antigen the IgG is synthesized to fight. Variable domains have a more complex structure, being related to the binding of the antibody with its specific antigen. Variable domains are built by a sequence of framework regions (FR) interleaved with the active residues segments that can be hypervariable regions (HVR) also called complementarity determining regions (CDR).

CDRs are the regions where the IgG complement an antigen's shape. Thus, CDRs determine the immunoglobulin affinity and specificity for specific antigens. The CDRs' residue sequences are the most variable part of the antibody allowing it to recognize a vast repertoire of antigens. The name hypervariable regions is also derived from the property.

Looking more in detail at the structure of IgGs domains, they are folded into a characteristic compact structure called the immunoglobulin fold. This structure consists of a sandwich of two β sheets each containing antiparallel β strands of amino acid residues, which are connected by loops of various lengths as shown schematically in Figure 2.40. The β strands within a sheet are stabilized by hydrogen bonds that connect the -NH groups in one strand with carbonyl groups of an adjacent strand. The β strands are characterized by alternating hydrophobic and hydrophilic amino acids whose side chains are arranged perpendicular to the plane of the sheet; the hydrophobic amino acids are oriented toward the interior of the sandwich, and the hydrophilic amino acids face outward. The two β sheets within an immunoglobulin fold are stabilized by the hydrophobic interactions between them and by the conserved disulfide bond.

Although variable and constant domains have a similar structure, there are subtle differences between them. The V domain is slightly longer than the C domain and contains an extra pair of β strands within the β-sheet structure, as well as the extra loop sequence connecting this pair of β strands (see Figure 2.40).

The resulting strips structure of an IgG is shown in Figure 2.41, where different chains are evidenced with dark gray and light gray. Figure 2.41 shows that the extreme end of the IgG arms form a sort of cup structure. This is an important conformational characteristic that helps to bind the designed antibody epitome by creating conformational adaptation [48].

We have also seen that immunoglobulins are glycoproteins, thus carbohydrate residues are found bonded to the different immunoglobulin chains. The carbohydrate chain wraps around one of the protein domains as shown in Figure 2.42 [47,49], preventing its contact with the adjacent

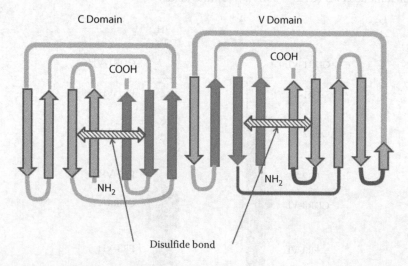

FIGURE 2.40 Arrangement of antiparallel β sheets in the CDR region of the variable heavy domain of an IgG.

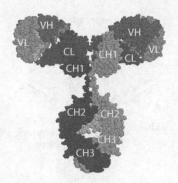

FIGURE 2.41   IgG immunoglobulin in the volume representation where the various chains constituting the proteins are evidenced.

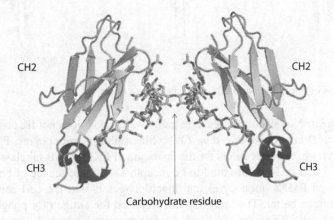

FIGURE 2.42   IgG tail showing the position of the carbohydrate residue preventing the two parts of the Y tail from touching.

domain. When the carbohydrate chain is removed, the domain could no longer perform its ordinary function. Because immunoglobulin function is determined to a large extent by its structure, the carbohydrate removing affected the structure of the molecule. At least one carbohydrate chain may also be required for high-affinity ligand binding to antigens.

2.4.2   Classification of Human Immunoglobulin

A table of the human antibody classification is reported in Figure 2.43. A brief discussion of the properties and the differences among various immunoglobulin classes is reported here below. All the different immunoglobulin classes share and replicate the same basic structure made by heavy and light chains bonded by disulfide bonds. Also antigen-binding mechanisms via active sites at the top of the immunoglobulin arms are similar, even if different immunoglobulin have affinity for different antigen classes.

- Immunoglobulin G (IgG)
  - *Structure:* The structures of the IgG subclasses are presented in Figure 2.43. All IgG's are monomers (7S immunoglobulin). The subclasses differ in the number of disulfide bonds and length of the hinge region.
  - *Properties:* IgG is the most versatile immunoglobulin because it is capable of carrying out all of the functions of immunoglobulin molecules. They are the major Ig in serum and in extra-vascular spaces—75% of serum Ig is IgG.

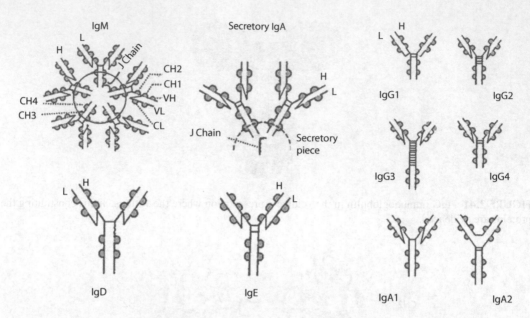

FIGURE 2.43   Types of immunoglobulin found in the human body.

- *Complement:* Not all subclasses fix equally well; IgG4 does not fix complement.
- *Binding to Other Immune System Cells:* Macrophages, monocytes, PMNs and some lymphocytes have Fc receptors for the Fc region of IgG. Not all subclasses bind equally well; IgG2 and IgG4 do not bind to Fc receptors. A consequence of binding to the Fc receptors on PMNs, monocytes and macrophages is that the cell can now internalize the antigen better. The antibody has prepared the antigen for phagocytosis by the phagocytic cells. The term opsonin is used to describe substances that enhance phagocytosis. IgG is a good opsonin. Binding of IgG to Fc receptors on other types of cells results in the activation of other functions.
- Immunoglobulin M (IgM)
  - *Structure:* The pentamer structure of IgM is presented in Figure 2.43. IgM normally exists in this form (19S immunoglobulin) but it can also exist as a monomer. In the pentameric form all heavy chains are identical and all light chains are identical. Thus, the valence is theoretically 10. IgM has an extra domain on the mu chain (CH4) and it has another protein covalently bound via a S–S bond called the J chain. This chain functions in polymerization of the molecule into a pentamer.
  - *Properties:* IgM is the third most common serum Ig. As a consequence of its structure, IgM is also a good agglutinating Ig. Thus, IgM antibodies are very good in clumping microorganisms for eventual elimination from the body.
  - *Complement:* As a consequence of its pentameric structure, IgM is a good complement fixing Ig. Thus, IgM antibodies are very efficient in leading to the lysis of microorganisms.
  - *Binding to Other Immune System Cells:* Surface IgM exists as a monomer, schematically shown in Figure 2.44, and lacks J chain but it has an extra 20 amino acids at the C-terminus to anchor it into the membrane. Cell surface IgM functions as a receptor for antigen on B cells.
- Immunoglobulin A (IgA)
  - *Structure:* Serum IgA is a monomer, but IgA found in secretions is a dimer as presented in Figure 2.43 besides the different subtypes of the monomer form. When IgA exits as a dimer, a J chain is associated with it.

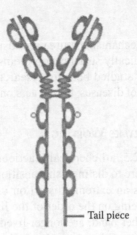

Tail piece

FIGURE 2.44   Scheme of an IgM in a monomer form.

When IgA is found in secretions it also has another protein associated with it called the secretory piece or T piece; in this case it takes the name of secretory IgA or sIgA and is sometimes referred to as 11S immunoglobulin.

Unlike the remainder of the IgA which is made in the plasma cell, the secretory piece is made in epithelial cells and is added to the IgA as it passes into the secretions. The secretory piece helps IgA to be transported across mucosa and also protects it from degradation in the secretions.

- *Properties:* IgA is the second most common serum Ig and it is the major class of Ig in secretions—tears, saliva, colostrum, and mucus. Since it is found in secretions, secretory IgA is important in local (mucosal) immunity.
- *Complement:* Normally, IgA does not fix complement, unless aggregated.
- *Binding to Other Immune System Cells:* IgA can bind to some cells—PMN's and some lymphocytes.
- Immunoglobulin D (IgD)
  - *Structure:* IgD exists only as a monomer.
  - *Properties:* IgD is quite rare in serum and its role as a free serum molecule, if any, is uncertain. IgD is primarily found on B cell surfaces where it functions as a receptor for antigen. IgD on the surface of B cells has extra amino acids at C-terminal end for anchoring to the membrane. It also associates with the Ig-α and Ig-β chains.
  - *Complement:* IgD does not fix complement.
  - *Binding to Other Immune System Cells:* IgD is mainly designed to bind with B cells.
- Immunoglobulin E (IgE)
  - *Structure:* IgE exists as a monomer and has an extra domain in the constant region.
  - *Properties:* IgE is the least common serum Ig since it binds very tightly to Fc receptors on basophils and mast cells even before interacting with antigen. As a consequence of its binding to basophils and mast cells, IgE is involved in allergic reactions. Binding of the allergen to the IgE on the cells results in the release of various pharmacological mediators that result in allergic symptoms.

    IgE also plays a role in parasitic helminth diseases. Since serum IgE levels rise in parasitic diseases, measuring IgE levels is helpful in diagnosing parasitic infections. Eosinophils have Fc receptors for IgE and binding of eosinophils to IgE-coated helminths results in killing of the parasite.
  - *Complement:* IgE does not fix complement.
  - *Binding to Other Immune System Cells:* Basophils and mast cells, see above.

2.5 ENZYMATIC CATALYSIS

As anticipated in Section 2.3.2, the mechanism nature used to accelerate complex biochemical reactions is catalysis via a class of specifically structured proteins called enzymes [24,25,50]. A very large number of enzymes have been studied both for research and for their relevance in analytic procedures and in medical treatment of diseases, but all acts on the ground of a general mechanism.

2.5.1 THE BASIC PRINCIPLE OF ENZYMES WORKING

As detailed in Sections 1.2.4 and 1.2.5, all chemical reactions transit through transition states or intermediate states. It is important here to distinguish transition states from intermediate states.

A transition state is envisioned as an extreme distortion of a bond, and thus the lifetime of a typical transition state is viewed as being on the order of the lifetime of a bond vibration, typically 0.1 ps. Intermediate states, on the other hand, are longer-lived, with lifetimes in the range of 1 ps up to 1 ms. In other words, reactions transiting through transition states are at all effects single-step reactions under a kinetic point of view and the transition state is simply a distortion of the stable state, and as such is characterized by a very high free formation energy.

However, reactions transiting through intermediate states are multi-step reactions that happens rapidly and the free energy barrier to overcome to realize the reaction is generally smaller due to the less unstable structure of the intermediate states. In a great number of biological reactions the main reagent, frequently called the substrate S, is converted into a product P by transiting through a transition state which we will call generically X. Under an energetic point of view such a reaction is very unfavorable, thereby being very slow or even not spontaneous. The reaction has to be written as

$$S + N_1 \rightarrow P + N_2 \tag{2.8}$$

where the composites N_1 and N_2 are generally simple molecules or ions. These small molecules are several times related to the solvent as in the case of hydrolysis that is a typical reaction of this kind. Elements N_1 and N_2 are almost always present in abundance with respect to the biological macromolecules. They are not involved in the action of the enzyme and their concentration at equilibrium in the solution is almost equal and it is not sensibly altered by the reaction due to the high dilution of biological macromolecules. This means that the concentrations of N_1 and N_2 simply eliminates in the law of mass action determining the reaction equilibrium (see Section 1.2.3) and have no impact in determining the reaction kinetic. Thus, when dealing with enzymatic catalysis, the presence of N_1 and N_2 is generally neglected and reaction (2.8) is synthetically written as

$$S \rightarrow P \tag{2.9}$$

Naturally, if we exclude reactions consisting simply in a change of aggregation state or of molecule configuration, expression (2.9) has no sense if we do not remember the presence of N_1 and N_2, even if their structure and concentration do not impact on the reaction characteristics, but for rendering it possible.

The catalytic role of an enzyme is, as in all catalysis processes, to reduce the energy barrier between substrate and transition state. This is accomplished through the formation of an enzyme–substrate (ES) complex. This complex is converted into product by passing through a different transition state, that we will call EX, that would not be possible without the presence of the enzyme as shown in Figure 2.45. Since the formation free energy of EX is much lower than that of X we could envision a standard catalysis mechanism, where the reaction acceleration happens due to a reduction of the free energy barrier.

In reality, even if this phenomenon has naturally an important role, the enzyme working mechanism is more complex. As a matter of fact from Figure 2.45 it is clear that the enzymes do not limit its own action in substituting X with EX while lowering the activation energy: it first creates a complex ES with the substrate, that allows this complex to transform to P + E via an intermediate state EX.

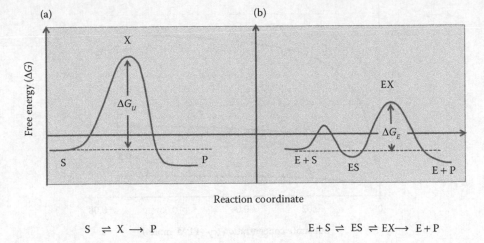

$$S \rightleftharpoons X \longrightarrow P \qquad\qquad E + S \rightleftharpoons ES \rightleftharpoons EX \longrightarrow E + P$$

FIGURE 2.45 Energy profile of a free organic reaction (a) and of the same reaction with a catalyzing enzyme (b) in the second case the free activation energy is much lower.

This description of the enzyme catalyzed reaction dynamic is called Michaelis–Menten hypothesis and it is very well verified in practice [24,51]. The energy barrier to be surmounted in the enzyme-catalyzed reaction, assuming that E is saturated with S, is the energy difference between ES and EX, thus reaction rate acceleration by an enzyme means simply that the energy barrier between ES and EX is less than the energy barrier between S and X. In terms of the free energies of activation,

$$\Delta G_E < \Delta G_U \tag{2.10}$$

The enzyme thus must stabilize the transition-state complex, EX, more than it stabilizes the substrate complex, ES, that is, it has to bind the transition-state structure more tightly than the substrate and the product. The equilibrium constant of the dissociation reaction of ES can be expressed through the law of mass action as

$$K_S = \frac{c_E c_S}{c_{ES}} \tag{2.11}$$

and the corresponding dissociation constant for the transition-state complex as

$$K_{ST} = \frac{c_E c_X}{c_{EX}} \tag{2.12}$$

Enzyme catalysis requires that $K_{ST} < K_S$.

2.5.2 Kinetics of Enzyme-Catalyzed Reactions

The plot of the reaction speed for a simple uni-molecular reaction A- > B versus the molecule concentrations result to be quite simple: a straight line. The more component A is available, the greater the rate of the reaction, v. This is easily forecasted by the general kinetic theory (see Section 1.2.4) assuming that the reaction is single step, so being a first-order reaction under a kinetic point of view.

Similar analyses of enzyme-catalyzed reactions involving only a single substrate yield remarkably different results as shown in Figure 2.46. At low concentrations of the substrate, the rate is proportional to the substrate concentration c_S, as expected for a first-order reaction; high values of c_S, it stabilizes on an almost constant value, that we can consider the maximum possible rate for the

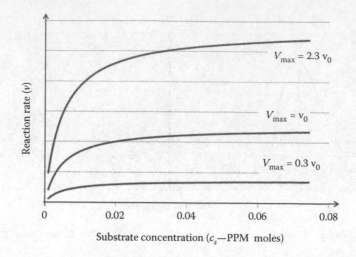

FIGURE 2.46 Reaction rate of an enzymatic catalyzed molecular decomposition for different values of the maximum possible rate V_{max} versus the substrate concentration in PPM moles.

reaction V_{max}; in other words, at high values of the substrate concentration the reaction is obeying zero-order kinetics; that is, the rate is independent of c_S.

The presence of saturation in the reaction kinetics can be interpreted assuming that every enzyme molecule has its substrate-binding site accommodating only one possible substrate molecule. When all the binding sites are occupied, no more increment of the reaction rate is possible, even if the substrate concentration is increased. This interpretation is not only confirmed by all experimental observation, also at a microscopic level, but is also completely in line with the general action of biological phenomena that is based on the concept of molecules complementarity (see Section 2.2.1.5). This situation is schematically shown in Figure 2.47.

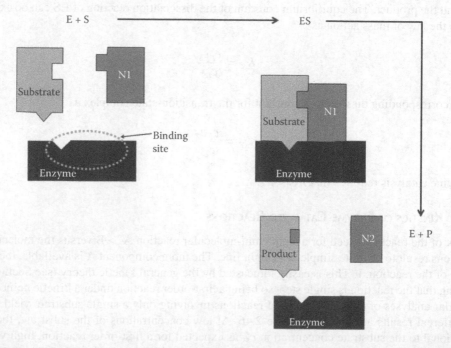

FIGURE 2.47 Schematic view of an enzymatic catalyzed reaction and of the role of the enzyme binding site.

2.5.2.1 The Michaelis–Menten Kinetic Model

The Michaelis–Menten theory is based on the Michaelis–Menten assumption that the enzyme, E, and its substrate, S, associate reversibly to form an ES complex:

$$E + S \underset{v_-}{\overset{v_+}{\rightleftharpoons}} ES \tag{2.13}$$

This association/dissociation is assumed to be rapid at thermodynamic equilibrium in every instant while the slower catalyzed reactions go on. The overall reaction thus assumes the form of a two-step reaction where the ES composite is an intermediate composite while the EX composite is a transition composite. As demonstrated in Section 1.2.4 through the kinetic theory, the ES dissociation constant K_s is related to the rates of Equation 2.13 so that we have

$$K_s = \frac{c_E c_S}{c_{ES}} = \frac{v_-}{v_+} \tag{2.14}$$

The second step of the reaction forms the product P by decomposing ES, thus the overall reaction can be written as

$$\begin{cases} E + S \underset{v_-}{\overset{v_+}{\rightleftharpoons}} ES \\ ES \overset{v_2}{\longrightarrow} E + P \end{cases} \tag{2.15}$$

E is then free to interact with another S molecule.

This model was refined and extended by Briggs and Haldane, by assuming the concentration of the ES complex quickly reaches a constant value in such a dynamic system. That is, ES is formed as rapidly from E + S as it disappears in two possible ways: dissociation to regenerate E + S, and reaction to form E + P. This means that the concentration of ES is always thermodynamically at equilibrium so that its derivative is always zero and the overall intermediate reaction is reversible.

This assumption is named the steady-state assumption and, on the ground of what previously observed, is expressed as

$$\frac{dc_{ES}}{dt} = 0 \tag{2.16}$$

This approximation makes very simple to evaluate the time evolution of the concentrations in Equation 2.15. As a matter of fact, since the overall number of molecules have to conserve and the catalyst number of molecules also conserves through the reaction, we can derive that the concentration of P follows without delay the variations of the concentration of S so that

$$\frac{dc_S}{dt} + \frac{dc_P}{dt} = 0 \tag{2.17}$$

The dynamic behavior of the concentrations is represented in Figure 2.48, in two different time scales: the first is the time scale of the overall reaction, where c_{ES} appears to be constant; and the second is the much faster time scale characteristic of the variation of c_{ES}, where there are the variations of c_S and c_P to be negligible.

The reaction starts from an initial reaction speed that does not depend on the concentration of P simply since P is not present, going on slower and slower up to stop in an equilibrium state where the direct and inverse rates are equal. To determine the exact values of the rates in every instant of the reaction, we have to solve the kinetic system typical of two-step reactions as detailed in Section 1.2.4. Due to the hypothesis on the stationary value of c_{ES} this is particularly simple assuming that the enzyme concentration is much greater that the substrate one so that we are far from saturation.

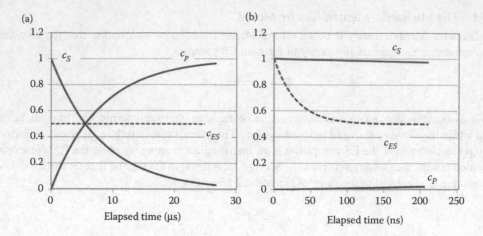

FIGURE 2.48 Concentration dynamics in an enzymatic catalyzed reaction on the reaction time scale (a) and on the evolution time scale of the intermediate composite (b).

If we call ΔG_0 the free energy difference between the initial state with $c_S = c_{S0}$ and $c_P = 0$ and the final state where $c_S = (1 - K_s)c_{S0}$ and $c_P = K_s c_{S0}$ we can write for the rates of the overall reaction, due to the stationary hypothesis

$$v_{2+} = v_{0+}c_S \tag{2.18a}$$

$$v_{2-} = v_{0-}c_P \tag{2.18b}$$

with

$$\frac{v_{0+}}{v_{0-}} = e^{-\frac{\Delta G_0}{\kappa T}} \tag{2.19}$$

Thus, the equation for $c_s = \zeta \, c_{S0}$, being ζ the substrate percentage converted into the product at the instant t, becomes

$$c_{s0}\frac{d\zeta}{dt} = -c_{s0}v_{0+}\left[\zeta - (1 - \zeta)e^{-\frac{\Delta G_0}{\kappa T}}\right] \tag{2.20}$$

where naturally

$$\lim_{t \to \infty} \zeta = K_s \tag{2.21a}$$

$$\lim_{t \to 0} \zeta = 1 \tag{2.21b}$$

Solving Equation 2.20 with conditions (2.21) is easy far from saturation so that increasing the concentration of the substrate causes an almost linear increase of the reaction speed.

In this condition, remembering the kinetic expression of K_s and writing $V_0 = v_{0+} \, e^{(\Delta G_0/\kappa T)} = v_{0+}(K_s/(1 - K_s))$, Equation 2.20 can be written as

$$c_s(t) = c_{s0}K_S\left[1 + \frac{1 - K_s}{K_s}e^{-V_0 t}\right] \tag{2.22a}$$

$$v_+(t) = \frac{dc_s(t)}{dt} = -\frac{c_{s0}V_0}{K_S} e^{-V_0 t} \tag{2.22b}$$

The qualitative trends of the substrate concentration and the reaction rate in linear regime are shown in Figure 2.49. If the enzyme is abundant, the acceleration due to the enzymatic catalysis depends on the concentration of the substrate and on the initial rate V_0. Thus, V_0 is a good measure of the enzymatic catalysis acceleration.

It is thus relevant to evaluate the initial P formation rate, that is, the reaction rate with $c_p = 0$, removing the linear approximation and assuming that the concentration of the enzyme is of the same order of magnitude of the concentration of the substrate. The total concentration of enzymatic molecules both recombined or free is in any instant equal to the initial enzyme concentration c_{E0}. Thus, we can write

$$c_{E0} = c_E + c_{ES} \tag{2.23}$$

The rate of ES formation is

$$v_f = v_+ \frac{c_E}{c_S} = v_+ \frac{c_{E0} - c_{ES}}{c_S} \tag{2.24}$$

while the rate of ES decomposition is

$$v_d = v_- c_{ES} + v_2 c_{ES} = (v_- + v_2)c_{ES} \tag{2.25}$$

Owing to the fact that the derivative of c_{ES} is zero the rates in the opposite directions have to be the same. Equaling Equations 2.24 and 2.25 and grouping all the rates on the right we have

$$\frac{c_T - c_{ES}}{c_{ES}} c_S = \frac{v_- + v_2}{v_+} \tag{2.26}$$

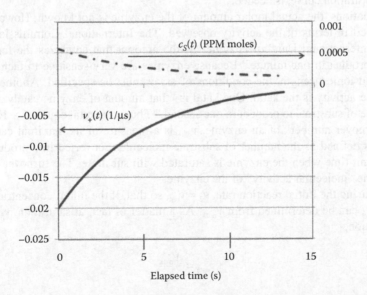

FIGURE 2.49 Substrate concentration and reaction rate versus time in the hypothesis that the enzyme concentration is much greater than the substrate concentration (linearized reaction model).

The constants $K_m = (v_- + v_2)/v_+$ is called the Michaelis constant. Owing to Equation 2.26 K_m is characteristic of each given reaction and has the units of a concentration. The initial ratio v_{p0} of formation of P is proportional through the corresponding rate v_2 to c_{ES}. Thus, calculating C_{ES} from Equation 2.26 and multiplying by v_2 we get

$$v_{p0} = \frac{v_2 c_T c_S}{K_m + c_S}$$ (2.27)

The product $v_2 c_T$ has a precise physical meaning. When c_S is high enough to saturate all of the enzyme, the velocity of the reaction, v_{p0}, is maximal. At saturation, the amount of ES complex is equal to the total enzyme concentration, c_T and initial rate of formation of P is $V_{max} = v_2 c_T$. Substituting this relationship into the expression for v_{p0} we obtain the original form of the Michaelis–Menten equation

$$v_{p0} = \frac{V_{max}}{K_m + c_S} c_S$$ (2.28)

from which we also immediately obtain a condition for the linearization of the process that is $K_m \gg c_S$.

Equation 2.28 depends only by two reaction-dependent constants, K_m and V_{max}, besides the concentration of substrate. Experimental values of the Michaelis constant for various human enzymes are presented in Table 2.7.

The Michaelis–Menten equation describes a curve known from analytical geometry as a *rectangular hyperbola*. In such curves, as c_S is increased, v_{p0} approaches the limiting value, V_{max}, in an asymptotic fashion. Experimentally, V_{max} can be approximated from a substrate saturation curve, and K_m can be derived setting $c_S = V_{max}/2$, so the two constants of the Michaelis–Menten equation can be obtained, in principle, by simply observing the asymptote of a curve like those reported in Figure 2.48.

If an accurate measure has to be performed, a statistical fitting of the two unknown parameters, for example, with a maximum likelihood method [52] starting from a certain number of measured points of the saturation curve, is needed.

In many situations, the actual molar amount of the enzyme is not known. However, its amount can be expressed in terms of the activity observed. The International Commission on Enzymes defines "One International Unit" of enzyme "as the amount that catalyzes the formation of one micromole of product in one minute." Because enzymes are very sensitive to factors such as pH, temperature and ionic strength, the conditions of assay must be specified. Another definition for units of enzyme activity is the katal. One katal is "that amount of enzyme catalyzing the conversion of one mole of substrate to product in one second." Thus, one katal equals 6×10^7 international units. The "turnover number" of an enzyme, v_{cat}, is a measure of its maximal catalytic activity. The turnover is defined as the number of substrate molecules converted into product per enzyme molecule per unit time when the enzyme is saturated with substrate. The turnover number is also referred to as the "molecular activity" of the enzyme.

When measuring the initial reaction rate, $v_2 = v_{cat}$, so that, if the initial concentration of enzyme c_T is known, v_{cat} can be determined from V_{max}. As a matter of fact, at saturation, $v_{p0} = V_{max} = v_2 c_T$. Thus, at saturation,

$$v_{cat} = \frac{V_{max}}{c_T}$$ (2.29)

The term v_{cat} represents the kinetic efficiency of the enzyme. Table 2.8 lists turnover numbers for some representative enzymes. Catalase has the highest turnover number known; each molecule

TABLE 2.7
Experimental Values of the Michaelis Constant for Various Human Enzymes

Enzyme	Substrate	K_m(mM)
Carbonic anhydrase	CO_2	12
Chymotrypsin	N-Benzoyltyrosinamide	2.5
	Acetyl-L-tryptophanamide	5
	N-Formyltyrosinamide	12
	N-Acetyltyrosinamide	32
	Glycyltyrosinamide	122
Hexokinase	Glucose	0.15
	Fructose	1.5
β-Galactosidase	Lactose	4
Glutamate dehydrogenase	NH_4^+	57
	Glutamate	0.12
	α-Ketoglutarate	2
	NAD^+	0.025
	NADH	0.018
Aspartate aminotransferase	Aspartate	0.9
	α-Ketoglutarate	0.1
	Oxaloacetate	0.04
	Glutamate	4
Threonine deaminase	Threonine	5
Arginyl-tRNA synthetase	Arginine	0.003
	RNA^{Arg}	0.0004
	ATP	0.3
Pyruvate carboxylase	HCO_3^-	1.0
	Pyruvate	0.4
	ATP	0.06
Penicillinase	Benzylpenicillin	0.05
Lysozyme	Hexa-N-acetylglucosamine	0.006

Source: Bender M. L., *The Bioorganic Chemistry of Enzymatic Catalysis*. August 23, 1984. 1st edition. Copyright Wilcy-VCH Verlag GmbH & Co. KGaA. Reproduced with permission.

TABLE 2.8
Values of the Enzyme Turnover for Representative Enzymes (in 1/s)

Enzyme	v_{cat} (s^{-1})
Catalase	4×10^7
Carbonic anhydrase	10^6
Acetylcholinesterase	1.4×10^4
Penicillinase	2×10^3
Lactate dehydrogenase	1×10^3
Chymotrypsin	100
DNA polymerase I	15
Lysozyme	0.5

Source: Bender M. L., *The Bioorganic Chemistry of Enzymatic Catalysis*. August 23, 1984. 1st edition. Copyright Wiley-VCH Verlag GmbH & Co. KGaA. Reproduced with permission; Morokuma K., Musaev G. D., *Computational Modeling for Homogeneous and Enzymatic Catalysis: A Knowledge-Base for Designing Efficient Catalysts*, March 25, 2008, 1st edition. ISBN-13: 978-3527318438. Copyright Wiley-VCH Verlag GmbH & Co. KGaA. Reproduced with permission.

TABLE 2.9

Kinetic Parameters of Selected Enzymes

Enzyme	Substrate	v_{cat} (s^{-1})	K_m (mol)	v_{cat}/K_m (s^{-1}mol^{-1})
Acetylcholinesterase	Acetylcholine	1.4×10^4	9×10^{-5}	1.6×10^8
Carbonic anhydrase	CO_2	1×10^6	0.012	8.3×10^7
	HCO_3^-	4×10^5	0.026	1.5×10^7
Catalase	H_2O_2	4×10^7	1.1	4×10^7
Crotonase	Crotonyl-CoA	5.7×10^3	2×10^{-5}	2.8×10^8
Fumarase	Fumarate	800	5×10^{-6}	1.6×10^8
	Malate	900	2.5×10^{-5}	3.6×10^7
Triosephosphate isomerase	Glyceraldehyde-3-phosphate*	4.3×10^3	1.8×10^{-5}	2.4×10^8
β-Lactamase	Benzylpenicillin	2×10^3	2×10^{-5}	1×10^8

Source: Bender M. L., *The Bioorganic Chemistry of Enzymatic Catalysis*. August 23, 1984. 1st edition. Copyright Wiley-VCH Verlag GmbH & Co. KGaA. Reproduced with permission; Fersht A., *Enzyme Structure and Mechanism*, W. H. Freeman & Co; 2nd edition (January 1985), ISBN-13: 978-0716716143.

of this enzyme can degrade 40 million molecules of H_2O_2 in 1 s. At the other end of the scale, lysozyme requires 2 s to cleave a glycoside bond in its glycan substrate.

Under physiological conditions, c_S is seldom saturating, the in vivo ratio of c_S/K_m usually falls in the range of 0.01–1.0, and v_{cat} itself, referring to the saturation condition, is not particularly informative. Nevertheless, we can derive a meaningful index of the efficiency of enzymes under in vivo conditions by noting that, in the quasi-linear condition, the concentration of the free enzyme molecules is approximately equal to its total concentration c_T and $c_S/K_m \ll 1$.

Using the equation $v_2 = v_{cat}$ and these approximations in the Michaelis–Menten equation in the form (2.27) we get

$$v_{p0} = \frac{v_{cat}}{K_m} c_E c_S \qquad (2.30)$$

That is, v_{cat}/K_m behave as a sort of second-order rate constant for the reaction of E and S to form a product. Because K_m is inversely proportional to the affinity of the enzyme for its substrate v_{cat} and is directly proportional to the kinetic efficiency of the enzyme, v_{cat}/K_m provides an index of the catalytic efficiency of an enzyme operating at substrate concentrations substantially below saturation amounts.

Table 2.9 [50,53] lists the kinetic parameters of several enzymes in this category. Note that v_{cat} and K_m show a substantial range of variation in this table, even though their ratio falls around 10^8 mol/s.

2.5.3 DEPENDENCY OF ENZYME KINETICS ON ENZYME TYPE AND ENVIRONMENT

2.5.3.1 Allosteric Enzymes

There is a category of enzymes, called allosteric enzymes, that do not follow the Michaelis–Menten equation, due to the fact that they are not simple catalysts, but perform a more complex role. Allosteric enzymes are enzymes that change their conformational ensemble upon binding an affine molecule at a determined binding site, which results in an apparent change in binding affinity at a different ligand binding site.

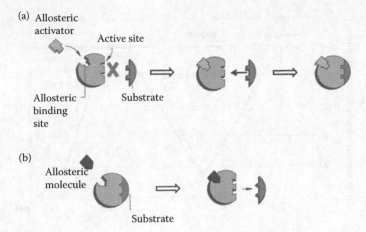

FIGURE 2.50 Allosteric effect in enzyme catalysis: effectors allosteric molecules (a) acts increasing the enzyme affinity to the substrate so that binding is enabled by the allosteric molecule presence; release allosteric molecules (b) allows a controlled quantity of the intermediate composite to decay when the enzyme binds with the allosteric molecule.

The property that the binding or free state of an active molecule site influences the affinity of a distant site for a different ligand, is the essence of the allosteric concept [54,55]. The allosteric effect allows allosteric enzymes to work not only as catalysis, but also as reaction controllers.

The binding sites affine molecules can be classified as effectors and substrates. In some cases, the same enzyme works also as effectors with a binding of two equal molecules, in other cases the effector is another, generally small, molecule. When the effector binds to the effector active site, the activity of the substrate binding site increases greatly so to increase the probability that a substrate molecule is bonded to the substrate binding site. In this way, small changes in the concentration of effectors regulates the active enzymes concentration and regulates the reaction kinetic.

Allosteric effect can drive reaction regulation also using different mechanisms, in any case related to the effect of binding another molecule to a binding site far from the substrate binding site. As an example, in few cases the binding energy of the intermediate composite ES is so strong that it results in more favorable of the reaction product P. In these cases, the enzyme very effectively binds to the substrate by forming a stable composite that does not decay. When a release allosteric element is bonded to the enzyme the substrate binding energy decreases causing the composite ES to decay so as to form the product P. In this way, the amount of composite P produced by the reaction is controlled by the amount of release allosteric element that is present. The effect of effectors allosteric molecules and release allosteric molecules is schematically described in Figure 2.50a and b.

Allosteric effect plays a crucial role in many fundamental biological processes, including cell signaling and the regulation of metabolism.

2.5.3.2 Effect of pH on Enzymatic Activity

ES recognition and the following catalytic effect are greatly dependent on pH. An enzyme possesses an array of ionizable side chains that not only determine its secondary and tertiary structure but may also be intimately involved in its active site. Further, the substrate itself often has ionizing groups, and one or another of the ionic forms may preferentially interact with the enzyme. Enzymes, in general, are active only over a limited pH range and most have a particular pH at which their catalytic activity is optimal [55,56].

Changes in pH may affect K_m or V_{max} or both. Figure 2.51 illustrates the relative activity of four enzymes as a function of pH. Although the optimum pH of an enzyme often reflects the pH of its

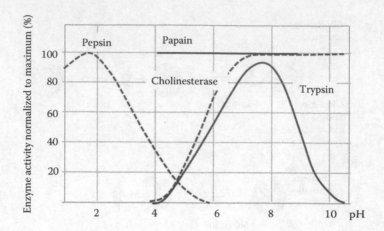

FIGURE 2.51   The pH activity profiles of four different enzymes. Trypsin, an intestinal protease, has a slightly alkaline pH optimum, whereas pepsin, a gastric protease, acts in the acidic confines of the stomach and has a pH optimum near 2. Papain, a protease found in papaya, is relatively insensitive to pHs between 4 and 8. Cholinesterase activity is pH-sensitive below pH 7 but not between pH 7 and 10. (Rosenthal M. D., *Medical Biochemistry: Human Metabolism in Health and Disease*. March 30, 2009. 1st edition. Copyright Wiley-VCH Verlag GmbH & Co. KGaA. Reproduced with permission; McGrath B. M., Walsh G., *Directory of Therapeutic Enzymes*, CRC Press; 1st edition (August 12, 2005), ISBN-13: 978-0849327148.)

normal environment, the optimum may not be precisely the same. This difference suggests that the pH-activity response of an enzyme may be a factor in the intracellular regulation. Optimum pH for selected enzymes is reported in Table 2.10.

2.5.3.3   Effect of Temperature on Enzymatic Activity

Like most chemical reactions, the rates of enzyme-catalyzed reactions generally increase with increasing temperature. However, at temperatures above 50–60°C, enzymes typically show a decline in activity, as it is qualitatively shown in Figure 2.52. Two effects determine this behavior: the increase in reaction rate and the thermal denaturation of protein structure.

Most enzymatic reactions double in rate for every 10°C rise in temperature as long as the enzyme is stable and fully active. The increasing rate with increasing temperature is ultimately offset by the instability of the protein structure at elevated temperatures, where the enzyme is inactivated.

TABLE 2.10
Optimum pH for Selected Enzymes

Enzyme	Optimum pH
Pepsin	1.5
Catalase	7.6
Trypsin	7.7
Fumarase	7.8
Ribonuclease	7.8
Arginase	9.7

Source: Bender M. L., *The Bioorganic Chemistry of Enzymatic Catalysis*. August 23, 1984. 1st edition. Copyright Wiley-VCH Verlag GmbH & Co. KGaA. Reproduced with permission; McGrath B. M., Walsh G., Directory of Therapeutic Enzymes, CRC Press; 1st edition (August 12, 2005), ISBN-13: 978-0849327148.

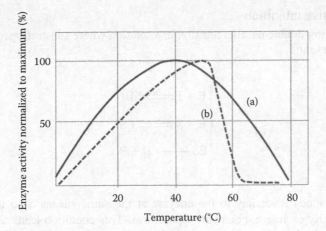

FIGURE 2.52 The effect of temperature on enzyme activity. Curves (a) and (b) correspond to different enzymes: in curve (a) a very complex enzyme is considered, whose denaturation with temperature happens progressively, while curve (b) refers to an enzyme with a much sharped denaturation threshold temperature.

The threshold temperature at which the maximum activity is achieved and denaturation starts to drive the decrease of enzyme activity is quite different for different enzymes. Many human and mammalian enzymes have the maximum activity to a temperature of the order of 40–45°C, but, for example, the enzymes of thermophilic bacteria found in geothermal springs retain full activity at temperatures in excess of 85°C.

2.5.4 ENZYME INHIBITION

Enzyme inhibition, that is, the action of chemical substances whose role is to prevent the catalysis action of enzymes, is also a frequent process both in nature and in artificial chemistry. In nature, several diseases are caused by pathogens that inhibit the action of key enzymes in the human body [56–58]. Enzymes inhibition is, on the other side, also a mechanism exploited by drugs to combat pathogens action when either they are enzymes catalyzed or in other ways exploit the enzymes action [59,60].

Enzyme inhibitors are classified in several ways. The inhibitor may interact either reversibly or irreversibly with the enzyme. Reversible inhibitors interact with the enzyme through noncovalent association–dissociation reactions. In contrast, irreversible inhibitors usually cause stable, covalent alterations in the enzyme.

Reversible inhibitors fall into two major categories: competitive and noncompetitive, although other more unusual and rare categories are known.

Competitive inhibitors are characterized by the fact that the substrate and inhibitor compete for the same binding site on the enzyme. Thus, increasing the concentration of S favors the likelihood of S binding to the enzyme instead of the inhibitor, I. That is, high c_S can overcome the effects of I.

Noncompetitive inhibition is generated by effects intrinsically lowering the enzyme activity, thus it cannot be overcome by increasing the substrate concentration.

The two types can be distinguished by the particular patterns obtained when the kinetic data are analyzed. A general formulation for common inhibitor interactions in the enzyme kinetic model would include, besides the enzymatic catalyzed reaction, the inhibitor related reaction in the form

$$E + I \rightleftharpoons EI \tag{2.31a}$$

$$ES + I \rightleftharpoons ESI \tag{2.31b}$$

2.5.4.1 Competitive Inhibition

Consider the following double parallel reaction in a solution where substrate, product, enzyme (E), and inhibitor are present:

$$
\begin{cases}
\mathrm{E + I} \underset{v_{i-}}{\overset{v_{i+}}{\rightleftharpoons}} \mathrm{EI} \\
\mathrm{E + S} \underset{v_{-}}{\overset{v_{+}}{\rightleftharpoons}} \mathrm{ES} \\
\mathrm{ES} \xrightarrow{v_2} \mathrm{E + P}
\end{cases}
\tag{2.32}
$$

where an inhibitor binds reversibly to the enzyme at the same site as S so that S-binding and I-binding are mutually exclusive, competitive processes. This condition leads us to anticipate that S and I must share a high degree of structural similarity because they bind at the same site on the enzyme. Also notice that, in our model, EI does not react to give rise to E + P. That is, I is not changed by interaction with E.

It is interesting to compare the equation for the uninhibited case, the Michaelis–Menten equation, with the equation for the rate of the enzymatic reaction in the presence of a fixed concentration of the competitive inhibitor, that can be deduced in a similar way and results to be

$$
v_{p0} = \frac{V_{\max} c_S}{c_S + K_m (1 + (c_I / K_I))}
\tag{2.33}
$$

The K_m term in the denominator in the inhibited case is increased by the factor$(1 + (c_I/K_I))$; thus,v_{p0} decreases in the presence of the inhibitor, as expected.

Figure 2.53 shows an initial ratio plot in the presence of competitive inhibition while Figure 2.54 presents the dependence of the initial reaction ratio on the inhibitor concentration.

When c_S becomes infinite, $v_{p0} = V_{\max}$, unaffected by I because all of the enzyme is in the ES form. The value $K_m(1 + (c_I/K_I))$ is often termed the *apparent* K_m(or K_{mapp}) because it is the K_m apparent under these conditions.

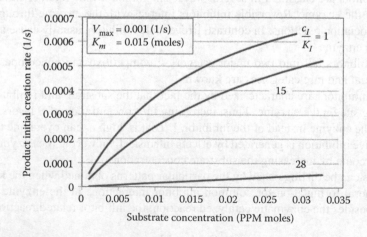

FIGURE 2.53 Starting product creation rate versus the substrate concentration in the presence of a competitive enzyme inhibitor.

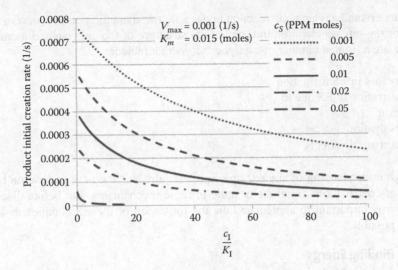

FIGURE 2.54 Starting product creation rate versus the competitive enzyme inhibitor normalized concentration for different values of the substrate concentration.

2.5.5 ENZYMATIC CATALYSIS THERMODYNAMICS

Enzyme-catalyzed reactions are typically 10^7–10^{14} times faster than their uncatalyzed counterparts as shown in Table 2.11. These large rate accelerations correspond to substantial changes in the free energy of activation for the reaction in question. The urease reaction, for example, that writes

$$H_2N - \overset{\overset{O}{\parallel}}{C} - NH_2 + 2H_2O + H^+ \rightarrow 2NH_4^+ + HCO_3^- \tag{2.34}$$

shows an energy of activation of about 84 kJ/mol smaller than the corresponding uncatalyzed reaction.

TABLE 2.11

Increase of Initial Reaction Speed by Enzyme Action with Respect to the Base Reaction without Catalysis

Reaction	Enzyme	Uncatalyzed Rate, v_u (s^{-1})	Catalyzed Rate, v_e (s^{-1})	v_e/v_u
$CH_3 - O - PO_3^{2-} + H_2O \rightarrow CH_3OH + HPO_4^{2-}$	Alkaline phosphatase	1×10^{-15}	14	1.4×10^{16}
$H_2N - \overset{\overset{O}{\parallel}}{C} - NH_2 + 2H_2O + H^+ \rightarrow 2NH_4^+ + HCO_3^-$	Urease	3×10^{-10}	3×10^4	1×10^{14}
$Glycogen_n + P_i \rightarrow Glycogen_{n-1} + Glucose\text{-}1\text{-}P$	Glycogen phosphorylase	$<5 \times 10^{-15}$	1.6×10^{-3}	$>3.2 \times 10^{11}$
$Glucose + ATP \rightarrow Glucose\text{-}6\text{-}P + ADP$	Hexokinase	$<1 \times 10^{-13}$	1.3×10^{-3}	$<1.3 \times 10^{10}$
$CO_2 + H_2O \rightarrow HCO_3^- + H^+$	Carbonic anhydrase	10^{-2}	10^5	1×10^7
$Creatine + ATP \rightarrow Cr\text{-}P + ADP$	Creatine kinase	$<3 \times 10^{-9}$	4×10^{-5}	$>1.33 \times 10^4$

Source: Adapted from Chang, *Handbook of Neurotoxicology (Neurological Disease and Therapy)*, Informa Healthcare; 1st edition (January 17, 1995), ISBN-13: 978-0824788735; Griffin J. P. Editor, *The Textbook of Pharmaceutical Medicine*, BMJ Books; 6th edition (December 15, 2009), ISBN-13: 978-1405180351; Koshland, D., *Journal of Cellular Comparative Physiology*, Supp. 1, pp. 217–224, 1956.

To fully understand any enzyme reaction under a thermodynamic point of view, it is important to account for the rate acceleration in terms of the structure of the enzyme and its mechanism of action. There are a limited number of catalytic factors that include:

- Entropy loss in ES formation
- Destabilization of ES due to
  - Strain
  - Desolvation
  - Electrostatic effects

A thorough understanding of any enzyme would require that the net acceleration be accounted for in terms of contributions from one or more of these mechanisms. But before discussing these mechanisms it is important to appreciate how the formation of the ES complex makes all these mechanisms possible.

2.5.5.1 ES Binding Energy

There are a number of important contributions to the free energy difference between the uncomplexed enzyme and substrate (E + S) and the ES complex, as shown in Figure 2.55. The favorable interactions between the substrate and amino acid residues on the enzyme account for the intrinsic binding energy, ΔG_b. The intrinsic binding energy ensures the favorable formation of the ES complex, but, if uncompensated, it makes the activation energy for the enzyme-catalyzed reaction unnecessarily large. As an example compare the two cases reported in Figure 2.56. Because the enzymatic reaction rate is determined by the difference in energies between ES and EX, the smaller this difference, the faster the enzyme-catalyzed reaction. Tight binding of the substrate with the enzyme deepens the energy well of the ES complex and actually lowers the rate of the reaction.

In the extreme case, catalysis does not occur if the ES complex and the transition state for the reaction are stabilized to equal extents, as in part (a) of Figure 2.56. Differently, catalysis will occur if the transition state is stabilized to a greater extent than the ES complex as in part (b) of Figure 2.56.

2.5.5.2 Entropy Loss and Destabilization of the ES Complex

Raising the energy of ES will increase the enzyme-catalyzed reaction rate. This can be accomplished both because the entropy of the complex ES is lower than those of the final state or because

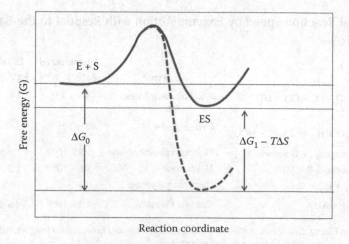

FIGURE 2.55 Compensation of the binding energy of the ES complex (ΔG_b) by entropy loss ($T\Delta S$) and by destabilization of ES (ΔG_d). Dashed line reports the formation of ES dynamics without free energy compensation mechanisms.

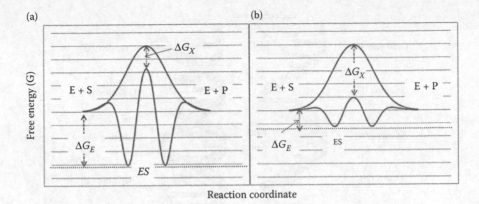

FIGURE 2.56 Effect of binding energy of the compose ES on the catalysis effect; catalysis does not occur if the ES complex and the transition state are stabilized to equal extents (a) while it occurs if the transition state is stabilized to a greater extent than the ES (b).

ES is destabilized by other configuration related or chemical effects. The entropy loss arises from the fact that the ES complex is a highly organized entity compared to E + S in solution. Molecules in solution generally increases their entropy due to the greater number of available configurations while entry of the substrate into the active site of the enzyme brings all the reacting groups and coordinating residues of the enzyme together with the substrate in just the proper position for reaction, with a net loss of entropy.

Destabilization of the ES complex can also involve structural strain, desolvation, or electrostatic effects. Destabilization by strain or distortion is usually just a consequence of the fact that the enzyme is designed to bind the transition state more strongly than the substrate. When the substrate binds, the imperfect nature of the fit results in distortion or strain in the substrate molecule, in the enzyme molecule, or both. This effect increases the energy needed to create the bond of the amount of energy needed to create deformation with respect to the minimum molecule energy configuration, so increasing the formation energy of ES.

Destabilization may also involve desolvation of charged groups on the substrate upon binding in the active site. Charged groups are highly stabilized in water. For example, the transfer of Na^+ and Cl^- from the gas phase to aqueous solution is characterized by a high enthalpy of solvation, namely −775 kJ/mol. When charged groups on a substrate move from water into an enzyme active site they are often desolvated to some extent, becoming less stable and therefore more reactive.

Moreover, when a substrate enters the active site, charged groups may be forced to interact with charges of the same sign. Also, in this case, energy has to be expended to counteract electrostatic repulsion and the free energy of formation of ES increases.

2.6 NUCLEIC ACIDS

The term nucleic acid is the overall name for deoxyribonucleic acids (DNA) and ribonucleic acids (RNA), two families of biopolymers [62,63] collectively called polynucleotides. Nucleic acids were named for their initial discovery within the nucleus, and for the presence of phosphate groups (related to phosphoric acid). Although first discovered within the nucleus of eukaryotic cells, nucleic acids are now known to be found in all life forms, including within Bacteria, Archaea, mitochondria, chloroplasts, viruses, and viroids.

Nucleic acids can vary in size, but are generally very large molecules. DNA molecules are probably the largest individual molecules known. Well-studied biological nucleic acid molecules range in size from 21 nucleotides (small interfering RNA) to large chromosomes (human chromosome 1 is a single molecule that contains 247 million base pairs [64]).

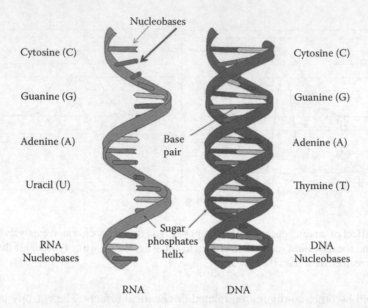

FIGURE 2.57 Graphical representation of the structure of a single-stranded RNA section and a double-stranded DNA section. The elementary bases that form the inner structure of these molecules are also reported.

In most cases, naturally occurring DNA molecules are double-stranded while RNA molecules are single stranded. A pictorial representation of such molecules' structure is presented in Figure 2.57, in which the elementary bases that compose the inner structure of DNA and RNA are also indicated. There are numerous exceptions, however: some viruses have genomes made of double-stranded RNA and other viruses have single-stranded DNA genomes (see Section 2.2.3) and, in some circumstances, nucleic acid structures with three or four strands can be formed.

Nucleic acids are linear polymers of nucleotides, whose structure formula and stereographic representations are depicted in Figure 2.58. Each nucleotide consists of three components: a nucleobase, a pentose sugar, and a phosphate group. The substructure consisting of a nucleobase plus sugar is termed a nucleoside.

Nucleic acid types differ in the structure of the sugar in their nucleotides–DNA contains 2′-deoxyribose while RNA contains ribose, where the only difference is the presence of a hydroxyl group. The nucleobases found in the two nucleic acid types are also different: adenine, cytosine, and guanine are found in both RNA and DNA, while thymine occurs in DNA and uracil occurs in RNA, as shown in Figure 2.57.

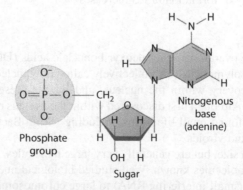

FIGURE 2.58 Nucleotide structure formula; adenine is represented as example of nucleobase.

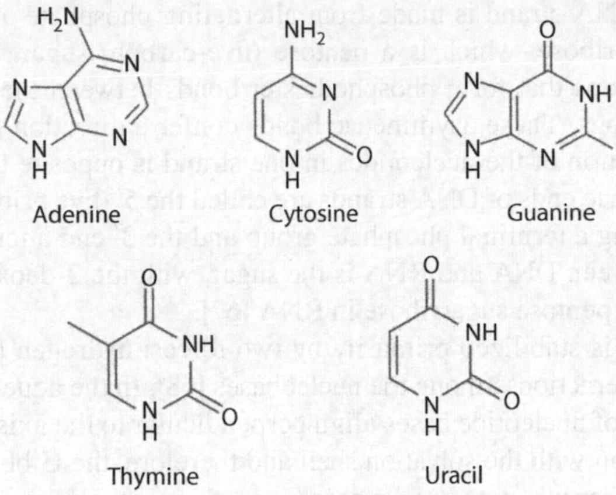

Adenine   Cytosine   Guanine

Thymine   Uracil

FIGURE 2.59 Structure formulas of the five nucleobases that are normally present in nucleic acids.

The nucleobases are classified into two families on the ground of the type of heterocyclic compounds they contain, that is, the kind of aromatic rings where one or more carbon is substituted by other atoms. In particular, the purines A and G present a structure containing connected five- and six-membered heterocyclic compounds, while the pyrimidines, C, T, and U present only a six-membered ring. The structure formulas of the five standard nucleobases are reported in Figure 2.59. Nonstandard nucleosides are also found in both RNA and DNA and usually arise from modification of the standard nucleosides. Transfer RNA (tRNA) molecules contain a particularly large number of modified nucleosides [65].

2.6.1 Deoxyribonucleic Acid

Deoxyribonucleic acid is a nucleic acid containing the genetic instructions used in the development and functioning of all known living organisms, with the exception of RNA viruses. The DNA segments carrying a specific genetic information, for example, the information needed for the synthesis of a protein or of an RNA strand, are called genes. Other DNA sequences have structural purposes, or are involved in regulating the use of this genetic information. Set of genes and structural sequences coding phenotypic characteristics, like hair color or blood type in human beings, are called alleles. Alleles composed by a single gene exist, as alleles formed by quite a number of genes.

Within cells, DNA is organized into long structures called chromosomes. A chromosome is an organized structure containing many genes, regulatory elements and other nucleotide sequences. Chromosomes also contain DNA-bound proteins, which serve to package the DNA and control its functions. During cell division, these chromosomes are duplicated in the process of DNA replication, providing each cell its own complete set of chromosomes.

Eukaryotic organisms (animals, plants, fungi, and protists) store most of their DNA inside the cell nucleus and some of their DNA in organelles, such as mitochondria or chloroplasts. In contrast, prokaryotes (Bacteria and Archaea) store their DNA only in the cytoplasm.

2.6.1.1 DNA General Structure

The structure of DNA of almost all species comprises two helical chains each coiled round the same axis, and each with a pitch of 34 Å and a radius of 10 Å. In living organisms DNA does not usually exist as a single molecule, but instead as a pair of molecules that are held tightly together [66,67]. These two long strands forms double helix, as depicted in Figure 2.57. The nucleotide repeats contain both the segment of the backbone of the molecule, which holds the chain together, and a nucleobase, which interacts with the other DNA strand in the helix.

The backbone of the DNA strand is made from alternating phosphate and sugar residues. The sugar in DNA is 2-deoxyribose, which is a pentose (five-carbon) sugar. The sugars are joined together by phosphate groups that form phosphodiester bonds between the third and fifth carbon atoms of adjacent sugar rings. These asymmetric bonds confer a direction to the DNA strand and in a double helix the direction of the nucleotides in one strand is opposite to their direction in the other strand. The asymmetric ends of DNA strands are called the 5′ (five prime) and 3′ (three prime) ends, with the 5′ end having a terminal phosphate group and the 3′ end a terminal hydroxyl group. One major difference between DNA and RNA is the sugar, with the 2-deoxyribose in DNA being replaced by the alternative pentose sugarribose in RNA [67].

The DNA double helix is stabilized primarily by two forces: hydrogen bonds between nucleotides and base-stacking interactions among the nucleobases [68]. In the aqueous environment of the cell, the conjugated bonds of nucleotide bases align perpendicular to the axis of the DNA molecule, minimizing their interaction with the solvation shell and therefore, the Gibbs free energy. The four bases found in DNA are adenine, cytosine, guanine, and thymine. Under an information point of view, the DNA can be seen as a message encoded into a sequence of characters from an alphabet of four elements. When this view is adopted, the four nucleobases are coded by their initial letters, C, G, A, and T, as presented in Figure 2.57. Using this code, a sequence on a DNA strand could be written as

$$\dots\dots\text{AAGCCTACCTGGTTA}\dots\dots \tag{2.35}$$

Since the nucleobases are bonded only in conjugate pairs, forming in particular the A–T and G–C pairs, the information contained on the second DNA strand is completely equivalent to that contained in the first one. The global chemical structure of a DNA double helix is represented in Figure 2.60, evidencing both backbone bonds and hydrogen bonds linking the base pairs.

Besides the main helicoid structure, another double helix may be found in the DNA structure by tracing the spaces, or grooves, between the strands as evidenced in Figure 2.61. These voids are adjacent to the base pairs and may provide a binding site. As the strands are not directly opposite

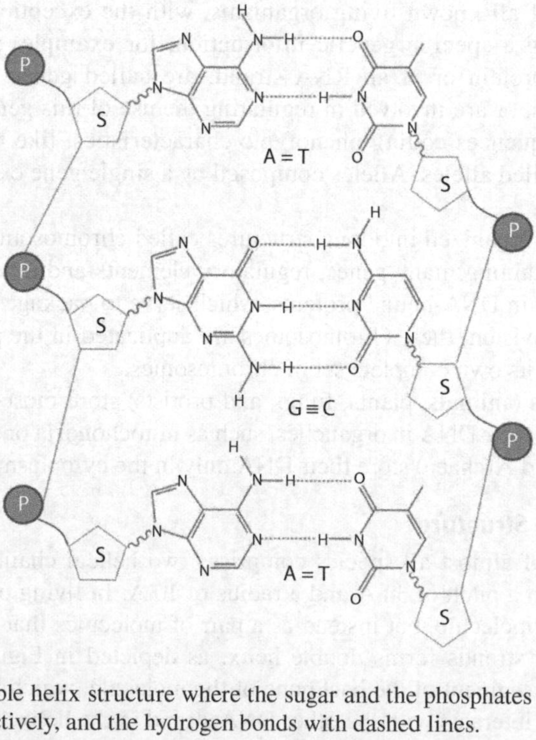

FIGURE 2.60 DNA double helix structure where the sugar and the phosphates in the backbone are represented with S and P, respectively, and the hydrogen bonds with dashed lines.

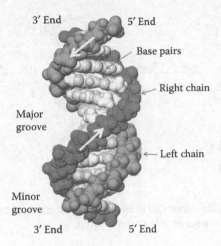

FIGURE 2.61 Major and minor grooves position: figure of eight formation as a consequence of the gain or the loss of a single helix twist.

each other, the grooves are unequally sized. One groove, the major groove, is 22 Å wide and the other, the minor groove, is 12 Å wide [69]. The narrowness of the minor groove means that the edges of the bases are more accessible in the major groove. As a result, proteins like transcription factors that can bind to specific sequences in double-stranded DNA usually make contacts to the sides of the bases exposed in the major groove [70].

This situation varies in unusual conformations of DNA within the cell (see below), but the major and minor grooves are always named to reflect the differences in size that would be seen if the DNA is twisted back into the ordinary B form.

2.6.1.2 DNA Supercoiling

In a relaxed double-helical segment of DNA, the two strands twist around the helical axis once every 10.4–10.5 base pairs. Adding or subtracting twists, as some enzymes can do, imposes strain to the structure. If a DNA segment under twist strain were closed into a circle by joining its two ends and then allowed to move freely, the circular DNA would contort into a new shape, such as a simple figure of eight. Such a contortion is a supercoil.

In practice, intermediate segments of a chromosome, due either to the chromosome dimension or to spatial constraints due, for example, to the presence of chromosome proteins, may act as if their ends were anchored. As a result, they may be unable to distribute excess twist to the rest of the chromosome or to absorb twist and may become supercoiled. In response to supercoiling, they will assume an amount of writhe, just as if their ends were fixed. Thus, DNA of most organisms is supercoiled.

The so-called figure of eight is the simplest supercoil, and is the shape a circular DNA assumes to accommodate one more or one less helical twist. The two lobes of the figure eight will appear rotated either clockwise or counterclockwise with respect to one another, depending on whether the helix is over or under twisted. This process is schematically shown in Figure 2.62. For each additional helical twist being accommodated, the lobes will show one more rotation about their axis.

In general, the number of writhes present in the topology of a DNA segment is defined as the number of times the helix crosses over itself; a number is also associated to each writhe: +1 for left or positive writhe and −1 for right or negative writhe. The global writhe number W is the sum of numbers associated to each writhe. Similarly, the number of twists that are present in a DNA segment is equal to the number of helix turns, to each twist +1 is associated if the twist is from left to right and −1 otherwise and the total twist number T of a DNA segment topology is defined as the sum of the numbers associated to each twist.

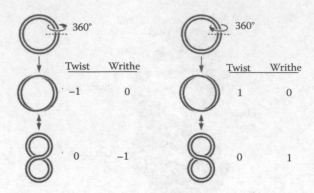

FIGURE 2.62 Simple supercoil formation due to addition or subtraction of an helical twist to a circular DNA topology: both positive and negative supercoils are considered.

If we consider the above definitions we can define for each DNA segment a base twist number T_0 equal to the twist number of the relaxed helix, while the writhe number for a relaxed helix is zero. The total supercoil SC of a DNA segment topology is then defined as

$$SC = T - T_0 + W \tag{2.36}$$

On the basis of this definition, subtracting twists creates a negative supercoil while adding them creates a positive supercoil.

Supercoiled DNA forms two main elementary structures or more complex combinations of them: a plectoneme or a toroid, whose schematic representations are reported in Figure 2.63. A negatively supercoiled DNA molecule will produce either a one-start left-handed helix, the toroid, or a two-start right-handed helix with terminal loops, the plectoneme. Plectonemes are typically more common in nature for small DNAs like those found in bacteria. For larger molecules it is common for hybrid structures to form a loop on a toroid can extend into a plectoneme. If all the loops on a toroid extend then it becomes a branch point in the plectonemic structure.

2.6.1.3 Genetic Code for Proteins Synthesis

The information code into the DNA is used to code all the processes happening in a living organism and needed to sustain its life. Proteins production is a particularly important class of such processes, due to the importance of proteins in the biological mechanism. Since a protein is essentially a sequence of 20 base amino acids, the codes driving protein synthesis inside the cell is a transcription of the amino acid sequence characterizing the protein. When the protein is produced in the controlled chemical environment inside the cell, the amino acids chain will configure in the correct stereographic structure driven by the need of minimizing the molecule free energy so as to constitute a functional biomolecule [66,67].

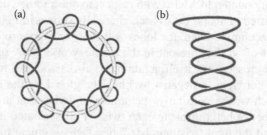

FIGURE 2.63 Schemes of torus (a) and plectomene (b) supercoil structures.

In eukaryotes, proteins are synthesized into the ribosomes, the specialized cell organelles. Even if the process is quite complex, in a first approximation it can be described as follows. The sequence of amino acids encoded in a DNA gene is translated into an mRNA that is used by the ribosome to assemble the correct sequence of amino acids while they are conveyed to the synthesis site by tRNA. Due to the specific role different types of RNA have in protein synthesis, the process will be analyzed in better detail in Section 2.5.3.1.

A DNA sequence is called "sense" if its sequence is the same as that of an mRNA copy that is translated into proteins. The sequence on the opposite strand is called the "antisense" sequence. Both sense and antisense sequences can exist on different parts of the same strand of DNA since it is composed by several genes coding different proteins.

A few DNA sequences in prokaryotes and eukaryotes, and more in viruses, blur the distinction between sense and antisense strands by having overlapping genes [67]. In these cases, some DNA sequences do double duty, encoding one protein when read along one strand, and a second protein when read in the opposite direction along the other strand.

Each amino acid is coded by a set of three nucleobases, called codon. Thus, the mRNA is read codon by codon during the protein synthesis. Specific codons, called START and STOP, are used to begin and to stop the synthesis. Since four nucleobases are available, there are 64 possible codons, so that each amino acid and the START and STOP signals are coded by more than one codon. The coding table used in protein synthesis is reported in Table 2.12.

TABLE 2.12
Protein Synthesis Genetic Code: Correspondence among Codons and Amino Acids

Amino Acid	Codons
Ala	GCT, GCC, GCA, GCG
Arg	CGT, CGC, CGA, CGG, AGA, AGG
Asn	AAT, AAC
Asp	GAT, GAC
Cys	TGT, TGC
Gln	CAA, CAG
Glu	GAA, GAG
Gly	GGT, GGC, GGA, GGG
His	CAT, CAC
Ile	ATT, ATC, ATA
Leu	TTA, TTG, CTT, CTC, CTA, CTG
Lys	AAA, AAG
Met	ATG
Phe	TTT, TTC
Pro	CCT, CCC, CCA, CCG
Ser	TCT, TCC, TCA, TCG, AGT, AGC
Thr	ACT, ACC, ACA, ACG
Trp	TGG
Tyr	TAT, TAC
Val	GTT, GTC, GTA, GTG
START	ATG
STOP	TAA, TGA, TAG

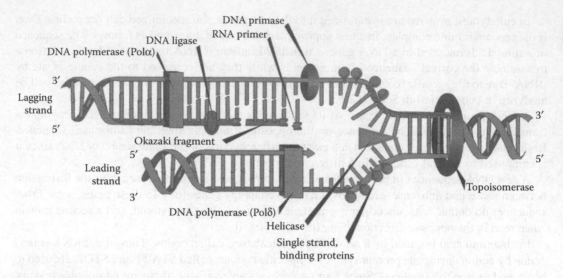

FIGURE 2.64 DNA replication process; the involved enzymes are indicated in correspondence of their role in the process.

2.6.1.4   DNA Replication

Cell division is essential for an organism to grow; when a cell divides, it must replicate the DNA in its genome so that the two daughter cells have the same genetic information as their parent. The double-stranded structure of DNA provides a mechanism for DNA replication, that is graphically shown in Figure 2.64.

Different enzymes participate in the process to accelerate and regulate it. First, the two DNA helixes are parallelized by an enzyme called topoisomerase, that changes the topological form of the double helix acting on the hydrogen bounds that causes the two helixes to turn one on the other. After the two DNA strands are parallelized, they are separated by interaction with another protein called helicase, so as to create two associated, but separated strands. The single strand is stabilized by binding it with single strand binding proteins, like protein A in humans, that prepare it for the successive phases of the replication process.

Owing to the complementary nature of the two strands, each of them carries all the DNA information and it can be used to create a barely new complete DNA.

The replication is carried out with two different processes for the two parent strands that during the replication are called leading strand and lagging strand. This is due to the fact that DNA polymerase (DNAase) can only extend a DNA strand in a 5′ to 3′ direction. In both the processes however, it is the old strand base that dictates which base appears on the new strand, so that a perfect copy of the original DNA is created in both cases.

The leading strand is replicated by assembly the needed material carried out by the RNA primer directly via DNA polymerase δ, that operating in the correct direction recreates the needed associate bases and positions them to recreate hydrogen bonds with the parent helix. Hydrogen bonds drive the helix–turn–helix tertiary DNA structure and a new DNA is formed.

As far as the lagging strand is created, an enzyme, called DNA primase, processes the parent helix so to allow the formation of a fragment of the complementary helix called Okazaki fragment. Okazaki fragments are united by another enzyme, called DNA ligase, so to allow to DNA polymerase to set up the hydrogen connection with the parent helix proceeding in the suitable direction.

2.6.1.5   DNA Interactions with Proteins

All the functions of DNA depend on interactions with proteins, as we have already seen in the above section. Several proteins are involved in the DNA replication, both enzymes and other kinds of proteins. Protein A, for example, is responsible in human beings to stabilize the single strand DNA and to prepare it for replication, while among the enzymes, DNA polymerase is responsible for the new DNA strand elongation during replication, as described in Section 2.5.1.4.

Both specific and nonspecific interactions between proteins and DNA exist, while in specific interaction the interacting protein binds to selected DNA sequences, in nonspecific interaction the protein can bind almost on all the parts of the backbone helix.

Examples of specific interaction between DNA and proteins are interaction with enzymes that drive, for example, the DNA replication process. Structural proteins that bind DNA are examples of nonspecific DNA–protein interactions.

Within chromosomes, DNA is held in complexes with structural proteins. These proteins organize the DNA into a compact structure called chromatin. In eukaryotes, this structure involves DNA binding to a complex of small basic proteins called histones, while in prokaryotes multiple types of proteins are involved [71,72]. The histones form a disk-shaped complex called a nucleosome, which contains two complete turns of double-stranded DNA wrapped around its surface. These nonspecific interactions are formed through basic residues in the histones making ionic bonds to the acidic sugar–phosphate backbone of the DNA, and are therefore largely independent of the base sequence [73]. These chemical changes alter the strength of the interaction between the DNA and the histones, making the DNA more or less accessible to transcription factors and changing the rate of transcription.

Other nonspecific DNA-binding proteins in chromatin include the high-mobility group proteins, which bind to bent or distorted DNA [http://en.wikipedia.org/wiki/DNA-cite_note-85]. These proteins are important in bending arrays of nucleosomes and arranging them into the larger structures that make up chromosomes [74].

2.6.2 RIBONUCLEIC ACID STRUCTURE

RNA differs from DNA in three main ways:

- Unlike double-stranded DNA, RNA is generally a single-stranded molecule in many of its biological roles and has a much shorter chain of nucleotides (for the exceptions in viruses see Section 2.2.3).
- While DNA contains deoxyribose, RNA contains ribose (in deoxyribose there is no hydroxyl group attached to the C_2 of pentose ring. This hydroxyl group makes RNA less stable than DNA because it is more prone to hydrolysis.
- The complementary base to adenine is not thymine, as it is in DNA, but rather uracil which is, an unmethylated form of thymine.

Most biologically active RNAs, including mRNA, tRNA, rRNA, snRNAs, and other noncoding RNAs, contain self-complementary sequences that allow parts of the RNA to fold and pair with itself to form double helices. Analysis of these RNAs has revealed that they are highly structured. Unlike DNA, their structures do not consist of long double helices but rather collections of short helices packed together into structures similar to proteins. An example of RNA stereographic structures are reported in Figure 2.65. In this fashion, RNAs can achieve chemical catalysis, like enzymes [75]. For instance, determination of the structure of the ribosome—an enzyme that catalyzes peptide bond formation—revealed that its active site is composed entirely of RNA [76].

Another important structural feature of RNA, consequence of the presence of a hydroxyl group in the ribose sugar, emerges when different parts of the same RNA strand or different RNA strands join to form a double helix. The double helix has a different shape with respect to that almost always adopted by DNA, exhibiting very deep and narrow major grooves and shallow and wide minor grooves [77]. A second consequence of the presence of the hydroxyl group is that in flexible regions of an RNA molecule that are not involved in the formation of a double helix, it can chemically attack the adjacent phosphodiester bond to cleave the backbone [78].

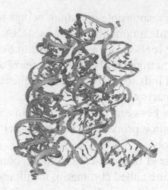

FIGURE 2.65 Example of stereographic structure of RNA. (Image from Wikimedia Commons, put in Public Domain by the author Miranker A D.)

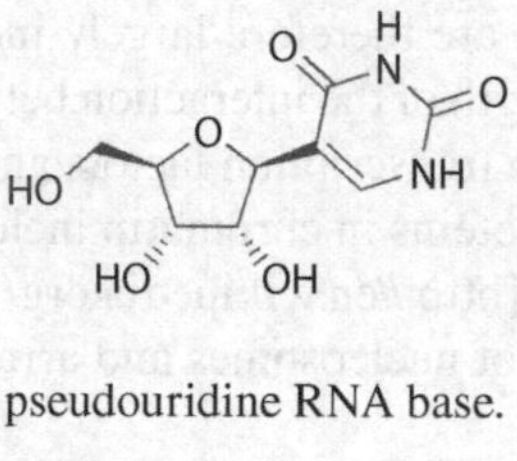

FIGURE 2.66 Structure formula of the pseudouridine RNA base.

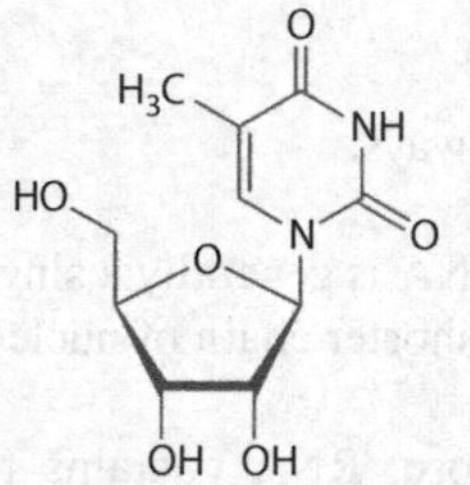

FIGURE 2.67 Structure formula of the ribothymidine RNA base.

However, other interactions are possible, such as a group of adenine bases binding to each other in a bulge [75], or the GNRA tetra-loop that has a guanine–adenine basepair [79,80].

RNA is generated with only four bases, but these bases and attached sugars can be modified in numerous ways as the RNAs mature, that is, while it is processed inside the cell that has produced it. Pseudouridine (Ψ) (see Figure 2.66), in which the linkage between uracil and ribose is changed from a C–N bond to a C–C bond, and ribothymidine (T) (see Figure 2.67) are found in various RNA types at different stages of their maturation [81]. There are nearly 100 other naturally occurring modified nucleosides, of which pseudouridine and nucleosides with 2′-O-methylribose are the most common [82]. The specific roles of many of these modifications in RNA are not fully understood. However, it is notable that, in ribosomal RNA, many of the post-transcriptional modifications occur in highly functional regions, such as the peptidyl transferase center, implying that they are important for normal function [83].

2.6.3 RNA TYPES AND ROLES

Messenger RNA (mRNA) is the RNA that carries information from DNA to the ribosome, the sites of protein synthesis, also called translation. The coding sequence of the mRNA determines the amino acid sequence in the protein that is produced. Many RNAs do not code for protein however: about 97% of the transcriptional output is nonproteincoding in eukaryotes. These so-called non-coding RNAs (ncRNA) can be encoded by their own genes (RNA genes), but can also derive from mRNA introns [63,67].

The most prominent examples of noncoding RNAs are transfer RNA (tRNA) and ribosomal RNA (rRNA), both of which are involved in the process of translation [67]. There are also noncoding RNAs involved in gene regulation, RNA processing and other roles. Certain RNAs are able to catalyze chemical reactions such as cutting and ligating other RNA molecules, and the catalysis of peptide bond formation in the ribosome; these are known as ribozymes.

2.6.3.1   RNA Role in Translation

Messenger RNA (mRNA) carries information about a protein sequence to the ribosomes, the protein synthesis factories in the cell. It is coded so that every three nucleotides (a codon) correspond to one amino acid. In eukaryotic cells, mRNA is not directly generated. Instead an immature form, called precursor mRNA (pre-mRNA) is transcribed from DNA, then it is fatherly processed to synthesize mature mRNA. This post-synthesis removes pre-mRNA introns, that are noncoding sections of the pre-mRNA, that are transcribed from the DNA besides the active section that will become the mature mRNA. After maturation, the mRNA is exported from the nucleus to the cytoplasm, where it is bound to ribosomes and translated into its corresponding protein form with the help of tRNA.

In prokaryotic cells, which do not have nucleus and cytoplasm compartments, mRNA can bind to ribosomes while it is being transcribed from DNA.

After a certain amount of time the mRNA degrades into its component nucleotides with the assistance of ribonucleases [84], the enzyme accelerating the decay reaction, so that new mRNA is always present in the cell, minimizing transcription errors due to unforeseen decay of an old molecule.

Transfer RNA (tRNA) is a small RNA chain of about 80 nucleotides that transfers a specific amino acid to a growing polypeptide chain at the ribosomal site of protein synthesis during translation. It has sites for amino acid attachment and an anticodon region for codon recognition that binds to a specific sequence on the mRNA chain through hydrogen bonding [84]. Thus, as graphically shown in Figure 2.68 the tRNA convey to the ribosome the material to grow the peptide chain in the form of amino acids and uses the mRNA as a model to assembly correctly the amino acids to form the desired peptide chain with the assistance of the ribosome environment. This translation is enabled

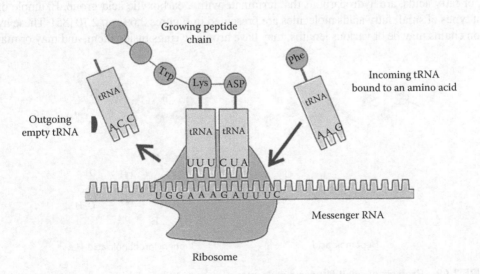

FIGURE 2.68   Protein synthesis in the ribosome by mRNA transcription in a new peptide chain.

by Ribosomal RNA (rRNA), that is, the engine that synthesize the ribosomes and also has a catalytic role inside the ribosomes themselves. Eukaryotic ribosomes contain four different rRNA molecules: 18S, 5.8S, 28S, and 5S rRNA. Nearly all the RNA found in a typical eukaryotic cell is rRNA.

2.6.3.2 Regulatory RNAs

Several types of RNA can downregulate gene expression by being complementary to a part of an mRNA or a gene's DNA. MicroRNAs (miRNA) that are 21–22 nucleotides long, are found in eukaryotes and act through RNA interference (RNAi), where an effector complex of miRNA and enzymes can cleave complementary mRNA, can block the mRNA so to avoid translation, or can accelerate its degradation [82,83].

Small interfering RNAs (siRNA), that are 20–25 nucleotids long, act through RNA interference in a fashion similar to miRNAs. Some miRNAs and siRNAs can cause genes they target to be methylated, thereby decreasing or increasing transcription of those genes. Many prokaryotes have CRISPR RNAs, a regulatory system similar to RNA interference.

2.7 LIPIDS

Lipids have a variety of biochemical roles [1,2]: lipids are widely used to store energy, they are key components of membranes and play a variety of roles in signal-transduction pathways. Unlike the three other classes of biomolecules (carbohydrates, amino acids, and nucleic acids), lipids do not form polymers.

Five classes of lipids can be individuated, different for their biological role and chemical structure:

- Free fatty acid, also called nonesterified fatty acids, commonly used to provide energy
- Triacylglycerols that mainly stores fatty acids
- Phospholipids that consist of fatty acids attached to a scaffold and are mainly used in membranes
- Glycolipids that are bound to carbohydrates and are important membrane constituents
- Steroids that differ from the other lipids in that they are polycyclic hydrocarbons and function as hormones that control a variety of physiological functions

2.7.1 FREE FATTY ACIDS

Fats, or fatty acids, are hydrocarbons that terminate with a carboxylic acid group. Example of different types of small fatty acids molecules are presented in Figures 2.69 and 2.70 [85]. These hydrocarbon chains may be of various lengths, may have aromatic rings inside them, and may or may not

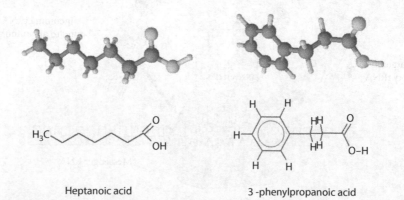

Heptanoic acid   3-phenylpropanoic acid

FIGURE 2.69 Example of small fatty acid molecules: a saturated linear fat is considered in (a) while a fat containing an aromatic ring is sketched in (b). UIPAC names are indicated for the molecules.

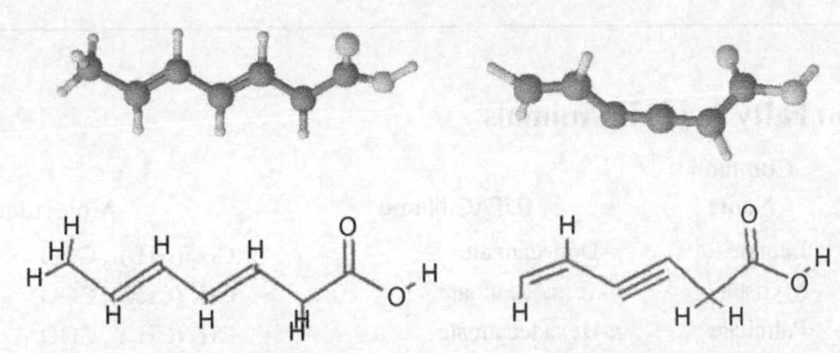

(3E,5E)-hepta-3,5-dienoic acid   (2R)-hexa-2,3,5-trienoic acid

FIGURE 2.70 Example of small fatty acid molecules: a linear fat with unsaturated double bonds is considered in (a) while a fat containing an unsaturated triple bond is sketched in (b). IUPAC names are indicated for the molecules.

present one or more double bonds, depending on the fat. Fatty acids with triple bonds exist in a few vegetables, but they are not so diffused as those presenting double bonds.

Two key roles for fatty acids are providing fuels and being building blocks for membrane-like cells or organelle membranes. Fats are good fuels because they are more reduced than carbohydrates; that is, the carbon atoms are bonded to hydrogen atoms and other carbon atoms rather than to oxygen atoms, as is the case for carbohydrates. Because of this greater reduction, fats yield more energy than carbohydrates when undergoing combustion to carbon dioxide and water.

Fats have almost all a common name, derived from naming use precedent to IUPAC conventions. Common names, however, can sometimes bring to confusion so that IUPAC has introduced a convention for systematic fats names. A fatty acid's systematic name is derived from the name of its parent hydrocarbon by the substitution of *oic* for the final *e*. For example, the saturated fatty acid known familiarly as stearic acid, is called octadecanoic acid because the parent hydrocarbon is octadecane. Fatty acids composed of single bonds only are called saturated fatty acids, coming from the correspondent saturated hydrocarbons (see Section 1.3.1); analogously fatty acids with one or more double or triple bonds are called unsaturated fatty acids. Oleic acid, a fatty acid with one double bond, is called octadecenoic acid; whereas linoleic acid, with two double bonds, is octadecadienoic acid; and linolenic acid, with three double bonds, is octadecatrienoic acid. The composition and structure of a fatty acid can also be designated by numbers. The notation 18:0 denotes a fatty acid with 18 carbon atoms with no double bonds, whereas 18:2 signifies that there are two double bonds.

When considering fatty acids, we often need to distinguish the individual carbon atoms. Fatty acid carbon atoms are numbered starting at the carboxyl terminus. Carbon atoms 2 and 3 are often referred to as α and β, respectively. The last carbon atom in the chain, which is almost always a methyl carbon atom, is called the ω-carbon atom. The position of a double bond is represented by the symbol Δ followed by a superscript number. For example, *cis*-Δ^9 means that there is a *cis* double bond between carbon atoms 9 and 10; *trans*-Δ^2 means that there is a *trans* double bond between carbon atoms 2 and 3. Just as in proteins, *cis* and *trans* designate the relative positions of substituents on either side of the double bond. Just like amino acids, fatty acids are ionized at physiological pH, and so it is preferable to refer to them according to their carboxylate form: for example, palmitate rather than palmitic acid.

Fatty acids in biological systems usually contain an even number of carbon atoms, typically between 14 and 24 with the 16- and 18-carbon fatty acids being the most common; the series of fatty acids with *n* carbon atoms is generally called C*n*, so that the fats with 18 carbons are called C18. The most common fatty acids in animals are listed in Table 2.13. The double bonds in polyunsaturated fatty acids are separated by at least one methylene group.

The physical properties of fatty acids and of lipids derived from them are dependent on chain length and degree of saturation. Unsaturated fatty acids have lower melting points than those of saturated fatty acids of the same length. For example, the melting point of stearic acid is 69.6°C, whereas that of oleic acid, which contains one double bond, is 13.4°C. The melting points of polyunsaturated

TABLE 2.13

The Most Common Fatty Acids in Animals

Carbons	Double Bonds	Common Name	IUPAC Name	Molecular Formula
12	0	Laurate	*n*-Dodecanoate	$CH_3 (CH_2)_{10} COO^-$
14	0	Myristate	*n*-Tetradecanoate	$CH_3 (CH_2)_{12} COO^-$
16	0	Palmitate	*n*-Hexadecanoate	$CH_3 (CH_2)_{14} COO^-$
18	0	Stearate	*n*-Octadecanoate	$CH_3 (CH_2)_{16} COO^-$
20	0	Arachidate	*n*-Eicosanoate	$CH_3 (CH_2)_{18} COO^-$
16	1	Palmitoleate	*cis*-Δ^9-Hexadecanoate	$CH_3 (CH_2)_5 CH{=}CH (CH_2)_7 COO^-$
18	1	Oleate	*cis*-Δ^9- Octadecanoate	$CH_3 (CH_2)_7 CH{=}CH (CH_2)_7 COO^-$
18	2	Linoleate	*cis, cis*-Δ^8- Δ^{12}- Octadecanoate	$CH_3 (CH_2)_4 (CH{=}CH\ CH_2)_2 (CH_2)_6 COO^-$

fatty acids of the C18 series are even lower. The presence of a double bond introduces a kink in the fatty acid and makes tight packing between the chains impossible. The lack of tight packing limits the van der Waals interactions between chains, lowering the melting temperature.

2.7.2 TRIACYLGLYCEROLS

Despite the fact that fatty acids are our principal energy source, the concentration of free fatty acids in cells or the blood is low because free fatty acids are strong acids. High concentrations of free fatty acids would disrupt the pH balance of the cells.

Fatty acids required for energy generation are stored in the form of triacylglycerols [86], which are formed by the attachment of three fatty acid chains to a glycerol molecule, as shown in Figure 2.71, where an example of triacylglycerol structure formula and stereographic model are presented. The fatty acids are attached to the glycerol through ester linkages, in a process known as esterification [2,86]. When energy is required the fatty acids are cleaved from the triacyglycerol and carried to the cells. The ingestion of food replenishes the triacylglycerol stores.

2.7.3 MEMBRANE LIPIDS

We have seen in Section 2.1 that lipids are not only energy providers for living organisms, but also constitutes the fundamental building block of cellular and organelles membranes [87–89].

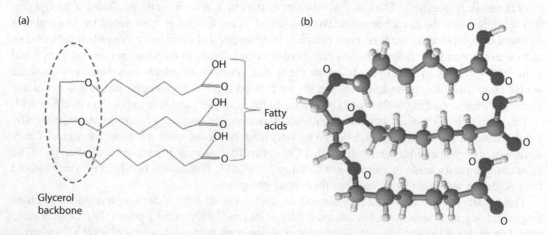

FIGURE 2.71 Example of triacylglycerol: (a) structure formula, (b) stereographic representation.

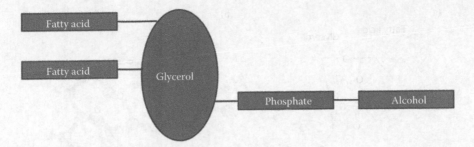

FIGURE 2.72   General structure of phospholipids.

The structure of a membrane is a complex one, and three main lipid types contribute to its main functionality, which is to insulate water solutions contained inside the membrane from water solutions of the outside environment: phospholipids, glycolipids, and cholesterol.

Phospholipids are abundant in all biological membranes. A phospholipid molecule, as shown in Figure 2.72 is constructed from four components: one or more fatty acids, a platform to which the fatty acids are attached, a phosphate, and an alcohol attached to the phosphate. The platform on which phospholipids are built may be glycerol, a three-carbon alcohol, or sphingosine, a more complex alcohol.

Phospholipids derived from glycerol are called phosphoglycerides and are composed of a glycerol backbone to which are attached two fatty acid chains and a phosphorylated alcohol. In phosphoglycerides, the hydroxyl groups at C-1 and C-2 of glycerol are esterified to the carboxyl groups of the two fatty acid chains. The C-3 hydroxyl group of the glycerol backbone is esterified to phosphoric acid.

When no further additions are made, the resulting compound is phosphatidate (diacylglycerol 3-phosphate), the simplest phosphoglyceride. Only small amounts of phosphatidate are present in membranes. However, the molecule is a key intermediate in the biosynthesis of the other phosphoglycerides as well as triacylglycerides.

The major phosphoglycerides are derived from phosphatidate by the formation of an ester linkage between the phosphoryl group of phosphatidate and the hydroxyl group of one of several alcohols. The common alcohols of phosphoglycerides are the amino acid serine, ethanolamine, choline, glycerol, and inositol. An example of phosphoglyceride is reported both in structure formula and in stereographic view in Figure 2.73.

Phospholipids built on a sphingosine backbone are called sphingolipids. Sphingosine is an amino alcohol that contains a long, unsaturated hydrocarbon chain. Sphingomyelin is a common sphingolipid found in membranes. In sphingomyelin, the amino group of the sphingosine backbone is linked to a fatty acid by an amide bond. In addition, the primary hydroxyl group of sphingosine is attached to phosphorylcholine through an ester linkage. Sphingomyelin is found in the plasma membrane of many cells but is especially rich in the myelin sheath of nerve cells. The structure formula and stereographic representations of sphingomyelin is reported in Figure 2.74, where all the parts of the molecule are evidenced.

Glycolipids, as their name implies, are sugar-containing lipids. Glycolipids are ubiquitous in all membranes, although their function is unknown. Like sphingomyelin, the glycolipids in animal cells are derived from sphingosine. The amino group of the sphingosine backbone is acylated by a fatty acid, as in sphingomyelin.

Glycolipids differ from sphingomyelin in the identity of the unit that is linked to the primary hydroxyl group of the sphingosine backbone. In glycolipids, one or more sugars (rather than phosphorylcholine) are attached to this group. The simplest glycolipid, called a cerebroside, contains a single sugar residue, either glucose or galactose as shown in Figure 2.75. More complex glycolipids, such as gangliosides, contain a branched chain of as many as seven sugar residues. Glycolipids are oriented in an asymmetric fashion in membranes with the sugar residues always on the extracellular side of the membrane.

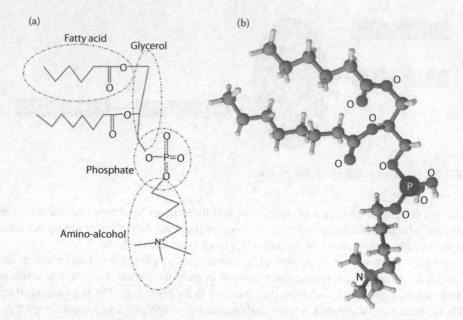

FIGURE 2.73 Structure formula (a) and stereographic representation (b) of a selected phospholipid.

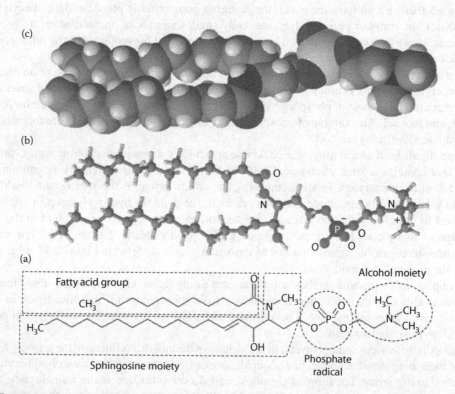

FIGURE 2.74 Structure formula (a), balls and sticks representations (b) and volume representation (c) of sphingomyelin. In the structure formula all the parts of the molecule are evidenced. The fatty acid group represented in the figure is only an example and other similar groups can be present.

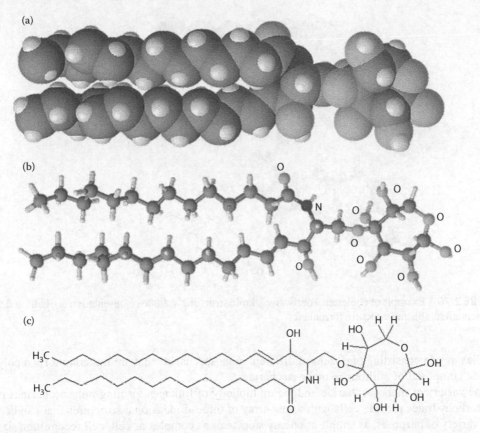

FIGURE 2.75 Glucose containing cerebroside: volume representation (a), balls and sticks representations (b), and (c) structure formula, the fatty acid group represented in the figure is only an example and other similar groups can be present.

2.7.4 STEROIDS

Steroids function as hormones, facilitate the digestion of lipids and are key membrane constituents. Unlike the other classes of lipids, steroids take on a cyclical rather than linear structure. All steroids have a tetracyclic ring structure called the steroid nucleus. The steroid nucleus consists of three cyclohexane rings and a cyclopentane ring joined together. The most common steroid, and the precursor to many biochemically active steroids, is cholesterol, whose structure is shown in Figure 2.76. A hydrocarbon tail is linked to the steroid at one end, and a hydroxyl group is attached at the other end. Cholesterol is important in maintaining proper membrane fluidity [88,89].

Cholesterol is absent from prokaryotes but is found to varying degrees in virtually all animal membranes. It constitutes almost 25% of the membrane lipids in certain nerve cells but is essentially absent from some intracellular membranes. Free cholesterol does not exist outside of membranes. Rather, it is esterified to a fatty acid for storage and transport.

2.8 CARBOHYDRATES

Carbohydrates are carbon-based molecules that are rich in hydroxyl groups (OH). Indeed, the molecular formula for many carbohydrates is $(C-H_2O)_n$—R literally, a carbon hydrate. Simple carbohydrates are called monosaccharide and many of them are also normally called sugars. Complex carbohydrates—polymers of covalently linked monosaccharide—are called polysaccharides. A polysaccharide can be as simple as one comprising two identical monosaccharides. Or it can be as

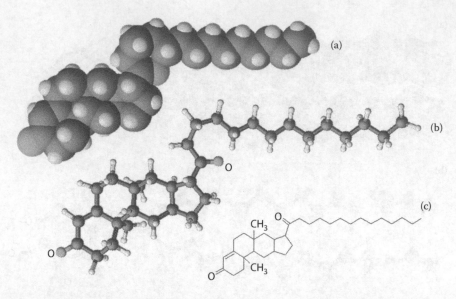

FIGURE 2.76 Example of cholesterol derivative steroid structure: volume representation (a), balls and sticks representations (b), and structure formula (c).

complex as one consisting of dozens of different monosaccharide that are linked to form a polysaccharide composed of millions of monosaccharides.

The variety of monosaccharide and the multiplicity of linkages forming polysaccharides mean that carbohydrates provide cells with a vast array of three-dimensional structures that can be used for a variety of purposes, as simple as energy storage or as complex as cell–cell recognition signals.

2.8.1 Monosaccharides

Monosaccharides are the simplest form of sugar and are usually colorless, water-soluble, crystalline solids. Some monosaccharides have a sweet taste. Examples of monosaccharides include glucose (dextrose), fructose (levulose), galactose, xylose, and ribose. With few exceptions (e.g. deoxyribose), monosaccharides have the chemical formula $C_n(H_2O)_m$, where n is at least 3. Monosaccharides can be classified by the number n of carbon atoms they contain as reported in Table 2.14.

Glucose, that is perhaps the most important monosaccharide, belongs to the hexose family. Examples of heptoses include the ketoses mannoheptulose and sedoheptulose. Monosaccharides with eight or more carbons are rarely observed as they are quite unstable.

TABLE 2.14

Suffixes of Monosaccharides as a Function of the Number of Carbon Atoms

Suffix	Carbons Number	Example
Triose	3	Glyceraldehyde
Tetrose	4	Erythrose
Pentose	5	Ribose
Hexose	6	Glucose
Heptose	7	Sedoheptulose

Monosaccharides are classified as aldehydes or ketones, whose general properties were discussed in Section 1.3.2. Simple monosaccharides have a linear and unbranched carbon skeleton with one carbonyl (C=O) functional group, and one hydroxyl (OH) group on each of the remaining carbon atoms, as shown in Figure 2.77.

Carbohydrates, due to the simplicity of their molecular formulae, that are constituted only by carbon, oxygen, and hydrogen atoms, give rise to several isometric forms. Constitutional isomers have identical molecular formulas but differ in how the atoms are ordered; stereoisomers are isomers that differ in spatial arrangement and are generally called by tagging the molecule name with a letter as D-glyceraldehyde and L-glyceraldehyde, where, according to convention, the D and L isomers are determined by the configuration of the asymmetric carbon atom farthest from the aldehyde or keto group. An asymmetric carbon is a carbon atom within the molecule that is attached to four different types of atoms or four different groups of atoms. A complete review of all the isomer types occurring among carbohydrates with examples and an indication of the naming convention is reported in Figure 2.78.

Even if in Figure 2.77 the linear form of the sugars is reported, that is a practically possible stereographic configuration for these molecules, more frequently sugars occur in one of several ring or cyclic structures. The chemical basis for ring formation is that an aldehyde can react with an alcohol to form a hemiacetal as represented in the following reaction:

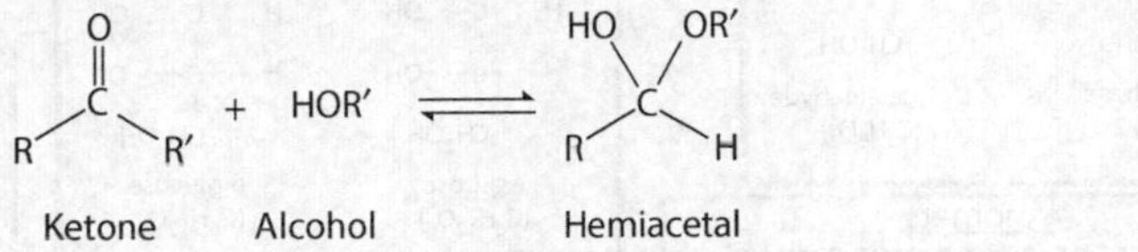

$$
\underset{\text{Ketone}}{\overset{\displaystyle O}{\underset{R}{\overset{\|}{C}}\diagdown R'}} + \underset{\text{Alcohol}}{HOR'} \rightleftharpoons \underset{\text{Hemiacetal}}{\overset{HO \quad OR'}{\underset{R}{\overset{\diagup \overset{|}{C} \diagdown}{\diagdown}}H}} \tag{2.37}
$$

(a)　　　　　　　　　　　　　　　(b)

Ribose

Glucose

Fructose

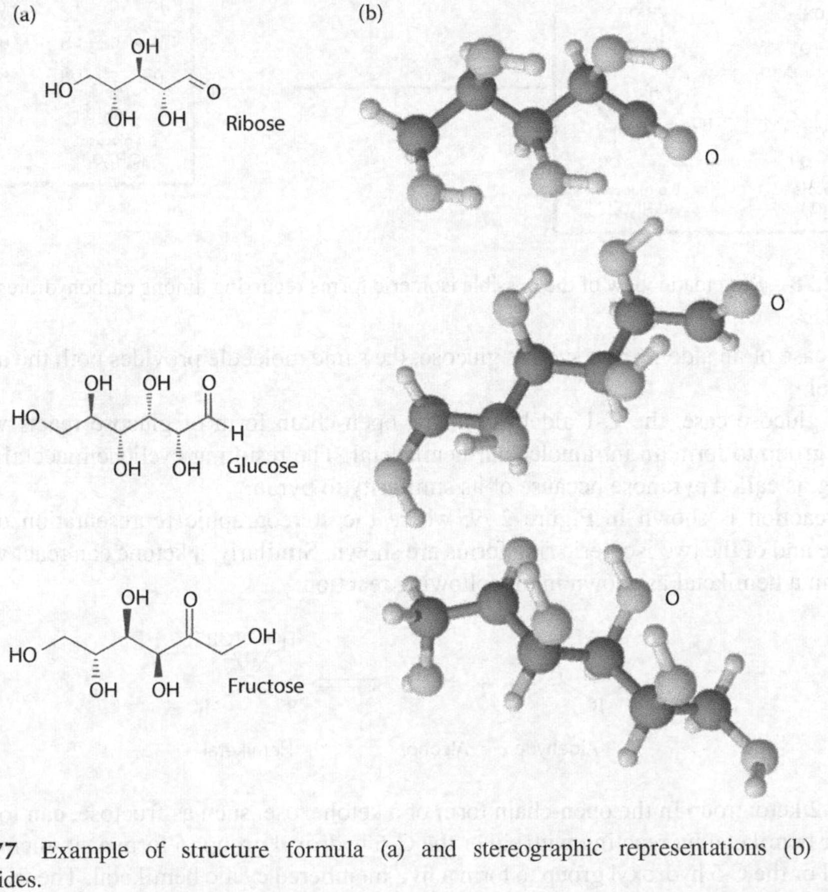

FIGURE 2.77 Example of structure formula (a) and stereographic representations (b) of simple monosaccharides.

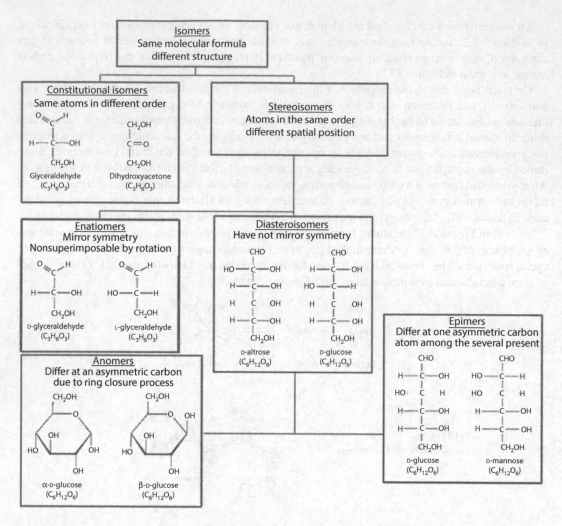

FIGURE 2.78 Systematic view of the possible isomeric forms recurring among carbohydrates.

In the case of an aldohexose, such as glucose, the same molecule provides both the aldehyde and the alcohol.

In the glucose case, the C-1 aldehyde in the open-chain form of glucose reacts with the C-5 hydroxyl group to form an intramolecular hemiacetal. The resulting cyclichemiacetal, a six-membered ring, is called pyranose because of its similarity to pyran.

This reaction is shown in Figure 2.79, where the stereographic representation of the linear D-glucose and of the two isomeric ring forms are shown. Similarly, a ketone can react with an alcohol to form a hemiketal as shown in the following reaction:

$$\text{Aldehyde} \quad \text{Alcohol} \qquad \text{Hemiketal} \tag{2.38}$$

The C-2 keto group in the open-chain form of a ketohexose, such as fructose, can form an intramolecular hemiketal by reacting with either the C-6 hydroxyl group to form a six-membered cyclic hemiketal or the C-5 hydroxyl group to form a five-membered cyclic hemiketal. The five-membered

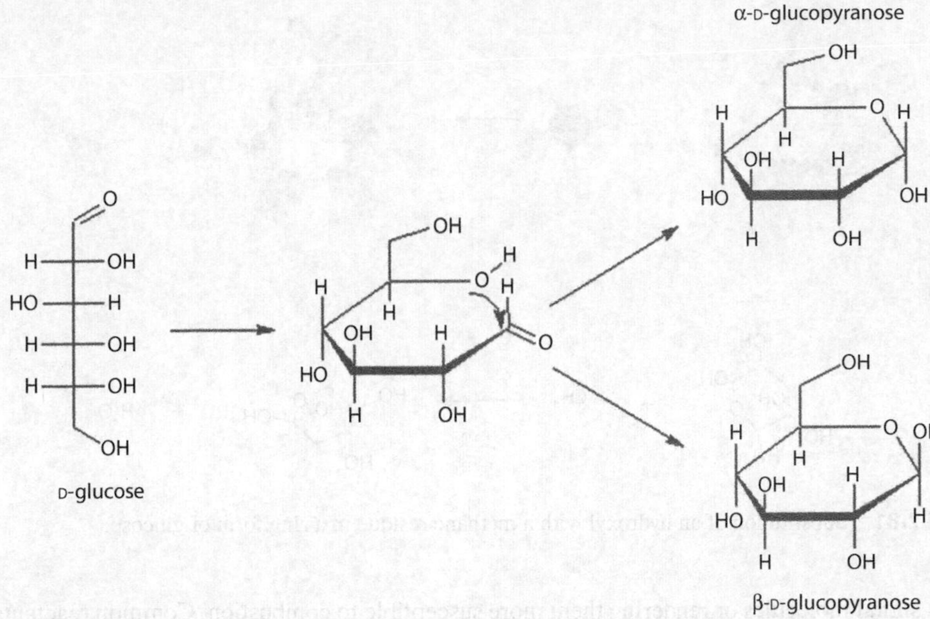

FIGURE 2.79 Formation reaction of the ring form of glucose: the C-1 aldehyde in the open-chain form of glucose reacts with the C-5 hydroxyl group to form an intramolecular hemiacetal.

ring is called a furanose because of its similarity to furan as indicated in Figure 2.80, where the reaction creating furanose from the linear form of fructose is shown.

Carbohydrates may contain many asymmetric carbon atoms. An additional asymmetric center is created when a cyclic hemiacetal is formed, creating yet another diastereoisomeric form of sugars called anomers. In glucose, C-1 (the carbonyl carbon atom in the open-chain form) becomes an asymmetric center. Thus, two ring structures can be formed: α-D-glucopyranose and β-D-glucopyranose. For D sugars, the designation α means that the hydroxyl group attached to C-1 is below the plane of the ring; β means that it is above the plane of the ring. The C-1 carbon atom is called the anomeric carbon atom, and the α and β forms are called anomers. An equilibrium mixture of glucose contains approximately one-third α anomer, two-thirds β anomer, and about 1% of the open-chain form. Because the α and β isomers of glucose are in an equilibrium that passes through the open-chain form, glucose has some of the chemical properties of free aldehydes, such as the ability to react with oxidizing agents.

The biochemical properties of monosaccharides can by modified by reaction with other molecules. These modifications increase the biochemical versatility of carbohydrates, enabling them to

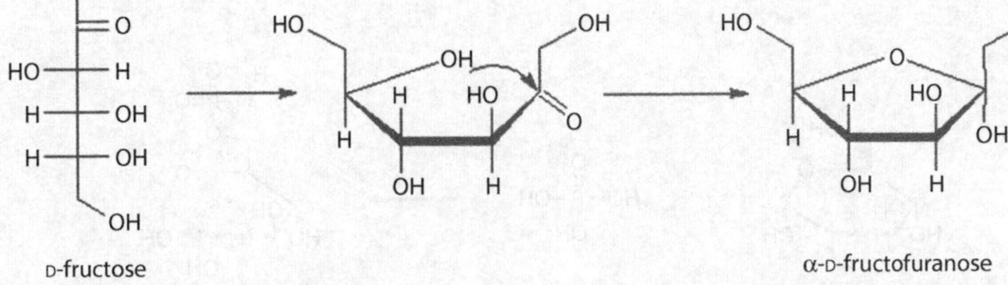

FIGURE 2.80 Reaction creating fructofuranose from the linear form of fructose.

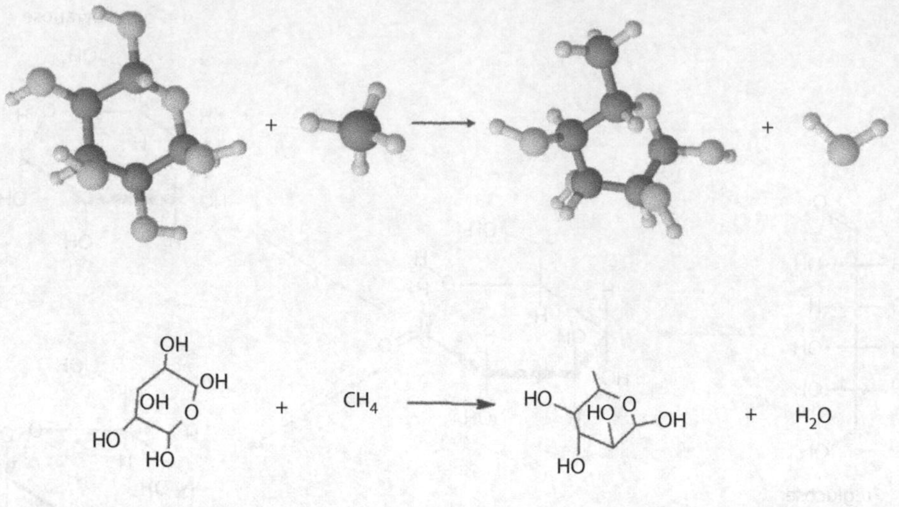

FIGURE 2.81 Substitution of an hydroxyl with a methane residue in a ring form of glucose.

serve as signal molecules or rendering them more susceptible to combustion. Common reactants are alcohols, amines, and phosphates. Examples of such reactions are provided in Figure 2.81, where the substitution of an hydroxyl with a methane residue is shown, in Figure 2.82, where an addition is performed appending an alcohol radical to a ring form of glucose and in Figure 2.83 where the molecules obtained after reaction of glucose with a phosphate radical are represented.

A bond formed between the anomeric carbon atom of glucose and the oxygen atom of an alcohol is called a glycosidic bond—specifically, an O-glycosidic bond. We have already encountered this kind of bond in DNA and RNA backbones, where sugars have a main role.

O-glycosidic bonds are prominent when carbohydrates are linked together to form long polymers and when they are attached to proteins, as in the case of immunoglobulin. In addition, the anomeric carbon atom of a sugar can be linked to the nitrogen atom of an amine to form an N-glycosidic bond. Carbohydrates can also form an ester linkage to phosphates, one of the most prominent modifications in carbohydrate metabolism.

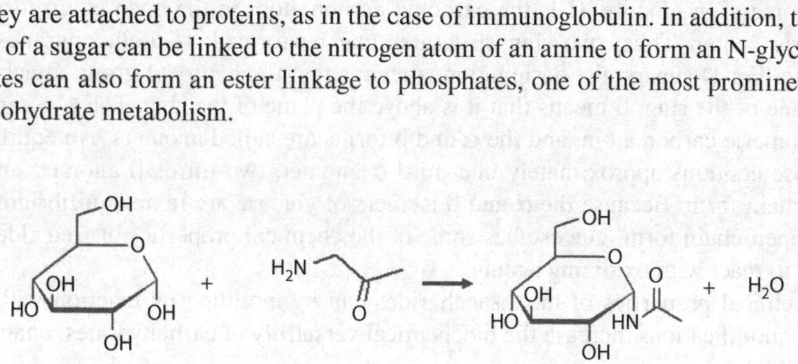

FIGURE 2.82 Additions of an alcohol radical in a ring form of glucose.

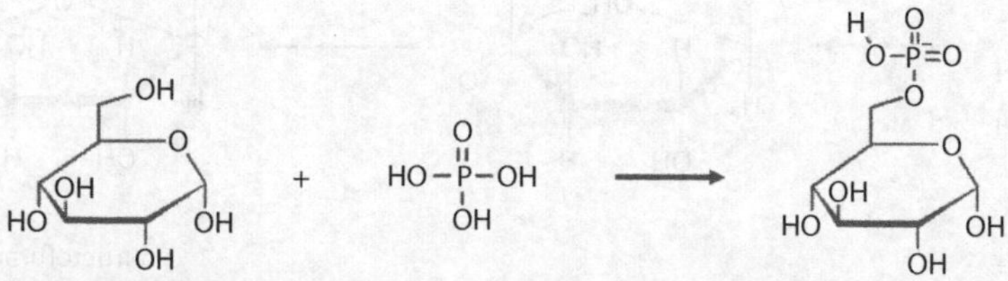

FIGURE 2.83 Addition of a phosphate radical to a ring form of glucose.

2.8.2 OLIGOSACCHARIDES

Because sugars contain many hydroxyl groups, glycosidic bonds can join one monosaccharide to another. Oligosaccharides are built by the linkage of two or more monosaccharides by O-glycosidic bonds maltose, for example, is built by two D-glucose residues joined by a glycosidic bond as shown in Figure 2.84. Such a linkage is called an α-1,4-glycosidic bond due to the fact that it links carbon 1 in a molecule with carbon 4 in the other if carbons are numbered in the conventional way (cf. Section 1.3.1).

The fact that monosaccharides have multiple hydroxyl groups means that many different glycosidic linkages are possible. For example, the three monosaccharides—glucose, mannose, and galactose—can be linked together to form more than 12,000 different stable molecules.

Oligosaccharides are synthesized through the action of specific enzymes, glycosyltransferases, which catalyze the formation of glycosidic bonds. Given the diversity of known glycosidic linkages, many different enzymes are required.

Three abundant disaccharides that are frequently encountered in nature are sucrose, lactose, and maltose, whose structures are represented in Figure 2.84.

Sucrose, that is the dominant component of common table sugar, is obtained commercially from sugar cane or sugar beets. The anomeric carbon atoms of a glucose unit and a fructose unit are joined in this disaccharide; the configuration of this glycosidic linkage is α for glucose and β for fructose. Sucrose can be cleaved into its component monosaccharides by the enzyme sucrose.

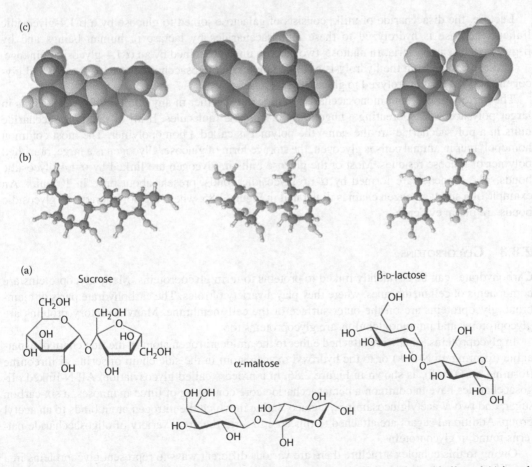

FIGURE 2.84 Structure formula (a) and stereographic representations (b) in sticks and balls and (c) in volumes representation of the most common disaccharides: sucrose, lactose, and maltose.

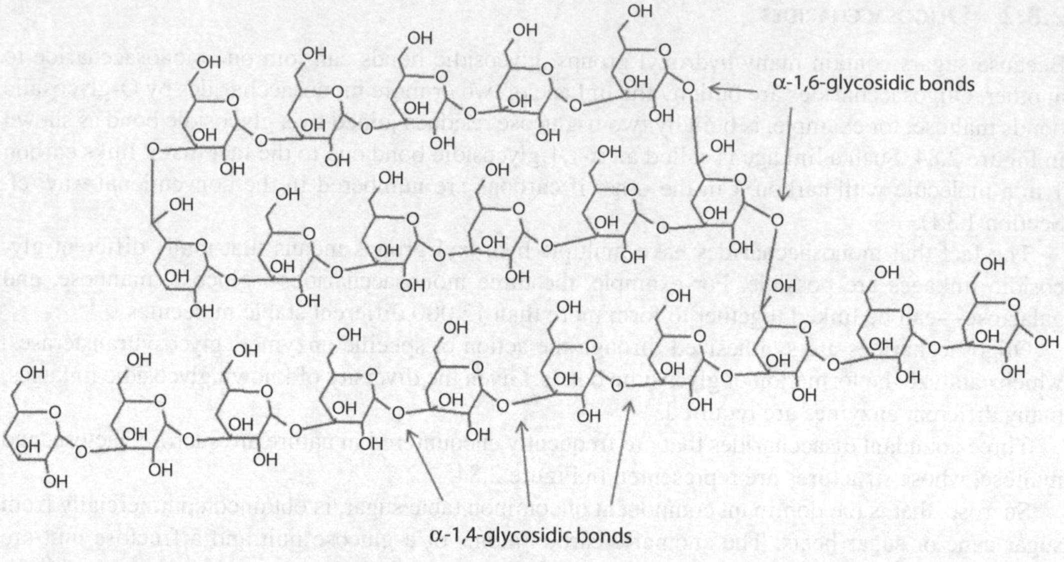

FIGURE 2.85 Structure formula of a small glycogen molecule composed by three glucose residues chains.

Lactose, the disaccharide of milk, consists of galactose joined to glucose by a β-1,4-glycosidic linkage. Lactose is hydrolyzed to these monosaccharides by lactase in human beings and by β-galactosidase in bacteria. In maltose, two glucose units are joined by an α-1,4-glycosidic linkage.

Maltose comes from the hydrolysis of large polymeric oligosaccharides such as starch and glycogen and is in turn hydrolyzed to glucose by maltase.

The variety of different monosaccharide can be put together in any number of arrangements in larger polysaccharides, creating a huge array of possible molecules. If all of the monosaccharide units in a polysaccharide are the same, the polymer is called a homopolymer. The most common homopolymer in animal cells is glycogen, the storage form of glucose. Glycogen is a large, branched polymer of glucose residues. Most of the glucose units in glycogen are linked by α-1,4-glycosidic bonds. The branches are formed by α-1,6-glycosidic bonds, present about once in 10 units. An example of a small glycogen chain is illustrated in Figure 2.85, where the polymerization glycosidic bonds are put in evidence.

2.8.3 GLYCOPROTEINS

Carbohydrates can be covalently linked to proteins to form glycoproteins. Many glycoproteins are components of cell membranes, where they play a variety of roles. The carbohydrate parts of membrane glycoproteins are on the outer surface of the cell membrane. Many secretory proteins are glycoproteins and immunoglobulins are glycoproteins too.

In glycoproteins, sugars are attached either to the amide nitrogen atom in the side chain of asparagine (forming an N-link) or to the hydroxyl oxygen atom in the side chain of serine or threonine (forming an O-link), as shown in Figure 2.86, in a process called glycosylation. All N-linked oligosaccharides have in common a pentasaccharide core consisting of three mannoses, a six-carbon sugar, and two N-acetylglucosamines, a glucosamine in which the nitrogen atom binds to an acetyl group. Additional sugars are attached to this core to form the great variety of oligosaccharide patterns found in glycoproteins.

Owing to this complex structure there are various different ways to represent glycoproteins in a simplified manner with respect to a structure formula or a stereographic representation. Generally, the structure is shown as a branched chain of blocks, each of which represents a residue and is

(a)
Asparagine
N-link
(b)
Serine
O-link

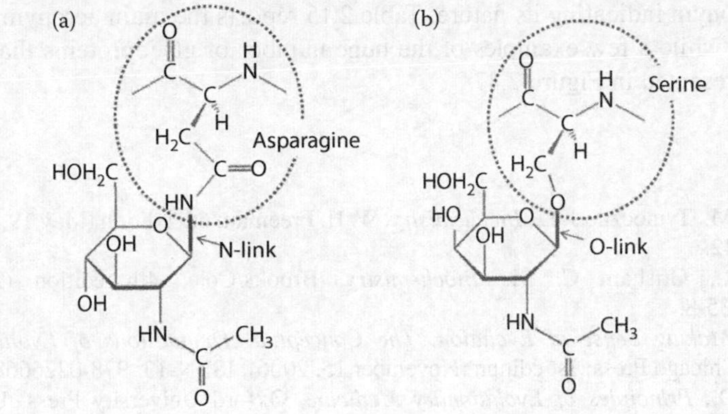

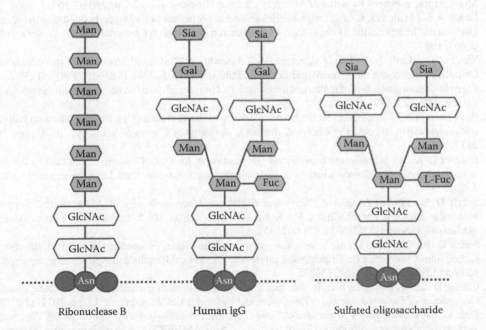

FIGURE 2.86 Possible covalent bonds forming glycoproteins: N-link (a) and O-link (b).

TABLE 2.15
Main Acronyms Used in Glycoproteins Representation

Acronym	Residue
GlcNAc	*N*-acetylgalactosamine (N-link block)
GalNac	*N*-acetylglucosamine (O-link block)
Man	Mannose
Gal	Galactose
Glc	Glucose
Fuc	Fucose
Sia	Sialic acid
Asn	Asparagine
Ser	Serine

Man
Sia
Gal
GlcNAc
Fuc
L-Fuc
Asn
Ribonuclease B
Human IgG
Sulfated oligosaccharide

FIGURE 2.87 Examples of glycoproteins.

tagged with an acronym indicating its nature. Table 2.15 reports the main acronyms used to represent glycoproteins, while a few examples of the huge number of glycoproteins that are present in living beings are presented in Figure 2.87.

REFERENCES

1. Berg J., Stryer M., Tymoczko J. L., *Biochemistry*, W. H. Freeman; 6th edition (May 19, 2006), ISBN-13: 978-0716787242.

2. Garreth H. R., Grisham C. M., *Biochemistry*, Brooks/Cole; 4th edition (2010), ISBN-13 978-0-495-10935-8.

3. Pigliucci M., *Making Sense of Evolution: The Conceptual Foundations of Evolutionary Biology*, University Of Chicago Press; 1st edition (November 15, 2006), ISBN-13: 978-0226668376.

4. Gluckman P. D., *Principles of Evolutionary Medicine*, Oxford University Press, USA; 1st edition (September 14, 2009), ISBN-13: 978-0199236398.

5. Luo Y.-L., *Comprehensive Handbook of Chemical Bond Energies*, CRC Press; 1st edition (March 9, 2007), ISBN-13: 978-0849373664.

6. Alberts B., Bray D., Hopkin K., Johnson A., *Essential Cell Biology*, Garland Science; 3rd edition (March 27, 2009), ISBN-13: 978-0815341291.

7. Dudek R. W., *High-Yield Cell and Molecular Biology (High-Yield Series)*, Lippincott Williams & Wilkins; 3rd edition (December 21, 2010), ISBN-13: 978-1609135737.

8. Phillips R., *Physical Biology of the Cell*, Garland Science; 1st edition (November 18, 2008), ISBN-13: 978-0815341635.

9. Bent H. A., *Molecules and the Chemical Bond*, Trafford Publishing (April 8, 2011), ISBN-13: 978-1426962998.

10. Abrikosov A. A., Gorkov L. P., Dzyaloshinsky I. E. 1963–1975. *Methods of Quantum Field Theory in Statistical Physics*. Dover Publications; 2nd edition (November 1975) ISBN-10: 0486632288.

11. Desirajiu G. R., Steiner T., *The Weak Hydrogen Bond: In Structural Chemistry and Biology*, Oxford University Press, USA (August 9, 2001), ISBN-13: 978-0198509707.

12. Larson J. W., McMahon, T. B. Gas-phase bihalide and pseudobihalideions. an ion cyclotron resonance determination of hydrogen bond energies in XHY- species (X, Y = F, Cl, Br, CN). *Journal of Inorganic Chemistry*, vol. 23, pp. 2029–2033, 1984.

13. Emsley J., Very strong hydrogen bonds. *Chemical Society Reviews*, vol. 9, pp. 91–124, 1980.

14. Monographic number of Journal of American Chemical Society, vol. 126, pp.16310–16311, 2004.

15. Legon A. C., Millen D. J. Angular geometries and other properties of hydrogen-bonded dimers: A simple electrostatic interpretation of the success of the electron-pair model. *Chemical Society Reviews*, vol. 16, p. 467, 1987.

16. Westhof E., Hardy N. editors, *Folding and Self Assembly of Biological Molecules*, Proceedings of the Deuxièmes Entretiens de Bures, World Scientific Publishing Co. (2004), ISBN-13: 978_9812385002.

17. Eigen M., Selforganization of matter and the evolution of biological macromolecules, *Naturwissenschaflen*, vol. 58, 465–523, 1971.

18. Root-Bernstain R., A modular hierarchy-based theory of the chemical origins of life based on molecular complementarity, *Accounts of Chemical Research, Accounts of Chemical Research*, vol. 45, pp. 2169–2177, 2012.

19. Buheler L. K., *An Introduction to Molecular Interaction in Biological Systems*, Published by the author in public domain, http://www.whatislife.com/reader/interaction-reader.html, last time accessed on March 5, 2012.

20. Searls D. B., *Formal Language Theory and Biological Macromolecules*, in Mathematical Support to Molecular Biology, Farach-Colton M., Roberts F. S., Vingron M., Waternam M., editors, American Mathematical Society; ISBN-13 978-0821808265.

21. Searls D. B., Gwynedd L., *Molecules, Languages and Automata*, Proceedings of the 10th International Colloquium Conference on Grammatical Inference: Theoretical Results and Applications, Springer; 1st edition (2010), ISBN-10:3642154875.

22. Chiang D., Joshi A. K., Searls D. B., Grammatical representations of macromolecular structure, *Journal of Computational Biology a Journal of Computational Molecular Cell Biology*, vol. 13, pp. 1077–1100, 2006.

23. Dhir V., *Denaturation of Protein Model Compounds (Adiabatic Approach): Amino Acids, Electrolytes, Various Temperatures, Adiabatic Compressibility*, LAP LAMBERT Academic Publishing (October 12, 2011), ISBN-13: 978-3846518410.

24. Kurzinski M., *The Thermodynamic Machinery of Life*, Springer; Reprint of 2006 1st edition (November 23, 2010), ISBN-13: 978-3642062841.

25. Swieger G. F., *Mechanical Catalysis: Methods of Enzymatic, Homogeneous, and Heterogeneous Catalysis*, Wiley-Interscience; 1st edition (September 29, 2008), ISBN-13: 978-0470262023.

26. Guzman N. A., *Prolyl Hydroxylase, Protein Disulfide Isomerase and Other Structurally Related Proteins*, CRC Press; 1st edition (September 23, 1997), ISBN-13: 978-0824798314.

27. Branden C. I., *Introduction to Protein Structure*, Garland Science; 2nd edition (January 3, 1999), ISBN-13: 978-0815323051.

28. IUPAC-IUB Commission on Biochemical Nomenclature, Abbreviations and symbols for the description of the conformation of polypeptide chains. *Journal of Biological Chemistry*, vol. 245, pp. 6489–6497, 1970.

29. Lovell S.C., Davis I.W.,Arendall W.B., De Bakker P.I.W., Word J.M., Prisant M.G., Richardson J.S., Richardson D.C. *Structure Validation by Cα Geometry: φ, ψ and Cβ Deviation*. Proteins: Structure, Function, and Genetics, vol. 50, pp. 437–450, 2003.

30. Buxbaum E., *Fundamentals of Protein Structure and Function*, Springer; 1st edition (September 18, 2007), ISBN-13: 978-0387263526.

31. Xu J., Xu D., Liang J., *Computational Methods for Protein Structure Prediction and Modeling: Volume 1: Basic Characterization*, Springer; Reprint 1st edition (November 29, 2010), ISBN-13: 978-1441922052.

32. Moroder L., Buchner J., *Oxidative Folding of Peptides and Proteins*, Royal Society of Chemistry; 1st edition (January 8, 2009), ISBN-13: 978-0854041480

33. Hutchinson E.G., Thornton J.M. The Greek Key Motif: Extraction, Classification and Analysis. *Protein Engineering*, vol. 6, pp. 233–245, 1993.

34. Rutt W. R., Butt T. D., Morris R., *Hormone Chemistry: Steroids, Thyroid Hormones, Biogenic Amines and Prostaglandins, Ellis Horwood Ltd*, Publisher; 2nd edition (May 25, 1977), ISBN-13: 978-0853120384.

35. Dratman M., Gordon J., Thyroid hormones as neurotransmitters. *Thyroid*, vol. 6, pp. 639–647, 1996.

36. Berbel P. et al. Role of late maternal thyroid hormones in cerebral cortex development: An experimental model for human prematurity. *Oxford Journal: Cerebral Cortex*, vol. 20, pp. 1462–1475, 2010.

37. Farach-Carson M. C., Davis Paul J., Steroid hormone interactions with target cells: Cross talk between membrane and nuclear pathways, *The Journal of Pharmacology and Experimental Therapeutics*, vol. 307, pp. 839–845, 2003.

38. Vasudevan N., Ogawa S., and Pfaff D. Estrogen and thyroid hormone receptor interactions: Physiological flexibility by molecular specificity. *Physiological Review*, vol. 82, pp. 923–944, 2002.

39. Johns E. R., Lopez K.H., *Human Reproductive Biology*, Academic Press; 3rd edition (March 31, 2006), ISBN-13: 978-0120884650.

40. Theil, E. Ferritin: Structure, gene regulation, and cellular function in animals, plants, and microorganisms. *Annual Review of Biochemistry*, vol. 56, pp. 289–315, 1987.

41. Andrews, S. C. et al., Structure, function, and evolution of ferritins. *Journal of Inorganic Biochemistry*, vol. 47, pp. 161, 1992.

42. Zhang, Y. A novel ferritin subunit involved in shell formation from the pearl oyster (Pinctadafucata). *Comparative Biochemistry and Physiology Part B: Biochemistry and Molecular Biology*, vol. 50, 2003.

43. Sadava, D. et al. Life, *The Science of Biology*, Macmillan Publishers; 9th edition (2009). ISBN-10 1429219629.

44. Gupta S.P. editor, *Ion Channels and Their Inhibitors*, Springer; 1st edition (July 8, 2011), ISBN-13:978-3642199219.

45. Parham, P., *The Immune System, Garland Science*; 3rd edition (January 19, 2009), ISBN-13: 978-0815341468.

46. Onjo T., Alt F., W., *Immunoglobulin Genes*, Academic Press; 2nd edition (October 26, 1995), ISBN-13: 978-0120536405.

47. Nezlin R. S., *The Immunoglobulins: Structure and Function*, Academic Press; 1st edition (April, 1998), ISBN-13: 978-0123887085.

48. Winkel J. G. J., Hogarth M. editors, *The Immunoglobulin Receptors and their Physiological and Pathological Roles in Immunity*, Springer; 1st edition (August 31, 1998), ISBN-13: 978-0792350217.

49. Kolenko P., Skalova T., Dohnalek, J. Hasek J., L-Fucose in crystal structures of IgG-Fc: Reinterpretation of experimental data. *Collection of Czechoslovak Chemical Communications*, vol. 73, pp. 608–615, 2008.

50. Bender M. L., *The Bioorganic Chemistry of Enzymatic Catalysis*, Wiley-Interscience; 1st edition (August 23, 1984), ISBN-13: 978-0471059912.

51. Morokuma K., Musaev G. D., *Computational Modeling for Homogeneous and Enzymatic Catalysis: A Knowledge-Base for Designing Efficient Catalysts*, Wiley-VCH; 1st edition (March 25, 2008), ISBN-13: 978-3527318438.

52. Pawitan J., *In All Likelihood: Statistical Modeling and Inference Using Likelihood*, Oxford University Press, USA; 1st edition (August 30, 2001), ISBN-13: 978-0198507659.

53. Fersht A., *Enzyme Structure and Mechanism*, W. H. Freeman & Co; 2nd edition (January 1985), ISBN-13: 978-0716716143.

54. Traut T. W., *Allosteric Regulatory Enzymes*, Springer; 2nd edition (November 4, 2010), ISBN-13: 978-1441944535.

55. Rosenthal M. D., *Medical Biochemistry: Human Metabolism in Health and Disease*, Wiley; 1st edition (March 30, 2009), ISBN-13: 978-0470122372.

56. McGrath B. M., Walsh G., *Directory of Therapeutic Enzymes*, CRC Press; 1st edition (August 12, 2005), ISBN-13: 978-0849327148.

57. Chang, *Handbook of Neurotoxicology (Neurological Disease and Therapy), Informa Healthcare*; 1st edition (January 17, 1995), ISBN-13: 978-0824788735.

58. Torday J. S., *Evolutionary Biology: Cell-Cell Communication, and Complex Disease*, Wiley-Blackwell; 1st edition (February 21, 2012), ISBN-13: 978-0470647202.

59. Griffin J. P. editor, *The Textbook of Pharmaceutical Medicine*, BMJ Books; 6th edition (December 15, 2009), ISBN-13: 978-1405180351.

60. Hoffmann E. J., *Cancer and the Search for Selective Biochemical Inhibitors*, CRC Press; 2nd edition (June 25, 2007), ISBN-13: 978-1420045932.

61. Koshland, D., Molecular geometry in enzyme action, *Journal of Cellular Comparative Physiology*, Supp. 1, pp. 217–224, 1956.

62. Blackburn G. M., Gait, M. J., Loakes D., Williams D., *Nucleic Acids in Chemistry and Biology*, Publisher: Royal Society of Chemistry; 1st edition (December 5, 2006), ISBN-13: 978-0854046546.

63. Bloomfield W. A., *Nucleic Acids: Structures, Properties, and Functions*, University Science Books; 1st edition (March 1, 2000), ISBN-13: 978-0935702491.

64. Gregory S. G. et al. The DNA sequence and biological annotation of human chromosome 1. *Nature*, vol. 441, pp. 315–321, 2006.

65. Rich A., Raj, Bhandary U. L., Transfer RNA: Molecular structure, sequence, and properties. *Annuals Reviews of Biochemistry*, vol. 45, pp. 805–860, 1976.

66. Micklos D. A., *DNA Science: A First Course*, Cold Spring Harbor; 2nd edition (September 30, 2010), ISBN-13: 978-1936113170.

67. Russell, P., *Genetics. Benjamin Cummings*; 1st edition (2001), ISBN-10 0805345531.

68. Yakovchuk P., Protozanova E., Frank-Kamenetskii M. D. Base-stacking and base-pairing contributions into thermal stability of the DNA double helix. *Nucleic Acids Research*, vol. 34, pp. 564–574, 2006.

69. Pabo C., Sauer R., Protein-DNA recognition, *Annuals Review of Biochemistry*, vol. 53, pp. 293–321, 1984.

70. Makalowska I., Lin C., Makalowski W., Overlapping genes in vertebrate genomes, *Computational Biological Chemistry*, vol. 29, pp. 1–12, 2005.

71. Sandman K., Pereira S., Reeve J., Diversity of prokaryotic chromosomal proteins and the origin of the nucleosome. *Cell Molecular Life Science*, vol. 54, pp. 1350–1364, 1998.

72. Dame R. T., The role of nucleoid-associated proteins in the organization and compaction of bacterial chromatin, *Molecular Microbiology*, vol. 56, pp. 858–870, 2005.

73. Luger K., Mäder A., Richmond R., Sargent D. Richmond T., Crystal structure of the nucleosome core particle at 2.8 a resolution. *Nature*, vol. 389, pp. 251–260, 1997.

74. Grosschedl R., Giese K., Pagel J., HMG domain proteins: Architectural elements in the assembly of nucleoprotein structures, *Trends in Genetics*, vol. 10, pp. 94–100, 1994.

75. Higgs P. G., RNA secondary structure: Physical and computational aspects. *Quarterly Reviews of Biophysics*, vol. 33, pp. 199–253, 2000.

76. Nissen P., Hansen J., Ban N., Moore P. B., Steitz T. A., The structural basis of ribosome activity in peptide bond synthesis. *Science*, vol. 289, pp. 920–930, 2000.

77. Hermann T., Patel D. J., RNA bulges as architectural and recognition motifs. *Structure*, vol. 8, 2000.

78. Mikkola S., Nurmi K., Yousefi-Salakdeh E., Strömberg R., Lönnberg H., The mechanism of the metal ion promoted cleavage of RNA phosphodiesterbonds involves a generalacid catalysis by the metal aquoion on the departure of the leaving group. *Perkin Transactions*, vol. 2, pp. 1619–1626, 1999.

79. Lee J. C., Gutell R. R., Diversity of base-pair conformations and their occurrence in rRNAStructure and RNA structural motifs. *Journal of Molecular Biology*, vol. 344, pp. 1225–1249, 2004.

80. Barciszewski J., Frederic B., Clark C., *RNA Biochemistry and Biotechnology*, Springer;1st edition (1999), ISBN-100792358627.

81. Yu Q., Morrow C. D., Identification of critical elements in the trnaacceptor stem and TψC loop necessary for human immunodeficiency virus type 1 infectivity. *Journal of Virology*, vol. 75, pp. 4902–4906, 2001.

82. Kiss T., Small nucleolar RNA-guided post-transcriptional modification of cellular RNAs. *The EMBO Journal*, vol. 20, pp. 3617–3622, 2001.

83. King T. H., Liu B., McCully R. R., Fournier M. J., Ribosome structure and activity are altered in cells lacking snoRNPs that form pseudouridines in the peptidyltransferasecenter, *Molecular Cell*, vol. 11, pp. 425–435, 2002.

84. Cooper G. C., Hausman R. E., *The Cell: A Molecular Approach*, Sinauer; 3rd edition (2004), ISBN_13 978-0878932.

85. Gunstone F. D, *Fatty Acid and Lipid Chemistry*, Springer Verlag; 1st edition (June 30, 1996), ISBN_13: 978-0834213425.

86. Gunstone F. D. *The Chemistry of Oils and Fats: Sources, Composition, Properties, and Uses*, Blackwell; 1st edition (July 14, 2004), ISBN-13: 978-0849323737.

87. Thompson Jr. G. A., *The Regulation of Membrane Lipid Metabolism*, CRC Press; 2nd edition (March 10, 1992), ISBN-13: 978-0849345616.

88. Mattson M. P., *Membrane Microdomain Signaling: Lipid Rafts in Biology and Medicine*, Humana Press; Reprint 1st edition from 2005 (November 5, 2010), ISBN-13: 978-1617375156.

89. Katsaras J., Gutberlet T., *Lipid Bilayers: Structure and Interactions*, Springer; Reprint of 2001; 1st edition (December 7, 2010), ISBN-13: 978-3642087028.

3 Biochemical Assays and Sequencing Techniques

3.1 INTRODUCTION

In this chapter, we will review a few key biochemical characterization techniques. In general, the goal of a biochemical characterization procedure is to either identify in a quantitative manner the presence and activity of a target substance in a sample or to determine the unknown structure of a target molecule that is present in the sample itself. In the first case, these techniques are commonly referred to as biochemical assays, in the second case, since biomolecules are generally polymers, they are referred to as sequencing techniques.

Common medical diagnostic analyses, like hemoglobin analysis in blood, are assays while the techniques to determine proteins or DNA structure and components are sequencing techniques.

Assays and sequencing techniques are commonly used in biochemical laboratories adopting macroscopic set-ups that can span from small and possibly high accurate research set-ups to large throughput and highly automatized analysis machines. These techniques are also used in labs on chip, since the scope of such microsystems is to carry out assay or sequencing in a microscopic arrangement.

In this chapter we will review mainly macroscopic techniques by focusing our attention on those aspects that will be relevant for labs on chip. Frequently, this will mean not to concentrate on large throughput technologies that frequently are not compatible with miniaturization.

The techniques we will review will be divided into three principal classes:

- Assay techniques, where we will provide an introduction to standard assays that are not based on the specific capacity of immune system proteins to bind complementary molecular sites.
- Immunoassays, exploiting synthetic antibodies to obtain a specific reaction with the target substance; in this part of the chapter we will also present a detailed review on the chemical action of antibodies, which is useful for an in-depth understanding on many immunoassays and their performances.
- Nucleic acids and proteins sequencing.

3.2 ASSAY PROCEDURE AND PREPARATION

Assays are, in general, designed to identify, and quantify the presence of a target substance in a biological sample [1,2]. The starting sample can be composed of different substances; however, the most common samples are either aggregates of cells that contain the target substance or biological solutions that, besides a large number of other elements, also contains the target substance. Example of the first type is the search of a specific intracellular enzyme, where the initial sample is a piece of tissue, that is an aggregate of cells, and an example of the second type is search of proteins in blood, where the blood sample is provided directly in liquid state.

Assays are very different from one another; however, a set of common steps can be recognized almost in all the assays. These steps can be described as follows:

1. Sample preparation and stabilization
2. Sample purification and/or amplification

3. Biochemical assay
4. Signal detection
5. Signal processing

In the first phase, the sample is prepared for the assay and, if degradation of the sample during the assay time is possible, it is also chemically stabilized. An example of sample preparation is the cell disruption, also called cell lysis, which is needed in assays looking for elements that are contained inside the cell, as selected proteins and nucleic acids. In this case, the initial cells that agglomerate have to be processed so as to break cell membranes and frequently also organelle membranes to create access to the target molecules. An example of sample stabilization is the need to avoid blood coagulation and oxidation adding anticoagulants and antioxidants in all assays starting from raw blood.

Generally the stabilized sample is not yet ready for the assay. Quite frequently, it contains several biomolecules that could interfere with the assay so that they have to be eliminated before the assay execution. This step is called sample purification; it can be carried out by physical procedures like centrifugation or filtering by diffusion, by chemical means, for example, by precipitation of the problematic species, or using both methods.

Another problem that could occur is related to the target concentration in the sample that can be too small to permit sufficient accuracy of the assay. In selected cases, it is possible to start from the small target concentration that is contained in the sample, even if it is unknown in structure, to generate new similar macromolecules, so increasing the target concentration. This procedure is called target amplification and it is frequently based on synthesis of the target starting from base biological materials driven by the complementarity between biomolecules. The best- known example of this kind is DNA amplification by polymerase chain reaction (PCR) that we will detail in Section 3.3.

After preparation and purification or amplification the assay can be performed. It is generally based on a biochemical reaction generating a detectable signal like light, heat generation, change of electrical properties of the sample, and so on. Assays can be classified in two main classes: unlabeled detection assays and labeled detection assays. Assays allowing unlabeled detection are characterized by a chemical reaction directly producing a detectable signal. For example, if the reaction of the target molecule with the assay reference species is exothermic, the produced heat could be detected by operating the assay in a calorimeter so as to estimate the number of target molecules that underwent a reaction; if after the assay a sample constituted by a solution undergoes a relevant change in the refractive index it could be detected by interferometry techniques. If the assay requires labeled detection, besides the assay reaction reagent, other chemical species are inserted in the assay chemical receipt in order to generate the signal to be observed. This frequently happens by inserting in the assay fluorescent species that are bonded to the reference species reacting with the target. When reaction happens either the fluorescent species is released and activated, or it becomes activated by the alteration of the reaction generated by the target in the complex with the reference assay species. In both cases, fluorescence is produced due to the assay reaction and detected by a suitable optical system.

Whatever mean is used to generate a detectable signal that is proportional to the concentration of the target composite, it has to be detected; detection is generally either electronic or optical. In both cases, the assay generated signal is converted into an electronic signal, filtered and amplified by a detection chain so to limit the influence of background and electronic noise and conveyed to the processing unit of the assay system.

The processing unit is almost always a digital system that performs sampling of the incoming electronic signal and operates all the transformations that are needed to extract the assay output information. Depending on the assay, electronic processing can be as simple as filtering plus rescaling or as refined as the application of a complex algorithm needed to extract with the required accuracy the necessary data from the detected signal.

In this section, we will focus our attention on the biochemical part of the assays we are going to consider, but signal detection and processing is frequently a key point to have effective assays. The reader interested on such techniques as applied in macroscopic assays can start the analysis from the following References [1,3–6].

3.2.1 CELLS LYSIS TECHNIQUES

The process of cells lysis is common in several biochemical processes, for example, for extraction of proteins in Western blot and in other protein assays. In the case of the extraction of nucleic acids cell lysis is particularly critical, due to the need to avoid damage to the delicate target molecules.

Several methods of cell lysis exist, based on different principles [7–9]. A first classification can be done dividing high-throughput industrial methods from typical laboratory methods. Industrial methods are used, for example, for large-scale production of biomolecules that are synthesized inside the cells; due to their nature these methods are generally not suitable to be applied in labs on chip. Thus, we will concentrate our attention on a few examples of laboratory-scale methods.

The choice of the most suitable method for the target cells depends on several factors. Among them we have

- *Sample size of cells to be disrupted*: If only a few milliliters or milligrams of sample are available, care must be taken to minimize loss and avoid cross-contamination. Disruption of microbial cells, when hundreds or even thousands of liters of material are being processed in a production environment, presents different challenges. Here, throughput, efficiency, and reproducibility are key factors.
- *Toughness of cells to be disrupted*: Some cells are relatively easy to disrupt, for example, *E. coli*, blood cells, brain tissue. More difficult samples, for example, yeast, fungi, animal connective tissue, often require increased mechanical power or more aggressive chemical treatments. The most difficult samples, for example spores, may require mechanical forces combined with chemical or enzymatic methods.
- *Stability of the molecule or component being isolated*: In general, the cell disruption method is closely matched with the material that is to be extracted from the cell, for example, specific methods have been devised as starters of nucleic acids processing. Moreover, the cell lysis does not produce directly the component to be processed, but a subsequent biochemical step is needed to insulate and purify it. Thus, the lysis method has not to immediately activate substance that could damage the target molecule and it has not to produce species that are difficult to eliminate in subsequent steps or that are highly probable to give unspecific positive results in the final assay. This is generally attained by using the less aggressive method that allows the lysis to be obtained.

3.2.1.1 Mild Lysis (Osmotic Lysis)

For easily disrupted cells such as blood cells and insect or animal cells grown in culture media, a mild osmosis-based method for cell lysis is commonly used. Quite frequently, simply lowering the ionic strength of the media will cause the cells to swell and burst. Assuming to have a total of N ions in sample, the total ionic I strength is defined as

$$I = \frac{1}{2} \sum_{j=1}^{N} c_j q_j^2 \tag{3.1}$$

where c_j is the concentration of the jth ion and q_j is its charge number, that is the charge of the ion divided by the proton charge.

In some cases, it is also desirable to add a mild surfactant and some mild mechanical agitation to completely disassociate the cellular components. Because these mild lytic methods are performed under chemically mild conditions, they are often used for nucleic acids and fragile proteins extraction.

3.2.1.2 Enzymatic Lysis Method

Most biological cells cannot be disrupted by a mild method. This includes most bacteria, yeast, algae, and many plant and animal tissues. Further, cost and relative effort to grow and harvest these cells, combined with the often small quantity of cells available to process, have favored cell disruption methods utilizing manual protocols based either on more aggressive chemical reactions or on manually generated mechanical forces.

The use of enzymatic methods [10,11] to remove cell walls is well established for preparing cells for disruption, or for preparation of protoplasts (cells without cell walls). The enzymes commonly used include lysozyme, lysostaphin, zymolase, cellulase, mutanolysin, glycanases, proteases, and mannase.

This method has the advantage to be purely chemical and to release substances that can be produced on large scale, so as to be suitable also to small dimension production systems. However, it is very sensible to the processing conditions so that its reproducibility is sometimes difficult. A frequent cause of performance fluctuations is the need of assuring enzymes stability by thermal and mechanical stabilization so to maintain the enzyme concentration under control. In addition, the susceptibility of the cells to a specific enzyme can be dependent on the state of the cells. For example, yeast cells grown to maximum density generate cell walls that are very difficult to remove, whereas cells in the intermediate growing phase are much more susceptible to enzymatic removal of the cell wall.

3.2.1.3 Bead Lysis Method

Bead method for cell disruption uses tiny glass, ceramic, or steel beads mixed with a sample suspended in aqueous media. The sample and bead mix is subjected to high-level agitation by stirring or shaking. Beads collide with the cellular sample, cracking open the cell to release intercellular components. Unlike other methods, mechanical shear is moderate during homogenization, resulting in excellent membrane or subcellular preparations. The method, often called *beadbeating*, works well for all types of cellular material from spores to animal and plant tissues. It has the advantage over other mechanical cell disruption methods of being able to disrupt very small sample sizes, process many samples at a time with no cross-contamination concerns, and does not release potentially harmful aerosols in the process.

In the simplest example of the method, an equal volume of beads are added to a cell or tissue suspension in a test tube and the sample is vigorously mixed in a common laboratory vortex mixer. In most laboratories, beadbeating is done in sealed, plastic vials, centrifuge tubes, or deep-well microtiter plates. The sample and tiny beads are agitated at about 2000 oscillations per minute in specially designed vial shakers driven by high-power electric motors. Cell disruption is complete in 1–3 min of shaking. Machines are available that can process hundreds of samples simultaneously inside deep-well microplates.

Successful beadbeating is dependent not only on the design features of the shaking machine, which take into consideration shaking oscillations per minute, shaking throw or distance, shaking orientation, and vial orientation, but also the selection of correct bead size, generally comprised between 0.1 and 6 mm diameter, bead composition, for example, glass, ceramic, steel, and bead load in the vial.

All high-energy beadbeating machines warm the sample about 10°/min. This is due to frictional collisions of the beads during homogenization. Cooling of the sample during or after beadbeating may be necessary to prevent damage to heat-sensitive molecules. Sample warming can be controlled by beadbeating for short time intervals with cooling on ice between each interval, by processing vials in pre-chilled aluminum vial holders or by circulating gaseous coolant through the machine during beadbeating.

3.2.1.4 Sonication Lysis

Sonication is another common method for cell lysis that relies on the application of ultrasound to the sample, typically with a frequency of 20–50 kHz. The high-frequency oscillation is electronically generated and transmitted to the sample via a metal probe. The probe is placed into the cell-containing sample and the high-frequency oscillation causes a localized low-pressure region resulting in cavitation and impaction, ultimately breaking open the cells [12]. Sonication systems permit cell disruption in smaller samples including multiple samples under 200 µL in microplate wells. As in the case of the bead method, ultrasonic action on the cell solution or tissue generates heat that has to be dissipated to avoid damaging the biomolecules; moreover, the method yield is difficult to be reproduced so that the efficiency of the method presents a high variability.

The sonication method has to also be taken under control carefully so as not to damage the target substance: ultrasound now and then also breaks weaker protein and other substances thereby producing free radicals that are extremely chemically active so that damaging of the target molecule by free radicals have to be somehow avoided.

3.2.1.5 Detergent Lysis Method

Detergent-based cell lysis is an alternative to physical disruption of cell membranes, although it is sometimes used in conjunction with homogenization and mechanical grinding. Detergents disrupt the lipid barrier surrounding cells by disrupting lipid–lipid, lipid–protein, and protein–protein interactions. The ideal detergent for cell lysis depends on cell type and source and on the downstream applications following cell lysis. Animal cells, bacteria, and yeast all have differing requirements for optimal lysis due to the presence or absence of a cell wall. Because of the dense and complex nature of animal tissues, they require both detergent and mechanical lysis to effectively lyse cells.

In general, nonionic and zwitterion detergents are milder, resulting in less protein denaturation upon cell lysis and are used to disrupt cells when it is critical to maintain protein function or interactions. CHAPS, a zwitterionic detergent, and the Triton X series of nonionic detergents are commonly used for these purposes.

CHAPS is an abbreviation for 3-[(3-cholamidopropyl)dimethylammonio]-1-propanesulfonate whose structure equation is reported in Figure 3.1a. A related detergent, called CHAPSO, has the same basic chemical structure with an additional hydroxyl functional group whose IUPAC name is 3-[(3-cholamidopropyl)dimethylammonio]-2-hydroxy-1-propanesulfonate.

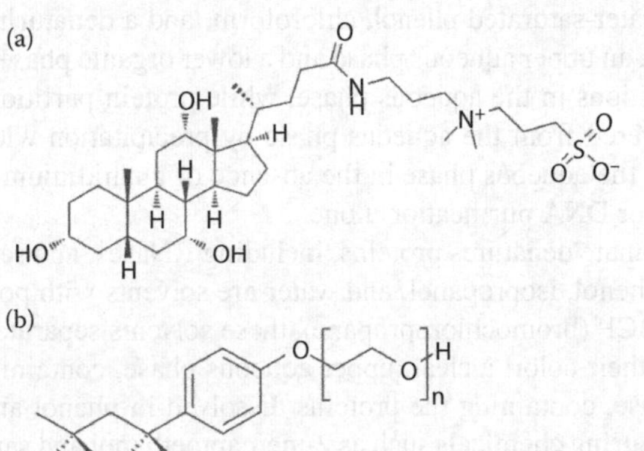

FIGURE 3.1 Structure formulas of two sample detergents frequently used in cell lysis: CHAPS (a) and Triton X-10 (b).

Triton X-100 is one of the most used Triton X series detergent, its brute formula is $(C_{14}H_{22}O(C_2H_4O)_n)$ while the structure formula is reported in Figure 3.1b. It is a nonionic surfactant which has a hydrophilic polyethylene oxide chain (on average it has 9.5 ethylene oxide units) and an aromatic hydrocarbon lipophilic or hydrophobic group. The hydrocarbon group is a 4-(1,1,3,3-tetramethylbutyl)-phenyl group.

Both detergents have low light absorbance in the ultraviolet region of the electromagnetic spectrum, which is useful for laboratory workers monitoring ongoing chemical reactions or protein–protein binding with UV/Vis spectroscopy.

In contrast, ionic detergents are strong solubilizing agents and tend to denature proteins, thereby destroying protein activity and function. In addition to the choice of detergent, other important considerations for optimal cell lysis include the used buffer, the pH, and ionic strength of the used solution and the process temperature.

3.2.1.6 Thermal Lysis Method

Thermal lysis is one of the more well-established lysis techniques in nucleic acid preparation, and is common in laboratory settings for its mild action and simple control. At high temperatures proteins within the cell membranes are denatured, irreparably damaging the cell and releasing the cytoplasmic contents. The most common method of inducing sufficient thermal damage in case of cells like animal cells obtained by artificial culture and blood cells is immersion of a sample tube in a boiling water bath for about half a minute. This short exposure at 100°C is sufficient to cause significant damage to the cell membrane without damaging the nucleic acids. Prolonged heat-treatment risks cause irreversible denaturation of supercoiled DNA.

3.2.2 Nucleic Acid Extraction from Cell Lysates

If the target substance is a nucleic acid, after cell lysis it has to be extracted while purifying the solution from other unwanted substances and preserving its integrity against all possible chemical and physical aggressions. Several procedures are available for extraction [13,14]; we limit ourselves to provide a few details for a selected number of them.

3.2.2.1 Guanidinium Thiocyanate–Phenol–Chloroform Extraction

After cell lysis, the target nucleic acid has to be extracted while purifying the solution from other unwanted substances and preserving its integrity against all possible chemical and physical aggressions. The most common process to attain this target is the so-called guanidinium thiocyanate–phenol–chloroform extraction [15,16].

This method relies on phase separation by centrifugation of a mix of the aqueous sample and a solution containing water-saturated phenol, chloroform, and a denaturing solution (guanidinium thiocyanate) resulting in an upper aqueous phase and a lower organic phase (mainly phenol). Nucleic acid (RNA, DNA) partitions in the aqueous phase, while protein partitions in organic phase. In a last step, RNA is recovered from the aqueous phase by precipitation with 2-propanol or ethanol. DNA will be located in the aqueous phase in the absence of guanidinium thiocyanate and thus the technique can be used for DNA purification alone.

Guanidinium thiocyanate denatures proteins, including RNases, and separates rRNA from ribosomal proteins, while phenol, isopropanol, and water are solvents with poor solubility. In the presence of chloroform or BCP (bromochloropropane), these solvents separate entirely into two phases that are recognized by their color: a clear, upper aqueous phase, containing the nucleic acids, and a bright pink lower phase, containing the proteins dissolved in phenol and the lipids dissolved in chloroform. Other denaturing chemicals such as 2-mercaptoethanol and sarcosine may also be used. The major downside is that phenol and chloroform are both hazardous and inconvenient materials, and the extraction is often laborious. A scheme working of this separation method performed using a typical kit is provided in Figure 3.2 in the example case of RNA extraction.

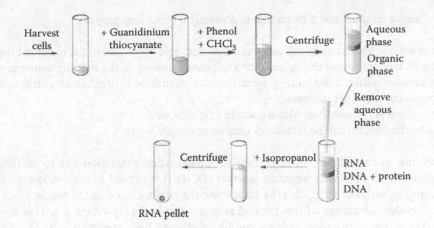

FIGURE 3.2 Schematic example of guanidinium thiocyanate–phenol–chloroform extraction in the case of RNA assay.

3.2.2.2 Spin Column-Based Nucleic Acid Extraction

Column-based nucleic acid purification is a solid-phase extraction method to quickly purify nucleic acids [17,18]. This method relies on the fact that the nucleic acid may absorb to silica surfaces depending on the pH and the salt content of the buffer. Although the absorption mechanism is not fully understood, one possible explanation involves reduction of the silica's surface's negative charge due to the high ionic strength of the buffer. This decrease in surface charge leads to a decrease in the electrostatic repulsion between the negatively charged DNA and the negatively charged silica. Meanwhile, the buffer also reduces the activity of water by formatting hydrated ions. This leads to the silica surface and DNA becoming dehydrated. These conditions lead to an energetically favorable situation for DNA to adsorb to the silica surface.

A further explanation of how DNA binds to silica is based on the action of guanidium HCl (GuHCl), which acts as a chaotrope. A chaotrope denatures biomolecules by disrupting the shell of hydration around them. This allows positively charged ions to form a salt bridge between the negatively charged silica and the negatively charged DNA backbone in high salt concentration. This mechanism is shown in Figure 3.3, in which sodium bridge is shown.

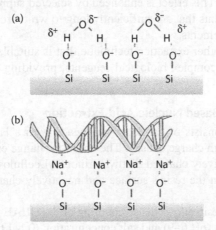

FIGURE 3.3 Mechanism of DNA absorption on a silicon surface via a sodium salt bridge: surface active coating (a) and DNA absorption (b).

The process of column-based extraction is generally a three-step process:

- The sample is added to the column and the nucleic acid binds due to the lower pH (relative to the silanol groups on the column) and salt concentration of the binding solution, which may contain buffer, a denaturing agent (such as guanidine hydrochloride), Triton X-100, isopropanol, and a pH indicator.
- The column is then washed with a suitable acid solution.
- Finally, the column can be eluted with buffer or simply water.

Spin column extraction has an important advantage when extraction has to be followed by DNA amplification by polymerase chain reaction (PCR): it is proved to remove many of the factors inhibiting an efficient PCR, thereby improving the performance of the whole DNA analytical chain. Another advantage of this method is that it can be easily adapted to labs on chip. As a matter of fact, the macroscopic column can be substituted by a microfluidic duct with suitable prepared walls where the result of cell lysing is injected. All the species in the solution traverse the duct while DNA or RNA attach to the duct walls. At the end a suitable buffer is sent into the duct to remove the nucleic acids and send them to the section where the subsequent processing is performed.

3.2.2.3   Magnetic Bead-Based Nucleic Acid Extraction

Another effective method for nucleic acids extraction that can be used either in macroscopic arrangements or in lab on chip relies on the use of magnetic beads.

A nucleic acid separation magnetic bead is a particle where magnetic dipoles are incorporated so that it can be moved by applying a magnetic field through the solution obtained after cell lysis so as to send them to a reservoir that is different from the waste where all the other substances are disposed. The difficult point of this procedure is that a magnetic bead has to be found that bind selectively either DNA or RNA, depending on the need.

Magnetic carriers with immobilized affinity ligands or prepared from biopolymer showing affinity to the target nucleic acid are used for the isolation process [19,20]. For example, magnetic particles that are produced from different synthetic polymers, biopolymers, porous glass, or magnetic particles based on inorganic magnetic materials such as surface modified iron oxide. Materials with a large surface area are preferred to be used in the binding of nucleic acids. Magnetic particulate materials such as beads are more preferable to be a support in isolation process because of their larger binding capacity. The nucleic acid binding process may be assisted by the nucleic acid wrapping around the support [21]. This effect is enhanced by selected supports that are demonstrated to bind only nucleic acid fragments that are sufficiently long to wrap around them so that they can be used to extract only great fragments.

Magnetic extraction is another extraction technique that is suitable to be used in a lab on chip; moreover, it has no need of complex biological reagents, providing both a reliability and a cost advantage.

3.2.2.4   Anion-Exchange-Based Nucleic Acid Extraction

The anion-exchange resin consists of defined silica beads with a large pore size, a hydrophilic surface coating, and has a high charge density. The anion-exchange extraction method is based on the interaction between positively charged diethylaminoethyl cellulose groups (DEAE, see structure formula in Figure 3.4) on the resin's surface and negatively charged phosphates of the DNA backbone.

The large surface area of resin allows dense coupling of the DEAE groups. The resin works over a wide range of pH conditions (pH 6–9) and salt concentration (0.1–1.6 M), which can optimize the separation of DNA from RNA and other impurities. Therefore, salt concentration and pH conditions of the buffers are one of the main factors that determine whether nucleic acid is bound or eluted

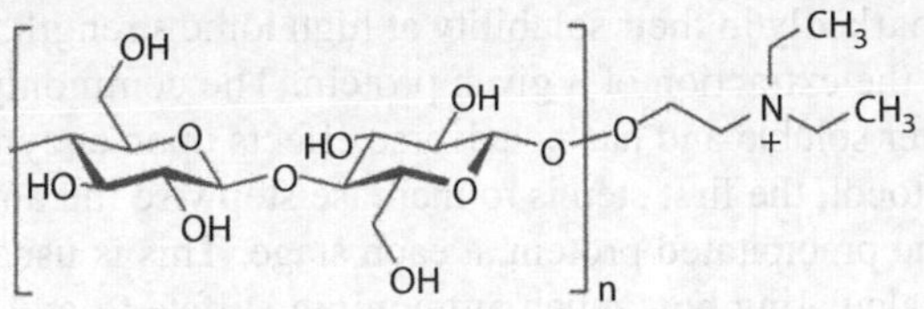

FIGURE 3.4 Structure formula of the diethylaminoethyl cellulose polymer (DEA) evidencing the positively charged N side element.

out from the column. DNA can bind to the DEAE group over a wide range of salt concentration. Impurities such as protein and RNA are washed from the resin by using medium-salt buffers, while DNA remains bound until eluted with a high-salt buffer [22–24].

3.2.3 PROTEIN EXTRACTION FROM CELL LYSATES

If the assay target is a cell protein, it has to be extracted from cell lysates as in nucleic acids assays. Some methods described in Section 3.2.2 can be used also in case of proteins once suitably modified. This is true, for example, for magnetic bead extraction and somehow also for anion-exchange extraction. Moreover, chromatography is extensively used for the first step of protein purification from the elements of the lysate having much higher or smaller mass. Since chromatography is one of the most-used methods to divide substances having different masses that are present in the same solution and many different chromatographic methods exist [25–27], we will devote a section to chromatography, namely Section 3.5. In this section, we will briefly review a method used specifically for protein separation from cell lysates.

3.2.3.1 Ammonium Sulfate Precipitation

A simple way of protein separation from the cell lysate is constituted by the so-called ammonium sulfate precipitation [28]. The solubility of proteins varies according to the ionic strength of the solution (see Equation 3.1), and hence according to the salt concentration. Two distinct effects are observed, as represented in Figure 3.5: at low salt concentrations the solubility of the protein increases with increasing salt concentration, that is increasing ionic strength, an effect called salting in. As the salt concentration and ionic strength increase, the solubility of the protein arrives to a maximum and starts to decrease. At sufficiently high ionic strength, the protein will be almost completely precipitated from the solution, a phenomenon that is generally called salting out.

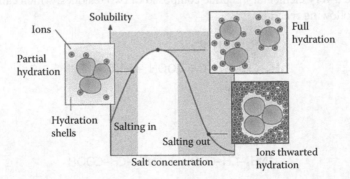

FIGURE 3.5 Qualitative behavior of protein solubility in water as a function of the salt concentration in the solution. Schematics of the main phenomena driving solubility in the salt-in and salt-out zones are also shown at the sides of the plot.

Since proteins differ markedly in their solubility at high ionic strength, salting-out is a very useful procedure to assist in the extraction of a given protein. The commonly used salt is ammonium sulfate, as it is highly water soluble and has no adverse effects upon enzyme activity.

In the purification protocol, the first step is to increase stepwise the ammonium sulfate concentration so as to recover the precipitated protein at each stage. This is usually done by adding solid ammonium sulfate, but calculating how much ammonium sulfate to add to a solution at one concentration to achieve a desired higher concentration is tricky, since addition of ammonium sulfate significantly increases the volume of the solution. The amount to add can be determined either from published nomograms or by using suitable formulas.

Each protein precipitate is dissolved individually in fresh buffer and it can be assayed for total protein content and amount of target protein. The aim is to find the ammonium sulfate concentration which will precipitate the maximum proportion of undesired protein, while leaving most of the desired protein still in solution or vice versa. The precipitated protein is then removed by centrifugation and then the ammonium sulfate concentration is increased to a value that will precipitate most of the target protein while leaving the maximum amount of protein contaminants still in solution. The precipitated target protein is recovered and dissolved in fresh buffer for the next stage of purification.

This technique is useful to quickly remove large amounts of contaminant proteins, as a first step in many purification schemes. It is also often employed during the later stages of purification to concentrate protein from dilute solution following procedures such as gel filtration.

After ammonium sulfate precipitation, generally further protein purification steps are needed in order to reach the sample quality required by a quantitative protein assay.

3.2.4 PROTEIN HYDROLYSIS

Protein hydrolysis is a method of dividing the amino acid residues composing the protein breaking the peptide links that create protein chains. This procedure is used during digestion to decompose proteins and in this case it is catalyzed by suitable enzymes. Protein hydrolysis can also be used for analytical methods, starting from a protein solution and producing a solution of the component amino acids in ionic form.

With an amide like ethanamide, the carbon–nitrogen bond in the amide group can be broken by hydrolysis to obtain carboxylic acid. The resulting reaction looks like

$$CH_3CONH_2 + H_2O + H^+ \rightarrow CH_3COOH + NH_4^+ \tag{3.2}$$

A similar reaction can be done to break a peptide chain into amino acid and analyze it.

Let us imagine a very elementary peptide composed of two residues, which can be decomposed as shown in the following reaction:

$$
\begin{array}{c}
\text{R} \quad\;\; \text{H R}' \\
|\quad\;\; |\; | \\
NH_2\text{–CH–C–N–CH–COOH} + H_2O + 2H^+ \\
\;\;\;\;\;\;\;\; || \\
\;\;\;\;\;\;\;\; O \\
\\
\downarrow \\
\\
\text{R} \quad\quad\quad\quad\;\; \text{R}' \\
|\quad\quad\quad\quad\;\; | \\
{}^+NH_3\text{–CH–COOH} + {}^+NH_3\text{–CH–COOH}
\end{array}
\tag{3.3}
$$

Instead of ammonium ions, positive ions made from the NH_2 groups reacting with hydrogen ions are produced. Moreover, an extra hydrogen ion is needed to allow the equation to work compared with the amide equation. It is needed to react with the NH_2 group on the left-hand end of the dipeptide, the so-called N end, the one not involved in the peptide link.

Scaling up to a polypeptide, each of the peptide links will be broken in exactly the same way. This means that a mixture of the amino acids that make up the protein is obtained although in the form of their positive ions because of the presence of the hydrogen ions from the hydrochloric acid.

Generally, hydrolysis is a slow reaction, and it can be catalyzed by the addition to the solution where the reaction involves a strong acid or a strong base. This allows faster creation of the needed ions by cooperating with the breaking of the peptide links with their high (or low) electronegativity. Even catalyzing the reaction in this way, however, several hours are needed to bring the reaction to equilibrium, demonstrating the exceptional stability of the protein structure, even one day or more in a few cases.

The reaction can be much more effectively catalyzed if the solution with the strong acid and the protein to hydrolyze is heated by microwave at about 200°C. It is possible to demonstrate that microwave interacts weakly with the organic molecules, provoking simply rotations of the peptide bonds that in any case weaken them. However, the strong acid ions are generally vaporized becoming much more active in reaching the protein molecules at a high energy and generating hydrolysis. In this way, a time gain of about a factor 100 can be obtained, reducing hydrolysis time in the order of minutes [29].

3.3 DNA AMPLIFICATION BY POLYMERASE CHAIN REACTION

This procedure is the most important amplification procedure, a key enabling technology for DNA assays and sequencing, due to the fact that frequently a very small quantity of a specific DNA is extracted from the available cell lysates.

Polymerase chain reaction (PCR) somehow mimics the natural DNA replication process (see Section 2.5.1) to replicate the target DNA molecules several times in order to obtain a DNA abundant sample suitable for successive processing. The PCR reaction requires the following components:

- *DNA template*: The sample DNA that contains the target sequence. At the beginning of the reaction, high temperature is applied to the original double-stranded DNA molecule to separate the strands from each other.
- *DNA polymerase*: The enzyme that synthesizes new strands of DNA complementary to the target sequence (see Section 2.5.1). Several different enzymes can work as DNAase. The first and most commonly used is Taq-DNA polymerase, when the probability of wrong DNA copy has to be minimized, the most commonly used enzyme is Pfu-DNA polymerase. Besides the characteristics of being able to replicate a DNA strand from the suitable primer, DNAase enzymes used in PCR have to be heat resistant, due to the fact that PCR is essentially based on thermal cycles.
- *Primers*: Short pieces of single-stranded DNA that are complementary to the target sequence. The polymerase begins synthesizing new DNA from the end of the primer.
- *Nucleotides (dNTPs or deoxynucleotide triphosphates)*: Single units of the bases A, T, G, and C, which are essentially "building blocks" for new DNA strands.
- *Buffer solution*: Providing a suitable chemical environment for optimum activity and stability of the DNA polymerase.
- *Divalent cations*: Magnesium or manganese ions; generally Mg^{2+} is used, but Mn^{2+} can be utilized for PCR-mediated DNA mutagenesis, as higher Mn^{2+} concentration increases the error rate during DNA synthesis [30].
- *Monovalent potassium ions*.

Typically, PCR consists of a series of 20–40 repeated temperature cycles, each cycle commonly consisting of discrete temperature steps, usually three. The cycling is often preceded by a single temperature step, called *hold*, at a high temperature (>90°C), and followed by one hold at the end for final product extension or brief storage. The temperatures used and the length of time they are applied in each cycle depend on a variety of parameters. These include the used DNAase, the concentration of divalent ions and dNTPs in the reaction, and the melting temperature of the primers.

- *Initialization step*: This step is required when the hot-start technique is used. Hot-start technique is a means to reduce nonspecific amplifications during the start phase of the PCR by adding to the system specialized enzymes that inhibit the amplification action at ambient temperature, either by the binding of an antibody [31] or by the presence of covalently bound inhibitors. Such substances dissociate or deactivate after a step at high temperature. Thus, an initialization step is needed in this case by heating the reaction components to the denaturation temperature (e.g., 95°C) before adding the polymerase.
- *Denaturation step*: This step is the first regular cycling event and consists of heating the reaction to 94°C–98°C for 20–30 s. It causes disruption of the hydrogen bonds generating the helix-turn-helix tertiary structure of the DNA (see Section 2.5.1) and yielding single-stranded DNA molecules.
- *Annealing step*: The reaction temperature is lowered to 50°C–65°C for 20–40 s allowing annealing of the primers to the single-stranded DNA template. Typically, the annealing temperature is about 3°C–5°C below the melting temperature of the primers used. Stable DNA–DNA hydrogen bonds are only formed when the primer sequence very closely matches the template sequence. The polymerase binds to the primer–template hybrid and begins DNA formation.
- *Extension/elongation step*: The temperature at this step depends on the DNA polymerase used; Taq polymerase has its optimum activity temperature at 75°C–80°C, [32,33] and commonly a temperature of 72°C is used with this enzyme. At this step, the DNA polymerase synthesizes a new DNA strand complementary to the DNA template strand by adding dNTPs that are complementary to the template in 5′–3′ direction, condensing the 5′-phosphate group of the dNTPs with the 3′-hydroxyl group at the end of the nascent, called extending, DNA strand. The extension time depends both on the DNA polymerase used and on the length of the DNA fragment to be amplified. As a rule of thumb, at its optimum temperature, the DNA polymerase will polymerize a thousand bases per minute.
- *Final elongation*: This single step is occasionally performed at a temperature of 70°C–74°C for 5–15 min after the last PCR cycle to ensure that any remaining single-stranded DNA is fully extended.
- *Final hold*: This step at 4°C–15°C for an indefinite time may be employed for short-term storage of the reaction.

A schematic representation of the global PCR processing is provided in Figure 3.6, where typical temperatures are reported for the different steps of the thermal cycle.

3.3.1 PCR Efficiency

From the process description it is clear that theoretically, if the primer concentration would be infinite and the replication would be perfect at each step, the number of DNA molecules will grow exponentially, increasing the DNA concentration very fast. This process is shown schematically in Figure 3.7. In a real PCR experiment, this is true only in the first part of the amplification.

Typical amplification curves for the PCR process are shown in Figure 3.8, while the experimental values of PCR efficiency is reported in Figure 3.9 via dots, where the process efficiency

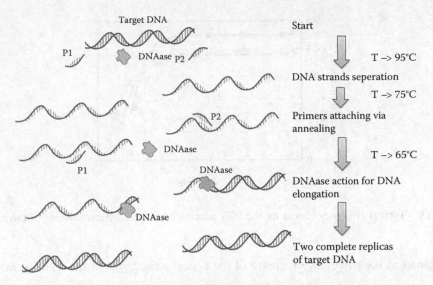

FIGURE 3.6 Scheme of the repetitive steps of a PCR process. P1 and P2 indicates two different primers.

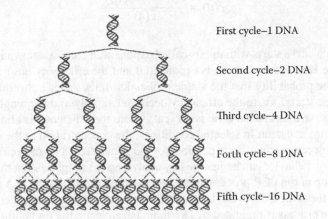

FIGURE 3.7 Exponential growth of the number of DNA helixes in the exponential phase of PCR.

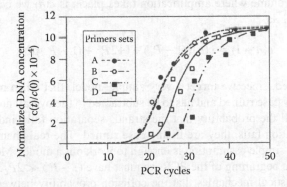

FIGURE 3.8 Typical amplification curves for the PCR process, curves for different sets of primers are reported, the type of primer set is not specified intentionally due to the need not to report names of commercial products. Dots and squares are experimental points and lines are obtained by best fitting (not all the experimental data are represented in the plot).

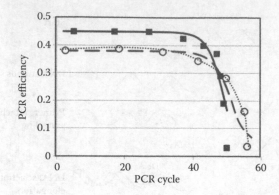

FIGURE 3.9 Typical efficiency curves for the PCR process where the different phases of the process are evidenced.

ϵ is evaluated as the percentage increase of the concentration $c(n)$ of the DNA at nth step, so that

$$\epsilon(n) = \frac{c(n+1) - c(n)}{c(n)} \tag{3.4}$$

The amplification curve starts with the so-called exponential zone, as shown in Figure 3.8, where the evolution of the DNA concentration is exponential and the efficiency has a constant value that only depends on the probability that the single replication fails. After a threshold concentration a subexponential zone starts, where the efficiency decreases rapidly and the amplification has a flex. At the end of the curve a saturation zone is present, where the efficiency is almost zero so that the concentration remains constant. In selected conditions, the concentration in the saturation zone can even decrease, if a decay mechanism is possible for the generated DNA molecules.

This amplification behavior can be justified by analyzing the amplification mechanism. It is reasonable, for the setup of the PCR process, to neglect the probability that a DNA molecule replicates more times during the same PCR cycle. Let us assume that the mechanism generating amplification at the jth step of the process is regulated by two main parameters: the probability P_c that a duplication mechanism is successful and the probability P_A that a specific DNA molecule undergoes an amplification at a certain stage. If the DNA concentration at stage n, which is the number of molecules divided by the volume where amplification takes place, is $c(n)$ we can write the number of molecules at stage $n + 1$ as

$$c(n+1) = c(n)\{(1 - P_A) + [+2P_C - (1 - P_c)]P_A\} \tag{3.5}$$

where we have imagined, since we target a very simple model, that when multiplication fails, the DNA molecule is in any case ruined and has to be subtracted to the overall number. This means that we consider almost null the probability that the strands separation fails and, once the strands are divided and the replication fails, they are in any case ruined. The real chemistry of PCR is much more complex, but this simple assumption is enough to work out a model. Moreover, since amplification takes place at the beginning of the PCR we must have $(1 - P_c) \ll 2P_C$.

We know from statistical mechanics that the collision probability between two molecules in a solution depends on the concentrations of both the molecules (see Section 1.6.4). Here we have two successive collisions needed: the collision with a primer and the collision with a polymerase molecule; the two collisions are located in different steps of the process. Thus it is possible to approximate them as independent processes. While the enzyme is not burned during amplification, the collision probability with the enzyme does not change in different cycles. This is not true for the primers. As a matter of fact, at the very beginning of the process the primers concentration is much bigger than the DNA concentration and we can imagine that qualitatively the collision of a DNA with a primer is almost sure in the step time, going on with DNA multiplication this starts to be no more true.

This means that we can set, in a first approximation, the probability P_A can be set proportional to the concentration $c_P(n)$ of the primers. Thus, we have

$$P_A(n) = K_A c_P(n) \tag{3.6}$$

This forces us to follow the primers concentration evolution. Primers are consumed by generating DNA amplification and are not recovered in our model if the amplification fails. Thus, the system of equations resulting from Equation 3.13 and the evolution equation for the primers concentration writes

$$c_P(n+1) = c_P(n)[1 - c(n)K_A] \tag{3.7a}$$

$$c(n+1) = c(n)\{(1 - c_P(n)K_A) + 2\pi_c c_P(n)K_A\} \tag{3.7b}$$

where we have set $\pi_c = P_C - (1 - P_c)/2$.

Equations 3.7a and 3.7b have been used to best fit changing the parameters K_A and π_c; the measured efficiency values reported in Figure 3.9. The theoretical curves correctly reproduce the qualitative behavior of the efficiency, while the correct shape of the transition from the exponential and the saturation regimes seems not to be correct. This is confirmed by the dotted line that is simply obtained by a high degree polynomial interpolation of experimental data, revealing a different shape of the transition.

This is due to the fact that, while decrease of the available concentration of primers is a main element determining PCR efficiency decrease, several other phenomena are also influent, that are not taken into account in the simple model of Equations 3.7a and 3.7b. Much more complex modeling have been carried out theoretically to determine the PCR efficiency by evaluating in detail the efficiency of each PCR phase [34–36] obtaining much more accurate results that have been demonstrated to reproduce with great accuracy the experimental results [37].

To obtain a very good fit of the efficiency curve, the following expression is often used [36]:

$$\epsilon(n) = \begin{cases} \dfrac{K}{K+S} & n < S \\[3mm] \dfrac{K}{K+n}\left(\dfrac{1 + e^{-C(n/S-1)}}{2}\right) & n \geq S \end{cases} \tag{3.8}$$

where S and C are fitting parameters. The ratio K/S can be determined by the constant value that the efficiency assumed during the exponential phase, while the other two parameters are determined by best fitting the transition between the exponential and the saturation phases.

3.3.2 PCR ALTERNATIVE PROCEDURES

Several protocols have been derived from the basic form of PCR with a variety of goals. In this section, we will review the two most common protocols used to monitor in real time the PCR efficiency and to recreate the single-stranded DNA conjugated to a target RNA to give rise to a sort of RNA amplification.

At the end of the section a list of other used protocols with a very brief description is provided for reference.

3.3.2.1 Real-Time PCR

Real-time PCR, also called quantitative real-time polymerase chain reaction (qPCR) or kinetic PCR is a modification of the PCR that allows to quantitatively evaluate the amount of DNA produced by the amplification techniques [38,39], and in reality experimental points both in Figures 3.8 and 3.9 are obtained using this technique.

The procedure follows the general principle of PCR; its key feature is that the amplified DNA is detected as the reaction progresses in real time. This is a new approach compared to standard PCR, where the product of the reaction is detected at its end. Two common methods for detection of products in real-time PCR are nonspecific fluorescent dyes that intercalate with any double-stranded DNA, and sequence-specific DNA probes consisting of oligonucleotides that are labeled with a fluorescent reporter, which permits detection only after hybridization of the probe with its complementary DNA target.

In nonspecific fluorescent dye-based real-time PCR, the first step is to bind the target DNA with a dye to all double strands. When the DNA is amplified, the dye that is present in the PCR solution binds new DNA also. Since the dyes emit fluorescence, an increase in DNA concentration leads to an increase in fluorescence intensity. It can be measured at each PCR cycle, thus allowing DNA concentrations to be quantified. However, dyes that bind to DNA such as SYBR Green will bind to all DNA like PCR products, including nonspecific PCR products, such as primer dimer. This can potentially interfere with, or prevent, accurate quantification of the intended target sequence.

Like other real-time PCR methods, the values obtained do not have absolute units associated with them, a comparison of a measured DNA/RNA sample to a standard dilution will only give a fraction or ratio of the sample relative to the standard, unless the standard dilution is very well known. Due to this fact, frequently this technique allows only relative comparisons between different tissues or experimental conditions.

Fluorescent reporter probes detect only the DNA containing the probe sequence; therefore, use of the reporter probe significantly increases specificity, and enables quantification even in the presence of nonspecific DNA amplification. Fluorescent probes can be used in multiplex assays—for detection of several genes in the same reaction—based on specific probes with different-colored labels, provided that all targeted genes are amplified with similar efficiency. The specificity of fluorescent reporter probes also prevents interference of measurements caused by primer dimers, which are undesirable potential by-products in PCR. However, fluorescent reporter probes do not prevent the inhibitory effect of the primer dimers, which may depress accumulation of the desired products in the reaction.

The method relies on a DNA-based probe with a fluorescent reporter at one end and a quencher of fluorescence at the opposite end of the probe. The close proximity of the reporter to the quencher prevents detection of its fluorescence; breakdown of the probe by the activity of the polymerase breaks the reporter–quencher proximity and thus allows unquenched emission of fluorescence, which can be detected after excitation with a laser. An increase in the product targeted by the reporter probe at each PCR cycle, therefore, causes a proportional increase in fluorescence due to the breakdown of the probe and release of the reporter. This procedure can be schematically described as in Figure 3.10.

The PCR is prepared as usual (see PCR), and the reporter probe is added.

- As the reaction commences, during the annealing stage of the PCR both probe and primers anneal to the DNA target.
- Polymerization of a new DNA strand is initiated from the primers, and once the polymerase reaches the probe, its activity degrades the probe, physically separating the fluorescent reporter from the quencher, resulting in an increase in fluorescence.
- Fluorescence is detected and measured in a real-time PCR machine, and its geometric increase corresponding to exponential increase of the product is used to determine the threshold cycle (CT) in each reaction.

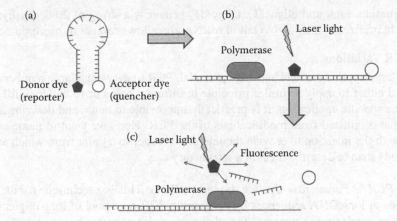

FIGURE 3.10   Principle of fluorescent reporter probes-based PCR; primer after DNA denaturation, donor and acceptor dyes are linked to the terminations of the primer (a); when the primer attaches to the DNA strand to be replicated the vicinity of the two dyes inhibit fluorescence (b); due to the polymerase action the primer is broken and the two dyes are divided; laser light can now cause florescence and the end of the replication operation is detected as shown in (c).

3.3.2.2   Reverse Transcriptase-Polymerase Chain Reaction

Up to now we have studied DNA amplification via PCR, but real-time PCR can also be used to amplify mRNA starting from a suitably selected specific primer and to study gene expression starting from a target RNA extracted from a cell [39,40]. The process comprises three steps:

1. Reverse transcription of RNA into the complementary DNA (cDNA) by the use of the enzyme reverse transcriptase
2. The obtained single-stranded cDNA divided by the RNA by denaturation
3. The cDNA strand is amplified by PCR to detect or sequence it

The first two steps are shown in Figure 3.11. The reverse transcription is carried out by maintaining the RNA in suitable buffer with the reverse transcriptase, triphosphate deoxyribonucleic primers

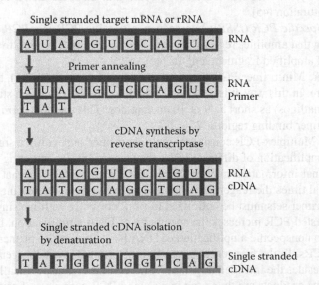

FIGURE 3.11   Derivation of a single-stranded cDNA from an RNA in reverse transcriptase PCR.

(dNTP), magnesium ions, and oligo(dT). Oligo(dT) primer is a string of 20 deoxythymidylic acid residues that hybridizes to the poly(A) tail of mRNA and allows reverse transcription of the RNA.

3.3.2.3 PCR Variations

Owing to its large application field and huge potential, PCR underwent a large number of modifications intended either to apply a similar principle in different cases or to better fulfill the requirements of some specific application. It is practically impossible to name and describe all analytical procedures that originated from modifications of the PCR. Here, we want to name only a few of them, more with the intention to provide the interested reader to a point from which to start a bibliographic study than to describe them in a satisfactory way.

Assembly PCR or Polymerase Cycling Assembly (PCA): This is a technique for the artificial synthesis of long DNA sequences by performing PCR on a pool of long oligonucleotides with short overlapping segments. The oligonucleotides alternate between sense and antisense directions, and the overlapping segments determine the order of the PCR fragments, thereby selectively producing the final long DNA product [41].

Asymmetric PCR: This technique is used when only one of the two complementary DNA strands has to be amplified. It is used in sequencing and hybridization probing where amplification of only one of the two complementary strands is required. PCR is carried out as usual, but with a great excess of the primer for the strand targeted for amplification. Because of the slow (arithmetic) amplification later in the reaction after the limiting primer has been used up, extra cycles of PCR are required [42]. A recent modification on this process, known as linear-after-the-exponential-PCR (LATE-PCR), uses a limiting primer with a higher melting temperature than the excess primer to maintain reaction efficiency as the limiting primer concentration decreases mid-reaction [43].

Dial-Out PCR: It is a highly parallel method for retrieving accurate DNA molecules for gene synthesis. A complex library of DNA molecules is modified with unique flanking tags before massively parallel sequencing. Tag-directed primers then enable the retrieval of molecules with desired sequences by PCR [44].

Helicase-Dependent Amplification: Helicase-dependent amplification is similar to traditional PCR, but uses a constant temperature rather than cycling through denaturation and annealing/extension cycles. DNA helicase, an enzyme that unwinds DNA, is used in place of thermal denaturation [45].

Intersequence-Specific PCR (ISSR): Intersequence-specific PCR is a PCR method for DNA fingerprinting that amplifies regions between simple sequence repeats to produce a unique fingerprint of amplified fragment lengths [46].

Miniprimer PCR: Miniprimer PCR uses a particular polymerase (S-Tbr), that is very stable in temperature. In this way, it is possible to obtain the DNA extension starting from primers (called smalligos) as short as 9 or 10 nucleotides. This method permits PCR targeting to smaller primer binding regions [47].

Multiplex-PCR: Multiplex-PCR consists of multiple primer sets within a single PCR mixture to produce amplification of different DNA sequences [48]. By targeting multiple genes at once, additional information may be gained from a single test-run that otherwise would require several times the reagents and more time to perform. Annealing temperatures for each of the primer sets must be optimized to work correctly within a single reaction.

Nested PCR: Nested PCR increases the specificity of DNA amplification, by reducing background due to nonspecific amplification of DNA [49]. Two sets of primers are used in two successive PCRs. In the first reaction, one pair of primers is used to generate DNA products, which besides the intended target, may still consist of nonspecifically amplified DNA fragments. The products are then used in a second PCR with a set of primers whose binding sites are completely or partially different from and located 3′ of each of the primers used in the first reaction. Nested PCR is often more successful in specifically amplifying long DNA fragments than conventional PCR, but it requires more detailed knowledge of the target sequences.

3.4 ENZYMATIC ASSAYS

Enzymes are often important elements in assays, both to catalyze the assay reaction and to facilitate detection of the assay product. The category of enzymatic assays is, however, generally restricted to assays measuring the rate at which a selected enzyme catalyzes the transformation of its substrate into the reaction product. This can be done either measuring the rate at which the substrate is consumed or the rate at which the product is created. Since almost all the important biochemical reactions are accelerated and controlled through enzymes, such assays have a large application field both in medicine and in other biotechnology areas.

Essentially, four different families of enzymatic assays exist [50].

- *Initial rate assays*: The initial rate of an enzymatic reaction provides several important information regarding the enzyme concentration and activity (see Section 2.5.1). As a matter of fact, due to the Michaelis–Menten relation, if the substrate concentration is much greater that the Michaelis–Menten constant the initial rate does not depend on the substrate concentration and it is equal to the maximum reaction rate achievable through catalysis with the selected enzyme. When it is possible to increase the substrate concentration as much as needed to reach this condition the enzyme–substrate intermediate builds up in a fast initial transient. Then the reaction achieves a steady-state kinetics in which enzyme substrate intermediates remains approximately constant over time and the reaction rate changes relatively slowly. Rates are measured for a short period after the attainment of the quasi-steady state, typically by monitoring the accumulation of product with time. Since the rate has to be measured over a short time with respect to the Michaelis–Menten dynamics characteristic time, enzyme degradation is not generally a problem in such assays.
- *Progress curve assays*: In these assays, the kinetic parameters are determined quantifying the evolution of the species concentrations as a function of time. The concentration of the substrate or product is recorded in time after the initial fast transient and for a sufficiently long period to allow the reaction to approach equilibrium. This allows the equilibrium ratio between the substrate and the product concentrations to be evaluated. As shown in Section 2.5.1, this measure allows the Michaelis–Menten constant to be determined.
- *Transient kinetics assays*: In these assays, reaction behavior is tracked during the initial fast transient as the intermediate reaches the steady-state kinetics period. Owing to the fact that the concentrations of the reaction products have to be observed with a good resolution in a very short time, a very fast detection technique is needed, thereby rendering these assays generally more complex than assays relying on steady-state or quasi-steady-state measurements.
- *Relaxation assay*: In these assays, an equilibrium mixture of enzyme, substrate, and product is perturbed, for instance, by a temperature, pressure, or pH jump, and the return to equilibrium is monitored.

3.4.1 DETECTION METHODS IN ENZYMATIC ASSAYS

Detection of the rate or of the reaction products in an enzymatic assay is inherently a time-dependent measurement that can be performed in two different ways, depending on the assay characteristics: continuous and sampled detection. If continuous detection is performed, the chemical reaction parameters, like concentrations and rates, are detected in real time while the reaction advances. This requires the possibility to observe some reaction produced observable, like emitted UV light, with a continuous time detector. Differently, if sampled detection is performed, a sample of the reacting blend is extracted from the reaction at selected instants in time. The reaction is stopped and the required quantities are measured. In this case, off-line measurement is performed.

3.4.1.1 Continuous Detection

There are many different types of continuous detection methods relying on the real-time observation of different quantities.

3.4.1.1.1 Spectrophotometric Detection

Spectrophotometric detection is based on the measurement of the spectrum of the electromagnetic radiation either absorbed or reflected before and after the assay reaction. Frequently, in order to have a measurable amount of radiation a suitable substrate has to be chosen for any considered enzyme. Thus, this technique is quite suitable for the characterization of the enzyme activity and for the quantification of the presence of an enzyme in a solution where the suitable substrate can be added.

If the reaction emits light in the visible spectrum it is also called a colorimetric assay. Colorimetric assays are very useful in that the presence and activity of the enzyme can be detected directly by observation, so that the assay can be rapidly tuned up to the correct equilibrium among its components before performing a real quantitative measurement.

UV light is also often used, since the common coenzymes nicotinamide adenine dinucleotide (NADH) and nicotinamide adenine dinucleotide phosphate (NADPH) absorb UV light in their reduced forms, but do not in their oxidized forms. The structure formulas of these synthetic substrates are shown in Figure 3.12. An oxidoreductase assay using NADH as a substrate could, therefore, be carried out by monitoring the reaction reported in Figure 3.13 by following the decrease in UV absorbance at a wavelength of 340 nm as it consumes the coenzyme. A typical output of the assay is reported in Figure 3.14 besides the UV spectrum of NADH and NAD^+.

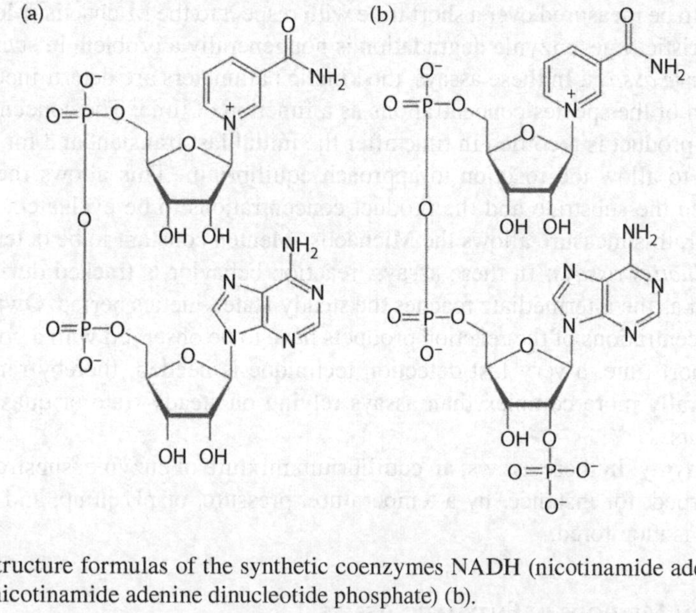

FIGURE 3.12 Structure formulas of the synthetic coenzymes NADH (nicotinamide adenine dinucleotide) (a) and NADPH (nicotinamide adenine dinucleotide phosphate) (b).

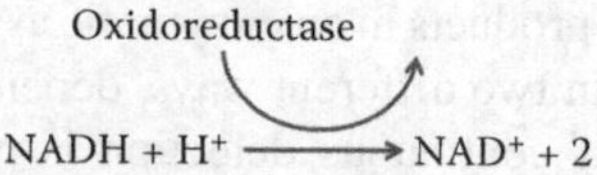

$$\text{NADH} + \text{H}^+ \xrightarrow{\text{Oxidoreductase}} \text{NAD}^+ + 2\,\text{H}^+$$

FIGURE 3.13 Oxidoreductase enzymatic assay using NADH.

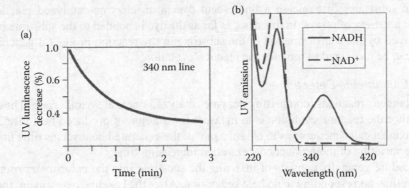

FIGURE 3.14 Oxidoreductase enzymatic assay using NADH: typical UV emission intensity versus time (a), UV absorption spectrum of NADH and NAD⁺ (b).

Even when the enzyme reaction does not result in a change in the light absorption, it can still be possible to use a spectrophotometric assay for the enzyme by using a coupled assay technique. In coupled assays, the product of one reaction is used as the substrate of a subsequent reaction that is easily detectable via spectrometry. An example of coupled assay is the colorimetric assay of a phosphatase by using p-nitrophenylphosphate (pNPP) as a substrate. The phosphate group of pNPP, that is colorless in solution, is cleaved by the enzyme to yield p-nitrophenol, as shown in Figure 3.15. The colorless p-nitrophenol, under alkaline conditions, is converted into the p-nitrophenolate anion, having a strong absorbance peak around 400 nm. This is at the blue edge of the electromagnetic spectrum, but since light reflected from an approximately white source is detected, the measured light is in the 570–590 nm bandwidth and the solution looks yellow.

3.4.1.1.2 Fluorometric Detection

Fluorometric assays use the difference in the fluorescence of substrate and product to measure the enzyme reaction. These assays are, in general, much more sensitive than spectrophotometric assays, but can suffer from interference caused by impurities and the instability of many fluorescent compounds when exposed to light. The nucleotide coenzymes NADH and NADPH can also be used for fluorescent assays since the reduced forms are fluorescent and the oxidized forms are nonfluorescent. Oxidation reactions can, therefore, be monitored by measuring the decrease in fluorescence and reduction reactions by measuring its increase.

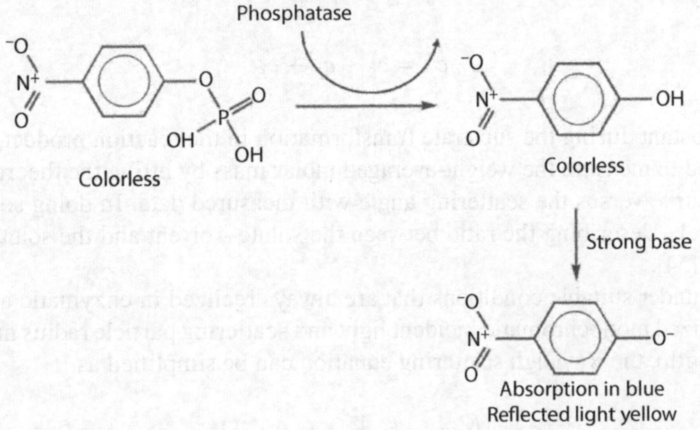

FIGURE 3.15 Coupled assay of phosphatase by p-nitrophenylphosphate (pNPP) substrate in basic solution.

Synthetic substrates that release a fluorescent dye in an enzyme-catalyzed reaction are also available for a variety of assays. In this case, as far as the dye is bonded to the substrate it is inactive, when it is freed by the transformation of the substrate in the reaction product it generates fluorescence that can be measured to monitor the reaction evolution.

3.4.1.1.3   Calorimetric Detection

Many spontaneous reactions, comprising enzyme catalyzed ones, are exothermic. Thus, a possible way to monitor the reaction evolution is to measure the amount of produced heat [51,52]. This can be done through a calorimeter so as to obtain a plot of the generated heat versus time that is proportional to the variation of the product concentration increasing time.

The procedure generally consists of inserting the substrate into the calorimeter room and measuring a baseline, corresponding to no heat generation. After the baseline assessment, the enzyme is inserted and the heat per unit time is measured at constant temperature up to the moment in which the curve reaches the baseline again. At that point no further heat is produced, which means that the reaction is arrived at a state in which no increase of product amount is further generated.

At constant temperature, the generated heat for unit time can be assumed proportional to the derivative of the product concentration in time, so that direct integration of the experimental curve provides a concentration curve suitable to derive the enzyme kinetic data.

3.4.1.1.4   Chemiluminescent Detection

Some enzyme reactions manifest the decrease of energy achieved by the creation of the product by emitting light that can be measured to detect product formation: these kind of reactions are called chemiluminescent.

3.4.1.1.5   Static Light Scattering

In static light scattering assays, a high-intensity monochromatic light, usually a laser, is launched in a solution containing the assayed macromolecules, in an enzymatic assay, the enzyme, the substrate, and the product. One or many detectors are used to measure the scattering intensity at one or many angles.

This measure can be used to evaluate the product of weight-averaged molar mass M_w (see Section 1.4.2) and overall concentration c_T of macromolecules in solution by using the Rayleigh scattering equation [53]. Having three components in the solution: the substrate S, the product P, and the enzyme E, M_w and c_T are defined as

$$M_w = \frac{c_S M_S^2 + c_P M_P^2 + c_E M_E^2}{c_S M_S + c_P M_P + c_E M_E} \tag{3.9}$$

$$c_T = c_S + c_P + c_E \tag{3.10}$$

Since c_T is constant during the substrate transformation in the reaction product, static light scattering can be used to measure the weight-averaged molar mass by fitting the theoretical form of the light scattering curve versus the scattering angle with measured data. In doing so, also the second virial coefficient A_2, describing the ratio between the solute–solvent and the solute–solute interaction is evaluated [54].

In particular, under suitable conditions that are always realized in enzymatic assay instruments (essentially focalized monochromatic incident light and scattering particle radius much smaller than the light wavelength), the Rayleigh scattering equation can be simplified as

$$\frac{K c_T}{R(\theta)} = \left(\frac{1}{M_w} + 2 A_2 c_T \right) \tag{3.11}$$

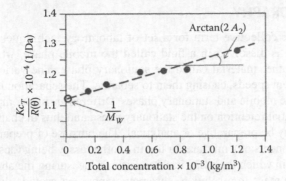

FIGURE 3.16 Example of Debye plot: points are experimental measures while the dashed line represents the linear interpolation.

where K is an optical coefficient depending only on the optical properties of the solutes and the solvent and on the inverse of the fourth power of the incident light [53] and $R(\theta)$ is the light intensity scattered at the angle θ normalized to the incident light intensity.

If Equation 3.11 is represented on the so-called Debye plot, representing the factor $Kc_T/R(\theta)$ versus the concentration c_T we obtain ideally a straight line, whose intercept with the ordinate axis is proportional to $1/M_w$ as shown in Figure 3.16.

Using such a plot and the fact that the total concentration of solutes remains constant during the catalyzed reaction, the time behavior of the weight-averaged mass M_w during the catalyzed reaction and consequently the concentration of the solutes, can be evaluated as follows.

Two or more assay sets are prepared with different concentrations of the substrate, so that the total concentration is different in the various cases. A detector is placed at a certain angle with respect to the incident light beam so as to determine the scattering angle. When the enzyme is added to the solution, the continuous measurement of the scattered light starts so that, in every instant, the Debye plot is obtained by linear interpolation of data coming from assays with different substrate concentration.

Each Debye plot is interpolated so to measure M_w; at this point the evaluation of the substrate and product concentrations with respect to time is trivial from the definition of M_w. Unfortunately, an unbiased direct measure can be achieved only if the constant K is exactly known, which means that all the characteristics of the detector are exactly known. Since this is an unpractical condition, the assay equipment has to be biased correctly before use. It can be achieved by using reference solutions with a known concentration of an isotropic scatters whose characteristics are completely known by direct measures. Generally, toluene is used for this procedure.

3.4.1.2 Discontinuous Detection

Discontinuous detection requires to take off samples from an enzyme reaction at regular intervals so as to measure the amount of product production or substrate consumption in these samples. Once the sample is extracted, standard methods can be used to measure concentrations, since they no more evolve in time. Besides standard chromatographic methods, radiometric detection is quite diffused in the field of enzymatic assays.

Radiometric detection measures the incorporation of radioactivity into substrates or its release from substrates. The radioactive isotopes most frequently used in these assays are ^{14}C, ^{32}P, ^{35}S, and ^{125}I. Since radioactive isotopes can allow the specific labeling of a single atom of a substrate, these assays are both extremely sensitive and specific. They are frequently the only way of measuring a specific reaction directly in the cell lysate without enzyme purification. Radioactivity is usually measured in these procedures using a scintillation counter [55].

3.5 CHROMATOGRAPHY

Chromatography is the collective term for a set of laboratory techniques for the separation of mixtures. The mixture is dissolved in a fluid called the mobile phase, which carries it through a structure holding another material called the stationary phase. The various constituents of the mixture travel at different speeds, causing them to separate. The separation is based on differential partitioning between the mobile and stationary phases. Differences in a compound's partition coefficient result in differential retention on the stationary phase and thus in changing the separation.

Chromatography may be preparative or analytical. The purpose of preparative chromatography is to separate the components of a mixture for use in another assay being thus a form of purification of the sample. In cases in which the assay itself consists in measuring the abundance of substances with a given molecular mass in a solution, chromatography can provide directly the essay result [56,57].

In the following sections we will analyze a few of the most diffused chromatographic techniques, but it is far to be a complete list of all the available chromatography variations. A much more complete list can be found in dedicated books.

3.5.1 LIQUID COLUMN CHROMATOGRAPHY

This was the first form of chromatography to be introduced and is still quite used [58]. The schematic illustration of the procedure used for column chromatography is shown in Figure 3.17. The assay's main instrument is a column constituted by a duct filled with a suitable porous material constituting, in this case, the chromatography solid phase. By far, the most used material is fine silica powder, with an average dimension of the particle generally greater than 10 μm and frequently around 50 μm. The dimension of the solid-phase particles is quite important since on one side they have to be small so as to allow a better separation of different targets, on the other side they have not to pose a so great obstacle to the flow of the moving phase to generate a too high separation time or, in the extreme case, no mobile phase elution from the chromatographic column.

In the simpler implementation, the column is placed vertically so that the solution under test is pushed through the column by gravity. The solution containing the substances to be divided is placed on top of the column after being concentrated sufficiently to obtain a correct work of the assay, but not so much to cause precipitation of the solutes on the column walls.

After insertion of the target solution different solvents are introduced in the system in controlled volume and at a controlled time. Since these solvents have different elution powers they cause the target solution to flow through the chromatographic column differently provoking the separation of the solutes on the ground of their mass and their affinity to the used moving and fixed phases. In the

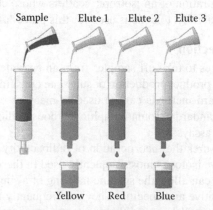

FIGURE 3.17 Scheme of the column chromatography procedure.

simpler chromatography implementation the different solvents are tagged with dyes so that they can be recognized at the output of the column due to their different color, from which the name of this separation technique. Typical solvents that are used in liquid-phase chromatography are listed in Table 3.1 besides a few of their characteristics.

While direct observation of the color of the eluted exiting from the chromatographic column allows direct inspection of the chromatography result, in order to have a quantization of the quantities of the individual targets the so-called chromatogram is used. A chromatogram is a plot where the solute masses exiting from the column is reported versus time. Since different times are associated to the elution of substances with a different mass, the chromatogram can also be read as a plot reporting the quantity of solute existing in the initial sample versus the solute mass. A sample chromatogram is reported in Figure 3.18.

To create a chromatogram a real-time measure of the quantity of matter exiting from the chromatographic column is needed: when the material that is contained into the target solution is known, optical absorption is frequently used. In this case, a white light source is used as signal source and the absorption of the solution exiting from the chromatographic column is continuously measured, in case using optical filters to opportunely shape the detector response so to better.

From the chromatogram of Figure 3.18, the effect causing a limitation in the chromatography capability of evaluating the presence of a well-defined quantity of a target substance results clearly. The chromatogram associates to each target substance a peak whose finite width is caused by several phenomena, such as diffusion of the solutes and nonhomogeneity of the stationary phase. If two or more peaks are substantially superimposed the corresponding substances quantities cannot be distinguished. For this reason, while a very precise measure of the quantity of linoleic acid can be performed starting from the chromatogram of Figure 3.18, this is not possible for arachidic acid, due to the interfering peak.

TABLE 3.1
Selected Characteristics of Common Solvents Used as Mobile Phases in Column Chromatography

Solvent	Refractive Index	Viscosity (nN s/m²)	Boiling Point (°C)
Cyclohexane	1.423	0.90	81
n-Hexane	1.372	0.30	69
1-Chlorobutane	1.400	0.42	78
Carbon tetrachloride	1.457	0.90	77
i-Propyl ether	1.365	0.38	68
Toluene	1.494	0.55	110
Diethyl ether	1.350	0.24	35
Tetrahydrofuran	1.405	0.46	66
Chloroform	1.443	0.53	61
Ethanol	1.359	1.08	78
Ethyl acetate	1.370	0.43	77
Dioxane	1.420	1.20	101
Methanol	1.326	0.54	65
Acetonitrile	1.341	0.34	82
Nitromethane	1.380	0.61	101
Ethylene glycol	1.431	16.5	182
Water	1.333	0.89	100

Note: A first idea of the elution capability is provided by the viscosity while the refraction index is important if optical detection is used. All data are at 25°C and the refraction index is at a wavelength of 300 nm.

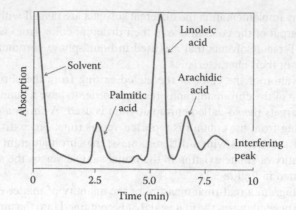

FIGURE 3.18 Absorption chromatogram for the analysis of a solution of organic acids.

To evaluate the resolution of the adsorption chromatography it is necessary to chemically describe the equilibrium of a specific target solute between the absorbed phase (ab) and the liquid phase into the flowing elute (liq). Generally, this equilibrium can be described simply as a single step reaction such as

$$X(\text{ab}) \rightleftharpoons X(\text{liq}) \tag{3.12}$$

where X is the target solute. The equilibrium constant of this reaction is called partition coefficient providing the percentage ratio between the quantities of the solute in absorbed and liquid phase. The time between sample injection and a target peak reaching a detector at the end of the column is called the target retention time (t_R). Different targets must have different retention times to be resolved by the chromatography. The time taken for the mobile phase to pass through the column is called t_M. The characteristic times t_R and t_M can be directly obtained from the chromatogram.

The characteristic pass through rate of a target through the chromatographic column is generally called retention factor k' and it is defined for the analyte X as

$$k'_x = \frac{t_R - t_M}{t_M} \tag{3.13}$$

When an analyte retention factor is less than 1, elution is so fast that accurate determination of the retention time is very difficult. High retention factors, greater than 20, mean that elution takes a very long time so that assay conditions are not easy to be maintained stationary unless particular care is taken. Generally, retention factors of the order of 2–5 are used in practice.

Since the capability of chromatography to clearly divide the peaks related to different analytes is greater and greater while the relative peaks are farther and farther on the chromatogram, the ratio between the retention factors of two different analytes X and Y is called selectivity factor α, and it is always calculated so to be greater than 1, dividing the retention factor of the slower target by the retention factor of the faster one so that

$$\alpha = \frac{k'_X}{k'_Y} \quad \text{with } k'_X > k'_Y \tag{3.14}$$

To evaluate the chromatography column resolution the so-called theoretical plates model is frequently used. The plate model supposes that the chromatographic column contains a large number of separate layers so that the equilibrium of the target between absorbed and liquid phase is independently realized in each individual plate.

In this model, the column is considered as a cascade of a finite number of mechanical filters, each constituted by an individual theoretical plate and each characterized by the same filtering efficiency and by the fact that equilibrium is instantly established between absorbed and liquid target phase. Since greater the filters number better the filtering capability of the column, the number of theoretical plates N_{pl} is also a quality index of the column selectivity.

This approximation can be justified by considering that in the real equilibrium taking place in the column, a correlation exists between infinitesimal layers of the stationary phase depending both on the stationary phase particles dimension and on their aggregation form. Filtration efficiency is greater if the typical correlation length through the column is small, so that adsorption and desorption phenomena in different column sections are as uncorrelated as possible, bringing naturally to define the ratio between the column height and the correlation length as a column quality parameter. This is exactly the number of theoretical plates. This interpretation also explains why the number of theoretical plates characterizing a certain chromatographic column is different for each target: this is due to the fact that correlation between processes taking place in different column sections depends not only on the stationary phase, but also on the target characteristics.

By adopting the discrete filters approximation and assuming Gaussian diffusion of the target solute through each plate, the number of theoretical plates of a chromatographic column can be determined for each considered target starting from the analysis of the corresponding peaks on the chromatogram obtaining

$$N_X = \xi \frac{t_R^2}{w^2} \tag{3.15}$$

where N_X is the number of theoretical plates for the target X and ξ is a constant, that is approximately equal to 5.55. If this calculation method would reflect exactly the target diffusion through the column, all the peaks at the output of the chromatogram should have a Gaussian shape, while in practice this is not true, being the peaks frequently strongly asymmetric also presenting slower tails with respect to the Gaussian distribution. Different alternative methods have been proposed to evaluate the number of theoretical plates starting from the real peaks of the chromatogram, different number of plates is obtained especially in the presence of long peak tails, but qualitative ratio of efficiency between different column and analytes is generally maintained.

On the ground of the number of theoretical plates concept, it is possible to arrive to a very useful definition of the selectivity of a chromatographic column as a function of its parameters. Taking into account the separation among different peaks α and the peaks width at half maximum w, it is natural to define on the ground of the chromatogram the resolution R_{XY} between the analytes X and Y as

$$R_{XY} = 2 \frac{t_{R,X} - t_{R,X}}{w_X + w_Y} \tag{3.16}$$

Assuming the hypothesis at the base of the plates theory and a pure Gaussian diffusion through the column, Equation 3.17 can be rewritten as a function of the three main column parameters as

$$R_{XY} = \frac{\sqrt{(N)}}{4} \left(\frac{\alpha - 1}{\alpha} \right) \left(\frac{k}{1 + k} \right) \tag{3.17}$$

where N and k are the average number of plates and retention factor between the two considered targets.

Although a somehow rough approximation, Equation 3.17 contains all the elements enabling to understand the dependence of the chromatographic resolution on the chromatography parameters: the number of plates N, the selectivity α, and the retention factor k.

The most sensible factor is the selectivity, due to the fact that the resolution is interesting in case of analytes with similar masses, where the retention ratios are not so different, the selectivity is not far from 1 and even a small increase in selectivity generates a great increase in the resolution. This is shown in Figure 3.18, in which the resolution is plotted versus the three relevant parameters varying one of them in a practical range and maintaining the other two at the center of their range.

In any case, increasing α can be achieved essentially by increasing the temperature of the column and by suitably selecting the eluent and the composition of the stationary phase. A limit naturally exists to the increase of the column temperature, related to the need of not damaging the molecules to be processed and not to provoke evaporation of the solvents, unless gas phase is used instead of liquid phase for chromatography. Both the opportune choice of the solvents and of the stationary phase composition critically depends on the substances to be assayed and a large variety of composites are used in practice for column chromatography.

The average retention factor also depends on temperature and on the mobile phase composition so that it can be optimized simultaneously to the selectivity by optimizing the column structure.

While the selectivity and the retention can be increased within a certain range, it could seem that the number of theoretical plates could be increased arbitrarily simply by increasing the column length. As a matter of fact, by increasing the column length the chromatography resolution increases, but the time needed for the solutes elution also increases. Since there is a practical limit both to the time a separation process can last and to the dimension a chromatography column has, this method cannot be used up to whatever value of the resolution.

The number of plates, however, can also be increased differently. As a matter of fact, the number of plates is practically given by the column length divided by the correlation length of the stationary mobile phase equilibrium, that is almost completely determined by the average size of the particles constituting the stationary phase. Thus, the number of equivalent plates can be greatly increased by decreasing the average stationary phase particles dimension. However, decreasing the average stationary phase particle dimension also increases the average opposition the static phase excerpt to the motion of the mobile phase so that the separation time gets longer and longer. This problem can be solved by inducing the mobile phase motion through the application of an external pressure much greater than that induced by gravity (Figure 3.19).

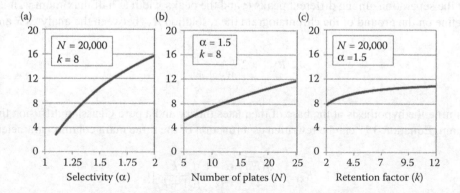

FIGURE 3.19 Dependence of the column chromatographic resolution on the column separation (a), on the number of theoretical plates (b) and on the retention factor (c). Number of theoretical separation and retention factor are averaged considering both the target that have to be resolved.

3.5.2 HIGH-PERFORMANCE LIQUID CHROMATOGRAPHY

High-performance liquid chromatography (HPLC) is basically a highly improved form of column chromatography. Instead of a solvent being allowed to drip through a column under gravity, it is forced through under high pressures of up to 400 atm so as to allow much smaller particles to be used and faster separation to be obtained [59,60].

Owing to the potential accuracy in the separation of very similar solutes, HPLC equipments are frequently associated with very sensitive optical detection systems, like systems based on UV absorption. The principle scheme of HPLC is presented in Figure 3.20. Design of chromatographic column used for HPLC essentially depends on the pressure they have to resist and on the required column length. Typically, the column length is of the order of 20–30 cm. In case of very high pressures, steel is used to fabricate the column, allowing pressures in excess of 40 MPa to be used in conjunction of a silica powder with average particle radius in the order of 1.5 μm or less. An example of structure of a stainless-steel HPLS column is provided in Figure 3.21. Stainless steel is not the best material if very good chemical neutrality is needed due to the need of separation of very reactive materials. In this case, lower pressures have to be used in order to adopt either glass or polymeric columns. A sample of possible performances that can be obtained by HPLC is reported in Table 3.2.

There are two variants of HPLC depending on the relative polarity of the solvent and the stationary phase. Normal-phase HPLC is characterized by the use of nonpolar mobile phase and polar stationary phase, like silica fine powder. In this case, polar compounds in the mixture passing through the column will stick longer to the polar silica than nonpolar compounds will. The nonpolar ones will, therefore, pass more quickly through the column.

In the case of reversed-phase HPLC the stationary phase is nonpolar, for example, incorporating long hydrocarbons to compensate silica polarity, while polar elute is used—for example, a mixture of water and an alcohol such as methanol. In this case, there will be a strong attraction between the polar solvent and polar molecules in the mixture being passed through the column. There would not

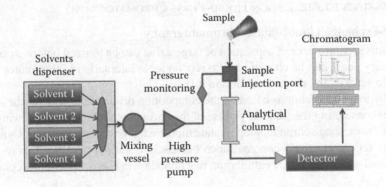

FIGURE 3.20 Principle scheme of an HPLC equipment.

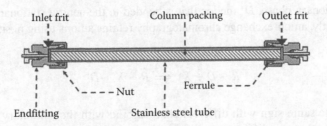

FIGURE 3.21 Structure of a stainless-steel column for HPLC.

TABLE 3.2

Pressures and Performances of an Example Reversed-Phase HPLC with Different Column Length and Average Stationary Phase Particle Diameter

Column Length (cm)	Particles Radius (mm)	Pressure (MPa)	Theoretical Plates (Thousands)	Retention Time (min)
15	5	0.87	10	17.5
15	1.5	33.10	33.2	5.25
15	0.75	25.65	66.4	2.5
25	5	1.45	25	35
25	1.5	55.16	83	10.5
25	0.75	427.49	166	5
50	5	2.90	83	70
50	1.5	110.32	166	21

Note: Data evaluated for an analyte with $k' = 2$ and a molecular mass of 6 kDa.

be as much attraction between the hydrocarbon chains attached to the silica (the stationary phase) and the polar molecules in the solution. Polar molecules in the mixture will, therefore, spend most of their time moving with the solvent. Nonpolar compounds on the contrary will tend to form attractions with the hydrocarbon groups because of van der Waals dispersion forces. They will also be less soluble in the solvent because of the need to break hydrogen bonds as they squeeze in between the water or methanol molecules, for example. They therefore spend less time in solution in the solvent and this will slow them down on their way through the column. That means that in reversed-phase HPLC, the polar molecules travel through the column more quickly.

3.5.3 ALTERNATIVES TO ADSORPTION LIQUID-PHASE CHROMATOGRAPHY

3.5.3.1 Ions-Exchange Liquid-Phase Chromatography

In the case of ions separation, or of separation of targets that can be ionized before chromatography, suitable stationary phase can be chosen so as to rely on ionic interaction of the solutes with the stationary phase to achieve an effective separation [61].

Separating by ionic interaction is based on the competition off different ions for the same binding sites of the fiber constituting the stationary phase of the chromatographic column. Owing to this fact, we can have cation-exchange chromatography, and anion-exchange chromatography. Cation-exchange chromatography retains positively charged cation because the stationary phase displays a negatively charged functional group so that the equilibrium reaction allowing separation in the column writes

$$R - D + X^+ \rightleftharpoons R - X + D^+ \tag{3.18}$$

where R is the stationary phase, D^+ the ion that is bonded to the neutral stationary phase, and X^+ the target ion. Differently, anion-exchange chromatography retains anions using positively charged functional group:

$$R - D + X^- \rightleftharpoons R - X + D^- \tag{3.19}$$

Since ions of the same sign with different charges bind with the stationary phase forming ion bonds with different energy, different targets can be separated on the ground of their charge. As

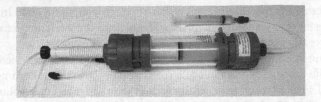

FIGURE 3.22 Photograph of a sample polymeric chromatographic column for protein ion-exchange chromatography.

a matter of fact, different eluents can establish either different pH in the column, so to move the equilibrium of the reaction (18) or (19) in the wanted direction, or can insert different types of ions in the column so as to cause the elution of target ions with suitable charge. For example, in cation-exchange chromatography, the positively charged analyte could be displaced by the addition of positively charged sodium ions.

In ion-exchange chromatography, the stationary phase is typically a resin or gel matrix consisting of agarose or cellulose beads with covalently bonded charged functional groups. To detect the presence of the target in the eluted mobile phase, besides standard optical methods, also a conductivity measure can be used since in this case the conductivity of the solution is proportional to the ions concentration due to the fact that ions charge is known.

Ion-exchange chromatography is one of the most used mean to separate proteins from a complex solution, due to the fact that proteins assume a charge that depends on the pH of the solute (see Section 2.3.1). Every protein has a specific pH-charge characteristic, thus using solutions with different pH for elution in different phases of the chromatography different proteins can be selected. Proteins chromatography is frequently performed with plastic columns that do not contaminate the protein solution when presenting a chemically inert surface. Moreover, a huge pressure is dangerous for proteins risking to denature them by mechanically changing their stereographic structure. The photograph of a sample column for ion-exchange protein chromatography is reported in Figure 3.22.

3.5.3.2 Size-Exclusion Chromatography

The principle of size-exclusion chromatography (SEC) relies on the fact that different molecules have different dimensions so that smaller analytes can enter the stationary phase particle pores more easily and spend more time in the pores, increasing their retention time. Conversely, larger analytes spend little if any time in the pores and are eluted quickly. If an analyte is too large or too small it will be either not retained or completely retained, respectively [62,63].

A key requirement for SEC is that the analyte does not interact with the surface of the stationary phases. Differences in elution time are based solely on the stationary phase volume the analyte experiences. A small molecule that can penetrate every corner of the pore system of the stationary phase experiences the entire pore volume and the inter-particle volume, generally about 80% of the column volume, and will elute late. Differently, a large molecule that cannot penetrate the pore system experiences only the inter-particle volume, generally about 35% of the column volume, and will elute earlier when this volume of mobile phase has passed through the column. This results in the separation of a solution of particles based on size. Provided that all the particles are loaded simultaneously or near simultaneously, particles of the same size should elute together.

However, as there are various measures of the size of a macromolecule, for instance, the radius of gyration and the hydrodynamic radius, a fundamental problem in the theory of SEC has been the choice of a proper molecular size parameter by which molecules of different kinds are separated. Experimentally, an excellent correlation between elution volume and the hydrodynamic volume of the molecules was found for several different chromatographic equipment architecture and chemical compositions of stationary and mobile phase. The observed correlation based on the hydrodynamic volume is currently accepted as the basis of universal SEC calibration.

The hydrodynamic volume is the volume that has to be used to determine hydrodynamic and electro-hydrodynamic properties of a molecule (see Chapter 7), and it takes into account the molecule hydration shell so as to result in generally greater than the molecular volume evaluated using different definitions [64]. The hydrodynamic volume is generally experimentally evaluated, but it can also be calculated with statistical mechanics models like implicit solvent models (see Section 1.2). The most direct way of evaluating the hydrodynamic volume of globular molecules is to measure the diffusion coefficient in a selected solvent, for example, water. If the molecule would be a rigid sphere without any interaction with the solvent the diffusion coefficient D would be provided by the Einstein formula (see Section 7.4.2):

$$D = \frac{\kappa_B T}{6\pi\eta R} = \frac{\kappa_B T}{3\eta\sqrt[3]{6\pi^2 V}} \qquad (3.20)$$

where
  κ_B is the Boltzmann constant
  T is the absolute temperature
  η is the solvent dynamic viscosity
  R is the particle radius
  V is the particle volume

If Equation 3.20 is used to evaluate, starting from a measure of the diffusion coefficient, the volume of a macromolecule, for example, a globular protein like hemoglobin, the result is found to depend on the solution characteristics like solvent viscosity temperature and so on. This result, depending on the hydration mechanism, is called hydrodynamic volume of the molecule. For molecules that have a clearly not globular shape, like antibodies, the same procedure can be applied, evaluating the diffusion coefficient for a rigid body with a suitable shape approximating the molecule shape, operation that frequently requires numerical evaluation.

Another way of determining the hydrodynamic volume starts from the solute partial specific volume when it is in solution (Figure 3.22).

Each size-exclusion column has a range of molecular weights that can be separated that result from the so-called column calibration curve, relating the elution volume to the molecular mass of the eluted targets. On such curves the exclusion limit (EL) defines the molecular weight at the upper end of this range and is identified by molecules too large to be trapped in the stationary phase, while the permeation limit (PL) defines the molecular weight at the lower end of the range of separation and is identified by molecules that can penetrate into the pores of the stationary phase completely: all molecules below this molecular mass are so small that they elute as a single band [64]. An example of SEC calibration curve in the case of a column designed to work with biochemical composites is presented in Figure 3.23.

Several factors limit the practical resolution of SEC. In practice, particles in solution do not have a fixed size, resulting in the probability that a particle that would otherwise be hampered by a pore passing right by it, moreover, both particles and pores of the stationary phase may vary in size. Moreover, any chemical interaction between the stationary phase and the target solute alters the retention time, generally increasing it so as to mimic a smaller molecular mass. Elution curves, therefore, resemble Gaussian distributions. If a continuous time detector is placed at the end of the elution column, we can construct a chromatogram whose shape is similar to the chromatograms associated to other forms of chromatography. An example is reported in Figure 3.24. In general, SEC is considered a low-resolution form of chromatography, adopted either when it is needed to

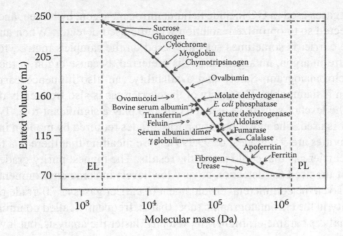

FIGURE 3.23 Example of SEC calibration curve in the case of a column designed to work with biochemical composites.

separate targets with very different molecular mass, as in the case of first processing of a cell lysate, or when accurate separation is not needed.

3.5.3.3 Gas Chromatography

Dealing with liquid chromatography, the fact that chromatography resolution increases with increasing temperature frequently is taken into consideration. This procedure is limited by the fact that the mobile liquid phase has to remain liquid for chromatography to work so that the liquid boiling point has not to be exceeded. The situation becomes different if the mobile phase is not liquid but gaseous, in this case much higher temperatures can be achieved in order to improve resolution. Such an analytical technique is called gas chromatography [65–67].

Gas chromatography is widely used in analyzing inorganic components or hydrocarbons and temperature-resistant polymers, in order, for example, to determine the relative mass composition of a polymer after a specific polymerization process (see Section 1.4.2). It is also widely used in biological compounds analysis, frequently with a careful tuning of its parameters due to the need not to denature the biomolecules.

In gas chromatography, while the mobile phase is a gas, the stationary phase is a liquid filling the chromatographic tube. To stabilize the separation procedure so to improve repeatability and resolution the chromatographic tube is placed in an oven that allows the process temperature to be stabilized. Other parameters that are used to tune the selection process during gas chromatography are temperature and gas flow rate.

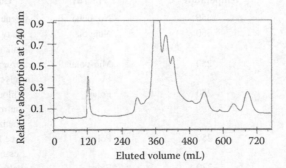

FIGURE 3.24 Example of SEC chromatogram.

Typical carrier gases used in GC include helium, nitrogen, argon, hydrogen, and air. The adopted gas is usually selected so to optimize resolution with the used detector. When analyzing gas samples, however, the carrier is sometimes selected based on the sample's matrix, for example, when analyzing a mixture in argon, an argon carrier is preferred, because argon in the sample does not show up on the chromatogram. Safety and availability can also influence carrier selection, for example, hydrogen is flammable. The purity of the carrier gas is also frequently determined by the detector, though the level of sensitivity needed can also play a significant role. Typically, purity of 99.995% or higher is used. The most common purity grades required by modern instruments for the majority of sensitivities are 5.0 grades, or 99.999% pure meaning that there is a total of 10 ppm of impurities in the carrier gas that could affect the results. The highest purity grades in common use are 6.0 grades, but the need for detection at very low levels in some environmental and biological applications has driven the commercial development of carrier gases at 7.0 grade purity. The carrier gas average velocity in the chromatographic tube, that is, frequently called column also in this case, is an important analysis parameter: higher the velocity, faster the analysis, but lower the separation between analytes.

To have a reasonable residence time in the column, a species must show some degree of solubility with the stationary phase. Generally, this requirement is fulfilled by adopting a stationary phase with a polarity similar to that of the target (see Section 1.3), that is, polar for polar targets and nonpolar for nonpolar targets. Polar stationary phases contain functional groups such as –CN, –CO, and –OH, polyester phases are highly polar. Hydrocarbon-type stationary phase and dialkyl siloxanes are nonpolar.

Other desirable properties for the immobilized liquid phase in a gas–liquid chromatographic column include:

- Low volatility: ideally, the boiling point of the liquid should be at 100°C higher than the maximum operating temperature for the column
- Thermal stability
- Chemical inertness

A list of selected stationary phases used in GC is reported in Table 3.3.

The schematic representation of a gas chromatography equipment is reported in Figure 3.25.

TABLE 3.3
Selected Stationary Phases for Gas Chromatography with Maximum Operating Temperature and Selected Applications

Stationary Phase	Maximum Operating Temperature °C	Polarity	Common Applications
Polydimethyl siloxane	350	Nonpolar	General purpose
5% Phenyl-polydimethyl siloxane	350	Nonpolar	Fatty acids, methyl esters, alkaloids, drugs
50% Phenyl-polydimethyl siloxane	250	Mid-polar	Drugs, steroids, pesticides, glycols
50% Trifluoropropyl-polydimethyl siloxane	250	Polar	Chlorinated aromatics, nitroaromatics, alkyl-substituted benzene
Polyethylene glycol	250	Polar	Free fatty acids, alcohols, ethers, essential oils
50% Cyanopropyl—polydimethyl siloxane	240	Polar	Polyunsaturated fatty acids, free acids, alcohols, rosin acids

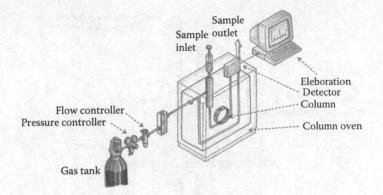

FIGURE 3.25 Schematics of a gas chromatography equipment.

Column efficiency requires that the sample be of suitable size and be introduced as a *plug* of vapor; too slow injection and/or oversized samples cause band spreading and poor resolution. The most common method of sample injection involves the use of micro-syringe to inject a liquid or gaseous sample through a self-sealing, silicone-rubber diaphragm or septum into a flash vaporizer port located at the head of the column. The sample port is ordinarily about 50°C above the boiling point of the least volatile component of the sample. A scheme of a micro-syringe injection system is reported in Figure 3.26.

Two general types of columns are encountered in gas chromatography, packed and open tubular, or capillary. Chromatographic columns vary in length from less than 2 to 50 m or more. They are constructed of stainless steel, glass, fused silica, or Teflon. To fit into an oven for thermal control they have usually a coil shape with a diameter of the order of 10–30 cm. Open tubular columns can be either wall-coated open tubular (WCOT) or support-coated open tubular (SCOT). Wall-coated columns are simply capillary tubes coated with a thin layer of the stationary phase. In support-coated open tubular columns, the inner surface of the column is lined with a thin film of a thickness around 30 μm of a support material, such as diatomaceous earth. This type of column holds several times as much stationary phase as does a wall-coated column and thus has a greater sample capacity.

A large variety of detectors is used in GC, depending both on the performance required and on the need of conserving the sample for further processing.

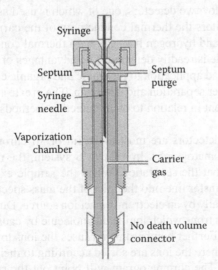

FIGURE 3.26 Scheme of a micro-syringe injection system for gas chromatography.

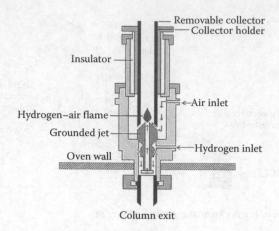

FIGURE 3.27 Scheme of a flame ionization detector for application in gas chromatography.

Flame ionization detectors (FID) are the most generally applicable and most widely used detectors. In an FID, the sample is directed at an air–hydrogen flame after exiting the column as shown in Figure 3.27. At the high temperature of the air–hydrogen flame, the sample undergoes pyrolysis, or chemical decomposition through intense heating. Pyrolyzed hydrocarbons release ions and electrons that carry current. A high-impedance pico-ammeter measures this current to monitor the sample's elution. It is advantageous to used FID because the detector is unaffected by flow rate, noncombustible gases and water. These properties allow FID high sensitivity and low noise. The unit is both reliable and relatively easy to use. However, this technique does require flammable gas and also destroys the sample.

Thermal conductivity detectors (TCD) are one of the earliest detectors developed for use with gas chromatography. The TCD works by measuring the change in carrier gas thermal conductivity caused by the presence of the sample, which has a different thermal conductivity from that of the carrier gas. Their design is relatively simple, and consists of an electrically heated source that is maintained at constant power. The temperature of the source depends upon the thermal conductivities of the surrounding gases. The source is usually a thin wire made of platinum or gold. The resistance within the wire depends upon temperature, which is dependent upon the thermal conductivity of the gas. TCDs usually employ two detectors, one of which is used as the reference for the carrier gas and the other which monitors the thermal conductivity of the carrier gas and sample mixture. Carrier gases such as helium and hydrogen has very high thermal conductivities so the addition of even a small amount of sample is readily detected. The advantages of TCDs are the ease and simplicity of use, the devices' broad application to inorganic and organic compounds, and the ability of the analyte to be collected after separation and detection. The greatest drawback of the TCD is the low sensitivity of the instrument in relation to other detection methods, in addition to flow rate and concentration dependency.

Mass spectrometer (MS) detectors are most powerful of all chromatography detectors and it is frequently used in gas chromatographs. In a GC/MS system, the mass spectrometer scans the masses continuously throughout the separation. When the sample exits the chromatography column, it is passed through a transfer line into the inlet of the mass spectrometer. The sample is then ionized and fragmented, typically by an electron-impact ion source. During this process, the sample is bombarded by energetic electrons which ionize the molecule by causing them to lose an electron due to electrostatic repulsion. Further bombardment causes the ions to fragment. The ions are then passed into a mass analyzer where the ions are sorted according to their mass-to-charge ratio. Most ions are only singly charged. The chromatogram will point out the retention times and the mass spectrometer will use the peaks to determine the kind of molecules that exist in the mixture.

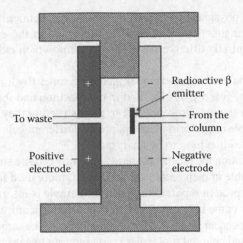

To waste

Positive electrode

Radioactive β emitter

From the column

Negative electrode

FIGURE 3.28   Scheme of the simpler implementation of electron-capture detector for gas chromatography.

Electron-capture detectors (ECD) are highly selective detectors commonly used for detecting environmental samples as the device selectively detects organic compounds with moieties such as halogens, peroxides, quinones, and nitro groups and gives little to no response for all other compounds. Therefore, this method is best suited in applications where trace quantities of chemicals such as pesticides are to be detected and other chromatographic methods are unfeasible. The simplest form of ECD, schematically shown in Figure 3.28, involves gaseous electrons from a radioactive β emitter in an electric field. As the analyte leaves the GC column, it is passed over this β emitter, which typically consists of nickle-63 or tritium. The electrons from the β emitter ionize the nitrogen carrier gas and cause it to release a burst of electrons. In the absence of organic compounds, a constant standing current is maintained between two electrodes. With the addition of organic compounds with electronegative functional groups, the current decreases significantly as the functional groups capture the electrons. The advantages of ECDs are the high selectivity and sensitivity toward certain organic species with electronegative functional groups. However, the detector has a limited signal range and is potentially dangerous owing to its radioactivity. In addition, the signal-to-noise ratio is limited by radioactive decay and the presence of O_2 within the detector.

Other adopted detection methods for gas chromatography include atomic emission detectors, chemiluminescence detectors, and photoionization detectors [65–67].

3.6   ELECTROPHORESIS

In general terms, electrophoresis is the motion of charged particles of a solute with respect to the neutral solvent due to the presence of an electrostatic field (see Section 7.5.1). This phenomenon is used in one of the most affirmed ways to separate and quantify charged molecules in a solution [68].

In biochemistry this is an important task, since peptides, proteins, and nucleic acids tend to acquire a net charge when in solution with a suitable pH so that all these species can be processes by electrophoresis. If electrophoresis has to be used to separate and quantify a particular type of molecules it is needed that, when the electrical field is applied, they move into the solution at a suitable speed so to be effectively separated without arriving in a very short time at the electrode. This allows to distinguish the position of different molecules at the end of the assay time. This condition is generally not reached in water solution, even if small electrical fields are applied, due to the high mobility of charged molecule in this low viscosity medium.

To slow the molecules movement when practical electrical fields are applied, electrophoresis is performed using a gel as solvent. Gels consist of a solid three-dimensional network that spans the volume of a liquid medium and ensnares it through surface tension effects. This internal network structure may result from physical bonds (physical gels) or chemical bonds (chemical gels), as well as crystallites or other junctions that remain intact within the extending fluid. Thus, gels can be defined as a substantially dilute cross-linked system, which exhibits no flow when in the steady state [69].

Virtually any fluid can be used as an extender including water (hydrogels), oil, and air (aerogel). Both by weight and volume, gels are mostly fluid in composition and thus exhibit densities similar to those of their constituent liquids. However, due to their structure they manifest much higher viscosity, so being quite suitable to perform electrophoresis. Different gels are used depending on the weight and type of molecules that have to be analyzed.

In its simpler implementation the electrophoretic apparatus is quite simple, as it is represented in Figure 3.29, in its two possible implementations: horizontal, more used for nucleic acids separation, and vertical, more used for protein separation. When the sample is inserted into the wells that have been created in the gel they come in contact with the gel pH and acquire a charge strictly related to the pH. Generally, the pH is chosen so as to have all molecules of the same charge. In this way, when the electrical field is activated charged molecules starts moving toward the opposite sign electrode, all on the same side of the starting well. The molecules velocity, after a very short initial transient, relax on a value proportional to the applied field due to the great hydrodynamic resistance of the gel (see Section 7.4.1): the proportionality constant between the velocity and the applied field is called molecules mobility.

In general, the molecules mobility is a complex function of their charge, their shape, and their molecular mass, so that it is not easy to foresee where the molecules will stop after the field is switched off. In any case, molecules with the same mobility stop at the same distance from the well so as to form the so-called electrophoresis bands. Bands have a width depending on the well dimension and on the diffusivity of the molecules in the gel (see Section 7.4.1). For each given gel composition, the mobility of different proteins, peptides, and nucleic acids can be measured using reference solutions so as to calibrate the system.

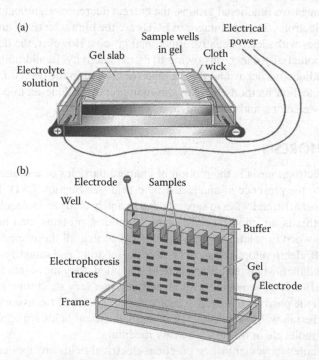

FIGURE 3.29 Scheme of the simpler electrophoresis implementation in its horizontal (a) and vertical (b) versions.

In selected cases, especially when dealing with proteins and RNA, whose secondary and tertiary structure can heavily influence the value of the electrophoresis mobility, it is opportune to denature the macromolecules before electrophoresis. For this use is adopted a so-called denaturing gel, in which chemical groups, generally detergents [70] causing the break of the weak bonds creating secondary and tertiary structure of proteins and RNA are incorporated. In this way, the macromolecules are reported to the linear chain structure and their mobility in electrophoresis depends, at least in a first approximation, only by the chain mass and charge.

The typical procedure to execute an electrophoresis test with a manual macroscopic equipment as shown in Figure 3.29 can be described as follows [71]:

- *Detection plate preparation*
  - The detection plates of the equipment must be soaked with the marker that will allow the detection of the presence of proteins.
  - After absorption of the buffer, the plates have to be placed in the suitable slot into the equipment.
- *Electrophoresis chamber preparation*
  - The side containers of the electrophoresis chamber has to be filled with the suitable buffer.
  - The chamber has to be covered with the buffer so as to eliminate air.
- *Sample application*
  - Each well has to be filled in the sample plate generally using a suitable microdispenser
  - Remove the wetted plates from the buffer.
- *Electrophoresis*
  - Place the plate in the electrophoresis chamber.
  - Cover the chamber securely and wait for a time interval of the order of half a minute depending on the specific equipment to equilibrate.
  - Electrophorese the plate for the prescribed time at the prescribed voltage. Time and voltage depends both on gel and on the type of molecules to process.
- *Visualization of the bands*
  - At the end of the electrophoresis time, the plate has to be removed from the chamber and placed in suitable stain.
  - After washing and drying the plates they have to be dehydrated (e.g., in methanol wash).
- *Evaluation of the bands*
  - The intensity of the electrophoresis bands is measured with a suitable detector. The simpler possible detector is a densitometer, detecting the density of the marker that has been added at the beginning in the individual bands. In this case, scan the plates in the densitometer using a suitable filter and read the densitometer measure.

3.6.1 ELECTROPHORESIS GEL TYPES

3.6.1.1 Agarose

Agarose gels are easily cast and handled compared to other matrices, because the gel setting is a physical rather than chemical change. Samples are also easily recovered. After the experiment is completed, the resulting gel can be stored in a plastic bag in a refrigerator.

Agarose gel electrophoresis can be used for the separation of DNA fragments ranging from 50 bp to several megabases (millions of bases) using specialized apparatus. The distance between DNA bands of a given length is determined by the percent agarose in the gel. The disadvantage of higher concentrations is the long run times (sometimes days). Instead, high percentage agarose gels should be run with a pulsed-field electrophoresis (PFE), or field inversion electrophoresis.

Agarose gels are also used for electrophoresis of proteins that are larger than 200 kDa [72].

3.6.1.2 Polyacrylamide

Polyacrylamide gel electrophoresis (PAGE) is used for separating proteins ranging in size from 5 to 2000 kDa due to the uniform pore size provided by the polyacrylamide gel. Pore size is controlled by controlling the concentrations of acrylamide and bis-acrylamide powder used in creating a gel. Typically, resolving gels are made in 6%, 8%, 10%, 12%, or 15%. Stacking gel (5%) is poured on top of the resolving gel and a gel comb (which forms the wells and defines the lanes where proteins, sample buffer, and ladders will be placed) is inserted. The percentage chosen depends on the size of the protein that one wishes to identify or probe in the sample. The smaller the known weight, the higher the percentage that should be used. Changes on the buffer system of the gel can help to further resolve proteins of very small sizes [73].

3.6.1.3 Starch

Partially hydrolyzed potato starch makes for another nontoxic medium for protein electrophoresis. The gels are slightly more opaque than acrylamide or agarose. Nondenatured proteins can be separated according to charge and size. Typical starch gel concentrations are 5–10%.

3.6.2 Protein Electrophoresis

Protein electrophoresis methods can be divided, as already introduced, in denaturing and native, that is not denaturing methods.

The most used denaturing methods for proteins gel electrophoresis is the so-called sodium dodecyl sulfate polyacrylamide gel electrophoresis (SDS-PAGE). The gel used in this technique, as usually in protein electrophoresis, is based on polyacrylamide, but in this case sodium dodecyl sulfate (SDS) is added to the sample before electrophoresis (Figure 3.30). Processing of the sample in SDS before electrophoresis with temperature increased up to 60°C or 100°C denatures secondary and nondisulfide-linked proteins tertiary structures, and applies a negative charge to each protein in proportion to its mass [74,75]. The negative charge imposed by SDS renders almost negligible the protein charge due to the solution pH so that the mobility is in a first approximation dependent only on the protein mass, being the charge proportional to the polypeptide chain length.

As far as native electrophoresis is concerned, we can distinguish protocols using a gel that while preserving the folded state of proteins also interact with them by charging them with a much higher charge with respect to the natural charge the protein tends to assume in the gel pH. In this case, the electrophoresis mobility does not depend on the charge, but since proteins maintain their secondary and tertiary structure it does not depend only on the protein mass, but also on its shape. A typical gel used in this application is polyacrylamide while the sample is treated before electrophoresis with Coomassie Brilliant Blue dye [76]. Coomassie Brilliant Blue is the name of two similar triphenylmethane dyes whose structure formula is shown in Figure 3.31 and that differs from the presence of two methyl groups. Coomassie Brilliant Blue dye provides the necessary charges to the protein complexes during the pretreatment. The disadvantage of this procedure is that the dye, in binding to proteins, can act like a detergent causing complexes to dissociate. Another drawback is the potential quenching of chemiluminescence or fluorescence. An example of electrophoresis plate reading after Brilliant Blue PAGE on several samples in vertical arrangement equipment is reported in Figure 3.32.

Pure native electrophoresis, that is, electrophoresis where proteins move on the effect of the field due to their charge is generally performed with polyacrylamide gel without any treatment. It is

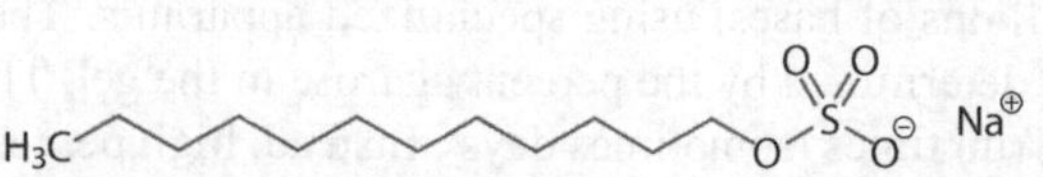

FIGURE 3.30 Structural formula of the detergent SDS.

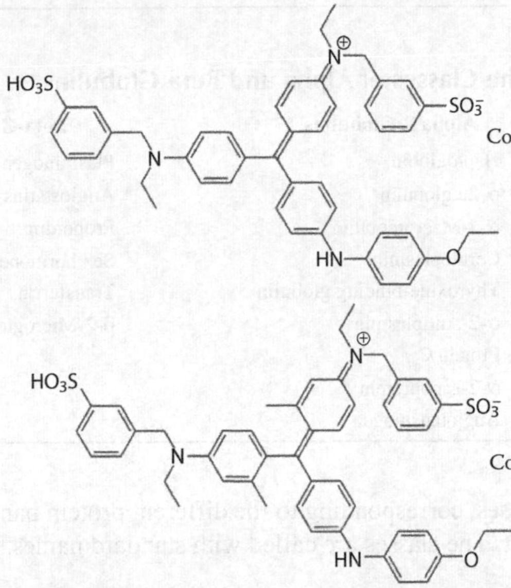

Coomassie Brilliant Blue R-250

Coomassie Brilliant Blue G-250

FIGURE 3.31   Structural formulas of Coomassie Brilliant Blue dyes. (The name "Coomassie" is a registered trademark of Imperial Chemical Industries.)

characterized by a lesser resolution with respect to electrophoresis protocols fixing the protein charge, but is much milder, preserving more fragile species with untouched structure for further assaying.

An interesting example of protein electrophoresis is the analysis of human blood proteins through the electrophoresis of blood serum, that is, of the blood liquid part remaining after elimination of blood cells. Generally, blood serum proteins electrophoresis is carried out at a pH of about 9.0 in cellulose gel so that all the proteins have a net negative charge. Agarose gel charged with positive ions is used since many heavy proteins are present in the serum and they have to be well resolved for a diagnostic use of this assay.

Since a large concentration of positive ions is needed to obtain a pH equal to 9.0, when electrophoresis begins positive ions migrate rapidly toward the negative electrode, causing a water flux in the same direction through the gel structure. This flux is generally so important that it carries along the most massive proteins, that are found to move toward the negative electrode even if they have a negative charge carried along by the electro-hydrodynamic flux. To read the electrophoretic curve,

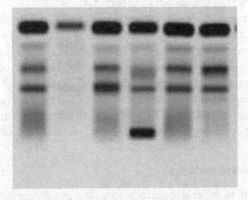

FIGURE 3.32   Example of electrophoresis plate reading after Brilliant Blue PAGE on several samples in a vertical arrangement equipment.

TABLE 3.4

Examples of Proteins Classified in the Classes of Alpha and Beta Globulins

Alpha 1 Globulins	Alpha 2 Globulins	Beta-Globulin
α1-Antitrypsin	Haptoglobin	Plasminogen
Alpha 1-antichymotrypsin	α-2u globulin	Angiostatins
Orosomucoid (acid glycoprotein)	α-2-Macroglobulin	Properdin
Serum amyloid A	Ceruloplasmin	Sex hormone-binding globulin
	Thyroxine-binding globulin	Transferrin
	α-2-Antiplasmin	β-2-Microglobulin
	Protein C	
	α-2-Lipoprotein	
	Angiotensinogen	

the blood proteins are collected in classes, corresponding to the different protein bands that can be recognized in the electrophoresis result. The classes are called with standard names.

- *Serum albumin* is the most abundant plasma protein in mammals. Albumin is essential for maintaining the oncotic pressure needed for proper distribution of body fluids between intravascular compartments and body tissues. It also acts as a plasma carrier by nonspecifically binding several hydrophobic steroid hormones and as a transport protein for hemin and fatty acids.
- *Alpha globulins* are a group of globular proteins in plasma that are highly mobile in electrophoresis and form an almost continuous band just on the right (lower mobility, higher molecular mass) of the albumin band. With high-resolution electrophoresis two secondary peaks can be distinguished in the α-globulin band, corresponding to α-1 and α-2 proteins. A list of blood proteins in the α-1 and α-2 groups is reported in Table 3.4.
- *Beta globulins* are a group of many different proteins, having practically in common only their position in the electrophoresis diagram. Examples of α-globulins are provided in Table 3.4.
- *Gamma globulins* are a class of globulins, identified by their position at the right extreme of the electrophoresis result. The most significant α- globulins are IgG immunoglobulin (see Section 2.4.1). However, a few immunoglobulin does not enter into this electrophoresis band and this band includes also other types of proteins.

A typical band set observed through a densitometer after the electrophoresis and staining of the proteins in normal human serum are shown in Figure 3.33.

The densitometer scan in Figure 3.33 is interpreted as follows: The numbers recorded under the various protein peaks are called integration units. These are recorded by the densitometer and represent, in simple terms, the area encompassed under each peak, which is proportional to the amount of protein present. This sample had a total of 140 integration units, 77 of which are represented by albumin. The percent of albumin in the serum is therefore 77/140, or 55%. The complete analysis of the serum proteins is accomplished by having the value of the total amount of protein in the serum determined by an independent method. The total serum protein in this case was 6.7 g/100 mL. Thus, the milligrams of albumin per 100 mL for this sample were calculated to be 3.7.

3.6.3 Nucleic Acid Electrophoresis

Nucleic acid electrophoresis is generally performed either in agarose gel or in polydimethylacrylamide (PDMA) gel, depending on the sample to be analyzed. Typical electrophoresis mobility curves for different kinds of nucleic acids in PDMA and in agarose gel are reported in Figure 3.34

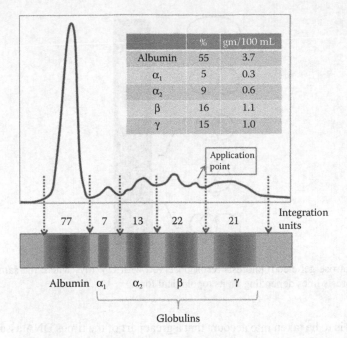

	%	gm/100 mL
Albumin	55	3.7
α_1	5	0.3
α_2	9	0.6
β	16	1.1
γ	15	1.0

FIGURE 3.33   A typical band set observed through a densitometer after electrophoresis of proteins in normal human serum.

[77]. From the curves in Figure 3.34, it can be observed that in both the cases an almost linear part of the curve exists in between two zones where the mobility slowly depends on the mass, the electrophoresis resolution is naturally maximum if the system is biased around the middle of the linear phase and, due to this fact, in laboratory practice the number of base pairs of a certain nucleic acid is approximately estimated relating linearly to the logarithm of the mobility with the logarithm of the number of base pairs.

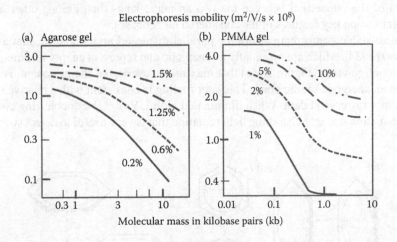

FIGURE 3.34   Dependence of the mobility on the number of base pairs in double DNA electrophoresis; (a) agarose gel electrophoresis of double-stranded DNA at 25°C, with different agarose concentrations in percentage of the electrophoretic gel and with a field of 6.4×10^{-3} V/m; (b) PMMA gel electrophoresis of single-stranded DNA with 4 mol of urea at 50°C and different PDMA concentrations. (Adapted from Stellwagen N. C., Stellwagen E., *Journal of Chromatography A*, vol. 1216, pp. 1917–1929, 2009.)

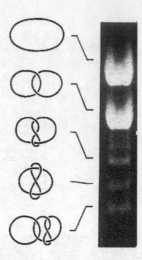

FIGURE 3.35 Agarose gel electrophoresis result observed with UV rays where the same molecule forms different electrophoresis lines depending on its topological form.

Additionally, it is to be taken into account that a great part of the times DNA assumes supercoiled structures, besides the linear helix-turn-helix form, that manifest themselves in several different forms when the DNA is insulated [78,79]. Supercoiled forms of DNA (often also called plasmid) migrate in agarose distinctly differently from linear DNAs of the same mass. A typical agarose gel electrophoresis result observed with UV rays is shown in Figure 3.35, in which the same molecule forms different electrophoresis lines depending on its topological form.

The most common detection method used to reveal electrophoresis results is based on UV spectroscopy [80]. Nucleic acids show a strong absorbance in the region of 240–275 nm. It originates from the π–π transitions of the pyrimidine and purine ring systems of the nucleobases [81,82]. This important transition is due to the aromatic rings that are present in these nucleobases. The most simple system with more than one aromatic ring is the so-called benzene dimer, that is formed by two benzene rings bonded by weak forces, that has been widely studied to investigate the important characteristics of the interaction between the two aromatic rings that, among other applications, allows to explain some key features of the considered nucleobases.

The two most stable conformations are the parallel displaced and T-shaped, that are shown in Figure 3.36b and c [34], which are essentially isoenergetic and represent energy minima. In contrast, the sandwich configuration (Figure 3.36a) that maximizes overlap of the pi system, is least stable, and represents an energetic saddle point. This later finding is consistent with a relative rarity of this configuration in x-ray crystal data. When illuminated with UV rays the double-ring configurations can create a transition strongly absorbing light radiation that is very useful to detect such molecules.

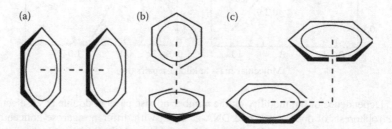

FIGURE 3.36 Three representative conformations of the benzene dimer: Sandwich configuration (a), T-shape configuration (b), and parallel displaced configuration (c).

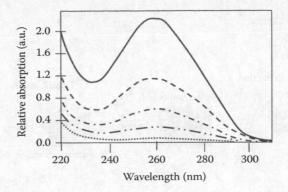

FIGURE 3.37 Absorption spectrum of different concentrations of calf thymus DNA.

The bases can be protonated, and therefore the spectra of DNA and RNA are sensitive to pH. At neutral pH the absorption maxima range from 253 nm (for guanosine) to 271 nm (for cytidine), and, as a consequence, polymeric DNA and RNA show a broad and strong absorbance near 260 nm. As an example, absorbance spectra of different concentrations of calf thymus DNA are shown in Figure 3.37.

In native DNA, the bases are stacked in the hydrophobic core of the double helix and accordingly their absorbance is considerably decreased relative to the absorbance of single-stranded DNA and even more so relative to short oligonucleotides in which the aromatic bases are exposed to the aqueous solvent. The decrease in absorbance upon base stacking in the interior of DNA or RNA double helices is called hypochromism. It provides a very sensitive and convenient probe for monitoring strand dissociation and unfolding of DNA double helices.

An important observation is that in order to have a real quantitative measure of the amount of DNA or RNA that is present in a sample, the sample has to be carefully purified. Not only both DNA and RNA, being built of the same nucleic bases, have a strong absorbance at 260 nm, but also many proteins have an important resonance at that frequency. This can be an important limitation of this detection method if the sample cannot be purified sufficiently.

Another detection method that has been introduced to overcome the limitations of UV detection is the fluorometric method that uses specific dyes to detect a certain type of nucleic acids that bind to that nucleic acid [83,84]. The sample is maintained in a dye solution at the required temperature, frequently the room temperature, for a few minutes in a solution containing the selected dye so that the dye binds to the DNA or RNA molecules. After that the obtained solution is placed in a fluorescence detector where the dye is activated and the fluorescence is revealed. For diluted solutions, the fluorescence is linear with the tagged nucleic acid concentration so that this allows the concentration to be evaluated.

Another high sensitivity and high specificity methods, somehow at the boundary between detection and sequencing methods is the so-called hybridization method. There are a great number of variants of this detection method, due to its intrinsic flexibility and to the different applications for which it is used [85–87]. In all the cases, it relies on a hybridization probe: a fragment of DNA or RNA of variable length, usually 100–1000 bases long, which is used in DNA or RNA samples to detect the presence of nucleotide sequences that are complementary to the sequence in the probe.

The most common procedure, inspired somehow by the Western blot that is used for protein immunoelectrophoresis, implies the DNA or RNA extraction, separation of different molecules by electrophoresis, and transfer of the electrophoresis separated molecules on a membrane, generally by applying an electrical field orthogonal to the membrane–electrophoresis chamber sandwich. After the transfer, the nucleic acids are hybridized with a suitable hybridization probe, carrying a suitable fluorescent dye that will have the role of detection tag. This procedure, that is schematically shown in Figure 3.38, is called Southern blot if tuned to detect DNA and Northern blot if tuned to detect RNA.

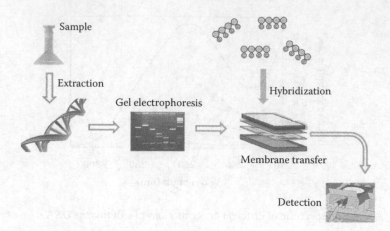

FIGURE 3.38 Schematic illustration of a Northern blot procedure for RNA quantification. (The Southern blot for DNA quantification is very similar.)

3.7 IMMUNOASSAYS

Immunoassays are a wide class of very important assays for the specific recognition of proteins and other kinds of macromolecules. All methods that we have analyzed up to now separate and quantify the amount of macromolecules that are present in a sample on the ground of some physical property like molecular mass, hydrodynamic volume, or electrophoretic mobility.

Immunoassays exploit the unique capability of antibodies to bind selectively to the molecule segment they recognize as the conjugate antigen epitope to identify a molecule presenting that specific arrangement of atoms. For this reason, immunoassays constitute one of the most powerful instruments for molecule identification. In the following, we will study in some detail the chemistry of antigen–antibody neutralization so as to be able to evaluate not only the qualitative behavior, but also the performance of selected immunoassays.

3.7.1 STRUCTURE AND THERMODYNAMIC OF ANTIGEN–ANTIBODY NEUTRALIZATION

The antigen-binding specificity of an antibody is defined by the physical and chemical properties of its CDR surface (see Section 2.4.1). These in turn are determined by the conformation of the antigens by varying the amino acid sequences of the CDR loops [88,89]. While the structure of the CDR loops might vary randomly, there are certain preferred conformations. Such preferred conformations can be deduced from the lengths and sequences of these regions.

Contrary to other molecular interactions, antibodies can recognize various foreign antigens, small molecules, soluble proteins, surface proteins on viruses, and so on, by varying the hypervariable regions.

The six CDR loops from the two chains at the rim of the eight-strand barrel provide an ideal arrangement for generating antigen-binding sites of different shapes depending on the size and sequence of the loops. These CDR structures can create flat, extended binding surfaces for protein antigens, a specific groove for a peptide, DNA, and carbohydrate, or specific deep binding cavities for small molecules called haptens. A hapten is a simple chemical molecule that has the ability to bind antibody and can induce specific antibody production when it is attached to a carrier molecule such as albumin (see Section 2.4.1).

It has been pointed out that the distribution of amino acids in variable domains seems to be biased, and certain residues (tyrosine—Tyr, tryptophan—Trp, and asparagine—Asn) seem to have a propensity for being in the CDRs, and for participating in antigen recognition. It seems that the aromatic side chains containing Tyr and Trp are more exposed to the solvent than in usual water-soluble proteins, and they are frequently found to be involved in the interaction with the ligand. This is explained by their large size causing hydrophobic effect, large polarization generating stronger van der Waals interactions, their ability to form hydrogen bonds and rigidity, characteristic of structure including several aromatic rings that decreases the loss of conformational entropy upon interactions.

Thus, the concentration of aromatic rings would give a certain "stickiness" to the CDRs and give diverse specificity to antibodies. Specificity for a particular antigen would arise from the complementarity of the shapes of the interacting surfaces created by the proper positioning of the aromatic rings and the correct location of polar and/or charged groups.

The contact site in antigen–antibody binding is generally quite big, involving from 10 to 25 residues and occupying an overall area of 500–1000 Å². However, the chemically active part of this contact surface, the true antigen epitope is not so large [90]: generally, no more that 5–8 side chains account for more than 80% of the overall bound free energy, constituting the most effective part of the epitope. The other parts of the contact surface, however, are not irrelevant to the specificity of the bound, contributing to the conformational complementarity, that is one element of the immunoglobulin specificity.

The strength of the antigen–antibody bound, determined by the sum of all forces contributing to the bound or opposing to it, is generally called antibody affinity to the specific antigen. Besides van der Walls forces, ion bound and hydrogen bound, the so-called salt-bridge bound has generally an important effect in antigen–antibody binding. This is a bound that forms when a charged residue like aspartate attracts its oppositely charged group (lysine in the aspartate example). From several observations [90], it seems that salt-bridge bonds have a determinant role in fixing antigen–antibody specificity when it is not determined by hydrogen bounds. In particular, hydrogen bound seems to be dominant in determining specificity in the case of protein antigens, where salt-bridge bond is generally not observed.

Using a monovalent antibody fragment in the reaction, the antigen–antibody reaction can be generally written as

$$A_n + A_b \rightleftharpoons A_{nb} \tag{3.21}$$

where A_n indicates the antigen, A_b the antibody fragment, and the A_{nb} antigen–antibody complex. The reaction is a single-step reaction, no intermediate complex is formed. Thus, it is also a first-order reaction under a kinetic point of view. As far as the free energy is considered, since this is a spontaneous process in the physiological conditions, it has to decrease due to the reaction. Studying the different contribution to the free energy, even if there are antigen–antibody combinations generating a negative entropy, generally the entropic contribution is positive [91,92]. This is due to the fact that the negative contribution due to the reduction of the solvated molecule species from two to one, with the relative reduction in a variety of possible configurations in the phase space, is more than compensated by the decrease of the molecule surface available to fix water molecules. This means that more water molecules return in a state similar to the standard water liquid state, where continuous changing of hydrogen bonds generate a great positive contribution to the solvent entropy.

This phenomenon is confirmed by observation of the complete absence of water molecules in between the contact surfaces between antigen and antibodies, where a real solvent exclusion volume is formed (see Section 1.5.1). When the entropy contribution is positive and dominant in determining a negative value of the free energy, the enthalpy can be negative, also if generally a small enthalpy positive contribution is also detected. When the negative entropy contribution is not present, a negative entropy has to be compensated by negative enthalpy. This frequently happens when the ion bond is dominant in the reaction. Typical antibody/antigen complexes with equilibrium constant from 10^2 to 10^{10} mol^{-1} have free enthalpies of about $30–100 \times 10^{-21}$ J/molecule that corresponds to 18–60 kJ/mol.

The force binding the complex can be directly evaluated by measurements with the atomic force microscope [93] resulting in forces from 20 to 200 pN, that combined with an estimate of the minimum energy distance between the centers of mass of the contact regions can be compared with the measured values of negative free energy.

The bound free energy ranges from 30 to 50 kJ/mol [93–95] that means about 6.6×10^{-20} J/molecule. Combining these data with the atomic force microscope observations, we arrive to a distance between ligands of the order of 6 Å, that is a figure also confirmed by direct observations [93].

Assuming that this reaction takes place in a diluted solution, the "macromolecules perfect gas" theory can be applied (see Section 1.4) and the free energy of the bond can be written as

$$\Delta G = -M R_g T \log(K_a) \tag{3.22}$$

where

R_g is the perfect gas constant

M the number of moles of the substance

T the temperature

K_a the equilibrium constant that appears in the mass action law for the reaction equilibrium (see Section 1.2.3).

So that the free energy of the bound can also be measured starting from the macroscopic observation of the reaction equilibrium constant. Experimental values of the equilibrium constants ranges from 10^5 to 10^{10} 1/mol, confirming the ranges of free energy evaluated by microscopic calculations. A set of measured values of antigen–antibody equilibrium constants are reported for blood cells antigens of the IgG type in Table 3.5 with the associated free energy for the antigen–antibody complex. The equilibrium constant can be related to the type of occurring reaction; thus to the type of antigen epitope. This has been done in simple cases and an interesting result is shown in Table 3.6 [88,91].

The strength of a single antigen–antibody bond is termed the antibody affinity or sometimes intrinsic affinity, and the equilibrium constant is sometimes also called affinity constant. Since each monoclonal antibody has at least two antigen-binding sites they can bind multiple antigenic epitopes. When an antigen carrying multiple copies of the antigenic epitopes combines with a multivalent antibody, the binding strength is greatly increased with respect to the intrinsic affinity

TABLE 3.5
Measured Values of Antigen–Antibody Equilibrium Constants are Reported for Blood Cell Antigens of the IgG with the Associated Free Energy for the Antigen-Antibody Complex

Antibody	K_a (1/mol)	ΔG (kJ/mol)
Anti-D	$2 \times 10^7 – 3 \times 10^9$	$-43 \rightarrow -56$
Anti-C	5×10^6	-39
Anti-c	$1.9 \times 10^7 – 5.6 \times 10^7$	$-43 \rightarrow -45.8$
Anti-E	4×10^8	-50.9
Anti-e	2.5×10^8	-49.7
Anti-K	$6 \times 10^9 – 2.5 \times 10^{10}$	$-57.8 \rightarrow -61.5$

Source: Adapted from Reverberti R., Reverberi L., *Blood Transfusions*, vol. 5, pp. 227–240, 2007.

TABLE 3.6

IgG Antigen Binding Energy versus the Antigen Epitope Structure

Epitope Structure	Equilibrium Constant (1/mol)
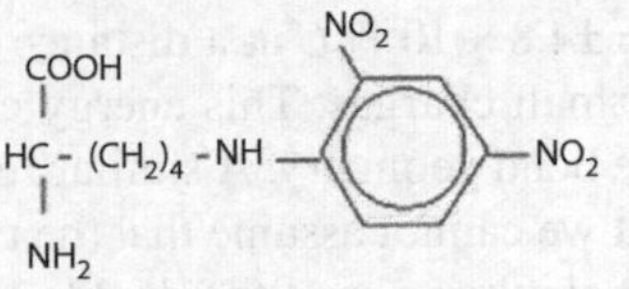	2×10^7
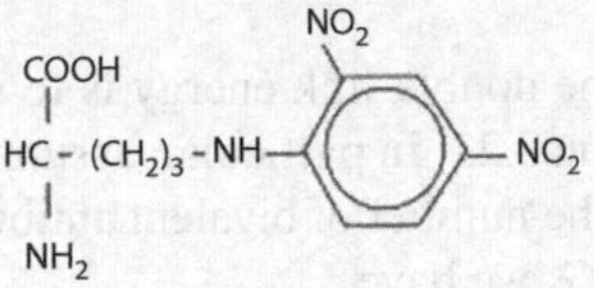	8×10^6
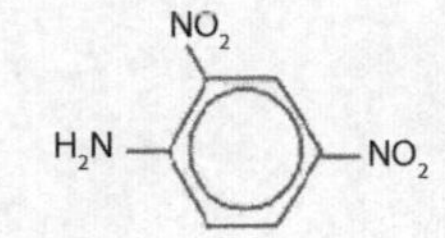	2×10^6
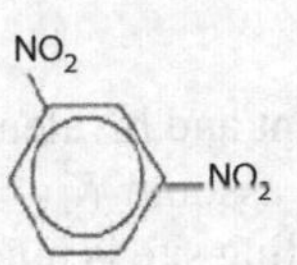	8×10^5
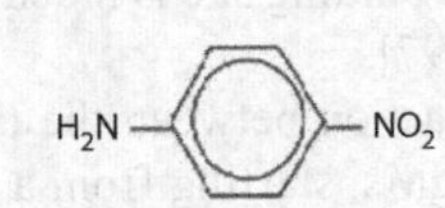	5×10^4

Source: Adapted from Nezlin R. S., *The Immunoglobulins: Structure and Function*, Academic Press; 1st edition (April 1998), ISBN-13: 978-0123887085; Jin L., Wells J. A. *Protein Science*, vol. 3, pp. 2351–2357, 1994.

because all of the antigen–antibody bonds must be broken simultaneously before the antigen and antibody can dissociate. Total binding energy between a multivalent antibody and more than one of the antigen-binding sites is greater than the summation of the affinities of each binding site. The strength with which a multivalent antibody binds a multivalent antigen is termed avidity, to differentiate it from the affinity.

The avidity of an antibody for its antigen depends both from the binding sites configuration and by the sum of all of the individual interactions taking place between individual antigen-binding sites of antibodies and epitopes on the antigens. Moreover, it naturally strongly depends on the affinities of the individual combining sites being a factor from 10^2 to 10^7 greater than the single affinity.

It could be natural to set

$$\Delta G_2 = 2\Delta H_1 - T\Delta S \tag{3.23}$$

where ΔH_1 is the single bond enthalpy and ΔS the total double bond entropy variation, that cannot be simply related to the entropy variation of the single bond.

Unfortunately, this simple theory does not give reason correctly of the observed energy and equilibrium constant values [97] and a much more complex calculation based on the microscopic analysis of the bond area has to be carried out in order to obtain quantitatively correct data.

An important factor determining the antibody avidity is the bond distance, that is, in general quite smaller with respect to the case of a single bond. To understand the relevance of this parameter, it is sufficient to consider the fact that a simple calculation of the electrostatic energy related to two atoms carrying a point charges of ± 0.3 a.u. $= \pm 4.8 \times 10^{-20}$ C at a distance of 1 nm gives about 12.54 kJ/mol: a quite substantial energy for two small charges. This energy critically depends on distance and, in case of distributed charges, on the bond geometry. A similar result can be obtained both for van der Walls and hydrogen bonds so that we cannot assume that the two bounds are independent, even under the point of view of the enthalpy term, and the double bound link has to be studied as a single structure [98].

The simpler way to obtain realistic values for the double link energy is to start from measured values of the equilibrium constant and from Equation 3.22. In particular, assuming to maintain constant the number of binding sites, thus having half the number of bivalent antibodies with respect to the monovalent segments, and defining $\gamma = \Delta G_2 / 2 \Delta G_1$ we have

$$\gamma = \frac{\ln(K_{a2})}{\ln(K_{a1})} \tag{3.24}$$

where K_{a1} and K_{a2} are the equilibrium constants for the monovalent and bivalent bond, respectively. As an example, following experimental values for IgGs, if we assume $K_{a2} = 10^{11}$ the value of γ results to be $\gamma = 1.38$. This confirms the result that the double binding site is much stronger than that of the simple theory based on Equation 3.23 would foresee [97].

Much bigger effects can be found if more effective interaction between the two bound sites or higher valence are considered. For example, in the case of IgMs, starting from a monovalent value of K_{a1} equal to 10^8, values as high as 10^{13} can be obtained for K_{a2}. In this case, $\gamma = 1.65$.

Thus, due to the logarithmic relationship between the equilibrium constant and the free energy, allowing small free energies increase to change the equilibrium constant orders of magnitude, even when each antigen binding site has only a low affinity antibodies can function effectively in the immune system.

3.7.2 KINETIC OF ANTIGEN–ANTIBODY NEUTRALIZATION

The kinetic of antigen–antibody binding has been widely studied, frequently using monovalent antibodies obtained by insulation of a single antibody-binding site [98–101]. In this case, the reaction is a classical first-order reaction without catalysis, thus the dynamic of the reaction is regulated by the following differential equations:

$$\frac{dc_B}{dt} = -v_+ \, c_B \, c_G + v_- \, c_N \tag{3.25a}$$

$$\frac{dc_G}{dt} = -v_+ \, c_B \, c_G + v_- \, c_N \tag{3.25b}$$

$$\frac{dc_N}{dt} = +v_+ \, c_B \, c_G - v_- c_N \tag{3.25c}$$

where c_B, c_G, and c_N are the antibodies, the antigens, and the neutralized complex concentrations, respectively. The forward and backward reaction rates v_+ and v_- are linked to the equilibrium constant by the classical formula

$$\frac{v_+}{v_-} = K_a \tag{3.26}$$

Reasonable values for v_+ in terms of 1/s/mol are 10^7–10^{10} and the values of v_- can be evaluated consequently [102,103].

Let us assume, as realistic in this kind of applications, that at the starting instant $c_{B0} = 0.05$ PPM mol (i.e., 2.7×10^{-6} mol/L), $c_{G0} = 0.001$ PPM moles (i.e., 5.55×10^{-8} mol/L), and $c_{N0} = 0$. Moreover, let us assume that $v_+ = 10^9$ 1/s/mol and $K_a = 10^8$ 1/mol. The starting reaction rate, that is, the value of

$$V_+(t = 0) = \frac{dc_G}{dt} \frac{1}{c_G}\bigg]_{t=0} \tag{3.27}$$

is given by $V_+(t = 0) = 5$ s^{-1}. Thus, the reaction starts with a fast pace. The complete time evolution has to be obtained by solving Equations 3.25 and taking into account that due to Equation 3.26 $v_- = 10$ s^{-1}.

These equations can be solved with elementary methods and the result can be written as follows:

$$c_N = c_{B0} - c_B \tag{3.28a}$$

$$c_G = c_B - c_{B0} + c_{G0} \tag{3.28b}$$

$$c_B = \frac{b_1 - b_2 b_0 e^{-t/\tau_B}}{1 - b_0 e^{-t/\tau_B}} \tag{3.28c}$$

where the four parameters b_0, b_1, b_2, and τ_B are related to the original reaction dynamics data with equations reported in Table 3.7, besides the specific values these parameters assume in the above example. The antigens and neutralized antigen concentrations and the neutralization rate are shown

TABLE 3.7
Equation Relating the Parameters of Equation 3.28 with the Data of the Original Reaction Dynamics

Parameter	Equation	Example Values Monovalent	Example Values Bivalent
a	$(-v_- + v_+ c_{B0} - v_+ c_{G0})$	-39.00 (1/s)	-49.00 (1/s)
b_1	$\frac{1}{2v_+}\left[-a + \sqrt{a^2 + 4v_+ v_- c_{B0}}\right]$	4.92×10^{-8} (mol/L)	4.90×10^{-8} (mol/L)
b_2	$\frac{1}{2v_+}\left[-a - \sqrt{a^2 + 4v_+ v_- c_{B0}}\right]$	-1.01×10^{-8} (mol/L)	-1.02×10^{-11} (mol/L)
b_0	$\dfrac{b_1 - c_{B0}}{b_2 - c_{B0}}$	0.014 (adim)	0.02
τ_B	$\dfrac{b_2}{b_1 - b_2}$	0.17 (1/s)	2.08×10^{-4} (1/s)

Note: Numerical values are from the example detailed in the text.

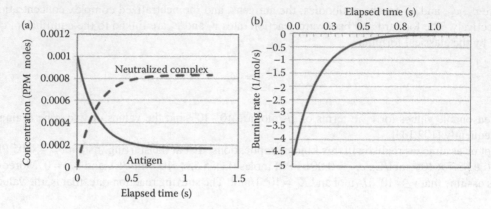

FIGURE 3.39 Antigens and neutralized antigens concentrations in PPM moles (a) and neutralization rate in 1/s/mol (b) for the monovalent antibody fragment fixing to an antigen example of the text.

in Figure 3.39a and b. The monovalent antibody segment is effective in reducing the concentration of the free antigen of about one order of magnitude, but it is much less effective with respect to real serum antibodies. Moreover, the reaction takes about 1 s to go to chemical equilibrium.

In Figure 3.40a and b, the antigens and neutralized antigen concentrations and the neutralization rate are shown in the case of bivalent bond considered in the previous section. The elapsed time for reaction equilibrium passes from about 1 s to about 1 ms, due to the much lower rate of neutralized antigen decay owing to the much stronger double bond. This causes the antigen concentration to be reduced below 2.1×10^{-7} PPM moles, that under a practical point of view is equivalent to zero.

While the dynamic expressed by Equations 3.25 is well suited to represent what happens in an artificial reaction, it is not equally suited to represent what happens during a real infection. As a matter of fact, during an infection, not only antigens are eliminated by the immune system neutralizing and then destroying them, but they are also multiplied by infected cells degradation. Moreover, several parallel mechanisms are activated by the immune system, all intended to eliminate antigens and infected cells before they give rise to new antigens.

Oversimplifying the situation we imagine the following situation:

- The infection rate is proportional to the antigens concentration through the available concentration c_T of target.

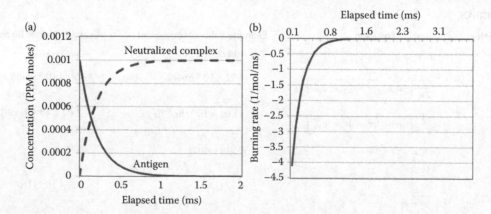

FIGURE 3.40 Antigens and neutralized antigens concentrations in PPM moles (a) and neutralization rate in 1/s/mol (b) for the antigen–IgG neutralization considered in the example of the text.

- An infected cell has a probability p_i to generate m new antigens before undergoing apoptosis or being destroyed by the immune system.
- A single antibody is present specifically synthesized for the considered antigen.
- The antigen is immune to the innate system, that in any case provides to eliminate infected cells and residues from cells and antigens destruction.

Calling the parameter $A_G = p_i\mu$ the antigen generation rate, the rate equations become

$$\frac{dc_B}{dt} = -v_+\, c_B\, c_G + v_-\, c_N \tag{3.29a}$$

$$\frac{dc_G}{dt} = -v_+\, c_B\, c_G + v_-\, c_N + A_G\, c_T\, c_G \tag{3.29b}$$

$$\frac{dc_N}{dt} = +v_+\, c_B\, c_G - v_-\, c_N \tag{3.29c}$$

$$\frac{dc_T}{dt} = -A_G\, c_T\, c_G \tag{3.29d}$$

These equations cannot be solved analytically and a numerical solution is needed. The result for the antigens concentration versus time is reported in Figure 3.41, where the concentration is shown in logarithmic scale for different values of the antigens activity. The parameters are all those of the bivalent model plus target cells' initial concentration of 0.1 PPM moles. As intuitive, up to reach activity near to the threshold value for which the antigen concentration does not change in time (in our example 6.28×10^5 L/mol), the antigen concentration decreases rapidly under the action of antibodies and the value of the activity is not so relevant.

When the threshold activity is overcome in the same way the antigens concentration increases rapidly and the antibodies action becomes less and less effective. Naturally, on the long run the target cells concentration decreases and it also causes a decrease of the antigens concentration, but in a real case this means a relevant biological damage to the tissue involved in the antigen aggression. When this happens the immune system tries both to increase the antibodies concentration and to

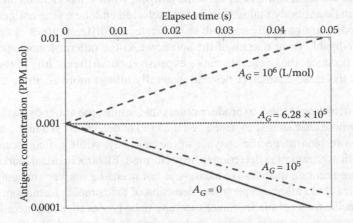

FIGURE 3.41 Antigen concentration for different values of the antigen activity in the simple immunity reaction model of the text.

decrease the antigen replication rate by increasing the immune cells destroying the infected cells so as to limit the antigens replication.

3.7.3 IMMUNOASSAY PROCESSES

Out of their role in living being bodies, antibodies are massively used in immunoassays, one of the assay technique most used both in traditional assay equipment and in labs on chip. An immunoassay is an assay using the quality of an antibody specific for the substance to be detected to label that molecule by binding specifically to it. This allows a sort of labeling of the molecule to detect that which distinguishes it from all the other molecules in the material under test and allows it to be recognized.

Immunoassays are used in the medical practice as support to medical decision in a large number of situations [104,105] as in hepatitis, HIV infection, strep throat disease, and therapeutic drug monitoring. Moreover, they are also used in industrial applications, like in food industry, agriculture, environmental, and water quality control and in many other applications.

Almost all immunoassays, whatever is the used technique, have three key components:

- *A pure antibody:* as specific as possible to the substance to be detected that is used to perform the assay
- *A detection element:* that provide observable results when the antibody is linked to the antigen
- *A substrate:* where the antibody is fixed so that the antibody–antigen complex will also be fixed to the substrate when it will be generated

In macroscopic assays the detection elements is frequently an enzyme or another marker that is tagged to the antibody so as to provide observable results when the antibody is linked to the antigen like light emission. This kind of detection is also called labeled detection [106]. When the observable parameter is directly related to the antigen–antibody reaction, without the need of another label molecule, the detection method is called unlabeled. In this case, very frequent in lab on chip immunoassays, detection is operated by observing the change of physical parameters like the refraction index of the solution and its dielectric constant or, when possible, with calorimetric methods [107,108].

Immunoassays can be carried out by using either monoclonal or polyclonal antibody solutions [104,109]. A polyclonal antibodies solution is a solution containing a set of different antibodies that are specific to different epitopes of the same antigen, while a monoclonal antibodies solution contains only a single antibody that is specific for a selected epitope on the antigen to be detected. Polyclonal antibodies are naturally easier to be generated by different lines of cells from serum, but are less reproducible from one lot of the solution and the other. Monoclonal antibodies are more difficult to produce, thus generally more expensive, but different lots of the antibody solution have always the same characteristics and generally allows more accurate measurements to be done.

When labeled detection is used, to produce observable results, the antibody has to be bonded to a specific marker, whose characteristics depend on the kind of detection used in the assay. Enzymatic detection requires to bind a specific enzyme to the antibody, while a fluorescent or radioactive marker allows optical or radiation detection to be performed. Electrochemical markers are also used and in cases where accurate quantitative measure is not needed a marker changing its color when the complex creates could allow simple visual detection of the complex formation.

Antibodies specific for a certain immunoassay have to be produced, and generally this is done by using animals to generate immune reaction to the antigen to be assayed. Polyclonal antibodies are produced by obtaining from selected mammals in whom the antigen has been injected. The natural immune reaction enriches the blood of the desired antigens, so that they can be obtained by purifying extracted blood. At this point, after suitable tests for efficiency and specificity, the antibodies can be used in the assay. The production of monoclonal antigens is more complex [110,111].

Several immunoassays have been designed and are effectively used in common laboratory practice. A brief list of a selected number of immunoassay with a brief description and comment is reported below [104,105].

- *Western blot (or immunoelectrophoresis)* is used to detect protein either in solution or, more frequently, in a given sample of tissue homogenate or extract. This technique utilizes gel electrophoresis to separate native proteins by shape and size. The proteins are then transferred out of the gel and onto a membrane, typically nitrocellulose or polyvinylidene fluoride (PVDF), where they are probed using antibodies specific to the protein.
- *Enzyme-linked immunosorbent assay (ELISA)* involves, in its common implementation, at least one antibody with specificity for a particular antigen. The sample with an unknown amount of antigen is immobilized on a solid support, usually a polystyrene microtiter plate, either nonspecifically, via adsorption to the surface, or specifically via capture by another antibody specific to the same antigen, in a sandwich ELISA. After the antigen is immobilized the detection antibody is added, forming a complex with the antigen. The detection antibody can be covalently linked to an enzyme, or can itself be detected by a secondary antibody which is linked to an enzyme through bio-conjugation.
- *Radioimmunoassay (RIA)* involves essentially four steps before the result measurement:
  - Insert in the test chamber a known quantity of radioactive antigen frequently labeled with γ-radioactive isotopes of iodine attached to tyrosine with antibody specific to that antigen
  - Adding unlabeled or *cold* antigen
  - Adding a secondary antibody
  - Precipitate free antigens
  - Measure the amount of labeled antigen displaced by measuring radiation from solution with fixed antigens and from the precipitate.

  Initially, the radioactive antigen is bound to the antibodies. When the unlabeled antigen is added, the two compete for antibody-binding sites—at higher concentrations of unlabeled antigen, more of it binds to the antibody, displacing the radioactive variant. A scheme of radioimmunoassay procedure is reported in Figure 3.42.
- *ELISpot (enzyme-linked immunosorbent spot assay)* is based on a modified version of the ELISA immunoassay. ELISpot assays were originally developed to enumerate B cells secreting antigen-specific antibodies, and have subsequently been adapted for various tasks. At appropriate conditions the ELISpot assay allows visualization of the secretory product of individual activated cells. Thus, the ELISpot assay provides both qualitative (type of immune protein) and quantitative (number of responding cells) information.
- *Immunoprecipitation assay (IP)* is the technique of precipitating an antigen out of solution using an antibody specific to that antigen. This process can be used to enrich a given protein to some degree of purity. Co-immunoprecipitation, also known as a "pull-down," can identify protein complexes present in cell extracts: by immunoprecipitating one protein believed to be in a complex, additional members of the complex can also be identified. The complexes are brought out of solution by insoluble antibody-binding proteins isolated initially from bacteria, such as protein A [112], protein G [113,114], and protein A/G [115]. These can also be coupled to agarose beads that can easily be isolated out of solution. After washing, the precipitate can be analyzed using gel electrophoresis, mass spectrometry,

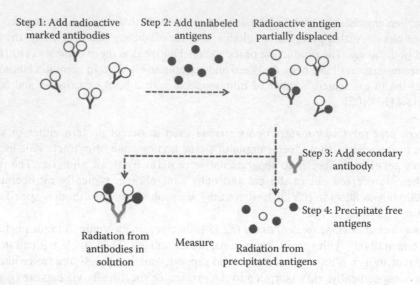

Step 1: Add radioactive marked antibodies

Step 2: Add unlabeled antigens

Radioactive antigen partially displaced

Step 3: Add secondary antibody

Step 4: Precipitate free antigens

Radiation from antibodies in solution

Measure

Radiation from precipitated antigens

FIGURE 3.42   Scheme of radioimmunoassay procedure.

Western blotting, or any number of other methods for identifying constituents in the complex.

- *Immunohistochemistry assay* refers to the process of localizing proteins in cells of a tissue section exploiting the principle of antibodies binding specifically to antigens in biological tissues [116]. Immunohistochemical staining is widely used in the diagnosis and treatment of cancer. Specific molecular markers are characteristic of particular cancer types. IHC is also widely used in basic research to understand the distribution and localization of biomarkers in different parts of a tissue. Visualizing an antibody–antigen interaction can be accomplished in a number of ways. In the most common instance, an antibody is conjugated to an enzyme, such as peroxidase, that can catalyze a color-producing reaction. Alternatively, the antibody can also be tagged to a fluorophore, such as FITC, rhodamine, or Texas Red. The latter method is of great use in confocal laser scanning microscopy, which is highly sensitive and can also be used to visualize interactions between multiple proteins [117,118]. A more indirect detection can also be performed, where specific antigens needed to detect the target biomarker are difficult to tag with suitable enzymes or fluorophores. In this case, after bonding the marker with the primary antigen a secondary antigen tagged with the suitable detection marker is inserted in the assay system. The secondary antigen binds to the primary one, generally to its tail, thereby allowing markers detection. Principle schemes of immunohistochemistry assay with direct and indirect detection are shown in Figure 3.43.

- *Immunocytochemistry assay (ICC).* Immunocytochemistry differs from immunohistochemistry in that the former is performed on samples of intact cells that have had most, if not all, of their surrounding extracellular matrix removed [119]. This includes cells grown within a culture, deposited from suspension, or taken from a smear. In contrast, immunohistochemical samples are sections of biological tissue, where each cell is surrounded by tissue architecture and other cells normally found in the intact tissue. There are many ways to prepare cell samples for immunocytochemical analysis. Each method has its own strengths and unique characteristics, so the right method can be chosen for the desired sample and outcome. Cells to be stained can be attached to a solid support to allow easy handling in subsequent procedures. This can be achieved by several methods: adherent cells may be grown on microscope slides, coverslips, or an optically suitable plastic

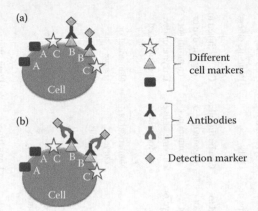

FIGURE 3.43 Scheme of the final arrangement of an immunohistochemistry assay with direct (a) and indirect (b) detection.

support. Suspension cells can be centrifuged onto glass slides (cytospin), bound to solid support using chemical linkers, or in some cases handled in suspension.

- *Flow cytometry assay (FLOW)* is a technique for counting, examining, and sorting microscopic particles suspended in a stream of fluid. It allows simultaneous multiparametric analysis of the physical and/or chemical characteristics of single cells flowing through an optical and/or electronic detection apparatus.
- *Cytometric bead array assay (CBA)* commonly referred to as a multiplexed bead assay, is based on spectrally discrete particles that can be used to capture a soluble analyte. The analyte quantity is then measured by detection of a fluorescence-based emission and flow cytometric analysis. The CBA generates data that are comparable to ELISA-based assays, but in a "multiplexed" or a simultaneous fashion [120,121].

A general comparison among different immunoassays is performed in Table 3.8. In the following, we analyze more in detail a selected number of these analytical techniques.

3.7.4 WESTERN BLOT OR IMMUNOELECTROPHORESIS

Western blot [105,106,109] is a very diffused analytical technique articulated in several subsequent steps allowing detection of specific proteins in solution or in a tissue sample. Assuming to start from a tissue sample, the steps of conventional Western blot are

1. Tissue preparation
2. Gel electrophoresis
3. Transfer
4. Blocking
5. Detection
6. Analysis

If the protein is directly present in solution, for example, in a biological fluid, the first step is not needed, frequently substituted by an opportune procedure of solution purification.

3.7.4.1 Tissue Preparation

This is generally a standard cell lysis process (see Section 3.2.1) followed, if necessary, from cell lysate purification. Sometimes, as in the case of proteins that are present on the surfaces of viruses, the cell lysis is not needed if the protein can be directly taken out from the cell, for example, by using suitable enzymes.

TABLE 3.8
Characteristics of Selected Immunoassays

Methods	Western Blot	ELISA	ELISpot	Immuno-Precipitation	Immuno-Cytochemistry	Immuno-Histochemistry	Flow Cytometry	Multiplex Assay
Target (analyte)	Proteins or polypeptide	Peptides, proteins, others	Cells	Proteins or complex	Cells	Tissue sections or tissue array	Cells	Proteins, others
Primary antibody	Binds antigen (can also be isotope-labeled)	Binds antigen, can be used for self-pairing	Can be linked to organic dye or quantum dot	Can be linked to beads	Can be linked to organic dye or quantum dot	Can be linked to organic dye or quantum dot	Can be linked to organic dye or quantum dot	Can be linked to organic dye or quantum dot
Secondary antibody	Used for signal generating	Enzyme-linked for generating signal	Enzyme or dye or dot linked	May be omitted	Enzyme or dye or dot linked	Enzyme or dye or dot linked	Enzyme or dye or dot linked	Enzyme or dye or dot linked
Data forms	Protein banding image	Numerical and curve	Image or numerical	Protein binding image	Image	Image	Numerical or curve	Numerical or curve
Sensitivity	ng/mL	pg/mL	pg/mL	ng/mL	ng/mL	ng/mL	$1/10^5$ cells	pg/mL
Reproducibility	Good	High	Good	Variable	Variable	Variable	Good	Good
Quantification	Semi	Yes	Semi	Semi	Semi	Semi	Yes	Yes
Applications	Protein analysis and identification	Antigen analysis	Antigen analysis	Protein analysis and identification	Protein analysis and identification	Protein analysis and identification	Antigen analysis	Antigen analysis
Assay development	Simple	Take time (days)	Take time (days)	Longer time (weeks)	Longer time (weeks)	Longer time (weeks)	Long time (month)	Long time (month)
Validation	Simple	Complicate	Difficult	Difficult	Difficult	Difficult	Complicate	Complicate
High-through-put	No	Possible with automation	No	No	No	Possible with automation	Yes	Yes

3.7.4.2 Gel Electrophoresis

The different proteins that are present in the sample are separated using gel electrophoresis (see Section 3.6.2) up to obtain electrophoresis bands. Electrophoresis is used in Western blot as a way of purifying the protein solution; however, densitometer or similar measures can be applied after electrophoresis for a first evaluation of the protein band intensity.

3.7.4.3 Transfer

To make the proteins accessible to antibody detection, they are moved from within the gel onto a membrane made of nitrocellulose or polyvinylidene difluoride (PVDF). The membrane is placed on top of the gel, and a stack of filter papers placed over that. The entire stack is placed in a buffer solution which moves up the paper by capillary action, bringing the proteins with it. This process, in its native form quite slow, is accelerated by using electric current to pull proteins from the gel into the PVDF or nitrocellulose membrane. The proteins move from within the gel onto the membrane while maintaining the organization they had in the gel. As a result of this process, the proteins are exposed on a thin surface layer for detection. The entire transfer process is schematically shown in Figure 3.34. Both varieties of membrane are chosen for their nonspecific protein-binding properties. Protein binding is based upon hydrophobic interactions, as well as charged interactions between the membrane and protein (Figures 3.43 and 3.44).

3.7.4.4 Blocking

Since the membrane is able to attach proteins in a nonspecific way it is needed to avoid that the antibodies that will be used to test the target proteins will be attached to the membrane. This will be done by saturating all the membrane attaching sites by other generic proteins that does not react with the antibodies that will be used. Suitable low concentration solutions of almost inert proteins are available for this scope.

3.7.4.5 Detection

In the traditional version of Western blot, detection is achieved by luminescence provoked starting by the target proteins fixed to a saturated membrane in two steps. In the first step, a specific antibody is bonded to the protein inserting the membrane in a suitable solution containing it. This process can take from 30 min to a few hours and sometimes is helped either by thermal cycles or by solution periodic moderate agitation. In a second step, a secondary antibody is used to link it to a species specific site of the primary one. The secondary antibody is complementary to a specific enzyme, like biotin or to a reporter enzyme such as alkaline phosphatase or horseradish peroxidase in such a way that when it binds with this specific enzyme the chemical reaction generates luminescence. In several cases, like in the case of biotin, the bond between the enzyme and the substrate is multivalent so that the signal results also amplified.

When the bonds between the primary and the secondary antibodies are completely formed, the activated membrane is exposed to the enzyme conjugated to the secondary antibody via insertion

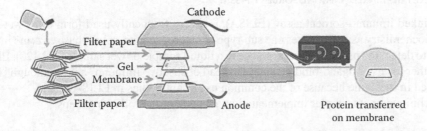

FIGURE 3.44   Schematic illustration of the transfer procedure in a Western blot immunoassay.

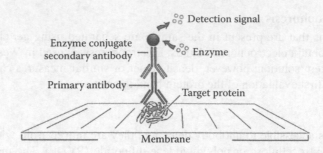

Detection signal

Enzyme conjugate
secondary antibody

Enzyme

Primary antibody

Target protein

Membrane

FIGURE 3.45   Schematic illustration of the two steps detection procedure in Western blot.

in a solution containing it. In this way, luminescence is generated by the reaction of secondary antibodies and their conjugated enzyme, whose intensity is proportional to the quantity of target protein fixed on the membrane. In alternative versions of the Western blot, instead of luminescent generating enzymes, the secondary enzyme can be conjugated with radioactive or IR luminescent molecules, allowing different types of detection to be performed. This procedure is schematically presented in Figure 3.45.

The above-described double-step process is diffused and quite flexible, due to the great number of elements that can be adapted to specific exigencies.

Recently, tests with a single-step process have also been introduced, where the primary antibody is directly conjugated to the enzyme causing luminescence. Such antibodies are more difficult to be produced, but the single-step procedure allows much higher throughput to be achieved via equipment designed for large laboratories or for industrial applications.

3.7.4.6   Analysis

Two main analysis techniques exist once the membrane is prepared: colorimetric detection and luminescence detection. The colorimetric detection method depends on incubation of the Western blot with a substrate that reacts with the reporter enzyme (such as peroxidase) that is bound to the secondary antibody. This converts the soluble dye into an insoluble form of a different color that precipitates next to the enzyme and thereby stains the membrane. Development of the blot is then stopped by washing away the soluble dye. Protein levels are evaluated through densitometry or spectrophotometry.

Luminescent detection methods depend on incubation of the Western blot with a substrate that will luminesce when exposed to the reporter on the secondary antibody. The light is then detected by photographic film, and more recently by CCD cameras which capture a digital image of the Western blot. The image is analyzed by densitometry, which evaluates the relative amount of protein staining and quantifies the results in terms of optical density. Newer software allows further data analysis such as molecular weight analysis if appropriate standards are used.

3.7.5   Enzyme-Linked Immunosorbent Assay

Enzyme-linked immuno-sorbent assay (ELISA), is a very frequently used form of a "wet-lab"-type analytic biochemistry assay that uses one sub-type of heterogeneous, solid-phase enzyme immunoassay (EIA) to detect the presence of a substance in a liquid sample or wet sample [122,123]. ELISA can perform other forms of ligand-binding assays instead of strictly "immuno" assays, though "immuno" is conserved in the name because of the common use of antibodies in ELISA assays.

The technique, in its simpler implementation, is made of the following steps:

- Dilute antigen solution in coating buffer that allows absorption in solid phase on the well surface.

- Coat each ELISA well with antigen in coating buffer solution.
- Cover each coated well with plastic film and incubate it for a few hours, often overnight, at standard cooler temperature, for example, 4°C. In some ELISA implementation incubation can be fasted by increasing the temperature up to physiological temperature around 36°C–37°C, depending on the implementation. Adhesion of the coated antigens to the well surface happens during incubation, typically through charge interactions; uncoated molecules does not adhere and remains in liquid phase.
- Shake coating solution out of wells and wash with distilled/deionized water. This is an important step to remove unwanted residues and impurities.
- Block wells by using a blocking solution. This has the role of saturating the wells surface capacity of absorbing molecules so as to avoid that antibodies are absorbed by the well surface too.
- Incubate the well containing the blocking solution for a time of the order of 1 h at physiological temperature around 36°C–37°C or at room temperature around 26°C depending on the implementation, wrapped in plastic or in a moist sealed container.
- Shake off blocking solution without any washing not to ruin the absorption in the well surface and add primary antibody preparation.
- Wrap and incubate at physiological temperature around 36°C–37°C or at room temperature around 26°C, depending on the implementation; a time of the order of 1 h.
- Shake off the antibody solution and wash, generally with distilled water, to eliminate any remaining free antibody and impurity. After this wash, only the ligand and its specific binding counterparts remain specifically bound or *immunosorbed* by antigen–antibody interactions to the solid phase, while the nonspecific or unbound components are washed away.
- Add antibody enzyme conjugate solution, wrap and incubate at physiological temperature around 36°C–37°C or at room temperature around 26°C depending on the implementation; a time of the order of 1 h.
- Shake off the antibody enzyme conjugate solution and wash with suitable washing solution or distilled water depending on the implementation.
- Add substrate solution.
- Develop at room temperature and reading. Reading can be performed either in a single step or periodically three or four times, for example, after 1 and 30 min and after 1 h. It is performed generally by optical means since development with suitable substrate generates a chemical reaction emitting luminescence. Accurate quantitative reading can be performed by a spectrometer, while less accurate results can be obtained by simple methods.

This schematic procedure admits many variations, like a different number of washing, but the main steps are always the same. These main steps are shown in Figure 3.46.

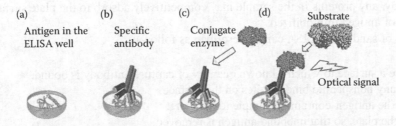

(a) Antigen in the ELISA well   (b) Specific antibody   (c) Conjugate enzyme   (d) Substrate

Optical signal

FIGURE 3.46 Main steps of direct ELISA immunoassay: antigen in coating buffer solution absorbed on the well surface (a); specific antibody bonded to the antigen after washing out of the impurities and unwanted residues (b); reaction between the antibody and the conjugate enzyme (c); reaction of the enzyme with the substrate generating the detected optical signal (d).

Several modifications of the ELISA direct procedure can be introduced either if the direct procedure is not possible, as in the case of antigens that cannot be coated to be absorbed on a solid surface, or to improve its performances, for example, to obtain a stronger signal so as to improve quantitative measure accuracy.

3.7.5.1 Indirect ELISA

In the case of indirect ELISA, a two-step process is performed to enhance the detection signal, similar to what is frequently done in other immunoassays as Western blot. The main steps of "indirect" ELISA are

- A buffered solution of the antigen to be tested for is added to each well of a microtiter plate, where it is given time to adhere to the ELISA well.
- A solution of nonreacting protein, such as bovine serum albumin or casein, is added to block any plastic surface in the well that remains uncoated by the antigen.
- Next the primary antibody is added, which binds specifically to the test antigen that is coating the well.
- Afterwards, a secondary antibody is added, which will bind the primary antibody. This secondary antibody often has an enzyme already attached to it, which has a negligible effect on the binding properties of the antibody. Other times the secondary antigen is combined with the conjugate enzyme in a second reaction after the binding to the primary antigen and suitable washing.
- A substrate for the enzyme is then added. Generally, this substrate is optically active upon reacting with the enzyme and this generates the detection signal.

Indirect ELISA is frequently also used to verify the reactivity of a donor with respect to a selected antigen, for example, to verify the immunity with respect to specific pathogens. In this case, the pathogen is absorbed in the well and the primary antigen comes from the serum of the donor. In this case, it is evident that indirect ELISA is needed, due to the fact that the primary antigen is not generally complementary to a suitable enzyme to perform detection. In this case, the test is generally used qualitatively, since presence or absence of selected antibodies has to be observed.

3.7.5.2 Sandwich ELISA

This variation of the ELISA technique is used mainly when the antigen to be detected cannot be directly absorbed on a solid surface. In this case a first antibody specific for the considered antigen is absorbed and the antigen is fixed by combining it with the absorbed antigen. This procedure is also used when the antigen to be revealed is available only in a solution with several other proteins, like serum, for example, and cannot be easily purified. In this case, without the first layer of "capture" antibody, any proteins in the sample may competitively adsorb to the plate surface, lowering the quantity of antigen immobilized.

The steps of sandwich ELISA can be described as follows:

- Prepare a surface to which a known quantity of capture antibody is bound.
- Block any nonspecific binding sites on the surface.
- Apply the antigen-containing sample to the plate.
- Wash the plate, so that unbound antigen is removed.
- A second specific antibody is added, and binds to antigen; this explains the sandwich name: the antigen is stuck between two antibodies.
- Apply enzyme-linked secondary antibodies as detection antibodies that also bind specifically to the second antibody's Fc region (nonspecific).

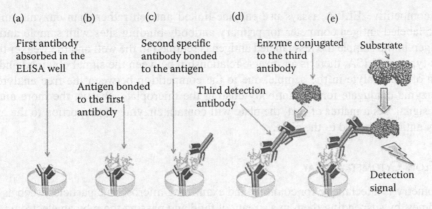

(a)

First antibody
absorbed in the
ELISA well

(b)

Antigen bonded
to the first
antibody

(c)

Second specific
antibody bonded
to the antigen

(d)

Third detection
antibody

Enzyme conjugated
to the third
antibody

Substrate

(e)

Detection
signal

FIGURE 3.47 Scheme of a sandwich ELISA assay: The first antibody is absorbed in the ELISA well surface (a), the antigen is bonded to the first antibody (b), a second specific antibody is bonded to the antigen (c), a third antigen is bonded to the second antigen and subsequently reacts with a suitable conjugate enzyme (d), the enzyme emits the detection signal upon reacting with the conjugate substrate (e).

- Wash the plate, so that the unbound antibody–enzyme conjugates are removed.
- Apply a chemical that is converted by the enzyme into a color or fluorescent or electrochemical signal.
- Measure the absorbency or fluorescence or electrochemical signal of the plate wells to determine the presence and quantity of antigen.

The above steps include a two-step detection process. Also, a single-step detection can be used, even if in practical applications the two-step process is more common. A scheme of the procedure of sandwich ELISA assay is reported in Figure 3.47.

3.7.5.3 Competitive ELISA

When the two *matched pair* antibodies needed for the sandwich ELISA are not available for a target, another option is the competitive ELISA. The advantage of competitive ELISA is that nonpurified primary antibodies may be used. Although there are several different configurations for competitive ELISA, in all of them one reagent must be conjugated to a detection enzyme. The enzyme may be linked to either the antigen or the primary antibody.

A step description of an implementation of competitive ELISA can be detailed as follows:

- An unlabeled antibodies solution is incubated with the solution to be assayed that contains the target antigen.
- The ELISA well is coated with antigens. The antigens that coat the well are the same type of the antigens present in the sample solution, but the coating solution is artificially prepared so as to contain sufficient number of antigens to saturate the well surface.
- The remaining antigens solution is washed out from the well.
- The solution containing bound antibody/antigen complexes created starting from the sample are added to the antigen-coated well. The name competitive ELISA is derived from the fact that, due to the well antigens coating, the more antigen in the sample, the less antibody is to bound to the antigens in the well.
- The well is washed, so that unbound antibodies are removed.
- The secondary antibody, specific to the primary antibody is added.
- The second antibody is coupled to the enzyme.
- A substrate is added, and remaining enzymes elicit a chromogenic or fluorescent signal.
- The reaction is stopped in order to prevent eventual saturation of the signal.

Some competitive ELISA assays use enzyme-linked antigen rather than enzyme-linked anti-body. The labeled antigen competes for primary antibody-binding sites with sample antigen. The more antigen in the sample the less labeled antigen is retained in the well and the weaker the signal.

In this type of ELISA, there is an inverse relationship between the signal obtained and the concentration of the analyte in the sample, due to the competition between the free analyte and the ligand–enzyme conjugate for the antibody coating the microplate, that is, the more analyte, the lower the signal. As a matter of fact, the plate will contain enzyme in proportion to the amount of secondary antibody bound to the plate.

3.7.6 FLOW CYTOMETRY ASSAY

Flow cytometry is a technique for counting and examining microscopic particles, such as cells and chromosomes, by suspending them in a stream of fluid and passing them by an electronic detection apparatus. It allows simultaneous multiparametric analysis of the physical and/or chemical characteristics of up to thousands of particles per second. Flow cytometry is routinely used in the diagnosis of health disorders, especially blood cancers, but has many other applications in both research and clinical practice.

A beam of coherent light generated by a laser is directed onto a fluid dynamically focused stream of liquid. A number of detectors are aimed at the point where the stream passes through the light beam: one in line with the light beam to collect forward scattered light (FSC) and several perpendicular to it to collect side scattered light (SSC). One or more fluorescence detectors are generally added to the detection apparatus to collect signals from fluorescent chemical species. Some types of flow cytometers do not collect fluorescence, being able to create a real image of the analyzed particles by the analysis of the scattered and transmitted light.

Each suspended particle from 0.2 to 150 µm passing through the beam scatters the ray, and fluorescent chemicals found in the particle or attached to the particle may be excited into emitting light at a longer wavelength than the light source. This combination of scattered and fluorescent light is picked up by the detectors, and, analyzing the fluctuations in detected power and the spectrum of the detected light, it is possible to derive information about the physical and chemical structure of individual particles.

FSC is related to the electromagnetic cross section of the analyzed particles. Therefore, giving information on their shape and dimension while SSC, being generated by photons entering inside the particle and scattered at great angles by its inner opaque components, depends on the inner complexity of the particle, like the shape of the nucleus, the amount and type of cytoplasmic granules or the membrane roughness, and so on. An example of graphical output data produced by a flow cytometer is schematically reported in Figures 3.48 and 3.49. In particular, in Figure 3.48, a diagram of the particle density detected as a function of the FSC and a particular SSC spectrum is reported, while in Figure 3.49, a particle counting diagram versus the peak of the fluorescence intensity is shown.

3.7.6.1 Particle Labeling in Flow Cytometry

Flow cytometry is listed among the immunoassay because specific particles to be detected and studied are generally marked with specific antibodies, so as to generate a characteristic fluorescence or scattered light that can be divided from all the other elements of the solution response to target the wanted particle specifically [124–127].

The fact that flow cytometers look for scattering and fluorescence in different parts of the optical spectrum allows also multiple antibody marking of different particles so as to obtain multiple characterizations in parallel during a single measure on the same flow.

A wide range of fluorophores can be used as labels in flow cytometry. Fluorophores, or simply "fluors," are typically attached to the antibody used as marker, but they may also be attached to a chemical entity with affinity for the cell membrane or another cellular structure. Each fluorophore

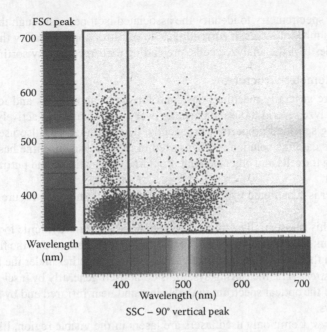

FIGURE 3.48 Diagram of the particle counts detected as a function of the FSC spectrum peak and of a particular SSC spectrum peak wavelengths.

has a characteristic peak excitation and emission wavelength, and the emission spectra often overlap. Consequently, the combination of labels which can be used depends on the wavelength of the lamps and lasers used to excite the fluorochromes and on the detectors available. The maximum number of distinguishable fluorescent labels is thought to be 17 or 18, and this level of complexity necessitates laborious optimization to limit artifacts, as well as complex deconvolution algorithms to separate overlapping spectra.

To ease signal processing, quantum dots are sometimes bonded to the marking antibodies in place of traditional fluorophores because of their narrower emission peaks [128,129]. Another approach to overcome the fluorescent labeling limit is to attach lanthanide isotopes to antibodies [130]. This method could theoretically allow the use of 40–60 distinguishable labels and has been demonstrated for 30 labels. Cells are introduced into plasma, ionizing them and allowing

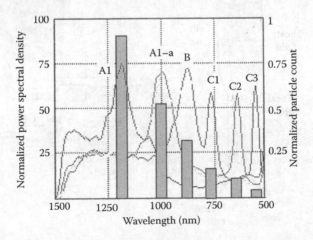

FIGURE 3.49 Histogram of detected fluorescence spectra and particle count for each spectrum.

time-of-flight mass spectrometry to identify the associated isotopes. Although this method permits the use of a large number of labels, it currently has lower throughput capacity than traditional flow cytometry. It also destroys the analyzed cells, precluding their recovery by sorting.

3.7.6.2 Flow Cytometer Structure

Flow cytometers are generally machines designed for great laboratories and for industries. Thus they are able to analyze several thousand particles every second and can actively separate and isolate particles having specified properties. Frequently, flow cytometry is also used to analyze parts of tissue, but in this case the solution to be inserted in the analysis machine has to be prepared in advance by dividing the cells and other elements contained in the tissue and putting them in solution in a suitable solvent.

A flow cytometer is constituted by five main components, as shown in Figure 3.50:

- *A flow cell:* This is essentially a filter structured to create fluid-dynamic focalization of the solution stream; it is formed by a set of very small tissue filters so that the flowing particles are aligned in the flux and passes practically one after the other under the light beam.
- *Measuring system:* The measuring system is composed generally by a set of lasers in different parts of the optical spectrum in the visible and near infrared and by a suitable set of optical sensors.
- *Optical sources:* Commonly used lasers are lasers in the visible region, like argon, krypton, and He–Ne lasers, spanning all the frequencies from green to red and semiconductor lasers spanning all the infrared region from 800 nm to beyond 1600 nm. In recent machines diode lasers emitting in the visible region, from the blue to the red wavelength are used both for the capability to provide light at high frequency without the complexity of optical multiplication and for the possibility to select with a certain accuracy the wanted frequency by small bandwidth tuning of the laser. Power spectral density measurements are obtained by high power lamps covering with a single incoherent beam all the wanted optical spectrum.
- *Detector and analog front end:* Generates FSC and SSC as well as fluorescence signals from light into electrical signals, filters them to limit noise, and converts it into digital signal that can be processed by a computer.
- *Computer* for signal processing and data analysis.

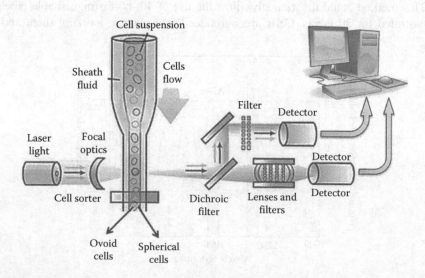

FIGURE 3.50 Principle scheme of a flow cytometric analysis equipment.

3.7.6.3   List of Measurable Parameters

To have an idea of the capability of flow cytometry, we report here a partial list of measurable parameters with industrial machines. This list depends both on the detection and analysis part of the equipment and on the availability of suitable markers to divide signals coming from different particles.

- Volume and morphological complexity of cells
- Cell pigments such as chlorophyll or phycoerythrin
- Total DNA content
- Total RNA content
- DNA copy number variation
- Chromosome analysis and sorting
- Protein expression and localization
- Protein modifications, phospho-proteins
- Transgenic products *in vivo*, particularly the green fluorescent protein or related fluorescent proteins
- Cell surface antigens (cluster of differentiation markers)
- Intracellular antigens
- Nuclear antigens
- Enzymatic activity
- pH, intracellular ionized calcium, magnesium, membrane potential
- Membrane fluidity
- Monitoring electropermeabilization of cells
- Oxidative burst
- Characterizing multidrug resistance (MDR) in cancer cells
- Cell adherence (for instance, pathogen–host cell adherence)

3.8   NUCLEIC ACID SEQUENCING

Even if several techniques for nuclei acids detection exist, they do not allow the structure of the molecule to be determined if it is not a priori known. To determine the exact nucleic base sequence and topology of a DNA or RNA molecule the so-called sequencing is needed. All the techniques allowing the exact sequence of nucleic bases of nucleic acids to be determined are classified under the wide category of sequencing methods [131–134].

To exactly realize the challenge posed by the complete sequencing of a complete DNA molecule it is to take into account that a human DNA, formed by 46 chromosomes, is composed by about 3 billion base pairs and a single human chromosome, the chromosome six, for example, is 225 million base pair long. This complexity is not a human characteristic, but it is shared by all the complex living beings, as it is shown in Table 3.9, where the complexity in terms of number of base pairs of selected chromosomes and genes of a few living species are reported and in Table 3.10 where the same quantity is reported for the genome of selected living beings and viruses, for which the genome is not a complete DNA, but either a part of the DNA or an RNA.

No single chemical method can perform the analysis of such a huge molecule as a genome, thus sequencing has to be performed by three steps:

- The genome or the genome part to be analyzed is divided into small pieces.
- Every piece of the original molecule is sequenced by a suitable chemical assay.
- The obtained sequences are assembled to obtain the final nucleic acid map.

The situation is complicated by the fact that it is not possible to be sure to break all the molecules belonging to a certain sample in the same point. Thus it is not possible to perform the sequencing by simply putting partial sequences one beside the other. Whatever method is used

TABLE 3.9
Complexity in Terms of Number of Base Pairs (bp) of a Few Genes and Chromosomes

Escherichia coli ferredoxin gene	333	bp
Bacillus subtilis ATP synthase (subunit a) gene	732	bp
Escherichia coli biotin synthetase gene	1038	bp
Human β-globin gene	1.5	kb
Human insulin gene	1.7	kb
Escherichia coli β-galactosidase gene	3.5	kb
Human thyroglobulin gene	300	kb
Drosophila melanogaster (fruit fly) chromosome 4	1.75	Mb
Mus musculus (mouse) chromosome 11	45	Mb
Drosophila melanogaster chromosome 3	50	Mb
Human chromosome 20	90	Mb
Human chromosome 6	225	Mb

Note: kb means kilo base pairs, and Mb mega base pairs.

TABLE 3.10
Complexity in Terms of Number of Base Pairs (bp) of a Few Genomes

Commelina yellow mottle virus	7.8	kb
Sulfolobus virus 1	15.5	kb
Lambda virus	48.5	kb
Smallpox virus	186	kb
Mosquito iridescent virus	440	kb
Escherichia coli genome	4.6	Mb
Streptomyces coelicolor (bacteria) genome	8	Mb
Plasmodium falciparum (malarial parasite) genome	25	Mb
Drosophila melanogaster genome	165	Mb
Oryza sativa (rice) genome	441	Mb
Musa sp. (banana) genome	873	Mb
Spinacia oleracea (spinach) genome	989	Mb
Gallus gallus (chicken) genome	1200	Mb
Zea mays (corn) genome	2500	Mb
Homo sapiens (human) genome	3000	Mb
Nicotiana tabacum (tobacco) genome	4434	Mb
Vanilla planifolia (vanilla) genome	7672	Mb
Avena sativa (oat) genome	11,315	Mb
Triticum aestivum (wheat) genome	15,966	Mb
Triturus cristatus (crested newt) genome	18,600	Mb
Necturus maculosus (mudpuppy) genome	50,000	Mb
Lilium longiflorum (Easter lily) genome	90,000	Mb
Fritillaria assyriaca (butterfly) genome	124,900	Mb
Protopterus aethiopicus (lungfish) genome	139,000	Mb

Note: Mb indicates a million base pairs.

TABLE 3.11

Comparison among Selected Sequencing Methods

Method	Single-Molecule Real-Time Sequencing	Ion Torrent Sequencing	Pyrosequencing	Sequencing by Synthesis	Sequencing by Ligation	Chain Termination Sequencing
Read length	2900 bp average	200 bp	700 bp	50–250 bp	50 + 35 or 50 + 50 bp	400–900 bp
Accuracy	87% (read length mode), 99% (accuracy mode)	98%	99.9%	98%	99.9%	99.9%
Reads per run	35–75 thousand	Up to 5 million	1 million	Up to 3 billion	1.2–1.4 billion	N/A
Time per run	30 min to 2 h	2 h	24 h	1–10 days	1–2 weeks	20 min to 3 h
Advantages	Longest read length; fast; detects 4 mC, 5mC, 6 mA	Less expensive equipment; fast	Long read size; fast.	Potential for high sequence yield	Low-cost per base	Long individual reads; useful for many applications
Disadvantages	Low yield at high accuracy; equipment can be very expensive	Homopolymer errors	Runs are expensive; homopolymer errors	Equipment can be very expensive	Slower than other methods	Expensive and impractical for large sequencing projects

Note: Data depend both on the nature of the sequenced molecule, on the application and on the used equipment, thus they have to be considered as indicative. Homopolymer errors refer to the particular situation in which the error probability in the sequence increases sensibly in the presence of a long sequence of the same base. For all methods both the approximated maximum length of a single sequence and the number of contemporary sequences are indicated.

to break the molecule into pieces they will be at least a bit different from molecule to molecule. Hence, the only possible way to perform the assembly of the partial sequences correctly is to break the molecules in overlapping pieces so to use the overlap to guide the assembly operation. Since this operation is not deterministic, that is, it is not possible to break all the molecules exactly in the same point, several fragments can have an overlap, even if they are not one after the other. This means that the assembly cannot be easily performed, but a suitable algorithm has to be devised so as to avoid assembly errors. In conclusion, sequencing of great nucleic acid molecules present a double difficulty: a chemical difficulty and an algorithmic difficulty, needed for a correct assembly of the sequencing results.

The most powerful among the presently used sequencing methods are able to sequence up to about 1 kb with a single read, as it is shown by Table 3.11, where the approximate capacity of selected sequencing methods in terms of single read length is shown. However, while a few methods have been developed up to their full potential, other methods shows a sensible improvement potentiality, so that it is possible to expect that this number will increase rapidly.

Depending on the used techniques and, not unimportant, of the sequencing cost, the sequencing methods are frequently classified in first-, second-, and third-generation methods [134]. First generation is essentially constituted by the chain termination or Sanger method and the Maxam–Gilbert method. They are consolidated methods of analysis and the first reported analysis of human genome was essentially obtained by the Sanger method. This analysis required 10 years of parallel work of several analysis centers, an intensive human work and a great cost, being a great research result, but also underlining the fact that those methods are not suitable if genome analysis has to become a practical method for diagnostic and biological investigation [135,136].

A second and third generation of sequencing methods have emerged after the end of the genome project driven by this target. Second-generation technologies can be classified roughly as a combination of a synchronized reagent wash of nucleotides (NTPs from Nucleoside triphosphates) with a synchronized optical detection method. Second-generation technologies also rely on sequencing by ligation or sequencing by synthesis, including pyrosequencing and reversible chain termination. However, this definition is not rigid, as several variations exist. A few third-generation technologies also rely on optical detection, while a tendency can be registered to eliminate such element to enhance the sequencing and to achieve more economic operation substituting it with novel approaches such as the use of scanning tunneling electron microscope (TEM) and fluorescence resonance energy transfer (FRET). Single-molecule detection, and protein nanopores have also been used.

In the following, we will review briefly a few methods for sequencing of single DNA/RNA fragments, starting from first-generation methods, still largely used being well known and consolidated technologies, up to leading to a few very new and promising methods. At the end we will consider two methods allowing to put together the result of the fragment sequencing to produce the sequence of a long nucleic acid, like a whole genome.

3.8.1 FIRST-GENERATION FRAGMENT SEQUENCING

3.8.1.1 Chain Termination Method (Sanger Method)

The classical chain-termination method (also called Sanger method by its inventor) [137,138] is the first and more diffused among first-generation sequencing methods. It requires the following components:

- Single-stranded DNA target, since the method required single-stranded DNA, denaturation is needed before sequencing
- DNA primer
- DNA polymerase
- Normal deoxynucleotidetriphosphates (dNTPs), all the four possible dNTPs are needed, corresponding to the four nucleic bases
- Modified nucleotides (dideoxyNTPs or ddNTPs), all the four possible ddNTPs are needed, corresponding to the four nucleic bases

The normal dNTP are suitable to replicate DNA under the action of the DNA polymerase; in particular, there are four nucleotides (dATP, dGTP, dCTP, and dTTP) that complementarily combine with the four nucleic bases to reply the DNA strand (see Figure 3.45). Modified dideoxyNTPs (ddATP, ddGTP, ddCTP, and ddTTP) are also nucleotides that complementarily combine with the DNA bases under the action of polymerase, but they lack a 3′-OH group. This group is required for the formation of a phosphodiester bond between two nucleotides, so that during DNA extension, the presence of such a nucleotide in the extended chain causes the extension to terminate, as shown in Figure 3.51. Moreover, ddNTPs may be radioactively or fluorescently labeled for detection in sequencing machines.

The chain termination method is based on the property of ddNTPs. The DNA sample is divided into four separate sequencing reactions, each of which contains all the dNTPs and the DNA polymerase. Moreover, to each reaction is added only one of the four ddNTPs.

This causes each of the reactions to stop where a different nucleic base is encountered in the DNA sequence. Following rounds of template DNA extension from the bound primer, the resulting DNA fragments are heat denatured and separated by size using gel electrophoresis. This is frequently performed using a denaturing polyacrylamide–urea gel with each of the four reactions run in one of four individual lanes (lanes A, T, G, C). The DNA bands may then be visualized, for

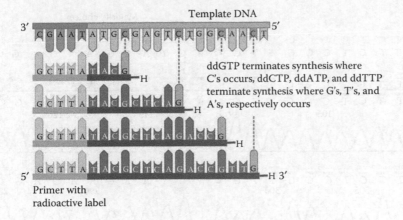

Template DNA

ddGTP terminates synthesis where C's occurs, ddCTP, ddATP, and ddTTP terminate synthesis where G's, T's, and A's, respectively occurs

Primer with
radioactive label

FIGURE 3.51 Principle of chain termination sequencing method.

example by UV light, and the DNA sequence can be directly read off the gel image as shown in Figure 3.52. The electrophoresis result is read from the 5′ to the 3′ terminal and the electrophoresis bands directly identify the sequence of the DNA bases.

In practice, the reading is not always clear as in the case of Figure 3.52; both because electrophoresis bands have a finite bandwidth and because errors can occur. The output of an automatized Sanger sequencer is reported in Figure 3.53, so as to show the effect of the finite electrophoresis bands. Generally, these bands are identified either by a color code or by some other tag, so that it is possible to associate each of them to a specific nucleic base. Nevertheless, it is possible that several bands superimpose, as in the case reported in the Figure 3.53. As in the case of other analytical methods this problem is solved by repeating the sequencing several times on the same sample and applying a majority criterion to decide what is the estimated value of the nucleic base in an uncertain position.

Technical variations of chain-termination sequencing include tagging with nucleotides containing radioactive phosphorus for radiolabeling, or using a primer labeled at the 5′ end with a fluorescent dye. Dye primer sequencing facilitates reading in an optical system for faster and more economical analysis and automation. A limitation of this sequencing method is constituted by the

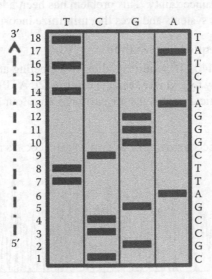

FIGURE 3.52 Principle of the DNA sequence reading after electrophoresis in the chain termination sequencing method.

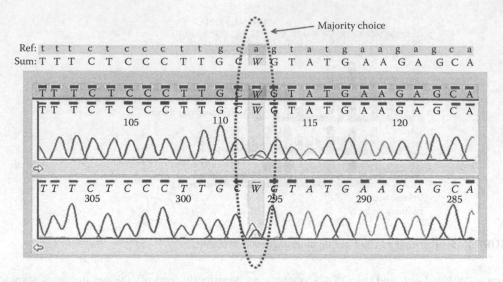

FIGURE 3.53 Principle of majority choice for conflict solving in the chain termination method.

fact that ddNTPs can also tag nonspecific DNA elongated by the polymerase, so affecting the accuracy of the sequencing.

Another important limitation of the Sanger method is the fact that it does not distinguish DNA strains with different topologies, so that coiled strains can affect accuracy of the sequencing too. An important step in improving the ease of use of the Sanger sequencing method was the introduction of dye-tagged ddNTPs. Using this type of ddNTPs the base pair detection can be performed by fluorescence electrophoresis, similar to the case of fluorescence-based quantification, since each ddNTP emits at a different frequency when the dye terminating it is activated [139].

The main limitation of the dye-based method resides in the differences in the incorporation of the dye-labeled chain terminators into the DNA fragment, resulting in unequal peak heights and shapes in the electronic DNA sequence trace chromatogram after electrophoresis. This effect tends to be particularly evident at the start of the sequence, as it is shown in Figure 3.54, so that the first estimated bases have a higher uncertainty. This problem has been addressed with the use of modified DNA polymerase enzyme systems and dyes that minimize incorporation variability.

3.8.1.2 Maxam–Gilbert Sequencing Method

Maxam–Gilbert sequencing [140,141] requires radioactive labeling at one 5′ end of the DNA fragment to be sequenced (typically by a kinase reaction using γ-32P ATP) and purification of the DNA. After this first step, four chemical treatments are carried out on four separated parts of the sample

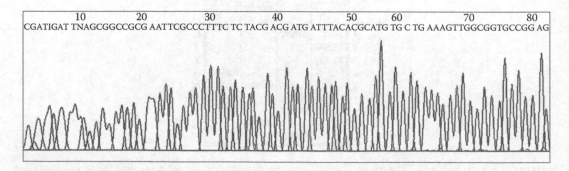

FIGURE 3.54 Example of fluorescence reading after dye-based Sanger sequencing.

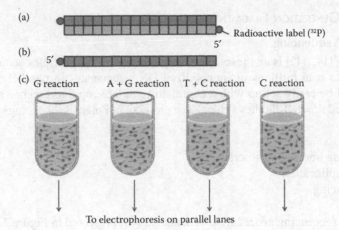

FIGURE 3.55 Maxan–Gilbert sequencing procedure: DNA radioactive labeling (a), DNA denaturation (b), base modification (c).

in order to modify one base in the DNA sequence. The following four modification reactions are carried out:

- *A + G reaction*: Purines are depurinated using formic acid.
- *G reaction*: Guanines and to some extent the adenines are methylated by dimethyl sulfate.
- *C + T reaction*: Pyrimidines are methylated using hydrazine. The addition of salt (sodium chloride) to the hydrazine reaction inhibits the methylation of guanines.
- *C reaction*: Cytosine is treated with hydrazine and sodium chloride so as to inhibit with the salt addition methylation of thymine.

The modified DNAs may then be cleaved by hot piperidine at the position of the modified base. Thus, a series of labeled fragments is generated, from the radiolabeled end to the first cut site in each molecule. This procedure is schematically reported in Figure 3.55.

The fragments in the four reactions are electrophoresed side by side for size separation. To visualize the fragments, the gel is exposed to x-ray film, yielding a series of dark bands each corresponding to a radiolabeled DNA fragment, from which the sequence may be inferred. The simpler method to do that is by visual inspection of the electrophoresis bands as shown in Figure 3.56. In reality, quite frequently, the electrophoresis bands are not so clear as in the Ffigure and signal analysis methods have to be used to distinguish nearby bands and to correct potential errors, as considered in the case of the chain termination method.

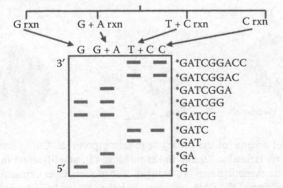

FIGURE 3.56 Reading procedure of the electrophoresis of a Maxan–Gilbert sequencing product.

3.8.2   Second-Generation Fragment Sequencing

3.8.2.1   Polony Sequencing

Polony sequencing [142,143] is an inexpensive, but highly accurate multiplex sequencing technique that can be used to read millions of immobilized DNA sequences in parallel. The hardware of this technique can be easily set up with a commonly available epifluorescence microscope and a computer-controlled flowcell/fluidics system. The protocol of Polony sequencing can be broken into three main parts:

- Paired end-tag library construction
- Template amplification
- DNA sequencing

The whole Polony sequencing procedure is schematically represented in Figure 3.57.

3.8.2.1.1   Paired End-Tag Library Construction

The first step of Polony sequencing has the scope of building up the primes library that will be used to perform the sequencing. This library is directly produced starting from the DNA under test. The procedure begins by randomly shearing the tested DNA into a tight size distribution. The sheared DNA molecules are then subjected to end repair and A-tailed treatment. The end-repair treatment converts any damaged or incompatible protruding ends of DNA to 5′-phosphorylated and blunt-ended DNA, enabling immediate blunt-end ligation. The A-tailing treatment adds an A to the 3′ end of the sheared DNA. At the end DNA molecules with a length of 1 kb are selected by an electrophoretic treatment.

In the next step, the DNA molecules are circularized with T-tailed 30 bp long synthetic oligo-nucleotides (T30), which contains two outward-facing MmeI recognition sites. The resulting circularized DNA undergoes rolling circle replication. The amplified circularized DNA molecules

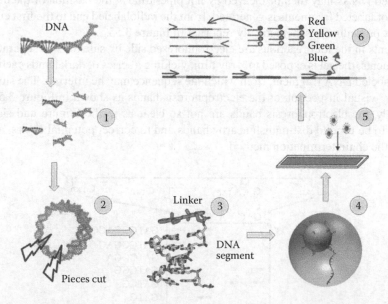

FIGURE 3.57   High-level scheme of the Polony sequencing protocol. Cut of the whole genomic DNA in small pieces (1), pieces circularization (2) and linker bonding (3), amplification of the obtained library into water droplet once fixed on magnetic beads (4), fixing of a bead monolayer containing amplifier library on an acrylamide matrix (5), marking of the DNA sequence with the obtained dye-tagged library and collection of the fluorescence for bases identification (6).

are then digested with MmeI (type IIs restriction endonuclease [144,145]), which will cut at a distance from its recognition site, releasing the T30 fragment flanked by 17–18 bp tags (~70 bp in length) that are the first step to obtain paired end tag molecules (PET). PETs are the short sequences at the 5′ and 3′ ends of a DNA fragment. These short sequences are called tags or signatures because they contain enough sequence information to be uniquely mapped to the DNA fragment, thus completely representing it. It was shown conceptually that 13 bp is sufficient to map small DNA fragments [146]; however, longer sequences are more practical for use in sequencing process.

The PETs need to be end-repaired prior to the ligation of emulsion PCR primer oligonucleotides to both their ends to perform the amplification step.

3.8.2.1.2   Paired End-Tag Library Amplification

The PETs library obtained with the first step of Polony sequencing contains all the PETs that are needed for sequencing, but it needs amplification in order to obtain a sufficient number of molecules. PETs amplification is obtained by a multi-step process.

- *Step 1—Emulsion PCR*: Beads coated with an emulsion of paramagnetic streptavidin are pre-loaded with dual biotin forward primer. Streptavidin has a very strong affinity for biotin, thus the forward primer will bind firmly on the surface of the beads. An aqueous phase is prepared with the pre-loaded beads, a PCR mixture, forward and reverse primers, and the paired end-tag library. This is mixed and vortexed with an oil phase to create the emulsion. Ideally, each droplet of water in the oil emulsion has one bead and one molecule of template DNA, permitting millions of noninteracting amplification within a milliliter-scale volume by performing PCR.
- *Emulsion breaking*: After amplification, the emulsion is broken using isopropanol and detergent buffer followed by a series of vortexing, centrifuging, and magnetic separation. The resulting solution is a suspension of empty, clonal, and nonclonal beads, which arise from emulsion droplets that initially have zero, one or multiple DNA template molecules, respectively.
- *Bead enrichment*: The enrichment of amplified beads is achieved through hybridization to a larger, low density, nonmagnetic polystyrene beads pre-loaded with a biotinylated capture oligonucleotides sequence. This is a DNA sequence complementary to ePCR amplicon sequence so that it can divide amplified from non-amplified beads. The beads capture DNA sequence that are complementary to PCR amplicon sequence. The mixture is then centrifuged to separate the amplified and capture beads complex from the unamplified beads. The amplified, capture bead complex has a lower density and thus will remain in the supernatant while the unamplified beads form a pellet. The supernatant is recovered and treated with NaOH which will break the complex. The paramagnetic amplified beads are separated from the nonmagnetic capture beads by magnetic separation.
- *Bead capping*: The purpose of bead capping is to attach a capping oligonucleotide to the 3′ end of both unextended PCR primers and the template DNA. The cap is an amino group that prevents fluorescent probes from ligating to these ends and at the same time, helps the subsequent coupling of template DNA to the aminosilanated flow cell coverslip.
- *Coverslip arraying*: First, the coverslips are washed and aminosilane-treated, enabling the subsequent covalent coupling of template DNA on it and eliminating any fluorescent contamination. The amplified, enriched beads are mixed with acrylamide and poured into a shallow mold formed by a Teflon-masked microscope slide. The aminosilane-treated coverslip is placed on top of the acrylamide gel and polymerized for a time of the order of 45 min. The silane-treated coverslips will bind covalently to the gel while the Teflon on the surface of microscope slide will enable the better removal of slide from the acrylamide gel. The coverslips then bonded to the flow cell body and any unattached beads will be removed.

5′ Cy5-NNNNNNNNT
5′ Cy3-NNNNNNNNA   First cycle nonamers
5′ TexasRed-NNNNNNNNC
5′ 6FAM-NNNNNNNNG

5′ Cy5-NNNNNNNTN
5′ Cy3-NNNNNNNAN   Second cycle nonamers
5′ TexasRed-NNNNNNNCN
5′ 6FAM-NNNNNNNGN

FIGURE 3.58 Polony sequencing: position of the querying bases in the test nonamers in the first and second cycle of the sequencing.

3.8.2.1.3 DNA Sequencing

The biochemistry of Polony sequencing mainly relies on the discriminatory capacities of polymerases and ligases. First, a series of anchor primers are flowed through the cells and hybridize to the synthetic oligonucleotide sequences at the immediate 3′ or 5′ end of the 17–18 bp proximal or distal genomic DNA tags. Next, an enzymatic ligation reaction of the anchor primer to a population of degenerate nonamers that are labeled with fluorescent dyes is performed. A nonamer is simply a chain with four elements, as shown in Figure 3.58.

The fluorescence dyes that are generally used are as follows:

- Cye3 that emits green fluorescence
- Cye5 that emits yellow fluorescence
- Texas Red that emits red fluorescence
- 6FAM that emits blue fluorescence

The fluorophore-tagged nonamers selectively ligate onto the anchor primer, providing a fluorescent signal that indicates whether there is an A, C, G, or T at the query position on the genomic DNA tag. After four color imaging, the anchor primer/nonamer complexes are stripped off and a new cycle is begun by replacing the anchor primer. A new mixture of the fluorescently tagged nonamers is introduced, for which the query position is shifted one base further into the genomic DNA tag. The query mechanism through nonamers is schematically represented in Figure 3.58.

Seven bases from the 5′ to 3′ direction and six bases from the 3′ end could be queried in this fashion. The ultimate result is a read length of 26 bases per run (13 bases from each of the paired tags) with a 4–5 bases gap in the middle of each tag.

3.8.2.2 Pyrosequencing

Pyrosequencing is a method of DNA sequencing based on the "sequencing by synthesis" principle [147–149]. Sequencing by synthesis involves taking a single strand of the DNA to be sequenced and then synthesizing its complementary strand enzymatically.

The pyrosequencing method is based on detecting the activity of DNA polymerase while it synthesizes the complementary strand of the single-stranded DNA target with another chemiluminescent enzyme one base pair at a time detecting which base was actually added at each step. The template DNA is immobile, and solutions of A, C, G, and T nucleotides are sequentially added and removed from the reaction. Light is produced only when the nucleotide solution complements the first unpaired base of the template. The sequence of solutions which produce chemiluminescent signals allows the determination of the sequence of the template.

The process steps can be described as follows:

1. The target DNA is denatured so as to obtain single-stranded DNA (ssDNA).
2. ssDNA template is hybridized to a sequencing primer and incubated with the enzymes DNA polymerase, ATP sulfurylase, luciferase, and apyrase, and with the substrates adenosine 5′ phosphosulfate (APS) and luciferin.
3. The addition of one of the four dNTPs initiates the second step. DNA polymerase incorporates the correct, complementary dNTPs onto the template, the incorporation releases pyrophosphate (PPi) stoichiometrically. Generally, dATPαS [150], which is not a substrate for a luciferase, is added instead of dATP.
4. ATP sulfurylase quantitatively converts PPi into ATP in the presence of adenosine 5′ phosphosulfate. This ATP acts as fuel to the luciferase-mediated conversion of luciferin into oxyluciferin that generates visible light in amounts that are proportional to the amount of ATP. The light produced in the luciferase-catalyzed reaction is detected by a camera and analyzed in a program.
5. Unincorporated nucleotides and ATP are degraded by the apyrase, and the reaction can restart with another nucleotide.

Currently, a limitation of the method is that the lengths of individual reads of DNA sequence are in the neighborhood of 300–500 nucleotides, shorter than the 800–1000 obtainable with chain termination methods. This can make the process of genome assembly more difficult, particularly for sequences containing a large amount of repetitive DNA.

3.8.2.2.1 Base Encoding Sequencing

The 2 base encoding sequencing is a type of sequencing by ligation procedure [151,152]. It can be used for traditional sequencing, but due to its characteristics it is particularly effective if mutations are to be found with respect to a known sequence and, in general, when information is already known on the sequence to be detected. In this technique, a pool of all possible oligonucleotides of a fixed length is labeled according to the sequenced position. Oligonucleotides are annealed and ligated; the preferential ligation by DNA ligase for matching sequences results in a signal informative of the nucleotide at that position. Before sequencing, the DNA is amplified by emulsion PCR. The resulting bead, each containing single copies of the same DNA molecule, is deposited on a glass slide. The 2 base encoding sequencing procedure is schematically shown in Figure 3.59.

The 2 base encoding procedure can be described dividing it into five steps as follows:

- *Step 1—Preparing a Library:* This step begins with shearing the genomic DNA into small fragments. Then, two different adapters are added, that we can call for reference A1 and A2. The resulting library contains template DNA fragments, which are tagged with one adapter at each end so as to form a sort of A1-template–A2 chain.
- *Step 2—Emulsion PCR (Figure 3.59a):* In this step, using the environment formed by a water emulsion in oil, emulsion PCR is performed using
  - DNA fragments from library
  - Two primers that complement to the previously used adapters, for example, P1 complementing A1 and P2 complementing A2
  - Other PCR reaction components
  - 1 μm beads coupled with one of the primers (e.g., P1).

In each droplet, DNA template anneals to the P1-coupled bead from its A1 side. Then, DNA polymerase will extend from P1 to make the complementary sequence, which eventually results in a bead enriched with PCR products from a single template. After PCR reaction, templates are denatured and disassociate from the beads [153].

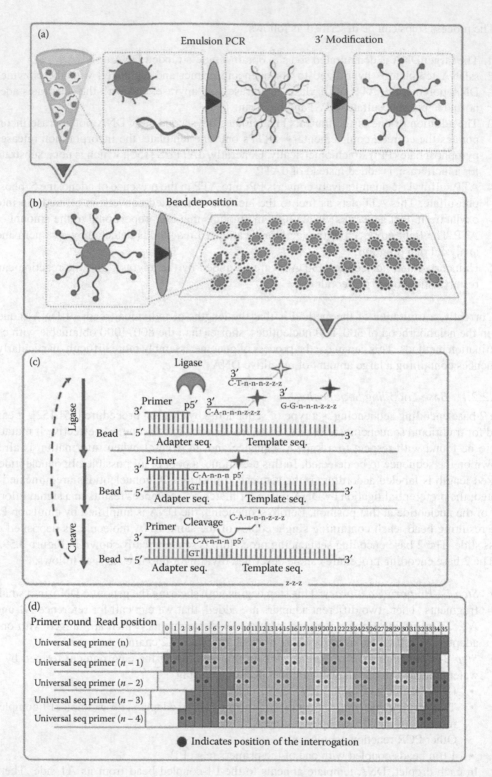

FIGURE 3.59 Phases of the 2 bases encoding sequencing method: emulsion PCR and bead enrichment (a), bead deposition (b) and sequencing by ligation (c), primer reset with two base read (d). (Reproduced under permission of AB Applied Biosystems Inc. from the corporate site at http://www.appliedbiosystems.com. Accessed on November 2013.)

- *Step 3—Bead Enrichment (Figure 3.59a):* In practice, only 30% of beads have target DNA. To increase the number of beads that have target DNA, large polystyrene beads coated with A2 are added to the solution. Thus, any bead containing the extended products will bind polystyrene bead through its P2 end. The resulting complex will be separated from untargeted beads, and melt off to dissociate the targeted beads from polystyrene. This step can increase the throughput of this system from about 30% before enrichment to about 80% after enrichment.

  After enrichment, the 3′-end of products (P2 end) will be modified which makes them capable of covalent bonding in the next step. Therefore, the products of this step are DNA-coupled beads with 3′-modification of each DNA strand.

- *Step 4—Bead Deposition (Figure 3.59b):* In this step, products of the last step are deposited onto a glass slide. Beads attach to the glass surface randomly through covalent bonds of the 3′-modified beads and the glass.

- *Step 5—Sequencing Reaction (Figure 3.59c and d):* As mentioned earlier, unlike next-generation methods which perform sequencing through synthesis, 2-base encoding is based on sequencing by ligation. The ligation is performed using specific 8-mer probes. These probes are eight bases in length with a free hydroxyl group at the 3′ end, a fluorescent dye at the 5′ end, and a cleavage site between the fifth and sixth nucleotide. The first two bases, starting at the 3′ end, are complementary to the nucleotides being sequenced. Bases 3 through 5 are degenerate and able to pair with any nucleotides on the template sequence. Bases 6–8 are also degenerate but are cleaved off, along with the fluorescent dye, as the reaction continues. Cleavage of the fluorescent dye and bases 6–8 leaves a free 5′ phosphate group ready for further ligation. In this manner, positions $n + 1$ and $n + 2$ are correctly base-paired followed by $n + 6$ and $n + 7$ being correctly paired, and so on. The composition of bases $n + 3$, $n + 4$, and $n + 5$ remains undetermined until further rounds of the sequencing reaction.

  The sequencing step is basically composed of five rounds and each round consists of about 5–7 cycles as shown in Figure 3.59d. Each round begins with the addition of a P1-complementary universal primer. This primer has, for example, n nucleotides and its 5′-end matches exactly with the 3′-end of the P1. In each cycle, 8-mer probes are added and ligated according to their first and second bases. Then, the remaining unbound probes are washed out, the fluorescent signal from the bound probe is measured, and the bound probe is cleaved between its fifth and sixth nucleotide. Finally, the primer and probes are all reset for the next round.

  In the next round a new universal primer anneals the position $n - 1$ whose 5′-end matches to the base exactly before the 3′-end of the P1 and the subsequent cycles are repeated similar to the first round. The remaining three rounds will be performed with new universal primers annealing positions $n - 2$, $n - 3$, and $n - 4$ relative to the 3′-end of P1. A complete reaction of five rounds allows the sequencing of about 25 bp of the template from P1.

In practice, direct translation of color reads into base reads is not effective in assuring reliable sequencing since a single error in the color results in a frameshift of the base calls. To best leverage the error robustness of two base encoding, the base reference sequence is converted into the color space by substituting the bases sequence with a color string. Considering the way the read is done, a color does not correspond to a particular value of the read base, but to the transition from that base to the subsequent one. The scheme is represented in Table 3.12.

There is only one unambiguous conversion of a base reference sequence into a color string, but there are four possible conversions of a color string into base strings. As a matter of fact, due to differential encoding the first base cannot be identified and, depending on the unknown value of the first base the differential color sequence translates into a different base sequence. For this reason, the first base of each fragment to be identified is inserted by the sequencing method so as to provide a fixed reference. Besides this property, the selected color coding has a set of important properties.

TABLE 3.12

Base Transition Color Coding Used in Two

Bases Encoding Sequencing

Base Transition	Color
A → A, C → C, G → G, T → T	Blue
A → C, C → A, G → T, T → G	Green
A → G, C → T, G → A, T → C	Yellow
A → T, C → G, G → C, T → A	Red

- The reverse of a base transition is marked with the same color, for example, A → T is marked red as T → A.
- The conjugate of a base transition is marked with the same color, for example, C → A is marked green as G → T.
- Combining the above properties it is also found that the inverse complementary of a base transition is marked with the same color, for example, C → A is marked green as T → G.

The differential color coding transforms a single color error in a multiple error in the sequenced fragment, so that it can be more easily identified if some property of the fragment is already known. But it is really very useful when mutations have to be identified in a known sequence.

Mutations are constituted more probably by a change in one base of the sequence, much less probable are mutations involving two adjacent bases while mutations involving two random bases along the chain are practically almost impossible. As far as errors are concerned, by far the most probable error is constituted by a single read error, more than one error is quite improbable in a relatively short sequence and, even if two errors occur, they are frequently located statistically along the chain, even if the error probability is not uniform since generally the start and the tail of the estimated sequence are more error prone.

If the single base is encoded with a single color and a direct read is performed converting colors in base pairs like in chain termination method the most probable error is almost undistinguishable from a mutation since it causes a single base change. Differently, if differential encoding is performed, a single read error is transformed in a complex alteration of a whole sequence that can be easily distinguished from a probable mutation. This mechanism is represented in Figure 3.60.

3.8.2.3 Other Second-Generation Sequencing Methods

The description of three second-generation sequencing methods allows to have a general idea of how the sequencing technique is evolved from first too second generation. The analysis will not

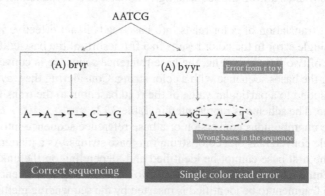

FIGURE 3.60 Effect of a single-color error in two bases encoding method.

be satisfactory, however, without at least citing a set of other methods having their own specificity and application field. They are not inferior or less used with respect to the three methods we have described in more detail. The fact that the following methods are almost only cited is due simply to the fact that a complete and detailed review of sequencing methods is beyond the scope of this chapter. Details can be found in the corresponding bibliographies and in several excellent reviews on sequencing methods like that reported in Reference [134].

3.8.2.3.1   Ion Semiconductor Sequencing

This method of sequencing is based on the detection of hydrogen ions that are released during the polymerization of DNA, as opposed to the optical methods used in other sequencing systems. A microwell containing a template DNA strand to be sequenced is flooded with a single type of nucleotide. If the introduced nucleotide is complementary to the leading template nucleotide it is incorporated into the growing complementary strand. This causes the release of a hydrogen ion that triggers a hypersensitive ion sensor, which indicates that a reaction has occurred. If homopolymer repeats are present in the template sequence multiple nucleotides will be incorporated in a single cycle. This leads to a corresponding number of released hydrogens and a proportionally higher electronic signal [154].

3.8.2.3.2   DNA Nanoball Sequencing

DNA nanoball sequencing is a type of high-throughput sequencing technology used to determine the entire genomic sequence of an organism. The method uses rolling circle replication to amplify small fragments of genomic DNA into DNA nanoballs. Unchained sequencing by ligation is then used to determine the nucleotide sequence [155]. This method of DNA sequencing allows large numbers of DNA nanoballs to be sequenced per run and at low reagent costs compared to other next-generation sequencing platforms [156]. However, only short sequences of DNA are determined from each DNA nanoball, which makes mapping the short reads to a reference genome difficult [157].

3.8.2.3.3   Heliscope Single-Molecule Sequencing

Heliscope sequencing is a method of single-molecule sequencing. It uses DNA fragments with added poly-A tail adapters which are attached to the flow cell surface. The next steps involve extension-based sequencing with cyclic washes of the flow cell with fluorescently labeled nucleotides, one nucleotide type at a time, as with the Sanger method. The reads are short, up to 55 bases per run, but recent improvements allow for more accurate reads of stretches of one type of nucleotides [158].

3.8.2.3.4   Single-Molecule Real-Time Sequencing

Single-molecule real-time (SMRT) sequencing is based on the sequencing by synthesis approach. The DNA is synthesized in zero-mode wave-guides (ZMWs)—small well-like containers with the capturing tools located at the bottom of the well. The sequencing is performed with the use of unmodified polymerase (attached to the ZMW bottom) and fluorescently labeled nucleotides flowing freely in the solution. The wells are constructed in a way that only the fluorescence occurring by the bottom of the well is detected. The fluorescent label is detached from the nucleotide at its incorporation into the DNA strand, leaving an unmodified DNA strand [159].

3.8.3   THIRD-GENERATION FRAGMENT SEQUENCING

A great amount of third-generation methods are still under research. Their main target is to accelerate the sequencing time and increase the length of the single strand that can be sequenced with respect to second-generation methods, while decreasing costs via both the amount of reagents reduction and the use of less expensive procedures. Here, we give a simple list of selected third-generation methods with a few comments, leaving to the interested reader a more complete exploration of this stimulating field starting from the provided bibliography.

3.8.3.1 Sequencing by Hybridization

Sequencing by hybridization is a nonenzymatic method that uses a DNA microarray. A single pool of DNA whose sequence is to be determined is fluorescently labeled and hybridized to an array containing known sequences. Strong hybridization signals from a given spot on the array identify its sequence in the DNA being sequenced [160].

3.8.3.2 Microscopy-Based Techniques

This approach directly visualizes the sequence of DNA molecules using electron microscopy. The first identification of DNA base pairs within intact DNA molecules by enzymatically incorporating modified bases, which contain atoms of increased atomic number, direct visualization, and identification of individually labeled bases within a synthetic 3272 basepair DNA molecule and a 7249 basepair viral genome has been demonstrated [161].

3.8.3.3 RNAP Sequencing

This method is based on use of RNA polymerase (RNAP), which is attached to a polystyrene bead. One end of DNA to be sequenced is attached to another bead, with both beads being placed in optical traps. RNAP motion during transcription brings the beads in closer and their relative distance changes, which can then be recorded at a single-nucleotide resolution. The sequence is deduced based on the four readouts with lowered concentrations of each of the four nucleotide types, similar to the Sanger method [162].

3.8.4 FRAGMENTING AND ASSEMBLY METHODS

The need of fragmenting long nucleic acid molecules to sequence the fragments and to reassemble the results of all the individual fragments sequencing was born contemporary to the first sequencing methods, due to the fact that genes and chromosomes are so long that they cannot be sequenced in a single operation. Even if the sequence that can be analyzed with a single process is getting increasingly longer while the technology proceeds, sequencing simultaneously a long chromosome or even a whole genome is still beyond the possibilities of known techniques.

Two principal segmenting and reassembling methods are widely diffused: primer walking, also called chromosome walking, which progresses through the entire strand, piece by piece, and shotgun sequencing, which is a faster but more complex process, and uses random fragments.

3.8.4.1 Primer Walking (Chromosome Walking)

Primer walking is a sequencing method of choice for sequencing DNA fragments between 1.3 and 7 kb. Such fragments are too long to be sequenced in a single sequence read. This method works by dividing the long sequence into several consecutive short ones. The term 'primer walking' is used where the main aim is to sequence the genome. The term 'chromosome walking' is used instead when we know the sequence but do not have a clone of a gene. For example, the gene for a disease may be located near a specific marker on the sequence [163].

The fragment is first sequenced as if it were a shorter fragment—sequencing will be performed from each end using either universal primers or primers designated by the customer. This should identify approximately the first 1000 bases. To completely sequence the region of interest, design and synthesis of new primers—complementary to the final 20 bases of the known sequence—is necessary to obtain contiguous sequence information.

The basic technique is as follows:

- A primer that matches the beginning of the DNA to sequence is used to synthesize a short DNA strand adjacent to the unknown sequence, starting with the primer.
- The new short DNA strand is sequenced using the chain termination method.
- The end of the sequenced strand is used as a primer for the next part of the long DNA sequence.

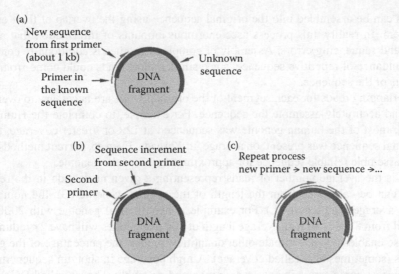

FIGURE 3.61   Scheme of the primer walking process: Start of the procedure with the first primer based on a known sequence and first unknown sequence read (a); seconds primer synthesized on the ground of the first sequence estimate and second sequence estimate (b); read of the whole fragment through second step repetition (c).

That way, the short part of the long DNA that is sequenced keeps *walking* along the sequence as it is schematically shown in Figure 3.61. The method can be used to sequence entire chromosomes (thus, chromosome walking), small genes or very small genomes.

3.8.4.2   Shotgun Sequencing

Shotgun sequencing, also known as shotgun cloning, is named by analogy with the rapidly expanding, quasi-random firing pattern of a shotgun. In shotgun sequencing [164], DNA is broken up randomly into numerous small segments, which are sequenced independently. Multiple overlapping reads for the target DNA are obtained by performing several rounds of this fragmentation and sequencing. Computer programs then use the overlapping ends of different reads to assemble them into a continuous sequence.

A very simple example of shotgun fragmentation and reconstruction is shown in Figure 3.62. In this extremely simplified example, none of the reads cover the full length of the original sequence,

Strand	Sequence
Original	AGATTCATCCATTGACTCCTAGGAGTCATCAGGA
First shotgun sequence	AGATTCA.. ..............TCCATTGACTCCTAGGA......................... ....GTCATCAGGA
Second shotgun sequence	AGATTCATCCATT... .............................GACTCCTAGGAGTCATCAGGA
Third shotgun sequence	AGATTCATCCATTGACTCCTAGGAGT............... ....CATCAGGA
Fourth shotgun sequence	AGATTCATCCATTG... ....ACTCC................................. ...................................TAGGAGTCATCAGGA
Reconstruction	AGATTCATCCATTGACTCCTAGGAGTCATCAGGA

FIGURE 3.62   Simplified example of shotgun fragmentation and reconstruction.

but the reads can be assembled into the original sequence using the overlap of their ends to align and order them. In reality, this process uses enormous amounts of information that are rife with ambiguities and sequencing errors. Assembly of complex genomes is additionally complicated by the great abundance of repetitive sequence, since similar short reads could come from completely different parts of the sequence.

Many overlapping reads for each segment of the original DNA are necessary to overcome these difficulties and accurately assemble the sequence. For example, to complete the Human Genome Project [135], most of the human genome was sequenced at 12× or greater coverage; that is, each base in the final sequence was present, on average, in 12 reads. Even so, current methods have failed to isolate or assemble reliable sequence for approximately 1% of the genome.

Coverage is the average number of reads representing a given nucleotide in the reconstructed sequence. It can be calculated from the length of the original genome (G), the number of reads (N), and the average read length (L). For example, a hypothetical genome with 2000 base pairs reconstructed from 8 reads with an average length of 500 nucleotides will have 2× redundancy. This parameter also enables one to estimate other quantities, such as the percentage of the genome covered by reads (sometimes also called coverage). A high coverage in shotgun sequencing is desired because it can overcome errors in base recognition and assembly. The so-called DNA sequencing theory [165,166] addresses the relationships of such quantities.

Sometimes a distinction is made between sequence coverage and physical coverage. Sequence coverage is the average number of times a base is read (as described above). Physical coverage is the average number of times a base is read or spanned by mate paired reads.

3.9 PROTEIN SEQUENCING AND STRUCTURAL ASSESSMENT

As in the case of nucleic acids, the determination of the amino acid sequencing that constitute a protein and of the protein structure is quite important to understand the active parts of the molecule and, at the end, its role.

The determination of the amount of each amino acid constituting the protein structure is generally obtained via a strong purification of solution containing the target protein followed by protein hydrolysis that not only denature the molecule by eliminating the weak bonds constituting the secondary and the tertiary structure, but also breaks the peptide link separating individual residues (see Section 3.2.4). Once a solution containing almost all the amino acids constituting the original protein is obtained, individual amino acids can be resolved either by electrophoresis or by chromatography so as to obtain a quantitative measure of their abundance. No information is provided, however, on the order in which the amino acid residues appear in the protein chain and on the high-level protein structure. To have more detailed information, different methods have to be used.

3.9.1 PROTEIN SEQUENCING

Traditional methods for protein sequencing are chemical methods that are methods used for nucleic acids sequencing rely on the progressive analysis of the polypeptide chain while either breaking or synthesizing it. If the DNA sequence used for the protein synthesis in the cell is easy to be obtained, a way to determine the protein sequence is to sequence the DNA and to use the genetic code (see Section 2.6.1) to determine the corresponding amino acid sequence. This method has the advantage of exploiting the huge quantity of results obtained in the field of DNA sequencing, but it cannot be used if the synthesis DNA is not at hand.

Other methods for protein sequencing are based on direct protein observation with a suitable microscope [167,168] frequently after protein denaturation allowing the polypeptide chain to be elongated. Direct observation methods are accurate, but they can analyze effectively only small peptides chains, like epitope sites, due to the long time needed to obtain a reliable observation.

Among the chemical methods, the so-called Edman degradation is largely the most used and effective.

3.9.1.1 Sequencing through Edman Degradation

The Edman degradation is a very important reaction for protein sequencing, because it allows the ordered amino acid composition of a protein to be discovered by starting from the N-terminal and eliminating them one by one from the chain [169,170]. Due both to the small error probability in the procedure of peptide identification, that is estimated in about 2% in automated machines, and to the long time needed for the identification, the Edman degradation method is suitable for the sequencing of small polypeptide chains. The maximum length of the chain that can be sequenced in this way is generally around 50 residues.

This causes the fact that, when a polypeptide chain is elongated and purified, it has to be broken into fragments, each fragment has to be sequenced and the sequencing results have to be composed to obtain the whole chain sequence. This procedure is generally carried out using a sort of shotgun method (see Section 3.8.4), where the chain is cleaved several times in different points so as to use computer programs to reconstruct the whole amino acid sequence. In the protein case however, the chain building blocks are 20 instead of four, as in the case of nucleic acids. This causes the reconstruction process to be much easier, due to the much smaller probability that the same sequence represents itself in the terminal of different fragments.

In the protein case, the fragmentation of the chain in small segments is done either via enzymes like endopeptidases (e.g., trypsin or pepsin) or by chemical reagents such as cyanogen bromide. Different enzymes give different cleavage patterns, and the overlap between fragments can be used to construct an overall sequence.

The general scheme of the Edman degradation sequencing method can be schematized as follows:

1. Break any disulfide bridge in the protein with a reducing agent such as 2-mercaptoethanol. A protecting group such as iodoacetic acid may be necessary to prevent the bonds from re-forming.
2. Separate and purify the individual chains of the protein complex, if there are more than one.
3. Determine the amino acid composition of each chain by hydrolysis and quantification.
4. Determine the terminal amino acids of each chain.
5. Break each chain into fragments under 50 amino acids long.
6. Separate and purify the fragments.
7. Determine the sequence of each fragment.
8. Repeat with a different pattern of cleavage.
9. Construct the sequence of the overall protein.

The procedure for the sequencing of a single polypeptide fragment is schematically shown in Figure 3.63.

The Edman degradation reaction that is the core of the sequencing method is, generally carried out by absorbing the peptide chain to be sequenced onto a solid surface such as glass fiber coated with polybrene. The Edman reagent, phenylisothiocyanate (PITC), is added to the adsorbed peptide, together with a mildly basic buffer solution of 12% trimethylamine. This reacts with the amine group of the N-terminal amino acid. The tagged terminal amino acid can then be selectively detached by the addition of anhydrous acid. The derivative then isomerizes to give a substituted phenylthiohydantoin which can be washed off and identified by chromatography (Figure 3.64).

3.9.1.2 Protein N-Terminus Identification

Determining which amino acid forms the N-terminus of a peptide chain is useful for two reasons: to aid the ordering of individual peptide fragment sequences into a whole chain, and because the

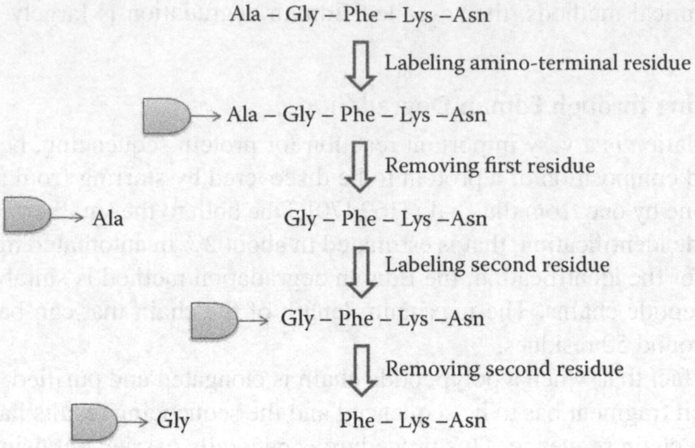

Ala – Gly – Phe – Lys –Asn

⇓ Labeling amino-terminal residue

→ Ala – Gly – Phe – Lys –Asn

⇓ Removing first residue

→ Ala   Gly – Phe – Lys –Asn

⇓ Labeling second residue

→ Gly – Phe – Lys –Asn

⇓ Removing second residue

→ Gly   Phe – Lys –Asn

FIGURE 3.63   Schematic illustration of polypeptide chain sequencing by Edman degradation.

first round of Edman degradation is often contaminated by impurities and therefore does not give an accurate determination of the N-terminal amino acid. A general method for the identification of the N-terminus amino acid can be described as follows:

1. React the peptide with a reagent which will selectively label the terminal amino acid
2. Hydrolyze the protein
3. Determine the amino acid by chromatography and comparison with standards

There are many different reagents which can be used to label terminal amino acids. They all react with amine groups and will, therefore, also bind to amine groups in the side chains of amino acids such as lysine—for this reason it is necessary to be careful in interpreting chromatograms to ensure that the right spot is chosen. Two of the more common reagents are Sanger's reagent (1-fluoro-2,4-dinitrobenzene) and dansyl derivatives such as dansyl chloride. Phenylisothiocyanate, the reagent for the Edman degradation, can also be used. The cheme of the N-terminus identification reaction using the Sanger reagent is shown in Figure 3.65.

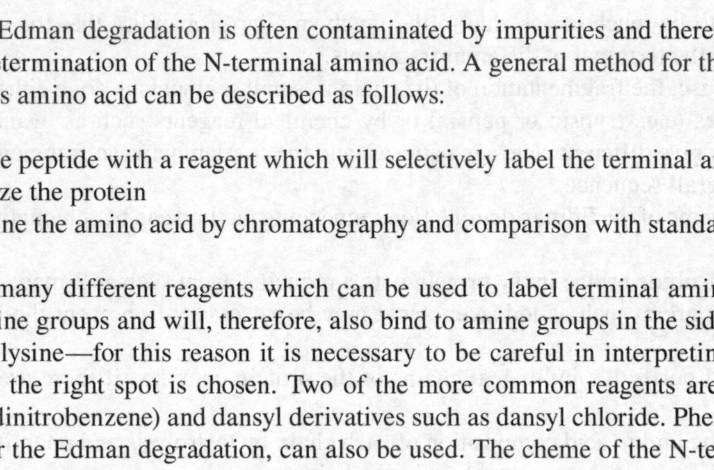

Chromatography

AZT amino acid

FIGURE 3.64   Scheme of the core reaction of the Edman degradation cycle.

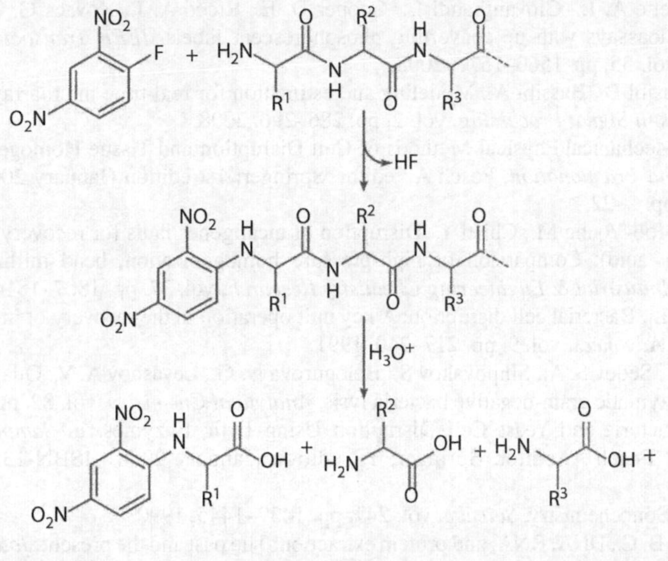

FIGURE 3.65 Base reaction for the polypeptide chain N-terminus identification using the Sanger method.

3.9.2 PROTEIN STRUCTURE ASSESSMENT

Perhaps, the most diffused method to access the folding structure of proteins is to generate a protein crystal from a concentrated protein solution [171,172] and investigate the crystal structure via x-ray diffraction [173,174].

This method has very good resolution due to the accuracy with which the spatial structure of the molecule at the crystal structure nodes can be determined, but has a main drawback. Owing to the fact that proteins interact with each other in a strong and regular way, that is, not present when they are in solution, it is not sure that the folding structure they assume once in the crystal is the same that they have when in solution. For this reason, the folding structure obtained by crystallization has always to be verified somehow before assuming it is the same that the active protein assumes [175–177].

A direct way for a partial verification of such a structure is to assess the capability of the crystallized protein to react with conjugate biomolecules in the same way it does when in solution. Since biochemical reactions are strongly affected by steric factors that can enable or disable interactions between binding sites, this test can be highly relevant to investigate if the structure is maintained or modified during crystallization.

The most important method of protein structure determination using proteins in solution is nuclear magnetic resonance (NMR) that allows the spatial structure of the molecule to be accurately identified [178–180]. This method is also quite effective in verifying whether the structure derived from protein crystal is maintained when proteins are in solution, being the investigation much eased by the fact that a reference structure to test is already known.

REFERENCES

1. Wu G., *Assay Development: Fundamentals and Practices*, Wiley; 1st edition (April 26, 2010), ISBN-13: 978-0470191156.
2. Fishbatch F. T., A Manual of Laboratory and Diagnostic Tests, Lippincott Williams & Wilkins; 8th edition (May 22, 2008), ISBN-13: 978-0781771948.
3. Polat K., Güneş S., A hybrid medical decision making system based on principles component analysis, k-NN based weighted pre-processing and adaptive neuro-fuzzy inference system, *Digital Signal Processing*, vol. 16, pp. 913–921, 2006.
4. Jitmanee K. et al., Enhancing chemical analysis with signal derivatization using simple available software packages, *Microchemical Journal*, vol. 86, pp. 195–203, 2007.

5. Li J. J., Ouellette A. L., Giovangrandi L., Cooper D. E., Ricco A. J., Kovacs G. T. A., Optical scanner for immunoassays with up-converting phosphorescent labels, *IEEE Transactions on Biomedical Engineering*, vol. 55, pp. 1560–1571, 2008.

6. Vikalo H., Hassibi B., Hassibi A., Modeling and estimation for real-time microarrays, *IEEE Journal of Selected Topics in Signal Processing*, vol. 2, pp. 286–296, 2008.

7. Goldberg S., Mechanical/Physical Methods of Cell Disruption and Tissue Homogenization, *in Sample Preparation and Fractionation*, Posch A., editor, Springer; 1st edition (January 2008), ISBN-13: 978-1588297228, pp. 2–22.

8. Tamer I. M., Moo-Young M., Chisti Y., Disruption of alcaligenes latus for recovery of poly(-hydroxybutyric acid): Comparison of high-pressure homogenization, bead milling, and chemically induced lysis, *Industrial & Engineering Chemistry Research*, vol. 37, pp. 1807–1814, 1998.

9. Harrison S. T. L., Bacterial cell disruption: A key unit operation in the recovery of intracellular products, *Biotechnology Advances*, vol. 9, pp. 217–240, 1991.

10. Levashov P. A., Sedov S. A., Shipovskov S., Belogurova N. G., Levashov A. V., Quantitative turbidimetric assay of enzymatic gram-negative bacteria lysis, *Analytical Chemistry*, vol. 82, pp. 2161–2163, 2010.

11. Salazar O., Bacteria and Yeast Cell Disruption Using Lytic Enzymes, in *Sample Preparation and Fractionation*, Posch A. editor, Springer; 1st edition (January 2008), ISBN-13: 978-1588297228, pp. 23–24.

12. Suslick K. S., Sonochemistry, *Science*, vol. 247, pp. 1439–1445, 1990.

13. Tan S. C., Yiap B. C., DNA, RNA, and protein extraction: The past and the present, *Journal of Biomedicine and Biotechnology*, vol. 2009, Article ID 574398, pp. 2–12, 2009.

14. Keer J. T., Birch L., editors, *Essentials of Nucleic Acid Analysis: A Robust Approach*, Royal Society of Chemistry; 1st edition (March 6, 2008), ISBN-13: 978-0854043675.

15. Chomczynski P, Sacchi N., The single-step method of RNA isolation by acid guanidinium thiocyanate–phenol–chloroform extraction: Twenty-something years on, *Natures Protocols*, vol. 1, pp. 581–585, 2006.

16. Siebert P. D., Chenchik A., Modified acid guanidinium thiocyanate–phenol–chloroform RNA extraction method which greatly reduces DNA contamination, *Nucleic Acids Research*, vol. 21, pp. 2019–2020, 1993.

17. Marko M. A., Chipperfield R., Birnboim H. C. A procedure for the large-scale isolation of highly purified plasmid DNA using alkaline extraction and binding to glass powder, *Analytical Biochemistry*, vol. 121, pp. 382–387, 1982.

18. Boom R., Sol C. J., Salimans M. M., Jansen C. L., Wertheim-van Dillen P. M., van der Noordaa J. Rapid and simple method for purification of nucleic acids, *Journal of Clinical Microbiology*, vol. 28, pp. 495–503, 1990.

19. Caldarelli R. S., Vago L., Bonetto S., Nebuloni M., Costanzi G., Use of magnetic beads for tissue DNA extraction and IS6110 mycobacterium tuberculosis PCR, *Molecular Pathology*, vol. 52, pp. 158–160, 1999.

20. Störmer M., Kleesiek K., Dreier J., High-volume extraction of nucleic acids by magnetic bead technology for ultrasensitive detection of bacteria in blood components, *Clinical Chemistry*, vol. 53, pp. 104–110, 2007.

21. Wang H., Yang R., Yang L., Tan W., Nucleic acid conjugated nanomaterials for enhanced molecular recognition, *ACS Nano*, vol. 3, pp. 2451–2460, 2009.

22. Khym J. X., An analytical system for rapid separation of tissue nucleotides at low pressures on conventional anion exchangers, *Clinical Chemistry*, vol. 21, pp. 1245–1252, 1975.

23. Murphy S. E., DNA isolation from small tissue samples using anion-exchange HPLC, *Carcinogenesis*, vol. 10, pp. 1435–1438, 1989.

24. Bergemann C., Müller-Schulte D., Oster J., à Brassard L., Lübbe A. S., Magnetic ion-exchange nano- and microparticles for medical, biochemical and molecular biological applications, *Journal of Magnetism and Magnetic Materials*, vol. 194, pp. 45–52, 1999.

25. Miller J. M., *Chromatography: Concepts and Contrasts*, Wiley-Interscience; 2nd edition (August 17, 2009), ISBN-13: 978-0470530252.

26. Snyder R. L., Kirkland J. J., Dolan J. W., *Introduction to Modern Liquid Chromatography*, Wiley; 3rd edition (December 9, 2009), ISBN-13: 978-0470167540.

27. McNair H. M., Miller J. M., *Basic Gas Chromatography*, Wiley-Interscience; 2nd edition (July 7, 2009), ISBN-13: 978-0470439548.

28. Harris D. C., *Quantitative Chemical Analysis*, W. H. Freeman; 8th edition (April 30, 2010), ISBN-13: 978-1429218153.

29. Lill J. R., Ingle E. S., Liu P. S., Pham V., Sandoval W. N., Microwave-assisted proteomics, *Mass Spectrometry Reviews*, vol. 26, pp. 657–671, 2007.

30. Sambrook J., Russel D. W, *Molecular Cloning: A Laboratory Manual, Spring Harbor Laboratory Press*; 3rd edition 2001, ISBN-13 978-0879695765.

31. Sharkey D. J., Scalice E. R., Christy K. G., Atwood S. M., Daiss J. L., Antibodies as thermolabile switches: High temperature triggering for the polymerase chain reaction, *Biotechnology*, vol. 12, pp. 506–509, 1994.

32. Chien A., Edgar D. B., Trela J. M., Deoxyribonucleic acid polymerase from the extreme thermophile thermus aquaticus, *Journal of Bacteriology*, vol. 127, pp. 1550–1557, 1976.

33. Lawyer F. et al., High-level expression, purification, and enzymatic characterization of full-length thermus aquaticus DNA polymerase and a truncated form deficient in 5 to 3 exonuclease activity, *PCR Methods and Applications*, vol. 2, pp. 275–287, 1993.

34. Booth S. C. et al., Efficiency of the polymerase chain reaction, *Chemical Engineering Science*, vol. 65, pp. 4996–5006, 2010.

35. Assibi A., Sharif M., Efficiency of Polymerase Chain Reaction Processes: A Stochastic Model, *Proceedings of IEEE International Workshop on Genomic Signal Processing and Statistics*, GENSIPS '06, pp. 35–36, 2006.

36. Lalam N., Estimation of the reaction efficiency in polymerase chain reaction, *Journal of Theoretical Biology*, vol. 242, pp. 947–953, 2006.

37. Louw T. M. et al., Experimental validation of a fundamental model for PCR efficiency, *Chemical Engineering Science*, vol. 66, 15 pp. 1783–1789, 2001.

38. Ferré F. et al., *Quantitative PCR: An Overview*, in The Polymerase Chain Reaction, Mullis K. B. Ferré F., Gibbs R. A., editors, Birkhäuser Boston; 1st edition (March 1, 1994), ISBN-13: 978-0817637507, pp. 67–89.

39. Dorak M. T. editor, *Real Time PCR*, Taylor & Francis; 1st edition (June 13, 2006), ISBN-13: 978-0415377348.

40. Chelly J., Kahn A., *RT-PCR and mRNA Quantitation*, in *The Polymerase Chain Reaction*, Mullis K. B., Ferré F., Gibbs R. A., editors, Birkhäuser Boston; 1st edition (March 1, 1994), ISBN-13: 978-0817637507, pp. 97–110.

41. Stemmer W. P., Crameri A., Ha K. D., Brennan T. M., Heyneker H. L., Single-step assembly of a gene and entire plasmid from large numbers of oligodeoxyribonucleotides, *Gene*, vol. 164, pp. 49–53, 1995.

42. Innis M. A., Myambo K. B., Gelfand D. H., Brow M. A., DNA sequencing with thermus aquaticus DNA polymerase and direct sequencing of polymerase chain reaction-amplified DNA, *Proceedings of the National Academy of Science of USA*, vol. 85, pp. 9436–4940, 1988.

43. Pierce K. E., Lj W., Linear-after-the-exponential polymerase chain reaction and allied technologies real time detection strategies for rapid, reliable diagnosis from single cells, *Methods in Molecular Medicine*, vol. 132, pp. 65–85, 2007.

44. Schwartz J. J., Lee C., Shendure J. Accurate gene synthesis with tag-directed retrieval of sequence-verified DNA molecules, *Nature Methods*, vol. 9, pp. 913–915, 2012.

45. Myriam V., Yan X., Huimin K., *Helicase-Dependent Isothermal DNA Amplification*, *EMBO Reports* 5, pp. 795–800, 2004.

46. Zietkiewicz E., Rafalski A., Labuda D., Genome fingerprinting by simple sequence repeat (SSR)-anchored polymerase chain reaction amplification, *Genomics*, vol. 20, pp. 176–183, 1994.

47. Isenbarger T. A., Finney M., Ríos-Velázquez C., Handelsman J., Ruvkun G., Miniprimer PCR, a new lens for viewing the microbial world, *Applied and Environmental Microbiology*, vol. 74, pp. 840–849, 2008.

48. Hayden M. J., Nguyen T. M., Waterman A., Chalmers K. J. Multiplex-ready PCR: A new method for multiplexed SSR and SNP genotyping, *BMC Genomics*, vol. 9, pp. 80–89, 2008.

49. Porter-Jordan K. et al., Nested polymerase chain reaction assay for the detection of cytomegalovirus overcomes false positives caused by contamination with fragmented DNA, *Journal of Medical Virology*, vol. 30, pp. 85–91, 1990.

50. Schnell S., Chappell M. J., Evans N. D., Roussel M. R., The mechanism distinguishability problem in biochemical kinetics: The single-enzyme, single-substrate reaction as a case study, *Comptes Rendus Biologies*, vol. 329, pp. 51–61, 2006.

51. Williams B. A., Toone E. J., Calorimetric evaluation of enzyme kinetic parameters, *The Journal of Organic Chemistry*, vol. 58, pp. 3507–3510, 1993.

52. Todd M. J., Gomez J., Enzyme kinetics determined using calorimetry: A general assay for enzyme activity? *Analytical Biochemistry*, vol. 296, pp. 179–187, 2001.

53. Schärtl W., *Light Scattering from Polymer Solutions and Nanoparticle Dispersions*, Springer; reprint 2007 edition (November 23, 2010), ISBN-13: 978-3642091087.

54. Moran M. J., Shapiro H. N., Boettner D. D., Bailey M. B., *Fundamentals of Engineering Thermodynamics*, Wiley; 7th edition (December 7, 2010), ISBN-13: 978-0470495902.

55. Huges K. T., Radiometric Assays, in *Enzyme Assays: A Practical Approach*, Eisenthal M., Dansom R. editors, Oxford University Press; 2nd edition (June 20, 2002), ISBN-13: 978-0199638208.

56. Miller J. M., *Chromatography: Concepts and Contrasts*, Wiley-Interscience; 2nd edition (August 17, 2009), ISBN-13: 978-0470530252.

57. Carta G., Jungbauer A., *Protein Chromatography: Process Development and Scale-Up*, Wiley-VCH; 1st edition (June 16, 2010), ISBN-13: 978-3527318193.

58. Snyder L. R., Kirkland J. J., Dolan J. W., *Introduction to Modern Liquid Chromatography*, Wiley; 3rd edition (December 9, 2009), ISBN-13: 978-0470167540.

59. Meyer V. R., Practical *High-Performance Liquid Chromatography*, Wiley; 5th edition (May 25, 2010), ISBN-13: 978-0470682173.

60. Lindsay S., High Performance Liquid Chromatography, Wiley; 2nd edition (May 11, 1992), ISBN-13: 978-0471931157-

61. Fritz J. S., Gjerde D. T., *Ion Chromatography*, Wiley-VCH; 4th edition (March 31, 2009), ISBN-13: 978-3527320523.

62. Mori S., Barth H. G., *Size Exclusion Chromatography*, Springer; Softcover reprint 1999 edition (December 3, 2010), ISBN-13: 978-3642084935.

63. Striegel A., Wallace W. Y., Kirkland J. J., Bly D. D., *Modern Size-Exclusion Liquid Chromatography: Practice of Gel Permeation and Gel Filtration Chromatography*, Wiley; 2nd edition (June 29, 2009), ISBN-13: 978-0471201724.

64. Chikazumia N., Ohta T., Estimation of hydrodynamic volume of proteins using high-performance size-exclusion chromatography and intrinsic viscosity measurement: An attempt at universal calibration, *Journal of Liquid Chromatography*, vol. 14, pp. 403–425, 1991.

65. McNair H. M., Miller J. M., *Basic Gas Chromatography*, Wiley; 2nd edition (July 7, 2009), ISBN-13: 978-0470439548.

66. C. Poole editor, *Gas Chromatography*, Elsevier; 1st edition (July 3, 2012), ISBN-13: 978-0123855404.

67. Blumberg L. M., Temperature-Programmed Gas Chromatography, Wiley-VCH; 1st edition (December 21, 2010), ISBN-13: 978-3527326426.

68. Bruus H., *Theoretical Microfluidics*, Oxford University Press, USA (November 17, 2007), ISBN-13: 978-0199235094.

69. Wright J. D., Sommerdijk N. A. J. M., *Sol–Gel Materials: Chemistry and Applications*, CRC Press (December 21, 2000), ISBN-13: 978-9056993269.

70. Norris J. L., Porter N. A., Caprioli R. M., Combination detergent/MALDI matrix: Functional cleavable detergents for mass spectrometry, *Analytical Chemistry*, vol. 77, pp. 5036–5040, 2003.

71. Shi Q., Jackowski G., *One Dimensional Polyacrylamide Electrophoresis*, in *Gel Electrophoresis of Proteins: A Practical Approach*, Hames P. D., editor, OUP Oxford; 3rd edition (October 1, 1998), ISBN-13: 978-0199636402.

72. Smisek D. L., Hoagland D. A., Agarose gel electrophoresis of high molecular weight, synthetic polyelectrolytes, *Macromolecules*, vol. 22, pp. 2270, 1989.

73. Schägger H., Tricine–SDS-PAGE, *Nature Protocols*, vol. 1, pp. 16–22, 2006.

74. Weber K., Osborn M., The reliability of molecular weight determinations by dodecyl sulfate-polyacrylamide gel electrophoresis, *Journal of Biological Chemistry*, vol. 244, pp. 4406–4412, 1969.

75. Laemmli U. K., Cleavage of structural proteins during the assembly of the head of bacteriophage T4, *Nature*, vol. 227, pp. 680–685, 1970.

76. Wittig I., Braun H. P., Schägger H., Blue native PAGE, *Nature Protocols*, vol. 1, pp. 418–428, 2006.

77. Stellwagen N. C., Stellwagen E., Effect of the matrix on DNA electrophoretic mobility, *Journal of Chromatography A*, vol. 1216, pp. 1917–1929, 2009.

78. Champoux J., DNA topoisomerases: Structure, function, and mechanism, *Annual Reviews of Biochemistry*, vol. 70, pp. 369–413, 2001.

79. Bates A. D., Maxwell A., *DNA Topology*, Oxford University Press, USA; New edition (April 2005), ISBN-13: 978-0198506553.

80. Schmid F.-X., *Biological Macromolecules: UV-Visible Spectrophotometry*, in *Encyclopedia of Life Sciences*, Macmillan Publishers Ltd, Nature Publishing Group; 1st edition (2001), ISBN-13: 978-1561592746.

81. Etinski M., Fleig T., Marian C. M., Intersystem crossing and characterization of dark states in the pyrimidine nucleobases uracil, thymine, and 1-methylthymine, *Journal of Physical Chemistry A*, vol. 113, pp. 11809–11816, 2009.

82. Hunter C. A., Sanders J. K. M., The nature of .pi.-.pi. interactions, *Journal of American Chemical Society*, vol. 112, pp. 5525–5534, 1990.

83. Downs T. R., Wilfinger W. W., Fluorometric quantification of DNA in cells and tissue, analytical, *Biochemistry*, vol. 131, pp. 538–547, 1983.

84. Labarca C., Paigen K., A simple rapid, and sensitive DNA assay procedure, *Analytical Biochemistry*, vol. 102, pp. 344–352, 1980.

85. Bridger J. M., Volpi E. V. editors, Fluorescence *in situ* Hybridization (FISH): Protocols and Applications, Humana Press; 2010 edition (September 2010), ISBN-13: 978-1607617884.

86. Gaylord B. S., Heeger A. J., Bazan G. C., DNA hybridization detection with water-soluble conjugated polymers and chromophore-labeled single-stranded DNA, *Journal of the American Chemical Society*, vol. 125, pp. 896–900, 2003.

87. Cai H., Xu Y., Zhu N., He P., Fang Y., An electrochemical DNA hybridization detection assay based on a silver nanoparticle label, *Analyst*, vol. 127, pp. 803–808, 2002.

88. Nezlin R. S., *The Immunoglobulins: Structure and Function*, Academic Press; 1st edition (April 1998), ISBN-13: 978-0123887085.

89. Winkel J. G. J., Hogarth M. editors, The Immunoglobulin Receptors and their Physiological and Pathological Roles in Immunity, Springer; 1st edition (August 31, 1998), ISBN-13: 978-0792350217.

90. Kumagal I., Tsumoto K. Antigen–Antibody Binding, in *Encyclopedia of Life Science*, 2010 Wiley on line library - http://www.els.net, last accessed March 27, 2012.

91. Jin L., Wells J. A. Dissecting the energetics of an antibody–antigen interface by alanine shaving and molecular grafting, *Protein Science*, vol. 3, pp. 2351–2357, 1994.

92. Hughes-Jones N. C., Nature of the reaction between antigen and antibody, *British Medical Bulletin*, vol. 19, pp. 171–177.

93. Dammer U. et al., Specific antigen/antibody interactions measured by force microscopy, *Biophysical Journal*, vol. 70, pp. 2437–2441, 1996.

94. Takamatsu J. et al., Binding free energy calculation and structural analysis for antigen–antibody complex, *AIP Conference Proceedings*, vol. 832, pp. 566–569, 2006.

95. Pellegrini M., Doniach S., Computer simulation of antibody binding specificity, *Proteins Structure, Function, and Genetics*, vol. 15, pp. 436–444, 1993.

96. Reverberti R., Reverberi L., Factors affecting the antigen–antibody reaction, *Blood Transfusions*, vol. 5, pp. 227–240, 2007.

97. Mach T. E. et al., Dependence of avidity on linker length for a bivalent ligand bivalent receptor model system, *Journal of the American Chemical Society*, vol. 2012, pp. 333–345, 2011.

98. Mason W. D., Williams A. S., The kinetics of antibody binding to membrane antigens in solution and at the cell surface, *Biochemical Journal*, vol. 187, pp. 1–20, 1980.

99. Garreth H. R., Grisham C. M., *Biochemistry*, Brooks/Cole (4th edition 2010), ISBN-13: 978-0-495-10935-8.

100. Kusnezow W. et al., Kinetics of antigen binding to antibody microspots: Strong limitation by mass transport to the surface, *Proteomics*, vol. 6, pp. 794–803, 2006.

101. Joergensen L. M. et al., The kinetics of antibody binding to plasmodium falciparum VAR2CSA PfEMP1 antigen and modelling of PfEMP1 antigen packing on the membrane knob, *Malaria Journal*, vol. 9, pp. 1–12, 2010.

102. Sadana, A. and Madugula, A., Binding kinetics of antigen by immobilized antibody or of antibody by immobilized antigen: Influence of lateral interactions and variable rate coefficients, *Biotechnology Progress*, vol. 9, pp. 259–266, 1993.

103. Sadana A., Ram A. B., Fractal analysis of antigen-antibody binding kinetics: Biosensor applications, *Biotechnology Progress*, vol. 10, pp. 291–298, 1994.

104. Gosling P. J. editor, Immunoassays: A Practical Approach, Oxford University Press, USA; 1st edition (August 31, 2000), ISBN-13: 978-0199637102.

105. Wild D. G. editor, *The Immunoassay Handbook*, Elsevier Science; 3rd edition (July 4, 2005), ISBN-13: 978-0080445267.

106. Deshpande S. S., *Enzyme Immunoassays: From Concept to Product Development*, Springer; 1st edition (January 15, 1996), ISBN-13: 978-0412056017.

107. Saltzman W. M., *Biomedical Engineering: Bridging Medicine and Technology*, Cambridge University Press; 1st edition (June 29, 2009), ISBN-13: 978-0521840996.

108. Iniewski K. editor, *Biological and Medical Sensor Technologies*, CRC Press (February 16, 2012), ISBN-13: 978-1439882672.

109. van Emon J. M., *Immunoassay and Other Bioanalytical Techniques*, CRC Press; 1st edition (December 19, 2006), ISBN-13: 978-0849339424.

110. Honjo T., Alt and Neuberger M., *Molecular Biology of B Cells*, Academic Press; 1st edition (March 4, 2003), ISBN-13: 978-0120536412.

111. Bowdler A. J., *The Complete Spleen*, Humana Press; 2nd edition (December 15, 2001), ISBN-13: 978-0896035553.

112. Graille M. et al., Crystal structure of a staphylococcus aureus protein a domain complexed with the fab fragment of a human IgM antibody: Structural basis for recognition of B-cell receptors and superantigen activity, *Proceedings of the National Academy of Science of USA.*, vol. 97, pp. 5399–5404, 1997.

113. Sjobring U. et al., Streptococcal protein G. gene structure and protein binding properties, *Journal of Biological Chemistry*, vol. 266, pp. 399–405, 1991.

114. Kmiecik S., Kolinski A. folding pathway of the b1 domain of protein G explored by multiscale modeling, *Biophysics Journal*, vol. 94, pp. 726, 2008.

115. Heelan A., *Purification of Monoclonal Antibodies Using Protein A/G*, in *Diagnostic and Therapeutic Antibodies*, George A. J. T., Urch T. E., editor, Humana Press; reprint of 2000 edition (November 9, 2010), ISBN-13: 978-1617371950.

116. Ramos-Vara J. A., Technical aspects of immunohistochemistry, *Veterinary Pathology*, vol. 42, pp. 405–426, 2005.

117. Lakowitcz J. R., *Principles of Fluorescence Spectroscopy*, Springer; 3rd edition (September 15, 2006), ISBN-13: 978-0387312781.

118. Gell C., Brockwell D., Smith A., *Handbook of Single Molecule Fluorescence Spectroscopy*, Oxford University Press, USA (October 12, 2006), ISBN-13: 978-0198529422.

119. Oliver C., Jamur M. C., *Immunocytochemical Methods and Protocols*, Humana Press; 3rd edition (December 23, 2009), ISBN-13: 978-1588294630.

120. Elshal F. S., McCoy J. P., Multiplex bead array assays: Performance evaluation and comparison of sensitivity to ELISA, *Methods*, vol. 38, pp. 317–323 2006.

121. Morgan E. et al., Cytometric bead array: A multiplexed assay platform with applications in various areas of biology, *Clinical Immunology*, vol. 110, pp. 252–266, 2004.

122. Kemeny D. M., Challacombe S. J. editors, *ELISA and Other Solid Phase Immunoassays: Theoretical and Practical Aspects*, Wiley; 1st edition (June 1988), ISBN-13: 978-0471909828.

123. Crowther J. R., *Elisa: Theory and Practice*, Humana Press; 1st edition (May 1, 1995), ISBN-13: 978-0896032798.

124. Sklar L. A. editor, *Flow Cytometry for Biotechnology*, Oxford University Press, USA; 1st edition (September 2, 2005), ISBN-13: 978-0195152340.

125. Tukin V. V. editor, *Advanced Optical Flow Cytometry: Methods and Disease Diagnoses*, Wiley-VCH; 1st edition (June 7, 2011), ISBN-13: 978-3527409341.

126. Javois C. L. editor, *Immunocytochemical Methods and Protocols*, Humana Press, Reprint of 1999; 2nd edition (November 10, 2010), ISBN-13: 978-1617370786.

127. Darzynkiewicz Z., Robinson J. P., Roederer M., editors, Essential Cytometry Methods Academic Press; 1st edition (November 9, 2009), ISBN-13: 978-0123750457.

128. Abrams B., Dubrovsky T., Quantum dots in flow cytometry, *Methods of Molecular Biology*, vol. 374, pp. 185–203, 2007.

129. Chattopadhyay P. K., Perfetto S. P., Yu J., Roederer M., The use of quantum dot nanocrystals in multicolor flow cytometry, *Wiley Interdisciplinary Reviews: Nanomedicine and Nanobiotechnology*, vol. 2, pp. 334–348, 2010.

130. Ornatsky O., Bandura D., Baranov V., Nitz M., Winnik M. A., Tanner S., Highly multiparametric analysis by mass cytometry, *Journal of Immunology Methods*, vol. 361 (1–2), pp. 1–20, 2010.

131. Wu W., Zhang H. H., Welsh M. J., Kaufman P. B., Gene Biotechnology, CRC Press; 3rd edition (May 18, 2011), ISBN-13: 978-1439848302.

132. Rodríguez-Ezpeleta N., Hackenberg M., Aransay A. M., editors, *Bioinformatics for High Throughput Sequencing*, Springer; 2012 edition (October 25, 2011), ISBN-13: 978-1461407812.

133. Kim S., Tang H., Mardis E. R., editors, *Genome Sequencing Technology and Algorithms*, Artech House; 1st edition (October 31, 2007), ISBN-13: 978-1596930940.

134. Niedringhaus T. P., Milanova D., Kerby M. B., Snyder M. P., Barron A. E., Landscape of next-generation sequencing technologies, *Analytical Chemistry*, vol. 83, pp. 4327–4341, 2011.

135. A complete information on the Human Genome Project is reported on http://www.ornl.gov/sci/techresources/Human_Genome/home.shtml last accessed on December 10, 2012.

136. Schmutz. et al., Quality assessment of the human genome sequence, *Nature*, vol. 429, pp. 365–368, 2004.

137. Smith L. M., Sanders J. Z. et al. Fluorescence detection in automated DNA sequence analysis, *Nature*, vol. 321, pp. 674–679, 1986.

138. Blazej R. G., Kumaresan P., Cronier S. A., Mathies R. A., Inline injection microdevice for attomole-scale sanger DNA sequencing, *Analytical Chemistry*, vol. 79, pp. 4499–4506, 2007.

139. Smith L. M., Fung S., Hunkapiller M. W., Hunkapiller T. J., Hood L. E., *The synthesis of oligonucleotides containing an aliphatic amino group at the 5′ terminus: Synthesis of fluorescent DNA primers for use in DNA sequence analysis, Nucleic Acids Research*, vol. 13, pp. 2399–2412, 1985.

140. Maxam A. M., Gilbert W. A new method for sequencing DNA, *Proceedings of the U.S. National Academy of Science*, vol. 74, pp. 560–564, 1997.

141. Boland E. J., Pillai A., Odom M. W., Jagadeeswaran P., Automation of the maxam–gilbert chemical sequencing reactions, *BioTechniques*, vol. 16, pp. 1088–1092 and 1094–1095, 1994.

142. Mitra R. D., Shendure J. et al. Fluorescent in situ sequencing on polymerase colonies, *Analytical Biochemistry*, vol. 320, pp. 55–65, 2003.

143. Shendure, J., Porreca G. J. et al. Accurate multiplex polony sequencing of an evolved bacterial genome, *Science*, vol. 309, pp. 1728–1732, 2005.

144. Tucholski J., Skowron P. M., Podhajska A. J., MmeI, a Class-IIS restriction endonuclease: Purification and characterization, *Gene*, vol. 157, pp. 87–92, 1995.

145. Morgan R. D., Dwinell E. A., Bhatia T. K., Lang E. M., Luyten Y. A., The MmeI family: Type II restriction-modification enzymes that employ single-strand modification for host protection, *Nucleic Acids Research*, vol. 37, pp. 5208–5221, 2009.

146. Fullwood M. J., Wei C. L., Liu E. T., Ruan Y., Next-generation DNA sequencing of paired-end tags (PET) for transcriptome and genome analyses, *Genome Research*, vol. 19, pp. 521–532, 2009.

147. Gharizadeh B. et al.; *Long-read pyrosequencing using pure 2′-deoxyadenosine-5′-O′-(1-thiotriphosphate) Sp-Isomer, Analytical Biochemistry*, vol. 301, pp. 82–90, 2002.

148. Fakhrai-Rad H. et al., Pyrosequencing: An accurate detection platform for single nucleotide polymorphisms, *Humans Mutations*, vol. 19, pp. 479–485, 2002.

149. Langaee T., Ronaghi M., Genetic variation analyses by pyrosequencing, *Mutations Research*, vol. 573, pp. 96–102, 2005.

150. Oras A., Kilk K., Kunapuli S., Barnard E. A., Järv J., Kinetic analysis of [35S]dATP alpha S interaction with P2y(1) nucleotide receptor, *Neurochemistry International*, vol. 40, pp. 381–386, 2002.

151. McKernan K. J. et al., Sequence and structural variation in a human genome uncovered by short-read, massively parallel ligation sequencing using two-base encoding, *Genome Research*, vol. 19, pp. 1527–1541, 2009.

152. Smith D. R. et al., Rapid whole-genome mutational profiling using next-generation sequencing technologies, *Genome Research*, vol. 18, pp. 1638–1642, 2008.

153. Dressman D., Yan H., Traverso G., Kinzler K. W., Vogelstein B., Transforming single DNA molecules into fluorescent magnetic particles for detection and enumeration of genetic variations, *Proceedings of the National Academy of Sciences of the USA*, vol. 100, pp. 8817–8822, 2003.

154. Rusk N., Torrents of sequence, *Nature Methods*, vol. 8, pp. 44–44, 2011.

155. Drmanac R. et al. Human genome sequencing using unchained base reads in self-assembling DNA nanoarrays, *Science*, vol. 327, pp. 78–81, 2010.

156. Porreca J. G., Genome Sequencing on Nanoballs, *Nature Biotechnology*, vol. 28, pp. 43–44, 2010.

157. Drmanac R. et al., Human genome sequencing using unchained base reads in self-assembling DNA nanoarrays, *Supplementary Material. Science*, vol. 327, pp. 78–81, 2010.

158. Thompson J. F., Steinmann K. E., *Single Molecule Sequencing with a HeliScope Genetic Analysis System*, in *Current Protocols in Molecular Biology* Ausubel F. M. et al. editors, Wiley (2010), ISBN-13 978-0471142720.

159. Flusberg B. A. et al., Direct detection of DNA methylation during single-molecule, real-time sequencing, *Nature Methods*, vol. 7, pp. 461–465, 2010.

160. Hanna G. J. et al. Comparison of sequencing by hybridization and cycle sequencing for genotyping of human immunodeficiency virus type 1 reverse transcriptase, *Journal of Clinical Microbiology*, vol. 38, pp. 2715–2721, 2000.

161. Bell D. C. et al., DNA base identification by electron microscopy, *Microscopy and Microanalysis: The Official Journal of Microscopy Society of America, Microbeam Analysis Society, Microscopical Society of Canada*, vol. 18, pp. 1–5, 2012.

162. Pareek C. S., Smoczynski, R., Tretyn A., *Sequencing technologies and genome sequencing, Journal of Applied Genetics*, vol. 52, pp. 413–35, 2011.

163. Cann A. *DNA Viruses: A Practical Approach*, Oxford University Press; 1st edition 1999, ISBN-13: 978-0199637180.

164. Staden R, A strategy of DNA sequencing employing computer programs, *Nucleic Acids Research*, vol. 6, pp. 2601–2610, 1979.

165. Waterman M. S., *Introduction to Computational Biology*, Chapman & Hall/CRC; 1st edition (1995), ISBN-13 978-0412993910.

166. Hall, P., *Introduction to the Theory of Coverage Processes*, Wiley; 1st edition (1988) ISBN-13 978-0471857025.

167. Galvin N. J., Dixit V. M., O'Rourke K. M., Santoro S. A., Grant G. A., Frazier W. A., Mapping of epitopes for monoclonal antibodies against human platelet thrombospondin with electron microscopy and high sensitivity amino acid sequencing, *Journal of Cell Biology*, vol. 101, pp. 1434–1441, 1985.

168. Donachy J. E., Drake B., Sikes C. S., Sequence and atomic-force microscopy analysis of a matrix protein from the shell of the oyster crassostrea virginica, *Marine Biology*, vol. 114, pp. 423–428, 1992.

169. Steen H., Mann M., The abc's (and xyz's) of peptide sequencing, *Nature Reviews Molecular Cell Biology*, vol. 5, pp. 699–711, 2004.

170. Smith B. J. editor, *Protein Sequencing Protocols*, Humana Press; 2nd edition (October 10, 2002), ISBN-13: 978-0896039759.

171. Ducruix A., Giegé R., editors, *Crystallization of Nucleic Acids and Proteins a Practical Approach*, Oxford University Press, USA; 2nd edition (January 20, 2000), ISBN-13: 978-0199636785.

172. Shah U. V., Williams D. R., Heng J. Y. Y., Selective crystallization of proteins using engineered nanonucleants, *Crystal Growth & Design*, vol. 12, pp. 1362–1369, 2012.

173. Rhodes G., *Crystallography Made Crystal Clear: A Guide for Users of Macromolecular Models*, Academic Press; 3rd edition (March 2, 2006), ISBN-13: 978-0125870733.

174. Sherwood D., Cooper J., *Crystals, X-rays and Proteins: Comprehensive Protein Crystallography*, Oxford University Press, USA (December 30, 2010), ISBN-13: 978-0199559046.

175. Brunger A, T. Free R value: A novel statistical quantity for assessing the accuracy of crystal structures, *Nature*, vol. 355, pp. 472–475, 1992.

176. Badger J., Hendle J., Reliable quality-control methods for protein crystal structures, *Acta Crystallographica D, Biological Crystallography*, vol. 58 (Pt 2), pp. 284–291, 2002.

177. Sahakyan A. B., Cavalli A., Vranken W. F., Vendruscolo M., Protein structure validation using side-chain chemical shifts, *Journal of Physical Chemistry B*, vol. 116, pp. 4754–4759, 2012

178. Wüthrich K., Protein structure determination in solution by NMR spectroscopy, *Journal of Biological Chemistry*, vol. 265, pp. 22059–22062, 1990.

179. Bax A., Ikura M., An efficient 3D NMR technique for correlating the proton and 15N backbone amide resonances with the alpha-carbon of the preceding residue in uniformly 15N/13C enriched proteins, *Journal of Biomolecular NMR*, vol. 1, pp. 99–104, 1991.

180. Spronk C. A., Nabuurs S. B., Krieger E., Vriend G., Vuister G. W., Validation of protein structures derived by NMR spectroscopy, *Progress in Nuclear Magnetic Resonance Spectroscopy*, vol. 45, pp. 315–337, 2004.

Section II

Lab on Chip Technology

4 Planar Technology

4.1 INTRODUCTION

This chapter is the first of the second part of the book, the part devoted to technologies for labs on chip. As a matter of fact, what renders microfluidics revolutionary in the field of biotechnologies is the possibility to produce millions of inexpensive circuits that perform complex operations.

This opens the opportunity for capillary diffusion of disease prevention and screening on the one hand, and environmental and food control on the other, with a potential social revolution even more profound than that caused by microelectronics and broadband communications.

This is due mainly to the transfer of mass production technologies in the field of microfluidics, to transform the cost model of analytical biochemistry from the current situation dominated by work and material costs to a microelectronics like situation, where extremely larger volumes correspond to lower costs [1,2].

The process allowing integrated circuits, which are electronic, optical, or fluidics [2–5], to be realized is essentially constituted by two steps called front end and back end. All the techniques required to fabricate several different circuits on a single substrate are collected under the name of front-end technologies. Thus, the output of a front-end fabrication cycle is a set of circuits fabricated on the same surface (a single wafer in case of silica on silicon).

All the procedures starting from the wafer in which integrated circuits have been fabricated and that arrives to a single integrated circuit enclosed in a suitable package and ready to be integrated into a more complex system are collected under the name of back end technologies.

Thus, technologies such as photolithography and dopant diffusion are part of the front end while the process of separating chips fabricated on the same wafer (generally called dicing) and of fabricating the suitable interfaces with the outside world are part of the back end.

As far as front-end processes are concerned, essentially two types of technologies are used to target mass production of labs on chips, depending on the kind of used material: planar technologies, essentially derived from microelectronics, and polymer-based technologies. These technologies have many common elements, in particular, the capability of processing chips with very small critical dimensions with automatic machinery, but have also relevant differences.

After a general introduction, we will devote this chapter to planar front-end technologies and Chapter 5 to polymer-based technologies. We will include in Chapter 4 a paragraph on cost models for different production technologies, so as to clarify the impact, the potentialities, and the limits of the different manufacturing technique. Back-end technologies are analyzed in Chapter 6, since they are common to both planar and polymer-based circuits, but for a few elements that will be detailed during the exposition.

As we will see, the very small aspect ratio of integrated circuits is instrumental in their low-cost characteristic, thus complex technologies have to be used to be able to fabricate the small details of the circuits and the presence of even very small impurities can completely ruin a whole circuit. For this reason, planar technology and polymer-based processes have to be carried out in a very clean environment, where the presence of impurities, both from the air and from the very presence of human operators, has to be strictly controlled. Such an environment is realized in the so-called "clean rooms" [1], the typical structures where planar integration is realized.

Clean-room technology is instrumental to the realization of integrated circuits of whatever kind and they condition the characteristics of the available processes. Thus, a brief introduction to

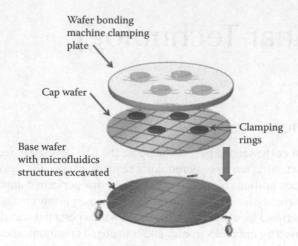

Wafer bonding
machine clamping
plate

Cap wafer

Clamping
rings

Base wafer
with microfluidics
structures excavated

FIGURE 4.1   Wafer bonding for microfluidics circuits.

clean rooms structure and functionalities is important to a full understanding of planar integration processes.

While the above considerations hold for whatever integrated circuit fabrication process, microfluidics has its own particular technologies and processes. On the one hand, if silicon and silicon oxide films on silicon are obliged materials for electronics and integrated optics, this is not true for microfluidics.

Even if microfluidics can be developed starting from traditional silicon wafers designed for microelectronics by exploiting the natural passivation of silicon surface by oxidation and, if needed, deposition of thick silicon oxide films, both polymeric materials and glass wafers have been used with success, thereby creating a set of specific processes for these kinds of materials. Moreover, in creating microfluidics circuits, exigencies that do not exist in microelectronics and integrated optics emerge, calling for specific processes or important modification of existing fabrication techniques.

As an example, since the fact that planar technology is able to excavate the wafer from the top, not to create ducts and chambers excavating it from the side, a duct has to be fabricated by creating a long hole in the wafer and then covering it with a roof. The roof cannot be obtained by deposition that will fill the hole, but has to be fabricated by placing on top of the hole a solid surface, that is another wafer (cf. Figure 4.1). Consequently, a technology called wafer bonding [6], consisting in placing two wafers one on top of the other with the top surfaces in contact is fundamental in the field of microfluidics, while it is a niche technology in the field of electronics and optics.

4.2   PLANAR PROCESS FLOW OF A LAB ON CHIP

The goal of this section is to present the whole fabrication process needed to build a microfluidics-based lab on chip with planar technologies [1,2,7]. A realistic fabrication process strongly depends on the structures to be implemented in the chip and in principle it is not possible to provide a generic process flow. Nevertheless, there are recurring operations and typical processes which have to be considered as steps of a complete fabrication cycle to be fully understood. Frequently, the most difficult challenge in fabricating a complex circuit is not to fabricate its individual parts, but to integrate them together in the same process flow. As a matter of fact, different processes require different conditions and it is not infrequent that performing process B after process A destroys the structures created by process A due to the conditions required to perform process B.

The most classic example is doping and annealing. To fabricate almost all the electronic structures doping is needed. This is a process that is required to give to silicon electrical characteristics suitable for electronic devices and consists in controlled diffusion of particular substance called

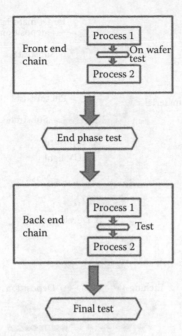

FIGURE 4.2   General scheme of the whole fabrication process for a microfluidics circuit.

dopants in the silicon crystal. Dopants generally substitute silicon atoms at the lattice nodes penetrating due to their mobility and high-temperature deep into the crystal [1,3]. Since integrated optics is generally constructed in a silica layer deposited over the silicon surface, it could seem possible to implement electronics on the silicon wafer, grow the silica layer, and then integrate optics in the silica.

To obtain good optical properties in terms of index uniformity and attenuation, the silica layer has to be annealed around 1000°C to uniform it before the optical waveguide fabrication [5]. Annealing the wafer at a high temperature completely destroys the underlying electronic structures, since it causes uncontrolled diffusion of the dopants. This is one of the major obstacles to the integration of electronics with silica-based optics and is still unresolved in single wafer circuits.

The case of dopant and annealing is quite extreme, even if practically important, but similar situations are common. Thus clarifying the need of looking at the fabrication process like a whole, instead like a set of sequential independent steps.

The chip production process is constituted by three main parts, as shown in Figure 4.2. Testing is a very important part of the process, having a great impact both on the end process quality, represented at first by the final product yield, and on the industrial cost. Under a cost point of view, testing is more expensive if located in the back-end section of the process, being performed chip by chip. The final test, in particular, is often one of the main contributions to the industrial cost due to the impact of testing time and labor cost. For this reason, in a steady-state process characterized by a very high fabrication yield, as it happens, for example, in electronic RAMs [3], a sampled final test can be operated; drastically decreasing the related cost.

4.2.1   FRONT-END PROCESS FLOW

The most basic procedure of planar technology is the series of steps that enable to transfer a planar shape designed on a mask on a wafer by modeling a film of the wanted material. This procedure is so common and important that often the complexity of a planar circuit is measured in "number of masks," that is, the number of consecutive times this procedure has to be repeated transferring on the wafer different superimposed forms to achieve the wanted structure.

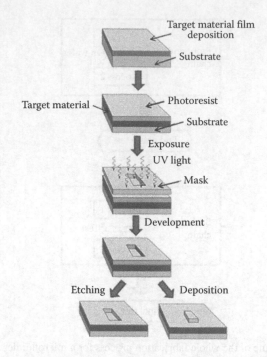

FIGURE 4.3   General scheme of the process of deposition, lithography, and etching (or deposition).

The procedure for the creation of a planar shape on the wafer is composed of the following steps, represented graphically in Figure 4.3.

1. The desired shape is created on a mask, that is, on a sheet of material suitable for the following process. The shape has to be planar, that is two dimensional, so as to be transferred on the wafer surface. Nevertheless, a depth is also associated to it, constant over all the shape. An example of mask is shown in Figure 4.4.
2. The material film over which the shape has to be transferred is growth on the wafer surface with one of the many growing techniques. The depth of the film will also be the depth of the shape that has to be realized.
3. A photoresist is deposited on the film; it is a material that will change suitably its chemical properties when exposed to ultraviolet light.
4. The mask is superimposed to the resist and aligned exactly to the wafer underlining structure. This is a critical operation due to the fact that the structure that has to be realized is to

FIGURE 4.4   Example of photolithographic mask.

be aligned with the already existing structures. In order to do that, when a particular structure is realized, also specific markers are present to allow subsequent structures alignment.

5. The wafer is lightened with ultraviolet light. Where the photoresist is protected by the mask it is not hit by light, while where the mask is not present it is impressed by it.

6. The mask is removed and the photoresist developed. Where the photoresist was impressed, its chemical structure changes due to the light and the development procedure.

7. The wafer with the photoresist on it is chemically attached by a photoresist etcher. In positive photoresists, the developed part is etched while the undeveloped part, which was protected by the mask, is not etched, while the contrary happens in negative photoresists. In this way, either the mask image or its negative photoresist is transferred to the resist.

8. The wafer is etched again with an etching process suitable to consume the film that was deposited at the start of the process, where it is exposed. Where the photoresist is still present the etching process does not reach the film and it is not consumed. In this way the image on the mask is transferred, via the photoresist, on the film that was grown on the wafer surface.

9. All the photoresists are chemically removed, by leaving the mask image transferred on the film, which was the desired result.

A possible variant of the process is substituting etching with deposition so that the holes left from the photoresist development and etching are filled by the new material and creates an image of the mask in relief with respect to the wafer surface.

Independently from the use of etching or deposition, a set of subprocesses are required: they are called

- Mask design
- Deposition
- Lithography
- Etching or deposition

These are the base processes of any planar technology, from microelectronics to integrated optics to microfluidics. As a first example, we want to present the schematic process flow that is needed to integrate silica on silicon optical waveguide, an optical element that is frequently present in labs on chip when optical detection is used.

The waveguide structure is presented in Figure 4.5: on the silicon substrate provided by a standard silicon wafer several silica layers with different diffraction indexes are fabricated, obtained by doping silica with different quantities of selected dopants, generally germanium [5]. The process

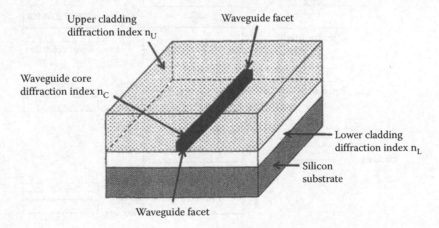

FIGURE 4.5 Scheme of a silica on silicon optical waveguide.

does not substantially change if the substrate is a glass wafer. The schematic process flow is shown in Figure 4.6. Here, the base operations that we have described in the above discussion can be recognized. Besides the basic processes of deposition, lithography, and etching, two new processes are shown, that are needed for this particular component. The first is silica annealing, as we have already discussed, to homogenize the property of silica and obtain good optical performances.

The second new process is planarization. This process is needed every time a planar surface has to be obtained after deposition on a surface where structures have been fabricated [1]. As the surface is not uniform and the deposition creates a uniform thickness film, the deposited film will follow somehow the profile of the underlining surface. To obtain a flat surface, a *flattening etching* has to be performed, that is called planarization. This is a key process in microfluidics devices, since a very good planarization is needed to achieve effective wafer bonding.

Let us now imagine to fabricate a more complex microfluidics circuit. We have to build a reaction chamber in which antibodies have to be trapped on the bottom surface to perform a sandwich immunoassay (cf. Section 3.7.5) having as target the solution that will be injected into the chamber.

Detection is performed by building an optical interferometer on top of the reaction chamber so to detect the refraction index change due to antigen–antibody neutralization. The planar scheme and the section of the structure we have to fabricate are represented in Figure 4.7. This is a very simplified scheme with respect to the realistic labs on chip design that we will discuss in later chapters, but here the point is not to show an effective design, but to define a simplified structure so as to imagine a fabrication process flow.

We have to work on two wafers. The first on top, we will use as the roof of our reaction chamber, where we will build the optical waveguide part of the detection interferometer. This wafer will need annealing to assure good optical performances, but since no other structure will be constructed upon it, this hides no problem. In any case, planarization will be needed after the annealing to assure an effective wafer bonding. On the other wafer, we will build the structures that will be needed for the reaction chamber, excavating it and constructing the structure that will capture the

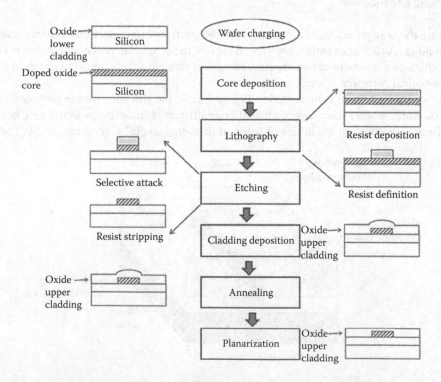

FIGURE 4.6 Schematic process flow for the silica on silicon waveguide fabrication.

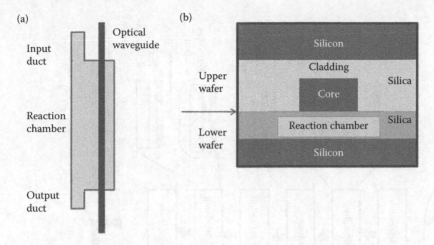

FIGURE 4.7 Planar scheme (a) and section (b) of the structure comprising an optical waveguide built upon a reaction chamber having antibodies fixed on the floor that is considered in the example of the text.

antibodies on its floor. This wafer will not be annealed, not to ruin the excavated reaction chamber. In any case, since etching will create inhomogeneous wafer surface, also in this case planarization will be performed before wafer bonding.

Antibodies will be added before wafer bonding by exposing the lower wafer to concentrated antibodies solution, waiting for the saturation of the reaction chamber floor and washing out the remaining antibodies with a suitable washing solution. Since the organic molecules will be bonded to the floor of the chamber from now on, we have to care that no high- or low-temperature processes are performed after antibodies bonding, not to cause molecules denaturation or detach from the activated surface.

Collecting all these considerations we can set up the process flow that is represented in Figure 4.8. From the figure it could seem that both the wafers experience a single mask process, but it is not true. As a matter of fact, we have synthesized the surface activation as a single step, but it is a quite complex procedure. There are several surface activation techniques: oversimplifying the process we have to follow the steps reported in Figure 4.9.

In this case, the mask is used to perform selective deposition on the floor of the reaction chamber and to protect the surface of the other parts of the circuit from the chemical attack that is needed to activate the reaction chamber surface. Thus, the process that is needed to fabricate the lower wafer is a two mask process and it renders it more complex. The two masks have to be suitably aligned not to create deposition and chemical attack in wrong places without activating a part of the reaction chamber floor. The mask alignment is obtained by lithographic marks that have to be realized on the wafer surface besides the integrated circuits and that are read by the lithographic machine when it places the mask.

Up to now we have considered processes that are able to transfer on the wafer surface pure planar structures; however, in labs on chips, more complex structures have to be realized. Suspended membranes, for example, are fundamental elements in many labs on chips both in microfluidics valves and in micro-pumps and movable surfaces are used in many biological applications (see Chapter 8). All these structures can be classified under the category of micro-electro-mechanical structures (MEMs) and when they are applied to labs on chip they are frequently called biomems [8,9].

Owing to the large use in microelectronics and to its very good mechanical properties, silicon is the main material used to fabricate MEMs, but sometimes other kinds of materials are also used, especially when a glass or polymer substrate is adopted. There are essentially two techniques that can be used to realize optical switches with silicon-based MEMs: bulk micromachining, and surface micromachining [10,11].

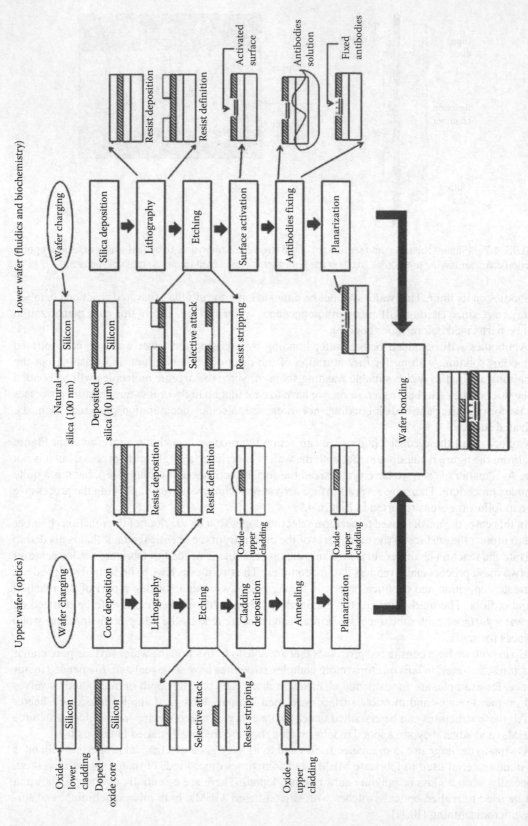

FIGURE 4.8 Process flow for the fabrication of the structure in Figure 4.7.

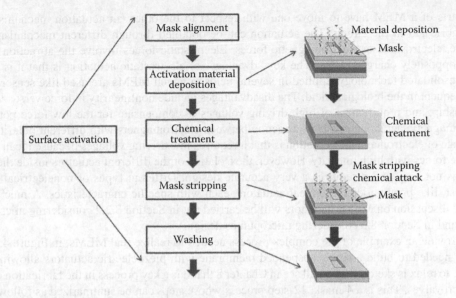

FIGURE 4.9 Details of a simplified process for the reaction chamber surface activation.

Bulk micromachining is the most mature and simple micromachining technology; it involves the removal of silicon from the bulk silicon substrate by etchants. Depending on the type of etchants that are used, etching can be isotropic, that is, oriented along one of the silicon crystal planes, or anisotropic, that is, oriented along a plane different from the crystal main planes.

Anisotropic etching is generally used to expose the silicon crystal planes in order to build non-planar structures like descendent ducts. In particular cases, these can be useful to exploit a small prevalence due to gravity without building a micro-pump or to devise three-dimensional microfluidics networks (see Section 8.4). Using bulk micromachining, the need of complex planar processes is reduced to the minimum, but only the simplest structures can be created.

Surface micromachining is a more advanced fabrication technique. It is based on the use of layers of sacrificial materials, that are destined to be etched out so to leave empty spaces between structural layers. An example is reported in Figure 4.10, shown as a sacrificial material layer is removed in order to create a suspended lever, often called a cantilever. The process is quite effective in obtaining complex structures, but it is also quite complex. The simple process sketched in Figure 4.10 requires two masks and it is only a small part of the fabrication of a practical MEMs.

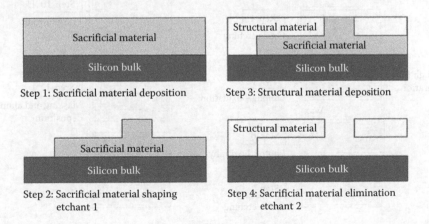

FIGURE 4.10 Schematic explanation of surface micromachining process.

If parts of a MEM have to move one with respect to the other, an actuation mechanism has to be fabricated in the circuit. The actuation can be obtained through different mechanisms, for example, electrostatic or electromagnetic forces. Electrostatic forces involve the attraction forces of two oppositely charged plates. The key advantages of electrostatic actuation is that it is a very well consolidated technology, applied in several fields in which MEMs are used like sensors, thus quite frequent in the biological field. The disadvantages include nonlinearity in force versus voltage relationship, and requirement of high driving voltages to compensate for the low force potential. Electromagnetic actuation involves attraction between electromagnets with different polarity. The advantage of electromagnetic actuation is that it requires low driving voltages because it can generate large forces with high linearity. However, the isolation of the different actuators inside the same switch is not easy and it requires a very accurate design. Different types of nonelectrical actuators exist, like pneumatic or chemical actuators, each with specific characteristics. A much more detailed discussion on MEMs actuators will be carried out in Section 8.2.2 considering microvalve design and in Section 8.3 considering micropumps design.

To provide an example of the complex process needed to realize real MEMs, in Figure 4.11 the process needed to build a single suspended membrane with piezoelectric actuators allowing it to curve or to relax is sketched. We will see in Chapter 8 that it is a key process in the fabrication of several microvalves. This is a 4-mask, 12-step process whose steps can be summarized as follows [9]:

Step 1.   p-Type wafers are cleaned.
Step 2.   Thermal oxidation to grow 200 nm oxide.
Step 3.   a. Photoresist is coated on the front surface of the samples and patterned.
          b. The back side of the wafer is coated with wax to prevent etching of back oxide.

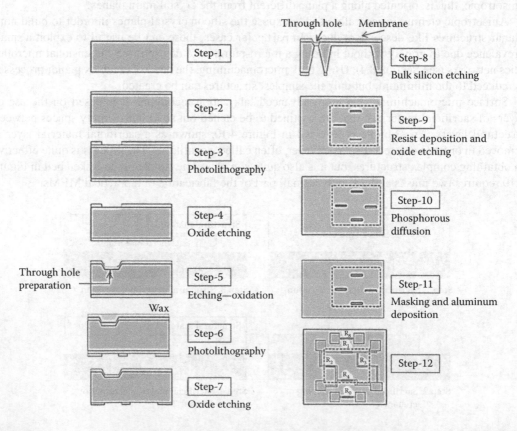

FIGURE 4.11   Possible process for the fabrication of a MEMs suspended membrane with piezoelectric actuators.

Step 4.   The front oxide is etched.
Step 5.   a. Etching of bulk silicon on the front side to obtain a 10 μm deep structure.
          b. The wafers are cleaned.
          c. The wafers are thermally oxidized to grow 1 μm oxide.
Step 6.   Photoresist is coated on the back surface of the samples and patterns are transferred with the help of alignment marks.
Step 7.   The back oxide is etched.
Step 8.   Etching of bulk silicon from back side is carried out in a two-step process.
Step 9.   Photolithography is done to transfer the patterns of piezoresistors on thermally grown oxide on the front side of the wafer. This is followed by oxide etching. The photoresist is removed followed by cleaning.
Step 10. Phosphorous diffusion is done to realize n-type piezoresistors.
Step 11. The native oxide is removed. This is followed by thermal evaporation of aluminum on the wafers to form the contacts of piezoresistors.
Step 12. The patterns for aluminum contacts are transferred through lithography and this is followed by aluminum etching. The photoresist is removed followed by cleaning. The wafers then undergo an annealing step.

4.2.2   BACK-END PROCESS FLOW

Although the front-end process is operated by very costly equipment, it works in parallel on all the chips fabricated on the same wafer. Back-end processes are almost all operated chip by chip, thus being critical under a cost point of view. Moreover, back-end processes are more influenced by the cost of materials acquired by suppliers, like the package, the cooling system, and so on. Thus, optimizing back-end processes is a key point in the case of labs on chip [12].

Even more than front-end flux, the back-end flux depends on the particular type of lab on chip we are dealing with. For example, some labs on chip are charged from the factory with reference chemical substances that are used when the chip works while others do not. When a reference substance is charged into the chip it is sometimes inserted at the wafer level during front-end processing, other times it is charged chip by chip in a back-end process [13].

A lot of the back-end process also depends on the type of adopted detection. For example, if optical detection is selected and the source and the detector are not on board of the chip, optical interfaces have to be provided, whose fabrication can be a difficult and costly back-end step [14].

Taking into account these observations, a possible back-end process flow for a lab on chip is represented in Figure 4.12 [12].

After the completion of the front-end working wafers are tested before dicing. This is a very important test whose scope is to avoid that wafers with important defects affecting the great majority of the chips are transferred to the back end causing a great number of defected chips to be worked one by one up to the first stage of back-end test.

After the test, the chips are separated in the process that is generally called dicing. Since in labs on chip wafer bonding is generally used, dicing is more critical than in standard integrated electronics processing, due to the need to not impact the superimposition between the two wafers [6].

Once separated, the dies are attached on the submount that will be the base of the final package with a process called die attach. This is needed also to allow easy handling of the single chip without the risk to damage it by scrapping the chip surface with the handling tools.

The surmount is also important for the chip thermal regulation. Depending on the requirement the surmount can be a simple base of thermal conducting material or it can be constituted, as shown in Figure 4.13, by superimposed layers of different materials to assure the required mechanical and thermal characteristics. If a cooler has to be placed below the chip to maintain a temperature control inside the package, it is placed on the surmount before die attach.

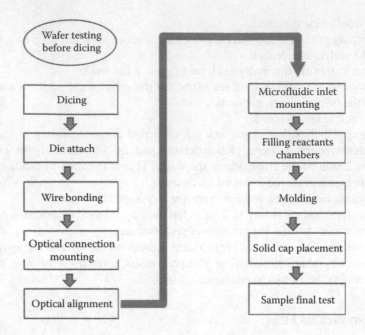

FIGURE 4.12   Possible back-end flux for a lab on chip.

After the die attach, the wires are fused on the electrical connections in order to be ready to connect the chip with the package pins during a process called wire bonding. Assuming that optical detection is used, optical interfaces have to be prepared in this phase.

In order to prepare optical interfaces, a groove has been constructed by lithography and etching in the place where the optical fiber has to interface the optical waveguide integrated in the chip (see Figure 4.14). The optical fibers that have to bring light out of the chip are inserted into the grove and aligned in order to optimize the coupling with the waveguide.

In the case of labs on chip, this operation is quite different from the same operation performed on standard integrated optics chips. On the one hand, the power budget of optical detection circuits is more favorable with respect to telecommunication-oriented optical interfaces, due to the possibility to integrate for several seconds the received signal to eliminate noise. Thus, a very small coupling loss is not needed and the so-called passive alignment is possible. This is constituted by fiber placing exploiting only the lithographic markers, without the help of real-time measurement

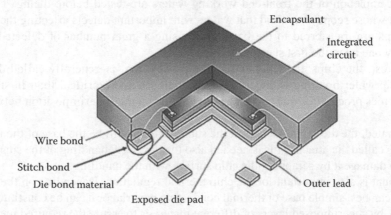

FIGURE 4.13   Example of package submount constituted by a set of superimposed layers of different materials.

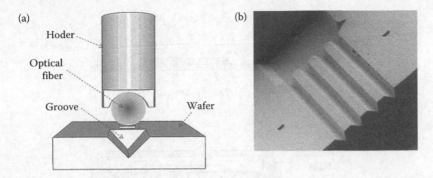

FIGURE 4.14 Passive alignment of a fiber optics in a V-groove in an integrated optics chip (a) and scanning electron microscope photo of a V-grooves array (b). ((b) Published under permission of Cyoptics Inc.)

of the coupling loss obtained injecting light in the waveguide during the coupling operation and measuring the fiber output power (active alignment).

Passive alignment can be automatized completely, thereby increasing the throughput and decreasing work cost. On the other hand, while in standard optical integrated circuits the groove is placed on the top of the wafer and no wafer bonding is adopted, in the case of labs on chip, wafer bonding oblige both to excavate a place for the fiber in both wafers and to place the fiber from the chip side. This is a much more complicated operation under a placing point of view and has an impact both on the cost and on the back-end yield. Different techniques have been devised for optical interface fabrication that are more suitable for labs on chip, as it will be discussed in some detail in Section 6.5.4; in any case, fabrication of optical interfaces remains a delicate process, to be realized with great care.

A possible alternative to the waveguide–fiber interface is to place both the laser source and the photodetectors on the chip. Depending on the cost of the two technologies and on the type of sources and detectors that are needed it can be a preferable solution or not. In this case, placing of lasers and photodiodes in suitable positions on the upper wafer are performed at the end of the front-end processing and it is a typical mixed front-end and back-end integration step.

As a matter of fact, on the one hand it is an operation performed on the whole wafer before dicing, while on the other, it involves discrete components like the photodiodes and the lasers to be integrated one by one. Due to the fact that the external chips will emerge from the surface of the upper wafer, also on the lower wafer suitable excavations have to be prepared for them.

After the preparation of the optical interfaces, fluidic interfaces have to be fabricated, by connecting suitable discrete elements to the inlets of the fluidic circuits. Since the inlets are on the lower wafer, suitable holes have to be done on the upper wafer to reach them. Selected inlets are prepared to be used during the lab on chip working, thus they have to be connected with suitable inlets prepared on the package itself to render possible liquid insertion from outside the chip when the chip is finished.

Other inlets are used only in factories to charge suitable reagents into the chip so that they have to be sealed after the charging of the reagents, a process located immediately after the fluidics inlets preparation. When all the interfaces of the chip, that is, electrical, optical, and fluidics are prepared, the chip is frequently molded. This means that the chip is immersed into a bit of specific glue or other suitable material to fix and to protect it. Molding is an important operation since the chip interfaces are not to be ruined by the molding. For this reason, when an external package is used, molding is not performed in every case.

Sometimes molding ends the back-end process: the chip is sufficiently protected by the mold and it is ready to be integrated. In other cases, the package also includes a solid upper cap that has to be placed after the molding on top of the surmount to form a case in which the chip is contained. This is naturally a much more robust solution, frequently adopted in nondisposable chips, but which

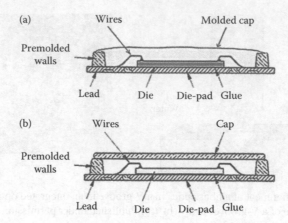

FIGURE 4.15 Purely molded (a) and solid cap closed (b) types of package.

implies higher costs both for the additional back-end step and for the additional solid cap, whose cost, even if minimal, is added to the overall cost of the chip. Purely molded and solid case package solutions are represented in Figure 4.15.

After the final test, the chip fabrication is ended and it is ready to exit from the fab.

4.2.3 PRODUCTION TESTING TECHNIQUES

4.2.3.1 On-Wafer Testing

All the testing techniques applied during front-end fabrication are called on-wafer testing due to the fact that the wafer is tested as a whole [15].

Owing to the fact that the circuits are not yet diced and the interfaces are not yet fabricated, a real functional test cannot be performed in this phase, and on wafer testing has the main scope of being eliminated as soon as possible from the production cycle. The wafer with extended defects probably will present a great number of nonfunctioning circuits. On-wafer testing results are also used to elaborate statistics on the front-end process so to monitor its overall quality and to individuate improvement areas.

Three types of on-wafer testing are generally conducted:

- Visual tests
- Optical tests
- Electrical tests

Visual tests are simply performed by looking systematically at the wafer surface with a microscope under different light conditions. Wafers containing integrated circuits of any kind has a periodical structure that under suitable light can be easily recognized, as it is evident, for example, in Figure 4.16, where the surface of the wafer containing integrated optical circuits is shown. A skilled operator, using an optical microscope can recognize nonuniform light reflection immediately; thus, identifying small defects on the wafer surface. The visual inspection station is essentially similar to a microscope whose construction is optimized for looking at a wafer surface, as shown in Figure 4.17.

When a defect is detected on a wafer surface it is generally looked at with the electron microscope to clearly define the defect characteristics and to try to individuate its cause. Systematic causes determining a recurring set of wafer defects are eliminated in this way. In many cases, the electron microscope is also used to look at samples of the production wafers to perform a better assessment of the front-end process.

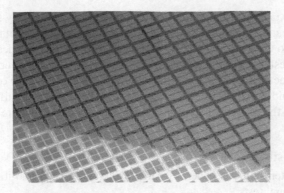

FIGURE 4.16 Photograph of the surface of a wafer evidencing the regular structure created by the periodic disposition of the chips. (Published under permission of Cyoptics Inc.)

Optical wafer tests are based on the same principle of visual tests, but for the fact that the reflected pattern generated when the wafer is lighted suitably are detected and analyzed by an optical system. This is able to detect the diffraction figure caused by monochromatic light incident on the wafer at different angles and with different frequencies and comparing them with the reference shapes obtained by a set of reference wafers.

This procedure, while more cumbersome with respect to simple visual inspection, is more effective in individuating small defects and in characterizing them. Sometimes this testing strategy is considered an integration of visual inspection used when defects are detected or on a sample basis.

Finally, electrical on-wafer tests consist of testing the electrical properties of the wafer. To execute this kind of tests specific elements are often constructed on the wafer, where point contacts are put to perform resistance or other kinds of electrical measures. These measures are then compared with the reference that is obtained from good wafers to characterize the wafer under test. Even if this is a less accurate measure with respect to the electrical one, it does not involve only the wafer surface, thus it is complementary and not alternative to it.

Electrical tests are more useful when conductive elements are present on the wafer, since if all the wafers are purely insulating, only capacity can be in case measured, thus effectiveness in case of microfluidic circuits depends on the particular circuit and on the working stage at which the measure is performed.

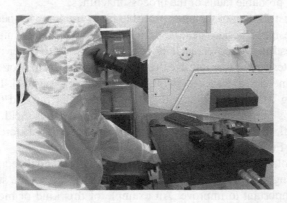

FIGURE 4.17 Visual inspection station in a front-end fab clean room. (Published under permission of Cyoptics Inc.)

On-wafer test is also performed with another technique, complementary to whole wafer testing: the test of specific test patterns built on the wafer. This is particularly useful in the case of microfluidic circuits to be able to use on-wafer testing developed for microelectronics.

Several electronics tests are meant to determine data on the layers depth or their doping through the measurements of electrical parameters linked to the conducting nature of the layer [16]. This is not the case of microfluidics, unless specific test-oriented structures are built on the wafer to allow such tests, especially in the case in which a silicon wafer is used as substrate for the construction of the microfluidics circuit.

4.2.3.2   Back-End Testing

Labs on chip testing after dicing is generally called back-end testing and it is generally composed of structure and functional tests.

Structure tests are analogue to on-wafer tests, but implemented chip by chip. They have the scope to verify, by some form of chip inspection, that the chip structure corresponds to the design, thus avoiding detectable errors in chip construction. Structure tests are generally located at the beginning of the back-end process chain, constituting a pass–fail test before entering the most costly part of the processing of the lab on chip.

While the back-end process goes ahead and the chip is more and more similar to the end product, that functional tests become needed; they are tests that assess the functionalities of the lab on chip by somehow simulating its working and looking to the result. The most complex functional test is the final test, in which the whole operation of the lab on chip is reproduced and its outcome compared with design requirements.

Functional tests are a particularly difficult part of the lab on chip fabrication due to two reasons: they are one of the most costly parts of the back-end process so that they have to be designed with great accuracy to obtain the better process quality with the smaller test effort, on the other, differently from microelectronics circuits, labs on chip are often disposable products, so that they can be used only once [17–19]. This means that many in-line and final functional tests destroy the device and they can be performed only on a small sample of the processed chips [18].

The complexity related to the back-end test is to be faced by systematic procedures: namely fault simulation [20,21] and design for testing [22,23].

4.2.3.3   Fault Simulation

To optimize testing it is important to know where defects tend to be generated and what are the most faulty steps of the fabrication process. This can be done by setting up simulators of the fabrication steps and of the labs on chip working. These simulators are mostly oriented to take into account phenomena generating malfunctioning and faults like the statistical distribution of the fabrication tolerances and the most probable faults of the process machines.

Once the type and distribution of the most probable faults are known, specific tests for the most probable fault can be designed besides generic performance tests, greatly improving the efficacy to cost ratio of back-end testing. Moreover, such modeling also allows to better individuate the placing of intermediate process tests so as to minimize the process steps performed on already failed circuits.

Suitable modeling is needed to place test points in an optimized way [24]. This procedure implies the back-end processing chain simulation with different tests placing and the comparison of the obtained results in terms of cost of the produced working chip versus yield. The outcome of such a modeling is, in general, the statistical distribution of chips suffering different types of defects, as schematically shown in Figure 4.18.

Another important role of testing modeling is to relate an observed defect to the possible causes so as to drive post-testing analysis of defected chips in order to detect the steps of the fabrication process that is more important to improve. An example of this kind of modeling is provided in Reference [24], where it was analyzed as the test of pins for the driving of droplet-based microfluidic circuits. A table of the main defects related to electrodes fabrication is reported in Table 4.1.

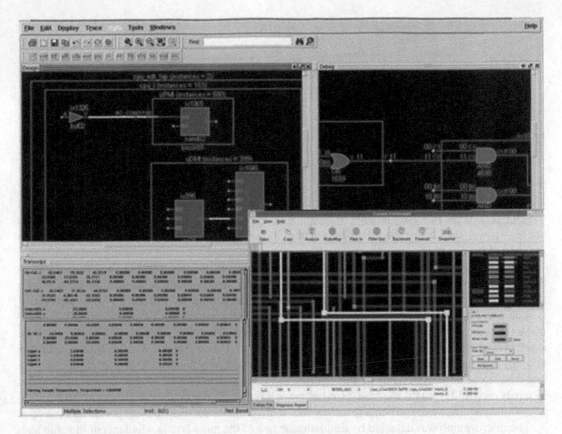

FIGURE 4.18 Screenshot from a simulation program aimed at the characterization of on chip defects at the end of the processing chain also considering the distribution of test points along the process chain. The program is developed for electronic circuits.

TABLE 4.1

Classification of the Main Defects Related to Electrode Fabrication in a Droplet-Based Microfluidics Circuit

Cause of Malfunction	Malfunction Type	Involved Cells	Fault Model	Observed Error
Electrode actuated for too long time	Irreversible charge concentration on the electrode	3	Droplet is dispensed but not separated by the reservoir	No droplet can be dispensed in the circuit
Electrode shape variation in fabrication	Electrode deformity	3	No overlap between droplet and electrode	Mixing failure
Electrode static property variation in fabrication	Unequal actuation voltage	3	Net static pressure in some direction	Unbalanced volume of split droplet
Bad soldering	Parasitic capacitance in the capacity sensing circuit	1	Oversensitive or insensitive capacity detection	False-negative or false-positive results

Source: Adapted from Chakrabarty K., *IEEE Transactions On Circuits and Systems—I: Regular Papers*, vol. 57, pp. 4–17, 2010.

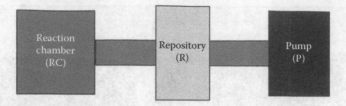

FIGURE 4.19 Scheme of the basic structure of a part of a microfluidics circuit considered in the example of Section 4.2.3.

4.2.3.4 Design for Testing

Design for testing is a design procedure that includes the design of testing procedure and includes in the chip structures that are intended to facilitate or enable specific testing techniques. This design strategy is well established for microelectronics circuits [22,23], while it is yet at research stage in the field of labs on chip.

However, the fact that several labs on chip are disposable devices, renders this approach even more necessary with respect to microelectronics, where it is considered a mandatory element of a successful circuit design. As an example, let us consider the simple part of a microfluidic circuit that is shown in Figure 4.19. The simple scope of this part of the circuit is to use a micro-pump (P) to move the solution stored in the repository (R) into a reaction chamber (RC) that, at this stage of the assay procedure is empty. The micro-pump can be operated several times without ruining its functionality, but the test solution in the repository can be moved only one time in the reaction chamber, and it has to be done at the right moment during the assay procedure. Moreover, the solution cannot be easily removed from the reaction chamber, since it is chemically reactive and a complete elimination would require washing with a specific wash solution that is not easy to incorporate into the chip.

The micro-pump was detected by simulation as one of the most critical elements of the chip and, while other elements could be tested only on a sample basis once the production process is at steady state, the micro-pump is to be tested at the beginning on every chip before releasing it and, also when the production is at its steady state, the sample test of the pump should be performed, more frequently, with respect to the complete final test.

To do that, the conceptual design represented in Figure 4.20 was adopted. A small secondary repository (SR) is created immediately after the micro-pump so as to be filled with a solution of water and a chemical neutral alcohol of about the same viscosity of the test solution (that in this

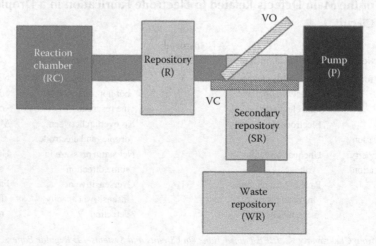

FIGURE 4.20 Scheme of the implementation of the functionality of the circuit reported in Figure 4.19, including a structure allowing nondestructive testing of the micropump.

case had a mixed alcohol–water solvent since it was needed to avoid jellification during the assay). A single opening valve VO (a valve that can be operated once starting closed and ending opened) was constructed besides a single close valve VC (a valve that can be operated once starting open and ending closed) to open and close at the right moment the access to the waste repository (WR). Just before the charging of the test solution into the repository, the neutral water–alcohol solution was charged in SR while VC is open VO closed. After that, the micro-pump testing starts: the pump is operated so that the water–alcohol solution is pushed up to WR, where a secondary testing system verifies both that no solution remains in SR after a certain time and that all the solution arrives in WR after the same time. At the end of the pump testing, VC is closed, VO opened and the chip is ready for charging the test solution in R.

This procedure is complex and requires construction of an elaborate structure (the design of Figure 4.19b is only conceptual, the real design is much more complex) only to allow the micro-pump test, but if the yield of the process essentially depends on the micro-pump yield and the valves are quite irrelevant in decreasing the yield itself, this can be needed to assure the correct industrial cost, that is attained only if a target yield is overcome.

The above example is somehow an extreme one: not always does design for testing require such an extended modification of the circuit layout, but it is quite significant of the effort that has to be put in designing, up to the very early stages of a project, the tests that will allow the production process to be correctly monitored.

Frequently, design for testing also consists of the construction on the chip of supplementary measurement devices that are used to test if different operations during the back-end process are executed correctly. For example, if during the front end it is necessary to charge an antibody solution in a reaction chamber whose floor surface has been activated to let the antibodies to be captured on this surface, after the washing needed to remove the remaining solution, verifying the effective saturation of the reaction chamber surface can be needed. This can be carried out, for example, with optical methods if the fabrication process is suitably designed.

4.2.4 In-Field Testing

Another field in which testing techniques, mainly fault simulation and design for testing, are a key for the success of a lab on chip project is the possibility of implementing operational tests.

When the chip is used, in order to assure that the performed measure is reliable, the chip has to have an internal self-test that is performed contemporary to the real measurement and has to be present, in case of a working chip, a predetermined result. If the result of the self-test is not correct, it is to be intended that the chip is not working and the result of the performed assay not reliable.

In medical and biological applications, the presence of such a self-test is mandatory to allow the assay to be accepted by local administrations so that it is a key point in the chip design and realization [25,26]. Also, in this case, since the chip is usually disposable, a suitable design for testing has to be realized, followed by the realization on the chip of test dedicated structures.

4.3   MICRO- AND NANO-FABRICATION FABS

Planar technologies require a specific manufacturing structure. In particular, all the manufacturing processes, both front end and back end, have to be executed in conditions of controlled environment and carefully planned action by the manufacturing people. This is required both to maintain a very low contamination degree, needed condition to assure an high yield process, and to assure the required security conditions in the presence of chemical and mechanical hazards. The environment in which these conditions are fulfilled is an artificially controlled site, generally called clean room, to underline the strict control of spurious elements present in the air and in all the materials here processed.

Under the point of view of the base material used for manufacturing, it is prepared in the form of standard wafers, as required by front-end processing machines. The kind of starting material that is used and the properties of the used wafers strongly influence the manufacturing process and the final industrial cost of the chips. A certain variety of possible materials exists even in microelectronics, for example, both pure silicon and SOI wafers can be used, not only of different radii, but also of different depth.

This variety is greatly enlarged in microfluidics and integrated optics wafers that are used to build labs on chip. Silicon wafers or SOI wafers can be both used as base, but also pure glass wafers are commonly adopted. Moreover, polymeric substances are frequency used in this field not only as process materials, but also for structural purposes, when they are deposed and directly polymerized on the base wafer [1,2].

4.3.1   CLEAN ROOMS

A clean room is "a room in which the concentration of airborne particles is controlled, and which is constructed and used in a manner to minimize the introduction, generation, and retention of particles and microbes inside the room and in which other relevant parameters, e.g. temperature, humidity, and pressure, are controlled as necessary" [27].

The importance of a strict control of the density of any kind of unwanted particle is clear if we consider the case in which only a total of 10^5 unwanted particles are present in a cubic meter of air. The average volume occupied by a particle due to its random motion is 10 cm^3 that we can approximate with a cube with 2.1 cm side. A standard pure Si wafer of a diameter of 8' has an equivalent area of about 0.125 m^2. Assuming to have 1500 chips on the wafer we can estimate that the number of particles that could deposit on the wafer in still air, for example, in a moment when the wafer is released on a support, is about 285.

If the probability that more than one particle hit a single chip is neglected and we assume that every chip with a particle deposited upon is ruined we have that up to 60 chips are ruined so that, this phenomenon only brings to a yield reduction from 100% to 81%. The hypothesis that every depositing particle creates a failure in a chip is not true in real clean rooms, due to the low speed at which depositing particles hit the wafer, causing a very weak link of the particle to the wafer surface and enabling an effective wafer surface cleaning. In any case, the above example is quite effective in showing the very strict requirements of clean rooms adopted for integrated circuits manufacturing. As a matter of fact, the average number of particles that are present in the air of an internal room that is kept clean with standard methods, for example, in a physician visiting room, is as high as 10^8 and 10-fold higher in normally clean external air.

4.3.1.1   Clean Room Classification

Owing to the paramount importance of controlling unwanted particles in the air, clean rooms are classified on the ground of the average number of spurious particles in the air for any given type of particle. As a matter of fact, it is intuitive that, bigger the particle, greater its energy for a constant air speed and greater the probability to damage the wafer surface.

The first universal classification of clean rooms was set-up in the United States with the different version of Federal Standard 209 [28]. From versions A to D, the clean room class number refers to the maximum number of particles of 0.5 μm size or bigger that would be allowed in 1 cubic foot of clean room air, generating a widely used way of referring to the quality of a clean room as a class N clean room. The table summarizing the clean rooms classification in standards 209A-D is reported in Table 4.2. In 1992, the standard 209 was updated to version E by introducing more classes and metric units, and also to create a table of comparison with the upcoming ISO standard for clean room classification.

Federal Standard 209E was used until the end of November 2001 to define the requirements for clean rooms. On November 29, 2001, these standards were superseded by the publication of ISO specification 14644 [27] that was de facto adopted all around the world; a summary of the clean room classes reported in ISO 14644 is reported in Table 4.3 in terms of number of unwanted particles of a

TABLE 4.2
U.S. Federal Standard 209A-D for Clean Room Classification

Clean Room	Number of Particles for Cubic Feet of Air for Particle Radius				
Class	0.1 μm	0.2 μm	0.3 μm	0.5 μm	5 μm
1	35	7	3	1	
10	350	75	30	10	
100	3500	750	300	100	
1000	1000	7			
10,000	10,000	70			
100,000	100,000	700			

Source: Adapted from U.S. General Services Administration, Federal Standard 209 A-D, 1992.

TABLE 4.3
ISO 14644-1 Clean Room Classification

Clean Room	Number of Particles for Cubic Meter of Air for Particle Radius					
Class	0.1 μm	0.2 μm	0.3 μm	0.5 μm	1 μm	5 μm
ISO 1	10	2				
ISO 2	100	24	10	4		
ISO 3	1000	237	102	35	8	
ISO 4	10,000	2370	1020	352	83	
ISO 5	100,000	23,700	10,200	3520	832	29
ISO 6	1,000,000	237,000	102,000	35,200	8320	293
ISO 7				352,000	83,200	2930
ISO 8				3,520,000	832,000	29,300
ISO 9				35,200,000	8,320,000	293,000

Source: Adapted from ISO 14644-1 Recommendation—*Cleanrooms and Associated Controlled Environments—Part 1: Classification of Air Cleanliness.*

certain dimension in a cubic meter of air. It is possible to establish a precise correspondence between the still quite diffuse language related to Standard 209 and the modern ISO classification as shown in Table 4.4 so that the ISO clean room class can be readily derived when the old 209 name is used.

4.3.1.2 Clean Room Structure and Procedures

Four basic components contribute to create and maintain the clean room controlled environment [29]:

- *Clean Room Architecture*—Materials of construction and finishes are important in establishing cleanliness levels and are important in minimizing the internal generation of contaminants from the surfaces.
- *The Heating, Ventilation, and Air Conditioning (HVAC) System*—The integrity of the clean room environment is created by the positive pressure difference between the clean room and adjacent areas and through the HVAC system. The HVAC system requirements include:
  - Supplying airflow in sufficient volume and cleanliness to support the cleanliness rating of the room.

TABLE 4.4

Correspondence between U.S. Federal Standard 209 and ISO 14644-1 Clean Room Classification

ISO	Federal Standard 209
ISO 3	1
ISO 4	10
ISO 5	100
ISO 6	1000
ISO 7	10,000
ISO 8	100,000

- Introducing air in a manner to prevent stagnant areas where particles could accumulate.
- Filtering the outside and recirculated air across high-efficiency particulate air (HEPA) filters.
- Conditioning the air to meet the clean room temperature and humidity requirements.
- Ensuring enough conditioned makeup air to maintain the specified positive pressurization.
- *Interaction Technology*—Interaction technology includes two elements:
  - The movement of materials into the area and the movement of people.
  - Maintenance and cleaning.
  Administrative instructions, procedures, and actions are necessary to be made about the logistics, operation strategies, maintenance, and cleaning.
- *Monitoring systems*—Monitoring systems is needed to continuously assess the correct clean room functioning. The variables monitored are pressure difference between the outside environment and the clean room, temperature, humidity, and, in some cases, noise and vibrations.

4.3.1.2.1   Clean Room Architecture

The clean room architecture greatly depends on the clean room class. In the case in which low class clean rooms are needed, like ISO 4 or ISO 5 rooms constructed for front-end manufacturing or even ISO 3 clean rooms where SOI wafers are fabricated, the general architecture tends simultaneously to minimize the space where the high controlled environment has to be maintained and to facilitate as far as possible both the HVAC system work and the execution of the needed internal procedures.

The most adopted architecture in this case is constituted by a shelf containing the clean rooms inserted inside the industrial building that has to be suitably prepared for that. An external view of this kind of architecture is provided in Figure 4.21. Typical height of the internal shell is 3 m, while the external roof has to be high about 8 m to host all the technical equipment needed to realize the HVAC. As a matter of fact, it is partially installed directly on top of the clean room while partially it has to be connected with the clean room rooftop with suitable pipes.

A possible internal plan of a low-class clean room is shown in Figure 4.22, where it is clear that the low-class clean areas are insulated so as to be better controlled and maintained. Moreover, the different areas can be specialized so as to be functional to the performed processes. For example, in clean room where high definition lithography equipment is located, like a submicron stepper or an electron beam lithography equipment, it is possible that a light with a controlled wavelength is needed not to interfere with the lithography process. In these cases, generally a yellow light is used. The bay architecture allows the yellow light to be used only in the bay where the sensitive equipment is located, without affecting the other areas of the clean room where it is not needed.

Where higher class clean rooms are needed, like ISO 8 or ISO 9 clean rooms, the bay architecture is less used and more commonly the clean room is a sort of open space where the machinery and

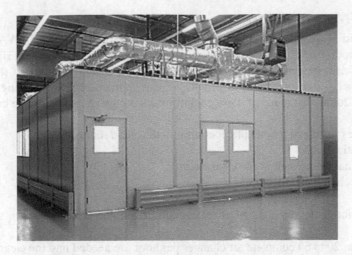

FIGURE 4.21 Plan of a modular clean room: clean areas (class ISO 4 and ISO 5) are located inside the structure as bays, the process and the exit corridors are class ISO 6 while interface areas like the in/out structure are class ISO 7. Air showers and other personal cleaning facilities are located in the in/out areas. (Published under permission of Cyoptics Inc.)

the test benches are located so as to allow the best possible circulation of materials and operators.

As far as the clean room floor is considered, it is always realized via a floating floor allowing the air flux to pass through so that the air, after entering from the ceiling and traversing the clean area is collected below the floor and sent back again to the HVAC system. When equipments that are greatly sensitive to vibrations are installed, it could be needed to build a specific support for the equipment providing vibration filtering. This is realized with alternating rigid and elastic layers of material so as to obtain the wanted mechanical filtering response.

Also, the materials that are used to build the structural parts of clean rooms (walls, floor, and roofs) have to be selected suitably. They have not to generate pollution, so that standard walls using paint are generally excluded.

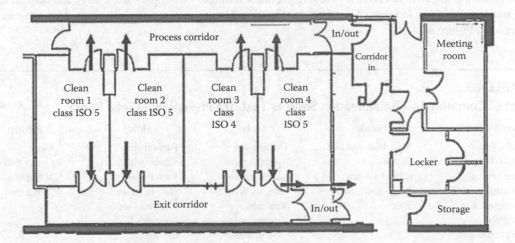

FIGURE 4.22 Plan of a modular clean room: areas in darker gray are clean areas (class ISO 4 and ISO 5—the clean rooms, class ISO 5—the corridors), light gray areas are transit and preparation areas (class ISO 6), white areas are interface areas (class ISO 7). Air showers and other personal cleaning facilities are located in the in/out areas.

4.3.1.2.2 The HVAC System

Owing to the need of maintaining a very high standard of air cleanness, the HVASC system of a low-class clean room is a very complex system collecting several equipment [30,31].

Spurious particles are generated in the clean room from several sources so that the airborne contamination level of a clean room is largely dependent on the particle-generating activities in the room. It has been found that many of these contaminants are generated from five basic sources:

1. The facilities itself and the people operating in the clean room
2. The fabrication tools
3. The fluids that are present in the clear room
4. The product being manufactured

A list of the more common sources of air contamination due to these elements is presented in Table 4.5.

Generally, from 20 to 60 complete air changes per hour are needed into the clean room, arriving at a requirement of 600 air changes per hour in ISO 4 and ISO 3 clean rooms. For comparison, in a normal air-conditioned environment, where a general comfort level has to be maintained through cleanness, humidity, and temperature control, only about five air changes per hour are needed.

The high-efficiency air cleaning needed in a clean room is attained by using of HEPA filters, specialized to filter different kinds of particles that purify the air that is injected into the clean room. These filters are generally placed on the clean room ceiling and in low-class clean rooms they fill almost all the ceiling area. The air flux inside the clean room has to be maintained as laminar as possible by an accurate design of the HVACS system, since vortices tend to spread randomly unwanted particles and render air cleaning very difficult near the vortex center.

Moreover, the air pressure into the clean room is maintained a bit higher with respect to the external air pressure, so as to favor particle removal from the clean room by pushing them toward the floor where the air is removed and transported out of the controlled environment, as shown in Figure 4.23. The air is maintained as laminar into the bay by a combination of a controlled air injection from ceiling and a system of air extraction from the floor. Frequently, this system is based on a vacuum pump placed directly under the ceiling collecting air extracted from the floor and used to maintain a constant pressure difference between the clean room internal volume and the space above the ceiling so as to increase pressure prevalence in the bottom part of the bays and contribute to maintain the flux laminar. A scheme of this arrangement in a set of clean room bays is represented in Figure 4.24.

TABLE 4.5

List of Common Air Contamination Sources That Are Present in a Clean Room

Facilities	People	Tools	Fluids	Product
Walls, floors, and ceilings	Skin flakes and oil	Friction and wear particles	Particulates floating in air	Chips
Paint and coatings	Spittle	Lubricants and emissions	Bacteria, organics, and moisture	Quartz flakes
Construction material	Clothing debris (lint, fibers, etc.)	Vibrations	Floor finishes or coatings	Aluminum particles
Air conditioning debris	Hair	Brooms, mops, and dusters	Cleaning chemicals	
Room air and vapors			Plasticizers (out-gases)	
Spills and leaks			Deionized water	

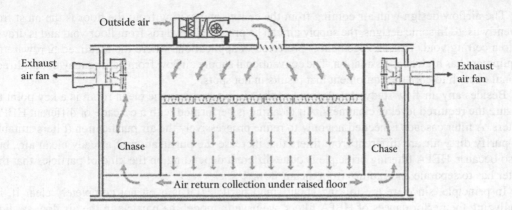

FIGURE 4.23   Laminar air flow in a clean room bay.

In the scheme of Figure 4.24, the low-class bays have 100% HEPA ceiling coverage. The make-up air handler (MAH) is a fresh air unit that provides the room pressurization and is designed for latent and sensible load of outside air. This unit feeds on two recirculation air handlers (RAH) that supply air into the clean room. The RAH are usually designed primarily to manage the sensible heat load generated indoors from the process equipment and occupancy.

Laminar airflow tends to become turbulent when it encounters obstacles such as people, process equipment, and workbenches. Placing these obstructions in a manner that prevents dead air spaces from developing will minimize turbulence. Use of workstations with perforated tabletops will allow the air to pass through them uninterrupted. Equipment shall also be raised on a platform (plinth) where possible to allow free air flows beneath it.

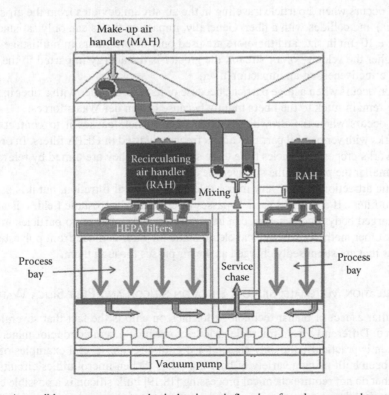

FIGURE 4.24   A possible arrangement to obtain laminar air flow in a few clean rooms bays.

The airflow design with air coming from the ceiling and exiting from the floor is the most frequently used. In some designs, the supply air can be projected upwards from floor void and is drawn into a ceiling void. This arrangement is preferred in applications where the localized hardware or equipment has high heat dissipation. The conventional supply airflow from ceiling may not be directional enough to cool the equipment that results in hot spots.

Besides any air flow study, the cleaning of the air injected into the clean room is a key point to assure the required level of cleanness. Air cleaning is performed with a cascade of different HEPA filters. A filter cascade is needed not only to refine progressively the air purification (filters suitable to purify dirty air are different from filters that increase the purification of already clean air), but also because HEPA filtering principle is quite different depending on the kind of particles that the filter has to separate and capture from the air flow.

In principle, since we are talking about small particles, it is even not completely clear if, in analyzing the performances of HEPA filters, we have to model the particle in the air flow as slide objects floating in a moving fluid or as a very diluted solution of many solutes in a gaseous solvent. The more suitable model to represent the phenomena happening during air purification and injection into the clean room critically depends on the average radius of the suspended particles. In the most common applications, a floating solid model is applied above a radius of 0.01 µm and a diluted solution below this radius. Filtration of particles relies on four main principles:

- Inertial impaction
- Interception
- Diffusion
- Electrostatic attraction

The first three of these mechanisms are mainly used in mechanical filters and are influenced by particle size.

Impaction occurs when a particle traveling in the air stream deviates from the air stream (due to particle inertia) and collides with a fiber. Generally, impaction filters can only satisfactorily collect particles above 10 µm in size and therefore are used only as pre-filters in multistage filtration systems. The higher the velocity of air stream, the greater is the energy imparted to the particles and greater is the effectiveness of an impaction filter.

Interception occurs when a large particle, because of its size, collides with a fiber in the filter. The particles then remain stuck to the fibers mainly because of van der Waals forces.

Diffusion occurs when the Brownian motion of a particle causes it to contact a filter fiber. Diffusion works with very small particles and is frequently used in HEPA filters. In order that a diffusion filter works properly, particles have to be so small that they are aimed by relevant Brownian motion: the smaller the particle, the stronger the effect.

Electrostatic attraction plays a very minor role in mechanical filtration, but it is used in specifically designed filters. If a charged particle passes through an electrostatic field, it is attracted to an oppositely charged body. Such charges can be generated and imparted to particles in an airstream by attrition or other methods. The typical electrostatic air filter is made from polyester or polypropylene strands that are supposedly charged as the air passes through them.

4.3.2 Fabrication Materials: Silicon, Silica on Silicon and Pure Silica Wafers

Another peculiar aspect of planar technology for labs on chip is the fact that several base materials can be used. Differently from microelectronics, for which a semiconductor material is mandatory and silicon is practically the only choice for digital circuits, several examples of microfluidic circuits have been built using a variety of base materials. When microfluidics circuits are used for applications that do not require chemical processing [18,19] bulk silicon is a possible choice. In this case, all the consolidated processes developed on this material for microelectronics can be used.

Moreover, wafer bonding is easier when it is performed to join crystal surfaces cut along the same crystal plane, due to the natural tendency of crystals to reproduce the crystal structure as possible to decrease the overall system energy.

When chemical processing is needed, generally pure crystal silicon cannot be adopted, due to its tendency to react with biological molecules and polymers and to absorb several organic structures. However, pure silicon when exposed to oxygen, also by a simple exposure to air, generates a thin surface silica layer. This layer is generally sufficient to passivize the surface under a chemical point of view so that silicon labs on chip can be realized simply allowing spontaneous silicon passivation.

An alternative choice for the chip base material is pure silica, which is one of the most inert materials when dealing with organic components and has very good mechanical properties. Silica can also be manufactured with well consolidated processes and it is also a common platform for integrated optics. Thick silica layers in excess of 10 µm can be grown on standard silicon wafers using different deposition techniques (see Sections 4.8) or whole silica wafers can be manufactured, thus providing a wide variety of alternatives.

The choice of the base material influences not only the fabrication processes and the industrial cost of the final product, but also the integration degree that can be attained in the final chip. At least in principle, using silica on silicon, microelectronics, microfluidics, and optics can be integrated together. Such a perspective is extremely interesting considering the possibility to integrate on a single chip a wide range of functionalities, thereby increasing more and more the advantage of planar processing. Developing such an ambitious technology presents, however, the great challenge of integrating all the processes needed to realize the different kinds of devices in a complete process flow. The use of pure glass wafers excludes the possibility of realizing electronics circuitry, but maintains the possibility to integrate microfluidics with optics.

4.3.2.1 Standard Silicon Wafers

Silicon wafers are produced in a wide variety and in huge volumes, thus they are a cheap substrate, even if the fabrication of a perfect silicon single-crystal wafer is a complex industrial process.

The standards for dimensions of silicon wafers, and mechanical and electrical characteristics are released by Semiconductor Equipment and Materials International (SEMI) [32], which is the collective organization of the microelectronics companies. The main SEMI standards for silicon wafers are listed in Reference [33]. Silicon wafers are available in a variety of sizes from 25.4 mm (1 in.) to 300 mm (11.8 in.).

The main standard diameters and relative thicknesses of crystal silicon wafers are listed below

- 1-in. (25 mm)
- 2-in. (51 mm); thickness 275 µm
- 3-in. (76 mm); thickness 375 µm
- 4-in. (100 mm); thickness 525 µm
- 5-in. (130 mm) or 125 mm (4.9 in.); thickness 625 µm
- 150 mm (5.9 in., usually referred to as "6 inch"); thickness 675 µm
- 200 mm (7.9 in., usually referred to as "8 inch"); thickness 725 µm
- 300 mm (11.8 in., usually referred to as "12 inch"); thickness 775 µm

A photograph of three 200 mm wafers is reproduced in Figure 4.25a, where the superficial structure of the wafers, incorporating different types of optical and electronics integrated circuits, is put in evidence.

The current state-of-the-art microelectronic fab is able to manufacture 300 mm wafers (commonly called 12 in. wafers), with the next standard projected to be 450 mm (18 in.). Even if there is formally an agreement to push the adoption of 450 mm wafers, there is a great resistance in the industry to afford the great research and development needed to reach this target in a short time, demonstrated by the fact that the original date stated for the first fab using 450 mm wafer was half

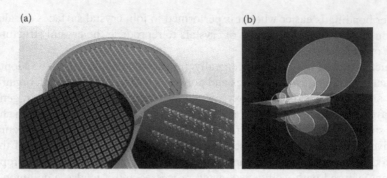

FIGURE 4.25 A photograph of three 200 mm wafers where the superficial structure of the wafers, incorporating different types of optical and electronics integrated circuits, is put in evidence (a) and comparison between 76, 100, 130, 150, and 200 mm wafers (b). ([a] Published under permission of Cyoptics Inc.)

2012, while in reality at that date this target seems quite far. In fact, moving to 300 mm wafers was a difficult operation even for the fabrication of very large volume ICs like RAMs and EPROMs, probably more difficult with respect to forecasts, and it happens during a hard industry crisis period. The general opinion is that recovering the investment that was done to transit to 300 mm is still far in time and in these conditions there is no means to plan another extremely costly transition.

The situation is completely different in the field of labs on chip. Labs on chip production has not yet arrived to the volume characteristics of microelectronics ICs and there is no reason pushing to set up an expensive fabrication structure as a 300 mm fab. Wafers with 200 or 150 mm diameter generally over-satisfy the needs of labs on chip production and research is frequently performed using smaller wafers.

Wafers grown using semiconductor materials other than silicon are also used for high-speed analog electronics [34,35] and active optical devices (like lasers or semiconductor amplifiers) [5] and they have different thicknesses than a silicon wafer of the same diameter. Wafer thickness is determined by the mechanical strength of the used material; the wafer must be thick enough to support its own weight without cracking during handling.

But for the case of silica, wafers are grown from crystals, mainly silicon having a diamond cubic structure with a lattice spacing of 5.43 Å [36]. To maintain a regular crystal structure of the wafer material, the wafer surface has to be aligned in one of the main crystallographic planes (see Figure 4.26). Orientation is important in electronics since crystal's structural and electronic properties are highly anisotropic.

Moreover, several processes are also influenced by the crystal orientation. For example, ion implantation depths depend on the wafer's crystal orientation, since each direction offers distinct paths for transport [37]. Wafers under 200 mm diameter have flats cut into one or more sides indicating the crystallographic planes of the wafer. In earlier-generation wafers a pair of flats at different angles additionally coded the doping type (see Figure 4.27). Wafers of 200 mm diameter and above use a single small notch to convey wafer orientation, with no visual indication of doping type.

Silicon wafers are generally not pure silicon, but are instead formed with an initial impurity doping concentration between 10^{13} and 10^{16} per cm^3 of boron, phosphorus, arsenic, or antimony which is added to the melt and defines the wafer as either bulk n-type or p-type [3]. However, compared with single-crystal silicon's atomic density of 5×10^{22} atoms per cm^3, this still gives a purity greater than 99.9999%. The wafers can also be initially provided with some interstitial oxygen concentration.

A last comment is needed regarding SOI wafers. In the most advanced microelectronics applications, in order to further improve the insulation of the superficial silicon film from the bulk wafer so decreasing spurious capacities in CMOS and bipolar transistors, silicon on insulator (SOI) wafers are used [38]. SOI wafers are constructed by dividing the superficial silicon layer where the electronics circuits have to be fabricated by the bulk silicon with an insulator layer, silica generally, or sapphire

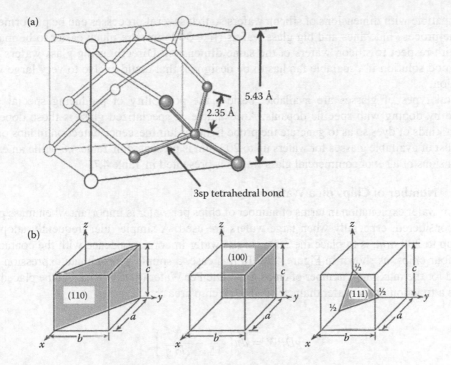

FIGURE 4.26 Silicon crystal elementary cell (a) and main crystal planes (b).

in high frequency and radiation-sensitive applications. SOI wafers however, up to now, find no application in the lab on chip field. Thus, we will not deal with this sort of wafer in more detail.

4.3.2.2 Glass Wafers

Several applications besides biotechnologies exploit wafers, thus the production of glass wafers is quite diffused and also if an official standard does not exist the production of such wafer reaches sufficient volumes to be suitable for mass production [39]. Dimensions of silica wafers

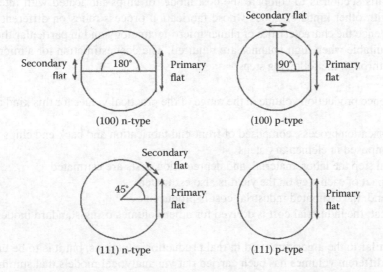

FIGURE 4.27 Standard placing of primary and secondary flats in wafers with a diameter smaller than 200 mm.

are compatible with dimensions of silicon wafers so that several processes can be performed with the same process machines and big glass wafers (like 300 mm) are much easier to be manufactured with respect to silicon wafers of the same dimension. Directly using glass wafers can be thus a good solution if a scalable fab has to be designed, that could evolve to very large volume production.

Several types of glasses are available, besides the possibility of producing special glasses obtained by doping with specific dopants. An example of specialized glass is those doped with different kinds of dyes so as to generate the probe light for luminescence detection in labs on chips [40]. A list of available glasses for wafers up to 200 mm is presented in Table 4.6 while an example of dimensions of a set of commercial glass wafers is presented in Table 4.7.

4.3.2.3 Number of Chips on a Wafer

Optimum wafer exploitation in terms of number of chips per wafer is important when mass production is considered, especially when large wafers are used. A simple rule, frequently adopted for wafers up to 200 mm, is to place the center of the wafer in correspondence with the contact point among four chips, as shown in Figure 4.28. In this case, a simple approximate expression can be obtained for the maximum number of chips gross Die Per Wafer (gDPW) that can be placed on the wafer as a function of the wafer diameter d and the chip area S:

$$gDPW = d\pi\left(\frac{d}{4S} - \frac{1}{\sqrt{2S}}\right) \tag{4.1}$$

In practice, the number of chips per wafer is smaller than gDPW due to the presence of the wafer of test sites and alignment markers that are needed both for mask aligners and for wafer bonding. This simple chip-placing rule, however, does not reflect a rigorous optimum chip-placing strategy. While the wafer dimension increases, the optimum placing becomes greatly important and several mathematical algorithms have been developed to attain this task [40,41].

4.4 PLANAR TECHNOLOGY COST MODEL

The goal of this section is to compare the cost model of chips fabricated with integrated planar technology with other kinds of goods whose fabrication process relies on different technologies. This will evidence the characteristics of planar micro-technology and in particular the fact that it is particularly suitable when high volumes are required. The cost estimation for a microfluidics chip is performed through the following steps:

- A reference production volume in the range of the practical values for this kind of products is fixed
- The fabrication process, composed of front-end fabrication and back-end chips processing is decomposed in elementary steps
- For each step the labor, material, and depreciation costs are estimated
- The impact of each step on the yield is also estimated
- At the end, the estimated industrial cost is produced
- After that, the industrial cost is derived for other volumes using standard models

This is similar to the algorithm used in real production situations, but it is to be underlined that expansion to different volumes has been carried out via analytical models that summarize average trends, completely neglecting effects due to negotiation or market fast fluctuations that are relevant in practical situations. Moreover, even if the reported estimates rely on the great experience that

TABLE 4.6

List of Different Kinds of Glasses Available to Be Manufactured in Glass Wafers with Characteristics and Potential Applications

	Density (g/cm³)	Thermal Expansion (1/°C)	Strain Point (°C)	Annealing Range (°C)	Softening Point (°C)	Refraction 435 nm	Index 635 nm	Dielectric Constant	Acid/Alkali Resistance
Soda lime (mirrors, microslides)	2.44	8.6×10^{-6}	490	480–575	575	1.523	1.513	7.75	–
Pyrex (filters, lenses)	2.23	32.5×10^{-7}	510	560	821	1468	1475	–	Class1/Class2
Alkaline earth aluminosilicate (flat panel displays)	2.54	37.6×10^{-7}	666	721	975	1.5290	1.5160	5.7	–
Lithium potash borosilicate (electrical applications)	2.13	32×10^{-7}	456	496	–	1.469 (589.3 nm)		4.0	Class2/_
Borosilicate (touch panel, LCD, electroluminescence)	2.51	8.6×10^{-6}	529	557	736	1.5230 (588 nm)		6.7	–

TABLE 4.7

Example of Parameters for a Set of Commercially Available Glass Wafers

Geometry (mm)	Geometry (")	Flats	Dimension First Flat	Dimension Second Flat
50.8 mm × 0.127 mm – 6.35 mm thick	2" × 0.005"–0.250" thick	With/without	0.625"	–
76.2 mm × 0.127 mm – 6.35 mm thick	3" × 0.005"–0.250" thick	With/without	0.875"	–
100 mm × 0.127 mm – 6.35 mm thick	3.937" × 0.005" – 0.250" thick	With/without	1.280"	–
100 mm × 0.127 mm – 6.35 mm thick	3.937" × 0.005" – 0.250" thick	1 flat	1.780"	–
125 mm × 0.127 mm – 6.35 mm thick	4.921" × 0.005" – 0.250" thick	With/without	1.670"	–
125 mm × 0.127 mm – 6.35 mm thick	4.921" × 0.005" – 0.250" thick	2 flats	1.670"	2.50"
150 mm × 0.127 mm – 6.35 mm thick	5.906" × 0.005" – 0.250" thick	1 flat	2.640"	–
200 mm × 0.127 mm – 6.35 mm thick	7.874" × 0.005" – 0.250" thick	Notch/no notch	N/A	–
300 mm × 0.127 mm – 6.35 mm thick	11.811" × 0.005" – 0.250" thick	Notch/no notch	N/A	–

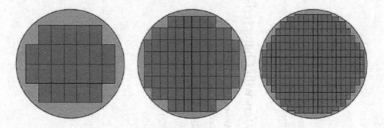

FIGURE 4.28 Placing of integrated circuits of different dimension on a silicon wafer with a simple rule: the center of the wafer coincides with an angle among four chips.

matured in microelectronics and integrated optics industry, the yield data have to be considered to be only indications of what would happen in a real production line.

4.4.1 INDUSTRIAL COST MODELS

In this section, we introduce the general cost models we will refer to in the rest of this section. We will introduce the models intuitively explaining their foundations. The interested reader can find a much detailed discussion in specialized publications [42–44].

4.4.1.1 General Expression of the Cost of Produced Goods

The main elements to consider modeling the cost of produced goods are the following:

- Cost of subparts that are acquired by suppliers to be mounted into the product. This is generally called bill of material (BOM) cost.
- Cost of work, both variable and structural.
- Production infrastructure depreciation.
- Fixed operating costs (e.g., maintenance and repair of production lines).

The different terms depend differently on the number of produced object (generally called production volume) and on how this volume increases with time.

Here, we call *volume* the number of produced items, both working and not working, so that the number of produced working items is the product between the volume and the yield. In literature, sometimes, the number of produced working items is called volume, and the total number of fabricated items is obtained by dividing the *volume* by the yield [3].

To determine the BOM cost, consider that a single product component has a unitary price that depends on the volume. At low volumes (where how much is low depends on the considered market), the cost strongly depends on the volume decreasing with it up to a critical volume; beyond the critical volume the cost stabilizes around a constant value. The asymptotic value is simply given by the bare high volumes' industrial cost of the component plus the suppliers' minimum survivability margin. A mathematical representation that can be adopted for the dependence of the BOM cost on the volume in a multi-supplier market is

$$C_{BOM} = \frac{C_\infty (V/V_0)^\alpha + C_0}{1 + (V/V_0)^\alpha} \tag{4.2}$$

where C_{BOM} is the BOM cost, V the produced volume, C_0 is the samples cost, C_∞ the asymptotic cost, V_0 the threshold volume, and α a parameter depending on a particular type of product.

The labor cost, different from the BOM, at the first order does not depend on V, but for a small part related to the service functions that have to be present in the factory (repair squads for example). Thus, in a first approximation labor cost marginally depends on volumes and it can be written as

$$C_{Labor} = C_{L0} + \frac{C_{L1}}{V} \quad \text{with } C_{L0} \gg C_{L1} \tag{4.3}$$

The last term, composed of infrastructure depreciation and all the maintenance and operational fixed costs, does not depend per se from the production volume, but it is a characteristic of the production infrastructure (the factory, the headquarter, and so on). Thus, when this cost is distributed among the produced items it contributes to the industrial cost of each individual item with a term inversely proportional to the volume as

$$C_{Dep} = \frac{C_{D0}}{V} \tag{4.4}$$

Equation 4.4 assumes that the factory is never saturated by the production volume: if factory saturation is considered, the model has to be changed to introduce the need or removing saturation bottlenecks via progressive investment in fabrication equipment. This is not a case relevant for our discussion, but it can be very important to analyze the overall performance of a realistic production structure.

Summarizing the industrial cost C_{ToT} of an item coming out from mass production is the sum of three terms, C_{BOM}, C_{Labor}, C_{Dep}, and each of these terms has a characteristic dependence on the produced volume.

4.4.1.2 Different Cost Models
Depending on the production process, different products have a different mix among the term constituting the industrial cost, so generating different cost models.

Example from different markets are provided in Table 4.8, where the reported figures have to be considered as general indications, since they can fluctuate also sensibly depending on the geographic area and on the specific company. From the table it is clear that in the first two considered industries costs are dominated by the materials (they are BOM driven), in the third case the industrial cost is dominated by the cost of labor (it is labor driven), and in the fourth case, the most typical case of very high volume planar chip industry, it is dominated by depreciation and fixed costs (it is depreciation driven). As a matter of fact, a modern 200 mm foundry costs about \$100–200 million, and a microelectronic factory based on 32 nm technology and on 12′ wafers requires an investment greater than \$1 billion.

TABLE 4.8

Example of Product Having Different Cost Models

		Cost Terms at Saturated Plant		
	Volumes (One Plant)	Labor Cost (%)	BOM–Materials Cost (%)	Depreciation and Fixed Costs (%)
Structural products manufacturing (plates and bars)	600,000 pieces	22	63 ($\alpha \approx 1$)	15
Optical access interface at 1.2 Gbit/s	2 million pieces	33	50 ($\alpha \approx 1.5$)	17
Clothes industry (far east)	1.3 million pieces	54	31 ($\alpha \approx 0.5$)	15
RAM memory chip	1 billion pieces	5	6	89

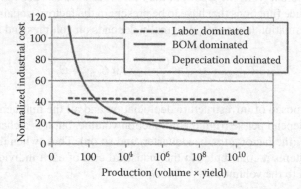

FIGURE 4.29 Industrial cost versus volumes for products having different cost models.

The dependence of the industrial cost on volumes is shown in Figure 4.29, for the different types of cost models we have introduced. In particular, planar integrated chips have a very high industrial cost for low volumes due to the great initial investment, but it scales much better than other technologies at the increase of the produced volume, up to allow the production of very high volumes with small prices. This is clear from the figure, even if the parameters have been changed a bit with respect to reality to be able to draw a clear plot (in the case of microelectronic the curve is much more steep, almost vertical in the scale of the graphic).

4.4.2 INDUSTRIAL COST ESTIMATION FOR MICROFLUIDIC-BASED LABS ON CHIP

To achieve a real cost estimation, in principle, we should exactly define the product we are dealing with. However, what we want to achieve here is not an impossible series of exact numbers, but a trend indication and in order to do that we will perform a set of hypothesis with the aim on one hand to simplify the evaluation, on the other, to maintain main trends by neglecting all the details that are specific of the single product and do not impact the general trend.

4.4.2.1 Industrial Cost Parameters

The lab on chip we are considering is a combination of two technologies: a detection technology (e.g., integrated optics if we perform optical detection) and microfluidics. Assuming for simplicity interferometry optical detection [4] the typical scale of both the technologies is the micron. As we will see in the next sections, in order to maintain the required definition at this kind of dimensions there is no need of critical technologies, but standard and well-experimented processes and machines can be used. On the other hand, complexity is introduced in the process by the need of integrating two different technologies and by the integration of specific technology steps, like wafer bonding, in the production flow.

The cost of the final product, a packaged chip ready to be integrated in a more complex system, is provided by the following equation:

$$C_{component} = \frac{C_{fixed}}{V_{produced}} + (BOM_{package} + W_{package} + C_{package}) + M_{operating}$$

$$+ \frac{2}{Y_{ield} N_{perwafer}} (C_{Wafer} + C_{wafer\,process} + W_{wafer\,fab}) + \frac{C_{Test}}{N_{cam}} \qquad (4.5)$$

where
- The fixed structure costs (administration, direction, R&D, and so on) divided for the volume is represented by the term $(C_{fixed}/V_{produced})$
- The cost of the back-end part of the fabrication, once eliminated the depreciation contribution, is constituted by the sum of three terms
  - The bill of materials $(BOM_{package})$ that takes into account all the elements that are acquired by external suppliers like the package itself, a heater where it is needed, and so on
  - The work cost $(W_{package})$ that is generally important in the packaging operations due to the fact that all the processes are executed chip by chip
  - The other variable costs (like the cost of technical gases and services) are represented by $C_{package}$
- The part of the cost due to the management of the production line that depends on the volume (like visual inspection of the produced wafers, in-line tests, and so on) are represented with $M_{operating}$
- The number of produced chips per wafer $(N_{perwafer})$ and the average wafer yield (Y_{ield}) are two important elements to evaluate the chip cost, since due to its nature the cost of the front-end fabrication depends on the number of wafer; thereby being lower and increasing the number of chips on a wafer and the yield
- The industrial cost of a wafer at the end of the front-end production line is made by three components:
  - A cost of the wafer itself (C_{Wafer}); here factor 2 reminds us to take into account the wafer bonding process
  - The cost of work and materials needed in the fabrication process $(C_{wafer\,process})$
  - And the impact of the facility depreciation $(W_{wafer\,fab})$
- The cost of the final test is indicated with C_{Test} and, if the final test is done on a reduced number of produced chip, this can be taken into account by assigning to N_{cam} a value greater than 1

Using what we have derived in the previous section regarding the expression of different cost terms, the cost of a chip can be rewritten starting from Equation 4.5 detailing the dependence of each term on the volume V as

$$C_{component} = \frac{C_{fixed}}{V_{produced}} + (BOM_{package} + W_{package} + C_{package}) + M_{operating} + \frac{C_{Test}}{N_{cam}}$$

$$+ \frac{2}{Y_{ield} N_{perwafer}} \left[\left(C_{W1\infty} + \frac{C_{W10}}{1 + N/N_0} + \frac{C_{w1lav}}{N/N_{0p}} \right) + \left(C_{W2\infty} + \frac{C_{W20}}{1 + N/N_0} + \frac{C_{w2lav}}{N/N_{0p}} \right) + \frac{C_{wbond}}{N/N_{0p}} \right] \qquad (4.6)$$

The meaning and the assumed value for all the parameters in Equation 4.5 and reasonable values deduced from a detailed process analysis on a certain number of different labs on chip using interferometry optical detection are reported in Table 4.9. The used material is assumed to be silica passivized silicon so that standard 200 mm silicon wafers are used as a starting point.

Moreover, in this example, we have assumed a relatively small chip considering a lab on chip, a chip that is only 1.0×1.0 cm. Working with wafers with a radius of 200 mm about 270 chips per wafer are usually fabricated. Scaling the cost with the chip dimension is in any case easy, taking into account the different situations that are the dominant cost factors. Using the parameter values reported in Table 4.9 it is possible to evaluate the chip cost dependence on selected parameters, the volume and the yield being perhaps the most important.

The details of the various cost contributions are reported in Figure 4.30. The first element clearly emerging from the figure is that, due to the different decreasing rate when volume increases, above a volume of about 900,000 good pieces, the dominant cost term is the back-end BOM, remaining from this volume on a level a bit below 1 in the adopted relative units. Below this threshold volume, the chip cost dominates, with a very important contribution of the back-end line depreciation.

The estimate of the final industrial cost is shown in Figure 4.31 for different areas of the lab on chip. In the example of the chip we have considered up to now, industrial cost is below 2.0

TABLE 4.9
Definition and Values of the Parameters Used in the Example of Cost Evaluation for a Microfluidics Biosensor

d	Chip side (the chip is assumed squared)	1.0 cm
$N_{potchipp}$	Wafer area divided chip area	315
$N_{perwafer}$	Number of chips per wafer (bad and good)	270
V_{ref}	Reference volume for the cost first calculation	1,000,000 chips
N	Number of wafer per year (8′ silicon wafers)	3700
$BOM_{package}$	Back-end BOM cost (at reference volume)	AU 1.3
$W_{package}$	Work cost per chip of the back-end process	AU 0.3
$C_{package}$	Other variable cost of the back-end per chip	AU 0.1
$M_{operating}$	Variable part of the production line management (cost per chip)	AU 0.1
C_{fixed}	Back-end fixed costs	AU 3,000,000
N_0	Threshold wafer number for suppliers	1000
N_{0p}	Threshold wafer number for depreciation scaling	100
N_{cam}	Final test period	500
M_{fab}	Fab margin on chips	60%
Y_{ield}	Yield (on the chip only, high volumes production)	80%
$C_{W1\infty}$	Wafer 1: wafer cost for infinite volume	AU 30
C_{W10}	Wafer 1: fluctuation of the wafer cost with volumes	AU 40
$C_{W2\infty}$	Wafer 2: wafer cost for infinite volume	AU 60
C_{W20}	Wafer 2: fluctuation of the wafer cost with volumes	AU 40
C_{w1lav}	Wafer 1: impact of fixed costs and depreciation	AU 1130
C_{w2lav}	Wafer 2: impact of fixed costs and depreciation	AU 2450
C_{wbond}	Cost of the bonded wafer minus cost of the two wafer components	AU 200
C_{Test}	Cost of an end-line chip test	AU 10

Note: AU indicates an arbitrary unit of measure for unit costs that is almost of the order of magnitude of a U.S. dollar or of an EU euro. This is used instead of a true monetary value to report results in terms of relative costs and values that are independent from economic conditions, change ratios, and the like.

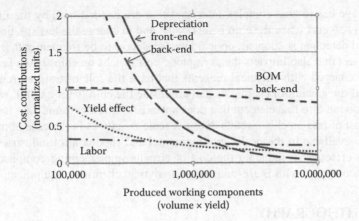

FIGURE 4.30 Industrial cost of the microfluidic circuit considered in the example in the text decomposed in the various cost contributions for different numbers of correctly working produced chips (volume × yield).

(in relative units) for a volume greater than 10 million pieces and below 1.5 above about 33 million pieces. The decrease rate is quite fast at the beginning, when the depreciation is important, and slow down for very large volumes where the cost is dominated by the BOM. By increasing the area the cost increases almost proportionally to the chip area in the region where depreciation dominates, while experiences a much smaller increase in the BOM-dominated region. The most important factor however is that, increasing the area, the threshold dividing the depreciation and the BOM-dominated regions moves toward upper volumes, thus it is more and more difficult to reach.

The industrial cost is also compared with an electronic IC built with the processes of a high-density RAM considering also in this case a 200 mm fab. The RAM has a lower cost even with respect to smaller labs on chip while it also decreases more with volumes, tending at a far lower limit. The first phenomenon is a combination of several elements: the use of two wafers due to wafer bonding, a greater variety of used processes and a less stabilized fabrication procedure causing a lower yield.

As far as the second phenomenon is concerned, it is a very important characteristic of labs on chip, where the back-end cost is always much more important than in the case of electronic circuits. This effect is essentially due to the back-end process. In electronic circuits, the package itself is a commodity, little more than a plastic case where the circuit is enclosed, and the contact with the outside world are simple electrical wires. The situation is completely different in labs on chips. Almost

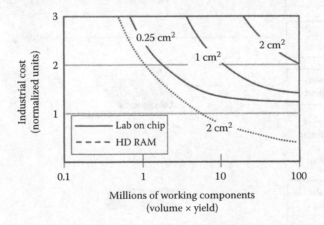

FIGURE 4.31 Overall industrial cost of the of the microfluidic circuit considered in the example in the text compared with similar microfluidics circuits with a greater area and with the cost of a high density RAM.

always the package has to host complex interfaces that are needed both by the fill chambers and repositories with reagents when the chip is fabricated and to charge the test solution when the chip is used. If optical detection is adopted, optical interfaces have to be frequently fabricated.

Another element that also impacts the asymptotic cost of labs on chips is the fact that they have to be frequently charged with chemical reagents that have the role of test, references, or washing solutions. Even if the amount of chemicals that are inside the chip is very small, when cents are to be taken into account, also this element that does not exist in the electronic case is important.

Even if the cost of labs on chip circuits does not scale exactly as in the case of microelectronics, the huge volume available in the health environmental and food control industries renders planar technology very effective in reducing the cost of circuits implementing complex functionalities, especially when compared with BOM-dominated analytical chemistry equipment.

4.5   PHOTOLITHOGRAPHY

Photolithography is the first fundamental step in planar front-end technology, allowing the transfer of patterns created on a mask on the photoresist layer placed on the wafer. Photolithography is a multistep process [1,3], starting from the wafer preparation and ending with the photoresist development.

A general scheme of a photolithography process is shown in Figure 4.32.

Photolithography, being essentially an optical process, has definition limits due both to the photoresist discrete nature and to the limited value of the used wavelength. Several other lithographic processes are industrially adopted or under study to overcome these limitations and high definition lithography processes based on particles beams or x-rays arrive to a sensitivity of the order of 2 nm. However, this extreme definition is not generally needed in labs on chip and the interested reader is

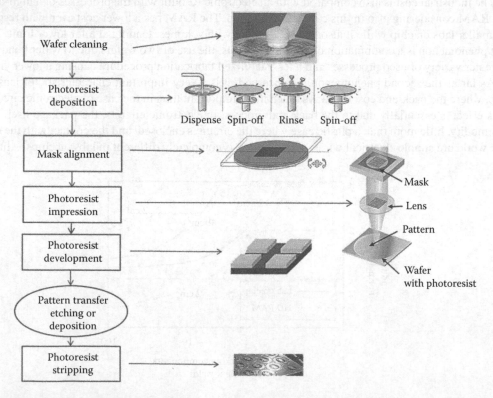

FIGURE 4.32   Photolithography process flow and subsequent transfer of the pattern on the wafer by etching or deposition.

encouraged to refer to the bibliography to start an analysis of such advanced lithography techniques [1,45–47].

4.5.1 Wafer Cleaning

Even if the wafer surface is protected from contaminants during all its history from production to the moment in which it starts the fabrication process, a preliminary wafer cleaning is needed before every mask around, that is, at the beginning of every lithography process. Various contaminants can be present on the wafer, residues of previous process steps or even from the wafer fabrication. Examples are solvents or other process chemicals, particles from operators and equipment, and other contaminants that could be present even in the air of a clean room. If left on the wafer surface, these contaminants can lead to serious problems during wafer processing, like compromising wafer planarity during lithography, creating unperfected adhesion of the resist on the wafer surface, or provoking unwanted chemical reactions.

All the clean room structure is built so as to cause particles that could hit the wafer surface not to exceed a limit energy so that wafer damage due to mechanical hit energy is not probable. Moreover, particle adhesion to the wafer surface is generally weak, so that an accurate cleaning process can remove the great part of the contaminants without damage.

Both wet and dry cleaning procedures are used in clean rooms. A well-known set of wet cleaning protocols called RCA1 and RCA2 [1] use mixtures of hydrogen peroxide mixed with various acids or bases to perform wet wafer surface cleaning combining chemical and mechanical processes. At the end of a wash with deionized water assures that no excess of the cleaning solution remains on the wafer surface. Other adopted procedures simply used vapor cleaning and high-temperature backing (up to 1000°C, depending on the resistance of the structures still on wafer to high temperature) in an atmosphere rich in oxygen. Alternatively, high-temperature backing can also be performed in vacuum, to favor contaminants detaching from the wafer surface.

Considering dry cleaning procedures, they use either ultrasonic beams, that are very good to remove particles from the wafer surface, but unfortunately are prone to the risk of damaging the surface itself, or simple wafer abrasion with suitable polishing compounds.

Generally, wet cleaning is preferred to dry cleaning that sometimes is used simply as a preliminary cleaning procedure before the more effective wet process.

As a last observation, it is to be noted that the wafer back also is generally cleaned, since several processes rely on the back planarity and the absence of defects, for example, to fix the wafer to the process machine plate, or for other reasons.

4.5.2 Photoresist Deposition

The photoresist deposition is the most expensive step of photolithography, both due to the cost of the resist itself and to the fact that almost all the deposition techniques have a relevant waste of material.

Thus, there are several used photoresist deposition techniques, both to adapt them at different kinds of resists and to optimize the process under a cost point of view.

4.5.2.1 Photoresist Spin Coating Deposition

Perhaps, the most used deposition technique is the spin coating [48]. Generally, before spin coating the cleaned wafer is protected by growing a thin silica film on it by oxidation. The film is annealed between 800°C and 100°C so as to homogenize its properties and it constitutes the base where the photoresist is deposited and, in selected cases, also the mask for subsequent processes like boron implantation.

After the oxidation the wafer is placed on a spinner plate and spin coating is performed (see Figure 4.33). An excess amount of a raw resist solution is placed on the substrate, which is then rotated at high speed in order to spread the fluid by centrifugal force. Rotation is continued while

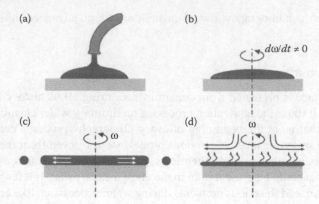

FIGURE 4.33 Photoresist spin coating; process phases (a) deposition of the coating fluid onto the wafer or substrate, (b) acceleration of the substrate up to its final, desired, rotation speed, (c) spinning of the substrate at a constant rate; fluid viscous forces dominate the fluid thinning behavior, and (d) spinning of the substrate at a constant rate causing solvent evaporation.

the fluid spins off the edges of the substrate, until the desired thickness of the film is achieved. The applied solvent is usually volatile, and simultaneously evaporates. So, the higher the angular speed of spinning, the thinner the film. The thickness of the film also depends on the concentration of the resist solute. In the case of standard UV photoresist, typical peak values of the spinner rotation speed are from 1500 to 6000 rounds per minute and the process duration is in the range of 10–100 s.

The spin coating process can be divided into steps, as shown in Figure 4.33.

1. The wafer is placed on the spinner plate, where it is fixed in position by a vacuum chuck. Here, the planarity of the wafer back is important like the absence of big contamination particles, in order to avoid a too weak force bonding the wafer to the chuck with the possibility that the wafer moves during the process and the coating results to be not homogeneous.
2. While the wafer rotation starts with a fast acceleration the resist solution is dispensed on the wafer near the wafer center through a dispenser. The dispenser characteristics in terms of uniformity of the solution flux and control of the flux variation in time are important to assure the wanted resist thickness to be realized by the spin coating process.
3. After the acceleration, the wafer is left to rotate at maximum speed while the solution arrives at the wafer borders and spill over the wafer borders. Contemporarily, the solution solvent tends to evaporate.
4. In a second phase, at maximum rotation speed the solvent evaporation is fastened, typically controlling the temperature inside the spinner or a small air flux toward the wafer. This is the phase in which the film has to reach the wanted thickness.
5. After the last phase, the spin plate is uniformly decelerated. This deceleration takes place when the film is almost solid; so generally it does not alter the film properties in a relevant way. At the end, when the plate stops, the film is formed.

The final film thickness can be defined only after a certain spin time, where the spillover of the resist solution from the wafer has eliminated at least 40% of the deposited initial material. Under this condition, the thickness depends on several parameters, mainly on the spin speed, on the photoresist solution viscosity, and on the time the spinner works after the film becomes almost uniform. An example of film thickness versus the spinning time for two commercial photoresists is provided in Figure 4.34, where it is evident as the thickness tends in any case to a limit value that cannot be further decreased while increasing the spinning time.

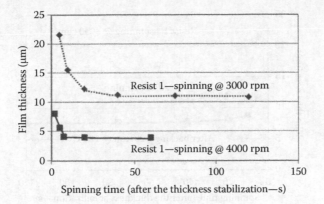

FIGURE 4.34 Example of film thickness versus the spinning time for commercial photoresists.

There are several theories trying to derive equations from the limit thickness δ of the film, but in general either they arrive to complex differential equation systems [49] or they introduce approximations that reproduce the phenomenon dynamics but do not allow to obtain accurate quantitative results. In practical processes, an empirical formula is often used that is given by [1,49]

$$\delta = K\,c^{\alpha_c}\,\mu^{\alpha_\mu/3}\,\omega^{-\alpha_\omega/2} \tag{4.7}$$

where
  K is a calibration constant depending on the specific equipment
  c is the initial photoresist solution concentration
  μ is the solution viscosity
  ω the stationary spinning rate
  α_c, α_μ, and α_ω are three empirical constants of the order of one that has to be determined
    experimentally

When the constants have been experimentally determined by a calibration set of measurements, Equation 4.7 is generally sufficiently accurate to allow the thickness of photoresist films to be correctly set by setting the spinner parameters.

After spin coating, the remaining unwanted solute is evaporated by wafer backing, that is generally performed at 90–100°C in a convection backing or at lower temperature (like 85°C) in a vacuum-backing chamber. The evaporation of the residual solvent reduces the film thickness to the final value, as shown, for example, in Figure 4.35.

Problems in spin coating can be due to several reasons, such as particles on the substrate at the moment of the spinning (causing streaks in the film like in Figure 4.36a), imperfect substrate wetting (causing nonuniform liquid expansion like in Figure 4.36b), or a too small initial amount of liquid (causing areas of the substrate to remain uncoated as in Figure 4.36c).

4.5.2.2 Alternative Photoresist Deposition Processes

Spin coating is not the only photoresist deposition used in micro-fabrication lithography, but several alternative techniques exist, that are reviewed in detail in References [1,3]. Here, we will briefly describe only two of them that are suitable in typical situations that could present during labs on chip manufacturing.

4.5.2.2.1 Spray Coating

In the so-called spray coating, the photoresist coating is created by passing the wafer under a spray of photoresist solution. In the spray equipment, the photoresist is pushed out of a pressurized tank

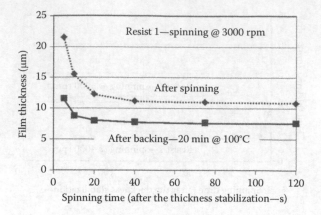

FIGURE 4.35 Resist film thickness before and after backing: example from a commercial photoresist.

via a supply pipe to a spray head that has a well-defined aperture and shape so as to form controlled droplets. Since the droplets are sprayed so that it attaches at the wafer where they hit it, the uniformity of the coating can be controlled by shaping the spray beam and suitably designing the motion of the spray head. In any case, the thickness control is not as good as in the case of spin coating and the spray head has to be maintained near the wafer (generally within 5 cm from the wafer surface).

While the film cannot be thin as in the case of spin coating, spray coating is particularly suitable for deposition on nonuniform surfaces, as it is the case of MEMs processing. In this case, the ability of the droplets to fill gaps and distribute so that a flat surface is created is important.

In cases in which such nonuniform surfaces are present, generally a low-speed spin is also added to the spray effect, for example at 30–60 rpm, to improve planarity of the outer surface of the photoresist film. Moreover, spray-coated films lack the internal stresses that are typical of spin-coated films so that the probability of film break after the coating process is lower. Finally, spray coating machine exists that can coat a wafer on the front and on the back, simultaneously. This operation very useful in both the front and the back of the wafer has to be processed as in the case of membranes fabrication shown in Figure 4.11—that is, a very important case in the field of labs on chip.

4.5.2.2.2   Electrophoresis Deposition (Electro-Deposition)

This is a technique used mainly when the substrate has relevant deviation from planarity, as it can be the case of microfluidics and MEMs fabrications. In the first case, excavations as deep as 50 μm can be conducted on silica in order to prepare reaction chambers and ducts so that, if successive lithography is needed, spin coating could not be usable due to the limited ability to produce a flat resist surface in this impervious conditions. In the second case, actuators and movable parts could not only have relevant vertical dimension, but they can also be fragile if a too strong force is applied to them in the horizontal direction.

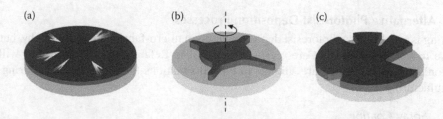

FIGURE 4.36 Selected possible defects in the resist film after spinning and backing: streaks in the film (a), nonuniform liquid expansion (b), and uncoated areas of the substrate (c).

To apply electrophoretic deposition, a conductive substrate is needed, besides an electrical biasing during the deposition process since the process is based on electrophoresis of the resist solution (see Sections 3.6 and 7.5.1). The coating solution is formed by charged micelles containing several components such as resist, solvent, dye, and photo-initiator molecules. When the electrophoretic field is established between a positively charged substrate and a negatively charged cathode, generally constituted by the wafer to be coated, the micelles migrate toward the cathode. When the micelles reach the cathode their positively charged surface is neutralized by hydroxyl ions produced by the electrolysis of water at the cathode and becomes unstable. After a very short transition time, the micelles coalesce on the surface of the cathode forming a self-limited resist film. Self-limitation happens due to the fact that the resist is not conductive. Thus when the film reaches a limit thickness the cathode results to be passivized by the resist film and electrophoresis ends, stopping the deposition of further resist on the substrate.

The coating thickness depends critically from the intensity of the electrophoretic field and on the process temperature that has to be maintained constant over all the substrate and for all the process time. Typical film thicknesses that are achievable with this method are 5–15 µm, but up to 35 µm thickness can be obtained with specific resist solutions.

Although the most important advantage of this deposition method is being compatible with relevant deviations from the substrate planarity, its main disadvantage is requiring an electrical biasing of the surface to be coated, that frequently means a metal coating of the same substrate before resist deposition, with additional process complications and costs. A comparison between spin coating, spray coating, and electrophoresis coating is reported in Table 4.10.

TABLE 4.10

Comparison between Spin Coating, Spray Coating, and Electrophoresis Coating for Resist Deposition

	Spin Coating	Spray Coating	Electrophoresis Coating
Process complexity	Simple	Simple	Complex
Process automation	Difficult	Possible (batch approach)	Possible (batch approach)
Key parameters	Viscosity, spin speed	Solution stoichiometry, spray speed, spray beam control, Scanning speed	Voltage, temperature
Needed photoresist solution	All types	Specific solutions with low viscosity	Specific prepared ED resist solution
Wasted material	More than 50%	20–35%	Depends on bath renewal, that is generally frequent
Planarity requirements	Very strict	Accept planarity deviations	Works with relevant deviations from planarity
Film uniformity	Difficult to control, need frequent equipment-specific calibration	Good control, depends on cavities position	Very good controls also without strong planarity
Film thickness before backing	Typical 5–20 mm	Typical 20–60 mm	Typical 5–20 mm, up to 35 mm possible
Applications	Transfer patterns on planar substrates or on the bottom of large cavities	Transfer patterns on substrates with geometrically similar cavities	Transfer patterns across and on the bottom of cavities, metal coating on substrate preferable
Cost	Intermediate	Intermediate	High

Source: Adapted from Madou M. J., *Fundamentals of Microfabrication and Nanotechnology*, Third Edition, Three-Volume Set, CRC Press; 3rd edition (August 1, 2011), ISBN-13: 978-0849331800.

4.5.2.3 Photoresist Types

A great part of the photolithography capability of producing small critical dimension patterns and of the related cost depends on the photoresist. The main components of a photoresist are

- A photo-sensible polymer
- A sensitizer
- A casting solvent

The polymer is the component that changes its state when exposed to light of a suitable wavelength, the sensitizer allows control of the chemical reaction in the polymeric phase, and the solvent allows resist deposition to form a thin film over the target substrate. Resist without a sensitizer also exist, called single component resist, while resist including a sensitizer are called double component resists.

A photoresist weakened by light exposure, so that the exposed part can be easily removed, is called positive resist (or also positive tone resist) while a resist that is reinforced by the exposure to light, so that it is the nonexposed part that can be easily removed, is called negative resist (or negative tone resist).

The weakening of the polymer in positive resists is obtained by photons-induced scission of polymeric chains, while the reinforcement in the case of negative resist is due to photon induced cross-links in the polymeric chains rendering them less reactive and more sturdy under a mechanical point of view (cf. Section 1.4.2).

Two widely used families of positive photoresists are the polymethylmethacrylate (also called PMMA) [50], that is available both in single and in double component versions, and the two components diazonaphtoquinone (DNQ) [51,52].

PMMA undergoes a photo-stimulated chain scission, whose reaction is sketched in Figure 4.37, if illuminated with deep UV light, with a maximum sensitivity around 220 nm. Above 220 nm, the sensitivity goes rapidly to zero and the resist becomes light insensitive. In single component resist the PMMA is a slow resist, requiring doses of UV light greater than 250 mJ/cm^2 to arrive to a satisfactory degree of impression, corresponding to several minutes of exposition using high-power UV lithography systems. By adding a suitable photosensitizer, the UV sensitivity of PMMA is greatly increased so as to reduce the impression dose up to less than 150 mJ/cm^2. A problem of PMMA is its poor adaptability to plasma etching (PE). As a matter of fact, the polymer residue changes the chemistry of the PE, frequently bringing to a spurious polymer film deposition on the substrate.

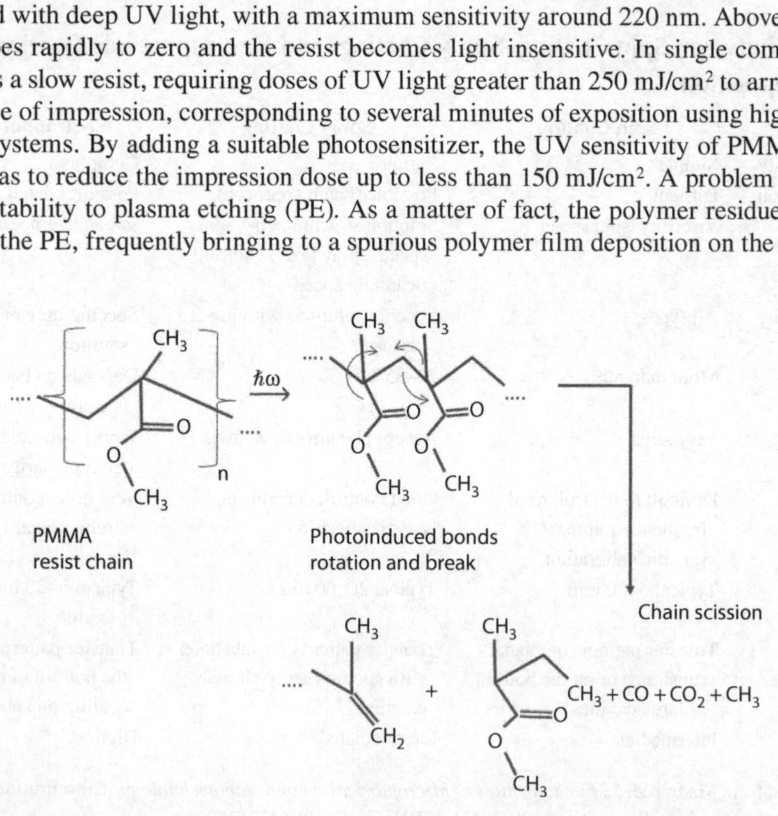

FIGURE 4.37   Photo-stimulated chain scission of PMMA resist.

The DNQ is a near UV resist that exists only in a two-component form and is widely used as far as its sensitivity is sufficient for the application. It is composed of the Novolak (N) resin, that in standalone form is a soluble alkali, and the diazonaphtaquinone (DQ), which is a hydrophobic compound. When the two components are joined together they form a practically insoluble and hydrophobic compound.

During exposition, photolysis eliminates the inhibition effect of DQ by breaking the composite and the resist develops a reaction forming a base-soluble carboxyl acid (see Figure 4.38). Typical UV wavelength used to expose DNQ are 365, 405, and 435 nm, that are emission lines of mercury lamps used in less performing lithographic equipment. Above 300 nm the DNQ becomes practically insensitive to UV light and cannot be used as resist. DNQ has the very good property that unexposed areas are practically unaltered by the development process, so that the shape of the mask is precisely transferred on the substrate and can be effectively used in conjunction with PE.

To conclude the discussion regarding positive resists, it is needed to underline that, in general, the adhesion of positive resists to the substrate, generally a silica film or, less frequently, pure silicon, is not sufficient for the greater part of the deposition processes to work properly. To improve adhesion, a primer has to be added before resist deposition [52].

In opposition to positive photoresists, negative resists becomes insoluble after UV exposition, so that the development allows the unexposed part of the film to be removed, while the exposed part remains in place. This can be achieved in one of two ways: either the resist increases its molecular weight by photo-stimulated cross-links so decreasing solubility or it undergoes photo-stimulated reactions that completely change its chemical structure to form a new insoluble molecule. This last mechanism is the most common in modern negative resists due to the absence of the so-called oxygen inhibition that typically happens in the first kind of resists.

This phenomenon, strictly related to the resist chemistry itself, consists in the presence of a side reaction involving oxygen that compete with the main reaction when the resist is developed and can completely ruin the pattern impressed on the resist by UV exposure. Thus, in order to avoid this side effect, exposure of this resist must be performed under a vacuum system or in nitrogen atmosphere. Oxygen inhibition is minimized when lithography is realized by putting the mask in strict contact with the resist film, since the mask itself protects the resist for oxygen residues that could be present in the atmosphere during development. In more performing photolithography machines, where the mask is not in contact with the resist, a very good atmosphere control is needed so complicating the process and increasing potential problems during development.

Another disadvantage of negative resist is that the film thickness limits the lithography resolution. This is due to the fact that resist hardness starts on the exposed surface, where the light hits

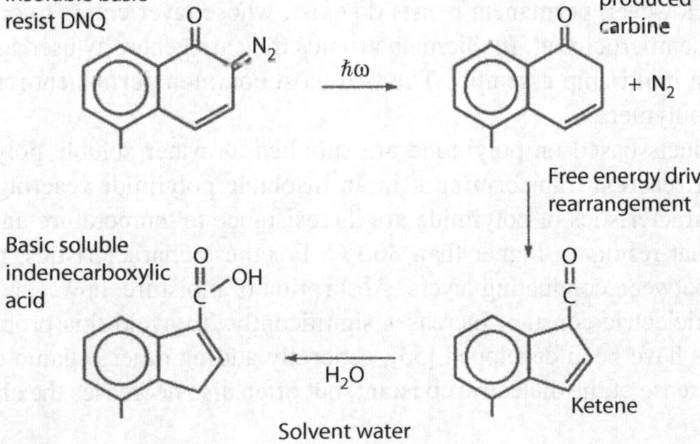

FIGURE 4.38 Photo-stimulated chain scission of DNQ resist.

TABLE 4.11

Synthetic Comparison between Positive and Negative Resists for Photolithography

	Positive Resist	Negative Resist
Adhesion to silicon	Primer generally needed	Primer not required
Backing	In air	In nitrogen or in vacuum
Contrast	High (e.g., 2.2)	Intermediate (e.g., 1.5)
Cost	High	Low
Developer	Temperature sensitive, water based	Temperature insensitive, based on organic solvents
Oxygen inhibition	Never	Frequent
Mask type	Dark field—higher performances	Clear field—lower performances
Photospeed	Slower	Faster
Pinhole count	Can be high	Have to be maintained small
PE resistance	Not very good	Very good
Residue after development	Mostly at <1 μm and at high-aspect ratio	Can be a problem
Resolution	High (lower than 1 μm)	Lower (greater than 1 μm)
Swelling in developer	No	Yes
Thermal stability	Good	Fair
Wet chemical resistance	Fair	Excellent

Source: Adapted from Madou M. J., *Fundamentals of Microfabrication and Nanotechnology*, Third Edition, Three-Volume Set, CRC Press; 3rd edition (August 1, 2011), ISBN-13: 978-0849331800.

the film, and a strong overexposure is needed to impress all the film thickness, whose time duration and needed dose depends on the film thickness. A greater over exposition, however, causes a great dose of scattered radiation that creates spurious exposure of different parts of the resist film thereby limiting lithography resolution. In a practical situation, a film with a depth of 1 μm does not permit a resolution better than 2 μm. In order to improve resolution thinner films have to be used, but when this solution is adopted pinholes can provoke problems.

A general comparison between positive and negative resists is synthetically presented in Table 4.11.

4.5.2.4 Permanent Resists

Generally, the resist is a sacrificial material used in the lithography step and then stripped out at the end of the process. However, permanent resists do exist, whose layer enters to constitute a permanent component of the microcircuit. In microelectronics they are generally used as insulating layers or as flexible layer in multi-chip assembly. The two most common permanent resists are based on polyimide and SU8 polymers.

Commercial products based on polyimide are supplied as water soluble polyamic acid which undergoes a thermal reaction transforming it in an insoluble polyimide reacting with the solvent water. Important characteristics of polyimide are its resistance to temperature and high glass transition temperature that results in higher than 300°C. For these characteristics, it is often used as insulating material between conducting layers. Absorption of moisture, however, causes polyimide to swell so that its dielectric constant increases significantly. To avoid this problem several similar permanent resists have been developed [53]; generally adding other organic components. This greatly limits the increase of the dielectric constant, but often also decreases the chemical resistance of the resist polymer.

Both photosensitive and nonphotosensitive polyimide exists. Photosensitive polyimides are impressed by UV light at 436 and 365 nm, having a strong sensitivity decrease generally above 300 nm.

These polymers can be used to reduce the number of process steps constituting contemporary the resist used for lithography and the permanent layer used for insulation or a stress relief layer.

The other different kinds of permanent resist categories are those based on the SU8 polymer: these are deep UV resist that can be deposited in extremely thick layers, like 100 μm or more, and are very used in MEMs and other lab on chip technologies where 3D structures have to be built using support layers that are electrical insulating, mechanically sturdy, and chemically inert. SU8 is an acid catalyzed negative photoresist made by dissolving SU-8 resin [54,55] in an organic solvent and adding a photo-initiator. The viscosity of the solution, and thus the thickness of the film, depends on the SU-8 concentration while the photo-initiator makes the role of catalyst in the photo-induced reaction.

4.5.3 Mask Alignment

Mask alignment is an important step of the photolithographic process: not only has the mask to be perfectly superimposed to the wafer area, but since every practical component requires several subsequent lithography steps, several subsequent masks and alignment of the mask with the structures already present on the wafer are needed. It derives that mask alignment is increasingly critical while the critical dimension of the structures fabricated on the wafer decreases.

Mask alignment is performed by building suitable alignment structures on the wafer during the previous lithography run, that are used to align the following mask. In low resolution lithography, alignment is simply performed by looking at the alignment patterns through similar patterns realized on the mask with a microscope. This technique has two drawbacks: the precision is limited by the accuracy of the observation and it cannot be automatized to process wafer batch without the intervention of the operator. Thus, in high throughput and low critical dimensions fabs mask alignment is performed by automatic machines using pattern recognition algorithms [56–58] to align the pattern on the mask with the reference on the wafer.

An example of the process of pattern recognition during mask alignment is reported in the scheme of Figure 4.39. Depending on the exposure technique, pattern recognition can exploit the resolution enhancement provided by the photolithography projection optics and achieve a huge precision that arrives to tens of nanometers in ultra-deep UV lithography adopting phase masks. Moreover, the feature on the mask used for mask alignment may be transferred to the wafer or not by the lithographic equipment. In the last case, it may be important to locate the alignment marks such that they do not affect subsequent wafer processing or device performance.

Alignment marks may not be arbitrarily located on the wafer, as the equipment used to perform alignment may have limited travel and therefore only be able to align to features located within a certain region on the wafer, as shown in Figure 4.40. Typically, two alignment marks are used to align the mask and wafer, one alignment mark is sufficient to align the mask and wafer in x and y, but it requires two marks, preferably spaced far apart, to correct for fine offset in rotation (cf. Figure 4.40).

4.5.3.1 Types of Masks for Planar Lithography

Normal lithography masks can be built in a variety of materials and are realized by means of computer high-definition methods so as to achieve the wanted resolution. They reproduce the pattern to be transferred to the resist by the UV exposure in a 1:1 geometric proportion in the case of proximity and contact exposure, or with an enhancement from 1:4 to 1:10 when projection exposure is adopted.

Corresponding to the existence of positive and negative resists, clear and dark masks exist, respectively, passing through the UV light where the mask pattern exists or blocking it in correspondence of the patterned areas.

The definition of a mask is defined as the standard deviation of the distance between the ideal position of a point of the contour of the profile that should be written on the mask and its real position. Thus, the mask definition is only one of the several terms contributing to limit the photolithography

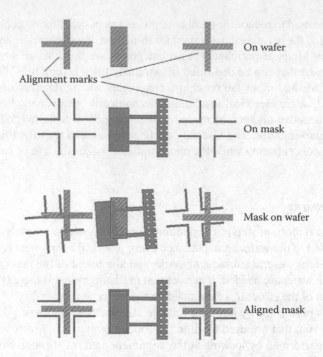

FIGURE 4.39 Example of the process of pattern recognition during mask alignment.

definition, and generally not the most important. Nevertheless, starting from a very good mask definition is important since in several lithography techniques the mask definition is not reduced by the definition enhancement technology, differently from other definition limiting factors. An example of this effect is found in projection exposure lithography, where the mask definition is multiplied by the exposure ration in the same manner of the nominal mask pattern.

Mask definition depends both on the mask writing technique and on the mask material. When high definition computer programs are used to write the mask the last factor is by far the most important.

Different processes can be implemented on the photo-mask to improve the pattern transfer precision. An example is proximity correction, which is a process that alters the image impressed on the mask to correct the distortion provoked by proximity exposure (see Section 4.5.4). An example of mask realized by using proximity correction is reported in Figure 4.41. The thicker dark areas on the mask constitute the pattern that has to be printed on the wafer. The thinner lines are assists that

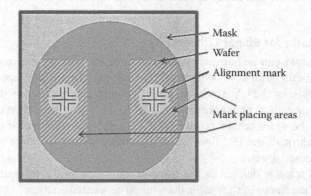

FIGURE 4.40 Example of placement of alignment marks on a mask and on the corresponding wafer.

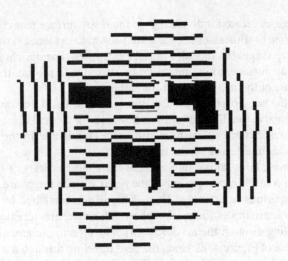

FIGURE 4.41 Example of photo-mask for proximity exposure corrected to enhance definition.

do not print themselves, but help the integrated circuit print better out of focus. The zig-zag appearance is due to optical proximity correction application.

A typical tolerance of glass masks is around ±0.8 μm, arriving to half this value if the pattern is carefully chosen to minimize the mask tolerance. Glass and quartz photo-masks are thus particularly suitable for applications requiring patterns smaller than 10 μm. Alternatively, if a less demanding process, the photo-mask can be built in a plastic film, achieving a typical mask resolution around 5 μm.

Particle contamination can be a significant problem if particles deposit on the photo-mask. Thus, generally, the mask is protected from particles by a pellicle—a thin transparent film stretched over a frame that is glued over one side of the photo-mask. The pellicle is far enough from the mask patterns so that moderate-to-small-sized particles that land on the pellicle will be too out of focus to be reproduced by lithography. Although they are designed to keep particles away, pellicles become a part of the imaging system and their optical properties need to be taken into account.

When the required lithography definition is very low, phenomena different from the mask resolution dominate the photolithography definition (see Section 4.5.7). One of them is the diffraction of the used UV light at the border of the mask pattern, whose effect is to project on the resist not a sharp image of the pattern border, but a thick diffraction figure, like it is shown in Figure 4.42.

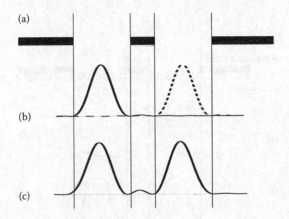

FIGURE 4.42 Effect of interference on lithography resolution if a normal mask is used; (a) mask pattern, (b) individual interference fringes of the two apertures on the mask pattern, and (c) overall optical power on the resist surface.

Here, the diffraction figures created individually on the resist surface from two apertures in a clear light mask (in a simplified bi-dimensional cases) are shown, to evidence how the light projected on the surface is not a sharp shape, but includes interference lines. The optical fields have to be added in amplitude on the resist surface taking into account that, due to the small details we are looking at on the mask, the phase of the field is almost the same.

Since in the figure the two apertures are 200 nm wide and the light wavelength is assumed to be 365 nm, we are still above the diffraction limit at which the critical dimension is half the wavelength, but the overall resolution is already insufficient. This is due to the lack of control of the phases of the optical fields interfering on the resist.

A phase mask is a mask built taking into account the characteristics of the lithography projection equipment so as to control in every point of the resist surface the phase of the interfering field in order to minimize spurious interference lines. This is accomplished by superimposing to the amplitude filtering characteristics of the mask a phase filtering characteristics that changes also the phase of the field traveling through the mask [59–61]. The effect is schematically shown in Figure 4.43, in the same example of Figure 4.42. Here, the field traveling through the second aperture of the mask is also inverted in phase, so that it subtract from the field coming from the first aperture once arrived on the resist surface. The effect on the final resist exposure is dramatically improved, not only does the intermediate spurious interference line disappear due to destructive interference but also the exposure is much more constant within the aperture area so that the resolution is completely sufficient for the resist exposure without defects.

Different types of phase masks exist. In alternating phase-shift masks, certain transmitting regions are made thinner or thicker. That induces a phase-shift in the light traveling through those regions of the mask creating a phase filter completely superimposed to the amplitude filter. When the thickness is suitably chosen, the interference of the phase-shifted light with the light coming from unmodified regions of the mask has the effect of improving the contrast on some parts of the wafer, which may ultimately increase the resolution on the wafer. The ideal case is a phase shift of 180°, which results in all the incident light being scattered. However, even for smaller phase shifts, the amount of scattering is not negligible. It can be shown that only for phase shifts of 37° or less will a phase edge scatter 10% or less of the incident light.

Attenuated phase-shift masks employ a different approach. Certain light-blocking parts of the mask are modified to allow a small amount of light to be transmitted through (typically just a few percent). That light is not strong enough to create a pattern on the wafer, but it can interfere with the light coming from the transparent parts of the mask, with the goal again of improving the contrast on the wafer.

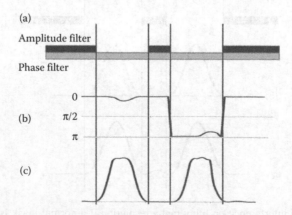

FIGURE 4.43 Effect of interference on lithography resolution if an optimized phase mask is used; (a) mask pattern, (b) phase filter characteristic, and (c) overall optical power on the resist surface.

4.5.3.2 Three-Dimensional Photolithography Masks

Up to now we have reviewed photolithography masks for planar pattern implementation. In microfluidics and MEMs technology, the realization of 3D structures is also very important. Creating vertical structures like chambers and ducts can be done via planar lithography and etching, but if inclined surfaces have to be created, using standard photolithography requires inhomogeneous etching techniques, like some types of wet etching (see Section 4.7.1) that imposes strong limits to the shapes that can be fabricated.

A possible alternative is the use of a specific type of photolithography based on a gradual exposure of the resist so that the subsequent etching is modulated by the remaining resist thickness and penetrates for a different depth into the wafer in different points. Current 3D photolithography technologies can be divided into three groups: multistep, direct-write, and grayscale mask photolithography.

Multistep photolithography utilizes several exposures using conventional optical masks [62,63], but each exposure produces a different gray level in the photoresist. With this technique, n masks have been demonstrated to produce $n + 1$ gray levels.

The maskless direct write process uses a writing beam to directly transfer a variable dose pattern into the photoresist [64–66], generally the beam is generated by an electron beam lithography equipment so that we will review this technique dealing with electron beam lithography.

Grayscale mask photolithography uses a conventional photolithography tool with a specialized grayscale optical mask [67,68]. Grayscale masks contain variable-transmission patterns that transmit part of the UV light intensity to create variable relief structures.

4.5.3.2.1 Multistep Lithography

This technique consists in using different masks to expose the photoresist varying the dose gradually along a certain direction. A schematic example of multistep lithography using a negative photoresist is reported in Figure 4.44. The key advantage of multistep lithography is to simply require a repetition of standard lithography steps: neither special lithography tool nor special masks are required. However, this simplicity corresponds to poorer performances with respect to the other methods of three-dimensional lithography.

Mask alignment is particularly critical in this technique; moreover, the limited contrast at the edge of each mask causes a deviation of the wanted dose profile on the resist that limit the critical dimension of the three-dimensional form to be realized. Last, but not least, deviations in booth alignment and exposure of each mask sums in the final result so that the overall process is quite less accurate than a single mask exposure using the same mask and the same lithography tool.

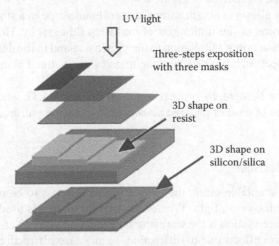

FIGURE 4.44 A schematic example of three-steps three dimensional lithography using negative photoresist.

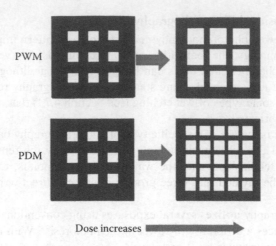

FIGURE 4.45   The structure of PWM and PDM masks for gray tone lithography.

4.5.3.2.2 *Gray Tone Lithography*

To overcome the limitations of the multistep process, gray tone lithography can be used, where different exposures are achieved using a single mask, called a gray tone mask. Ideally, a gray tone mask must have a different UV light transparency in different areas so as to create exposure of different points of the resist at different UV doses.

This is generally obtained using three possible methods:

1. In pulse width modulation (PWM) the transparent area of the mask is created by a grid of squared holes, with different widths so as to modulate the transmitted UV dose.
2. In pulse density modulation (PDM) the transparent area of the mask is also created by a grid of squared holes, but it is their density that is varied in order to modulate the transmitted UV dose.
3. Finally, in pulse width and density modulation (PWDM) both the dimension and the density of the holes are changed to have a better control of the dose in each area of the resist.

An example of PWM and PDM gray tone masks is reported in Figure 4.45, while the relative dose of UV light on the resist versus the relative side of the holes and the number of holes in the length of the exposed area is reported in Figure 4.46.

Gray tone lithography allows to obtain a three-dimensional shape in a single lithography exposition, thus overcoming some of the limitations of multistep lithography. However, the lithography exposure system diffraction poses a limitation to the dimension and to the density of the holes on the mask and this limits reflects in a limit on the roughness of the inclined planes that can be obtained by gray tone lithography.

A result of a gray tone lithography process is shown in Figure 4.47, where a scanning electron microscope (SEM) image of a set of inclined planes built on a wafer surface by gray tone lithography is shown.

4.5.4 PHOTORESIST EXPOSURE

After the fabrication of a suitable mask, the fabrication pattern has to be used to expose selected areas of the resist to the incoming light. Whatever exposure system is used, it is intuitive that the final limit to lithography resolution is the wavelength of the used light. Even if phase masks allow a great reduction of negative effects due to diffraction, in any case diffraction cannot be completely eliminated and it poses the ultimate limit to the critical dimension of photolithography systems.

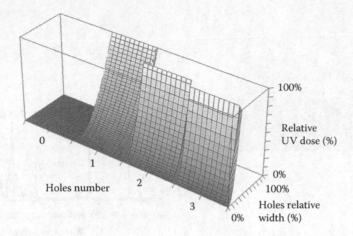

FIGURE 4.46 Relative dose of UV light on the resist versus the relative side of the holes and the number of holes in the length of the exposed area.

If extreme resolution is not required, a UV lamp can be used to generate the lithography light. High-pressure Hg vapor lamps are typically used in these cases. A photograph of one of these lamps with the corresponding UV spectrum is reported in Figure 4.48. Here, the Hg lines, generally, used for lithography at 365, 404.7, and 407.7 nm and the more powerful line at 436 nm are evidenced. Lamps add to the diffraction limit the fact that the large spectrum linewidth also contributes to degrade the contrast on the resist, also rendering practically impossible to control it by controlling the phase of the scattered light. Thus, if sub-micron resolution is to be achieved, lamps have to be substituted by UV lasers. For structures with a critical dimension of the order of 120 nm an argon or krypton fluoride laser is used, for smaller structures a nitrogen laser can be used exploiting the emission line at 157 nm.

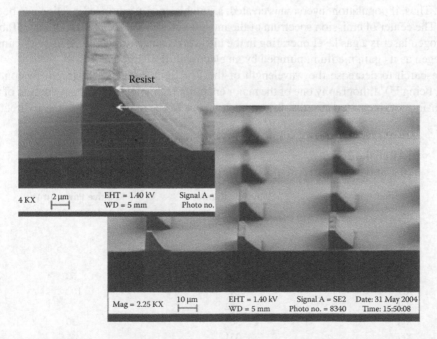

FIGURE 4.47 SEM image of a set of inclined mirrors built on a wafer surface by gray tone lithography. (Published under permission of Cyoptics Inc.)

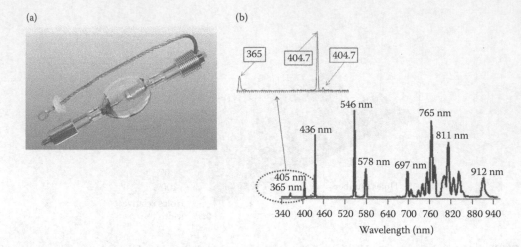

FIGURE 4.48 Photograph of an high pressure Hg lamp used for photolithography (a) and Hg infrared spectrum where the lines used for photolithography are evidenced (b).

Argon or krypton fluoride laser are examples of excimer lasers. Such lasers use a combination of a noble gas (argon, krypton, or xenon for example) and a reactive gas (generally, fluorine or chlorine). Under the appropriate conditions of electrical stimulation and high pressure, a pseudo-molecule called an excimer is created, which can only exist in an energized state.

Noble gases, such as xenon and krypton, are highly inert at normal conditions (temperature 25°C, pressure 100 kPa), but when in the excited state induced by an electrical discharge or an high-energy pulsed electron beams, they can form temporarily diatomic molecules or two atoms compounds with halogens, such as fluorine and chlorine. The excited compound has a strongly unstable ground state and in a characteristic time of a few picoseconds dissociates back in two unbound atoms. The excess energy associated to such dissociation is released via photons both by spontaneous and stimulated emission. Thus, if population inversion is created, a suitable energy pump laser action can be obtained [69–71]. The center of emission spectrum of the most used excimer lasers is reported in Table 4.12.

A nitrogen laser is a gas laser operating in the ultraviolet range (typically 337.1 nm) using molecular nitrogen as its gain medium, pumped by an electrical discharge [72,73].

The research to decrease the wavelength of the UV light used in lithography is continuously evolving, being UV lithography one of the major enabling technologies for the reduction of the critical dimensions of integrated circuits. Information on one of the main subject in these directions, the

TABLE 4.12
Wavelength and Typical Emitted Power of Selected Excimer Lasers

Excimer	Wavelength (nm)	Relative Power (mW)
Ar_2	126	
Kr_2	146	
Xe_2 (first line)	172	
Xe_2 (second line)	175	
ArF	193	60
KrF	248	100
XeBr	282	
XeCl	308	50
XeF	351	45
KrCl	222	25

use of the so-called extreme UV, the UV light with wavelength of the order of 15 nm, can be found in References [74–76].

Whatever light source is used, a way to project the image printed on the mask onto the resist have to be designed. Three strategies are used to do that, whose principle schemes are reported in Figure 4.49: contact exposure, proximity exposure, and projection exposure.

Contact exposure has been the first solution to be adopted: in this case, the mask is put at direct contact with the resist surface with a slow process of simultaneous approach and alignment. The best property of this exposure technique is that diffraction coming from the mask edges does not travel a long path and forms small fringes on the resist. However, the contact between the mask and the resist provoke both mask and resist contamination. Resist particles remaining on the mask have to be cleaned before reuse of the mask with a different wafer. This cleaning procedure shortens the mask life and, in case of imperfect cleaning of the mask, can cause contamination of the next wafer. On the resist side, the mask contact can create unwanted shapes on the resist, thereby causing potential defects in resist exposure.

These drawbacks do not exist in proximity lithography, where the mask is maintained in close proximity of the wafer by a set of proximity halters at least 10 μm high. This avoids mask contact with the wafer and increases dramatically the yield of the process without introducing more complexity. However, due to the fact that the distance between the mask and the wafer is much larger of the UV light wavelength (generally from 30 to 100 times), the contrast of the mask image on the wafer is heavily degraded so as to cause an overall resolution worsening of one order of magnitude or greater. Several mask pre-processes have been introduce to compensate for this problem by trying to pre-compensate the diffraction effect, but in any case resolutions of the order of that reached with contact exposure are almost impossible to reach.

By far the most common method of exposure is projection printing. Projection lithography derives its name from the fact that an image of the mask is projected onto the wafer by an UV optical system. Projection lithography is enabled by very high-quality UV lenses and mirrors, designed using complex computer-aided design tools, so that lenses aberrations play only a marginal role in determining the quality of the image. The optical systems used in projection lithography are thus diffraction-limited projectors, since it is diffraction and not lenses aberrations that determine the final definition limit.

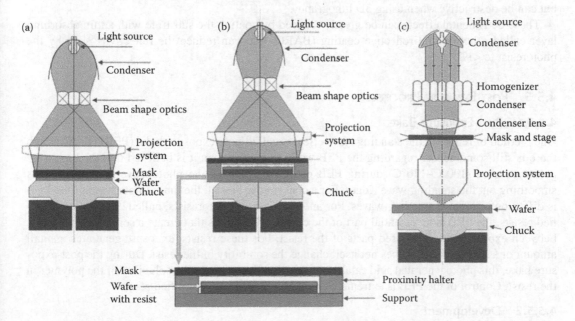

FIGURE 4.49 Schematics of the main photolithography exposure equipment: (a) contact exposure, (b) proximity exposure, and (c) projection exposure.

There are two major classes of projection lithography tools—scanning and step-and-repeat systems. Scanning projection printing [1,3], employs mirrors, to project a slit of light from the mask onto the wafer as the mask and wafer are moved simultaneously by the slit. Exposure dose is determined by the intensity of the light, the slit width, and the speed at which the wafer is scanned. These scanning systems, which generally use mercury lamps, reproduce the mask image on the wafer in 1:1 ratio so that the structures on the mask have the same dimensions of the structures that are to be reproduced on the wafer.

Step-and-repeat exposure systems, generally called simply steppers, expose the wafer one rectangular section at a time (the exposed section is frequently called the image field). Stepper can project the mask image on the wafer with an N:1 dimension ratio, where generally N varies from 1 in direct reproduction systems, up to 10 in very high definition systems.

The most advanced projection lithography equipment is a combination of the step-and-scan approaches. It uses a fraction of a normal stepper field, for example, a rectangular field of 25×8 mm^2, then scans this field in one direction to expose the entire $N \times 1$ mask, where N is rarely greater than 4. The wafer is then stepped to a new location and the scan is repeated. The smaller imaging field simplifies the design and manufacture of the lens, but at the expense of a more complicated reticle and wafer stage. Step-and-scan technology is the technology of choice today for below 250 nm manufacturing.

An important aspect tending to limit the resolution of photoresist exposure when laser UV light is used in conjunction with high-resolution steppers is the standing wave effect. Monochromatic light, when projected onto a wafer, strikes the photoresist approximating as a set of plane waves arriving from slightly different angles. These waves travel through the photoresist and, if the substrate is reflective, are reflected back up through the resist. The incoming and reflected light interferes to form a standing wave pattern of high and low light intensity at different depths in the photoresist. This pattern is replicated in the photoresist, causing ridges in the sidewalls of the resist feature. As pattern dimensions become smaller, these ridges can significantly affect the quality of the feature. The interference that causes standing waves also results in a phenomenon called swing curves, the sinusoidal variation in the resolution of a single width of a line on the resist pattern with changing resist thickness. Swing curves affect all types of projection lithography with monochromatic light, but can be destructive when using 3D lithography.

These detrimental effects can be greatly reduced by coating the substrate with a thin absorbing layer called a bottom antireflective coating (BARC) that can reduce the reflectivity seen by the photoresist to <1%.

4.5.5   Post-Exposure Processes

4.5.5.1   Post-Exposure Bake

One method of reducing the standing wave effect is called post-exposure bake (PEB) [1]. Although there is still some debate regarding the PEB working mechanism, it is believed that the high temperatures used (100°C–130°C) during PEB cause diffusion of the photoactive compound, thus smoothing out the standing wave ridges. For a conventional resist, the main importance of the PEB is diffusion to remove standing waves. For another class of photoresists, called chemically amplified resists, the PEB is an essential part of the chemical reactions that create a solubility difference between exposed and unexposed parts of the resist. For these resists, exposure generates a small amount of a strong acid that does not itself change the solubility of the resist. During the post-exposure bake, this photogenerated acid catalyzes a reaction that changes the solubility of the polymer in the resist. Control of the PEB is extremely critical for chemically amplified resists.

4.5.5.2   Development

Once exposed, the photoresist must be developed [1,77,78]. Most commonly used photoresists use aqueous bases as developers. In particular, frequently diluted solutions of tetra-methyl ammonium

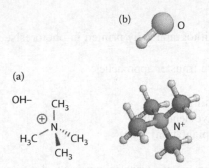

(a)

(b)

FIGURE 4.50 Tetra-methyl ammonium hydroxide structure formula (a) and stereographic representation in the balls and sticks convention (b).

hydroxide (TMAH—see Figure 4.50) are used. Development is a critical step in the photoresist process. The characteristics of the resist–developer interactions determine to a large extent the shape of the photoresist profile.

The method of applying developer to the photoresist is important in controlling the development uniformity and process latitude. In fabs manufacturing chips with critical dimensions in the micron range, batch development is the predominant development technique. A boat of 10–30 wafers is developed simultaneously in a large beaker, usually with some form of agitation. If the critical dimensions are lower, like in sub-micron fabs, and the throughput has to be maintained high without decreasing the yield, other kinds of development processes have to be used, such as spin development and spray development.

During spin development wafers are spun, using equipment similar to that used for spin coating, and developer is poured onto the rotating wafer. The wafer is also rinsed and dried while still spinning. Spray development has been shown to have good results using developers specifically formulated for this dispense method. Using a process identical to spin development, the developer is sprayed, rather than poured, on the wafer by using a nozzle that produces a fine mist of developer over the wafer. This technique reduces developer usage and gives more uniform developer coverage.

Another development strategy is called puddle development. Using developers specifically formulated for this process, the developer is poured onto a stationary wafer that is allowed to sit motionless for the duration of the development time. The wafer is then spin rinsed and dried.

Spin, spray, and puddle development processes can be generally performed by the same piece of equipment, with minor modifications, that allows to adapt the development process to the used resist and to the rest of the lithography process without using different equipment for every different development technique.

4.5.5.3 Postbake

Postbaking is used to harden the final resist image after development so that it will withstand the harsh environments of implantation or etching. The high temperatures used (120°C–150°C) cross-link the polymer in the photoresist, thus making the image more thermally stable.

However, if the postbaking temperature is too high, the resist flows causing degradation of the image. The temperature at which flow begins is related to the glass transition temperature of the polymer and it is a measure of the thermal stability of the resist. In addition to cross-linking, the postbake can remove residual solvent, water, and gases and will usually improve adhesion of the resist to the substrate.

Other methods have been proposed to harden a photoresist image. Exposure to high intensity deep-UV light crosslinks the resin at the surface of the resist forming a tough skin around the pattern [3,79]. Deep-UV hardened photoresist can withstand temperatures in excess of 200°C without dimensional deformation.

4.5.5.4 Pattern Transfer

After the patterns have been lithographically printed in photoresist, they must be transferred into the substrate.

There are three basic pattern transfer approaches:

- Subtractive transfer (etching)
- Additive transfer (selective deposition)
- Impurity doping (ion implantation)

Etching is the most common pattern transfer approach. A uniform layer of the material to be patterned is deposited on the substrate. Lithography is then performed such that the areas to be etched are left unprotected by the photoresist. Etching is performed either using wet chemicals such as acids, or more commonly in a dry plasma environment. The photoresist "resists" the etching and protects the covered material. When the etching is complete, the resist is stripped leaving the desired pattern etched into the deposited layer.

When selective deposition is adopted the lithographic pattern is used to open areas where the new layer is to be grown. Stripping of the resist then leaves the new material in a negative version of the patterned photoresist.

Doping involves the addition of controlled amounts of contaminants that change the properties of the host layer material. Ion implantation uses a beam of dopant ions accelerated at the photoresist-patterned substrate. The resist blocks the ions, but the areas uncovered by resists are embedded with ions, creating the selectively doped regions.

We will analyze in more detail these techniques, fundamental in the construction of labs on chip, in Sections 4.8 through 4.10.

4.5.5.5 Photoresist Stripping

After the imaged wafer has been processed the remaining photoresist must be removed. There are two classes of resist-stripping techniques: wet stripping using organic or inorganic solutions, and plasma dry stripping.

Most organic strippers are phenol based and are designed to avoid scum formation on the wafer after stripping. However, the most common wet strippers for positive photoresists are inorganic acid-based systems used at elevated temperatures [1,3]. Wet stripping has several inherent problems. Although the proper choice of strippers for various applications can usually eliminate gross scumming, it is almost impossible to remove the final monolayer of photoresist from the wafer by wet chemical means. It is often necessary to follow a wet strip by a plasma descum to completely clean the wafer of resist residues. Photoresist which has to undergone extensive hardening like deep-UV hardening to be suitable to resist at harsh processing conditions, for example, high-energy ion implantation, can be almost impossible to strip chemically. For these reasons, plasma stripping has become the standard in most semiconductor processing.

4.5.6 Photolithography Definition

The definition of a whole photolithography process depends on many factors, a few of them related to specific details of the process.

As far as the resist is concerned, the resist quantum efficiency is an important factor entering in the determination of the final resolution photolithography resolution. The resist quantum efficiency Φ is defined as the ratio between the photons absorbed by a unit resist area and the number of photon-stimulated processes that are generated, like break of polymer chains in positive resists. By its definition, the resist quantum efficiency enters in a fundamental way in the expression of the percentage of the resist exposure caused by the exposure process. The percentage of resist exposure ε, that is the number of resist molecules undergoing photo-induced transformation N_{PT} divided by the overall number of molecules in a unit resist volume, is given by

$$\varepsilon = \Phi DP(N_A)m_M \frac{A}{\xi} \qquad (4.6a)$$

where

Φ is the resist quantum efficiency.

D is the dose (power per unit time) emitted by the light source.

$P(N_A)$ is the percentage of the dose captured by the focusing system and directed over the wafer. $P(N_A)$ is an increasing function of the numeric aperture N_A, representing the product between the index to the lens material and the sin of half the acceptance angle [80,81]. The numerical aperture is linked to number of diffraction modes present at the output of each mask transmitting area that are captured by the optical system and directed to the wafer. The exact form of $P(N_A)$ depends on the particular type of optical system, a possible shape is reported in Figure 4.51.

m_M is the molecular weight of the resist polymer.

A is the Avogadro number.

ξ is an empirical configuration factor relating molar weight and molar volume. Since ξ depends on the molecular shape it is of the same order of magnitude for all the polymers, even if its specific value changes from molecule to molecule.

Increasing the mass of the polymer chain, the percentage of the exposed resist increases, due essentially to the fact that less photo-induced phenomena are needed. The same happens when increasing the resist quantum efficiency, due to the better exploitation of the incoming photons, and the optical system numerical aperture, due to the best exploitation of the power emitted from the light source. Ideally, the exposure efficiency have to be as near to 100% as possible, to avoid a nonuniform development of the resist, mainly in correspondence of the edges of the exposed area, causing contrast degradation near the edge of the transferred pattern.

The mask definition is another important element for the photolithography final definition: it is defined as the overall aberration of the optical system collecting the light from the source and focusing it on the resist surface.

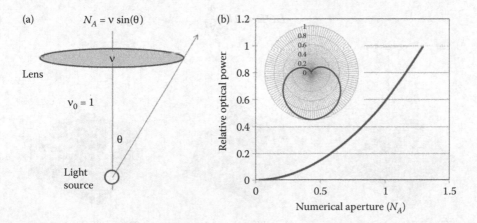

FIGURE 4.51 Definition of numerical aperture of a lens (a) and example of the dependence of the fraction of UV power emerging from a mask clear area that is focused on the resist surface from the optical system numeric aperture (b). The insert represents the wave front exiting from the mask clear area.

Resist quantum efficiency, mask definition, and other similar factors must be carefully engineered to obtain a high-performing photolithography system. However, high-quality photolithography machines are so carefully designed, that all these factors are near their optimum value, so that the main element determining the lithography resolution is the diffraction characteristics of the optical system. Let us consider as a reference a stepper projection system, where requirements for definitions are more stringent. We can represent the definition as the minimum width w of a line that can be resolved on the photoresist (also called the system linewidth) and write [1,81]

$$w = k \frac{\lambda}{N_A} \tag{4.7a}$$

where system constants and the effects of phenomena different from diffraction depending on the resist, lenses aberration, development technique, and so on, are collected in a process constant k. Typical values of k are of the order of 0.6–0.8 for excimer laser lithography systems; if a bi-dimensional phase mask is used, k is greatly reduced, arriving up to an order of 0.2.

The presence of the light wavelength λ at the numerator of Equation 4.7a is obvious, due to the fact that the diffraction fringes have a depth proportional to the wavelength, thus smaller the wavelength greater the contrast on the resist. As far as the numeric aperture is concerned, its influence can be understood considering the fact that, higher the percentage of the emitted light captured by the optical system, greater the number of diffraction orders that are collected to form the final image. This effect is evidenced in Figure 4.52.

Substituting realistic numbers, with $k = 0.55$, $\lambda = 193$ nm, $n = 1.5$, and $\theta = 110°$ so that $N_A = 0.86$ we achieve 124 nm resolution and with a bi-dimensional phase mask as low as about 40 nm.

From Equation 4.7a it could seem that greater the numerical aperture better the performances of the lithography. This is true in terms of resolution, but resolution is not the only performance parameter that characterizes a good lithographic process. The resist has a finite thickness, and if exposure has to be uniform all along the thickness of the photoresist, the incident light beam should be focused over all its depth. Even if theoretically there is a well-defined focus distance between a mask transparent area and the corresponding resist area, the beam defocusing is very small in a certain interval around the focus distance, called depth of focus (DOF), while out of this interval its increases abruptly completely defocusing the beam [80]. Thus, the optical system DOF has to be at least equal to half the resist film thickness to generate uniform resist exposure. The DOF also depends on the numerical aperture and on the wavelength following the equation [80,81]:

$$DOF = 2k' \frac{\lambda}{N_A^2} \tag{4.8}$$

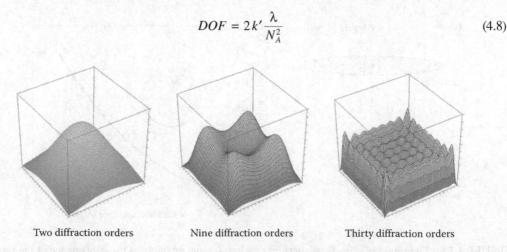

Two diffraction orders   Nine diffraction orders   Thirty diffraction orders

FIGURE 4.52 Diffraction image from a square aperture with a side equal to twice the incident plane wave wavelength versus the number of collected diffraction orders.

where k' is another process-related constant whose value is around 0.5 for the most performing excimer laser steppers. From Equation 4.8, it results that all the steps increasing the photolithography definition operating on the wavelength or on the numerical aperture also reduces the DOF, so that a trade-off have to be found. The DOF with the data of the previous example results to be about 260 nm, that means a resist thickness before backing of about 1 μm, at the limit of what can be done with a standard PMMA resist.

4.6 ELECTRON BEAM LITHOGRAPHY

Electron beam (e-beam) lithography is a very high-resolution lithography technique that uses electron beams instead of UV light beams to impress the photoresist. The typical energy of electron beams used in e-beam lithography is 10–50 keV, so that the corresponding De Broglie wavelength is of the order of 50 Å, so small that any diffraction effect disappears. The e-beam resolution is limited by factors different from diffraction, like electrons scattering in the resist and electrons optics aberration. In any case, resolutions smaller than 10 nm can be attained by electron beam techniques. An example of the structure fabricated using electron beam lithography is shown in Figure 4.53. It is a ring optical resonator fabricated directly in silicon. Light coupling between the resonator and the in/out waveguide is regulated by the distance between these structures, that in the case of the figure is as low as 120 nm and that has to be carefully controlled to match the resonator specifications. The resonator was fabricated using e-beam lithography and the estimated resolution was 7 nm, sufficient to achieve a good control of the coupling distance [46,82,83].

A schematic representation of the architecture of a direct writing e-beam lithography equipment is represented in Figure 4.54: a narrow bean of high-energy electrons is directly focused on the resist deposited on the wafer with a focus and scanning system similar to that of a scanning electron microscope. Two possible scanning techniques can be adopted: sequential scanning and vector scanning. In sequential scanning machines the electron beams scan the wafer surface sequentially following a grid trajectory that is the same for each wafer. When the resist is to be exposed the beam is empowered, while when it does not have to be exposed it is shut off almost completely. If vector scanning is used, the electron beam is driven by the software mask charged into the e-beam control system to scan and impress only the areas on the wafer that has to be exposed. Generally, control software for vector scanning is more complex, but allows a certain reduction of the scanning speed.

E-beam lithography has several advantages with respect to UV lithography, besides its definition: no mask is required (in some sense a software mask is charged into the e-beam control), the exposure of the resist is accurately controlled over very small areas, and focus can be adjusted during the electron beam scan so as to obtain large DOF. In particular, the combination of the ability to

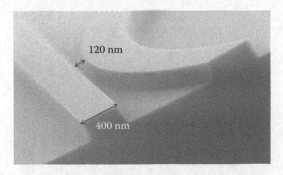

FIGURE 4.53 Scanning electron microscope image of a particular of an optical ring interferometer fabricated using e-beam lithography; the critical dimension is the minimum distance between the straight waveguide and the ring resonator, that is as small as 120 nm. The estimated e-beam lithography resolution was 7 nm. (Published under permission of Cyoptics Inc.)

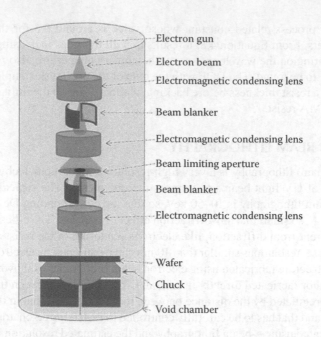

Electron gun
Electron beam
Electromagnetic condensing lens
Beam blanker
Electromagnetic condensing lens
Beam limiting aperture
Beam blanker
Electromagnetic condensing lens
Wafer
Chuck
Void chamber

FIGURE 4.54   Schematic representation of the e-beam equipment architecture.

accurately change the dose of electrons of the beam and the possibility to obtain a very large DOF renders e-beam lithography suitable for three-dimensional lithography of very small structures. An example of such structure is reported in Figure 4.55, where an SEM photograph of two superimposed optical waveguide fabricated with high-contrast index silicon core is shown [84].

E-beam lithography has also disadvantages with respect to photolithography. The resolution advantage, that was enormous when this technique was invented in the 1960s, is now quite reduced and, even the most complex photolithography machines are simpler in terms of structure with respect to an e-beam. This is due both to the fact that electrons require to be processed in vacuum and to the more complex and costly structure of the electron optics and the scanning system.

The fundamental limit of the e-beam lithography is, however, the low throughput with respect to photolithography. Exposure through the electron beam is slow and the processing of a 120 mm wafer can require sensibly more than an hour [46]. The throughput limit has in practice confined e-beam lithography to research and to niche applications where extreme resolution is needed for circuits that have not to be reproduced in huge numbers.

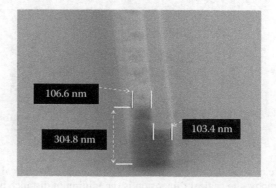

106.6 nm

304.8 nm

103.4 nm

FIGURE 4.55   SEM photograph of two superimposed optical waveguide fabricated with high contrast index silicon core. (Published under permission of Cyoptics Inc.)

Another common application of the electron beam lithography is the preparation of phase mask for steppers. On the one hand, a mask can be used to process a huge number of wafers, thus the fact that mask fabrication process is slow is not important even in very high-throughput fabs. On the other hand, if a resolution of the order of 40 nm or less is to be obtained with optical lithography, the mask accuracy is in any case critical. This is especially true when two-dimensional phase masks or when gray lithography masks have to be fabricated: in the first case, the control of the mask transmission phase requires very high definition and extremely accurate dose control and in the second case the critical size of the mask is generally quite smaller than the critical dimension of the final circuit.

An attempt to overcome the throughput limitation of e-beam lithography is the use of much larger electron beams [85] that illuminate large areas of the wafer. Naturally, in this case, a mask is required to reproduce the pattern on the wafer, similar to the case of photolithography. Even if the limitations implicit in proximity printing, that is generally the technique used to set the mask in this kind of e-beam machines, can be overcome in great part with optical corrections [86] (see Figure 4.41), this technique at present is not widely used.

4.7 ETCHING

Besides lithography, the most important planar processes are subtractive and additive processes. Subtractive technologies, also called etching, allows selected patterns to be removed from a superficial film on a wafer, while additive technologies allow similar patterns to be added in form of thin superficial film.

Under the general name of etching are collected a set of very different techniques that can be divided into two great families: wet and dry etching. Processes relying on the consumption of the film to be etched through chemical reaction with a suitable etchant are called wet etching processes, due to the fact that they are generally performed by immersion of wafers in an etchant solution. Dry etching on the contrary is the family of all the etching technique relying on mechanical elimination of a selected pattern from the wafer surface, generally through particle bombardment in case sustained by chemical action of the particles with the film to be removed.

Even if quite a variety of different techniques can be collected under the two etching families, they have common traits that are in part collected in Table 4.13. From the table it is evident that wet and dry etching are complementary techniques, not competitive once. They are both used widely for different applications and frequently coexist in the same processes stream.

TABLE 4.13

Qualitative Comparison between Wet and Dry Etching Techniques

	Dry	Wet
Environment	Vacuum	Atmosphere
Equipment	Vacuum chamber	Chemical bath
	Particles gun	
	Particles beam optics	
Advantages	Small feature sizes (<100 nm)	Low cost
		Good selectivity
		High etching rate
Implementation	More difficult	Easier
Disadvantages	High cost equipment	No features under 1 μm
	Low throughput	Wafer contamination possible
	Smaller selectivity (for selected techniques)	
Directionality	Anisotropic	Isotropic for amorphous materials (like SiO_2)
		Anisotropic etching possible for crystals (like Si)

4.7.1 Wet Etching Techniques

Wet etching techniques are used essentially in two different applications: to transfer a pattern on the wafer surface through a suitably exposed and developed resist or to create three-dimensional structures. In the first case, wet etching is often used in conjunction with dry etching, for example, to smooth too sharp corners where stress tends to accumulate creating potential failure due to material breaking.

Another possible application of wet etching in conjunction of dry etching is damage removal from the wafer surface by etching up a very thin film.

In application with critical dimensions greater than 1 μm, wet etching can be used also for pattern transfer. An example is given by the excavation of trenches between different devices or group of devices of the same circuit to create better electrical or thermal insulation. Also, lithographic structure like V grooves (see Section 6.5.4) and microfluidics ducts can be obtained by wet etching.

4.7.1.1 Wet Etching Characteristics

The most used wet etching process uses etch insensitive masks, that is masks that are not chemically attached by the etchant. In this way, the etching process happens under the mask, but it does not affect it. Etching mask of this type can be constituted either by photoresist after exposure, development and strong hardening (frequently using UV), or by a previously selectively etched film, like SiO_2 over silicon.

A first important characteristic of wet etching is the isotropy degree. Let us define a reference system where the x–y plane is the wafer surface under the resist and the z-axis is perpendicular to the wafer. Considered a direction θ, the etching rate along this direction, called r_θ, can be defined as

$$r_\theta = \frac{d\,H_\theta(t)}{dt} \tag{4.9}$$

where $H_\theta(t)$ is the etch depth reached along θ in the interval $[0, t]$. If wet etching is applied to a uniform amorphous film, the etching rates r_x and r_y in all the horizontal directions, that are the directions parallel to the wafer surface, is necessarily the same, while the etching rate r_z in the vertical direction is potentially different. In this case, the isotropy rate is defined as

$$\rho = \frac{r_x}{r_z} = \frac{r_y}{r_z} \tag{4.10}$$

Due to its definition $0 \leq \rho \leq 1$, where in the case of perfect isotropic etching $\rho = 1$ and in case of perfectly anisotropic etching $\rho = 0$. If wet etching is performed using normal etchants on amorphous films the etching isotropy rate is always quite near to one, since the etch tends to be isotropic.

The effect of different values of the etching isotropy rate is shown in Figure 4.56. In the figure, the fact that wet etching generally creates the so-called under-cut above the mask is also evidenced. The under-cut dimensions u is given by

$$u = \rho H_x(t) = \frac{1}{2}\,\frac{d\,H_x^2}{dH_z} \tag{4.11}$$

so as to be maximum in case of isotropic etching and minimum, equal to zero, in case of perfectly anisotropic etching. In case of normal etchants for amorphous films the etching isotropy rate is always quite near to one, since the etch tends to be isotropic. Small degrees of anisotropy could be created either by nonhomogeneity of the etched film (e.g., if the density increases with depth), or by the presence of hydraulic pressure in the etchant bath.

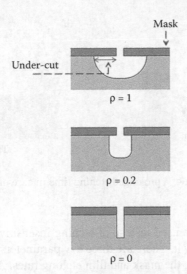

FIGURE 4.56 Effect of different values of the etching isotropy on the etched shape in an amorphous film. The under-cut created by the wet etching is also defined. The etching mask can be either photoresist after exposure, development and strong hardening (frequently using UV) or a previously selectively etched film, like SiO_2 over silicon.

An interesting example of anisotropic wet etching of a thick SiO_2 substrate is shown in Figure 4.57, where an isotropy rate of about 0.5 in Figure 4.57a and of 1.25 in Figure 4.57b (etch rate in horizontal direction greater than in the vertical direction) are achieved by ion implantation before etching. Ion implantation defines a material volume that can be etched at a higher rate-generating anisotropy. The scope in the specific case was to achieve a flat inclined surface to generate a mirror after suitable metallization.

Anisotropic etching can be obtained in a well-controlled way in the case of crystal films, since the effect of the etchant in this case depends on the crystal orientation so that anisotropy spontaneously rises. Since wet etching is generally highly selective, the etcher used for the surface film does not etch the substrate. Thus, when the etching depth reaches the substrate, etching in vertical dimension stops, while etching in horizontal dimension goes on, creating the so-called over-etching of the film (cf. Figure 4.58).

Over-etching allows a better definition of the pattern to be transferred, since the lateral wall gets more and more vertical, but also causes an increase in the dimension of the under-cut, that can cause problems in the phase of resist stripping (e.g., the break of the resist film). This is the reason, in particular, if thick films are considered, over-etching cannot be pushed for a too long time.

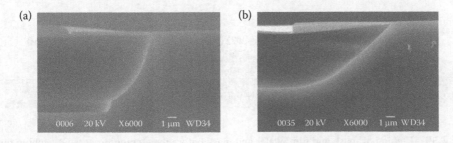

FIGURE 4.57 Example of anisotropic wet etching of a thick SiO_2 substrate, where an isotropy rate of about 0.5 in (a) and of 1.25 in (b) are achieved by ion implantation before etching. (Published under permission of Cyoptics Inc.)

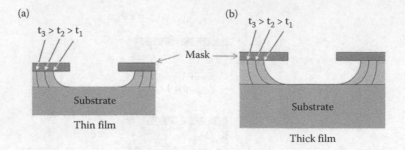

FIGURE 4.58 Over-etching effect of a prolonged etching time in case of a thin (a) or thick (b) etched film.

If etching sensitive masks are used instead of etching insensitive once, the mask is also etched contemporarily to the film below it. There are three key parameters for this kind of etching process that can be defined starting from the mask and film etching rates. Assuming the mask and the film to be amorphous materials, these parameters are called etching selectivity S_m, horizontal etching relative rate R_R and mask relative etching rate ρ_m, and they are defined as

$$S_m = \frac{r_{m,z}}{r_{f,z}} \tag{4.12}$$

$$R_{mR} = \frac{r_{m,x}}{r_{f,x}} \tag{4.13}$$

$$\rho_m = \frac{r_{mx}}{r_{m,z}} \tag{4.14}$$

where the subscript m identify mask etching rates and the subscript f film etching rates.

During the etching process, the etching mask is profiled as in Figure 4.59a, so as to present a lateral flat shape inclined of an angle (say θ) with respect to the horizontal plane. Two different etching regimes can be realized, generating different etching shapes: mask-dominated etching (where $R_{mR} > 1$) and film-dominated etching (where $R_{mR} < 1$). The relative etching profiles are reported schematically in Figure 4.59b and c.

In mask-dominated etching regime no under-cut is generated, while under-cut is still present in film-dominated etching regime. The so-called etching bias, defined in Figure 4.59, can be evaluated in both cases starting from the etch process parameters obtaining

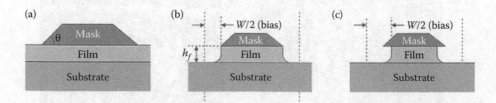

FIGURE 4.59 Etching of mask and film: wafer and mask before the etching process (a), etching result of a mask driven etching (b), and etching result of a film driven etching (c). The etching mask can be either photoresist after exposure, development and strong hardening (frequently using UV) or a previously selectively etched film, like SiO_2 over silicon.

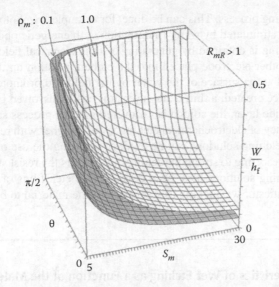

FIGURE 4.60 Bias to film thickness ratio versus etching selectivity and mask edge angle for different etching isotropy ratio on the mask inn the mask dominated etching regime.

$$W = \frac{2h_f}{S_m}\left(\frac{1}{\cos\theta} + \rho_m\right) \quad R_{mR} > 1 \tag{4.15a}$$

$$W = 2h_f\rho_m \quad R_{mR} < 1 \tag{4.15b}$$

In Figure 4.60, the ratio W/h_f is shown versus θ and S_m in a practical range of parameters in the case $R_{mR} > 1$ and isotropic mask etch ($\rho_m = 1$).

4.7.1.2 Wet Etching Equipments

The wet etching equipment is constituted by a chemical bath embedded in a machinery allowing both operators protection from chemical hazards and automatic wafer loading besides regulation of the process parameters. In large equipment, batch processing is possible by loading a set of wafers and leaving the machine to manage them one after the other.

The wet etching process is quite sensitive to a few process parameters that are specific of the individual equipment. The first of these parameters is the agitation of the bath. Agitation is generally performed to continuously renew the etching bath on the wafer surface, but the final etching result is quite dependent on the agitation parameters like frequency, continuous or discontinuous agitation, and so on.

In the case of crystal etching, mainly in the etching of silicon, part of this problem can be overcome by the use of suitable anisotropic etchant that by minimizing the lateral etching also minimizes the variability due to the effect of agitation. This is not possible when etching amorphous films such as glasses or polymers and a careful process calibration is needed for a good reproducibility.

The final etching result is also temperature sensitive and different equipment realizes the process at different temperatures.

Frequently, mainly when dealing with crystals, the wet etching process is supported by an electrical field that is generated in the etching bath. Such system is called electrochemical etching. Electrochemical etching requires positive charges (holes in semiconductors) in the wafer. Thus, while a p-doped silicon wafer can be used as it is, an n-doped wafer has to be inverted near the surface to allow the etching process. This can be done, for example, by photo-generation of positive charges near the surface stimulated by wafer illumination with energetic photons.

Electrochemical etching is obtained by generating a static electrical field between an electrode on the substrate and another electrode placed into the etchant solution on the floor of the etching bath. Holes are attracted at the surface of the wafer by the field and promote easy oxidation of the surface wafer layers. Once created, a thin oxide layer, it is easily dissolved by the etching solution; after etching the first oxide layer, the silicon is uncovered and the process starts again with oxidation. The etching efficiency of electrochemical etching is quite higher with respect to standard etching processes and mild etching solutions can be used, so allowing the use of simple photoresist as etching masks, without resorting to strong hardening that renders the resist stripping quite difficult.

Several different etching solutions have been developed to etch films of different materials. A review of the characteristics of wet etching as a function of the material to be etched is reported in Table 4.14.

TABLE 4.14
Review of the Characteristics of Wet Etching as a Function of the Material to be Etched

Material	Application	Etchant	Etchant Concentrations	Etching Rate (Vertical)	Notes
SiO_2	Microfluidics, integrated optics	HF	48%	20/2000 nm/min	Also Si substrate etched—0.3 Å/min for n-type with (111) wafer and E = 0.002 Ω m
SiO_2	Microfluidics, integrated optics	$HF:NH_4F$ (28 mL HF, 170 mL H_2O, 2113 g NH_4F)	28 mL–170 mL–2113 g NH_4F	100–500 nm/min	@25°C
Si (all planes)	General etching	$HF–HNO– CH_2COOH$	Volume 8%–75%–17%	5 μm/min	@25°C
Si (111)	Delineates defects	$HF–(5M–CrO_3)$	1:1		Needs agitation, do not reveal etch pits on (100) well
Si (100)–(111)	Delineates defects	$HF–HNO_3–(5M– CrO_3)–Cu(NO_3)– CH_2COOH–H_2O$	60 mL–30 mL–2 g– 60 mL–60 mL		Requires agitation
Si (100)	Heavy doped layers	$HF–(1M–CrO_3)– H_2O$	44%–22%–33% Volume		
Titanium	Metal definition	$HF–H_2O_2$		880 nm/min	
Tungsten		H_2O_2		20/100 nm/min	
Chromium		HCl–glycerine	1 mL–1 mL	80 nm/min	
Gold	Define contacts	$HCl–HNO_3$	75%–25% Volume	25–50 mm/min	Requires solution in aqua regia
Organic layers		$H_2SO_4–H_2O_2$		>1 mm/min	
Organic layers		Acetone		>4 mm/min	
Aluminum		$H_2PO_3–HNO_3– HC_2H_3O_2$		660 nm/min	40–50°C

Source: Adapted from Madou M. J., *Fundamentals of Microfabrication and Nanotechnology*, Third Edition, Three-Volume Set, CRC Press; 3rd edition (August 1, 2011), ISBN-13: 978-0849331800; With kind permission from Springer Science+Business Media: *Technology of Integrated Circuits*, Reprint of 2000 edition, December 15, 2010, Widman D., Mader H., Friedrich F.

4.7.2 Plasma Characteristics and Plasma Generation for Planar Processes

Wet etching has limits if used in transferring patterns from an etching mask. This happens especially when the film to be etched is a uniform, amorphous film like SiO_2, situation that is often characteristics of labs on chip micro-fabrication. In this case, only small deviations from perfect etching isotropy can be realized in a controlled way so that sharp shapes cannot be realized and the vertical dimension of the transferred path is always about equal to the horizontal dimension. In order to obtain vertical walls, high-aspect ratio shapes, and in general strong etching anisotropy, dry etching has to be used [1,87].

Dry etching techniques can be roughly divided into two categories: plasma-assisted dry etching and dry etching without use of plasma. In the first case, the etching is either obtained by a simple mechanical operation of high-speed particles of plasma incident on the film surface or via a combination of chemical and mechanical action. In the second case, purely chemical etching is realized, by means of accurately directed etching particles, so as to obtain a selective etching action.

PE is by far the most used form of dry anisotropic etching, so that plasma generation and processing is a key technology in designing dry etching machines.

This is one of several application of plasma in planar fabrication: plasma is also used in deposition processes (see Section 4.8.2), in wafer bonding processes (see Section 4.9.3), and even in few surface activation techniques. For this reason, before describing plasma dry etching, we will revise the plasma generation and management techniques that are applied in the field of microfabrication.

4.7.2.1 Plasma Characteristics and Generation

Plasma is defined as an electrically neutral medium made by chemically unbound positive and negative particles, generally positive ions and free electrons, even if also a plasma of negative and positive ions is conceivable [88,89].

Although the plasma particles are unbound, they do not constitute a sort of perfect gas; that is, they are not mechanically free. On the contrary, in order to talk about a plasma state, three conditions must hold:

1. *The plasma approximation:* When charged particles move they generate electrical currents and magnetic fields. In a plasma the charged particles density must be high enough that each particle influences many nearby particles so as to generate collective effects. These collective phenomena due to many body interactions are a distinguishing feature of a plasma. The plasma approximation is valid when the number of charge carriers within the sphere of influence of one of them is higher than unit.

    In a plasma, the sphere of electromagnetic influence of a single plasma particle is often called Debye sphere and its radius the Debye screening length L_D [90]. The average number of particles in the Debye sphere is given by the plasma parameter, generally indicated as Λ. This terminology is due to the affinity of classical plasma theory with the theory of electrolytes in a solution of neutral particles that we will review in some detail in Section 7.5. As a matter of fact, the definition of Debye length and Debye layer are completely analogous to the same definition in the electrochemical case and they can be found in Section 7.5.2.

2. *Bulk interactions:* In order to consider a set of charged particles a plasma, the Debye screening length has to be much shorter than the physical size of the plasma. This means that surface effects arising at the plasma boundaries through the creation of the Debey layer have to be negligible with respect to bulk effects and that the volume of the sphere of influence of a single charged particle, that is defined by the Debye layer arising around its surface, is negligible with respect to the whole plasma volume.

3. *Plasma frequency:* The electron plasma frequency, measuring plasma oscillations of the electrons [89] has to be large compared to the electron–neutral collision frequency,

measuring frequency of collisions between electrons and neutral particles. When this condition is valid, electrostatic interactions dominate over the processes related to ordinary gas kinetics.

The electron plasma frequency, when the thermal electron energy can be neglected with respect to their electrostatic energy, can be expressed as

$$f_{el} = \frac{1}{2\pi} \sqrt{\frac{\rho_e q^2}{m_e \varepsilon_0}} \tag{4.16}$$

where q and m_e are the electron charge and mass, respectively, and ρ_e is the electron density, that is generally called plasma density. Since the plasma frequency depends only on the plasma density and on physical constants the plasma frequency conditions can be simply reduced to a condition on the density of particles in the plasma. This is quite intuitive, since qualitatively it requires the plasma to be as far as possible from the condition of a perfect gas.

For plasma to exist, ionization is necessary to produce free charges. To characterize the effectiveness of the ionization process, besides the plasma density, the plasma ionization parameter α_p is introduced.

The plasma ionization is defined starting from the densities n_i of ions and n_a of the neutral atoms as

$$\alpha_p = \frac{n_i}{n_i + n_a} = \frac{n_i}{n} \tag{4.17}$$

where $n = n_i + n_a$ is the total number of particles containing a nucleus in the plasma. The plasma density and ionization are related by the ionization charge Z of the ions, indicating the number of electrons that each atom lost during plasma formation by ionization. In particular, it results

$$\rho_e = Z n \alpha_p \tag{4.18}$$

Another typical plasma parameter is the so-called plasma temperature, which is defined as the average energy of a free plasma electron. Generally, unless extremely violet phenomena are generated, that is not the case of artificially generated plasmas, the electron portion of the plasma can be described under a statistical point of view as a charged gas in a quasi-equilibrium state (see Section 1.2.1.4). In this situation, since a very high number of electrons are contained in a volume where statistical variables' variations are negligible, local thermodynamic potentials and variables can be defined, as the electron gas temperature. Local thermodynamic variables changes over macroscopic distances and times, depending on the plasma state. Moreover, the velocity electrons distribution can differ greatly from the Maxwell distribution due to external elements like UV fields, RF fields, or magnetic fields. Similar quasi-static approximations can be done for the ion population and the neutral atoms population, so defining relative local temperatures.

Because of the large difference in mass, the electrons come to thermodynamic equilibrium among themselves much faster than they come into equilibrium with the ions or neutral atoms. For this reason, the ion temperature may be very different, usually lower, than the electron temperature. This is especially common in weakly ionized technological plasmas, where the ions are often near the ambient temperature.

Based on the relative temperatures of the electrons, ions, and neutral atoms, thermal and nonthermal plasmas are defined. Thermal plasmas have electrons and heavy particles in thermal equilibrium, that is, at the same temperature. Nonthermal plasmas, however, have the heavy particles at a much

TABLE 4.15

Typical Ion Energy Requirements for Different Applications in the Field of Planar Technologies

Ion Energy (eV)	Planar Process
1–3	Physical absorption
4–10	Low-energy surface sputtering
10–5000	Sputtering
10,000–20,000	Ion implantation

lower temperature, frequently near room temperature, with respect to the much hotter electrons. On the ground of these definitions, a plasma is sometimes referred to as being hot if it is nearly fully ionized, so to have a high hot electrons density, or cold if only a small fraction molecules are ionized.

Plasmas used in dry etching processes are cold in this sense, even if the electron population is still at several hundred Celsius degree. Typical ions energy requirements for different applications in the field of planar technologies are reported in Table 4.15.

Since plasmas are very good conductors, electric potentials play an important role. The potential as it exists on average in the space between charged particles is called the plasma potential, or the space potential.

If an electrode is inserted into a plasma, its potential will generally lie considerably below the plasma potential due to the so-called Debye sheath, that is the plasma version of the Debye layer shielding that is present in electrolytic solutions. A Debye sheath arises when a conductive surface is inserted inside the volume occupied by the plasma. It is generated by the fact that electrons usually have a temperature on the order of magnitude or greater than that of the ions and are much lighter. Consequently, they are much faster than the ions. When a conduction interface is thus inserted into the plasma, electrons fly fast and absorb into it charging the interface with negative charges, while the surrounding plasma volume is charged positively due to the electrons lost. New electrons coming in near the surface due to diffusion of electrical attraction by local ions are reflected by the charged surface up to the moment in which an equilibrium is created.

In the equilibrium state there is a transition layer around the conducting surface, whose thickness is equal to the Debye length, comprises between the negatively charged surface and the overall neutral bulk plasma, where the plasma is positively charged. This transition region is called Debye sheath of Debye layer. Similar physics is involved between two plasma regions that have different characteristics; the transition between these regions is known as a double layer, and features one positive, and one negative layer (not to be confused with the double layer arising in electrochemical cells).

These and other similar effects result in the important concept of quasi neutrality of the plasma, that means that the plasma is overall neutral if a volume much greater than L_D^3 is considered, while locally, that is between points whose distance is of the order or smaller than the Debye distance, relevant potentials can be present.

Plasma with a magnetic field strong enough to influence the motion of the charged particles is said to be magnetized. A common quantitative criterion is that a particle on average completes at least one gyration around the magnetic field before making a collision, that is, $\omega_{ce}/\nu_{coll} > 1$, where ω_{ce} is the electron gyrofrequency [91] due to the magnetic field and ν_{coll} is the electron collision rate [92]. It is often the case that the electrons are magnetized while the ions are not. Magnetized plasmas are anisotropic, meaning that their properties in the direction parallel to the magnetic field are different from those perpendicular to it.

4.7.2.2 DC Glow Plasma Generation

Plasmas are generated by supplying energy to a neutral gas causing the formation of charge carriers. Electrons and ions are produced in the gas phase when electrons or photons with sufficient energy collide with the neutral atoms and molecules [93]. There are various ways to supply the necessary energy for plasma generation to a neutral gas. One possibility is to supply thermal energy, for example in flames, where exothermic chemical reactions of the molecules are used as the prime energy source. Adiabatic compression of the gas is also capable of gas heating up to the point of plasma generation. Yet another way to supply energy to a gas reservoir is via energetic beams that moderate in a gas volume.

The most commonly used method of generating and sustaining a low-temperature plasma for technological applications is by applying an electric field to a neutral gas. Any volume of a neutral gas always contains a few electrons and ions that are formed, for example, as the result of the interaction of cosmic rays or other radiations with the gas. These free charge carriers are accelerated by the electric field and new charged particles may be created by collisions with neutral atoms. This leads to avalanche of charged particles that is eventually balanced by charge carrier recombination, so that a steady-state plasma develops. In planar technologies, plasma is generated, for example in dry etching machines, mainly by using electrical fields: DC, pulsed DC, or RF and microwave frequencies. Nonthermal plasma in DC discharges is generally created in closed discharge vessels using interior electrodes, as shown in Figure 4.61 [90,93].

Low-pressure, normal glow discharges between planar electrodes in a cylindrical glass tube exhibit characteristic luminous structures as evidenced in Figure 4.61. The brightest part of the discharge is the negative glow, which is separated from the cathode by the cathode dark space (called "Crookes" or "Hittorf dark space"). The cathode dark space is a region of the discharge where the electrical potential drops drastically, as shown in Figure 4.61b. The negative glow is separated from the cathode dark space by a well-defined boundary and it is followed by a diffuse region in the direction toward the anode. The negative glow, where the electric field is close to zero, and the positive column are separated by the "Faraday dark space." The homogenous or striated positive column stretches all the way to the anode, which may be covered by a characteristic anode glow. The variations of plasma potential along the length of the discharge tube are shown schematically in Figure 4.61b.

The microscopic processes in such a discharge can be described as follows. A positive ion from the negative glow is accelerated by the electric field in the cathode fall and directed toward the cathode surface. The collision of the energetic ion with the surface produces secondary electrons, which are subsequently accelerated in the cathode fall to comparatively high energies. These energetic electrons transfer most of their energy to heavy particles like atoms or molecules in inelastic

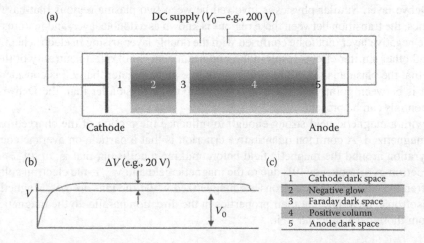

FIGURE 4.61 Schematic representation of the system for plasma generation via DC glow (a) and of the potential inside the void tube during the glow (b). Number labels from part (a) indicate the different plasma regions as reported in part (c).

TABLE 4.16

Minimum Breakdown Voltage (V_{min}) and the Product between the Gas Pressure P and the Discharge Chamber Length in the Direction of the Glow L for Various Gases

Gas	V_{min} (V)	$P\,L$ (kPa cm)
Ar	137	6.75
H_2	273	8.625
He	156	30
CO_2	420	3.825
N_2	251	5.025
N_2O	418	3.75
O_2	450	5.25
SO_2	457	2.475
H_2S	414	4.5

collisions. Such collisions generate excitation and ionization of the heavy particles primarily in the cathode fall and in the negative glow region thereby creating additional charge carriers [89,90].

The cathode regions of the discharge play a crucial role in sustaining the glow discharge. The positive column is formed only in the presence of a long, narrow discharge gap with charge carrier losses to the wall. In the homogenous positive column, a constant longitudinal electrical field is maintained. The electrons gain energy in this field and form an electron energy distribution with an appreciable number of energetic electrons that allows a sufficiently large number of ions and electrons to be generated and charge carrier losses due to walls absorption and recombination to be balanced. The minimum breakdown voltage needed to generate a glow and the product between the gas pressure and the chamber length in the direction of the glow are reported in Table 4.16 for various gases. These values are useful to have a first idea of the field and the pressures that have to be created to obtain and sustain DC generated plasma.

4.7.2.3 RF Plasma Generation

To generate the plasma both the cathode and the anode have to be conducting materials. Looking at Figure 4.61, it is clear that it is possible to exploit the high acceleration the ions undergo near the cathode hitting the electrode at high speed to generate dry etching. This is not, however, possible if the surface to be etched is not a conducting surface. As a matter of fact, if an insulating film is present upon the conduction cathode, the incoming ions are frequently captured into the insulating film by positively charging it. This creates near the cathode a positive film that tends to deflect other incoming ions and, at last, to extinguish the plasma. A possible solution to this problem, that is frequently adopted in dry etching systems, is to use alternate current.

If the polarity of the plasma generating field changes periodically, the ions that are absorbed in an half period by the insulating film to be etched are freed in the other half period, where the electrical field tends to launch them again into the plasma. Thus, if the variation frequency is sufficiently rapid, the screening effect due to charge absorbed into the insulating film can be made negligible.

Different system for plasma generation corresponds to different frequencies of the electrical field and from the way in which it is prevalently coupled with the plasma, exploiting a capacity of an inductive effect [93]. Capacity coupled RF plasmas are still the most common plasmas used in dry etching. The scheme of a typical reactor chamber for capacity coupled RF plasma generation is shown in Figure 4.62. The power is applied to the lower or the upper electrode. In general, the frequency of the applied field is 13.56 MHz. A so-called dark sheath is formed in the neighborhood of all surfaces in the reactor, electrodes, and walls. This dark sheath can be considered as some kind

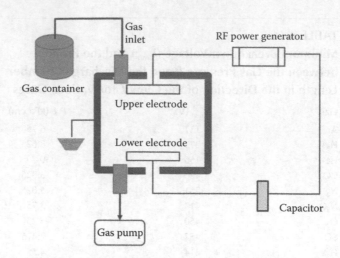

FIGURE 4.62 Scheme of a typical reactor chamber for capacity coupled RF plasma generation.

of dielectric or a capacitor, similar to what happens for Debye capacity in electrolytic cells. Thus, the applied power is generally considered as transmitted to the plasma through a capacitor.

At frequencies between 1 and 100 MHz, the free electrons are able to follow the variations of the applied electric field and, unless they suffer a collision, can gain considerable energy, of the order of some hundred eV. However, in this frequency range, the movement of the much heavier ions is very little influenced by these electric fields: their energy comes completely from the thermal energy of the environment and is of the order of a 0.01 eV so that the plasma is of the nonthermal type.

In the pressure range of these plasmas, from about 10 Pa to a few kPa, the electrons will travel much longer distances than the ions, and in this way, they will much more frequently collide with the reactor walls and electrodes and consequently be removed from the plasma. This would leave the plasma positively charged. However, in order to optimize etching by maintaining the plasma quasi-neutrality, a DC electric field has to be formed in such a way that the electrons are repelled from the walls.

The capacitor between the power generator and the electrode shown in Figure 4.62 helps to form the DC charge. During the first few cycles, electrons generated in the plasma escape to the electrode and charge the capacitor negatively. In this way, a negative DC bias voltage is formed on the electrode, which repels the electrons. The RF voltage becomes then superimposed on this negative DC voltage whose behavior is similar that typical of DC plasma generators. Thus, in the initial transitory electrons are absorbed in the electrodes and charged; this process arrives at an equilibrium when the field so generated repels other electrons avoiding the further capacitor charging and generating the DC field that maintain plasma quasi-neutrality and allows an efficient etching process to happen in the plasma chamber.

Although capacity coupled RF plasma generation is easy to design and control, it has also a certain number of limitations. The first limitation is that the reactive particle density is directly coupled to the ion energy. If a dense plasma is desired, rich in free atoms that are in general the particles which chemically react with the surface undergoing etching, the plasma is also rich in high energy ions. Moreover, to obtain high densities of reactive particles, the power in the plasma has to be increased. This increase of power will also increase ion density and energy. Increasing the pressure can increase the reactive particle density and decrease ion density and energy somewhat, but not to a great extent: in general, the effect of increasing the pressure is much lower than the effect of increasing the power.

Thus if highly reactive plasma is required, to attain a mainly chemical action with little bombardment, these types of plasma are not suitable. They will also not be very useful for the "inverse" type of plasma: a plasma with a low density of neutral and reactive atoms and a very high energetic ion density.

A second drawback is that it is not possible to generate plasmas at low pressures: typically, the lowest pressure at which a plasma can be sustained is of the order of 70 Pa. At lower pressures, there are not enough collisions to generate enough free electrons to sustain the plasma. Low-pressure plasmas are required in most advanced PE machines to obtain very high-aspect ratio structures. These can only be obtained if the ions collide with the wafer surface at a nearly perpendicular angle. To obtain this condition, little or no collisions should take place in the dark sheath, thus a large mean free path is needed. Therefore, the pressure must be reduced as much as possible.

In order to overcome these limitations, inductive coupling plasma generation can be used. There exist two types of inductively driven sources: using cylindrical or using planar geometries, as shown in Figure 4.63. The use of multipole permanent magnets is not indispensable, but their presence will increase the plasma density and mainly the uniformity of the plasma. An RF voltage is applied to the coil, resulting in an RF current which induces a magnetic field in the reactor. Therefore, the wall has to be a dielectric.

It is also possible to apply an extra (RF, low frequency, or DC) bias voltage to the substrate holder, as shown in both figures, to increase the ion bombardment on the substrate. This voltage is, in general, small and does not affect the plasma characteristics: the ions and electrons are mainly generated by the inductive coupling. In this way, it is possible to control independently the plasma density and the energy of the incoming ions. This gives the process engineer an extra parameter with which to optimize the process characteristics.

The preferred dielectric material for the reactor walls is alumina, which has excellent electric characteristics, is not etched by the most commonly used etchants, but is hard and expensive to manufacture. If no plasma is formed, the magnetic field generated by the coil, enters the etching reactor. If plasma is generated, an electric field can be formed in the reactor, because of Faraday's law. This electric field creates a current in the plasma, and the resulting total magnetic field will be null in the reactor. The absorbed power in the plasma is then proportional to the real part of the product of the current and electrical field vectors in the plasma. Ion densities of the order of 10^{17}–10^{18} ions/m^3 at pressures lower than 140 Pa, can be obtained in these discharges. This is one to two orders of magnitude higher than for traditional capacity coupled plasmas. However, an RF power of at least 100 W is needed to sustain the inductively coupled plasma.

Besides the inductive coupling, there is also a small capacitive coupling: the dielectric serves as the dielectric of a capacitor formed between the lower part of the coil and the plasma. At the high voltage end of the coil, RF voltages of the order of 2000 V have been measured. Therefore, a capacity coupled plasma is also formed. This capacitive coupling can help to strike and sustain the plasma. However,

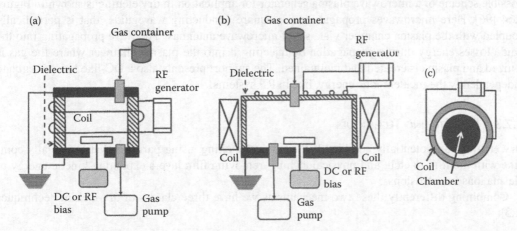

FIGURE 4.63 Schemes of the two types of inductively driven plasma sources: source with planar geometry (a) and with cylindrical geometry (b). A schematic top view of the cylindrical geometry system is represented in (c).

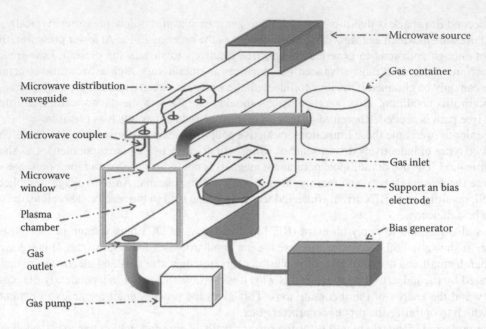

FIGURE 4.64 Scheme of a possible architecture for a microwave plasma generator.

a local DC voltage can be formed, which results in sputtering of the dielectric. The presence of dielectric material in the plasma can induce serious contamination on the wafer, or chemical changes in the plasma, and has to be avoided. Therefore, it is necessary that the dielectric plate is thick enough to reduce the capacitive coupling. Another way to decrease the capacitance of the coil is to place it a few millimeter above the dielectric, although this makes the manufacturing a little more difficult.

The principle of RF plasma generation can be extended also up in frequency to arrive to microwave frequencies. Microwave plasma generation is peculiar under various points of view. Microwaves have to be guided by some sort of waveguide to avoid dispersion of the microwave power. Thus, a simple structure like those represented in Figure 4.63 cannot be used. Several different structures have been implemented for microwave plasma generators [93–95], all operating in microwave resonant cavities under maser threshold and in traveling wave microwave guides. A possible scheme of a microwave plasma generator for application in dry etching is shown in Figure 4.64 [96]. Here microwaves propagate into a square conducting waveguide, that is periodically coupled with the plasma chamber via a set of microwave antennas. The wave propagating into the guide losses energy during propagation by injecting it into the plasma chamber where the gas is ionized and plasma is created and maintained. The support presents also a DC-like bias to regulate independently the incident ions energy, like in RF systems.

4.7.3 Dry Etching Techniques

Dry etching can potentially combine both chemical etching, using particles that chemically combine with the film to etch, and physical etching, removing film layers exploiting kinetic energy of plasma ions via collisions.

Combining differently these two mechanisms we have three classes of dry etching techniques [1,3]:

- Sputtering etching: purely mechanical
- Reactive ion etching: mixed chemical and mechanical
- Chemical dry etching: purely chemical

Depending on the etching machine architecture and on the used materials each dry etching family is composed of a great number of different techniques, sometimes simply different variations of the same base idea, other times exploiting completely different arrangements.

4.7.3.1   Sputtering Etching (Ion Milling)

The simpler form of dry etching technique is the sputtering etching, also called ion milling. This etching technique can be directly implemented by exploiting the fact that ions are accelerated in the dark zone around the cathode of a DC or RF glow so as to hit the cathode at high energy. Thus, if the wafer is placed on the cathode its surface is etched by incoming ions. A better control of the process, however, is attained by dividing the plasma generation and the etching process. In this case, ions are extracted from the plasma and focused as a beam on the wafer. This technique is also called ion beam etching.

A possible architecture of a sputtering dry etching machine using a combination of DC and RF plasma generation is reported in Figure 4.65. The plasma chamber is divided by the etching chamber: the plasma is generated in the plasma chamber by a circular inductive coupled RF plasma generator, the ions are extracted so as to obtain an ion beam that is focused in a different chamber on the substrate. Electrons are maintained out of the etching chamber by filtering them using conductive grids, vacuum in the etching chamber is maintained by a vacuum pump that also removes low-energy ions that either are scattered or do not hit the substrate. The target is exposed to the ion beam with a certain angle θ with respect to the beam average direction so as to have a further control variable to regulate the process. Due to its energy any incoming ion can extract one or more atoms from the surface of the wafer, so etching it.

Sputtering etching is purely mechanical and has generally good anisotropy characteristics. The typical profile of a pattern transferred from the mask to the underlying film via sputtering etching is reported in Figure 4.66. The angle that the etched area walls form with the vertical is due to the scattering of ions and extracted particles from the surface. Scattering takes place with a random

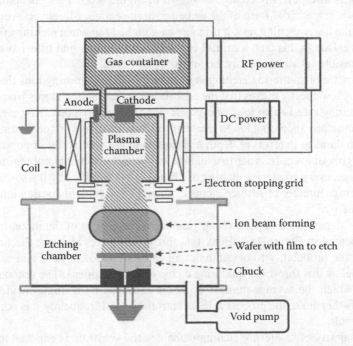

FIGURE 4.65 Possible architectures of a sputtering dry etcher that used both DC and RF plasma generation with separated plasma and etching chambers. An inductive coupled cylindrical plasma RF generator is used and electrons are maintained out of the etching chamber using a conductive grid.

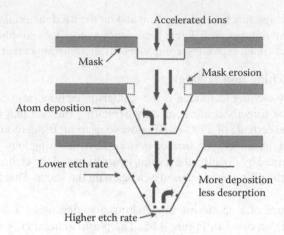

FIGURE 4.66 Schematic of the sputtering etching process evidencing the characteristic section of the etched pattern and the phenomenon of mask erosion.

deviation with respect to the vertical, causing both etching of the lateral walls due to deflected ions and deposition of deflected particles that build new layers on the wall itself.

The second phenomenon is by far prevalent with respect to the first since deflected ions have low energy due to the small collision angle. Since the deposition probability is higher if the impact energy of the deposited particles is higher, the phenomenon is greater near the bottom of the etched area, from which the characteristics form that is shown in Figure 4.66.

Sputtering etching is not very selective due to its purely mechanical nature. The first effect of this fact is that the etching mask, both in case it is constituted by hardened resist or by a protecting film like SiO_2 over Si, is also partially etched, as shown in Figure 4.66. This phenomenon contributes to the characteristic trapezoidal form of the etched pattern section. Moreover, even if generally the substrate has a quite lower etching rate, it is in any case etched too when etching arrives at the film–substrate interface. Due to this fact, a careful control of etching rate and time has to be maintained not to provoke sensible substrate damage below the etched area.

One key parameter of sputtering etching is the energy of the incoming ions that has to be carefully controlled. A low energy means that the probability for extracting atoms from the film surface is low and the etching rate is also low, or even etching does not happen. However, a too high ion energy causes almost any incoming ion to create an extended damage on the film surface. The characteristics of such damage in terms of depth and extension are practically impossible to control, so that etching is highly uneven. In order to avoid the two extreme detrimental regimes of no etching and surface damage, every sputtering etching machine is characterized by the so-called yield curve, providing the average number of surface atoms extracted by a single incoming ion versus the average ion impact energy.

An example of dependence of the etching yield from the energy of the incoming ions (argon in this case) is presented in Figure 4.67. Here, two thresholds are evidenced: the first is the threshold above which the probability to obtain an atom extraction is near zero and extractions almost never happens. Below this threshold sputtering etching do not happens. The second threshold is the threshold above which the average number of atoms extracted by a single incident ion is greater than 1. Above this threshold, the process is less controllable and frequently it is not possible to have a good etching result.

In the great majority of sputtering etching machines the substrate is exposed to the etching ion beam at a certain angle θ with respect to the beam axis (cf. Figure 4.65). This angle is another important control parameter of the etching process regulating in particular the etching rate. A typical behavior of the etching rate versus the substrate angle is reported in Figure 4.68. The yield, or

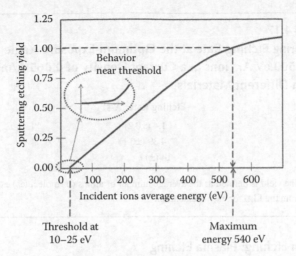

FIGURE 4.67 Example of yield of a sputtering etching process designed to etch (111) silicon after masking with UV hardened PMMA resist.

equivalently the sputter etching rate, varies from one material to another, but its fluctuations generally do not exceed one order of magnitude. Using Ar^+ ions with energies of the order of 500 eV the yield is generally of the order of 1, as shown Table 4.17, with the exception for Al_2O_3, that is, an extremely low etching material.

This fact causes the difficulty to provide a large difference of etching rate between the etching mask material and the film material to reduce the V shape of the etched form. Moreover, due to the dependence of the etching rate on the exposure angle, the lateral walls of the etching mask layer after the first etching phase are also etched at a different rate with respect to the underlying film, creating the facet effect, which is schematically shown in Figure 4.69a. This effect, besides the fact that the etched material also deposits after extraction from the film on the side walls of the etching mask, tending to form surface defects when the etching mask is removed (see Figure 4.69b), renders the achievement of high anisotropy pattern transfer and high flat surface after etching and mask removal difficult to achieve using sputtering etching.

These limitations are in great part overcome by the use of reactive ion etching, that is, a mixed physical and chemical form of PE.

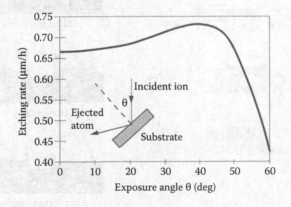

FIGURE 4.68 Example of dependence of the sputtering etching rate from the exposure angle. The definition of the exposure angle is reported in the insert of the plot.

TABLE 4.17

Sputtering Etching Rate at the Optimum Exposure Angle Using 500 eV Ar⁺ Ions at a Current Density of 0.065 A/m² to Etch Different Materials

Material	Etching Rate (Å/s)	Yield
Al_2O_3	1.4 ($\pm$0.2)	0.08
Si (111)	4.39 ($\pm$0.1)	0.54
GaAs	14 ($\pm$1)	0.76

Note: The yield is defined as the average number of atoms (or molecules) extracted from the film for each incident ion.

4.7.3.2 Reactive Ion Etching: Plasma Etching

Under the name of reactive ion etching several different techniques are collected, all of them having in common the use of plasma and the presence of a chemical etching effect on the surface of the etched film. Generally, the chemical etching effect due to neutral particles that are pushed by the plasma toward the wafer surface is combined with a physical etching effect due to bombardment with high-energy ions. However, PE is also widely used, where etching is uniquely due to chemical effect and the presence of plasma is only used to generate the etchant species and sometimes to enhance their chemical activity. The main reason to resort to PE is to avoid surface damages due to ions physical etching and contemporarily to avoid the use of very aggressive chemical etchants like those used in wet etching.

PE is generally composed by the following steps:

- The etchant species is formed by plasma in the plasma chamber.
- While the plasma is confined in the plasma chamber the neutral etchant diffuses through a neutral gas layer into the etching chamber and arrives to the wafer surface.
- Etching happens on the wafer surface due to the formation of a volatile compound by the combination of the etchant molecules and the superficial plasma film.

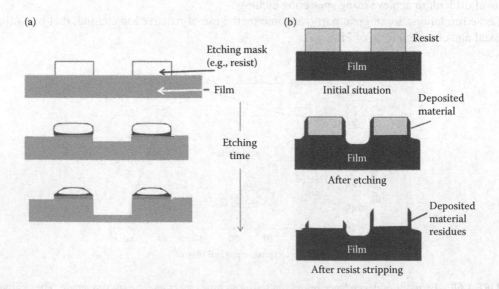

FIGURE 4.69 Facet effect (a) and side deposition on the etching mask (b) in sputtering etching.

- The volatile compound leaves the surface allowing deeper and deeper etching to be performed.

Two types of PE reactors are used: the first is very similar to the reactor shown in the previous section in the case of sputtering etching. Plasma is formed in a plasma chamber separated by the etching chamber. While plasma is confined by two separated sets of electrical charged rings into the plasma chamber, neutral elements that are meant to generate chemical etching are allowed to diffuse into the etching chamber where they arrive on the wafer surface. In this case, differently from the case of sputtering etching, the wafer is exposed to etchants diffusion horizontally, to optimize uniformity. The etching chamber is connected to the vacuum pump that both removes the results of the etching reaction and the unused etchant molecules, maintaining a low pressure in the etching chamber.

Besides this type of vertical reactor, the barrel reactor is also used for PE, whose principle scheme is shown in Figure 4.70. The reactor is formed by two coaxial cylinders: the inner cylinder is perforated to allow the diffusion of neutral particles and charged so as to confine plasma. Plasma is generated, generally by RF or microwaves, in the space between the two barrels, where also the gases that have to react to form the etching composite are injected. The inner cylinder allows the diffusion of neutral etching particles versus the inner part of the reactors, where a batch of wafers is present, while plasma is maintained in the space between the cylinders. A vacuum pump assures low pressure in the inner barrel at every moment of the process.

Since PE is a purely chemical etching it has the same isotropy properties of wet etching and the profiles of the etched patterns are quite similar to wet etching profiles.

A relevant effect in PE is loading effect. While in the case of wet etching the number of etchant particles is much greater that the number of particles of the film to be etched, this is not true in the case of PE. Here, the etching process depletes the etchants population causing two different effects called microscopic and local loading.

Macroscopic loading is because of the depletion in the etchant population due to the overall wafer etching. Due to this effect the etching rate is almost proportional to the area to be etched on the wafer. This also means that small variations in the etchant flux also cause a variation in the etchant rate, provoking an extreme difficulty in controlling process uniformity on similar wafers. The gas flow rate, generally of the order of 5–200 cm^3/min at standard conditions, is the most important parameter to be controlled in PE so as to assure uniformity. To prevent problems due to lack of etchant molecules, the gas flow utilization U is maintained generally greater than 0.1. The gas flow utilization is defined as the rate between the etching product formation rate and the inner gas flow rate.

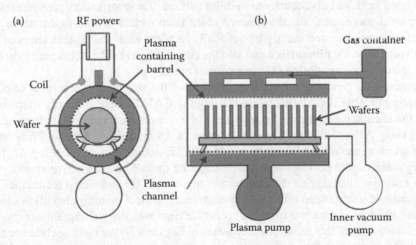

FIGURE 4.70 Principle scheme of a barrel reactor for PE: front section (a) and side section (b).

TABLE 4.18

List of Commonly Used Etchant for Different Materials in PE Reactors and Associated Etch Ratios in Å/min

Etchant	Material to Be Etched					Reference
	Si	Al	Resist	Quartz	SiO$_2$	
Ar	124	166	185	159		[1]
CCl$_2$F$_2$	2200	1624	410	533		[1]
CF$_4$	900	200	50	75		[1]
C$_2$F$_6$–Cl$_2$	600 (undoped)				100	[1]
CCl$_3$F	1670					[1]
CF$_3$CF=CFCF$_3$ [*]					5630	[97]
CF$_3$CF=CF$_3$ [+]					5380	[97]

Note: [*] indicates perfluoro-2-butene and [+] indicates hexafluoropropene.

Also, a local loading effect can happen, due to the nonuniformity of the etchant distribution on the surface of the same wafer so that larger etching areas are etched at a lower etching rate. This effect also has to be limited by a constant and sufficient gas flow during the etch process. A list of commonly used etchant for different materials and the associated etch ratios is reported in Table 4.18.

4.7.3.3 Reactive Ion Etching: Physical plus Chemical Etching

The most flexible and powerful family of dry etching processes is a combination of sputtering and PE, that is a combination of physical and chemical etching [1,98]. A first example of this type of process is the reactive ion beam etching (RIBE). In this case, the ions used to bomb the wafer surface are also reactive and colliding at high energy on the wafer surface combined with the etched film atoms generating volatile composites.

Even if RIBE can produce quite performing processes, more frequently mixed dry etching is realized using the chemically assisted reactive ion beam etching (CARIBE). In this case, ions are not reactive, performing a purely physical etching. Chemical etching is performed by another reactive composite diffusing in the atmosphere of the etching chamber. Frequently, ion bombing also increases the reactivity of the etched film surface by creating a cooperative effect with the chemical etchant. As a matter of fact, ion bombing, besides extracting atoms from the wafer surface, also provoke damages in terms of bond beak and dislocations in the film surface. These structures present exposed active sites and are much more reactive in the presence of the neutral etchant with respect to the film itself.

Since defects are generated mainly by vertically incident ions, the defects tends to be mainly vertical with respect to the film surface and also the chemical part of the etching tends to be strongly anisotropic, creating the possibility of strong overall anisotropy.

This characteristic generates a large improvement of the etch rate with respect of pure chemical or sputtering etching if CARIBE is used, being the CARIBE rate generally much higher than the sum of the chemical and the pure physical etching rates. As an example, sputtering etching of (111) silicon using Ar$^+$ ions reaches a rate of the order of 0.8 nm/min, while pure PE using chemical etchant can attain a rate around 0.5 nm/min. If CARIBE etching is used adopting Ar$^+$ plasma and neutral XeF$_2$ molecules to provide chemical etching, the overall rate can arrive up to a steady state value of 5.7 nm/min, much higher than the sum of the rates of the individual techniques [1].

The presence of a combined effect of physical and chemical etching also allows lateral etching inhibitors to be used, that are intended to further increase the etching anisotropy. A scheme explaining the working of this technique is reported in Figure 4.71: the etching chamber atmosphere contains, besides plasma and the chemical etchant, another composite driving the inhibition process. When particles of the film to be etched are extracted they combine with the inhibitor forming

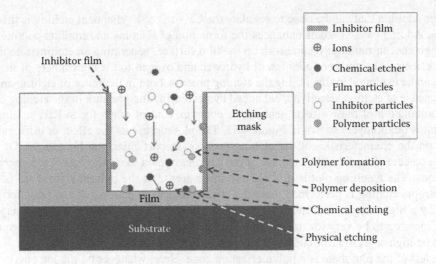

FIGURE 4.71 Inhibitor-driven anisotropy process scheme.

generally an inert polymer that deposits on the vertical walls of the etched area coating them with an inert polymer film. Due to this process, the chemical effect happens only on the horizontal surfaces and atoms or molecules extracted by the ion bombing cannot redeposit on the lateral walls due to the presence of the inhibitor film that does not absorb them.

The presence of the inhibition effect besides the natural anisotropy of the CARIBE allows high-aspect ratios to be achieved by this technique also with very small critical dimensions patterns. A typical example of inhibitor-driven anisotropy is provided by the addition of H_2 to a RIE process for Si etching by CF_4 plasma also causing chemical etching.

The bottom of the etched area results to be biased electrically by ions absorption while the lateral silicon is not biased due to the good focus of the ion beam realizing physical etching. Thus, a difference exists in the etching rate due to electrical bias between the bottom and the lateral walls, as shown in Figure 4.72a. Adding hydrogen to the etching chamber both the floor and the walls etching rates decreases at the same pace so that there is a well-defined hydrogen concentration at which the rate on the lateral walls is zero and the etching is ideally perfectly anisotropic, as shown in Figure 4.72b.

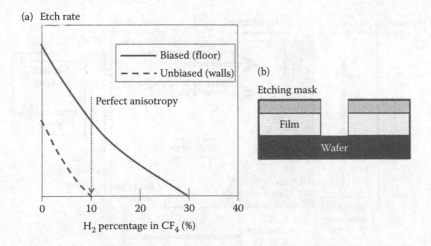

FIGURE 4.72 Hydrogen addition to Si RIE via CF_4 plasma. Effect on the biased (bottom of etched areas) and unbiased (walls of the etched areas) parts of the wafer (a) and perfect anisotropic etching result (b).

Another addition that can be done to regulate the CF_4-driven Si chemical etching is that of oxygen atoms. Adding oxygen atoms enhances the formation of F atoms and inhibits polymerization. At very high concentration oxygen absorb on the film surface, generating an etching rate decrease. Thus, the effects of a combined addition of hydrogen and oxygen to the atmosphere of the etching chamber can be exploited to fine tuning the etching process, both in the sense of etching anisotropy and in the sense of etching selectivity, enhanced by decreasing the pressure in the etching chamber.

The combination of these effects generates a complex control graph for Si RIE etching in CF_4 plasma that is qualitatively shown in Figure 4.73. The plot represents the effect of different control variables on the characteristics of the etching process. In particular, the H_2 and the O_2 addition effect are considered, besides the increase of the gas pressure on the wafer and of the energy of the incident ions. The resulting plot is divided into three areas: on the bottom right there is the area where isotropic etching is performed, here the chemical etching dominates and polymerization is inhibited by a high oxygen concentration. To make chemical etching dominant, the energy of the incoming ions has to be very low (or no incoming ions have to be present) and the pressure of the gas has to be high so as to favor chemical etching.

On the left of the plot there is a polymerization zone. Here, whatever be the ion energy and the gas pressure, a very high hydrogen concentration provokes a massive polymer formation that covers all the wafer, inhibiting etching. Naturally, higher the ions energy, higher the hydrogen concentration needed to reach this regime, so that higher the gas pressure, more efficient the polymerization process.

In the middle, between the two extreme regime, there is the RIE regime, where anisotropic etching happens due to a combination of physical and chemical etching. Chemical etching is favored by increasing the gas pressure, so that anisotropy decreases in this case. Similarly, physical etching is favored by increasing the ion energy so that in this case a more anisotropic etching is achieved. Anisotropy is also favored by hydrogen addition due to the inhibition-driven process and reduced by oxygen addition.

RIE Si etching is only a possible example of how the performances of an RIE can be tuned by regulating conditions in the etching chamber and composition of its atmosphere. Similar control charts exist for all widely industrial used etching processes, such as SiO_2 and Si_3N_4 RIE etching.

An example of strongly anisotropic RIE etching in SiO_2 is reported in Figure 4.74, where a SEM photograph of a grating excavated in SiO_2 by strongly anisotropic CARIBE is shown. The grating aspect ratio is 6.5 with a critical dimension of the order of 400 nm. The structure was defined by direct write e-beam lithography.

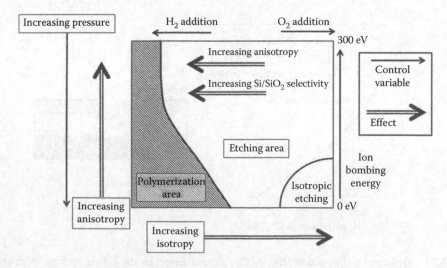

FIGURE 4.73   Control graph for Si RIE etching in CF_4 plasma.

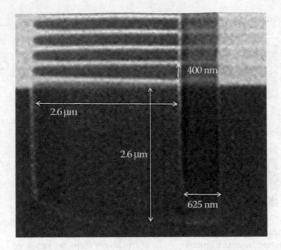

FIGURE 4.74 SEM photograph of a grating excavated in SiO$_2$ by strongly anisotropic CARIBE. The Grating aspect ratio is as high as 6.5 with a critical dimension of the order of 350 nm. The structure was defined by e-beam direct write lithography. (Published under permission of Cyoptics Inc.)

4.7.3.4 Deep Reactive Ion Etching

Deep RIE process is a variation of RIE whose goal is to generate structures with a very high-aspect ratio. In principle, RIE technologies are able to reach very high-aspect ratios, especially if physical etching is prevalent. However, a certain number of phenomena limits the maximum reachable aspect ratio. A first limitation is constituted by local loading. Even if this phenomenon in not so important in RIE as in PE, due to the contemporaneous presence of ion bombing, it is anyway present. If a great-aspect ratio is wanted local loading can become important.

If loading makes chemical etching less effective, physical etching is thwarted by the fact that the ion beam focus is not perfect. Increasing the etched trench depth, the probability that an incoming ion collide with the walls of the trench instead with the flood greatly increases. Walls collision generally do not generate walls etching, due to the small collision angle, but slower the ions rendering less effective the successive collision with the trench bottom. This effect is clearly shown in Figure 4.75, where the relative average ion beam energy generating etching on the trench bottom is shown versus the ion beam percent angle aperture and the trench aspect ratio. The ion beam is supposed to be a Gaussian beam, as it is frequently true. It is clear that increasing the trench aspect ratio the effectiveness of the physical etching decreases rapidly reaching very small values.

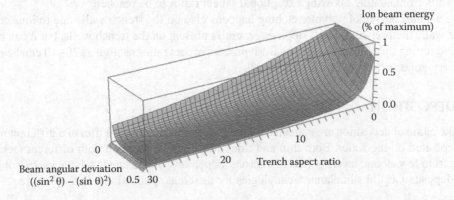

FIGURE 4.75 Relative average ion beam energy generating etching on the trench bottom is shown versus the ion beam percent angle aperture and the trench aspect ratio. The ion beam is supposed to be a Gaussian beam.

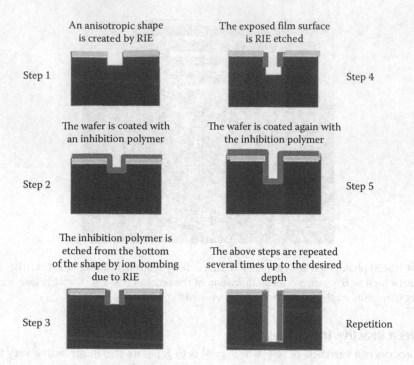

FIGURE 4.76 Scheme of the Bosh DRIE etching process.

The effect is still worse if hydrogen is added to the etching chamber atmosphere, since by decreasing the energy of the ion beam, the risk of entering the polymerization zone and completely inhibiting the etching is higher.

The capability of RIE to achieve high-aspect ratios can be improved by improving the quality of the ion beam (the focus in particular) and increasing pressure of the chemical etchant However, if very high-aspect ratios like 20 or 30 have to be attained, the process has to be changed more radically.

RIE processes modified for high-aspect ratios are called deep RIE or DRIE. The most diffused DRIE process is the so-called Bosh process, from the industry that patented it. The scheme of the Bosh DRIE etching is reported in Figure 4.76. This process is based on a succession of polymer deposition, polymer etching, and trench deepening. Since the polymer is etched only by ion bombing while it is inert to the chemical etchant, it is consumed only on the trench floor and protect the trench walls from etching allowing exceptional aspect ratios to be reached.

Since a small degree of polymer etching happens also on the trench walls due to ions colliding with the walls themselves, a small ripple is generally present on the trench walls, but it can be well-controlled tuning the process. Using the Bosh process aspect ratios as high as 20–40 can be reached with a very good verticality of the trench walls.

4.8 DEPOSITION

Under the name of deposition are collected all the processes that allows a film of a different material to be deposited on the wafer. Both thin and thick films can be realized with different techniques, starting from few atomic layers to tens of microns, depending on the need. A large variety of materials are deposited as films in planar technologies for different applications. Examples are

- Semiconductors as Si, for example, in SOI wafer realization, SiN_4, and many others
- Inorganic insulating films such as sapphire and SiO_2 with different doping

- Metals such as gold, platinum, aluminum, and copper
- Polymers such as SU8, PDMS, PMMA, and many others

Essentially, we can classify deposition techniques into three classes [1,3]:

- Chemical deposition techniques, where the film is formed by a surface chemical reaction between the wafer material and a suitable reagent
- Physical deposition techniques, where the film material is directly deposited on the surface of the wafer in its final form
- Molecular deposition techniques, where the physical deposition is controlled at molecular level so as to have a very fine control of the thickness and uniformity of the deposited film

Both chemical and physical deposition techniques can be plasma enhanced, if plasma is used to improve either the film quality control or the deposition rate.

4.8.1 Chemical Vapor Deposition

Chemical deposition is generally performed using a reagent in vapor phase; hence called chemical vapor deposition (CVD) [99,100]. Almost all types of layers can be produced by CVD; crystals, synthetic diamantes are manufactured by CVD too, so also amorphous and epitaxial.

An epitaxial film is a crystal film that is deposited on a crystal substrate in such a way as to match the two interfacing crystal planes to minimize stresses at the interfaces. The film thus grows following the substrate crystal structure and only in case of very thick films slowly relax on the standalone crystal structure. This, unless the film is made of the substrate material. In this case a continuous crystals formed by the so-called homo-epitaxy. Epitaxial films grow along preferential crystal directions depending on the crystal structures of the film and of the substrate and require similar structures of the two crystals [101–103]. Typical epitaxial growths are GaAlAs on a GaAs substrate or InGaAsP over an InP substrate, but many other examples are used in micro-fabrication technology.

A wide variety of CVD processes exists, that differ by the way the reaction is initiated and by the condition under which reaction is performed.

4.8.1.1 CVD Process Types and CVD Reactors

Considering the operating pressure, CVD processes can be classified as follows:

- *Atmospheric pressure CVD (APCVD)*—CVD processes performed at atmospheric pressure. Reactors for APCVD are generally made by a continuous wafer flow under a set of gas dispersers. The temperature of the wafer is either stabilized at the clean room temperature, or set at an higher value to enhance the deposition rate. Depending on the presence of a single gas dispenser or of a set of subsequent dispensers the APCVD reactors can be classified as gas injection or plenum-type reactor as shown schematically in Figure 4.77. In both cases, when more than one reagent is needed, an inert gas separation is used to avoid reagent mixing in gaseous phase.

  Several types of APCVD process exist, depending on the characteristics of the used vapor and on the structure of the vapor preparation unit. For example, in an APCVD based on aerosol vapor, the vapor preparation unit is composed of an aerosol generator.
- *Low-pressure CVD (LPCVD)*—CVD processes at low pressures [104]. Reduced pressures tend to reduce unwanted gas-phase reactions and improve film uniformity across the wafer. Reactors for LPCVD use vacuum pumps to lower the pressure in the deposition chamber and to remove unused chemicals. A widely used reactor architecture is the barrel-type architecture that is shown in Figure 4.78. The barrel-type LPCVD reactor can be charged with containers that can accommodate many wafers and are suitable for large batches.
- *Ultrahigh vacuum CVD (UHVCVD)*—CVD processes at a very low pressure, typically below 10^{-6} Pa. Most CVD processes used in high-volume fabrication are either LPCVD or UHVCVD.

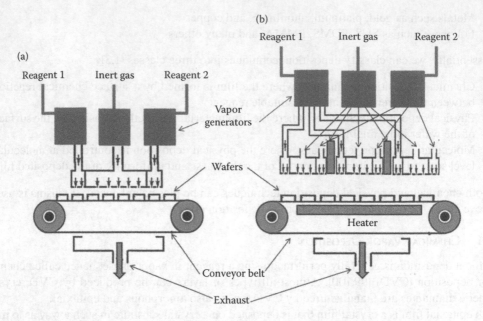

FIGURE 4.77   Gas injection (a) and plenum type (b) APCVD reactors schemes.

As far as the physical characteristic of the vapor used for the deposition we can individuate three CVD classes:

- CVD using neutral vapor
- Plasma-assisted CVD
- Other CVD types

These three families of CDV techniques collect several processes that differ in the way in which deposition is performed. The most used of these processes can be classified as follows.

4.8.1.1.1   Neutral Vapor-Based CVD Techniques

- *Aerosol-assisted CVD (AACVD)* is a CVD process in which the reagents are transported to the substrate by means of a liquid/gas aerosol, which can be generated ultrasonically. This technique is suitable for use with nonvolatile reagents.

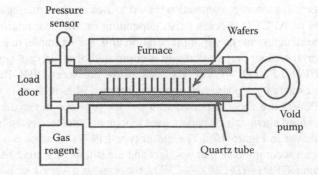

FIGURE 4.78   Barrel type LPCVD architecture using the so called hot-walls system to create high temperature inside the deposition chamber.

- *Direct liquid injection CVD (DLICVD)* is a CVD process in which the reagents are either in liquid form or solid dissolved in a convenient solvent. Liquid solutions are injected in a vaporization chamber toward injectors. Then, the vapors containing the reagents are transported to the substrate as in classical CVD process. This technique is suitable for use on liquid or solid precursors. High growth rates can be reached using this technique.

4.8.1.1.2 Plasma-Enhanced Methods

Somehow these methods are similar to the PE methods, but for the fact that ion energy is not sufficient to generate sensible etching of the wafer surface and the chemical reaction happening in the chamber do not generate volatile composite, but solid composites that deposits on the wafer surface creating a superficial film.

The most important advantage of plasma-enhanced CVD is the possibility to perform deposition at lower temperatures due to the fact that the plasma enhances the chemical reactivity of the CVD reagents.

As a matter of fact, even if the ions energy is not sufficient to provoke sensible etching of the wafer surface, it produces local defects and break chemical bonds on the wafer surface. This exposes reactive sites on the surface, rendering the reaction that gives rise to the film formation much faster. As in the case of dry etching (see Section 4.8.2), plasma can be created by DC, RF or by microwave. When plasma is generated by microwave, the deposition method is often called microwave plasma-assisted CVD (MPCVD).

Essentially, two types of plasma-enhanced CVD method exist, depending on the structure of the CVD reactor:

- *Plasma-enhanced CVD (PECVD)* is the name generally used for the technique using a simple glow reactor with the wafer where the film has to grow placed on the cathode. This method uses the fact that ions are accelerated mainly in the dark region around the cathode to generate an ion flux versus the wafer surface. The chemical reaction can happen either because the ions are directly chemically active or by insertion of an external reagent.

  An example of PECVD reactor scheme is reported in Figure 4.79. Here, the plasma is created via capacity coupled RF power and assisted by a DC bias. The wafer is on the plasma chamber cathode and two gas reagents different from the plasma particles are injected at controller pressures in the chamber. To avoid unwanted etching, the plasma is controlled via a control grid that is connected to the electrical ground.

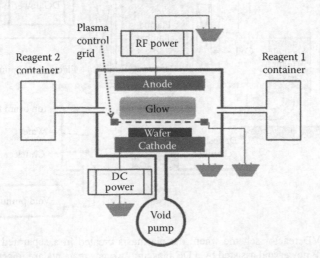

FIGURE 4.79 PECVD reactor scheme where the plasma is created via capacity coupled RF power and assisted by a DC bias and two gas reagents are injected at controller pressures in the CVD chamber.

- *Remote plasma-enhanced CVD (RPECVD)* uses reactors similar to that used in RIE where the CVD chamber is separated by the plasma chamber and an ion beam is extracted from the plasma chamber to be used in the CVD process besides the chemical precursor needed for the film growth, if it does not coincides with the plasma material itself.

  An example of RPECVD reactor scheme is reported in Figure 4.80. Here, the plasma is created via capacity inductively coupled RF power and assisted by a DC bias in a separated plasma chamber. An ion beam is derived by the plasma glow and focused on the wafer in the deposition chamber where two gas reagents are injected at controller pressures in the chamber.

  In similar reactors, if the plasma ions are of the same type of material to be deposited, or in a few cases if impurities have to be included in the film, sputtering (see Section 4.9.3.1) can be performed in parallel to RPECVD by allowing ion bombing of the wafer surface.

4.8.1.1.3 Other Types of CVD Techniques

- *Atomic layer CVD (ALCVD)* deposits successive layers of different substances to produce layered, crystalline films. ALCVD introduces two complementary reagents alternatively into the reaction chamber. Typically, one of the reagents will adsorb onto the substrate surface until it saturates the surface and further growth cannot occur until the second reagent is introduced. Thus, the film thickness is controlled by the number of reagent cycles rather than the deposition time as is the case for conventional CVD processes. ALCVD allows for extremely precise control of film thickness and uniformity.
- *Combustion chemical vapor deposition (CCVD)* is an open-atmosphere, flame-based technique for depositing high-quality thin films. In the CCVD process, a precursor compound, usually a metal-organic compound or a metal salt, is added to the burning gas. The flame is moved closely above the surface to be coated while wafers slowly pass through the deposition zone. The high energy within the flame converts the precursors into highly

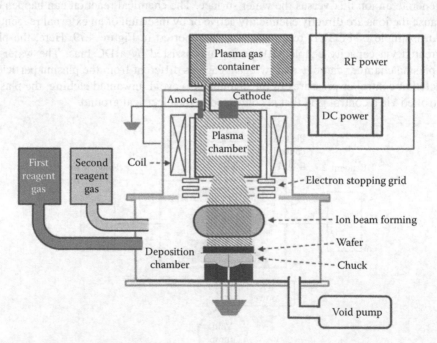

FIGURE 4.80 PECVD reactor scheme where the plasma is created in a separated plasma chamber via inductively coupled RF power and assisted by a DC bias and two gas reagents are injected at controller pressures in the deposition chamber.

reactive intermediates, which readily react with the substrate, forming a firmly adhering deposit. The microstructure and thickness of the deposited layer can be controlled by varying process parameters such as speed of substrate or flame, number of passes, substrate temperature, and distance between flame and substrate. CCVD can produce layers less than 10 nm thick.

- *Hot-wire CVD (HWCVD)*—also known as catalytic CVD (Cat-CVD) or hot filament CVD (HFCVD) uses a hot filament to chemically decompose the source gases.
- *Metalorganic chemical vapor deposition (MOCVD)* is a chemical vapor deposition method of epitaxial growth of materials, especially compound semiconductors, from the surface reaction of organic compounds or metal organics and hydrides containing the required chemical elements. For example, indium phosphide could be grown in a reactor on a substrate by introducing trimethylindium $((CH_3)_3In)$ and phosphine (PH_3). Formation of the epitaxial layer occurs by final pyrolysis of the constituent chemicals at the substrate surface. In contrast to molecular beam epitaxy (MBE) the growth of crystals by MOCVD is by chemical reaction and not physical deposition. This takes place not in a vacuum, but from the gas phase at moderate pressures (2–100 kPa). As such, this technique is preferred for the formation of devices incorporating thermodynamically metastable alloys, and it has become a major process in the manufacture of optoelectronic active devices like lasers and semiconductor amplifiers.
- *Hybrid physical–chemical vapor deposition (HPCVD)* is a thin-film deposition technique that combines physical vapor deposition (PVD, see Section 4.9.2) with CVD. For example, to grow magnesium diboride (MgB_2) thin film, HPCVD process uses diborane (B_2H_6) as gas reagent, but unlike conventional CVD which only uses gaseous sources, the Mg source is constituted by heated bulk magnesium pellets. Since the process involves chemical decomposition of precursor gas and physical evaporation of metal bulk, it is named as hybrid physical–chemical vapor deposition.
- *Rapid thermal CVD (RTCVD)* is a CVD process that uses heating lamps or other methods to rapidly heat the wafer substrate. Heating only the substrate rather than the gas or chamber walls helps reduce unwanted gas phase reactions that can lead to particle formation.

A synopsis of the characteristics of different CVD processes is reported in Table 4.19.

4.8.1.2 CVD Deposition of Different Materials

A great number of different materials are deposited via CVD in planar technologies. Each deposition receipt exploits a different chemical reaction or reaction chain to achieve the film of the wanted material with the wanted characteristics. In this section, a list of basic chemical receipts regarding common materials deposited in different planar technology fabrications is reported.

4.8.1.2.1 Polysilicon

Polycrystalline silicon is deposited from silane (SiH_4), using the following reaction:

$$SiH_4 \rightarrow Si + 2H_2 \tag{4.19}$$

This reaction is usually performed in LPCVD systems, with either pure silane feedstock, or a solution of silane with 70–80% nitrogen. Temperatures between 600°C and 650°C and pressures between 25 and 150 Pa yield a growth rate between 10 and 20 nm/min. An alternative process uses a hydrogen-based solution. The hydrogen reduces the growth rate, but the temperature is raised to 850°C or even 1050°C to compensate this effect. Doped polysilicon may be grown directly using CVD, if gases such as phosphine, arsine, or diborane are added to the CVD chamber. Diborane increases the growth rate, but arsine and phosphine decrease it.

TABLE 4.19

Synopsis of the Characteristics of Different CVD Processes

Process	Advantages	Disadvantages	Applications	Pressure	Temperature	Deposition Rate (SiO_2)	Epitaxy Rate
APCVD	Simple, high rate, low temperature	Poor step coverage, particle contamination	Thick oxides	10–100 kPa	250–450°C	700 Å/min	
LPCVD	Purity, uniformity, conformable step coverage, large batch capacity	High temperature, low rate	Oxides, silicon nitride, polysilicon, W, WSi_2	100 Pa	550–650°C	150 Å/min (from TEOS)	48 nm/min (Si on Si [105])
ULPCVD			Epitaxy and crystal films	1.3 Pa	550–650°C	—	137 nm/min (Si on Si [105])
LP-MOCVD	Very good epitaxy on large areas	High toxic and very expensive materials	Compound semiconductors (e.g., GaAs, InAsP, InGa AsP), quantum wells	100 Pa	800–1200°C	—	24–36 nm/min (InGaAsP on InP [106])
PECVD	Low temperature, high rate, good adhesion, good step coverage	Chemical and particle contamination, plasma damage	Insulators over metal, passivation films	266–650 Pa	200–600°C	3000 Å/min [107]	—

Source: Data from Madou M. J., *Fundamentals of Microfabrication and Nanotechnology*, Third Edition, Three-Volume Set, CRC Press; 3rd edition (August 1, 2011), ISBN-13: 978-084931800; With kind permission from Springer Science+Business Media: *Technology of Integrated Circuits*, Reprint of 2000 edition, December 15, 2010, Widman D., Mader H., Friedrich F.

4.8.1.2.2   Silicon Dioxide

Silicon dioxide (SiO_2) may be deposited by several different processes. Common source gases include silane and oxygen, dichlorosilane ($SiCl_2H_2$) and nitrous oxide (N_2O), ortetraethylorthosilicate (TEOS; $Si(OC_2H_5)_4$). The reactions are as follows:

$$SiH_4 + O_2 \rightarrow SiO_2 + 2H_2 \tag{4.20a}$$

$$SiCl_2H_2 + 2N_2O \rightarrow SiO_2 + 2N_2 + 2HCl \tag{4.20b}$$

$$Si(OC_2H_5)_4 \rightarrow SiO_2 + \text{by-products} \tag{4.20c}$$

The choice of source gas depends on the thermal stability of the substrate; for instance, aluminum is sensitive to high temperature. Silane deposits between 300°C and 500°C, dichlorosilane at around 900°C, and TEOS between 650°C and 750°C, resulting in a layer of *low-temperature oxide* (LTO). However, silane produces a lower-quality oxide than the other methods (lower dielectric strength, for instance), and it deposits nonconformal.

Any of these reactions may be used in LPCVD, but the silane reaction is also done in APCVD. CVD oxide has lower quality than thermal oxide, but thermal oxidation can only be used in the earliest stages of IC manufacturing, not to ruin other process results with high temperature. Doped oxide may also be directly grown with LPCVD, for example, to tune its refraction index in the fabrication of optical waveguides.

Another use of doped dioxide is indirect doping of lower layers during further process steps that occur at high temperature. In this case, the impurities may diffuse from the oxide into adjacent layers and dope them. Oxides containing 5–15% impurities by mass are often used for this purpose. In addition, silicon dioxide alloyed with phosphorus pentoxide ("P-glass") can be used to smooth out uneven surfaces. P-glass softens and reflows at temperatures above 1000°C. This process requires a phosphorus concentration of at least 6%, but concentrations above 8% can corrode aluminum. Phosphorus is deposited from phosphine gas and oxygen:

$$4PH_3 + 5O_2 \rightarrow 2P_2O_5 + 6H_2 \tag{4.21}$$

Besides these intentional impurities, CVD oxide may contain by-products of the deposition process. TEOS produces a relatively pure oxide, whereas silane introduces hydrogen impurities, and dichlorosilane introduces chlorine.

Lower temperature deposition of silicon dioxide and doped glasses from TEOS using ozone rather than oxygen has also been exploited (350–500°C). Ozone glasses have excellent conformality but tend to be hygroscopic: they absorb water from the air due to the incorporation of silanol (Si-OH) in the glass.

4.8.1.2.3   Silicon Nitride

Silicon nitride is often used as an insulator and chemical barrier in manufacturing integrated circuits. The following two reactions deposit nitride from the gas phase:

$$3SiH_4 + 4NH_3 \rightarrow Si_3N_4 + 12H_2 \tag{4.22a}$$

$$3SiCl_2H_2 + 4NH_3 \rightarrow Si_3N_4 + 6HCl + 6H_2 \tag{4.22b}$$

Silicon nitride deposited by LPCVD contains up to 8% hydrogen. It also experiences strong tensile stress, which may crack films thicker than 200 nm. However, it has higher resistivity and dielectric strength than most insulators commonly available in micro-fabrication (about 10^{16} Ω cm and 10 MV/cm, respectively).

Another two reactions may be used in plasma to deposit SiNH:

$$2SiH_4 + N_2 \rightarrow 2SiNH + 3H_2 \tag{4.23a}$$

$$SiH_4 + NH_3 \rightarrow SiNH + 3H_2 \tag{4.23b}$$

These films have much less tensile stress, but worse electrical properties (resistivity from 10^6 to 10^{15} Ω cm, and dielectric strength from 1 to 5 MV/cm).

4.8.1.2.4 *Metals*

Some metals (notably aluminum and copper) are seldom or never deposited by CVD. However, CVD processes for molybdenum, tantalum, titanium, nickel, and tungsten are widely used. These metals can form useful silicides when deposited onto silicon. Mo, Ta, and Ti are deposited by LPCVD, from their pentachlorides. Nickel, molybdenum, and tungsten can be deposited at low temperatures from their carbonyl precursors. In general, for an arbitrary metal M, the reaction is as follows:

$$2MCl_5 + 5H_2 \rightarrow 2M + 10HCl \tag{4.24}$$

4.8.2 PHYSICAL VAPOR DEPOSITION

The family of physical vapor deposition (PVD) techniques collects all the thin film deposition processes based on condensation of vapor particles on the wafer surface [108,109]. Evaporation is the most common method of physical thin film deposition. The source material is evaporated in a vacuum; vacuum allows vapor particles to travel directly to the target substrate, where they condense back to a solid state.

At a typical pressure of 10^{-4} Pa, a 0.4 nm particle has a mean free path of 60 m [92]. Poor vacuum can produce hot objects in the evaporation chamber, such as heating filaments, thereby generating unwanted vapors that limit the quality of the vacuum. Moreover, evaporated atoms that collide with foreign particles may react with them; for instance, if aluminum is deposited in the presence of oxygen, it will form aluminum oxide. They also reduce the amount of vapor that reaches the substrate, which makes the thickness difficult to control.

Evaporated materials do not deposit uniformly if the substrate has a rough surface as integrated microfluidics circuits often do. Because the evaporated material attacks the substrate mostly from a single direction, protruding features block the evaporated material from some areas. This phenomenon is called shadowing and it is qualitatively illustrated in Figure 4.81.

The deposition rate in thermal PVD process is generally good especially for metals; for example, in the case of Al films, a typical evaporation rate is 0.1–0.5 μm/min.

Different evaporation methods exist, using different energy sources to obtain the target evaporation.

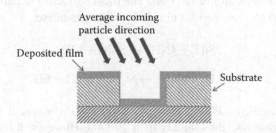

FIGURE 4.81 Schematic illustration of shadow effect in PVD.

4.8.2.1 Thermal PVD

In thermal PVD, a metal wire is fed onto a heated ceramic evaporator known as "boats" due to their shape. A pool of melted metal forms in the boat cavity and evaporates into a cloud above the source. Alternatively, the source material is placed in a crucible, which is radiatively heated by an electric filament, or the source material may be hung from the filament itself in the so-called filament evaporation.

Resistors designed to work as heaters in thermal PVD systems are made by materials with a very high melting temperature (T_m) so that high temperatures can be reached on the resistor surface without melting it. Typical resistors materials are tungsten (W, $T_m = 3380°C$), tantalum (Ta, $T_m = 2980°C$), and molybdenum (Mo, $T_m = 2630°C$).

Advantages of thermal evaporation is the simplicity of the related equipment and the low cost of the process, besides the possibility of shaping the process characteristics like the uniformity of the film and the coated area by simply changing the resistor and the target material forms and the vapor temperature.

A first problem of this technique is that evaporation of a small quantity of the resistor material at such a high temperature is not avoidable, so generating reactions between the film and the resistor materials in vapor phase and inducing pollution of the deposited film. This problem can be faced by coating the resistor with a ceramic layer that do not evaporate even at extreme temperatures, but this architecture exploits less effectively the resistor temperature due to the isolation nature of ceramic materials. Moreover, while metals are easily evaporated through thermal PVD, dielectric films are difficult to obtain since the evaporating temperature of isolators is too high. For example, the silicon oxide melting temperature is as high as 1703°C; in order to obtain such a high temperature on the target the resistor should be pushed too near to its melting temperature causing excessive resistor material evaporation. It is also difficult to deposit compound targets, since they may be decomposed by high temperature. Finally, the quality of film adhesion is poor with respect to other deposition methods.

Owing to these limitations, thermal PVD is used only in low-performance processes, where extremely good film qualities are not required and the cost of the process is a key issue.

A notable exception is the so-called thermal oxide layer that is generated by thermal oxidation on the surface of silicon wafers. In this process, evaporation of low-pressure oxygen provokes oxidation of the surface of the Si wafer generating silica. This technique is not suitable to deposit thick SiO_2 layers, due to the passivation role of the layer itself that above a certain thickness inhibits the further penetration of oxygen and the oxidation of the silicon substrate. Generally, layers up to 500 nm are grown in this way. However, under the point of view of uniformity, dielectric and optical properties and absence of embedded stress, thermal silica is superior to silica layers deposited with other techniques.

4.8.2.2 Electron-Beam PVD

In electron-beam PVD, high-speed electrons hit the target material, to create a high temperature on its surface and cause its evaporation. The electron beam is generally produced by an electron gun, which uses the thermionic emission of electrons produced by a tantalum cathode. Emitted electrons are accelerated toward an anode with very high speed. For example, at 10^4 eV energy electrons average speed is about 16.6 km/s; thus creating on the target surface a temperature in the range of 5000–6000°C.

The crucible which puts the target acts as the anode. A magnetic field is also applied to bend the electron trajectory. Avoiding the gun blocks the evaporation path. Via the control of the magnetic lens, similar to those used in an electron beam lithography equipment, the electron beam can be focalized and change its impact point on the target surface to obtain a very localized heating on the material to evaporate.

It also allows a precise control of the evaporation rate, from low-to-very high values. Most important of all, it could deposit the materials with high melting point such as W, Ta, C, dielectric

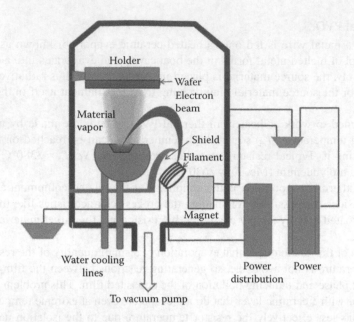

FIGURE 4.82 Schematic architecture of an e-beam evaporation PVD equipment.

oxide. Effective water cooling to crucible can avoid contamination problems inherent to heating and degasification of undesired material coming from the coater. A schematic representation of an electron beam PVD reactor is provided in Figure 4.82.

E-beam PVD produces films much purer with respect to thermal PVD, also because target contamination by the crucible particle evaporation is eliminated completely by water cooling of the crucible. Moreover, most dielectric oxide layers could be deposited by this method.

Multilayer depositions can be realized by disposing different crucibles into the deposition chamber and directing the electron beam toward one or the other depending on what layer is to be deposited, the fact that the electron beam has a small spot size, thus heating only a small part of the crucible surface avoids contamination completely between the targets devoted to different layers.

The film thickness can be controlled by both changing the electron beam spot size and its intensity, thus achieving a very good control. The film uniformity is also very good, since the film thickness can be controlled during deposition, for example, with interferometry methods and the electron beam illumination time over different wafer surfaces can be regulated on the run to maintain the better uniformity.

The only relevant source of contamination due to the deposition itself is the so-called x-ray contamination due to spurious x-rays generated by the electron source that can damage the deposited film during deposition.

4.8.2.3 Other PVD Techniques

In flash evaporation PVD, a fine wire of source material is fed continuously onto a hot ceramic bar, and evaporates on contact. This is accomplished by passing a large current through a resistive wire or foil containing the material to be deposited. The heating element is often referred to as an evaporation source. Wire type evaporation sources are made from tungsten tantalum, molybdenum, or ceramic-type materials capable of withstanding high temperatures. They can be formed into filaments, baskets, heaters, or point sources. Boat-type evaporation sources are more frequently made by tungsten.

Cathode arc deposition is a physical deposition technique based on the phenomenon of arc evaporation [110]. The arc evaporation process begins with the striking of a high-current, low-voltage arc on the surface of a cathode (the target) that gives rise to a small, usually a few micrometers wide, highly energetic emitting area known as a cathode spot. The localized temperature at the cathode spot is extremely high (~15,000°C), which results in a high velocity (10 km/s) jet of vaporized cathode material, leaving a crater on the cathode surface. The cathode spot is only active for a short period of time, then it self-extinguishes and re-ignites in a new area. This behavior causes the apparent motion of the arc.

As the arc is basically a current-carrying conductor it can be influenced by the application of an electromagnetic field, which in practice is used to rapidly move the arc over the entire surface of the target, so that the total surface is eroded over time. The arc has an extremely high power density resulting in a high level of ionization (30–100%), multiple charged ions, neutral particles, clusters, and macro-particles. If a reactive gas is introduced during the evaporation process, dissociation, ionization, and excitation can occur during interaction with the ion flux and a compound film will be deposited.

4.8.3 OTHER PHYSICAL DEPOSITION TECHNIQUES

There is a group of physical film deposition techniques that are not based on evaporation of the target, but have their specific principles. Here, we will describe plasma deposition, generally called sputtering, and MBE.

4.8.3.1 Physical Plasma Deposition (Sputtering)

As we have seen in Section 8.2, the generic term of sputtering indicates a process in which a target is bombed with high-energy ion coming from a plasma glow to extract particles from it. In sputtering etching the target is the film to be etched, in sputtering deposition, also called plasma-assisted PVD, the target is formed by the material to be deposited. The particle extracted from the target in this case travels through a low-pressure sputtering room up to the surface of the wafer and deposit on it forming the film to be deposited.

An important advantage of sputter deposition is that even materials with very high melting points are easily sputtered while evaporation of these materials in other PVD techniques is problematic or impossible. Sputtering can be used also to deposit composite films and the sputter deposited films have a composition close to that of the source material. The difference is due to different elements spreading differently because of their different mass. Due to the deterministic nature of this effect, this difference can be determined accurately and the target composition can be biased suitably.

Examples of materials that are frequently deposited by sputtering are [111–115]

- Metals (Al, Cu, Zn, Au, Ni, Cr, W, Mo, Ti)
- Alloys (Ag–Cu, Pb–Sn, Al–Zn, Ni–Cr)
- Nonmetals (graphite, MoS_2, WS_2)
- Refractory oxides (Al_2O_3, Cr_2O_3, Al_2O_3–Cr_2O_3, Y_2O_3, SiO_2, ZrO_2)
- Refractory carbides (TiC, ZrC, HfC, NbC)
- Refractory nitrides (TiN, Ti_2N, ZrN, TiN–ZrN, HfN, TiN–AlN–ZrN)
- Refractory borides (TiB_2, ZnB_2, HfB_2, CrB_2, MoB_2)
- Refractory silicides ($MoSi_2$, WSi_2, Cr_3Si_2)

Sputtered films typically have a better adhesion on the substrate than evaporated films. Sputtering sources contain no hot parts since to avoid heating they are typically water cooled and are compatible with reactive gases such as oxygen.

Sputtering sources are usually inductively coupled RF or microwave sources that utilize strong electric and magnetic fields to trap electrons close to the surface of the target. Because of the strong magnetic field due to inductive coupling, the electrons follow helical paths around the magnetic field lines undergoing more ionizing collisions with gaseous neutrals near the target surface than would otherwise occur [116].

The gas used to generate the plasma glow in sputtering systems is generally an inert gas, more frequently argon. Sputtering yield, or the number of atoms ejected per incident ion, is an important factor in sputter deposition processes, since it affects the sputter deposition rate. Sputtering yield primarily depends on three major factors:

- Target material
- Mass of the bombarding particles
- Energy of bombarding particles

In the energy range where sputtering occurs (10–5000 eV), the sputtering yield increases with particle mass and energy. A rage of typical sputtering yields for different materials when Ar^+ ions at 500 eV are used is reported in Table 4.20.

Different types of sputtering processes exist, depending on the sputtering conditions and the reactor structure. Two basic sputtering deposition processes are described here.

Ion-beam sputtering (IBS) is a method in which the sputtered target is bombed by an ion beam extracted from a plasma glow in an external reactor chamber, called sputtering chamber. Such reactors are also called Kaufman reactors. The source ions are generated in a plasma chamber, generally, via RF or microwave generation. Plasma electrons are confined in the plasma chamber while ions are extracted and accelerated by the electric field emanating from a grid toward a target.

As the ions leave the source they are neutralized by electrons from a second beam external to the plasma glow. Thus, the flux that hit the target is not composed of ions, but by neutral atoms so that either insulating and conducting sputtering targets can be used and no superficial charge accumulation on the target happens.

A pressure gradient between the ion source and the sample chamber is generated by placing the gas inlet at the source and shooting through a tube into the sample chamber. This saves gas and reduces contamination. The principal drawback of IBS is the large amount of maintenance required to keep the ion source operating [117].

Typical deposition rates that can be realized with ion beam sputtering deposition are reported in Table 4.21. A scheme of an ion beam sputtering reactor is reported in Figure 4.83; here, the secondary electron source used to neutralize the ion beam is evidenced, a target selection support is mounted to be able to alternate different targets to deposit composite films and a wafers rotating drum is present to process several wafers in the same batch.

In *ion-assisted deposition* (IAD), the substrate is exposed to a secondary ion beam operating at a lower power than the sputter gun. Usually, a Kaufman source like that used in IBS supplies the secondary beam. IAD can be used, as an example, to deposit carbon in diamond-like form on a substrate. Any carbon atoms landing on the substrate which fails to bond properly in the diamond crystal lattice will be knocked off by the secondary beam.

TABLE 4.20
**Typical Sputtering Yields for Different Materials
When Ar^+ Ions at 500 eV Are Used**

Target	Sputter Yields
Aluminum	1.05
Chrome	1.18
Gold	2.4
Nickel	1.33
Platinum	1.4
Titanium	0.51

Note: The sputtering yield is defined as the average number of extracted target particles per colliding ion.

TABLE 4.21
Sputtering Deposition Rate for Various Materials

	Deposition Rate (nm/min)	
Material	1 kW	3.5 kW
Al	18	63
Cu	34	119
Au	36	126
Ni	22	77
Pt	23	80.5
Ag	52	182
Ti	8	28
Ta	9	31.5

Note: An ion beam sputtering is considered and the rate is reported for different powers of RF source.

Besides this basic implementation, several variations exist to improve the target utilization [118], the reactor architecture [119], or to study the structure of sputtering generated films [119,120] and sputtering is still today one of the most used deposition techniques in micro-fabrication industry.

4.8.3.2 Molecular Beam Epitaxy

MBE is the better method today available to grow high crystal quality epitaxial layers. As such it is not of great importance in microfluidics circuits, but it is widely used to deposit epitaxial films of alloys such as InGaAsP or GaAsP that are used in active optical devices like lasers and amplifiers or in optical detectors [121–123].

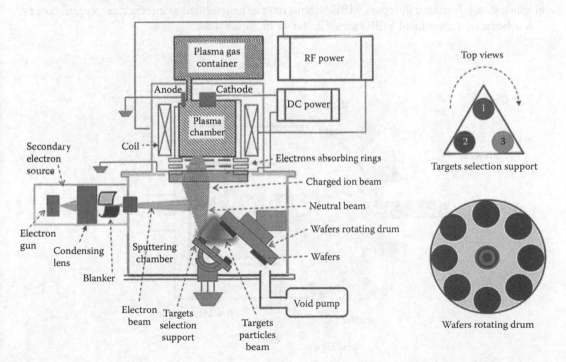

FIGURE 4.83   Scheme of an ion beam sputtering reactor.

MBE takes place in high vacuum or ultra-high vacuum (10^{-8} Pa). The most important aspect of MBE is the slow deposition rate (typically <20 nm/min), which allows the films to grow epitaxially. The slow deposition rates require proportionally better vacuum to achieve the same impurity levels as other deposition techniques.

In solid-source MBE, elements such as gallium and arsenic, in ultra-pure form, are heated in separate effusion cells until they begin to slowly sublimate. The gaseous elements then condense on the wafer, where they may react with each other. In the example of gallium and arsenic, single-crystal gallium arsenide is formed. The term beam means that evaporated atoms do not interact with each other or vacuum chamber gases until they reach the wafer, due to the long mean free paths of the atoms caused by the extremely low concentration.

During operation, reflection high-energy electron diffraction (RHEED) is often used for monitoring the growth of the crystal layers. A computer controls shutters in front of each furnace, allowing precise control of the thickness of each layer, down to a single layer of atoms.

Intricate structures of layers of different materials may be fabricated this way. Such control has allowed the development of structures where the electrons can be confined in space, giving quantum wells or even quantum dots.

In systems where the substrate needs to be cooled, the ultra-high vacuum environment within the growth chamber is maintained by a system of cryopumps, and cryopanels, chilled using liquid nitrogen or cold nitrogen gas to a temperature close to −196°C. Cryogenic temperatures act as a sink for impurities in the vacuum, so vacuum levels need to be several orders of magnitude better to deposit films under these conditions. In other MBE implementations, the wafers on which the crystals are grown may be mounted on a rotating platter which can be heated to several hundred degrees Celsius during operation.

MBE is also used for the deposition of some types of organic semiconductors. In this case, molecules, rather than atoms, are evaporated and deposited onto the wafer. Other variations include gas-source MBE, which resembles chemical vapor deposition.

Recently, MBE has been used to deposit oxide materials for advanced electronic, magnetic, and optical applications. For these purposes, MBE systems have to be modified to incorporate oxygen sources.

A scheme of a traditional MBE reactor is shown in Figure 4.84.

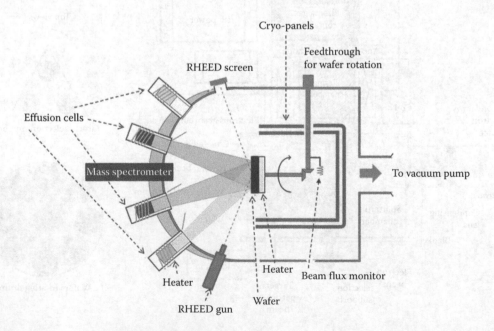

FIGURE 4.84　Scheme of a MBE growth chamber.

4.9   WAFER BONDING

In microfluidics-based labs on chip, one of the key elements in the circuit fabrication is the realization of closed chambers and ducts forming the microfluidic system. In the above sections we have seen that the standard procedure of planar technologies is not able to excavate closed areas below the surface of the wafer. On the contrary, open trenches or chambers can be created, that can be transformed into the elements that are needed in a microfluidics circuit by adding a top cover. The top cover can be realized by the technique of wafer bonding, consisting of superimposing two wafers one on top of the other, putting in contact and fixing the upper wafer surfaces.

This process was not created for microfluidics, but for MEMs and other applications requiring three-dimensional structures or closed rooms. Its application in microfluidics circuit is in any case almost obliged if standard planar techniques are to be adopted, so it became a key process in microfluidics-based labs on chip.

Several different techniques are adopted to realize wafer bonding, both in case of adhesion of crystal surfaces of the same or different materials and in case of adhesion of amorphous surfaces. In any case, the two surfaces to be put in contact has to be flat within a very small tolerance, due to the fact that lack of flatness, even by a very small amount, can completely ruin the bonding or create points of weakness causing later circuit failures.

This is the reason because planarization, that is, the process used to flatten the surface of a wafer after a fabrication cycle is a structural part of the wafer-bonding process.

Planarization was not originally introduced for microfluidics too, and it is still mainly used at the end of lithography processes to flatten the wafer surface, remove the uneven features that could be present due to resist stripping, and prepare the wafer for successive fabrication steps. When the successive step is a wafer bonding, the planarization requirements are quite tight and it is the reason why we have inserted the planarization process under the general cap of the wafer bonding technique.

4.9.1   PLANARIZATION

Planarization is not a process adopted only in planar fabrication, since several fabrication techniques need to flatten surfaces even at the nanometer level (e.g., optical lenses fabrication). A standard process used to obtain surface flattening is lapping, that if applied in successive steps can achieve a good degree of planarity. The main limitation of lapping process is the lack of selectivity that renders difficult to control the process if the underlying film has not to be consumed. Moreover lapping, due to the intrinsic need of lapping powder, imply a strong contamination risk that is difficult to control in a clean room where planar fabrication is performed.

This is the reason why, when a high degree of flattening and absence of contamination are needed, planarization is performed generally with the chemical–mechanical planarization (CMP) process [124,125]. Typical CMP tools, such as the ones represented in Figure 4.85, consist of a rotating and extremely flat platen which is covered by a pad. The wafer that is being polished is mounted upside-down in a carrier/spindle on a backing film. The retaining ring keeps the wafer in the correct horizontal position. During the process of loading and unloading the wafer onto the tool, the wafer is held by vacuum by the carrier to prevent unwanted particles from building up on the wafer surface.

A slurry introduction mechanism deposits the slurry on the pad. Both the platen and the carrier are then rotated and the carrier is kept oscillating as well. A downward pressure/down force is applied to the carrier, pushing it against the pad. The required amount of down force depends on the contact area which, in turn, is dependent on the structures of both the wafer and the pad. Typically, the pads have a roughness of 50 μm; contact is made by asperities, which typically are the high points on the wafer, and, as a result, the contact area is only a fraction of the wafer area.

The base mechanism of CMP is shown in Figure 4.86. The slurry has a chemical action that softens the surface of the wafer to be flattened. The inhomogeneous structure of the polishing pad

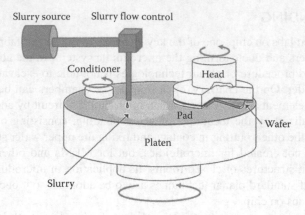

FIGURE 4.85   Scheme of a CMP (chemical mechanical planarization) equipment.

and the presence of abrasive particles tend to consume the surface of the wafer efficiently since it is so softened. Since adhesion of the wafer to the polishing pad happens first and with a higher pressure when an asperity is present, asperities are more efficiently consumed and the film is flattened. Moreover, the softening chemical reaction is selective, thus if a layer of a different material is found, it is not softened and the flattening effect is negligible.

Typically, SiO_2 films are flattened by softening them by hydration through the following reaction:

$$SiO_2 + H_2O \rightleftharpoons Si(OH)_4 \tag{4.25}$$

This reaction, breaks the Si–O bonds and softens the film. Besides allowing effective ablation, it also permits, in case it is needed, further chemical etching using a KOH solution. Thus, frequently, a very low-concentration KOH solution is adopted by allowing hydration and successive mixed ablation and chemical etching. In this case, however, requirements on the control of PMC time and slurry flow are much more stringent if the final film depth is to be well controlled.

In CMP, the mechanical properties of the wafer itself are important parameters. If the wafer has a slightly bowed structure, the pressure will be greater on the edges than it would on the center, which causes nonuniform polishing. To compensate for the wafer bow, pressure can be applied to the wafer's backside which, in turn, will equalize the center-edge differences.

The pads used in the CMP tool should be rigid in order to uniformly polish the wafer surface. However, these rigid pads must be kept in alignment with the wafer at all times. Therefore, real pads are often stacks of soft and hard materials that conform to wafer topography to some extent. Generally, these pads are made from porous polymeric materials with a pore size between 30 and

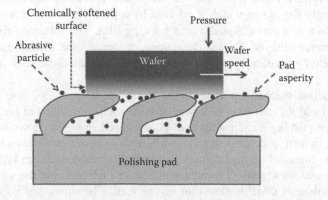

FIGURE 4.86   Schematic illustration of the principle of the CMP process.

TABLE 4.22

Main Process Parameters and Performances of CMP

Planarization of a Silicon Oxide Layer

Pressure on wafer	14–48	kPa
Platen rotation	20–60	rpm
Carrier rotation	20–80	rpm
Slurry flow rate	0.1–0.2	L/min
Etching rate	0.28	μm/min

50 μm and due to their characteristics they are consumed in the process so that regular reconditioning is needed.

Typical parameters of a CMP process on an oxide layer are reported in Table 4.22.

The CMP planarization process is not without problems. In case of oxide, planarization problems arise from a large set of phenomena, for example [126,127],

- Particle contamination either of the surface or of the film bulk, when the particles are absorbed in the film during the process.
- Stress accumulation on the film surface due to ablation.
- Imperfect slurry washing, leaving residual slurry on the film surface.
- Micro-scratches and deep defects on the surface due to ablation.
- Imperfect film edges that are present especially when trenches are fabricated on the chip. This is a very frequent situation in microfluidic chips, where deep trenches are present to prepare the ducts and chambers.

4.9.2 ADHESIVE WAFER BONDING

Wafer bonding process has a great number of applications and depending on the material that has to be bonded together different processes are necessary. In MEMs and electronic ICs applications it is frequent to require bonding between crystals, either semiconductors like silicon or GaAs or metals [6]. When crystals are involved, besides the great difference in bonding similar or dissimilar crystals, the ordered property of the surfaces to be bonded can be exploited. Moreover, if the wafers have a metal film on the surface, metal bond has also peculiar characteristics.

The most common case in microfluidics labs on chip is, however, the case in which the surfaces to be bonded are coated either with oxides or with polymers. We will deal with polymer technologies in the next chapter; thus, here we will consider wafer bonding where oxides coating is present at least on one of the wafer surfaces, considering in more detail coating with SiO_2 film. In this case, essentially two methods are possible: adhesive wafer bonding and direct wafer bonding [128,129].

4.9.2.1 Adhesive Wafer Bonding Principle

The basic principle that all bonding techniques have in common is that two materials adhere to each other if they are brought in sufficiently close contact. The cohesion of atoms and molecules within a solid material as well as the adhesion of atoms and molecules in between different solid materials is ensured by four basic bond types, which are covalent bonds, van der Waals bonds, metallic bonds, and ionic bonds.

Covalent bonds and van der Waals bonds are the dominant bonding mechanisms for oxide wafers that cannot exploit either metallic or ionic characteristics. To accomplish covalent and van der Waals bonds, the atoms of two opposing surfaces must be less than 0.3–0.5 nm apart, as it can be easily deduced from the characteristics of van der Waals and covalent bonds detailed in Chapter 2.

Macroscopically flat surfaces, such as the surfaces of polished SiO_2 surfaces, have a root-mean-square roughness of 0.3–0.8 nm. Nevertheless, the profile depth peak to valley of these surfaces is

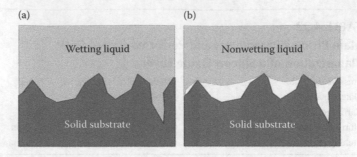

FIGURE 4.87 Microscopic view of a solid surface covered by a wetting (a) and a nonwetting (b) liquid.

several nanometers, which typically prevents bonding over larger surface areas. In order to bring two material surfaces in sufficiently close contact to achieve bonding at least one material surface must deform to fit the other. This deformation may be accomplished by plastic or elastic deformation, by diffusion of a solid material or by wetting of a surface with a liquid material. Practically, all wafer-bonding techniques use one of these mechanisms to establish bonding between different surfaces.

In adhesive wafer bonding, a polymer adhesive is placed in between the wafer pair to be bonded: the polymer adhesive deforms to fit the surfaces to be bonded so as to create a very close contact among the polymer molecules and the two surfaces. Polymer adhesives are typically in a liquid or semiliquid phase during part of the bonding process and wet the surfaces to be bonded by flowing into the troughs of the surface profile. The liquid polymer adhesive must then harden into a material that is capable of bearing the forces involved to hold the surfaces together.

Wetting of the surfaces by the liquid or semiliquid polymer adhesive (see Section 7.3.5) is critical in adhesive bonding. As a matter of fact, if wetting does not happen [128], the polymer remains suspended on the surface and leave spaces preventing a good bonding to take place (see Figure 4.87). For wetting to occur, the solid surface must have a greater surface energy than the liquid (see Section 7.3.5). The surface energy is a result of unbalanced cohesive forces at the material surface. A higher cohesive force between the atoms or molecules of a material correlates to a higher surface energy. Examples of surface energies for several materials when the surface is exposed to air are reported in Table 4.23.

The degree of wetting of a surface with a liquid adhesive can be reduced by surface contaminants, such as the weakly adsorbed organic molecules or by condensed moisture. The degree of wetting can also be influenced by the microscopic surface profile and by dust particles on the surface.

The more complete the polymer adhesive flows into and fills the troughs of a surface profile the better is the resulting bond quality and the long-term stability of the bond. Polymer adhesives that have low viscosity and low shrinkage during hardening generally achieve better filling of the troughs of a surface profile which decreases the amount of unfilled space at the bond interface.

4.9.2.2 Bond Quality of Adhesive Wafer Bonding

An important characteristic of all wafer bonding techniques is the bond force. As a matter of fact, even a local lack of bond brings to the circuit failure. In general, we can define the bond force as the maximum mechanical force needed to divide the bonded wafers. Assuming the bond homogeneous in the horizontal plane, at least on sufficiently large areas, the bond force can be defined both considering a shear test force and a pressure test force, even if generally the pressure bond force is deemed more important due to the fact that in normal applications it is the most common stress to which the circuit will be subject during use.

Another possible definition of the bond force is related to the surface energy at the bond. As a matter of fact, bonding takes place due to the energy reduction caused by the bonding of the two surfaces with respect to the surface energy of both of them exposed to air or vacuum. Thus, in order

TABLE 4.23

Examples of Surface Energies for Several Materials When the Surface Is Exposed to Air

Material	Physical Status	Surface Energy (mJ/m²)
Tungsten	Solid crystal	5800
Diamond	Solid crystal	4300
Platinum	Solid crystal	2800
Silicon	Solid crystal	1800
Aluminum	Solid crystal	900
Tin	Solid crystal	600
Glass	Solid amorphous	350
Ice	Solid crystal	85
Water	Liquid	80
Glycerol	Liquid	72
Polyurethanes	Liquid	34
Cyanoacrylates	Liquid	28
Polyethylene	Solid amorphous	22
Ethanol	Liquid	15
Methanol	Liquid	15
Teflon	Solid amorphous	12

to restore the situation in which the two wafers are divided, the energy difference has to be provided to the system by a suitable force.

If the wafer separation is performed by a purely normal force, there is a relationship between the bonding force (F_B) and the bonding energy (E_B). Let us imagine to apply a uniform force to the upper wafer for a time τ up to divide the two wafers and bring it to a speed v. This speed for sufficiently low values of v is small and can be easily measured.

If the wafers would not be joined, all the applied force would be transformed in kinetic energy, arriving at a speed v_0, while in our case $v < v_0$ due to the need of overcoming the bond energy. Thus, the bond energy can be evaluated by the following equation, where ρ is the average density of the upper wafer, r_w its radius, and d the wafer thickness.

$$E_B = \frac{F_B}{\pi r_w^2 \, d\rho}\tau - \frac{1}{2}\pi r_w^2 \, d\rho v^2 \approx \frac{P_B}{d\rho}\tau \qquad (4.26)$$

where P_B is the bound pressure and the approximation holds as far as the kinetic energy at the second member is negligible with respect to the bound energy, that is a reasonable assumption in this case. The bound energy has to be sufficiently high both to sustain post-processing steps and to assure sufficient operating life to the final product: generally, a value of 1 J/m² is considered as a good target [130].

Naturally, the bond energy is not the only parameter that is important in evaluating the bond quality. The Joung module, giving a measure of the compressive resistance of the bonded wafers, is another important parameter. Target values are above 1.5 GPa.

Under a chemical point of view, the bond has to resist to chemical actions that could be required in post-processing steps. Moreover, it has to be sufficiently stable to assure the required operating life of the final product.

The thermal expansion coefficient has also to be controlled, due to the fact that generally the upper and lower wafers do not expand at the same pace and the bond has to resist the stress introduced by this differential expansion.

TABLE 4.24

Adhesive Wafer Bonding Parameters for SiO$_2$–SiO$_2$ Bond Using SU8 Polymer

Spinning deposited layer	10–15 μm
Hardening temperature	65–90°C
Temperature hardening time	2 min + 10 min
Hardening UV exposure	100 mJ/cm^2
Glass temperature	>200°C
Young's modulus	2–4 MPa
Thermal expansion coefficient	52 PPM/°C [139]
Chemical stability	Class 3 w/acids
Shear bond strength	18–25 MPa

Source: Data from Yu L. et al., *Journal of Physics: Conference Series*, vol. 34 pp. 776–781, 2006, but when explicitly indicated.

Besides these parameters, that are typical of all the bonding techniques, if the polymer adhesive bond is used, other parameters have to be under consideration related to the specific technique.

As we have seen, the polymer is introduced as a solution, where generally the monomers or very short polymer chains are present. The real polymer is formed during hardening, where the long chains are formed. Thus, the degree of polymerization is an important parameter: higher the degree better is the bond.

Also, the glass transition temperature of the polymer is important, that is, required to be higher than the higher operating temperature of the final product and of all the post-processing steps.

Last, but not least, one of the advantages of the adhesive bonding is to require low temperatures with respect to other techniques that, after a room temperature prebonding, require annealing at more than 1000°C. Thus, the temperature at which the polymer hardening is performed is another important parameter of the process.

Characteristics of typical Si–SiO$_2$ adhesive wafer bonding processes are reported in Table 4.24, in correspondence to the use of SU8 (see Section 4.5.2) as adhesion polymer [131] and in the case of SiO$_2$–SiO$_2$ bonding.

4.9.2.3 Adhesive Wafer Bonding Process and Reactor Structure

A first element to be considered in designing the processing for adhesive wafer bonding of two wafers during the fabrication of a microfluidic circuit is that the bonding polymer has not to invade the trenches that have to constitute the ducts and chambers of the microfluidics circuit.

This is particularly important when activated surfaces are present, since the activation can be ruined by simple interaction with a different material. If the upper layer is flat, that is, no trenches are present, the deposition of the polymer solution can be done on the upper layer by spinning (see Section 4.5.2) and, after hardening, the bond can be done with the wafers in the inverse position (the upper wafer below). In this situation, gravity thwarts the falling of polymer particles on the floor of the trenches.

Frequently, however, this simple solution is not sufficient, either because trenches are present on both the wafers, or because the upper wafer for other reasons cannot be coated with the polymer before hardening (e.g., the polymer solution could contaminate the upper wafer surface).

In these cases, different solutions have to be found. The most used processes to deposit the polymer solution on a wafer with trenches without contaminating the trenches bottom surfaces are contact imprinting [131] and roller imprinting, whose principles are represented in Figure 4.88.

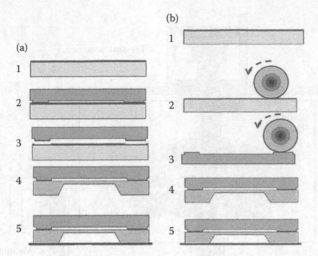

FIGURE 4.88 Operating principle scheme of contact imprinting (a) and roller imprinting (b) in adhesive wafer bonding process. The different steps of the two processes are described in the text.

In contact imprinting a dummy wafer is coated with the contact polymer solution (step 1), that is generally treated to obtain a hydrophilic characteristic so as to improve the adhesion to the final surface. The wafer with trenches is then put in contact under pressure with the dummy wafer so as to transfer the contact polymer to the upper wafer of the final assembly only on the exposed surfaces, without contaminating the trenches (step 2). The upper layer is then pressed onto the lower wafer in the wafer-bonding reactor so as to create contact only in areas where the polymer was present in the lower wafer (step 3). A final polymer hardening at the suitable temperature creates the wafer bonding without contaminating the structures that are present on the two wafers.

Also, in the case of roller imprinting the polymer solution is coated over a dummy wafer and undergoes a suitable treatment (step 1). After that, a roller collects the treated polymer solution (step 2) from the dummy wafer and rolling over the upper wafer of the final assembly deposits it only on the contact surfaces, without contamination of the trenches (step 3). The last steps of the process are similar to that of the imprinting technique.

A complete scheme of the adhesive wafer-bonding technique is reported in Table 4.25, while a scheme of an adhesive wafer-bonding chamber architecture is plotted in Figure 4.89.

TABLE 4.25
Summary of the Steps of a Typical Adhesive Wafer Bonding Process

No.	Process Steps	Observations
1	Cleaning and drying of the wafers	Remove particles and moisture from the wafer surfaces
2	Treating the wafer surfaces with an adhesion promoter	Adhesion promoters enhance the adhesion between the wafer surfaces and the polymer adhesive. In some cases, this step is not needed
3	Applying the polymer solution to one wafer	Suitable application process has to be used. Sometimes, the polymer is applied to both wafers (when trenches are not present)
4	Precuring of the polymer	Solvents and volatile substances are removed from the polymer coating. Partial polymerization could occur in this phase
5	Placing wafers in bond chamber and joining them	Wafers are joined in a vacuum environment to prevent voids and gases from being trapped at the bond interface
6	Applying pressure to the wafer stack	
7	Hardening the polymer while pressure is applied	Polymer hardening is typically performed by heating the system; sometimes, additional UV hardening is needed (as in the case of SU8)

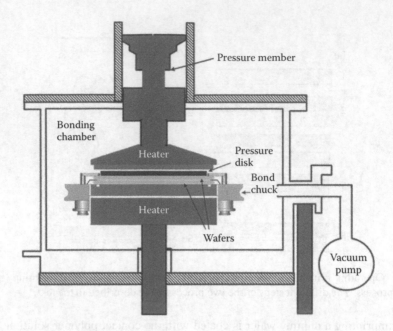

FIGURE 4.89 Bonding chamber scheme.

4.9.3 Direct Wafer Bonding

Adhesive wafer bonding is able to produce bonding strength sufficient for almost all the applications and works at relatively low temperature; moreover, due to the good bonding characteristics of adhesive polymers, the required wafer flatness is in the range of normal values attained after CMP at the end of any lithography cycle.

However, adhesive bonding has the disadvantage to require an intermediate bonding layer. The presence of an intermediate polymer is both a potential cause of contamination, both when the polymer is deposited and when, after bonding, the dice are separated. As a matter of fact, polymer particles can create even internally to the chip, at the edges of microfluidics chambers, due to stress and applied strength and contaminate the chip.

Thus, bonding techniques that does not require an intermediate bonding layer are quite desirable. Collectively, these techniques are called direct bonding, due to the fact that no intermediate layer is required between the wafers to be bonded [6]. The price to pay to get rid off the adhesive layer is the need of a much more flattened surface with respect to the adhesive bonding and the presence of a process meant to activate the surfaces to be put in contact in order that they can create bonding.

As far as the activation process is concerned, direct wafer bonding techniques can be divided in thermal techniques, where activation takes place due to high temperature, and ion-enhanced techniques, where activation occurs due to ion bombing.

4.9.3.1 Direct Wafer Bonding Principle

The phenomenon of wafer direct bonding originates from the intermolecular forces of attraction between two contacting surfaces. Therefore, the first step in the wafer bonding process is appropriate wafer surface preparation for bonding using no adhesive or external forces.

If two molecules are within the so-called van der Waals radius (see Section 2.1), they are attracted to each other by van der Waals intermolecular interactions that ubiquitously exist between almost all substances [129,132]. The force acting between two macroscopic bodies is the result of many-body effects. The pairwise summation of all of the interatomic forces acting between all of the atoms of the two bodies plus any additional medium can be considered as a first approximation of the force acting between the two bodies.

The surface force F_S between two bodies decreases rapidly with distance. Considering two flat and parallel surfaces at distance d, it can be written in a first approximation

$$F_S = \frac{F_0}{d^3} \tag{4.27}$$

where F_0 is the so-called limit bonding force, that is the force that would ideally bond the two surfaces if perfect contact at zero distance would be possible.

Two solid-state plates of almost any material can be bonded to each other even at room temperature provided that their surfaces are sufficiently smooth to allow the surface molecules of two plates to get close enough and the van der Waals forces between atoms on the touching surfaces to be sufficiently strong. The smoothness of wafer surfaces required for successful bonding mainly depends on the type and strength of the forces of interaction at the bonding interface. Bonding by the dispersion force, that is the van der Waals force acting between nonpolar molecules due to charge distribution fluctuations and exists between any substances, requires extremely smooth surfaces, which may only be achieved by expensive optical polishing. However, in many cases hydrogen bonding, in which the hydrogen atom in a polar molecule interacts with an electronegative atom of an adjacent molecule, can be generated.

A hydrogen atom can participate in a hydrogen bond if it is bonded to oxygen, nitrogen, or fluorine because H–F, H–O, and H–N bonds are strongly polarized, leaving the hydrogen atom with a partial positive charge. This electrophilic hydrogen has a strong affinity for nonbonding electrons so that it can form intermolecular attachments with an electronegative atom such as oxygen, nitrogen, or fluorine.

In this way, a longer range intermolecular force can be realized and the requirement of surface smoothness for direct bonding is greatly eased. To understand whether the above principle is practically applicable, it is needed to derive quantitative requirements for the surface flatness and to compare it with practically achievable values.

This requires a deep theoretical and experimental analysis of the contact between two nominally flat surfaces [133] whose major results can be summarized as follows. Let us assume that both the surfaces have the same mechanical properties, they are nominally flat and parallel, that is the average value of the surface is a plane and the two planes are parallel, and that the distribution of the roughness is uniform. In particular, let us assume that on an area A_S, much larger than the footprint of the average roughness, there is an average of N_S zones where the surface height deviates from the average, so that the average surface density of roughness is $\eta_S = N_S/A_S$. Let us also assume that the height of the roughness is a Gaussian variable with zero average and variance σ_S^2 and that the cap of each roughness can be approximated with a round surface whose average radius is R_S. In this condition, due to the small roughness dimension, when a force pushes the two surfaces one on the other the cap of each protruding roughness is elastically deformed so that the surface adherence force in that microscopic area can be written as $F_M = 2\pi w R_S$.

In this condition, the key parameter to define the possibility of generating direct bonding and its properties is the so-called adhesion parameter Θ that is given by

$$\Theta = \frac{E'}{w} \sqrt{\frac{\sigma_S^3}{R_S}} \tag{4.28}$$

where E' is the reduced Young module of the material constituting the surface.

Since all the parameters appearing in Equation 4.27 can be measured by a microscopic analysis of the surface, this equation can be used to determine the degree of polishing that is needed to achieve a certain bonding quality.

Defining the equilibrium pressure as the pressure that is needed to maintain the two surfaces attached with zero bonding energy, it results to be a function of the average surfaces distance d

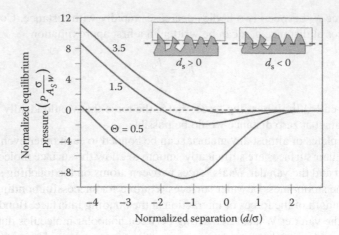

FIGURE 4.90 Normalized equilibrium pressure for the direct contact between a rough and an ideal surface versus the normalized surfaces distance. The definition of the normalize surfaces distance is reported in the figure insert, where the dashed line is the average surface of the rough wafer in the absence of elastic deformation. (After Gui C. et al., *Journal of Applied Physics*, vol. 85, pp. 7448–7454, 1999.)

and of Θ. If the equilibrium pressure is positive, it means there is no bond and if the surfaces are released, they spontaneously separate. If the equilibrium pressure is negative, its inverse is exactly the bond pressure. A reference graph of the equilibrium pressure for the contact between a rough and an ideal surface is shown in Figure 4.90.

A first observation is that, as it results from the insert in the figure, since the distance between the wafers is evaluated not considering the elastic deformation, but maintaining the average surface before the bond, it can also be smaller than zero. This is due to the elastic deformation of the two surfaces that brings the wafers in such a position that the trace of the nondeformed average surfaces switch as if a wafer was entering into the other. The second observation, and the most important one, is that for each value of the adhesion parameter, a threshold normalized distance exists, dividing a bond region from a region where bonding cannot be performed. To move as right as possible the threshold distance, that means to relax wafer planarity requirements, and to achieve higher bonding energies, the parameter Θ has to be as small as possible.

An extended measurement campaign on thermal oxides wafers is reported in Reference [133] to assess the values of Θ achievable with different flattening processes and the quality of bonding by pressure at room temperature. A simple CMP cycle, repeated CMP cycles with different slurries and pads, and a combination of CMP and wet chemical etching has been considered as flattening processes. The result is that the adhesion parameter achievable with practical flattening processes is in a range between 17 and 0.1 when realistic wafers and flattening processes are used, and the consequent bonding characteristics are reported in Figure 4.91.

From the definitions of the parameters and Figures 4.90 and 4.91 it is evident that to achieve a good direct bond the following actions are effective:

- Increase the wafers flatness: this decreases the adhesion coefficient; however, to achieve the above values like 0.1 very expensive optical methods have to be used that are not suitable for microcircuits mass production.
- Increase the bond pressure; however, the bond pressure cannot be increased too much, not to risk wafer damage since, when wafer bonding is performed, structures have been already fabricated on the wafer.
- Increase the Young module, but generally this is not possible since the material choice is dictated by other constraints than wafer bonding efficiency.

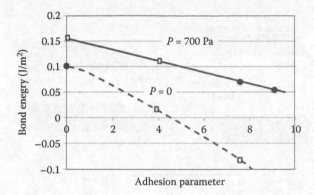

FIGURE 4.91   Bond energy versus the adhesion parameter for 3 inch Si–SiO$_2$ (spontaneous oxide) wafers and different values of the bond pressure P. Black round points are experiments from [133], square white points are calculated and the curves are interpolations. Where the bond energy is negative no bond is possible.

- Increase microscopic bond force: this means increasing w by somehow preconditioning the surfaces to be bonded. This is the most practical way to obtain direct bonding with bonding energies of the order of 1 J/m^2, as it is needed for practical purposes.

4.9.3.2   Thermal Direct Wafer Bonding

All the considerations we have done up to now assume to work at room temperature. The bonding energy has, however, a strong dependence on temperature, as shown in Figure 4.92 in the case of two Si–SiO$_2$ wafers [129].

The reason for the strong increase of the bond energy at high temperature is due to the fact that the hydrogen SiOH–SiOH bond that generates adhesion at room temperature are replaced more and more by siloxane covalent bonds (see Figure 4.93a) that has about 10 times the energy at each individual bond.

As a consequence, if the adhesion parameter is kept sufficiently low (let us say 0.1) the bond energy passes from a value of 0.1 J/m^2 at room temperature to an asymptotic value of more than 2 J/m^2. Thus, raising the temperature.

Once the siloxane bonds are formed, due to their high energetic nature, they remain stable decreasing the temperature if the excessive water is removed from the interface, thus temperature

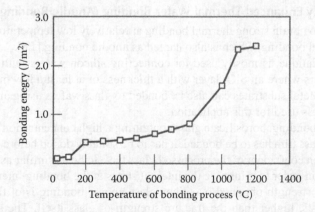

FIGURE 4.92   Surface bonding energy for direct wafer bonding of two SiO$_2$ surfaces with adhesive parameter equal to 0.1 versus the temperature of the bonding process. A pressure of 500 Pa is also applied during the bonding. (After from Yu L. et al., *Journal of Physics: Conference Series*, vol. 34 pp. 776–781, 2006.)

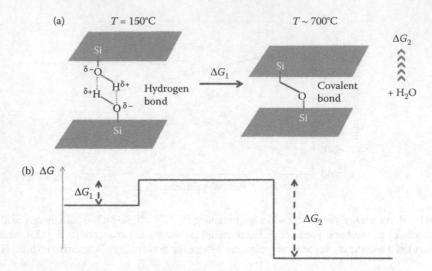

FIGURE 4.93 Chemical mechanism causing the bonding energy increase versus the bonding process temperature. Chemical scheme of the bonding and its transformation with temperature (a) energy diagram of the heath stimulated reaction (b).

direct wafer bonding is a very effective way of realizing wafer bonding without an adhesion intermediate film. Water can be removed, for example, by annealing at low temperatures such as 150–200°C after the bonding process.

The limit of thermal treatment is that no structure or composite has to be present on wafer that is ruined by high temperature. In the field of electronic structures, doping generally cannot stand so high temperatures, unless the doping composites are physically insulated into the doped areas by trenches or other systems. As a matter of fact, very high temperature causes diffusion of the dopant, changing the doping profile and probably ruining the circuit working.

In the biological field, if organic molecules have been already charged in the circuit, for example, in chambers with activated surfaces, they are probably denatured by high temperature losing their functionality. Last, but not least, if the wafers to be bonded are not made of the same material, differential thermal expansion can render high-temperature bonding impossible. Thus, there is a strong interest in using a surface conditioning method that does not require high temperatures.

4.9.3.3 Electrically Enhanced Thermal Wafer Bonding (Anodic Bonding)

A largely used way to obtain strong thermal bonding at relatively low temperatures is to use electrically assisted thermal bonding, which is also named as anodic bonding [1,6].

This bonding technique, is mostly used for connecting silicon wafers with either glass wafers or other silicon wafers where an SiO_2 layer with a thickness of at least a few microns is deposited, generally by CVD. Metal substrates can also be bonded to glass wafers using anodic bonding, even if this technique is less used for this application.

To obtain anodic bonding, borosilicate glass containing a high concentration of alkali ions has to be used. Thus, if a glass film has to be bonded, it has to be suitably doped before bonding. Moreover, the thermal expansion coefficient of the processed glass have to be as similar as possible to those of the bonding partner in order to minimize the internal stress at the bonding interface.

The typical bond strength obtained by silicon/glass anodic bonding is of the order of 15 MPa according to pull tests, higher than the fracture strength of glass itself. The scheme of a typical anodic bonding equipment is shown in Figure 4.94.

At the start of the bonding process the wafer to be bonded, after suitable surface polishing and planarization, are put in close contact by a pressure of the order of 50 kPa. After the contact creation

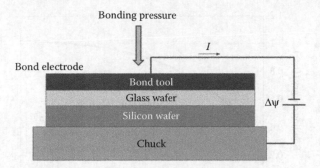

FIGURE 4.94   Scheme of a device for anodic bonding.

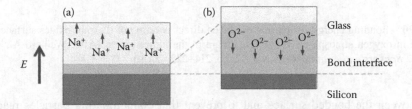

FIGURE 4.95   Ion drifting during anodic bonding between a silicon and a silica wafers: formation of depletion zone through Na^+ drifting (a) and drift of O^{2-} ions in the depletion zone (b).

the temperature is increased to a value between 200°C and 500°C, depending on the type of glass to be bonded, and a large potential, of the order of 1000 V, is applied at the electrodes so as to create an electrical field-oriented toward the glass wafer (see Figure 4.95a). This causes a diffusion of sodium ions (Na^+) out of the bond interface to the backside of the glass to the cathode. Drifting of the positive ions is continuously supported by high electrical field and facilitated by high temperature.

Combined with humidity and high temperature this phenomenon causes formation of NaOH in a thin layer near the wafers interface with the effect that free O^{2-} ions remain in the layer giving it a negative charge.

The negative charges in the glass layer causes a depletion of negative charges in the adjacent silicon layer due to electrostatic repulsion and a high impedance interface forms. This means that almost all the applied potential, after a very brief transition time, falls around a very small interface layer.

The electrical field intensity in the depletion region is so high that the oxygen ions drift to the bond interface and pass out to react with the silicon to form SiO_2 (see Figure 4.95b). The thin formed siloxane (Si–O–Si) layer between the bond surfaces ensures the irreversible connection between the wafers since Si–O–Si is formed by covalent bonds.

After the bonding process, slow cooling over several minutes has to take place. This can be supported by purging with an inert gas. The cooling time depends on the difference between the thermal expansion temperatures of the bonded materials: the higher the difference, the longer the cooling period.

4.9.3.4   Plasma-Enhanced Direct Wafer Bonding

In cases where thermal bonding is not possible, surface conditioning can be attained by ion bombing in high vacuum [129,134]. Plasma interacts with the surface mainly physically in the bonding process, creating surface defects that break bonds between the surface atoms and molecules, leaving chemically active sites that more effectively form chemical bonds with atoms or molecules of the other surface. Absolute absence of contamination is needed both to avoid the formation of void

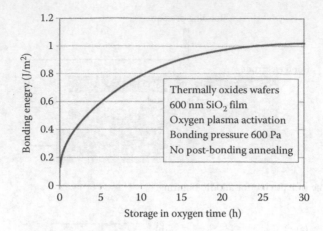

FIGURE 4.96 Bonding energy for plasma enhanced direct bonding of thermal oxides surfaces versus the storage time in oxygen atmosphere. Bonding data are in the figure insert. (After Weinerd A., Amirfeiz P., Bengtsson S., *Sensors and Actuators—A*, vol. 92, pp. 214–222, 2001.)

areas in between the bonded surface and to prevent that contaminating particles react with the chemically active sites forming spurious composites that both weakens the bonding and alter the chip functionalities.

This renders the vacuum requirements quite stringent if plasma-enhanced direct wafer bonding is performed, so that the equipment used to condition the surfaces before wafer bonding is somehow similar to an RIE equipment (see Figure 4.65).

Typical gases used to create the plasma are argon and oxygen. The process for plasma-enhanced wafer bonding can be schematically summarized as follows:

1. The wafers are polished and flattened using alternative cycles of PMC and wet etching
2. Both wafers are inserted in an RIE machine and bombed with ions
3. The wafer surface is washed with deionized water
4. Storage in oxygen-rich atmosphere is performed to enrich the surface of oxygen-active sites
5. Wafers are inserted in a bonding chamber and pressed to create bonding
6. Low-temperature annealing is performed (if necessary)

The process results to be very sensitive to the time the wafer is stored in contact with oxygen, due to the great role of interface oxygen-active sites in creating a strong bonding force. Generally, hours of storage are needed and the maximum bonding force is obtained after an optimum storage period, frequently about 24 h. After this period, further storage does not improve the bonding quality.

The bonding energy obtained by plasma-enhanced direct bonding of thermal oxide surfaces versus the storage time in oxygen atmosphere are reported in Figure 4.96, demonstrating the suitability of this technique for practical applications.

4.9.4 WAFER ALIGNMENT

Whatever technique is used to bond wafers, wafer alignment is a critical step in the bonding process [135]. Misalignment risks to ruin both wafers and, in general, unbonding and bonding again is not possible without ruining the fabricated structures.

The alignment accuracy has to be of the order of a fraction of the fabricated circuits' critical dimension, so that even if critical dimensions of the order of 5 μm are required, as typical of

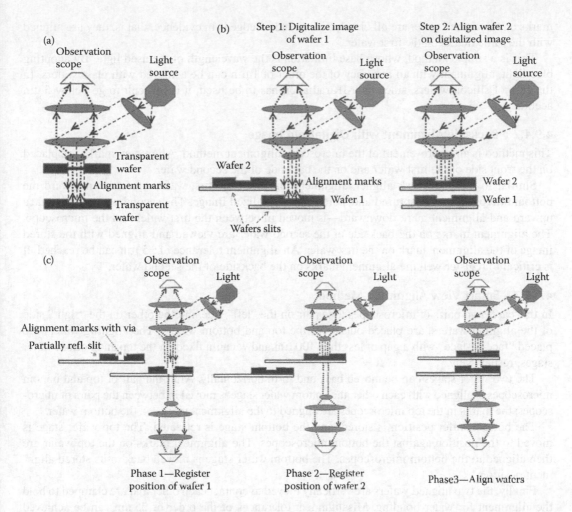

FIGURE 4.97 Different wafers alignment techniques: (a) optical microscopy alignment method, (b) backside alignment with digitalized image, and (c) smart view alignment method.

microfluidics circuits, a wafer alignment with sub-micron precision is required. Several techniques have been studied and industrially applied to align wafers to be bonded, a selected set of them is shown in Figure 4.97.

4.9.4.1 Optical Microscopy Alignment Method

Frequently, in microfluidic applications the substrates are transparent to a suitable wavelength. Not only is glass naturally transparent to visible wavelengths, but silicon is also transparent in the near IR. Under these conditions, the transparency can be used to align the two wafers. In particular, a set of reference lithography marks are fabricated in correspondent positions on the two wafers. These are similar to the marks that are used for mask alignment in lithography (see Section 4.5.3).

One of the two wafers is etched on the front and on the back in correspondence with the alignment marks so as to leave a very thin film, that has a small absorption at the frequency that is chosen for the alignment. On the other wafer, the marks are etched so as to be able to distinguish the mark edge.

At this point, the procedure is exactly similar to that used for mask alignment, where the first wafer takes the place of the mask. An optical microscope is focused through the first wafer on the marks bottom surface, on the second one and the first wafer is moved up to the moment in which the marks on the second wafer are all clearly visible and no edge is in evidence, that is, they are aligned with the same marks on the first wafer.

This is a simple method, whose base limitation is the wavelength of the used light. By adopting blue light, alignment with an accuracy of the order of 1 μm can be achieved with glass wafers. In the case of silicon wafers, since near-IR radiation has to be used, it is difficult to go below 5 μm accuracy.

4.9.4.2 Backside Alignment with Digitalized Image

This method is an improvement of the microscopy alignment method. Alignment marks are placed on the front side of the first wafer and on the backside of the second wafer.

Similar to a digital mask aligner, alignment marks on the first wafer—face down toward the bottom microscope—is captured and stored as a digitalized image. The second wafer—bond face upward and alignment mark downward—is moved in between the first wafer and the microscope. The alignment marks on the backside of the second wafer are viewed and aligned with the stored image of the alignment mark on the first wafer. An alignment tolerance of ±5 μm can be reached. It is critical to register well the alignment marks on the backside of the second wafer.

4.9.4.3 Smart View Alignment Method

In this case, two pairs of microscopes (one pair on the "left" side and the other on the "right" side of the aligning wafers) are placed outside of the top and bottom wafers. The aligning wafers are placed "face-to-face" with a gap of less than 100 μm and vacuum fixed on the top and bottom wafer stages, respectively.

The two wafer stages can be moved back and forth horizontally. After the pair of top and bottom microscopes is aligned with each other, the bottom wafer stage is moved in between the pairs of microscopes; the marks in the top microscopes are aligned to the alignment marks on the bottom wafer.

The bottom wafer position is stored, and the bottom stage is retreated. The top wafer stage is moved to the position against the bottom microscopes. The alignment marks on the top wafer are then aligned to the bottom microscopes. The bottom wafer stage is moved back to its stored alignment position.

Finally, the two aligned wafers are vertically moved to contact each other and are clamped to hold the alignment for wafer bonding. Misalignment tolerances of the order of 25 nm can be achieved with this method that results to be quite effective when sub-micron alignment precision is required.

REFERENCES

1. Madou M. J., *Fundamentals of Microfabrication and Nanotechnology*, Third Edition, Three-Volume Set, CRC Press; 3rd edition (August 1, 2011), ISBN-13: 978-0849331800.
2. Melin J., Quake S. R., Microfluidic large-scale integration: The evolution of design rules for biological automation, *Annual Review of Biophysics and Biomolecular Structure*, vol. 36, pp. 213–231, 2007.
3. Widman D., Mader H., Friedrich F., *Technology of Integrated Circuits*, Springer; Reprint of 2000 edition (December 15, 2010), ISBN-13: 978-3642085475.
4. Mayer M. G., Grey P. R., *Analysis and Design of Analog Integrated Circuits*, Wiley; 5th edition (January 20, 2009), ISBN-13: 978-0470245996.
5. Coldren L. A. Corzine S. W., Mashanovitch M. L., *Diode Lasers and Photonic Integrated Circuits* (Wiley Series in Microwave and Optical Engineering), Wiley; 2nd edition (March 27, 2012), ISBN-13: 978-0470484128.
6. Ramm P., Lu J.-Q., Taklo M. M. V., Editors, *Handbook of Wafer Bonding*, Wiley-VCH; 1st edition (March 13, 2012), ISBN-13: 978-3527326464.
7. Zeng J., *Design Automation Methods and Tools for Microfluidics-Based Biochips*, Springer; 1st edition (October 19, 2006), ISBN-13: 978-1402051227.
8. Richards Greyson A. C. et al., A BioMEMS review: MEMS technology for physiologically integrated devices, *Proceedings IEEE*, vol. 92, pp. 6–21, 2004.

9. Ziaiea B., Baldi A., Lei M., Gu Y., Siegel R. A., Hard and soft micromachining for BioMEMS: Review of techniques and examples of applications in microfluidics and drug delivery, *Advanced Drug Delivery Reviews*, vol. 56, pp. 145–172, 2004.

10. Liu, Ai-Qun. *Photonic MEMS Devices: Design, Fabrication and Control*. CRC Press, 2009. ISBN-13 9781420045600.

11. Korvink J. G., Paul O., *MEMS: A Practical Guide to Design, Analysis, and Applications*, Springer Verlag & William Andrew; 1st edition 2006. ISBN-10: 0815514972.

12. Peroziello G., *Microfluidics System Interfacing*, Lambert Academic Publishing; 1st edition, 2011, ISBN-13 9783844327700.

13. Gulliksen A. et al., Real-time nucleic acid sequence-based amplification in nanoliter volumes, *Analytical Chemistry*, vol. 76, pp. 9–14, 2004.

14. Hunsperger R. G., *Integrated Optics: Theory and Technology*, Springer, Reprint of 2009; 6th edition (October 29, 2010), ISBN-13: 978-1441928023.

15. Zhao Y., *Design and Testing of Microfluidics Circuits*, Springer; 2012 edition (May 31, 2012), ISBN-13: 978-1461403692.

16. Bahukudumbi S., Chakrabarty K., *Wafer-Level Testing and Test During Burn-In for Integrated Circuits*, Artech House Publishers; 1st edition (February 2010), ISBN-13: 978-1596939899.

17. Kornaros G., Meidanis D., Papaeystathiou Y., Chantzandroulis S., Blionas S., Architecture of a Consumer Lab on chip for Pharmacogenomics, International Conference on Consumer Electronics 2008, 9–3 Jan. 2008, Proceedings pp. 1–2.

18. Ghallab Y. H., Badaway W., *Lab-On-A-Chip: Techniques, Circuits, and Biomedical Applications*, Artech House (June 30, 2010), ISBN-13: 978-1596934184.

19. Li P. C. H., *Fundamentals of Microfluidics and Lab on a Chip for Biological Analysis and Discovery*, CRC Press; 1st edition (February 24, 2010), ISBN-13: 978-1439818558.

20. Chakrabarty K., Design automation and test solutions for digital microfluidic biochips, *IEEE Transactions On Circuits And Systems— I: Regular Papers*, vol. 57, pp. 4–17, 2010.

21. Mitra D., Ghoshal, S., Rahaman, H., Chakrabarty, K., Bhattacharya, B. B., Testing of Digital Microfluidic Biochips Using Improved Eulerization Techniques and the Chinese Postman Problem, Proceedings of 19th IEEE Asian Test Symposium (ATS), pp. 111–116, 2010.

22. Wuang L-T., Wu C-W., Wen X., *VLSI Test Principles and Architectures: Design for Testability*, Morgan Kaufmann; 1st edition (July 21, 2006), ISBN-13: 978-0123705976.

23. Wang L-T., Stroud C. E., Touba N. A., *System-on-Chip Test Architectures: Nanometer Design for Testability*, Morgan Kaufmann; 1st edition (December 4, 2007), ISBN-13: 978-0123739735.

24. Myers T. O., Bell I. M., Test Metric Assessment of Microfluidic Systems through Heterogeneous Fault Simulation, Proceedings of IEEE 16th International Workshop on Mixed-Signals, Sensors and Systems Test (IMS3TW), pp. 10, 2010.

25. Device Approvals and Clearances: USA Food and Drugs Administration, http://www.fda.gov/MedicalDevices/ProductsandMedicalProcedures, last accessed on April 12, 2012.

26. New guidance documents on Medical Devices: European Commission Administration, General Direction Health & Consumers, Section Public health—Februray 1–2010, http://ec.europa.eu/health/medical-devices/documents/guidelines/index_en.htm, last accessed April 12, 2012.

27. ISO 14644-1 Recommendation—Cleanrooms and associated controlled environments—Part 1: Classification of air cleanliness.

28. U.S. General Services Administration, Federal Standard 209 A-D, 1992.

29. Whyte W., *Cleanroom Technology: Fundamentals of Design, Testing and Operation*, Wiley; 2nd edition (March 9, 2010), ISBN-13: 978-0470748060.

30. Bell A., *HVAC Equations, Data, and Rules of Thumb*, McGraw-Hill Professional; 2nd edition (September 26, 2007), ISBN-13: 978-0071482424.

31. Angel W. L., *HVAC Design Sourcebook*, McGraw-Hill Professional; 1st edition (October 5, 2011), ISBN-13: 978-0071753036

32. The Official SEMI home page is http://www.semi.org/en/: All SEMI standards can be acquired here (last accessed on April 16, 2012).

33. Main SEMI standards for silicon wafer for microelectronics industry
    a. Standard for 2 inch Polished Monocrystalline Silicon Wafers, (SEMI M1.1-89, Re-approved 0299)
    b. Standard for 3 inch Polished Monocrystalline Silicon Wafers, (SEMI M1.2-89, Re-approved 0299)
    c. Standard for 100 mm Polished Monocrystalline Silicon Wafers (525 um thickness), (SEMI M1.5-89, Re-approved 0699)

d. Standard for 100 mm Polished Monocrystalline Silicon Wafers (625 um thickness), (SEMI M1.6-89, Re-approved 0699)

e. Standard for 125 mm Polished Monocrystalline Silicon Wafers, (SEMI M1.7-89, Re-approved 0699)

f. Standard for 150 mm Polished Monocrystalline Silicon Wafers, (SEMI M1.8-89, Re-approved 0699)

g. Standard for 200 mm Polished Monocrystalline Silicon Wafers, (Notched), (SEMI M1.9-89, Re-approved 0699)

h. Standard for 200 mm Polished Monocrystalline Silicon Wafers, (Fatted), (SEMI M1.9-89, Re-approved 0699)

i. Standard for 100 mm Polished Monocrystalline Silicon Wafers Without Secondary Flat (525 um thickness), (SEMI M1.11-90, Re-approved 0299)

j. Standard for 125 mm Polished Monocrystalline Silicon Wafers Without Secondary Flat, (SEMI M1.12-90, Re-approved 0299)

k. Standard for 150 mm Polished Monocrystalline Silicon Wafers Without Secondary Flat (625 um thickness), (SEMI M1.13-0699)

l. Guidelines for 350 and 400 mm Polished Monocrystalline Silicon Wafers, (SEMI M1.14-96)

m. Standard for 300 mm Polished Monocrystalline Silicon Wafers, (Notched), (SEMI M1.15-0302)

34. Ashby C., Baca A., *Fabrication of GaAs Devices*, The Institution of Engineering and Technology (September 30, 2005), ISBN-13: 978-0863413537.

35. Razeghi M., *The MOCVD Challenge: A Survey of GaInAsP-InP and GaInAsP-GaAs for Photonic and Electronic Device Applications*, CRC Press; 2nd edition (August 17, 2010), ISBN-13: 978-1439806982

36. O'Mara, W. C., Herring R. B., Hunt L. P., *Handbook of Semiconductor Silicon Technology*, William Andrew Inc.; 1st edition (1990), ISBN-13: 978-0815512376.

37. Yoshio N., *Handbook of Semiconductor Manufacturing Technology*. CRC Press; 1st edition (2000), ISBN-13: 978-0824787838

38. Kuo J. B., Su K-W., *CMOS VLSI Engineering: Silicon-on-Insulator (SOI)*, Springer; reprint of 1998 edition (December 3, 2010), ISBN-13: 978-1441950574.

39. Narayan R. Editor, *Biomedical Materials*, Springer; 1st edition (June 22, 2009), ISBN-13: 978-0387848716.

40. Chien C-F., Hsu S-C., Deng J-F., A cutting algorithm for optimizing the wafer exposure pattern, *IEEE Transactions on Semiconductor Manufacturing*, vol. 14, pp. 157–161, 2001.

41. Fukagawa Y., Shinano Y., Wada T., Nakamori M., Optimum Placement of a Wafer on a Rectangular Chip Grid, Proceedings of 6th World Congresses of Structural and Multidisciplinary Optimization, Rio de Janeiro, 2005.

42. Foussier P. M. M., *From Product Description to Cost: A Practical Approach: Volume 1: The Parametric Approach*, Springer; reprint of 2006 edition (November, 2011), ISBN-13: 978-184996982

43. Seuring S., Gooldbach M., *Costs Management in Supply Chain*, Physica-Verlag HD; reprint of 2002 edition (November 19, 2010), ISBN-13: 978-3790825152.

44. Stewart R. D., *Cost Estimating*, Wiley-Interscience; 2nd edition (January 2, 1991), ISBN-13: 978-0471857075.

45. Soh T. H., Guarini K. W., Quate C. F., *Scanning Probe Lithography*, Springer; Reprint of 2001 edition (December 8, 2010), ISBN-13: 978-1441948946.

46. Utke I., Moshkaleys F., Russel P. Editors, *Nanofabrication Using Focused Ion and Electron Beams: Principles and Applications*, Oxford University Press, (May 1, 2012), ISBN-13: 978-0199734214.

47. Levison H. J., *Principles of Lithography*, SPIE Press; 3rd edition (January 21, 2011), ISBN-13: 978-0819483249.

48. Martin P. M., *Handbook of Deposition Technologies for Films and Coatings*, William Andrew; 3rd edition (December 3, 2009), ISBN-13: 978-0815520313.

49. Meyerhofer D., Characteristics of resist films produced by spinning, *Journal of Applied Physics*, vol. 49, pp. 3993, 1978.

50. Myer K., *Handbook of Materials Selection*. Wiley; 1st edition (2002), ISBN-13: 978-0471359246.

51. Chemical Information Review Document for Diazonaphthoquinone Derivatives Used in Photoresists, Supporting Nomination for Toxicological Evaluation by the National Toxicology Program, January 2006, in public domain and downloadable for free at http://ntp.niehs.nih.gov/files/Photoresists_DNQcmpds2.pdf. Retrieved April 21, 2012.

52. Bradley D., Fahlman D., *Material Chemistry*, Springer; 2nd edition, 2011, ISBN-13: 978-9400706927.

53. Studt T., Polymides: Hot stuff for 90's, *IBM Journal of Research in Devices*, vol. 39, pp. 3031, 1992.

54. Liu J., Cai B., Zhu J., Ding G., Zhao X., Yang C., Chen D., Process research of high aspect ratio microstructure using SU-8 resist, *Microsystem Technologies*, vol. 10, pp. 265, 2004.

55. Hong G., Holmes A. S., Heaton M. E., Su8 Resist Plasma Etching and Its Optimisation, Proceedings of Symposium on Design, Test, Integration & Packaging of MEMS/MOEMS, France, pp. 268–271, 2003.

56. Theodoridis S., Koutroumbas K., *Pattern Recognition*, Academic Press; 4th edition (November 3, 2008), ISBN-13: 978-1597492720.

57. Liu Y., Xu D., Tan M., A new pre-alignment approach based on four-quadrant-photo-detector for IC mask, *International Journal of Automation and Computing*, vol. 4, pp. 208, 216, 2007.

58. Kwon S., Hwang J., Kinematics, Pattern recognition, and motion control of mask–panel alignment system, *Control Engineering Practice*, vol. 5, pp. 883–892, 2011.

59. Tritchkov A., Jeong S., Kenyon C., Lithography enabling for the 65 nm node gate layer patterning with alternating PSM, *Proceedings SPIE*, vol. 5754, pp. 215–225, 2005.

60. Perlitz S. et al., Novel solution for in-die phase control under scanner equivalent optical settings for 45-nm node and below, *Proceedings SPIE*, vol. 6607, pp. 1–5, 2007.

61. Rai-Choudhury, P., Editor. *Handbook of Microlithography, Micromachining, and Microfabrication, Volume 1: Microlithography*. SPIE Optical Engineering Press (1997), ISBN-13: 978-0852969066.

62. Yao P., Schneider G. J., Prather D., Three-dimensional lithographical fabrication of microchannels, *Journal of Microelectromechanical Systems*, vol. 14, pp. 799–805, 2005.

63. Yao P., Schneider G. J., Prather D., Wetzel E., O'Brein D., Fabrication of three-dimensional photonic crystals with multilayer photolithography, *Optics Express*, vol. 13, pp. 2370–2376, 2005.

64. Kim J., Joy D. C., Lee S.-Y., Controlling resist thickness and etch depth for fabrication of 3D structures in electron-beam grayscale lithography, *Microelectronics Engineering*, vol. 84, pp. 2859–2864, 2007.

65. Vivien L., Roux X. L., Laval S., Cassan E., Marris-Morini D., Design, realization, and characterization of 3-D taper for fber/microwaveguide coupling, *IEEE Journal on Selected Topics in Quantum Electronics*, vol. 12, pp. 1354–1358, 2006.

66. Hu F. Lee S.-Y., Dose control for fabrication of grayscale structures using a single step electron-beam lithographic process, *Journal of Vacuum Science Technology B, Microelectronics Processes Phenomena*, vol. 21, pp. 2672–2679, 2003.

67. Waits C. M., Modafe A., Ghodssi., R., Investigation of gray-scale technology for large area 3D silicon MEMS structures, *Journal of Micromechanical Microengineering*, vol. 13, pp. 170–177, 2003.

68. Morgan B., Ghodssi R., Vertically-shaped tunable MEMS resonators, *Journal of Microelectromechanical Systems*, vol. 17, pp. 85–92, 2008.

69. Jain K., *Excimer Laser Lithography*, SPIE Publications; 1st edition (February 1, 1990), ISBN-13: 978-0819402714.

70. Phamduy T. B., Abdul Raof N., Corr, D. T., Xie Y., Chrisey D. B., Laser Forward Transfer: Direct-Writing Arrays of Single Microbeads, Proceedings of 2011 IEEE 37th Annual Northeast Bioengineering Conference (NEBEC), pp. 1–2, 2011.

71. Chen J., Chen J.-C., Lin S.-Y., Yeh C.-H., Liu C.-Y., High Power Ultra-Short Pulse UV Laser System, Supplement to Proceedings of IEEE 2009 Asia Communications and Photonics Conference and Exhibition (ACP), pp. 1–6, 2009.

72. Hotta E., Sakai Y., Qiushi Zhu, Bin Huang, Kumai H., Watanabe M., EUV and SXR Sources Based on Discharge Produced Plasma, Proceedings of 2011 Academic International Symposium on Optoelectronics and Microelectronics Technology (AISOMT), pp. 4–7, 2011.

73. Lee S., Kwek K. H., Ali Jalil. Prabhakar M. V. H. V., Shishodia Y. S., Warmate A. G., Sequenced nitrogen lasers, *Journal of Applied Physics*, vol. 65, pp. 4133–4137, 1989.

74. Palmer K. M., An extremely fine line, *IEEE Spectrum*, vol. 49, pp. 47–50, 2012.

75. Mai J., Tsai R.-Y., Yang C.-T., Low-cost nanolithography, *IEEE Nanotechnology Magazine*, vol. 5, pp. 25–28, 2011.

76. Sivakumar S., EUV Lithography: Prospects and Challenges, Proceedings of 2011 16th Asia and South Pacific Design Automation Conference (ASP-DAC), pp. 402, 2011.

77. McKean D. R., Russell T. P., Hinsberg, W. D., Hofer D., Renaldo A. F., Willson C. G., Thick film positive photoresist: Development and resolution enhancement technique, *Journal of Vacuum Science & Technology B: Microelectronics and Nanometer Structures*, vol. 13, pp. 3000–3006, 1995.

78. Mach C., Stochastic approach to modeling photoresist development, *Journal of Vacuum Science & Technology B: Microelectronics and Nanometer Structures*, vol. 27, pp. 1122–1128, 2009.

79. Romig T., Chao K., Rendon M. J., Azrack M., Implant Charging Dependence on Photo Resist Bake and Electron Flood Gun, Proceedings of 2000. Conference on Ion Implantation Technology, pp. 558–560, 2000.

80. Fisher R. E., *Optical System Design*, McGraw-Hill Professional; 2nd edition (January 24, 2008), ISBN-13: 978-0071472487

81. Wong A. K.-K., *Optical Imaging in Projection Microlithography*, SPIE Publications (March 9, 2005), ISBN-13: 978-0819458292.

82. Molovski S. I., Sushkov A. D., *Intense Electron and Ion Beams*, Springer; Reprint of 2005 edition (November 9, 2010),

83. Chen J. J. H., Krecinic F., Chen J.-H., Chen R. P. S., Lin B. J. Future Electron-Beam Lithography and Implications on Design and CAD Tools, Proceedings of 2011 16th Asia and South Pacific on Design Automation Conference (ASP-DAC), pp. 403–404, 2011.

84. Grasso G., Galli P., Romagnoli M., Iannone E., Bogoni A., Role of integrated photonics technologies in the realization of terabit nodes [Invited], *IEEE/OSA Journal of Optical Communications and Networking*, vol. 1, pp. B111B119, 2009.

85. Harriott L. R., SCALPEL: Projection electron beam lithography, *Proceedings of the 1999 Particle Accelerator Conference*, vol. 1, pp. 595–599, 1999.

86. Kojima, S., Stickel W., Rockrohr J. D., Gordon M., Electron optical image correction subsystem in electron beam projection lithography, *Journal of Vacuum Science & Technology B: Microelectronics and Nanometer Structures*, vol. 18, pp. 3017–3022, 2000.

87. Van Roosmalen A. J., Baggerman J. A. G., Braden S. J. H., *Dry Etching for VLSI*, Springer; 1st edition (March 31, 1991), ISBN-13: 978-0306438356.

88. Fridman A. A., *Plasma Physics and Engineering*, CRC Press; 2nd edition (February 22, 2011), ISBN-13: 978-1439812280.

89. Bellan P. M., *Fundamentals of Plasma Physics*, Cambridge University Press; 1st edition (September 15, 2008), ISBN-13: 978-0521528009.

90. Clemmow P. C., Dougherty J. P., *Electrodynamics of Particles and Plasmas*, Addison-Wesley; 1st edition (1969), ISBN-13: 978-0201479869.

91. Griffiths D. J., *Introduction to Electrodynamics*, Benjamin Cummings; 3rd edition (January 9, 1999), ISBN-13: 978-0138053260.

92. Phillies G. D. J., *Elementary Lectures in Statistical Mechanics*, Springer; 1st edition (December 28, 1999), ISBN-13: 978-0387989181.

93. Conrads H., Schmidt M., Plasma generation and plasma sources, *Plasma Sources Science and Technology*, vol. 9, pp. 441–454, 2000.

94. Yagi H., Ide T., Toyota H., Mori Y., Generation of microwave plasma under high pressure and fabrication of ultrafine carbon particles, *Journal of Materials Research*, vol. 13, pp. 1724–1727, 1988.

95. Kim H. J., Choi J. J., Hong J. M., Uniform long-slit microwave plasma generation from a longitudinal-section electric mode coupling, *IEEE Transactions on Plasma Science*, vol. 34, pp. 1576–1578, 2006.

96. Mathew J. W., Microwave guiding and intense plasma generation at subcutoff dimensions for focused ion beams, *Applied Physics Letters*, vol. 91, pp. 041503–041503-3, 2007.

97. Li X., Hua X., Ling L. Oehrlein G. S., Barela M., Anderson H. M., Fluorocarbon-based plasma etching of SiO_2: Comparison of C_4F_6/Ar and C_4F_8/Ar discharges, *Journal of Vacuum Science and Technology A*, vol. 28, pp. 2052–2061, 2002.

98. Haruhiko Abe H., Yoneda M., Fujiwara N., Developments of plasma etching technology for fabricating semiconductor devices, *Japanese Journal of Applied Physics (in English)*, vol. 47, 2008, pp. 1435–1455, 2008.

99. Dobkin D. M., Zuraw M. K., *Principles of Chemical Vapor Deposition*. Springer; 1st edition (2003). ISBN-13: 978-1402012489.

100. Pierson H. O., *Handbook of Chemical Vapor Deposition: Principles, Technology and Applications*, William Andrew; 2nd edition (December 31, 1999), ISBN-13: 978-0815514329

101. Fukuda T., Scheel H. J., *Crystal Growth Technology*, Wiley; 1st edition (June 28, 2004), ISBN-13: 978-0471495246.

102. Herman M. A., Richter W., Sitter H., *Epitaxy: Physical Foundation and Technical Implementation*, Springer; 1st edition (September 20, 2004), ISBN-13: 978-3540678212.

103. Suo Z., Zhang Z., Epitaxial films stabilized by long-range forces, *Physical Review B*, vol. 58, pp. 5116–5120, 1998.

104. Jaeger R. C. *Introduction to Microelectronic Fabrication*, Prentice-Hall; 2nd edition (October 27, 2001), ISBN-13: 978-020144494-7.

105. Cheong W. S., Optimization of selective epitaxial growth of silicon in LPCVD, *ETRI Journal*, vol. 25, pp. 503–509, 2003.

106. Guillon S. et al., Low-pressure organometallic vapor phase epitaxy of coherent InGaAsP/InP and InGaAsP/InAsP multilayers on InP(001), *Journal of Vacuum Science and Technology A*, vol. 16, pp. 781–786, 1998.

107. Morimoto N. I., Swart J. W., Development of a cluster tool and analysis of deposition of silicon oxide by TEOSO2 PECVD, *Material Research Society Proceedings*, vol. 429, pp. 263–265, 1996.

108. Mattox D. M., *Handbook of Physical Vapor Deposition (PVD) Processing*, William Andrew; 2nd edition (May 19, 2010), ISBN-13: 978-0815520375.

109. Mahan J. E., *Physical Vapor Deposition of Thin Films*, Wiley-Interscience; 1st edition (February 1, 2000), ISBN-13: 978-0471330011.

110. Anders A., *Cathodic Arcs: From Fractal Spots to Energetic Condensation*, Springer; 1st edition (December 31, 2007), ISBN-13: 978-0387791078.

111. Purandare Y. P., Ehiasarian A., Hovsepian P. Eh., Deposition of nanoscale multilayer CrN/NbN physical vapor deposition coatings by high power impulse magnetron sputtering, *Journal Vacuum Science Technology A (AVS)*, vol. 26, pp. 288–296, 2008.

112. Hovsepian P. Eh, Reinhard C., Ehiasarian A. P., CrAlYN/CrN superlattice coatings deposited by the combined high power impulse magnetron sputtering/unbalanced magnetron sputtering technique, *Surface Coating Technology*, vol. 201, pp. 4105–4110, 2006.

113. Konstantinidis S., Dauchot J. P., Hecq M., Titanium oxide thin films deposited by high-power impulse magnetron sputtering, *Thin Solid Films*, vol. 515, pp. 1182–1186, 2006.

114. Konstantinidis S., Hemberg A., Dauchot J. P., Hecq M., Deposition of zinc oxide layers by high-power impulse magnetron sputtering, *Journal of Vacuum Science & Technology B*, vol. 25, pp. L19–L21, 2007.

115. Sittinger V., Ruske F., Werner W., Jacobs C., Szyszka B., Christie D. J., High power pulsed magnetron sputtering of transparent conducting oxides, *Thin Solid Films*, vol. 516, pp. 5847–5859, 2008.

116. Yusupov M., Bultinck E., Depla D., Bogaerts A., Behavior of electrons in a dual-magnetron sputter deposition system: A monte carlo model, *New Journal of Physics*, vol. 16, pp. 033018 033024, 2011.

117. Bernhard W., *Handbook of Ion Sources*, CRC Press; 1st edition (1995), ISBN-13: 978-0849325021.

118. Chow R., Ellis A. D., Loomis G. E., Rana S. I., Characterization of Niobium Oxide Films Deposited by High Target Utilization Sputtering Sources, Proceedings of International Conference on Metallurgical Coatings and Thin Films (ICMCTF), 2007.

119. Thornton J. A. Influence of apparatus geometry and deposition conditions on the structure and topography of thick sputtered coatings, *Journal of Vacuum Science Technology*, vol. 11, pp. 666–670, 1974.

120. Windischman H. Intrinsic stress in sputter-deposited thin film, *Critical Review of Solid State Material Science*, vol. 17, pp. 547–553, 1992.

121. McCray W. P. MBE deserves a place in the history books, *Nature Nanotechnology*, vol. 2, pp. 259–261, 2007.

122. Shchukin V. A., Dieter B., Spontaneous ordering of nanostructures on crystal surface, *Reviews of Modern Physics*, vol. 71, pp. 1125–1171, 1999.

123. Stangl J., Holý V., Bauer G., Structural properties of self-organized semiconductor nanostructures, *Reviews of Modern Physics*, vol. 76, pp. 725–783, 2004.

124. Liu A. Q., Surface planarization process, in *RF MEMS Switches and Integrated Switching Circuits*, Liu A. Q. Editor, Springer; 1st edition (2010), ISBN-13: 978-0387462615.

125. Sikder A. K., Giglio F., Wood J., Kumar A., Anthony M., Mechanical and tribological properties of interlayer films for the damascene-cu chemical-mechanical planarization process, *Journal of Electronic Materials*, vol. 30, pp. 1520–1526, 2001.

126. Fan S. S.-K., Quality improvement of chemical-mechanical wafer planarization process in semiconductor manufacturing using a combined generalized linear modelling—nonllinear programming approach, *International Journal of Production Research*, vol. 38, pp. 3011–3029, 2000.

127. Hurwitz M. A., Identifying sources of variation in a wafer planarization process, in *Statistical Case Studies for Industrial Processes Improvement*, Czitrom V., Spagon P. D., Editors, Society for Industrial and Applied Mathematics Press (1997), ISBN-13: 9780898713947.

128. Niklaus F., Stemme G., Lu J.-Q., Gutmann R. J., Adhesive wafer bonding, *Journal of Applied Physics*, vol. 99, pp. 031101-1-28, 2006.

129. Tong Q.-J., Göesel U. M., Wafer bonding and layer splitting for microsystems, *Advanced materials*, vol. 11, pp. 14091425, 1999.

130. Dicioccio L. et al., Direct Bonding for Wafer Level 3D Integration, Proceedings of International Conference on IC Design and Technology, 2010, pp. 110–113.

131. Yu L. et al., Adhesive bonding with Su-8 at wafer level for microfluidic devices, *Journal of Physics: Conference Series*, vol. 34 pp. 776–781, 2006.

132. Cannavo' M., van Zeijl H. W., Pandraud G., Driel J. V., Alan T., Sarro P. M., Oxide to Oxide Wafer Bonding for Three Dimensional (3D) IC Integration Technologies, Proceedings of Semiconductor

Advances for Future Electronics Workshop. SAFE 2007, Printed by STW, Veldhoven, The Netherlands, pp. 509–512, 2007.

133. Gui C., Elwenspoek M., Tas N., Gardeniers J. G. E., The effect of surface roughness on direct wafer bonding, *Journal of Applied Physics*, vol. 85, pp. 7448–7454, 1999.

134. Weinerd A., Amirfeiz P., Bengtsson S., Plasma assisted room temperature bonding for MST, *Sensors and Actuators—A*, vol. 92, pp. 214–222, 2001.

135. Li S. H., Chen K. N., Lu J. J.-Q., Wafer-to-wafer alignment for three-dimensional integration: A review, *Journal of Microelectromechanical Systems*, vol. 20, pp. 885–898, 2011.

5 Polymer Technology

5.1 INTRODUCTION

We have seen in Chapter 4 as micro-fabrication technologies originally introduced for microelectronics and integrated optics are a suitable set of techniques to obtain labs on chip starting from SiO_2 on Si or fully SiO_2 wafers. The excellent mechanical and chemical properties of glass, the large number of planar structures, and MEMs that can be built from silicon, besides the wide and complex set of techniques at the designer disposal, allow complex labs on chip to be developed with a fabrication cost model suitable for very large-scale production.

This technology reveals its limits when very large-scale production is not needed, and in any case in the research phase, when a very complex technology infrastructure has to be set up even to produce samples. Generally, this problem is solved by planar technology companies by sharing the same fabrication infrastructure between production and research, so also getting the advantage of directly developing new products on the production line. In any case, the problem of the high cost of manufacturing infrastructure remains and it is frequently an early problem for companies or research institutions starting an activity in this field.

A way of getting around this problem is to use less expensive processes that require to change the fabrication material if the same performances in terms of technology scaling with volumes and ability to deal with small critical dimensions have to be attained. Suitable materials do effectively exist: they are artificial polymers (see Section 1.4). Polymers can be used as base materials for the final product, accessing to simpler and less expensive process during the fabrication phase and as fast prototype materials, to develop lower cost research prototypes of structures that are meant to be fabricated with standard planar technologies in the industrial phase.

In several industrial applications, where a long product operating life is required, a few concerns still survive related to the intrinsic stability of selected polymeric materials when subject to continuous mechanical and thermal solicitation due to long-lasting use. It is remarkable that these concerns generally do not apply to labs on chip designed for biological or medical applications. As a matter of fact, they are generally design to be disposable chip, thus durability under repeated use is generally not required. Moreover, due to the fact that almost all the systems of this kind are charged with organic test solutions or organic molecules absorbed in suitably activated surfaces, the limit of duration in storage and the resistance to temperature fluctuations are not fixed by the polymers characteristics, but by the biological molecules stored inside the chip.

Thus, labs on chip application seems really suited to exploit the good properties of polymeric materials and the availability of low cost processes to fabricate polymers based chips.

Polymeric technologies have also another very interesting application field in the area of labs on chip. As a matter of fact proteins, DNA and RNA, and other biological molecules are natural polymers and, while frequently more complex in structure with respect to artificial polymers, share many of their characteristics. Thus, micro-fabrication technologies designed for artificial polymers are also suitable for deposition and patterning of many biological macromolecules, so opening a wider field of opportunities.

Under the industrial point of view, while a wide set of technologies has been developed up to research and testing stage for polymers based micro-fabrication, nothing similar to the experience that exists in the field of Si and SiO_2 technologies is still there. The fabrication process allowing to produce billions of microelectronics circuits and several millions of integrated optics elements has no correspondence in the field of polymers micro- and nano-fabrication technologies, where experimentation and research are still dominant over large volumes production. In any case, very large volume production is attained with similar techniques applied to macroscopic objects and small doubt exist that, if the market will require it, this scaling will be possible also in the micro-fabrication area.

Several variations are present almost for all the fabrication technologies we will present in this chapter: we will not focus our attention on describing all possible arrangement of the fabrication process or of the fabrication equipment, but we will try to clarify the key principles and control parameters besides the expected process performances.

5.2   SOFT LITHOGRAPHY

If polymers are selected as structural material to realize a lab on chip, it is possible either to maintain the conceptual structure of the fabrication process we have seen in Chapter 4, or change drastically the fabrication process sequence by exploiting polymers properties to device processes that has no analog in the planar technology.

In the first case, as a first step a substrate has to be prepared by polymerization of the wanted material. The substrate has to be polished and prepared for the subsequent fabrication steps. After substrate preparation a sequence of deposition, pattern transfer, and etching phases are carried out to define on the substrate the wanted patterns. In this case, what make polymer technology deeply different from $Si–SiO_2$ technology is the different material characteristics. As a matter of fact, if several traditional processes can be used also when dealing with polymers, the particular nature of these materials put at the designed disposal a completely new family of processes. The great majority of these processes are based on the property of polymers to assume, depending on the temperature, solid and viscous states so to be molded or deposited in such a way as to fill also small features on the underlying frame.

Soft lithography, in particular, refers to a set of different techniques that uses an elastomer as a stamp, a mold or a mask to reproduce micro-patterns or microstructures instead of a rigid mask as done in traditional photolithography [1,2]. An elastomer is a polymer exhibiting the viscoelasticity property, that is, it behaves as solids below a threshold stress and like high viscous liquids above the threshold stress (see Section 7.3.6.3 for more details). When the elastomer is forced in the pseudo-liquid behavior by an applied stress and the stress is removed it returns to the pseudo-solid behavior without any permanent structural modification, from which the name elastomer. Generally, such polymers have low Young's modulus in solid form and high yield strain compared with more rigid polymeric materials. The most used elastomer in this applications is PDMS (see Section 1.4 and Table 1.12), but several elastomers exist like Polysiloxanes, commonly called silicone rubber, whose molecule formula is $(SiC_2H_2O)_n$.

The viscoelastic behavior is generally derived from the ability of the polymer long chains with a high degree of covalent cross-links to reconfigure themselves to distribute an applied stress. The covalent cross-linkages ensure that the elastomer will return to its original configuration when the stress is removed. As a result of this extreme flexibility, elastomers can reversibly extend from 5% to 700%, depending on the specific material. Without the cross-linkages or with short, uneasily reconfigured chains, the applied stress would result in a permanent deformation. Temperature effects are also present in the demonstrated elasticity of elastomers.

A wide class of different techniques are generally collected under the name of soft lithography, being micro-contact printing (μCP), micro-transfer molding (μTM), micro-molding in capillaries (MIMIC), and micro-replica molding (μRM) the most diffused, even if a great number of other processes, small or great variations of these base four processes, have been introduced, generally in research works, for different applications. All these techniques have a general process in common and differ for the particular way in which the polymer stamp obtained at the end of the process is used to replicate its form.

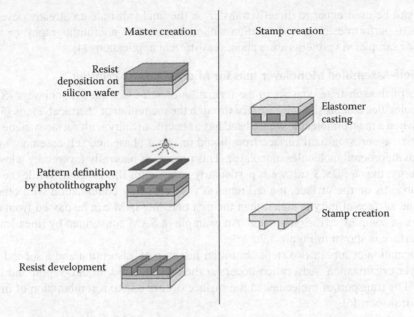

Master creation · Stamp creation

Resist deposition on silicon wafer

Elastomer casting

Pattern definition by photolithography

Stamp creation

Resist development

FIGURE 5.1 General scheme of a soft lithography process.

The general soft lithography process is represented in Figure 5.1. As a first step a master is generated on a rigid and durable support by standard lithography and etching or deposition. Often the master is generated by a silicon wafer or by a glass film deposited on a silicon wafer. Other times the master is simply created by developing a resist film deposited on a silicon wafer, without the need of transferring the pattern on the wafer. Hard resists are generally used for this process, like SU8 or Polyimide. After the master preparation pre-polymerized PDMS (or another suitable elastomer) is poured on the master.

PDMS has several properties rendering it suitable for this application [3]:

- PDMS has an interface free energy quite low, allowing easy contact with other interfaces. Standard surface energy of polymerized PDMS is as low as 21.6 mJ/m^2.
- It is chemically inert.
- It does not swell with high humidity.
- Has a good permeability to gasses.
- Has a good thermal stability up to temperatures as low as −186°C in air.
- PDMS is optically transparent from UV down to 300 nm infrared.
- PDMS is isotropic and homogeneous, differently from other polymers that has a preferential direction due to a preferential orientation of polymeric chains.
- PDMS is very durable; stamps can be used in harsh conditions up to more than 50 times without degradation.

Once the stamp is obtained, it is used to replicate its form on the substrates where the final circuits will be built.

5.2.1 Micro-Contact Printing

In micro-contact printing the PDMS stamp is coated with a special ink composed by the molecules that are to be transferred in specific patterns on the final substrate. These molecules are either artificial organic components or biomolecules that it has to be patterned on the final substrate. This technique can be used either to directly transfer on the final substrate an already developed resist mask so as to perform etching or deposition without the need of photolithography, or to activate a surface, for example, via proteins absorption, for different applications [4].

5.2.1.1 Self-Assembled Monolayer Inks for Micro-Contact Printing

The inking of the substrate consists in the formation of self-assembled monolayers (SAM) of the required molecules coating the solid surface through the formation of chemical bonds [5,6]. A SAM generates when a macro-molecule whose head has a specific affinity with surfaces made from a specific material, absorbs on such surface from liquid or vapor phase and self-assembly after absorption to form an ordered molecules monolayer. This process is naturally favored by a low absorbing surface energy, thus a PDMS surface is particularly suitable for this process. While the head of the molecule absorbs on the surface, the tail remains free, allowing combination with other surfaces. If the second surface affinity is higher than the first one, the SAM can be passed from a surface to the other via a complex diffusion process. An example of SAM constituted by linear molecules on a PDMS surface is shown in Figure 5.2.

SAM formation occurs in two steps, an initial fast step of adsorption and a second slower step of monolayer organization. Adsorption occurs at the liquid–liquid, liquid–vapor, and liquid–solid interfaces. The transport of molecules to the surface occurs due to a combination of diffusion and convective transport [6].

Under a chemical point of view, the formation phase of a SAM can be described as the equilibrium between different phases of the material that has to constitute the monolayer, that is moved during the formation more and more towards the existence of the monolayer phase only [5,7].

In the simplest cases three phases can be individuated during the SAM formation: the liquid or vapor phase, depending on the kind of formation process used, the phase constituted by the SAM material deposited onto the surface in a horizontal arrangement (sometimes called stripped phase), and the monolayer phase, where the macromolecule has one extreme absorbed onto the surface and the other as far as possible from the surface itself. Generally, also an intermediate phase can be individuated. The nature of this intermediate phase strictly depends on the involved material and the growing process and several different intermediate phases have been individuated: a few examples are a sort of super-cooled 2D fluid of the material on the surface [8] or a nucleation phase constituted by several disordered micro-layer in thermodynamic equilibrium [6]. The qualitative form of a kind of phase diagram for a SAM that is generated by a starting liquid phase is reported in Figure 5.3. Here, different phases and phase transition characteristics are represented on the

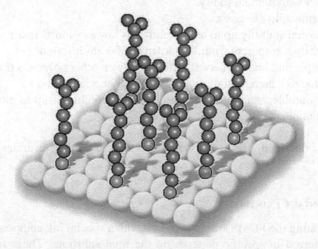

FIGURE 5.2   Principle scheme of a SAM of organic molecules on a surface.

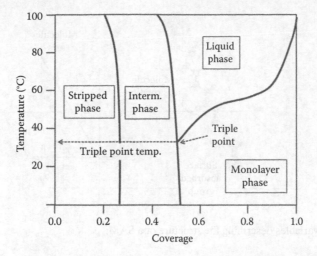

FIGURE 5.3 Phase diagram for the formation of a SAM from liquid phase in the coverage-temperature plane (numerical data refer approximately to the growth of decanethiol SAM on Au(111). (Adapted from Pruzinski S. A., Braun P. V., *Advanced Functional Materials*, vol. 15, pp. 1995–2004, 2005.)

coverage–temperature plane, where the coverage is defined as the number of available bonding sites on the surface that are saturated by the complementary extreme of the macromolecule.

As shown in Figure 5.3, the stripping phase, where the molecules are horizontally laying on the surface, is possible only for small values of the coverage that can be stable only for low temperatures, where the thermal energy is not sufficient to provoke a phase change. As a matter of fact, the molecule chain length is generally greater than the distance of active sites on the surface, so that even when the molecules are all aligned, the coverage is limited by the ratio between the maximum distance between adjacent bonding sites and the molecule chain length. By increasing the temperature this phase becomes unstable, since a greater coverage assures lower surface energy, starting the very complex process of monolayer formation.

The phase transitions in which the SAM forms depend on the ratio between the environment temperature and on the triple point temperature. Many different theories have been presented to completely explain the monolayer formation and it is quite possible that the process mechanism also depends on the involved materials and on the process. One of the most diffused interpretations of the SAM growth is based on a nucleation model, somehow similar to the nucleation process giving rise to crystals [10].

At temperatures below the triple point the growth goes from the stripped phase to the intermediate phase where many islands form with the final SAM structure, but are surrounded by random molecules. Similar to nucleation in metals, as these islands grow larger they intersect forming boundaries until they end up in the monolayer phase. At temperatures above the triple point the growth is more complex and can take two paths. In the first path the heads of the SAM organize to their near final locations with the tail groups loosely formed on top. Then as they transit to the monolayer phase, the tail groups become ordered and straighten out. In the second path the molecules start in a laying down position along the surface in the stripped phase. These then form into islands of ordered SAMs, where they grow into monolayers.

The nature in which the tail groups organize themselves into a straight ordered monolayer is dependent on the inter-molecular attraction, or van der Waals forces, between the alkyl and tail groups. To minimize the free energy of the organic layer the molecules adopt conformations that allow high degree of van der Waals forces with some hydrogen bonding. The small size of the SAM molecules are important here because van der Waals forces arise from the dipoles of molecules and are thus much weaker than the surrounding surface forces at larger scales. The assembly process

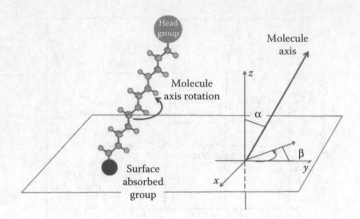

FIGURE 5.4 Angle variables describing the structure of a SAM.

begins with a small group of molecules, usually two, getting close enough so that the van der Waals forces overcomes the surrounding force.

The forces between the molecules orientate themselves so that they are in their straight, optimal, configuration. Then, as other molecules come close by they interact with these already organized molecules in the same fashion and become a part of the conformed group. When this occurs across a large area the molecules support each other into forming their SAM shape as seen in Figure 5.2.

The orientation of the molecules can be described with two parameters, α and β, as shown in Figure 5.4 where α is the angle of tilt of the backbone from the surface normal. In typical applications α varies from 0 to 60° depending on the substrate and type of SAM molecule. β is the angel of rotation along the long axis of the molecule. β is usually between 30° and 40° [11]. Many of the SAM properties, such as thickness, are determined in the first few minutes of the growth process. However, it may take hours for defects to be eliminated via annealing and for final SAM properties to be determined. The exact kinetics of SAM formation depends on the adsorbate, solvent, and substrate properties [11].

Once formed, the SAM is transferred from the stamp to the substrate by puttying the inked stamp surface in contact with the substrate.

5.2.1.2 Micro-Contact Printing Properties

When used as a lithography technique, that is to transfer a mask on the final substrate, the micro-contact printing has several interesting properties. The flexibility of the PDMS stamp allows to transfer the SAM mask also on rough surfaces and planarity of the final substrate is not required to obtain a good lithography result, but it is sufficient to limit the local curvature ratio below a critic value that, in general, is quite small.

Thus, potential spurious curvature of the substrate is not a problem, while they risk to seriously compromise standard photolithography due to the deep of field requirements, and lithography can be done also on curve surfaces, like an optical fiber or a lens substrate [11].

Although a very promising technique, μCP has a set of critical aspects that has to be well controlled to obtain a good result.

During direct contact the stamp can easily be physically deformed causing printed features that are different than the original stamp features. Horizontally stretching or compressing the stamp will cause deformations in the raised and recessed features. Also, applying too much vertical pressure on the stamp during printing can cause the raised relief features to flatten against the substrate. These deformations can yield submicron features even though the original stamp has a lower resolution.

Deformation of the stamp can occur during removal from the master and during the substrate contacting process. When the aspect ratio of the stamp is high buckling of the stamp can occur,

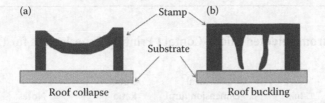

FIGURE 5.5 Deformation processes during micro-contact printing due to a too low (a) or too high (b) aspect ratio.

while when the aspect ratio is low roof collapse can occur. These two possible problems are shown schematically in Figure 5.5.

The curing process occurring after the stamp realization to harden the PDMS is a particularly critical phase of the whole process. During the curing process some fragments can potentially be left uncured and contaminate the process depositing on the substrate during printing.

During curing the stamp can also shrink in size leaving a difference in desired dimensions of the substrate patterning. Typical shrink percentage arrives to 1% [11] and can be partially compensated by biasing the process once the statistics of the particular fabrication considered is known.

Swelling of the stamp may also occur. Most organic solvents induce swelling of the PDMS stamp. Ethanol in particular has a very small swelling effect, but many other solvents cannot be used for wet inking because of high swelling. Because of this the process is often considered to be limited to nonpolar inks that are soluble in ethanol.

Last, but not least, ink diffusion from the PDMS bulk to the surface occurs during the formation of the patterned SAM on the substrate. This mobility of the ink can cause lateral spreading to unwanted regions. Upon transfer this spreading can influence the desired pattern.

Different variations can be done to the base μCP process to improve its performances or to face its limitations. Stability is greatly increased by submerging the stamp in a liquid medium. By printing hydrophobic long-chain thiols underwater the common problem of vapor transport of the ink is greatly reduced. PDMS aspect ratios of 15:1 can be achieved using this method that seems not to be possible by performing the process in air [12].

As opposed to wet inking, contact inking technique does not permeate the PDMS bulk. The ink molecules only contact the protruding areas of the stamp that are going to be used for the patterning. The absence of ink on the rest of the stamp reduces the amount of ink transferred through the vapor phase that can potentially affect the pattern. This is done by the direct contact of a feature stamp and a flat PDMS substrate that has ink on it [13].

Table 5.1 summarizes selected laboratory results obtained using μCP for different applications.

5.2.2 MICRO-TRANSFER MOLDING

In the case of micro-transfer molding (μTM) the pattern from the stamp on a substrate, either an Si wafer or a polymer substrate, for made by PDMS, using a different method [1]. The stamp is filled with a polymer precursor, once filled it is pushed against the substrate and the polymer precursor cached in between the stamp and the substrate is cured so as to harden it. At this time, the stamp is peeled and the form on the stamp is transferred as in a negative mask lithography technique on the substrate. This process is shown in Figure 5.6.

Micro-transfer molding has been demonstrated to be particularly suitable for fabrication of 3D structures on polymer substrates.

An example is reported in Figure 5.7 [21], where the technique of the polymer walls is used to build both a set of two concatenated rings where the inner ring can be moved with respect to the outer one, and a quite high-aspect ratio structure (with the form of the capital A). The PDMS walls

TABLE 5.1

Research Results from Selected Micro-Contact Printing Experiments for Different Applications

Substrate	Ink	Critical Dimension (μm)	Aspect Ratio	Notes	Reference
Silica on silicon	Alkane phosphoric acid	6	0.15	—	[14]
Silica with SU8 mask	ZnO NP	5	—	Deposition to start nanowire growth	[15]
Gold	Alkanethiol	0.8	1	—	[16]
PLL-g-PEG[a]	SbpA, SbpA-EGFP, SbpA-STV[b]	9	—	—	[17]
Chemically modified porous silica	Rabbit IgG solution	Large surface pores 4–6 nm radius 96–200 nm depth	—	IgG trapping for immunoassay	[18]
Au film on silicon	IgG solution	30	From 0.5 to 0.16	IgG trapping in ducts for immunoassay, permanent PDMS as roof of the micro-reactor	[19]
Thermal oxide on silicon	IgG solution	30	0.5	IgG trapping in ducts for immunoassay, permanent PDMS as roof of the micro-reactor	[19]
HDMS[c] patterns over SiO$_2$	Goat IgGs	30	—	Trap IgGs for immunoassay	[20]

a   Poly-L-lysine grafted polyethylene glycol.
b   Three bacteria S-layer (fusion) proteins.
c   Hexamethyldisilazane.

technique can be appreciated by looking at Figure 5.7a, where the stamp pattern realized on the PDMS stamp of the two ring structure is shown. Here, areas that have to result to be void in the final pattern, are occupied by very thin walls of PDMS polymer. When the intermediate polymer is cured and the stamp removed, the PDMS walls remain attached to the original stamp due to the PDMS surface adhesion, leaving the wanted holes on the final structure.

Even curved structures can be obtained with high-aspect ratio by pouring the polymer precursor in between two PDMS stamps and, during curing, deforming the two stamps with the polymer in between a curved surface (e.g., a curved cylinder) [22].

In general, problems that could arise when performing μTM are not different in nature from those encountered in μCP and are mainly related to the intrinsic tendency of polymer structure to release from the target form during curing or in high temperature processes.

5.2.3   Micro-Molding in Capillaries and Micro-Replica Molding

Micro-molding in capillaries (MIMC) is a technique for fabricating patterned microstructures of various organic polymers on a variety of solid substrates, frequently also made by polymers [23,24]. In this technique, the PDMS stamp is prepared by imprinting a network of small channels on it.

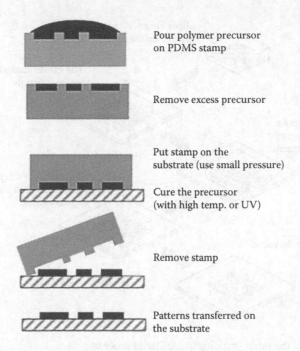

Pour polymer precursor
on PDMS stamp

Remove excess precursor

Put stamp on the
substrate (use small pressure)

Cure the precursor
(with high temp. or UV)

Remove stamp

Patterns transferred on
the substrate

FIGURE 5.6 Scheme of the micro-transfer molding process.

When it is placed on the surface of a substrate it makes conformal contact with that surface; as a result, a network of closed ducts is formed between the mold and the substrate. When a low-viscosity liquid polymer precursor is placed at the open ends of the network of channels, the liquid spontaneously fills in the channels by capillary action. After filling the channels and curing the precursor with thermal cycles or UV exposition into a solid, crosslinked polymer, the PDMS mold is removed, and a network of polymeric material remains on the surface of the substrate. The overall process is schematically represented in Figure 5.8.

In order to ease or homogenize the process in cases of very complex ducts networks, the opposite part of the stamp with respect to the position of the precursor can be placed in contact with a

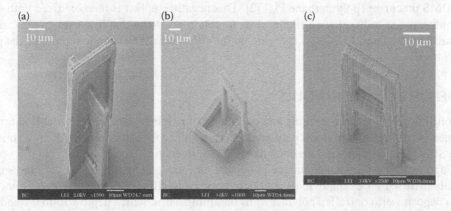

FIGURE 5.7 Examples of 3D structures with a high-aspect ratio fabricated with micro transfer molding (SEM photographs). Master form of interlocked rings on PDMS with PDMS walls (a), movable rings obtained by transferring the pattern in (a) on a polymer substrate (b) and (c), other 3D forms built with micro-transfer molding having an aspect ratio up to 6. (Published under permission, Copyright 2006 National Academy of Sciences, USA)

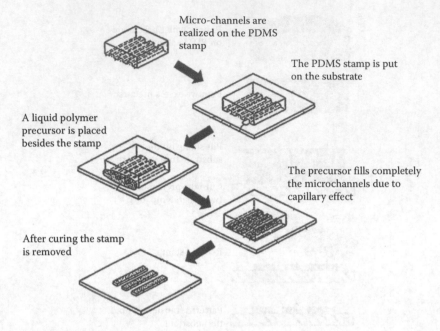

Micro-channels are realized on the PDMS stamp

The PDMS stamp is put on the substrate

A liquid polymer precursor is placed besides the stamp

The precursor fills completely the microchannels due to capillary effect

After curing the stamp is removed

FIGURE 5.8 Scheme of the micro-molding in capillaries process.

vacuum pump, so that the pressure resulting in the duct network enhances the liquid penetration. Pressure can also be created with standard pumps, or the liquid can be attracted through all the ducts network using electro-osmosis (see Section 7.5.4).

A variety of liquid precursors such as polyurethane (PU), polyacrylate, and epoxy can be used in this process. These polymeric microstructures can be released by dissolving the underlying substrates to form free-standing polymeric membranes.

For its own nature, this kind of process cannot be used to fabricate 3D structures, but it can be easily adapted to fabricate structures on curved surfaces. It has been successfully used to fabricate polymers transistors [2], that are interesting structures if a bit of electronic control is to be added to a disposable circuit like a lab on chip.

In micro-replica molding (μRM), PDMS stamp is replicated using PDMS itself via the curing of the PDMS precursor (polyurethane PU) [2]. This negative replica is then oxidized with oxygen plasma and exposed to fluorinated silane, so as to obtain a surface that has a very small adhesion to standard PDMS. Thus, PDMS is cast again on the cured negative stamp to reproduce the pattern in PDMS itself.

5.3 DEPOSITION TECHNIQUES

While soft lithography allows forming and deposition of polymer patterns on suitable substrate, it is often needed to deposit a uniform polymer layer on a solid substrate, either made by a solid polymer like SU8 or by another solid material like glass. Spin coating (see Section 4.5.2) is a very performing and well-consolidated technique to deposit uniform polymer layers on very flat surfaces, universally diffused for example to deposit polymeric resist films on silicon wafers. Spin coating is able to deposit well-controlled polymer films obtaining a film with a depth within 0.1 and 4 μm.

In several applications however, either the film has to be much thick (as in many 3D applications) or much thin (like in surface activation, where a macromolecules monolayer is needed). Moreover, the substrate is not always sufficiently flat to assure suitable performance of spin coating, either due to a wanted 3D form or to the intrinsic tolerance on flatness, that can be much greater for polymeric substrates with respect to silicon wafers.

In these cases, different techniques have to be used. Spray coating and electrophoresis deposition, that we also analyzed in Section 4.5.2, are frequently used in alternative of spin coating when a polymer layer has to be deposited on a flat surface whose flatness is not so well controlled to allow a good spin coating.

In different applications it is necessary to deposit a thin monolayer of natural or artificial polymers. In this case micro-contact printing can be an option, but also other deposition techniques exist, that are based on the same principle of SAM formation.

5.3.1 Polymer Film Deposition through Spray Coating

Spray coating is suitable to fill the surface roughness of many materials, obtaining absence of point of no contact between the deposited film and the surface with a very good film planarity on the air exposed surface.

Spray coating is frequently used for polymers that can be solved by a solvent suited to be sprayed through a small orifice. After solving the polymer into the solvent, this is either vaporized by pressure with a spray gas and pushed through the spray orifice, or directly pushed in liquid form against the orifice so as to be mechanically vaporized while passing through.

Aldo insoluble polymers can be sprayed using the so-called thermal spraying. In this case, the polymer is dissolved by high temperature while simultaneously mixing it to a spray gas. After creation, the gaseous hot mix is pushed through the orifice to be sprayed. When thermal spray is used, frequently more than one substance is dissolved in the spray, so that they react while arriving on the surface to be coated and, in case after further curing, they form a particular substance that is frequently achievable only through spray coating.

Several variations of thermal spraying can be distinguished:

- Plasma spraying [25–27]
- Detonation spraying [25]
- Wire arc spraying [25]
- Flame spraying [25]
- High-velocity oxy-fuel coating spraying (HVOF) [28]
- Warm spraying [29]
- Cold spraying [30]

In flame spraying and wire arc spraying, a high-temperature flame or a glow arc are used to vaporize the material to be sprayed and to mix it at high temperature with the spray gas. In this case, the particle velocities are generally low, frequently smaller than 150 m/s. While flame or arc spray are still widely used, especially micro-fabrication applications, plasma spraying, using a high-temperature plasma jet generated by arc discharge, is probably the most used spray coating technique.

5.3.1.1 Plasma Spray Coating

In plasma spraying, the material to be deposited, often called feedstock, is typically provided as a powder, a liquid suspension [26], or a solid wire [27]. The feedstock is introduced into the plasma jet, emanating from a plasma glow chamber. In the jet, where the temperature is in the order of 10^4 K, the material is melted and propelled toward a substrate, mixed if needed with a carrier spraying gas. On the substrate, the molten droplets flatten, rapidly solidify and form a deposit. Commonly, the deposits remain adherent to the substrate as coatings; free-standing parts can also be produced by removing the substrate.

There are a large number of technological parameters that influence the interaction of the particles with the plasma jet and the substrate and therefore the deposit properties. These parameters include feedstock type, plasma gas composition and flow rate, energy input, orifice distance from

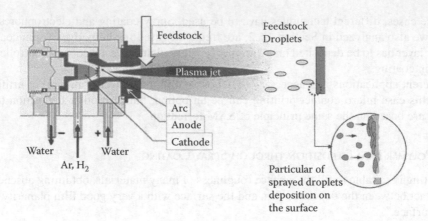

FIGURE 5.9 Schematic representation of a plasma spray equipment based on Ar plasma.

the substrate, substrate cooling, and so on. The schematic representation of a plasma spray equipment based on Ar plasma is reported in Figure 5.9.

The deposits obtained through plasma spray coating consist of a multitude of lamellae frequently called splats, formed by flattening of the liquid droplets projected by the plasma jet onto the substrate surface. As the feedstock powders more frequently used in such equipment typically have sizes from 10 to above 100 µm, the lamellae have thickness in the micrometer range and lateral dimension from several to hundreds of micrometers. Due to the random lamellae deposition, small voids are present among them, such as pores, cracks, and regions of incomplete bonding. As a result the deposits can have properties significantly different from bulk materials. Generally, a lower strength and elastic modulus are observed, besides higher strain tolerance and lower thermal and electrical conductivity. Due to the rapid solidification, metastable phases can be present in the deposits too.

Plasma spray can be performed in air and in this case it is called air plasma spraying (APS). In this way the complexity of the plasma spray equipment is minimized, but the deposited film can be contaminated not only from air particles moved by the spray up to the surface, but also by spurious components created by the reaction of the sprayed material with air particles like O_2 molecules in the high temperature environment of the process.

In order to avoid as much as possible this contamination source the spray can be operated in a chamber where a controlled atmosphere is maintained. Such a process is called controlled atmosphere plasma spraying (CAPS). The controlled atmosphere is generally constituted by a low pressure inert gas to avoid as much as possible chemical interaction of the material to be sprayed with the atmosphere both by decreasing the number of intercepted atmosphere particles during the fly of a spray droplet and rendering chemical interaction very difficult. In extreme cases, plasma spray can be carried out in high vacuum to further decrease contamination of the deposited surface.

Vacuum plasma spraying (VPS) is frequently used to create porous layers with high reproducibility. These layers can improve properties such as frictional behavior, heat resistance, surface electrical conductivity, lubricity, cohesive strength of films, or dielectric constant, or it can make materials hydrophilic or hydrophobic. This last property can be used in labs on chip as a way to prepare surface activation.

The process typically operates at 39°C–120°C to avoid thermal damage of the substrate and of the deposited film. In this way, when the suitable precursors are inserted into the plasma jet, non-thermally activated surface reactions can be generated, causing surface changes which cannot occur with molecular chemistries at atmospheric pressure.

5.3.1.2 Polymers for Spray Deposition

Two main classes of materials can be deposited through spray coating: thermosetting and thermoplastic coatings.

In thermosetting coatings, the small molecules that are coated create the polymer while baking after the spray deposition. This polymerization generally is very rich in inter-chains links so that the coating forms a sort of single giant molecule that is firmly fixed to the substrate and cannot melt or flow.

In the case of thermoplastic films, the spray creates sufficiently mobile molecules on the substrate surface that they bind strictly one to the other in the first phase after deposition and during subsequent curing. Although thermoplastic films can still be softened so as to allow them to flow on the surface of the substrate, and at high temperature they melt, the softening and melting temperatures are generally quite elevated.

Electrostatic spray coating is a variation of spray coating where the polymer powder to be deposited is electrostatically charged, generally with negative charge due to electrons absorption, in the spray gun.

When deposition on the grounded surface starts, the negative charged particles uniformly deposit on the surface due to the electrostatic repulsion avoiding superficial density fluctuations.

When a uniform film is created, since this is negatively charged, it starts to repel further incoming particles and the deposition ends.

5.3.2 POLYMER KNIFE COATING

This coating technique is based on the application of a coating polymer on the substrate and then the mechanical film formation by passing the substrate through a slit between a knife and a roller, also offering support for the moving substrate. The coating principle is shown in Figure 5.10. The schematic process described in Figure 5.10, if applied as it is shown, results to be inaccurate both due to the fact that the film cannot be more thin than the lower limit of the controllable blade precision and due to the fact that, once out of the slit, the polymer relaxes itself to assume the final position with a certain degree of random variability.

The last problem is due to the fact that the polymer chains are positioned in a random way inside the polymeric material and, especially for particularly long chains, it impacts local relaxation of the polymer.

There are, however, several modifications of the base process that tends to face its limits and try to improve its performances without losing its peculiar simplicity and suitability to be used

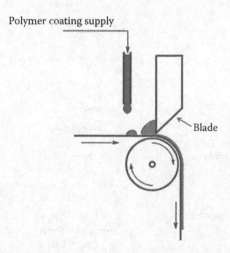

Polymer coating supply

Blade

FIGURE 5.10 Schematic representation of a knife polymer film deposition equipment.

for batch fabrication. For thick films, within the limits attainable with the process, the distance between the blade and the roller can be adjusted with great precision, thus the film thickness can be controlled and easily changed from support to support or also within the same support if needed.

5.3.3 PLASMA-ENHANCED POLYMERIZATION

This is a specific type of PECVD (see Section 4.9.1) in which monomers in gaseous phase deposits on a plasma-activated surface pushed by the plasma itself and create an highly interlinked polymer [31,32]. The key difference from plasma spray deposition is that in the spray case the plasma jet does not touch the surface where the film has to be deposited, working only as propulsion for the spray of the film material droplets. In this case on the contrary, the interaction between the plasma jet and the surface is a key element of the deposition technique.

Many monomers can be polymerized in a plasma deposition reactor, and one of the advantages of these techniques is that even molecules that generally do not give rise to polymerization, can be structured in plasma polymers. A selection of monomers used frequently in plasma polymerization and deposition is reported in Table 5.2 [33].

The ability of polymerized molecules that generally do not assembly in polymeric form is one of the consequences of the fact that the properties of plasma polymers differ greatly from those of conventional polymers. While both types of polymers are dependent on the chemical properties of

TABLE 5.2
Common Monomers Used in Plasma Polymer Deposition

Thiophene

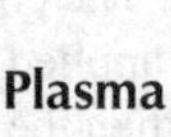

Pyridine

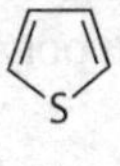

Acrylonitrile

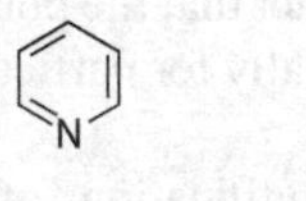

Furan

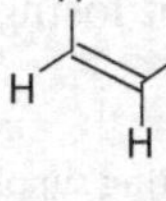

Styrene

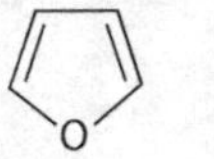

Acetylene $H-C{\equiv}C-H$

2-Methyloxazoline

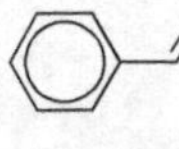

Tetramethyldisiloxane

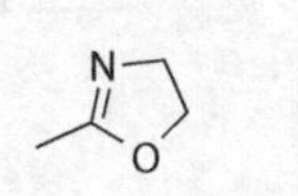

the monomer, the properties of plasma polymers depend greatly on the design of the reactor and the chemical and physical characteristics of the substrate on which the plasma polymer is deposited [32]. The location within the reactor where the deposition occurs also has an effect on the resultant polymer's properties. In fact, by using plasma polymerization with a single monomer and varying the reactor, substrate, and so on a variety of polymers, each having different physical and chemical properties, can be prepared [32].

The large dependence of the polymer features on these factors make it difficult to assign a set of basic characteristics, but a few common properties that set plasma polymers apart from conventional polymers do exist. The most significant difference between conventional polymers and plasma polymers is that plasma polymers do not contain regular repeating units. Due to the fact that interaction of monomers with the plasma discharge creates different assembly of the same monomers that propagates in the plasma and deposition chamber; moreover other species, like ions and free electrons are present in the plasma that could contribute to the polymerization process. The resultant polymer chains are highly branched and are randomly terminated with a high degree of cross-linking [32]. An example of a part of the structure of plasma deposited PDMS [34] demonstrating a large extend of cross-linking and branching is shown in Figure 5.11.

Other specific properties of plasma polymers are the following:

- *Free Radicals.* All plasma polymers contain free radicals as well. The amount of free radicals present varies between polymers and is dependent on the chemical structure of the monomer. Because the formation of the trapped free radicals is tied to the growth mechanism of the plasma polymers, the overall properties of the polymers directly correlate to the number of free radicals.
- *Internal Stress.* Plasma polymers also contain an internal stress. If a thick layer of a plasma polymer, for example 1 μm thick, is deposited on a glass slide, the plasma polymer will buckle and frequently crack. The curling is attributed to an internal stress formed in the plasma polymer during the polymer deposition. Most plasma polymers are insoluble and infusible. These properties are due to the large amount of cross-linking in the polymers too, so that these properties can be controlled to a point.
- *Permeability.* The permeability of plasma polymers also differ greatly from those of conventional polymers. Because of the absence of large-scale segmental mobility and the high degree of cross-linking within the polymers, the permeation of small molecules does not strictly follow typical mechanisms of standard polymers, that are either solution-diffusion or molecular-level sieve. In the solution-diffusion case, either ideal diffusion of small molecules happen inside the polymer or diffusion happens like solutes diffusion, where weak

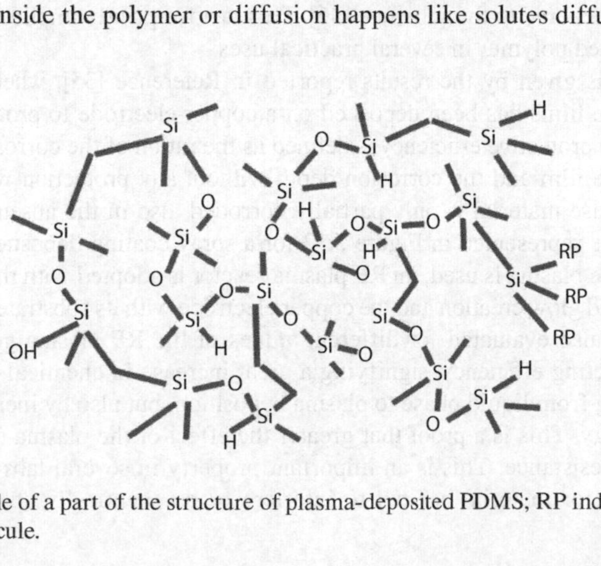

FIGURE 5.11 Example of a part of the structure of plasma-deposited PDMS; RP indicates bonds with other parts of the macromolecule.

links between polymer chains and the diffusing molecules influence the diffusion coefficient. In the second case, as far small molecules permeation is concerned, the polymer matrix can be modeled not as a continuous medium, but as a micro-porous material, a molecular-level sieve, whose pores have a sufficient dimension to let molecules under a critical dimension pass and to block molecules above the critical dimension. The real permeability characteristics of plasma polymers cannot be modeled with one of these models, but rather falls between these two ideal cases [32].

- *Adhesion ability*. The adhesion ability of plasma polymer is also generally quite different from standard polymers and few generalizations can be made.

Owing to the dependence of the polymer structure on the polymerization process, that is, on the plasma reactor used, several types of plasma reactors are adopted, to obtain different kinds of polymers even when using the same monomer. The simpler type of glow reactor used for plasma polymerization is the DC or AC reactor where the deposition chamber coincides with the plasma chamber (see Section 4.8.2). In this case, the cathode is also the support for the substrate where the film has to be deposited. While the polymerization happening when plasma is used seems to be mainly a radical polymerization process, the fact that it happens on the cathode, where a sensible ion bombing happens, seems to change its characteristics, generating specific polymers.

Alternatively, reactors where the plasma chamber is separated from the deposition chamber (see Section 4.8.2) and the monomers are injected into the plasma in the deposition chamber after the extraction of an ion beam from the plasma are also used. These reactors are somehow similar to those used for PECVD (see Figure 4.80). Finally, microwave plasma reactors are also adopted, generally in the configuration in which the plasma chamber and the deposition chamber are separated and an ion beam is extracted from the plasma chamber to generate polymer formation and deposition.

Under the point of view of the final result, plasma polymers deposition is a technique that offers several advantages. Plasma-enhanced polymers film deposition is not slow, taking into account the particular deposition methods. Deposition rates vary widely with the process characteristics, in particular with the rate of ion bombing on the surface of the substrate. The upper limit to the deposition speed is posed frequently from the maximum ion collision rate before the creation of diffused damage on the substrate/film surface. In any case, deposition rate in the order of 30–50 nm/min can be attained with many polymers [35,36].

The performances of the deposited polymers are, in general, superior to those deposited with other methods. They are more uniform, practically pinhole free, more chemically and mechanically resistant and better anchored to the substrate [36]. This fact frequently implies the best performance of the plasma deposited polymer in several practical uses.

A good example is given by the results reported in Reference [35], where a plasma polymerized ethylcyclohexane films has been deposited on a copper electrode to protect it from corrosion. Typically, a corrosion protective efficiency is defined as the ration of the corrosion depth in the presence of the protective film and the corrosion depth without any protection when a corrosion time is fixed so that the base material is only partially corroded also in the absence of protection. The corrosion efficiency is represented in Figure 5.12 for a spray coating-deposited film and a plasma-deposited film. In case plasma is used, an RF plasma reactor is adopted with the same chamber used both for deposition and glow creation and the copper electrode with its substrate is put on the cathode.

The efficiency is also evaluated for different values of the RF plasma generating power. The increase of the protecting efficiency, signifying a great increase in chemical resistance to acids, is clear not only passing from liquid phase to plasma deposition, but also by increasing the RF power, that is the glow energy. This is a proof that greater the effect of the plasma on the deposited film, better the chemical resistance. This is an important property in several labs on chip applications, where the micro-reactor material has not to interfere or be chemically changed by the ongoing reactions.

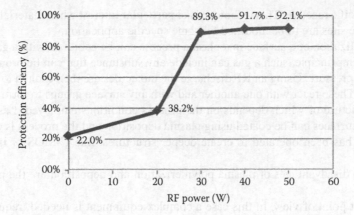

FIGURE 5.12 Polymerized ethylcyclohexane films deposited over a copper electrode efficiency evaluated for different values of the RF plasma generating power; no RF means spray deposition.

The better adhesion to the substrate induced by plasma deposition is evident from Figure 5.13, where the load needed to detach a pc-VTES 1 μm thin film from a substrate of glass is considered where the film is either plasma deposited using an RF plasma chamber with RF power of 5 W or wet deposited after surface pretreatment with acetone [37]. The effect of cold and boiling water has also been investigated. The adhesion improvement due to plasma deposition and the better resistance of the obtained film to water effect is clear from the measured results.

Also optical and electrical properties of plasma-deposited films can be improved with respect to other deposition methods [38] with the further advantage that they can be tuned to the desired result with a careful tuning of the deposition process parameters and with the suitable choice of the architecture of the deposition reactor.

Under the point of view of the dimensions of the film and of the chemical composition of the deposited material, plasma deposition has also several advantages. Polymer films with a wide range (from 200 Å to more than 100 μm) [2] can be obtained by plasma deposition having a very good control of the film thickness. Plasma polymerization is an effective way to functionalize polymer

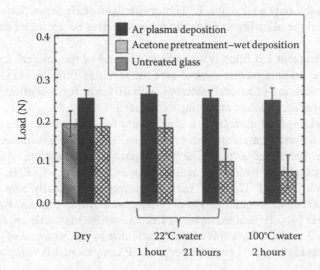

FIGURE 5.13 The load needed to detach a pc-VTES 1 μm thin film from a substrate of glass is considered where the film is either plasma deposited or wet deposited after surface pretreatment with acetone.

surfaces with specific reactive. This technique is of particular interest when materials whose surface contains no active sites are to be modified for some specific application.

The functionalization of a surface in a plasma process can be achieved with a gas giving rise to polymerization. In principle, such a gas can include any substance that can be brought into the gas phase at reduced pressure. Using an RF discharge the molecules are then excited to form a range of reactive species. These react with one another and with any surface groups to form a polymer film, the chemical structure of which depends on the process conditions employed. Last, but not least, highly irregular surfaces can be coated using plasma deposition and the process is compatible with any process that has been operated to create deeper structures, like C-MOS or integrated optics processes.

The main two disadvantages of plasma polymerization and deposition are the process cost and complexity.

Under the cost point of view, in this case a complex equipment is needed, requiring a vacuum chamber, a glow system and, in case of ion beam extraction, an ion beam control system. It is apparent that it is much more expensive than a simple spray coating or a well-controlled spin coating. The process is also quite complex, requiring generally a long time to be correctly set up and calibrated. If it is inserted in an overall fabrication infrastructure where silicon and silica processes are done, like photolithography and RIE (see Chapter 4) plasma polymerization has the same degree of complexity and fit well in the overall system. However, frequently polymer technology is adopted also for its simplicity and fast implementation with respect to typical silicon-related technologies, in this case plasma polymerization is probably by far the most complex process that is implemented in the whole fabrication chain.

Moreover, the specific chemistry at the base of plasma polymerization renders difficult to forecast a priori the characteristics of the polymer that will be deposited, and frequently a long process calibration is needed to achieve the wanted results.

5.3.4 LANGMUIR–BLODGETT DEPOSITION

In several applications, like surface activation, a film composed by a single molecule layer, or a few molecules layers, often composed by different molecules, has to be deposited on a substrate. Micro-contact printing is a viable technique to deposit SAMs (see Section 5.3.1.1) and it can be used for this task.

However, it is not the only alternative. Langmuir–Blodgett (LB) deposition of the so-called LB films is another technique allowing to reach the same objective being, under some points of view, is simpler [39,40].

The appealing feature of LB films is the intrinsic control of the internal layer structure down to the molecular level and the precise control over the resulting film thickness. Sophisticated LB troughs allow the processing of several materials with different functionalities and offer the possibility to tune the layer architecture according to the need.

In order to form a Langmuir monolayer, it is necessary for a substance to be water insoluble and soluble in a volatile solvent like chloroform or benzene. LB compatible materials consist of two fundamental parts, a "head" and a "tail." The "head" part is a hydrophilic, typically with a strong dipole moment, and capable of hydrogen bonding. Groups like $-OH$, $-COOH$, $-NH_2$ are typically present in the hydrophilic head. The "tail" part is hydrophobic, typically consisting of a long aliphatic chain. Such molecules, containing spatially separated hydrophilic and hydrophobic regions, are called amphiphiles [41]. Typical examples of LB compatible materials are fatty acids and their salts, but also selected proteins have this characteristic due to the presence of $-COOH$ and $-NH_2$ groups in the polypeptide C and N ends, respectively. Examples of LB compatible molecules are shown in Figure 5.14.

If amphiphile molecules arrive at the air–water interface with its hydrophobic tails pointing toward the air and its hydrophilic group toward water, the initial high energy interface is replaced

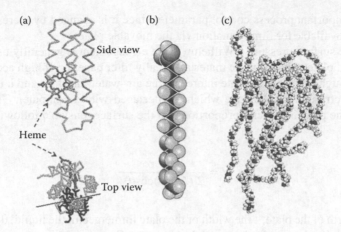

FIGURE 5.14 Different amphiphiles: (a) a protein helix (cytochrome 562 from *E. coli*); (b) a saturated fatty acid (palmitic acid); (c) an artificial polymer chain. (Adapted from Lee L. M. et al., *Lab Chip,* vol. 6, pp. 1080–1096, 2006.)

by lower energy hydrophilic–hydrophilic and hydrophobic–hydrophobic interfaces, thus lowering the total energy of the system. Hence, the molecules at the interface are anchored, strongly oriented normal to the surface and with no tendency to form a layer more than one molecule thick.

Different systems exists to deposit an LB film on a substrate, but all starts with the so-called LB trough, or Langmuir film balance, containing an aqueous phase amphiphilic molecules arrangement, as shown in Figure 5.15. Movcable barriers that can skim the water surface control the surface area available to the floating monolayer.

To form a Langmuir monolayer film, the molecules of interest is dissolved in volatile organic solvents such as chloroform, hexane, or toluene, that will not dissolve or react with the water or with the film molecules. The dilute solution is then minutely placed in the LB trough with a microliter syringe. The solvents evaporate quickly and the surfactant molecules spread over the water surface. As noted, when the Langmuir film is formed the surface free energy is reduced from the value it has for a free water surface in contact with air to a lower value. This corresponds to a decrease of the surface pressure, since the overall volume and temperature remains constant. This pressure

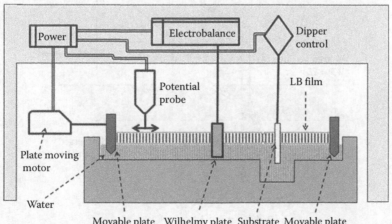

FIGURE 5.15 Scheme of an LB trough.

difference is an important process control parameter since it is changed by increasing or reducing the water surface available for film formation via the movable plates.

To measure the surface pressure a Wilhelmy plate arrangement is generally used. This method is based on a small plate of hydrophilic material, usually filter paper or, if high accuracy is needed, platinum with a rough surface. The plate intercepts the air–water interface and it is supported from the arm of an electronic microbalance which is interfaced with a computer. The force F vertically exerted on the plate is directly proportional to the surface tension γ following the Wilhelmy equation

$$\gamma = \frac{F \cdot z}{2\,(L + \tau)\cos(\theta)} \tag{5.1}$$

where L is the length of the plate, τ the width of the plate immerged in the liquid, θ the contact angle between water and the plate, and z the vertical unit vector. Equation 5.1 can be easily demonstrated by a simple equilibrium of the forces acting on the plate starting from the general theory of the surface tension detailed in Section 7.3.5. From Equation 5.1 it is deduced that an accurate measure of $F \cdot z$ results in an accurate measure of γ. From Equation 5.1 it is also evident why the use of platinum, whose contact angle with water is zero increases the measurement sensitivity. The principle scheme of the Wilhelmy plate is shown in Figure 5.16.

The dependence of surface pressure Π on the available film area divided by the number of film molecules A when the temperature is maintained constant is known as the isotherm characteristics of the film. A conceptual illustration of the general behavior of the isothermal characteristic of a LB film is provided in Figure 5.17.

As the pressure increases, the 2D monolayer goes through different phases that have some analogy with the 3D gas, liquid, and solid states. If the area per molecule is sufficiently high, then the floating film will be in a 2D gas phase where the film molecules are not interacting. As the monolayer is compressed, the pressure rises signaling a change in phase to a 2D liquid expanded (LE) state, which is analogous to a 3D liquid. Upon further compression, the pressure begins to rise more steeply as the liquid expanded phase gives way to a condensed phase, or a series of condensed phases. This transition, analogous to a liquid–solid transition in three dimensions, does not always

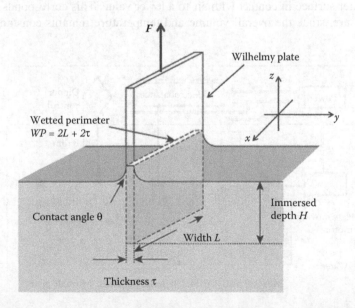

FIGURE 5.16 Scheme of surface tension measurements through the Wilhelmy plate method.

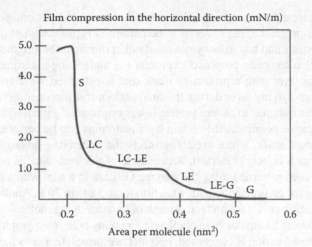

FIGURE 5.17 Typical isothermal characteristics of a Langmuir film; S indicates 2D Solid, LC condensed liquids, LE expanded liquid, and G indicates 2D perfect gas.

result in a true 2D solid. Rather, condensed phases tend to have short-range structural coherence and are called liquid condensed (LC) phases. If the surface pressure increases much further the monolayer will ultimately collapse or buckle, not still being a single molecule in thickness everywhere. This is represented by a sudden dip in the surface pressure as the containment area is decreased further, such as shown in Figure 5.17.

From the water surface the film can be transferred onto a substrate surface. The substrate can be made of almost anything. However, the most common choices are as glass, silicon, mica, and quartz. Vertical deposition is the most common method of LB transfer; however, horizontal lifting of Langmuir monolayers onto solid supports, called Langmuir–Schaeffer deposition, is also possible. In principle, the LB deposition method simply consists of dipping and pulling a solid substrate, orientated vertically, through the coating monolayer while keeping the surface pressure constant at a desired value (cf. Figure 5.15). It is also a common practice to coat the substrate with a highly hydrophobic or hydrophilic material. The rate at which the substrate is dipped or pulled through the monolayer must also be precisely controlled and kept constant at a very low value, typically 1–5 mm/min.

The surface pressure for film deposition is normally chosen to be in the solid like region. However, at any pressure film can be deposited. The transfer of monolayer film occurs via hydrophobic interactions between the alkyl chains and the substrate surface or the hydrophilic interaction between the head groups of the molecules and the hydrophilic substrate surface. Subsequent dipping or pulling deposits a second layer on top of the first, the process simply being repeated until the desired number of layers has been deposited.

5.4 PATTERNING TECHNIQUES

Besides deposition, patterning is the other base process for fabrication of polymer-based microcircuits.

The first option is naturally patterning through photolithography, having the advantage to leverage a well-known and diffused technology. A large number of artificial and natural macromolecules can be patterned using a lithography method, very similar to that used to transfer patterns from a rigid mask to a silicon or silica surface [2].

In case of an underlying organic film however, the process has generally to be modified to face problems that do not arise in the more traditional application. The first problem is related to the fact that organic molecules, especially proteins and nucleic acids, are much more fragile that traditional resist chains. Thus, if a dense solution of biomolecules is used instead of a traditional resist, measures have to be adopted not to ruin the film properties during the pattering operation. If an artificial polymer is to be processed, the material to be patterned is probably not directly available for deposition on the substrate and has to be synthesized either during or before the patterning process.

A first technique that has been proposed to protect the underlying macromolecules during patterning is to cover the layer with a protective mask that is patterned via standard method and is suitable to shield the underlying layer during the final pattern transfer operation.

This can be done, for example, to pattern protein layers by protecting them with a low melting point agarose layer. After agarose definition, the protein layer patterning can be performed by using a digestive enzyme. The agarose mask, where present, protects the underlying proteins so that the activity of the obtained patterns is largely preserved. An example of this technique is reported in Reference [42] where IgGs have been patterned using the enzyme GELase in a film with a critical dimension of 125 μm and preserving the IgGs activity in the final film for more than 70%. Another similar technique uses crystallized proteins to create the protective mask of the underlying molecules layer. In this case, a critical dimension as low as 10 nm has been obtained by making holes on a graphite surface [43].

As far as the polymer creation is concerned, polymerization can be performed during the lithography. Photosensitive materials can be created starting from high-purity precursors during the photolithography process; for example, polyvinyl alcohol, a water soluble polymer, can be treated by adding a photosensitizer like $(NH_4)_2 Cr_2O_7$. After spin coating on a flat surface, the polymer is crosslinked by UV exposition through a mask. Where the exposition hardens the polymer it becomes a water insoluble hydrogel so that a subsequent warm water bath can remove the unexposed polymer and perform patterning.

5.4.1 INKJET PRINTING

A method allowing simultaneous patterning and deposition of polymeric solutions is the inkjet print system [44–46]. It cannot reach the small critical dimensions typical of photolithography, but it is much less expensive. Depending on the used ink expulsion method and the related ink temperature, a wide range of both artificial and natural polymers, like proteins, can be deposited.

In an inkjet printer, either if it is used to print a document from a computer or to pattern a polymer solution in a micro-fabrication process, the substrate to be coated is placed on the x–y stage of the printing system and the ink is injected into a nozzle. Ink injection creates, due to the accurately designed nozzle profile, the creation of well-controlled drops, generally with a diameter in the range of 50 μm, that are expelled through the nozzle onto a well-controlled spot of the underlying substrate. Parallel nozzle can contemporaneously print different inks, to create more complex patterning constituted by different components.

Essentially three different technologies can be used to design an inkjet system: thermal technology, piezoelectric technology, and continuous inkjet technology.

Thermal ink jet printers work by having a print cartridge with a series of tiny electrically heated chambers constructed by photolithography. To produce a pattern, the printer runs a pulse of current through the heating elements. A steam "explosion" in the chamber forms a bubble, which propels a droplet of ink onto the paper. The ink's surface tension pulls another charge of ink into the chamber through a narrow channel attached to an ink reservoir. This mechanism is shown in Figure 5.18a.

Several orifices can be put in series in the head of an inkjet thermal printer up to arrive to a density of 120 orifices in one cm in a column. Several columns can then be put one besides the other so as to achieve a very dense and fast patterning capacity. Thus, typical values can be even overcome if a particularly dense patterning is needed and thermal inkjet printers with 250 orifices per cm per line do exist.

In thermal inkjets used for patterning, the ink is generally a water polymer solution that sometimes is cured after printing to improve its properties. Thermal technology is the less costly inkjet system and dominates the market of consumer and low cost industrial inkjet systems, but it is not suitable for patterning applications where high temperatures cannot be reached. These is frequently

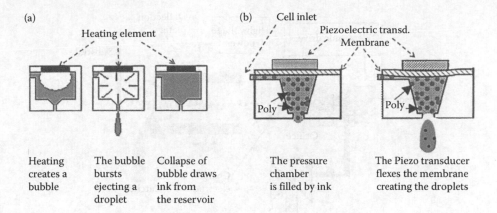

FIGURE 5.18 Thermal (a) and piezoelectric (b) inkjet printer head working principle.

true for applications involving natural polymers like proteins or nucleic acids, that can be denatured if a threshold temperature of the order of the organic temperature of 310 K is overcame.

Alternatively to a heater, a piezoelectric crystal can be used in each nozzle. When current is applied, the crystal changes shape or size, forcing a droplet of ink from the nozzle. Piezoelectric ink jets allow a wider variety of inks than thermal or continuous ink jet once, but are generally more expensive. Moreover, the need of a piezoelectric actuator makes it more difficult to reach a high density of nearby orifices and a typical value of the density of one orifices line is 35 per cm.

The great advantage of this technology in the field of polymers patterning is that high temperature is never reached and also more delicate molecules solutions can be patterned. A scheme of a piezoelectric inkjet head while patterning a polymeric solution is reported in Figure 5.18b.

In continuous inkjet technology, a high-pressure pump directs liquid ink from a reservoir through a microscopic nozzle, creating a continuous stream of ink droplets. A piezoelectric crystal causes the stream of liquid to break into droplets at regular intervals. The ink droplets are subjected to an electrostatic field created by a charging electrode as they form. The field is varied according to the degree of drop deflection desired. This results in a controlled, variable electrostatic charge on each droplet. Charged droplets are separated by one or more uncharged guard droplets to minimize electrostatic repulsion between neighboring droplets. The charged droplets are then deflected from straight drop direction to the substrate by electrostatic deflection plates, or are allowed to continue on without deflection to a collection gutter for reuse. The more highly charged droplets are deflected to a greater degree.

Continuous ink jet is one of the oldest inkjet technologies in use and is fairly mature. One of its advantages is a very high velocity of the ink droplets, which allows the ink drops to be thrown a long distance to the target. Another advantage is freedom from nozzle clogging because the jet is always in use. Volatile solvents like ketones and alcohols can therefore be used, giving the ability of the ink to dry quickly once on the substrate. The schematic working of a continuous inkjet printer is shown in Figure 5.19. Examples of PLGA patterns obtained by piezoelectric inkjet printing from Reference [47] are reported in Figure 5.20, showing typical critical dimensions attainable with this technology.

5.4.2 MICRO-STEREO-LITHOGRAPHY

Similar to the conventional process for rapid prototyping called stereolithography [48,49] the micro-stereolithography process (μSTL) fabricates complex 3D microstructures in a layer-by-layer fashion [50,51].

The first step of micro-stereo lithography is to create an accurate computer 3D (CAD) representation of the structure to be created. The digital model is divided into layers with vertical lateral

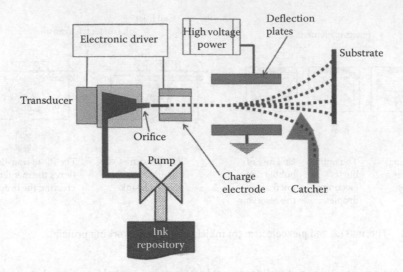

FIGURE 5.19   Continuous flow inkjet working principle.

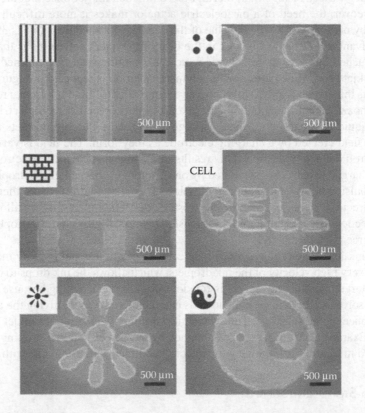

FIGURE 5.20   Optical micrographs of inkjet-printed PLGA patterns. Scale bars represent 500 μm. (With kind permission from Springer Science+Business Media: *Additive Manufacturing Technologies: Rapid Prototyping to Direct Digital Manufacturing*, 2009, Gibson I., Rosen G. W., Stucker B., Springer; 1st edition, ISBN-13: 978-1441911193.)

walls, which can be realized with a single μSTL step. The layers are individuated by slashing the model with equally spaced horizontal planes and correcting the walls between two adjacent planes with the best fitting vertical surface. The sliced layer in the electronic format are then used to drive the creation of a series of dynamic masks, one for each layer, as bitmap images on a computer-programmable array of digital micro-mirrors.

Either liquid crystal (LCD) or dot mirror (DMD) [52] chips can be used for this scope [50]. Nevertheless, if high resolution is required, LCD dynamic masks have several disadvantages with respect to DMD systems. An LCD display has not the ability to have so small pixels as a DMD display, moreover the space between pixels is greater, even with the same pixel dimension. Thus an overall smaller resolution is attained. The switching of LCD displays is slower since a switch time faster than 20 ms is difficult to obtain.

Under an optical point of view, the LCD cell is to be inserted between four layers of glass, two to contain the LCD itself and two to form the cell support in the equipment. Glass layers absorb UV, so that the use of LCD is practically restricted to blue visible light, where less photo-sensible resins are available and diffraction effects are more evident.

The dynamical mask is used to create all the layers constituting the shape to be fabricated, starting from the lower to the upper. In particular, a UV photo-sensible resin is used for the fabrication. Light from a flood UV source is either transmitted through or reflected off the dynamic mask and the beam containing the image is focused on the surface of a UV curable polymer resin through a projection lens, which reduces the image to the desired size. Once a layer is polymerized, the stage drops the substrate by a predefined layer thickness, and the dynamic mask displays the next image for the polymerization of the next layer on top of the preceding one. This proceeds iteratively until all the layers are complete. The process can create polymer layers on the order of 400 nm.

A scheme of a μSTL is represented in Figure 5.21 and an example of results obtained using DMD dynamical masks based μSTL is reported in Figure 5.22 [50].

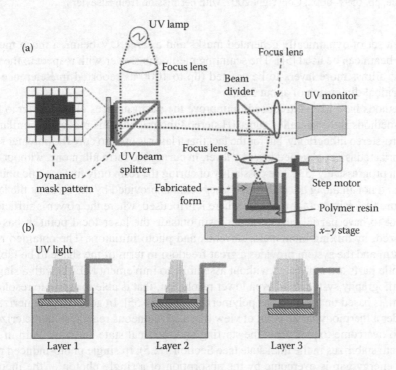

FIGURE 5.21 Scheme of a dynamic mask-based μSTL system (a) and process steps (b).

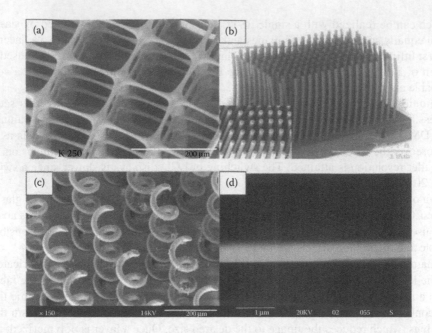

FIGURE 5.22   3D complex microstructures fabricated by micro-stereo lithography process: (a) micro matrix with suspended beam diameter of 5 μm; (b) high-aspect ratio micro rod array consists of 21 × 11 rods with the overall size of 2 × 1 mm. The rod diameter and height is of 30 μm and 1 mm, respectively; (c) micro coil array with the coil diameter of 100 μm and the wire diameter of 25 μm; (d) suspended ultra fine line with the diameter of 600 nm. (Reprinted from *Applied Surface Science*, vol. 15, Ovsianikov A., Ostendorf A., Chichkov B. N., Three-dimensional photofabrication with femtosecond lasers for applications in photonics and biomedicine, pp. 6599–6602, Copyright 2007, with permission from Elsevier.)

Instead of a set of dynamically generated masks and a large UV beam, a much more focused, scanning UV beam can be used [51]. The scanning method is slower with respect to the mask based method, but it allows more layers to be created (up to 1000 as reported in Reference [2]) with a single layer critical dimension of about 3 μm.

Several methods have been introduced to improve the performances of micro-stereo lithography. One of these methods is the so-called super IH stereo lithography. This process is similar to the conventional micro-stereo lithography, but for the fact that a laser is used to cure the polymer resin and the form to be fabricated is not obtained layer by layer, in curing the form all in one, without submerging it into the resin progressively [53]. The possibility of curing the resin only in a specific point below the resin surface and not all along the path of the laser beam is provided by the fact that the laser beam is too weak to cure the resin, but for the point where it is focused, where the power is sufficient.

In order not to have partial curing of the resin outside the laser focal point, it has to be carefully synthetized, by mixing monomers, solvents, and photo-initiators. The obtained resolution is lower than 1 μm and the system provides a great freedom in term of the shape to be fabricated. For example, mobile parts are fabricated without assembly, to implement MEMs with a single process.

A stereo lithography system with even lower resolution, that is able to arrive to resolutions of the order of 10 nm, is based on two photons polymerization [9,54,55]. In general, polymerization can be described under a thermodynamic point of view like a spontaneous reaction, characterized by a free energy wall to overcome to pass from the starting and the final state and a net gain in free energy when the system stabilizes in the final state (see Section 1.2.5). In single photo-induced polymerization, the free energy gap is overcome by the absorption of a single photon of the incoming light. This has to be done using a wavelength where absorption by the resin to be cured is high, so that polymerization happens efficiently.

However, two photons polymerization happens when two photons are simultaneously absorbed in a single location of the resin so as to add their energies allowing the reaction barrier to be overcome. In order for this effect to happen, the resin has to be transparent to the original wavelength to allow it to propagate up to the point where the laser is focused and the two photons polymerization has to happen. Generally, UV resins are transparent at IR frequencies, where the frequency is about one half the UV needed to cure the resin itself. Thus, under this point of view they are suitable for two photons polymerization.

The main reason that two photons effects are not important in standard processes is that they are much less probable than single photons effects. Interpreting the light absorption in a length dx as the probability that a photon combines with the material where light is propagating in this length, the single photon polymerization efficiency is proportional to a factor f_{sp} given by

$$f_{sp} = -\alpha P \, dx \qquad (5.2)$$

where α is the material absorption, that is big in case of standard photostimulated polymerization, and P the light power. If two photons polymerization is considered, the efficiency is proportional to a factor f_{tp} that is given by

$$f_{tp} = -\alpha^2 P^2 \, dx \qquad (5.3)$$

Apart from the fact that, since α is lesser than one $\alpha^2 < \alpha$, in order to have two photons polymerization, the material has to be transparent to the radiation, thus the absorption has to be much smaller than 1.

Reasonable orders of magnitude of the attenuation are $\alpha = 33W^{-1}$ in the UV region and $\alpha = 1.1W^{-1}$ in the IR region. The gap ranging from 10^2 to 10^3 between the efficiency of straight photo-polymerization and two photons polymerization has to be recovered by increasing the instantaneous light power. This cannot be done by increasing the power of a CW laser so much, but can be achieved by using pulsed lasers, simply paying a price term of polymerization speed.

As a matter of fact, using a laser emitting 100 ps pulses with a duty rate of 0.1 µs increases the pulse instantaneous power of a factor about 10^3 with respect to the time averaged power, simultaneously slowing about of the same factor the curing speed. This slow down can be partially recovered by carefully choosing the adopted resin and adding suitable photoinitiators that works well for this process so that a submicron stereo lithography system can be realized using this principle.

An example of a complex 3D form attainable with this technique including submicron details is presented in Figure 5.23 [56].

5.5 MICRO-MOLDING

Injection molding (IM) technique is a standard technique used in industry to form cheap plastic parts in large volumes. The scheme of a standard molding process equipment is shown in Figure 5.24 [57,58].

Several different polymers can be used for standard molding, with the constraint that the glass and the melting temperatures are sufficiently apart so that the molding machine can work sufficiently above the glass temperature, but not near the melting temperature. In this region of temperatures the polymer viscosity is reduced and its ability to fill all the details of the mold is enhanced, but it is not melted. As a matter of fact, if a good reproduction of the mold has to be obtained, getting too near the melting points can create temperature induced defects.

Very small plastic parts can be fabricated by using standard molding, up to critical dimensions below 1 mm. An application of high-performance IM characterized by huge volumes of fabricated objects is the manufacturing of highly demanding CD formats such as CD-R, involving features

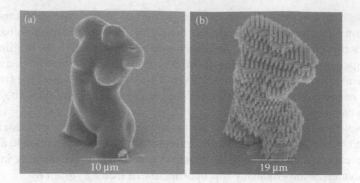

FIGURE 5.23 SEM photos of a Venus model realized using two-photons stereo lithography: (a) model with a smooth surface, (b) model with a composite surface to evidence sub-micron details. (Reprinted from *Applied Surface Science*, vol. 253, Ovsianikov A., Ostendorf A., Chichkov B. N., Three-dimensional photofabrication with femtosecond lasers for applications in photonics and biomedicine, pp. 6599–6602, Copyright 2007, with permission from Elsevier.)

with a depth of about 0.1 µm and a minimum lateral dimension of 0.6 µm, that is, an aspect ratio of 0.16 [59].

One of the most important factors for replication fidelity in IM is the thickness of the skin, which forms on the mold surface during filling of the cavity. The injection pressure must penetrate this skin so as to replicate the shape of the master accurately. The faster the injection, the thinner the skin on the insert mold surfaces and better the reproduction for a given injection pressure.

The upper shapes of the master forming the bottom of the parts are usually perfectly formed. It is the bottom of the master and especially inner corners that cause problems. Since, in conventional injection molding, the mold is kept closed during the entire mold-filling process, high clamping forces on the mold parts are required so that parts fabricated using IM often have high internal stress.

To obtain a good molding, the mold material has to resist at high temperatures and pressures so as not to deform, thus the principal attributes required of a stamper substrate are toughness, thermal shock resistance, thermal conductivity, and hardness. Thermal shock resistance is the product of a material's modulus of rupture or tensile strength and its thermal conductivity, divided by the product of its coefficient of thermal expansion and its modulus of elasticity. Selected materials used in practical molds for several applications are compared under this point of view in Table 5.3. Nickel compact disk stampers are normally 138 mm in diameter and 0.3 mm thick with an average roughness lower than 10 nm. For ceramic stampers, a thickness of 0.9 mm is generally selected

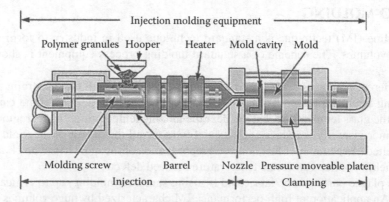

FIGURE 5.24 Scheme of an industrial injection molding equipment.

TABLE 5.3
Selected Parameter Values Relative to Mold Materials Used in Practice for Mass Production Applications

		Nickel	Al$_2$O$_3$	SiC	Glassy Carbon
Hardness	kg/mm^2	100	2000	2500	500
Fracture thoughness	MPa m$^{1/2}$	≈100	4	3	2
Thermal shock resist	kW/m	7.1	3.2	19.	135.5
Thermal conductivity	W/m/°K	80	30	90	120
Surface quality		Poor	Very good	Excellent	Excellent

Source: Adapted from Madou M. J., *Fundamentals of Microfabrication and Nanotechnology*; Third Edition, Three-Volume Set, CRC Press; 3rd edition (August 1, 2011), ISBN-13: 978-0849331800.

TABLE 5.4
Typical Process Conditions for Industrial Injection Molding and Possible Conditions for Thin Walls Injection Molding

	IM	Thin Walls IM
Mold temperature (°C)	85	85
Polymer temperature (°C)	350	350
Injection speed (cm/s)	1	5
Mold clamping force (kN)	500	1600
Injection time (s)	1	0.5
Cooling time (s)	1.5–3	100–180

Source: Adapted from Madou M. J., *Fundamentals of Microfabrication and Nanotechnology*; Third Edition, Three-Volume Set, CRC Press; 3rd edition (August 1, 2011), ISBN-13: 978-0849331800.

in order to avoid fracture in injection molding. Typical IM process conditions are summarized in Table 5.4.

All these characteristics render this process a good candidate for micro-manufacturing of very small polymer parts in MEMs and microfluidics applications [60,61]. As a matter of fact, very precise molds, incorporating even submicron elements, can be constructed with standard planar technologies, for example, using the characteristic of the e-beam direct writing lithography to be able to produce very high definition 3D structures.

5.5.1 THIN WALL INJECTION MOLDING

In several applications, frequently in labs on chip too, the main challenge to the micro-molding process consists in being able to reproduce structures with a high-aspect ratio allowing a complete filling of the flowing polymer during the injection into the mold.

A great number of experimental works [2,62] shows that the molds need to fill rapidly the mold to prevent early freezing. Moreover, this condition guarantees the polymer to remain above the no-flow temperature all the time needed to fill the mold and reduces considerably the polymer skin on mold surface, thereby improving the mold quality. For this reason, very fast IM processes, generally called thin walls IM, are used in cases where very small features are implemented in the mold and the aspect ratio of these features is higher than 0.2–0.25.

Shape deviation and damage of the fragile mold walls occur quite easily, possibly due to shrinkage of the polymer or defective filling and release. Since the mold cavity is filled at a mold temperature that exceeds the glass transition temperature of the polymer, the mold needs to be cooled down to obtain a sufficient molded part strength before ejection [63]. Conventional venting of the cavity is not feasible due to the presence of micro-features in the mold inserts so that a more complex cooling system has to be devised. Moreover, in order to avoid as much as possible temperature-induced defects, the process is generally carried out under low pressure conditions. Conventional IM equipment has to be modified for the molding of micro-sized parts or parts with high-aspect ratio [2,62]. The machine has to include a vacuum unit for the evacuation of the mold cavity in the molding tool and a temperature control unit for the molding tool.

Restoration of low pressure after ejection can be quite long in time so that, even if the molding itself results in a fast process, the overall cycle is generally quite longer than a standard IM, sometimes of the order of a few minutes. To keep the cycle time as short as possible, the thermal mass of the tool sections to be heated is minimized and thermally insulated from the adjacent assemblies. The guiding mechanisms of the tool halves and the ejector system should not be fitted too loosely, as small transverse movements might damage the microstructures during detach of the fabricated piece from the back half of the mold and the machines and tools to be evacuated have to comply with tolerances in the micrometer range.

With respect to other techniques for micromachining of polymers shapes, the injection molding has several advantages. It works well both with very low (~0.1) and with moderately high (~2) aspect ratio structures and is suitable for complex 3D shapes. The dimensional control of the created structures is very good, since the mold can be manufactured with high precision techniques and a good selection of the processed polymer assures a very good filling of small features. Moreover, the process itself is expandable to large volume automatic production. Just to give an idea, plastic syringes for private and hospital use are produced in a volume of about 600 million pieces a year, of which about 150–200 million are fabricated using injection molding.

However, only a selected set of polymers satisfy the properties that enable the reproduction of small feature size, high-aspect ratio features. Among them polycarbonate (PC), polymethyl-methacrylate (PMMA), polystyrene (PS), polyvinylchloride (PVC), polypropylene (PP), polyethylene (PE), and polyacrylnitrilbutadientyrol (ABS) are the most common. Commonly used and high-performance polymers such as PI, SU8, and others cannot be used in injection molding of small parts.

The equipment that is needed to mold small feature parts is costly, especially if it has to be used for research or for a limited volume production, and in any case its structure allows cyclic process to be performed, while continuous process cannot be performed and parallel process needs parallel machines.

The duration of the master is limited by the high residual stress remaining on the master after each molding process due to high pressure and temperature. If the master has to be produced with a sophisticated, high precision technology it can be quite expensive [63]. Last, but not least, a high residual stress generally also remains in the fabricated form, constituting a potential reason for an operating life reduction [63].

5.5.2 Hot Embossing

The principle of hot embossing (also called compression molding or relief imprinting) is a bit different from that of the injection molding. Differently from IM, hot embossing provides relatively low costs for embossing tools, a simple process, and high replication accuracy for small features.

In hot embossing a polymer substrate is first heated above its glass transition temperature. A mold is then pressed against the substrate, fully transferring the pattern onto it. After a certain time of contact between the mold and the substrate, the system is cooled below the glass temperature and, after a relaxing time, the mold is separated by the substrate [64,65].

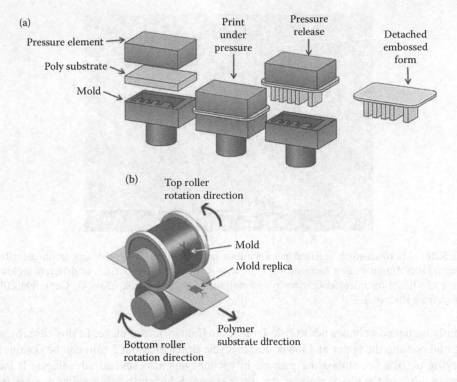

FIGURE 5.25 Schemes of hot embossing equipment: cyclic process equipment (a) and continuous process equipment (b).

The hot embossing process can be achieved in either a cyclic or continuous process. The setup of an equipment for cyclic hot embossing process is shown in Figure 5.25a: a metal master is put in a hydraulic press, and a heated polymer sheet is stamped by applying the appropriate force, thus replicating the structure from the master to the polymer. For mass production a continuous process can be devised [66]. Several different methods have been proposed, a schematic representation of the so-called 'roll-to-roll' hot embossing [67,68] is represented (Figure 5.25b). Here, a polymer sheet is mounted on a roll and forced to pass in between a support and a molding roll. On the molding roll a continuous series of identical molds are fixed so that continuous molding is realized. All the system is placed in a thermal chamber that assures the maintenance and stabilization of the process temperature and, after embossing, the continuous polymer sheet is sent to an automatic pieces separation stage.

The embossing force delivered on the embossing mold to obtain a correct replication of the structure is generally between 50 and 200 kN, the temperature difference between embossing and de-embossing, the separation of the form from the mold, ranges from 25°C to 40°C and higher the needed temperature difference, higher the time needed for the process thermal cycle.

The de-embossing temperature is an important parameter of the process that has to be carefully optimized. On one extreme the structure could cool down to room temperature before the separation of the formed shape from the mold, on the other end, smaller the de-embossing temperature, higher the risk to increase the stress embedded into the fabrication forms due to the great temperature difference. On the other extreme, if speeding the process and reducing the stress are high priorities, the separation could happen just below the glass temperature of the polymer. In this temperature region, however, the polymer is not completely hardened and the extraction from the mold can ruin the realized shape if it is not performed very carefully.

A compromise solution is generally adopted selecting the smaller possible temperature difference between the emboss temperature and the extraction temperature allowing to extract a

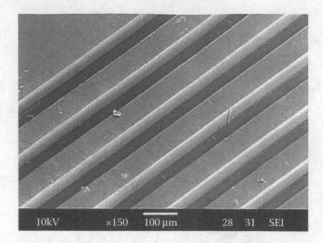

FIGURE 5.26   Micro-channels realized in a polymeric substrate using hot-embossing technique. (Reprinted from *Sensors and Actuators B: Chemical*, vol. 163, Jena R. K. et al., Comparison of different molds (epoxy, polymer, and silicon) for microfabrication by hot embossing technique, pp. 233–241, Copyright 2012, with permission from Elsevier.)

sufficiently hardened polymer not to risk damages to the fabricated piece. In this case, by actively heating and cooling the upper and lower bosses, cycle times of about 5 min can be obtained.

Carrying out the hot embossing process in vacuum has also several advantages. It increases the operating life of the mold, absorbs any water released during the embossing process from the polymer material preventing the humidity in the embossing chamber to contaminate successive processes and prevents bubbles from entrapped gases.

Several structures have been realized using hot embossing having micrometric critical dimensions and either high- or very-low-aspect ratios. A first example is provided in Figure 5.26, showing a set of micro-channels excavated by hot embossing in a polymer substrate. Each channel is about 75 μm wide and 40 μm deep, for an overall aspect ratio of 0.53. These dimensions are typical as order of magnitude of several labs on chip realizations, thus this is a relevant demonstration of the capabilities of these technology.

Entire sensors for application in labs on chips have been also realized using hot embossing as reported in Reference [69], where a compact integrated optical sensor system for a large variety of different (bio-) chemical applications using hot embossing replicated sensor chips is described.

5.6   LITHOGRAPHIE, GALVANIK UND ABFORMUNG

Lithographie, Galvanik, und Abformung (LIGA) is the German acronym for lithography, electroplating, and molding [2,70]. Even if primarily LIGA-process provides high-aspect ratio micro-structures in polymers like PMMA, via electroplating, these structures can be replicated in metals such as gold, nickel, magnetic nickel–iron alloys, or copper. Even replications in ceramics are possible. The LIGA process includes these principal steps that are represented in Figure 5.27:

1. Deposition of a thick PMMA layer on a metal plate
2. X-ray lithography on the PMMA of the shape to be replicated
3. PMMA development by polymerization
4. PMMA electroplating
5. Final metal form separation from the PMMA frame

The LIGA process as represented in Figure 5.27 is mainly aimed at the construction of small metal parts with submicron details and very high-aspect ratio: it is a very high performance and an

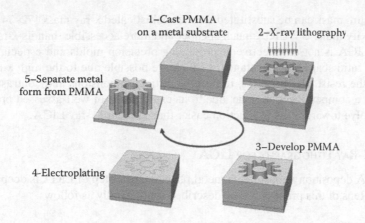

FIGURE 5.27 Main steps of the LIGA process up to the electroplated metal form. (From MEMSnet, http://www.memsnet.org/mems/fabrication.html, public domain image. Accessed on August 2013.)

expensive process due to the use of x-ray lithography and to the high number of subsequent steps. However, in polymer technology LIGA is a powerful tool to build very high accuracy molds to be used in subsequent polymer parts manufacturing. This is generally done by using the LIGA created shape as the master for a nickel mold that can be created by further electroplating. The so-obtained nickel mold can be then used for large volume fabrication of polymer parts by hot embossing.

When using to fabricate molds, low-cost reproduction of very precise polymer is possible since both the LIGA x-ray mask and the produced mold can be used a great number of times. Thus, the very high cost of the equipment and the first steps of the process is distributed onto a very large number of easily replicated elements, much like that happens in standard microelectronics (see Section 4.4). However, with respect to the other polymer-based processes LIGA requires quite a large initial investment for a low-class clean room, x-ray lithography, and a very skilled team to manage the infrastructure.

This was the reason why, after LIGA introduction, simpler methods were searched to manufacture high-precision polymer structures.

The main characteristics of the LIGA process can be summarized as follows:

- Large layout freedom in the mask geometry
- High-aspect ratios of up to >100 achievable
- Parallel side walls with flank angle very close to 90° (deviation: about 1 μm for 1 mm high structures)
- Smooth side walls (roughness in the 10 nm range or even smaller) suitable, for example, for optical micro-mirrors
- Lateral precision in the few microns range over distances of several centimeters
- Structural details on side walls in the 30 nm range possible
- Different side wall angles via double exposure possible

The base version of LIGA underwent several variations, mainly with the aim of simplifying the process and renders it easier to set up. Among them, UV LIGA is the LIGA variation that has been implemented more times [71]. Probably, the most important obstacle for the wide diffusion of LIGA process is the need of a very complex x-ray lithography equipment, which frequently links the LIGA facility to the availability of an external managed synchrotron, whose radiation is used by the LIGA x-ray equipment as by other x-ray-enabled processes. UV LIGA utilizes an inexpensive ultraviolet light source, like a mercury lamp, to expose a polymer photoresist, typically SU-8, instead of x-ray lithography. Because heating and transmittance are not an issue in optical masks, a simple chromium mask can be substituted for the sophisticated x-ray mask [72–74]. These reductions in complexity make UV LIGA much cheaper and more accessible than its x-ray counterpart. However, UV LIGA is not as effective at producing precision molds and especially in fabricating high-aspect ratio shapes that in standard LIGA are possible due to the high x-ray penetration capability into the resist. Nevertheless, if extreme critical dimensions and contrast ratios are not required, this is a competitive technique, due to its exploitation of well-assessed processes and its capability to evolve toward mass production easier than standard x-ray LIGA.

5.6.1 DEEP X-RAY LITHOGRAPHY FOR LIGA

After the PMMA deposition on a suitable metal plate, the first step of LIGA is deep x-ray lithography. The main steps of this process can be described synthetically as follows:

1. Fabrication of an intermediate mask (IM)
2. Fabrication of a working mask with x-ray lithography (WM)
3. Deep x-ray lithography

Naturally this is a general scheme, various modifications can be carried out to the process steps and the parameters we will indicate in the following description are not standard values, but more an order of magnitude reference.

5.6.1.1 Fabrication of an Intermediate Mask

Since x-ray lithography is used in LIGA, an x-ray mask has to be created. This is not an easy task, since it has to absorb x-rays sufficiently to have high masking performances and not to be too thick or too heavy to introduce further complications in the process. This means that the x-ray mask has to be created in high absorbing metals, so that a complex process is needed to have a sufficiently precise mask in the right material. The steps of this part of the LIGA process are represented schematically in Figure 5.28.

The starting point is a very flat surface, generally a silicon wafer, due to the high flatness and relatively low cost. The first step is to coat the wafer first with carbon, leaving an external part of the wafer uncoated. Over the carbon coating a thick titanium coating is applied (generally about

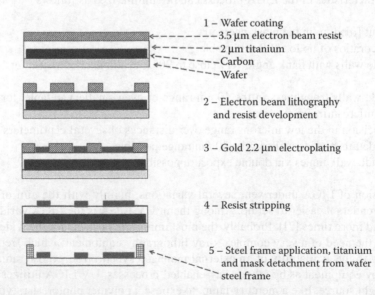

FIGURE 5.28 Schematic representation of the process for the intermediate mask fabrication.

TABLE 5.5

Comparison among Different Materials That Are Used as Membranes in X-Ray Lithography Masks for LIGA Process

Material	Thickness for 50% Absorption (μm)	Thermal Exp. Coefficient (×10⁶ 1/°C)	Young's Modulus (×10¹¹ Pa)	Aggregation	Breakage Resistance
Si	5.5	2.7	1.3	Crystal	Intermediate
SiN$_x$	2.3	2.7	3.36	Amorphous	High
SiC	3.6	4.7	3.8	Polycrystal	High
Diamond	4.6	1.0	11.2	Polycrystal	High
Ti	—	8.6	1.16	Crystal	Intermediate

2 μm thick), that will be the lower metal of the final intermediate mask. The titanium will not stick to the carbon layer, but to the silicon wafer where the silicon is visible. This prevents the titanium layer to lift off from the wafer by internal stress. Titanium is used, because of its good transparency for x-rays due to its low atomic number. Other membranes can be adopted as alternative to titanium, having similar properties. A summary of performances of different materials that can be used as membranes in the x-ray masks preparation (both in IM and WM) is presented in Table 5.5.

The resist is finally coated, generally by spin coating, on the titanium film. Generally, PMMA coating of 3.5 μm thickness is used. The resist is then impressed by direct writing e-beam lithography so as to obtain the wanted form on the resist. Even when very high-aspect ratio is required, this is not to be obtained during this step by e-beam. The intermediate mask has to report the surface pattern of the form to be reproduced. The creation of a deep form is due to the penetration of deep x-ray lithography.

The resist is developed and electroplating of a gold film is performed on the resist so that, after resist stripping, the pattern will remain impressed in the gold film. At least 2.2 μm of gold are needed to assure correct performances of the intermediate mask. Other materials can also be used as alternatives to gold to absorb x-rays during lithography, a selected set of them is compared under a physical point of view in Table 5.6. In this step, the thickness of the gold is critical: when the gold is overgrowing the resist layer, the wanted geometry of the mask is lost and it becomes useless.

The gold film is surrounded by a thick invar steel frame that will have the role of being the intermediate mask frame. Due to the high-precision requirements of the intermediate mask, the invar is needed, not to transfer to the IM stresses and not to create deformations due to the different

TABLE 5.6

Materials That Can be Used as Absorption Materials in X-Ray Lithography Masks Used in the LIGA Process

Material	Thickness for 10 dB Absorption (μm)	Thermal Exp. Coefficient (×10⁶ 1/°C)	Internal Stress due to Process	Possible Processes	Stability
Gold	0.7	4.5	Low	Electroplating	Intermediate
Tungsten	0.8	14.2	Potentially high	Dry etching CVD	High
Alloys	Order of 5	—	Low	Dry etching CVD	High

temperatures of the subsequent processes. Since the invar frame is glued on the gold film, also the glue process has to be carefully designed, using adaptable glues that do not create stresses at the contact between the frame and gold film and that resist with practically no deformation to all the processes the intermediate mask will have to undergo.

At this point, the IM is cut along the frame and the titanium layer is detached from the carbon layer so as to obtain the final mask: a support of 2 µm of titanium on which is deposited a patterned 2 µm gold film, all within an invar frame. The x-ray absorption contrast of the intermediate mask fabricated with the parameters indicated in this section is sufficient to produce structures of up to about 70 µm thickness by x-ray lithography. If higher depth is needed, the IM process parameters have to be tuned consequently.

5.6.1.2 Fabrication of a Working Mask

The steps of the second part of the LIGA process, the fabrication of the x-ray working mask, are represented schematically in Figure 5.29.

The starting point is an invar steel plate that is thinned at the back side to reach the wanted thickness, while the external frame is leaved at full thickness to provide mechanical resistance. On the front side the plate is coated with a titanium coating (thickness of the order of 22 µm). On top of the titanium layer a thick x-ray resist layer (50–70 µm) is deposited.

At this point the, IM is used as x-ray lithography mask to transfer the pattern on the x-ray resist exploiting the transparence of titanium to x-rays while the thick Au film, that is x-ray opaque, brings the pattern to be transferred. After resist development and a new electroplating with a very thick gold layer (of the order of 20–30 µm) the x-rays resist can be stripped and the gold film brings the pattern to be transferred.

It is important to notice that the gold film of the IM was not so thick, due to the fact that this first x-ray lithography can be performed with a low x-ray power, due to the fact that the mask has to be created with a not so high-aspect ratio; thus x-ray have not to penetrate too deep in the resist. The WM on the contrary will be used for deep x-ray lithography to obtain the final aspect ratio. Since in deep x-ray lithography the beam has to penetrate deeply in the resist it has to be much more powerful and a much thicker gold film is needed to block it in the black areas of the mask.

The last step in the creation of the working mask is to etch the back of the steel plate to reach the titanium layer, so that the invar remains as a frame and the thick x-ray mask, composed of a gold layer deposited on an x-ray transparent titanium layer is now ready to be used.

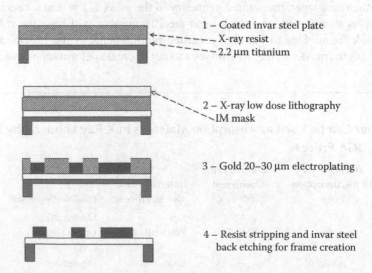

1 – Coated invar steel plate
X-ray resist
2.2 µm titanium

2 – X-ray low dose lithography
IM mask

3 – Gold 20–30 µm electroplating

4 – Resist stripping and invar steel
back etching for frame creation

FIGURE 5.29 Scheme of LIGA working mask preparation process.

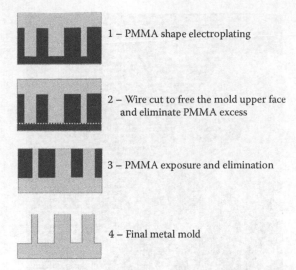

1 – PMMA shape electroplating

2 – Wire cut to free the mold upper face
and eliminate PMMA excess

3 – PMMA exposure and elimination

4 – Final metal mold

FIGURE 5.30 Scheme of final molding fabrication in the LIGA process.

5.6.1.3 Deep X-Ray Lithography

This is the step where the high-aspect ratio structure is created starting from the pattern registered on the working mask. This is made by using the working mask for deep x-ray lithography on a suitable thick resist film deposited on x-ray-resistant substrate. X-rays have the property to penetrate deep into the resist so as to impress it very far from the surface. For example, a cut 500 nm wide can be created by impressing the resist up to a depth of 50 μm, creating a structure with an aspect ratio of 100 and submicron critical dimension. This process requires a careful resist selection and process, since the resist film has to be quite thick to allow this process to be correctly performed.

5.6.1.4 Electroforming of Metal Mold: Hot Embossing

After x-ray lithography and development of the photoresist the final form is fabricated in the photoresist material, frequently PMMA. At this point, either the final metal part or a high accuracy metal mold (frequently fabricated from nickel, see Section 5.5) for subsequent polymer parts fabrication can be manufactured. The process is schematically shown in Figure 5.30.

The photoresist shape is embedded in a metal block by electroplating it for a sufficiently long time, so that it impresses in the inner part of the block the shape to be reproduced. The substrate on which the resist was deposited and the excess of metal are cut away, frequently with a wire cutting technology, and the contact surface between the resist and the original substrate is put in evidence. Here a negative form is printed in the metal, filled of developed resist. The resist filling the negative form in the mold is softened by a suitable exposure process and removed from the metal mold, so as to leave the pattern impressed in the mold with great precision. The mold is now ready for a mass replication of the shape, generally via hot embossing.

An example of a complex structure realized by LIGA using a polymeric material is represented in Figure 5.31. Here, a double W sensor is represented besides its balance structure. The critical dimension of the system, the width of the single W sensor blade, is around 8 μm and the aspect ratio is 4, for a depth around 32 μm [75].

5.6.2 X-Ray Lithography

X-ray lithography works on the same principle of deep UV lithography. A mask allows to harden a polymeric resist via x-rays only in certain areas [76,77]; after development, the hardened areas

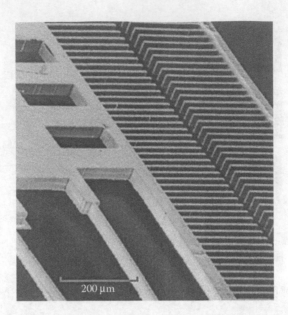

FIGURE 5.31 Example of a complex micromachining realized in nickel by LIGA: electroplated finger-style electrodes (220 μm long, 10 μm wide, and 40 μm thick). (Reprinted from *Journal of Micromechanics and Microengineering*, vol. 20, Joie C. D. et al., UV-LIGA microfabrication of 220 GHz sheet beam amplifier gratings with SU-8 photoresists, pp. 125016, Copyright 2010, with permission from Elsevier.)

remains on the wafer while the other resist areas are removed so that an etching or deposition process can transfer the pattern on the mask directly on the film under the resist.

Originally, x-ray lithography was introduced to achieve smaller critical dimensions with respect to UV photolithography by maintaining the typical photolithography nature of parallel process, a characteristic that is lost if direct writing e-beam is used (see Section 4.6). Even with a relatively simple x-ray lithography, based on contact between the mask and the photoresist, critical dimensions of about 15 nm can be achieved, and better can be done with projection x-ray lithography, since x-ray optics can be developed with suitable materials.

However, while standard UV photolithography seemed not to be able to go below micrometric structures, the use of phase masks and the stepper principle has removed this limitation, so that present days submicron steppers are able to reach a line-width of the order of 20 nm and it seems not to be the ultimate limit. Moreover, the introduction of x-ray lithography in Integrated circuits fabrication has been continuously delayed by the high cost and complexity of the process with respect to UV lithography.

If the ability to reach smaller critical dimensions has not been the winning characteristic of this technology, x-ray lithography has been found very useful for another characteristic that differentiates it from photolithography: the ability of the x-rays to penetrate deep in the resist so as to be able to impress with a single exposure even resist films 70–80 μm thick. This feature is partially due to the fact that the attenuation of standard resists at x-ray frequencies are smaller than those at UV frequencies, partially to the high energy and naturally collimated nature of the synchrotron radiation that is generally used as source in x-ray lithography.

Mainly for this reason x-ray lithography has been adopted in process, like LIGA, that requires the excavation of high-aspect ratio shapes in polymeric materials.

It remains in any case that several elements render x-ray lithography more complex and costly with respect to standard photolithography:

- The x-ray synchrotron-derived source, while intrinsically quite efficient, is much more difficult to manage than UV laser;
- X-ray mask are to be constructed with suitable materials that results opaque to x-rays and have a thickness much greater than UV masks;
- The process to build x-ray masks is more complex and they are much more expensive with respect to UV masks;
- The whole plant operating procedure is more complex with respect to photolithography, for the potential risk constituted to prolonged exposure to x-rays.

5.6.2.1 X-Ray Source

Several x-ray sources exist, used for a variety of applications in the industrial and medical field. In the case of x-ray lithography the emitted power and the beam collimation are key factors for the source effectiveness, thus synchrotron orbital radiation (SOR) is used [78,79].

A synchrotron, whose scheme is reported in Figure 5.32, is an electron accelerator with the form either of a large torus or, for more recently fabricated systems, of a round corners rectangle. The specificity of the synchrotron is that the relativistic mass change of accelerated electrons is compensated by a suitable time variation of the guiding magnetic and electromagnetic fields so that the electron trajectory remains always the same while the particle is accelerated.

The relativistic nature of the electrons in a synchrotron is also evident in the shape of the emitted radiation, that instead of a typical dipole characteristic of classical emitting particles, is a front-shaped cone, with an high degree of directionality and collimation (see Figure 5.33).

Another dramatic effect of the relativistic nature of the electrons accelerated in a synchrotron is that x-rays are emitted while the resonance frequency of the synchrotron cavity is in the GHz range. As a matter of fact the radiation emitted in the proper electrons reference system (the system where the electrons are still) is effectively in GHz range. Passing to the fixed system, where the synchrotron structure is still and the electrons move at relativistic speed, the relativistic Doppler effect multiply the emitted frequency by the relativistic factor γ, depending on the ratio between the electron speed and the light speed. Relativistic Lorentz time contraction amplifies the frequency by another factor of γ, so that the radiation emitted in the GHz range in the proper electron reference, is a radiation in

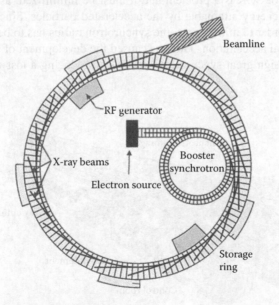

FIGURE 5.32 General diagram of a synchrotron.

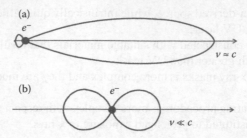

FIGURE 5.33 Emission profile of synchrotron orbital radiation emitted by a relativistic electron (a) and of a cyclotron radiation emitted by a classical electron (b) for which the relativistic factor γ is about 1.

the x-ray region in the fixed reference where the SOR is used. At a synchrotron facility, electrons are usually accelerated by a synchrotron, and then injected into a storage ring, in which they circulate, producing synchrotron radiation, but without gaining further energy. The radiation is projected at a tangent to the electron storage ring and captured by beamlines; an example of beamline structure is shown in Figure 5.34. These beamlines may originate at bending magnets, which mark the corners of the storage ring; or insertion devices, which are located in the straight sections of the storage ring. The spectrum and energy of x-rays differ between the two types. A possible scheme of a beamline of a great synchrotron is reported in Figure 5.35.

The beamline includes x-ray optical devices which control the bandwidth, photon flux, beam dimensions, focus, and collimation of the rays. The optical devices include slits, attenuators, crystal monochromators, and mirrors.

The mirrors may be bent into curves or toroid shapes to focus the beam. A high photon flux in a small area is the most common requirement of a beamline. The design of the beamline will vary with the application. At the end of the beamline is the end station, for example, an x-ray lithography machine or an x-ray crystal characterization system.

Depending on the application of the synchrotron, the emission of SOR is a either a problem or a wanted effect. If the synchrotron is built to study nucleus properties via collision with high-energy particles, the emission of SOR is a problem and it must be minimized, as a matter of fact it is a limit to the maximum energy attainable by the accelerated particles. Since SOR depends on the radial acceleration, in order to minimize it, the synchrotron radius has to be as great as possible so as to minimize the radial acceleration. This has caused the development of synchrotron techniques whose target was to design great synchrotrons without introducing a loss of efficiency due to the greater electrons orbit.

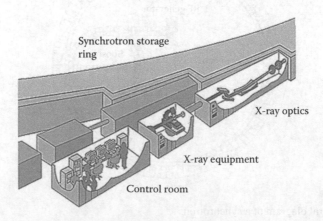

FIGURE 5.34 Possible structure of a big synchrotron beamline.

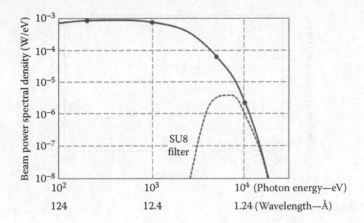

FIGURE 5.35 Typical SOR spectrum generated by a small synchrotron after x-ray filtering, as it arrives at an x-ray lithography system. The insert shown the final filter adopted if a SU8 resist is used for x-ray lithography.

If the synchrotron is intended to generate SOR, it has to be optimized both under a power and under a beam properties point of view. This creates the need of designing small synchrotrons, with the possibility to extract SOR in different points so as to have radiation beams with different characteristics. The technology to build small synchrotrons for SOR generation has been mainly enabled by the introduction of superconducting magnets that allow very small radii to be realized. For example, small synchrotrons to be used for x-ray lithography can be a ring of 2 m diameter and can be enclosed to the x-ray equipment, accommodated in the same clear room bay where the lithography equipment is located.

The main element generating both a management problem in the clean room and an additional cost when small synchrotrons are used is the liquid helium that is needed to maintain the magnets and the electrical field conductors in a superconducting state. Generally, liquid helium is not used in semiconductor clean rooms, thus adding it requires adding a new management element to the clean room, since the liquid helium has to be stored and distributed by a specifically designed low-temperature circuit due to its huge vapor pressure causing almost instantaneous evaporation if exposed to air.

The spectrum of a small synchrotron SOR is very wide, starting at UV and arriving at soft x-rays. Generally, the spectrum is filtered and shaped in the beamline at the synchrotron output so as to insulate the desired frequencies. A typical SOR spectrum after filtering, as it arrives at an x-ray lithography system, is presented in Figure 5.35. In a synchrotron for x-ray lithography all the system where electrons are accelerated, the initial accelerator, the ring and the beamline, are kept in high vacuum by a vacuum pump. The sample exposure chamber on the contrary is generally kept in helium atmosphere. The inner atmosphere is needed to prevent corrosion by oxygenated chemical components of the lithography chamber, the mask and the sample. Moreover, heat removal is easier in helium than in air since He has a comparatively higher heat conductivity.

5.6.2.2 X-Ray Resists

A resist that has to be used to fabricate high-aspect ratio structure with the LIGA process using x-ray lithography has to fulfill a series of requirements that are partially more strict or completely different from those of a normal UV resist [2].

These requirements can be summarized as follows:

- High x-ray sensitivity
- High resolution
- Resistance to dry and wet etching
- Thermal stability up to a temperature greater than 140°C

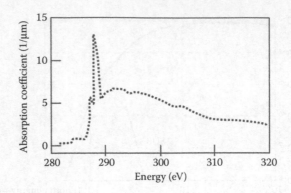

FIGURE 5.36   PMMA x-ray sensitivity.

- A bulk absorption of less than 0.35 mm^{-1} at the illumination wavelength (generally near 2 Å)
- To be absolutely inert with respect to the development process when not exposed (any residual solubility or change of shape has to be avoided)
- Very high adhesion to the substrate also for very thick resist films
- Resistance to electro-deposition also before development, that means to have a glass temperature higher than the temperature used for the electro-deposition of the considered metal, for example, around 60°C for gold
- Very low internal stress to avoid damage during processing

Moreover, in many LIGA applications, the resist developed structure is the process outcome, in this case application specific requirements can be added to the above list, for example, to be transparent at a given frequency or to have a selected dielectric constant.

Considering all the above conditions PMMA is frequently the resist of choice for x-ray lithography-based process. Not only does PMMA behave very well under the lithography process, but it is also transparent at IR and visible frequencies, presenting suitable optical properties for the great majority of optical applications. The only requirements that are not completely fulfilled by PMMA are the high sensitivity at x-rays and the lack of internal stresses after development.

As far as the sensitivity is concerned, it is represented in Figure 5.36. At wavelength of 8.34 Å the sensitivity of PMMA is about 2 J/cm^2, that is a not so high value. This means a quite high processing time, sometimes about 2 h for a 500 μm thick film, with the consequent high power consumption due to the long use of the synchrotron. This long exposure time, besides the tendency of PMMA to accumulate surface cracks, also renders stresses dangerous for further processing.

Several variations of PMMA, especially based on copolymerization (see Section 1.4.1) have been explored to improve both these characteristics, but results are not always positive. Another possible approach to improve PMMA sensitivity is to dope the polymer with high atomic number atoms, so as to increase sensitivity to x-rays, or to use photosensitizers at the suitable wavelength in the resist solution that is deposited on the wafer before exposition.

Also completely different resists have been used, like poly(lactides), for example PLGA, whose structure formula is reported in Figure 5.37 or polymetacrylide (PMI). PLGA is synthesized by

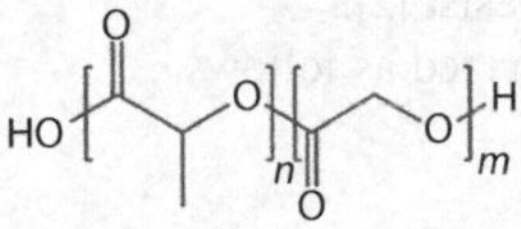

FIGURE 5.37   Molecule structure of PLGA. It is to note that the structure of PLGA depends on two chain numbers, *n* and *m* in the scheme of the figure.

copolymerization of two different monomers, the cyclic dimers of glycolic acid (1,4-dioxane-2,5-diones) and lactic acid. During polymerization, successive monomeric units (of glycolic or lactic acid) are linked together in PLGA by ester linkages, thus yielding a linear, aliphatic polyester as a product [80]. Depending on the ratio of lactide to glycolide used for the polymerization, different forms of PLGA can be obtained: these are usually identified in regard to the monomers' ratio used; for example, PLGA 75:25 identifies a copolymer whose composition is 75% lactic acid and 25% glycolic acid. All PLGAs show a glass transition temperature in the range of 40°C–60°C.

It is interesting to note that a strong correlation has been observed for all the polymers that have been considered for resist application between their sensitivity to x-rays and to e-beam so that processes for the new x-rays resist are already known from their use in e-beam lithography.

5.6.3 ELECTROPLATING

Electroplating, a fundamental step of the LIGA process, is a plating process in which metal ions in a solution are moved by an electric field to coat an electrode. The process uses electrical current to bring cations of a desired material from a solution and coat a conductive object with a thin layer of metal [81,82]. The process used in electroplating is called electrodeposition.

The part to be plated is the cathode of the circuit, the anode can be made of the metal to be plated or it can be inert and the plating metal can be present in the cell solution. The electrodes are immersed in a solution containing one or more dissolved metal salts as well as other ions that permit the flow of electricity.

A power supply supplies a direct current to the anode, oxidizing the metal atoms that comprise it if it directly provides the plating metal and allowing them to dissolve in the solution. At the cathode, the dissolved metal ions in the electrolyte solution are reduced at the interface between the solution and the cathode, such that they plate out onto the cathode. The rate at which the anode is dissolved is equal to the rate at which the cathode is plated since the ions in the electrolyte bath are continuously replenished by the anode.

For its characteristic to deposit atom after atom on the target the electroplating is particularly suitable to treat the small elements created with the LIGA process since it is able to reproduce very small details in a precise way. The scheme of a nickel electroplating system used for LIGA is schematically represented in Figure 5.38, where also the chemistry of the related electro-deposition process is detailed.

Other electroplating processes may use a nonconsumable anode such as lead. In these techniques, ions of the metal to be plated must be periodically replenished in the bath as they are drawn out of the solution.

The anode and cathode in the electroplating cell are both connected to an external supply of direct current commonly, a rectifier. The anode is connected to the positive terminal of the supply, and the cathode (the piece to be plated) is connected to the negative terminal. When the external power supply is switched on, the metal at the anode is oxidized from the zero valence state to form cations with a positive charge. These cations associate with the anions in the solution. The cations are reduced at the cathode to deposit in the metallic, zero valence state. For example, in an acid solution, copper is oxidized at the anode to Cu^{2+} by losing two electrons. The Cu^{2+} associates with the anion SO_4^{2-} in the solution to form copper sulfate. At the cathode, the Cu^{2+} is reduced to metallic copper by gaining two electrons. The result is the effective transfer of copper from the anode source to a plate covering the cathode.

The plating is most commonly a single metallic element, not an alloy. However, some alloys can be electrodeposited, notably brass and solder. Many plating baths include cyanides of other metals, such as potassium cyanide, in addition to cyanides of the metal to be deposited. These free cyanides facilitate anode corrosion, help to maintain a constant metal ion level and contribute to conductivity. Additionally, nonmetal chemicals such as carbonates and phosphates may be added to increase conductivity.

When plating is not desired on certain areas of the substrate, stop-offs are applied to prevent the bath from coming in contact with the substrate. Typical stop-offs include tape, foil, lacquers, and waxes.

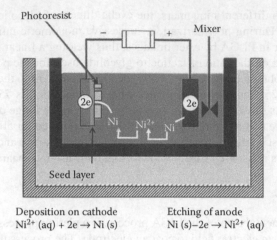

FIGURE 5.38 Scheme of nickel electroplating system used for LIGA. The chemistry of the related electro-deposition process is also detailed.

Initially, a special plating deposit called a *strike* or *flash* may be used to form a very thin (typically <0.1 μm thick) plating with high quality and good adherence to the substrate. This serves as a foundation for subsequent plating processes. A strike uses a high current density and a bath with a low ion concentration. The process is slow, so more efficient plating processes are used once the desired strike thickness is obtained.

5.7 LASER ABLATION

Laser ablation is the process of removing in a controlled way material from a solid surface by irradiating it with a laser beam. This process has several applications in fabrication of diverse objects, mainly made from metals or polymers [83,84]. This technique has been used to fabricate labs on chip for its excellent ability of work with selected polymers [85,86].

5.7.1 LASER ABLATION BASICS AND MECHANISM

Laser ablation is divided into two different kinds of techniques, depending essentially on the type of adopted laser energy flow. If a CW laser is used, we have CW laser ablation, otherwise if a pulse laser is adopted, we have pulsed laser ablation. Even if very powerful lasers exist, CW laser ablation suffers of the fact that the substrate heating is maximized, so that it is mainly applicable to situations where the surface to be ablated is thermally conductive and it can be easily cooled. This is possible in selected applications where macroscopic elements are to be ablated, but almost never applies to polymer-based labs on chip. Thus, we will mainly deal with pulsed laser ablation.

The basic mechanism of the laser ablation relies on the fact that when the laser emitted power interacts with the material to be ablated the inherent energy transfer causes a material state change causing its extraction from the surface. At low laser flux, the material is heated by the absorbed laser energy and evaporates or sublimates. At high laser flux, the material is typically converted to a plasma. Thus, a fundamental requirement for an effective process is that the surface absorbance is high at the adopted laser wavelength.

Another important element of the laser ablation process is the correct management of the material that is extracted from the ablated surface. As a matter of fact, atoms, molecules, cluster, and even material greater fragments are expelled during the interaction with the laser beam and care has to be taken to avoid damaging other parts of the surface where other structures can be present.

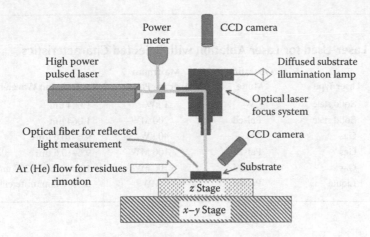

FIGURE 5.39 Scheme of laser ablation equipment for microfabrication.

The scheme of a laser ablation process machine is shown in Figure 5.39. The substrate to be processed is placed on a micrometric x–y–z stage that is used for the rough substrate positioning, while fine determination of the ablated zone position is performed by optical focusing of the laser beam. The laser beam is focused onto the substrate using an optical focusing system that is also designed to illuminate the substrate with a visible light coming from an illumination lamp thereby allowing direct ablation observation through CCD cameras. Residues created by ablation are removed by a high-speed flux of noble gas, generally either argon or helium, to avoid contamination of the surface and both reflected and scattered light is measured using a fiber optics system. All the process is carried out into a low pressure chamber.

Even if the ablation principle seems quite simple, the process depends on several parameters, mainly dependent on the selected laser. The following laser parameters are probably the most important to be controlled during laser ablation for labs on chip applications:

Average power (P): It influences mainly the substrate process temperature and the process throughput through the impact on the possible damage of the surface.

Laser wavelength (λ): It influences all the main optical properties, like absorption, transmission, and reflection, besides being responsible in selected cases of the presence of photochemical effects; the main types of lasers used in laser ablation are listed with their characteristic emission bands in Table 5.7.

Spectral linewidth (Δλ): It influences essentially the ablation efficiency.

Beam size (Δr): It influences the ablation critical dimension and the precision in the ablation depth.

Lasing mode distribution: It influences the ablation critical dimension and the precision in the ablation depth determining substantially the intensity distribution along the laser spot on the surface and its uniformity, the presence of the speckle phenomenon can be a problem in case of multimode lasers; generally an high-quality process is easier to obtain using a single mode laser.

Peak power (P_M): Determines essentially the instantaneous maximum temperature of the substrate influencing the stress accumulated during ablation and the possibility to damage the surface, at very high peak powers nonlinear effects can arise in the matter–light interaction rendering the process more difficult to be controlled.

Pulse width (τ): It is one of the most important characteristics of the process, controlling the interaction time between the substrate and the light beam; its influence will be detailed in the following discussion.

TABLE 5.7
Main Types of Laser Used for Laser Ablation with Selected Characteristics

Laser Element	Laser Type	Operation Mode	Maximum Average Power	Emission Wavelength
Nd:YAG	Solid state	CW	1 kW	1.064 µm
Nd:YAG	Solid state	Pulsed	200 MW	1.064 µm
CO_2	Gas	CW	40 kW	9.6–10.6 µm
CO_2	Gas	Pulsed	100 MW	9.6–10.6 µm
Excimer	Gas	Pulsed	100 nW	193, 248, and 308 nm (most common)
Dye	Liquid	Pulsed	1 MW	0.38–1 mm (different dyes)

As other thermal treatments, laser ablation is characterized by the fact that it leaves on the substrate a heat-affected zone (HAZ) all around the ablated area. This zone is formed by material that was melted by the light beam, but not abandoned the substrate so as to solidify after the end of the beam. This process creates a metastable material status that frequently results in embrittlement of the HAZ. The different phenomena occurring during laser ablation are shown graphically in Figure 5.40.

5.7.2 Parameters of Laser Ablation

Since several parameters influence the ablation process it is important to understand more in detail their effect in order both to determine the performances that can be attained by the process and how the process can be tuned by regulating these parameters.

5.7.2.1 Substrate Absorption and Reflection of the Laser Wavelength

Unless a strongly multimode laser is used, the laser beam appears, as far as absorption is considered, as a monochromatic source. Two main elements depend critically on the laser wavelength: the ablation mechanism and the laser beam penetration in the substrate.

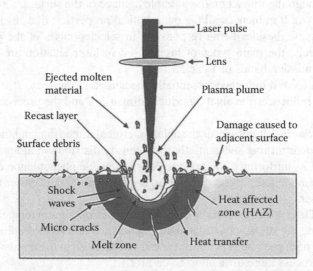

FIGURE 5.40 Graphical illustration of the laser ablation mechanism; several side phenomena are also shown as the creation of an heat-affected zone, the possible damage to nearby surfaces and the plasma plum creation. (Extracted from Shaheena M. E. et al. *Chemical Geology*, vol. 330–331, pp. 260–273, 2012.)

As far as the ablation mechanism is concerned, if the photons energy is sufficiently high, that is the photons wavelength sufficiently short, single photon photochemical breakage of the polymeric bonds seems to be the main process causing ablation. This creates small and high-energy fragments of the material that leave the surface either as sublimated gas or as plasma, depending on the breakage conditions. If single photon process dominates, double or multiple photons processes have a marginal part in the ablation, due to their much smaller efficiency. Single photon regime is dominant, for the most common polymers used in ablation processes, around a wavelength of 200 nm in the UV region. Thus it is generally attained using excimer lasers.

For longer wavelength, typically above 300 nm or even in the infrared region, single photon cleavage is no more relevant since photons have not sufficient energy, and double or multiple photons phenomena drive the ablation and therefore, the process is slower and requires higher laser energy. A qualitative model of the ablation process can help to understand the great impact of the substrate absorption coefficient.

The probability $p_a(x)$ that a single photon is not yet absorbed as a distance x from the surface can be readily derived from the absorption characteristics of the material, being

$$p_a(x) = e^{-\alpha(\lambda)x} \tag{5.4}$$

where $\alpha(\lambda)$ is the wavelength dependent absorption of the material, that is also the average penetration length of the photons of a given wavelength. Considering that a bond break causes a small material fragment to leave the surface when it happens at a small distance δ from the surface and when the photon energy is not dissipated in other ways (like high-energy phonons or spurious photoreaction), the probability $p_b(x)$ that a certain bond is broken near the surface by a photon results in

$$p_b(x) = \beta(1 - e^{-\alpha(\lambda)\delta}) \tag{5.5}$$

where β is the probability which the bond is broken once the photon is absorbed. If we want to obtain the ablated depth L per unit time we have to divide by the density of bonds per unit area ρ, multiplying by the photons flux per unit area and, remembering the expression of the beam intensity I (energy per unit time and unit area), we obtain

$$L = A(1 - R_f)\lambda I(1 - e^{-\alpha(\lambda)\delta}) \approx A(1 - R_f)\lambda I\alpha(\lambda)\delta \tag{5.6}$$

where A is a process variable, that in this simple approximation results to be given by $A = \beta/(2\pi \hbar \rho)$, R_f is the surface reflectivity and the approximation holds if the depth δ is much smaller than the penetration depth $1/\alpha(\lambda)$.

Equation 5.6 clearly indicates the fact that higher the absorption coefficient and higher the beam intensity, higher the ablation velocity. It could seem that also a higher wavelength causes an efficiency increase, provided that absorption does not decrease with increasing wavelength, but this is not completely true. As a matter of fact, Equation 5.6 is valid only if ablation is driven by single photons phenomena, thus the wavelength cannot be smaller than the wavelength allowing a single photon to break the polymer chain bond. Below this threshold wavelength (5.6) is simply not valid.

The behavior of the ablation above the threshold wavelength should be much rapidly decreasing while increasing the wavelength if a single bond with a precise bond energy was present, due to the increasing difficulties of phonons far from resonance to interact with the bond. In reality, a complex polymeric chain has a great number of bonds with nearby energies, so that in a wide wavelength range photons can in any case couple with the polymer via different bonds. In this situation, the dependence of the ablation rate from the wavelength, that is given in our simple model from the term $\lambda e^{-\alpha(\lambda)\delta}$ can be quite complex.

Reflection of the laser wavelength on the surface has to be avoided as far as possible, since it practically limits the amount of laser energy interacting with the surface. Refraction depends on the polymer material to be ablated, but also on the surface characteristics. A rough surface reduces net reflection increasing the ablation efficiency.

5.7.2.2 Laser Spot Size

The laser spot size is the footprint of the laser beam on the ablated surface, assuming vertical surface incidence of the laser beam. The spot size is a key factor for the determination of the laser ablation critical dimension. The first step in assuring a small and well-controlled spot size is to use a single mode laser. If many modes are present, the spot size is randomly influenced by phenomena like speckles and modal distribution fluctuations [93] so that a good control is impossible.

If a single mode laser is used, the beam shape far from the laser can be considered Gaussian so that the beam expression can be written as [93]

$$I(r) = \frac{2P}{\pi w^2(z)} e^{-2r^2/w^2(z)} \tag{5.7}$$

where P is the beam total power, z is the beam axial coordinate, and $w(z)$ is the transversal beam radius at the distance z from the source at which the beam intensity $I_M(z)/e^2$, being $I_M(z)$ the maximum beam for a given value of the axial coordinate. The expression of $w(z)$ can be written as

$$w(z) = w_0 \sqrt{1 + \left(\frac{\lambda z}{\pi w_0}\right)^2} = w_0 \sqrt{1 + \left(\frac{z}{z_R}\right)^2} \tag{5.8}$$

where w_0 is the beam width at the source, depending on the source emitting characteristics and z_R is the so-called confocal parameter, also called Rayleigh length, determining essentially the beam divergence rate. The so-called divergence angle $\Theta(z)$ is also often used to measure the divergence of a Gaussian beam at a distance z from the source, being

$$\Theta(z) = arctg\left(\frac{w(z)}{z}\right) = arctg\left(\frac{w_0}{z}\sqrt{1 + \left(\frac{z}{z_R}\right)^2}\right) \approx \frac{w(z)}{z} = \frac{\lambda}{\pi w_0} \tag{5.9}$$

where the approximation holds if the divergence is small. After the collimation length, the beam divergence experiences a transient growth to arrive at a stable value Θ_M when the beam is in the linear divergence zone. The value Θ_M is frequently called simply divergence. A picture of a Gaussian beam is presented in Figure 5.41.

From the above equations it can be seen that a Gaussian beam traverses two distinct regimes: as far as the longitudinal coordinates, in our case the distance between the beam origin and the target, is smaller than the Rayleigh length the beam radius is almost constant, while for a longitudinal coordinate much greater than the Rayleigh length Equation 5.8 can be linearized and we find that the beam radius grows almost linearly with the longitudinal coordinate. The growth ratio in the linear zone results to be equal to $\lambda/\pi w_0$ so that the longer the wavelength greater the divergence, but also smaller the initial beam radius, greater the divergence. Thus, more beam collimation at the origin means a longer length where the beam radius is constant, but also a greater divergence thereafter.

If we focus a laser beam with a perfect lens placed in the constant radius beam zone the situation depicted in Figure 5.42 is created and, after the lens, the beam is still Gaussian, having its minimum radius at the lens focus length. In this case, calling z_f the focal distance of the lens and D the lens

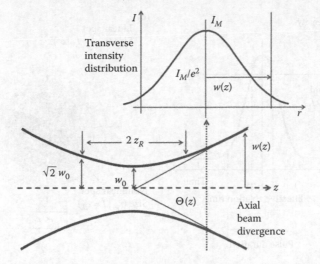

FIGURE 5.41 Longitudinal divergence and transversal shape of a Gaussian beam.

diameter we have that the beam diameter d_B at the lens focal length (i.e., in this case equivalent to $2 w_0$) is given by

$$d_B = \frac{\lambda z_f}{\pi D}$$ (5.10)

Thus, as expected, the main way to reduce the beam spot and increase the process critical dimension is to decrease the laser wavelength. An increase of the lens diameter is also useful in order to reduce the diffraction spot, as it is a decrease of the focus distance.

The results obtained up to now essentially assume linear propagation of the beam and linear absorption of the beam into the substrate. If an ultra-short pulses laser is used, the intensity near the pulse peak can be huge; so high that nonlinear ablation phenomena drive the process. In this case, effective ablation happens only when the pulse intensity is above a threshold that is, during a period shorter than the whole pulse duration, as depicted in Figure 5.43a. This reflects also on the spot size. As a matter of fact this means that only the part of the beam above the intensity threshold generates effective ablation, causing a nonlinear reduction of the spot size, as shown in Figure 5.43b.

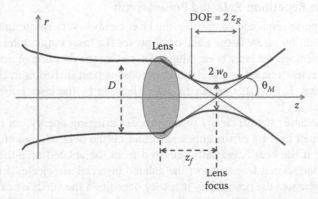

FIGURE 5.42 Scheme of the focalization of a Gaussian beam using a lens, DOF represents the depth of focus.

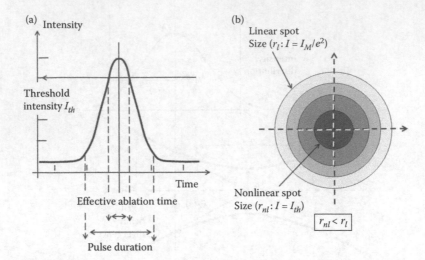

FIGURE 5.43 Nonlinear reduction of the spot size in ultra-short pulse laser ablation: (a) ablation period compared with the pulse duration; (b) nonlinear reduction of the ablation spot size.

5.7.2.3 Depth of Focus

The depth of focus (DOF), also called depth of field, of the beam after concentration through a length is the length where the beam radius practically does not change so that it is equal to twice the Rayleigh length. For long focal lengths the numerical aperture (NA) of the lens can be written as

$$NA = \Delta n_l \sin(\Theta_M) \approx \frac{D}{2z_f} \tag{5.11}$$

so that we can rewrite the DOF starting from Equation 5.8 as

$$DOF = \frac{4}{\pi} \frac{\lambda}{NA^2} \tag{5.12}$$

The required DOF depends essentially on the flatness of the surface to be ablated: as a matter of fact all the surface must be within the DOF if the ablation has to be effective.

5.7.2.4 Laser Pulse Repetition Rate and Pulse Length

The structure of the pulse sequence composing the laser beam is very important to define the ablation criteria. The repetition rate ν is the number of pulses the laser emits in a second and the duty rate σ is the time percentage the laser is emitting light, so that the duration of a single pulse is given by $\tau = \sigma/\nu$. A key element related to the ablation process is heat diffusion in the substrate during the laser pulse duration. Heat diffusion during active heating by the laser pulse has to be avoided for different reasons.

Heat diffusion decreases the efficiency of the process bringing energy out of the ablation area while causing unwanted heating of the zones surrounding the ablated area creating brittle material areas. Moreover, if the heat is partially removed from the ablated area the local temperature is lower during ablation so that fragments of the ablated material are ejected from the surface at a lower energy. This increases the probability that they deposit on the surface nearby the heated area causing defects. Last, but not least, heat diffusion is sometimes associated with the so-called shock waves, constituted by the propagation through the material of the density perturbation caused by the rapid material heating. Shock waves can damage nearby material, leave internal stress in the material when ended and even delaminate multilayer materials.

The length scale d of heat diffusion in the material can be deduced from the general diffusion rules (see Section 7.4) and it is given by

$$d = \sqrt{D_T\, t_{eff}} \qquad (5.13)$$

where t_{eff} is the pulse effective length that coincides with the pulse duration if linear coupling between light and substrate material happens, while it is determined from the characteristics of nonlinear interaction for very high energy power pulses (see Figure 5.43). The substrate thermal diffusion coefficient is indicated as D_T. The thermal diffusion coefficient is provided by the equation

$$D_T = \frac{\kappa}{\rho\, c_p} \qquad (5.14)$$

where κ is the thermal diffusion coefficient, ρ is the polymer density, and c_p is the constant pressure heat capacity (see Equation 7.59).

If we consider that the order of magnitude of D_T is 10^{-7} m²/s for many polymers used for laser ablation and a pulse duration of 10 ns we get $d = 1$ nm. An HAZ of the order of 1 nm all around the ablated structure is a relevant side effect of the ablation process and in general is considered a sort of threshold for the pulse length. When the HAZ is greater than 1 nm the used pulse is considered long with respect to the ablation process and the effects due to heat diffusion have to be considered in evaluating the ablation quality. When the HAZ is much smaller than 1 nm, for example 0.1 nm, the used pulse is considered short and heat diffusion is assumed to have a negligible impact on the process.

These considerations have pushed the use of very short pulse lasers for laser ablation, with low duty rate and very high pulse energy. This is possible using picosecond or even femtosecond lasers. Picosecond pulses can be obtained by several lasers, like CO_2, Nd:Yag and copper vapor lasers, while femtosecond high power lasers are generally excimer lasers (see Section 4.5.4). Recently, rare earth-doped fiber lasers with femtosecond pulses have been introduced, having lower power with respect to excimer lasers, but much easier to manage as part of an industrial process [94]. Performances of selected short pulse lasers compatible with laser ablation of polymers are shown in Table 5.8.

TABLE 5.8
Performances of Selected Short Pulse Lasers Compatible with Laser Ablation of Polymers

Laser	Wavelength (μm)	Pulse Duration (ps)	Average Power (W)	Duty Rate (Hz)	Pulse Energy (J)	Reference
CO_2	10.27 or 10.59	160	—	1	150	[87]
CO_2	10.3	3	4.5×10^5	10	3×10^{-4}	[88]
Nd:Yag	1.064	20	0.33	10	0.033	[89]
Nd:Yag	1.064	100	4.6	20	0.23	[89]
Ti:Sapphire	0.785	130	0.46	20	30×10^{-6}	[90]
Ti:Sapphire	From 0.76 to 0.84	0.15	2.25×10^3	10	225	[91]
Yb fiber laser	0.78	0.1	0.065	10^7	6.5×10^{-9}	[92]
Yb fiber laser	1.060	0.09	0.15	100	1.5×10^{-9}	[92]

Another interesting feature of ultrashort low duty rate laser ablation is the possibility to control the depth of ablation with a great accuracy simply by controlling the number of pulses that hit the substrate.

5.7.3 LASER ABLATION ALTERNATIVE PROCESSES

Several variations have been introduced to render the laser ablation process either more efficient or more suitable for particular applications. Here, we will deal with two of them that have been introduced also for polymers machining for labs on chip.

The need for avoiding excessive heating of the substrate during ablation prevents the use of very high-power IR lasers for laser ablation where small critical dimensions are involved. IR light directly couple with thermal phonons of the substrate material heating it quite efficiently.

Water jet-guided laser machining [95,96] is a method to locally cool the ablated material during ablation itself, thereby allowing high power lasers and IR wavelength to be used. The general scheme of a water jet-guided laser ablation system is reported in Figure 5.44. Purified water is injected at a pressure of the order of 10 MPa in a small water chamber with a hole in the floor placed on top of the substrate. From the hole in the water chamber a water flux continuously flows from the water chamber to the substrate forming a continuous water fillet. The laser light enters in the water chamber from a hole in the center of the roof, exiting from the chamber from the same hole forming the water fillet.

The light entering the water chamber is guided into the water filet with a guiding mechanism similar to optical fibers and maintains through all the space from the water chamber to the substrate about the same mode radius, determined essentially from the water fillet, that is, from the exit hole.

Laser ablation thus happens under a continuous water flow, allowing fast removal of debris and cooling of the substrate. More important, water flow goes on in the interval among laser pulses, allowing substrate cooling and avoiding heat from different pulses to accumulate.

Laser-induced chemical etching is another technique allowing clean laser ablation to be performed by avoiding debris to deposit on the substrate surface and provoke damage. It consists in executing laser ablation in an atmosphere containing elements that combine with the surface debris forming a gas that spontaneously leaves the ablation area.

A good example of this technique is silicon ablation in chlorine atmosphere. When silicon hot debris evaporates from the substrate surface they combine with chlorine by forming silicon chloride ($SiCl_4$) that is a gas, and spontaneously leave the ablation area.

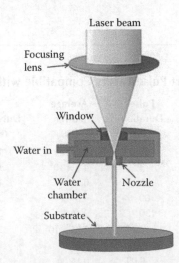

FIGURE 5.44 Principle scheme of a water jet-guided laser ablation system.

REFERENCES

1. Xia Y., Whitesides G. M., Soft lithography, *Annual Review of Material Science*, vol. 28, pp. 153–184, 1998.
2. Madou M. J., *Fundamentals of Microfabrication and Nanotechnology*; Third edition, Three-volume set, CRC Press; (August 1, 2011), ISBN-13: 978-0849331800.
3. Callister W. D., Rethwisch D. G., *Fundamentals of Materials Science and Engineering: An Integrated Approach*, Wiley; 4th edition (November 22, 2011), ISBN-13: 978-1118061602.
4. Renault J. P., Bernard A., Bietsch A., Michel B., Bosshard H. R., Delamarche E., Fabricating arrays of single protein molecules on glass using microcontact printing, *Journal of Physical Chemistry B.*, vol. 107, pp. 703–711, 2003.
5. Birdi K. S., *Self-Assembly Monolayer Structures of Lipids and Macromolecules at Interfaces*, Springer; 1st edition (October 1, 1999), ISBN-13: 978-0306460999.
6. Schwartz D. K., Mechanisms and kinetics of self-assembled monolayer formation, *Annual Review of Physical Chemistry*, vol. 52, pp. 107–137, 2001.
7. Schreiber F., Self-assembled monolayers: From 'simple' model systems to biofunctionalized interfaces, *Journal of Physics: Condensed Matter*, vol. 16, pp. R881–R900, 2004.
8. Poirier G. E., Coverage-dependent phases and phase stability of decanethiol on Au(111), *Langmuir*, vol. 15, pp. 1167–1175, 1999.
9. Pruzinski S. A., Braun P. V., Fabrication and characterization of two-photons polymerized features in colloidal crystals, *Advanced Functional Materials*, vol. 15, pp. 1995–2004, 2005.
10. Mendez-Villuendas E., Bowles R. K., Surface nucleation in the freezing of gold nanoparticles, *Physical Review Letters*, vol. 98, pp. 185503–185505, 2007.
11. Estroff L. A., Kriebel J. K., Nuzzo R. G., Whitesides G. M., Self-assembled monolayers of thiolates on metals as a form of nanotechnology, *Chemical Review*, vol. 105, pp. 1103–1170, 2005.
12. Bessueille F., Mateu Pla-Roca C. A., Mills E., Martinez J. S., Abdelhamid E., Submerged microcontact printing (SμCP): An unconventional printing technique of thiols using high aspect ratio, elastomeric stamps, *Langmuir*, vol. 21, pp. 12060–12063, 2005.
13. Libioulle L., Bietsch A., Schmid H., Michel B., Delamarche E., Contact-inking stamps for microcontact printing of alkanethiols on gold, *Langmuir*, vol. 15, pp. 300–304, 1999.
14. Goetting L. B., Deng T., Whitesides G. M., Microcontact printing of alkanephosphonic acids on aluminum, pattern transfer by wet chemical etching, *Langmuir*, vol. 15, pp. 1182–1191, 1999.
15. Kang W. H. et al., Simple ZnO nanowires patterned growth by microcontact printing for high performance field emission device, *Journal of Physical Chemistry C*, vol. 115, pp. 11435–11441, 2011.
16. Wilbur J. L., Kumar A., Biebuyck H. A., Kim E., Whitesides G. M., Microcontact printing of self-assembled monolayers: Applications in microfabrication, *Nanotechnology*, vol. 7, pp. 452–457, 1996.
17. Saravia V., Küpcü S., Nolte M., Huber C., Pum D., Fery A., Sleytr U. B., Toca-Herrera J. L., Bacterial protein patterning by micro-contact printing of PLL-g-PEG, *Journal of Biotechnology*, vol. 130, pp. 247–252, 2007.
18. Blinka E. et al., Enhanced microcontact printing of proteins on nanoporous silica surface, *Nanotechnology*, vol. 21, pp. 5302–5318, 2010.
19. Foley J., Schmid H., Stutz R., Delamarche E., Microcontact printing of proteins inside microstructures, *Langmuir*, vol. 21, pp. 11296–11303, 2005.
20. Li N., Ho J.-M., Patterning functional proteins with high selectivity for biosensors applications, *Journal of Laboratory Automation*, vol. 13, pp. 237–242, 2008.
21. LaFratta N., Li L., Fourkas J. T., Soft-lithographic replication of 3D microstructures with closed loops, *Proceedings of National Academy of Science of United States*, vol. 103, pp. 8589–8594, 2006.
22. Brittain S. T., Whitesides G. M., Fabrication of glassy carbon microstructures by soft lithography, *Sensors and Actuators A*, vol. A72, pp. 125–139, 1999.
23. Kim E., Xia Y., Whitesides G. M., Micromolding in capillaries: Applications in materials science, *Journal of American Chemical Society*, vol. 118, pp. 5722–5731, 1996.
24. Kim E., Xia Y., Whitesides G. M., Micromolding of polymers in capillaries: Applications in microfabrication, *Chemistry of Materials*, vol. 8, pp. 1558–1567, 1996.
25. Pawlowski L., *The Science and Engineering of Thermal Spray Coatings*, Wiley; 2nd edition (2008), ISBN-13: 978-0471490494.
26. Paulussen S., Rego R., Goossens O., Vangeneugden D., Rose K., Plasma polymerization of hybrid organic–inorganic monomers in an atmospheric pressure dielectric barrier discharge, *Surface and Coatings Technology*, vol. 200, pp. 672, 2005.

27. Leroux F., Campagne C., Perwuelz A., Gengembre L., Fluorocarbon nano-coating of polyester fabrics by atmospheric air plasma with aerosol, *Applied Surface Science*, vol. 254, pp. 3902, 2008.

28. Sobolev V. V., Guilemany J., Nutting J., Editors, *High Velocity Oxy-Fuel Spraying*, Institute of Materials, Minerals and Mining Publisher; 1st edition (2004), ISBN-13: 978-1902653723.

29. Xu Y., Hutchings I. M., Cold spray deposition of thermoplastic powder, *Surface and Coatings Technology*, vol. 201, pp. 3044–3050, 2006.

30. Kuroda S., Kawakita J., Watanabe M., Katanoda H., Warm Spraying—A novel coating process based on high-velocity impact of solid particles, *Science and Technology of Advanced Materials*, vol. 9, pp. 033002, 2008.

31. Mattox M. D., *Handbook of Physical Vapor Deposition (PVD) Processing*, William Andrew; 2nd edition (May 19, 2010), ISBN-13: 978-0815520375.

32. Yasuda H., *Plasma Polymerization*. Academic Press; 1st edition (year 1985). ISBN-13 978_0127687602.

33. Inagaki N., *Plasma Surface Modification and Plasma Polymerization*, CRC Press; 1st edition (March 6, 1996), ISBN-13: 978-1566763370.

34. Ayral A., Julbe A., Rouessac V., Roualdes S., Durand J., Microporous silica membrane: Basic principles and recent advances, *Membrane Science and Technology*. vol. 13, pp. 33–79, 2008.

35. Cho S.-H., Park Z.-T., Kim J.-G., Boo J.-H., Physical and optical properties of plasma polymerized thin films deposited by PECVD method, *Surface and Coatings Technology*, vol. 174–175, pp. 1111–1115, 2003.

36. Wang J. G., Neoh K. G., Kang E. T., Comparative study of chemically synthesized and plasma polymerized pyrrole and thiophene thin films, *Thin Solid Films*, vol. 446, pp. 205–217, 2004.

37. Prikryl R., Cech V., Kripal L., Vanek J., *Plasma Polymer Adhesion and Interfacial Hydrolytic Stability*, Proceedings of the 16th International Symposium on Plasma Chemistry, 2003.

38. Sajeev U. S. et al., On the optical and electrical properties of rf and a.c. plasma polymerized aniline thin films, *Bulletin of Material Science*, vol. 29, pp. 159–163, 2006.

39. Cerro L. M., Diaz M. E., *Physic-chemistry and Hydrodynamics of Langmuir–Blodgett Depositions*, VDM Verlag (October 23, 2008), ISBN-13: 978-3639088748.

40. Petty C. M., *Langmuir–Blodgett Films*, Cambridge University Press; 1st edition (year 1996), ISBN:13-978-0521424509.

41. Nagarajan R, editor, *Amphiphiles: Molecular Assembly and Applications*, American Chemical Society (March 20, 2012), ISBN-13: 978-0841226500.

42. Lee L. M., Heimark R. L., Guzman R., Baygents J. C., Zohar Y., Low melting point agarose as a protection layer in photolithographic patterning of aligned binary proteins, *Lab Chip*, vol. 6, pp. 1080–1096, 2006.

43. Douglas K., Deavaud G., Clark N. A., Transfer of biologically derived nanometer scale patterns to smooth substrates, *Science*, vol. 257, pp. 642–644, 1992.

44. Tekin E., Smith P. J., Schubert U. S., Inkjet printing as a deposition and patterning tool for polymers and inorganic particles, *Soft Matter*, vol. 4, pp. 703–713, 2008.

45. De Gans B.-J., Duineveld P. C., Schubert U. S., Inkjet printing of polymers: State of the art and future developments, *Advanced Materials*, vol. 16, pp. 203–213, 2004.

46. Singh M. et al., Inkjet printing—process and its applications, *Advanced Materials*, vol. 22, pp. 673–685, 2010.

47. Kim J. D., Choi J. S., Kim B. S., Choi J. C., Cho Y. W., Piezoelectric inkjet printing of polymers: Stem cell patterning on polymer substrates, *Polymer*, vol. 51, pp. 2147–2154, 2010.

48. Gibson I., Rosen G. W., Stucker B., *Additive Manufacturing Technologies: Rapid Prototyping to Direct Digital Manufacturing*, Springer; 1st edition (December 14, 2009), ISBN-13: 978-1441911193.

49. Bàrtholo P. J., editor, *Stereolithography*, Springer; 1st edition (April 6, 2011), ISBN-13: 978-0387929033.

50. Ovsianikov A., Ostendorf A., Chichkov B. N., Three-dimensional photofabrication with femtosecond lasers for applications in photonics and biomedicine, *Applied Surface Science*, vol. 15, pp. 6599–6602, 2007.

51. Ikuta K., Hirowatari K., *Real Three Dimensional Micro Fabrication Using Stereo Lithography and Metal Molding*, Proceedings of IEEE Micro-electro-mechanical-systems, pp. 42–47, 1993.

52. Younse J. M., Mirrors on a chip, *IEEE Spectrum*, vol. 30, pp. 27–31, 1993.

53. Ikuta K., Maruo S., Kojima S., New Micro Stereo Lithography for Free Movable Micro Structure—Super IH Process with Sub-Micron Resolution, Proceedings of IEEE Workshop on Micro-electro-mechanical-systems, pp. 290–295, 1998.

54. Lee K.-S. et al., Two-photon stereolithography, *Journal of Nonlinear Optical Physics and Materials*, vol. 16, pp. 59–73, 2007.

55. Park S. U. et al., Improvement of spatial resolution in nano-stereolithography using radical quencher, *Macromolecular Research*, vol. 14, pp. 559–564, 2006.
56. Ovsianikov A., Ostendorf A., Chichkov B. N., Three-dimensional photofabrication with femtosecond lasers for applications in photonics and biomedicine, *Applied Surface Science*, vol. 253, pp. 6599–6602, 2007.
57. Osswald T., Turnq L. S., Gramann P., *Injection Molding Handbook*, Hanser Publications; 2nd edition (June 1, 2008), ISBN-13: 978-1569904206.
58. Kulkarni S., *Robust Process Development and Scientific Molding: Theory and Practice*, Hanser Publications (September 1, 2010), ISBN-13: 978-1569905012.
59. Kang S., *Micro/Nano Replication: Processes and Applications*, Wiley; 1st edition (April 3, 2012), ISBN-13: 978-0470392133.
60. Zahn J. D., editor, *Methods in Bioengineering: Biomicrofabrication and Biomicrofluidics*, Artech House; 1st edition (October 31, 2009), ISBN-13: 978-1596934009.
61. Giboz J., Copponnex T., Mélé P., Microinjection molding of thermoplastic polymers: A review, *Journal of Micromechanics and Microengineering*, vol. 17, pp. R96–R109, 2007.
62. Liu A.-C., Chen R.-H., Injection molding of polymer micro- and sub-micron structures with high-aspect ratios, *The International Journal of Advanced Manufacturing Technology*, vol. 28, pp. 1097–1103, 2006.
63. Sha B., Dimov S., Griffiths C., Packianather M. S., Investigation of micro-injection moulding: Factors affecting the replication quality, *Journal of Materials Processing Technology*, vol. 183, pp. 284–296, 2007.
64. Worgull M., *Hot Embossing: Theory and Technology of Microreplication*, William Andrew; 1st edition (July 7, 2009), ISBN-13: 978-0815515791.
65. Jena R. K., Yue C. Y., Lam Y. C., Tang P. S., Gupta A., Comparison of different molds (epoxy, polymer and silicon) for microfabrication by hot embossing technique, *Sensors and Actuators B: Chemical*, vol. 163, pp. 233–241, 2012.
66. Velten T. et al., Roll-to-roll hot embossing of microstructures, *Microsystem Technologies*, vol. 17, pp. 619–627, 2011.
67. Liu Y., Liu W., Zhang Y., Wu D., Wang X., A novel extrusion microns embossing method of polymer film, *Modern Mechanical Engineering*, vol. 2, pp. 35–40, 2012.
68. Velten T., Schuck H., Haberer W., Bauerfeld F., Investigations on reel-to-reel hot embossing, *The International Journal of Advanced Manufacturing Technology*, vol. 47, pp. 73–80, 2010.
69. Zahng D., Men L., Chen Q., Microfabrication and applications of opto-microfluidic sensors, *Sensors*, vol. 11, pp. 5360–5382, 2011.
70. Menz W., Mohr J., The LIGA microfabrication technique, in *Microsystems Technology: Fabrication, Test & Reliability*, Boussey J., editor, ISTE Publishing Company (October 2003), ISBN-13: 978-1903996478.
71. Saile, V. et al. editors, *LIGA and its Applications*, Wiley; 1st edition (2009), ISBN-13: 978-3527316984.
72. Lawes L. A., Manufacturing tolerances for UV LIGA using SU-8 resist, *Journal of Micromechanics and Microengineering*, vol. 15, pp. 2198–2203, 2005.
73. Joie C. D., Calame J. P., Garven M., Levush B., UV-LIGA microfabrication of 220 GHz sheet beam amplifier gratings with SU-8 photoresists, *Journal of Micromechanics and Microengineering*, vol. 20, pp. 125016, 2010.
74. Jeong S. J., Wang W., Design and UV-LIGA microfabrication of an electro-statically actuated power relay, *Microsystem Technologies*, vol. 13, pp. 279–286, 2007.
75. Spearing S. M., Materials issues in microelectromechanical systems (MEMS), *Acta Materialia*, vol. 48, pp. 179–196, 2000.
76. Celler G. K., Maldonado J. R., editors, *Materials Aspects of X-Ray Lithography: Volume 306 (MRS Proceedings)*, Materials Research Society (October 27, 1993), ISBN-13: 978-1558992023.
77. Lercel L. J. editor, *Emerging Lithographic Technologies X (Proceedings of Spie)*, Society of Photo Optical (March 10, 2006), ISBN-13: 978-0819461940.
78. Willmott P., *An Introduction to Synchrotron Radiation: Techniques and Applications*, Wiley; 1st edition (August 30, 2011), ISBN-13: 978-0470745786.
79. Duke P. J., *Synchrotron Radiation: Production and Properties*, Oxford University Press, USA (February 15, 2009), ISBN-13: 978-0199559091.
80. Astete C. E., Sabliov C. M., Synthesis and characterization of PLGA nanoparticles, *Journal of Biomaterials Science—Polymer Edition*, vol. 17, pp. 247–289, 2006.
81. Schlesingher M., Paunovic M., editors, *Modern Electroplating*, Wiley; 5th edition (October 19, 2010), ISBN-13: 978-0470167786.

82. Kanani N., *Electroplating: Basic Principles, Processes and Practice*, Elsevier Science; 1st edition (January 25, 2005), ISBN-13: 978-1856174510.

83. Black E. S. editor, *Laser Ablation: Effects and Applications*, Nova Science Publishing Inc. (January 2011), ISBN-13: 978-1611224665.

84. Phipps C. editor, *Laser Ablation and its Applications*, Springer; reprint 2007 edition (December 1, 2010), ISBN-13: 978-1441940278.

85. Sugioka K., Cheng Y., Midorikawa K., Three-dimensional micromachining of glass using femtosecond laser for lab-on-a-chip device manufacture, *Applied Physics A*, vol. 81, pp. 1–10, 2005.

86. Wang L., Kodzius R., Yi X., Li S., Hui Y. S., Wen W., Prototyping chips in minutes: Direct laser plotting (DLP) of functional microfluidic structures, *Sensors and Actuators B: Chemical*, vol. 168, pp. 214–222, 2012.

87. Tochitsky S. Ya., Narang R., Filip C., Clayton C. E., Marsh K. A., Joshi C., Generation of 160-ps terawatt-power CO_2 *Laser Pulses, Optics Letters*, vol. 24, pp. 1717–1719, 1999.

88. Haberberger D., Tochitsky S., Joshi C., Fifteen terawatt picosecond CO_2 laser system, Optics Express, vol. 18, pp. 17865–17875, 2010.

89. Data from Photonics Solutions inc., www.photonicssolutions.uk, last accessed January 17, 2013.

90. Shaheena M. E., Gagnona J. E., Fryera B. J., Femtosecond (fs) lasers coupled with modern ICP-MS instruments provide new and improved potential for in situ elemental and isotopic analyses in the geosciences, *Chemical Geology*, vol. 330–331, pp. 260–273, 2012.

91. Svanberg S. et al., Lund high-power laser facility—systems and first results, *Physica Scripta*, vol. 49, pp. 187–192, 1994.

92. Data from Thorlabs inc., http://www.thorlabs.com, last accessed January 17, 2013.

93. Born M., Wolf E., *Principles of Optics*, Cambridge University Press; 7th edition (October 13, 1999), ISBN-13: 978-0521642224.

94. Ilday F. Ö., Buckley J., Kuznetsova L., Wise F. W., Generation of 36-femtosecond pulses from a ytterbium fiber laser, *Optics Express*, vol. 11, pp. 3550–3554, 2003.

95. Richerzhagen B., Water-guided laser processing, *Industrial Laser Review*, vol. 10, pp. 8–10, 1997.

96. Li C.-F., Johnson D. B., Kovacevic R., Modeling of waterjet guided laser grooving of silicon, *International Journal of Machine Tools & Manufacture*, vol. 43, pp. 925–936, 2003.

6 Back-End Technologies

6.1 INTRODUCTION

The family of front-end technologies collects all the technologies that are meant to build a chip, or a three-dimensional structure in MEMs case, that has to perform a well-defined function. Back-end processes are, on the contrary, all the processes that start from the final chip to condition it, so as to allow its practical use. This kind of conditioning is, for example, constituted by closing the chip in a suitable package so as to protect it from environmental damages, creating through the package the interfaces to connect the chip to external sources and sinks of chemical substances and signals (both optical and electrical), providing suitable chip thermal stabilization, and so on.

We have seen in Chapter 4 that in the semiconductor industry, independent from the type of application, electronic, optical, or microfluidic, front-end processes are performed in parallel on all the chips belonging to the same wafer, whereas back-end processes have to be performed necessarily chip-by-chip in a serial fashion. For this reason, a correctly designed back-end processes flow, especially if microfluidics or integrated optics are involved, is a key point in achieving a suitable cost for integrated components.

In considering labs on chip applications, in which microfluidics interfaces almost always exist, and are also accompanied by optical interfaces, important factors arise that do not exist in the case of electronics chips back-end [1,2]. In the electronic technology, back-end processes present a high complexity almost only when very high frequency and/or very high power signals are involved. High-frequency contacts require adapted lines, both internal and external to the chip package. High dissipated power conversely requires an accurate design of the package thermal properties and almost always the presence of an active thermal regulation system, like a Peltier junction.

Out of the above cases, almost all consumer microelectronics are characterized by the fact that the back-end processing is a very low-cost fabrication step whose cost is dominated by inline tests, the used materials being high-volume commodities, the related processes are well known and highly automatized.

This is completely not true in the case of labs on chips. Microfluidics connections imply small elements to be included into the chip package to guide external fluids into the chip: they are miniaturized parts that are external to the chip and are in no case still a commodity. Their placing needs a great accuracy that can be obtained in several cases only by exploiting pre-designed lithography marks provided during the front-end processing. In other cases, microfluidics interfaces are lateral to the chip and requires alignment and fixing of internal chip ducts with external ones, which is a nonconventional back-end operation [3].

Moreover, since labs on chip are disposable components, the back-end testing has to be carefully designed and in several cases specific structures have to be added to the basic chip structure so as to allow these tests to be performed without ruining the chip functionalities. Regarding the chemical reagents that have to be added inside the lab on chip, they can be inserted into the chip during front-end processing using different techniques, but this choice poses several limitations to the component fabrication process.

Once an organic solution is filled into a reaction chamber or a biological molecule is fixed to an activated surface, its functionality has to be maintained through the following process steps. High-temperature processes, like temperature-enhanced wafer bonding (see Section 4.10.3), cannot be performed in order not to denature organic molecules. Ion bombing is generally impossible too, due to the damage it implies on activated surfaces, so that ion-enhanced direct wafer bonding (see Section 4.10.3) and reactive ion etching (RIE, see Section 4.8.3) have to be avoided. Last, but not the least, aggressive chemical processes also have to be avoided.

Activated surfaces and charged micro-reactors can be shielded by masks during front-end processes to avoid de-functionalization of the biomolecules, but this is not always possible or convenient and in any case adds a further complication to the already very complex front-end processes. Thus, the biomolecules are charged into reaction chambers and repositories or fixed to the activated surfaces during the back-end process. This adds chemically sensible back-end steps that are all but a commodity at the state of the technology.

Besides microfluidics interfaces, optical interfaces call for complex back-end processes too. Depending on the kind of interface, toward an outgoing fiber, a transmitter, or a receiver, different requirements and techniques are used. In any case, the control of the optical beam shape and alignment between the optical waveguide integrated onto the chip and the outgoing fiber are not trivial operations, even if they are sometimes simplified by power budget requirements less stringent with respect to optical chips for other applications like telecommunications.

6.2   BACK-END REQUIREMENTS AND PROCESS FLOW

The back-end flow of labs on chip is quite different from microelectronics under the performance point of view [1,4]. On one side, labs on chip components are generally single-use elements, mainly due to the fact that a limited amount of reagent is stored into the chip and in any case, once the reaction chamber and the rest of microfluidics circuit is used, it has to be considered contaminated. This means that the duration through a long operating life is generally not required to these components [5–7].

However, the fact that organic molecules are stored inside the chip can pose a limitation to the storage time and conditions. In their main applications, labs on chip are destined to be stored in standard conditions in hospitals, biological institutes, or even pharmacies. In this condition, the package structure has to assure a sufficiently long storage time, protecting as much as possible the inside chip from environmental problems.

While under operation, the fact that biochemical reactions happen in the chip calls for a rigorous temperature control. The main biochemical reaction parameters, like reaction rates and diffusion coefficients (see Sections 1.2.4 and 1.6.3), are highly temperature-sensitive. Moreover, because of a tight temperature range, the activity of the biomolecules is severely hampered so that the reaction does not even happen at all.

Another characteristic element of several labs on chip is the need to be hosted into pluggable shells, that is, to be easily inserted into the final equipment that contains components that are not of single use, like optical receivers and transmitters, and performs data elaboration and presentation [2,3]. An example of this system architecture is shown in Figure 6.1, where the complete system is shaped like a computer, with an external satellite hosting the labs on chip, or a set of different labs on chip depending on the test to be performed. In Figure 6.1, the different packaging layers of a system incorporating a lab on chip for biochemical assays are shown. The lab on chip is first enclosed in a package to protect it from environment and to provide suitable interfaces with the outer system. The packaged chip is fixed on a board whose role is both to provide mechanical stability and suitable mechanical fixing points and to integrate selected parts of control electronics. The board is finally integrated into a chassis that provides suitable mechanical elements to be plugged into the corresponding plug of the system [8,9].

The selection of which electronics parts have to be integrated in the disposable board and which in the system is an important step. Electronic drivers that are inexpensive but have to be near to the lab on chip are integrated in the disposable board, while more expensive elaboration subsystems are part of the external system of a long-lasting equipment.

The system itself can be shaped in several ways, depending on the use. A PC-like system can be suitable for use in laboratories or medical studies [10], while smaller electronic appliances like

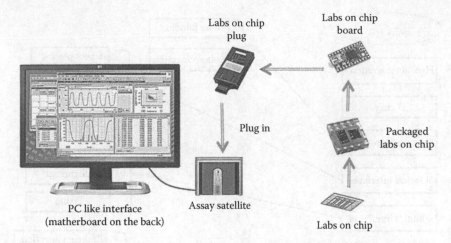

FIGURE 6.1 Different layers of a system incorporating a lab on chip for biochemical assays.

smartphones and tablets allow portable lab on chip use. Specific, portable systems can also be conceived, for example, including elements like optical components, for specific uses like emergency or environmental control [11,12].

Still different architectures have to be designed for systems that are subparts of more complex machines, like control subsystems of processing machines or high-throughput analysis equipment used in medical analysis centers. In this case, the function and architecture of the whole equipment dictate the most suitable architecture of the lab on chip subsystem.

In any case, after the chip fabrication, a complex back-end fabrication step is still required to obtain the final lab on chip based subsystem.

The back-end process flow depends on the structure and application of the considered lab on chip, due to both different requirements and different cost targets, but common elements can be identified that are almost always present [4,13]. In Figure 6.2, we depict a generic process flow, aimed to identify the role of all the main back-end steps. In specific cases, it is possible that not all the processes in the figure are present, while additional steps can appear if more specific needs emerge.

After wafer acceptance at the beginning of the back-end line, which is performed by means of specifically designed tests, the first back-end process, before dicing of single chips, can be hybrid integration. Hybrid integration is the process allowing the fixing of other chips, like electronic integrated circuits (ICs) or optical elements, on suitably prepared hosting sites on the surface of the lab on chip, so as to interface them with selected lab on chip parts. This is generally performed when the chips are still on the wafer, but it is a back-end process since it is performed on the single chip in a sequential manner.

A typical example of hybrid integration is the addition of infrared (IR) laser sources on silicon- or polymer-based chips. IR lasers are realized using III–V alloys like InGaAsP deposited in epitaxial layers on an InP substrate. Since III–V alloys epitaxial growth on a silicon substrate is almost impossible at the state of the art, even if many researches are obtaining results in this direction, lasers have to be realized separately from the main chip. During front-end fabrication, a suitable structure is prepared to interface the laser with the rest of the circuit and, before dicing, a laser is added to each chip on the wafer by a hybrid integration process called flip-chip mounting, due to the fact that the laser is generally mounted *head down* on the hosting chip. Similar processes can be used to integrate electronic parts on polymeric chips or polymer parts on Si–SiO$_2$ chips. In any case, the hybrid integration is prepared by a front-end micromachining process and realized during the back-end stage.

After hybrid integration, the chips are separated with a process called dicing. If wafer bonding has been used to create the microfluidics part of the chip, dicing has to be carried out carefully,

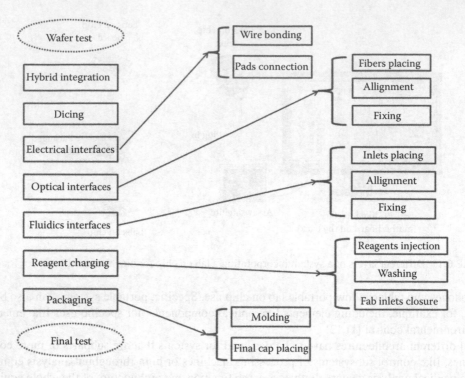

FIGURE 6.2 Back-end process flow scheme. Selected steps may not be present in specific cases, as further processes can be inserted if needed.

avoiding the accumulation of too much stress in the interface between wafers and the possibility to break the contact between them.

Single chips realized from silicon wafers are difficult to handle in the following processes, thus before any other back-end step they are individually fixed on a base, that is intended to provide mechanical resistance, ease handling and constitute the floor of the final chip package. This step is performed using a wide variety of techniques depending on the chip base material and the kind of functionality the chip is designed to perform. Sometimes, the chip presents the need of building interfaces both on the top and on the back, so that die attach has to be performed preserving the possibility to access the back of the chip where these interfaces have to be built, or it is even delayed after the interface fabrication process.

In other cases, especially for polymeric chips, either the chip is sufficiently sturdy that it does not need a base for mechanical reinforcement or they are directly packaged by immerging the original chip into a polymer block, that is then worked so as to perform the other back-end processes.

After the die attach, the core of the back-end processes regards the construction of the interfaces that will allow the lab on chip to exchange materials and data with the environment. In the most general case, we will have three kinds of interfaces: fluidic interfaces, optical interfaces, and electronics interfaces.

Fluidic interfaces are used to insert fluids under test and, in some cases, to extract fluids from the chip. They can be permanent interfaces, that are fabricated to be used at the moment of the lab on chip operation, or fab interfaces, that are used during the back-end process to insert reagent inside the chip and are then closed before the final chip package.

Optical interfaces are generally related to the onboard detection system and can either interface internal waveguides with external transmitters/receivers or allow the chip to present an optical output in the form of a fiber pigtail, interfacing the monolithic waveguide end with an optical fiber.

Finally, electronic interfaces allow both data extraction from the chip and control signal to be inserted and extracted from the chip. Internal control can be needed, for example, to assure a correct temperature control or to command the operation of active elements like valves and pumps.

The order in which interfaces are realized depends on the particular chip and the related back-end process starts from suitable structures realized during the front-end phase, like V-groove for fiber accommodation, metal pads for wire bonding, or suitable vias to convey electrical wires from the back of the chip to the front and to accommodate fluidic connections.

A specific element of lab on chip interface realization during the back-end process is related to the insertion into the microfluidic circuit of chemical reactant. This can be an easy operation, for example the injection of a small quantity of solution in a micro-funnel. In other cases, it is a complex procedure like fixing a specific molecule to an activated surface. In this case, the solution containing the molecule has to be inserted into the microfluidics part of the chip and reach the activated surface. After an opportune time the system has to be washed, for example, with an alcoholic mix, so as to remove the liquid part of the solution and leave inside the chip only with the molecules that have been captured by the activated surface. In order to allow such a complex operation, probably a specific microfluidic subsystem has to be built in the chip and fab microfluidic interfaces have to be fabricated, which have to be closed after the operation.

Charging the chip with chemical reagents can be a critical operation to be done in a back-end line both due to the need of managing potentially dangerous and in any case delicate chemical substances and due to the complex automation of such operations that require the development of dedicated machines. Moreover, after the insertion of organic solutions into the chip, a series of constraints for the subsequent processes arises, due to the need of preserving the activity and structure of such substances. This is the reason the charging of organic substances into the chip is delayed as much as possible in the process flow.

After the realization of all the interfaces, the chip is inserted into the final package. This is sometimes realized with an operation called molding (not to be confused with the process used to shape polymers and discussed in Section 5.4.1), which consists of the inclusion of the chip and all the interface structures in a drop of polymer that is then hardened so as to fix the final configuration. The hardening of the polymer implies a mechanical adjustment of its parts so that if the relative positions of the elements to be molded have to be preserved with great precision, they have to be previously fixed in case with a suitable bias to compensate the polymer change of shape. For this and other reasons, molding introduces stresses in the system that have to be taken into account and minimized as much as possible.

Sometimes molding is the last step of the process regarding the single chip, since the molding polymer also has the role of protecting the chip from the environment and to allow it to be used in its real operative conditions. In other cases, a solid package cap is also added for further protection.

In some applications, it is useful that different chips are enclosed in the same package, either to avoid extra packaging operations that would affect the final product cost or to allow the chips to be as near as possible whenever required. In this case, a possible solution is to mold more than one chip together after connecting them via common interfaces. It is useful that inter-chip interfaces have a certain degree of flexibility to adapt themselves to the following back-end operations. In this case, internal interfaces are realized either directly by polymeric structures, like SU8 or PMI microfluidic ducts, or protected using a polymeric structure, like electrical connections realized by aluminum wires and embedded in a polymeric strip.

Some important elements of all the back-end process flow is the nature and the position of the partial tests and the type of final test that has to be designed to assess both the whole process quality and the single-chip functionality. Tests are performed on each chip sequentially, so that, if complex and frequent tests allow failures to be immediately identified avoiding further processing of non-working pieces, an excessive number of too complex tests can easily become the main cost driver of the whole process. A trade-off has to be found, mainly based on the cost target of the system.

To address a correct trade-off design for testing and the careful identification of the main sources of process, errors have to be used as discussed more in detail in Section 4.2.3.

6.3 HYBRID INTEGRATION

The name hybrid integration collects a large number of technologies used to assemble together different chips before the final package has been realized. In general terms, hybrid integration technologies can be divided into two broad families: chip-on-chip integration and multi-chip packaging [14–16].

Chip-on-chip integration is used to mount together one or more chips by gluing, welding, or soldering one onto the other and contacting them. Multi-chip packaging, however, consists of placing more than one chip into the same package and connecting them in such a way as to interface the external system like a single subsystem.

The two processes are generally located at different points of the back-end process flow: chip-on-chip integration in the very early part, before dicing, multi-chip packaging at the end of the flow, when the final package is fabricated.

6.3.1 CHIP-ON-CHIP INTEGRATION

Chip-on-chip integration indicates a family of techniques all intended to connect two raw chips that have to be functionally integrated before the final package is operated. In this way, the connected chips are packaged together and are seen by the external system like a single subsystem. This technique was used for the integration of components that have to be fabricated using different materials in such a way that they cannot be fabricated using the same front-end process. In the field of electronics, this happens for example when a CMOS controller has to be integrated with a very high-frequency RF amplifier realized with HEMT technologies on InP or GaAs platform [14]. Chip-on-chip integration is also used in integrated optics where passive optical components are realized in Si-SiO$_2$ technology, while detectors and laser sources are realized using III–V alloys like InGaAsP over an InP substrate.

Due to its wide application in integrated optics, this technique is also useful when optical detection is used in the lab on chip and sources or detectors have to be integrated on the chip too [14]. This solution is pushed by the low cost of near IR lasers around 800 nm and the corresponding detectors are today produced in huge volumes for consumer applications. In this case, the chip-on-chip integration increases the chip cost a little, while avoids the need of creating optical interface with external components, which is a much more costly process.

A similar technique can also be used to integrate 3D elements fabricated from polymers with planar microfluidic chips realized on an Si-SiO$_2$ platform. A typical operation of this kind is the realization of a microfluidic interface via a micro-funnel realized from a suitable polymer that is inserted into an inlet of the underlying chip and fixed. To complete the interface, after molding, the funnel emerges from a suitable opening in the final package in such a way as to accept for example the input through a standard pipette.

In all cases the chip-on-chip integration is a mixed front-end/back-end process. In order to align and fix the parts that have to be plugged onto the chip, an opportune placing structure has to be fabricated during front-end processing. During back-end processing the external piece is aligned with the lithographic structure via a microscope and soldered or glued into it.

The process is different depending on the kind of considered external component; for example, we will consider the case of optical chip-on-chip process to integrate a laser into a silica-on-silicon optical structure [17]. While high-performance lasers, like those adopted in telecommunications, are costly elements, lasers designed for consumer applications are very cheap and their integration onboard of a lab on chip allows optical interfaces to be avoided, which could be more expensive in terms of back-end processing with respect to laser hybrid integration.

TABLE 6.1

Example Characteristics of a Low-Cost VCSEL for Consumer Applications; All Data Are for Continuous Wave Operation

Parameter	Symbol	Conditions	Value	Unit
Threshold current	I_{th}	$T = 25°C$	3	mA
Operating current	I_{op}	$T = 25°C$	4	mA
Optical output power	P_{out}	$I_{op} = 4$ mA	300	μW
Operating voltage	U_{op}	$I_{op} = 4$ mA	3.5	V
Differential resistance	R_d	$I_{op} = 4$ mA	250	Ω
Emission wavelength	λ	$I_{op} = 4$ mA	758	nm
Spectral bandwidth	$\Delta\lambda$	$I_{op} = 4$ mA	20	MHz
Beam divergence	Θ	$I_{op} = 4$ mA		
		Full-width half maximum	13	°
Slope efficiency	η	$I_{op} = 4$ mA	0.3	W/A
Maximum emitted power	P_{max}	$I_{op} = 6$ mA	0.6	mW

Two classes of semiconductor low-cost lasers exist: VCSELs and edge-emitting lasers. Examples of performances of lasers for very low-cost applications are provided in Table 6.1 for VCSELs and in Table 6.2 for edge-emitting lasers. If a VCSEL [18] is selected, the laser emission happens from the laser front face, while in the edge-emitting case it is generated from the laser side (see Figure 6.3). Different integration problems not only arise from the way in which the laser beam is emitted from the diode, but also from the beam form itself. As a matter of fact, as it is evident from data on beam divergence, while the VCSEL beam is quite circular, edge-emitting lasers generate a very elliptical beam, with the principal axis about 10 times greater than the secondary one.

In the VCSEL case, integration can be performed by realizing a micro-mirror at the end of the waveguide to be coupled with the laser, as shown in Figure 6.4a. A square hole is realized to uncover the guide facet so as to collect the light emitted by the laser. The mirror can be realized with different techniques, for example, by gray tone lithography or by direct e-beam writing (see Sections 4.5 and 4.6) on a silicon chip. Examples of realization of such mirrors by wet etching and gray tone lithography are reported in Figure 6.5a and b, respectively.

TABLE 6.2

Example Characteristics of a Low-Cost Edge-Emitting Laser; All Data Are for Continuous Wave Operation at 25°C

Parameter	Symbol	Conditions	Value	Unit
Threshold current	I_{th}	$T = 25°C$	22	mA
Operating current	I_{op}	$T = 25°C$	72	mA
Optical output power	P_{out}	$I_{op} = 72$ mA	50	mW
Operating voltage	U_{op}	$I_{op} = 72$ mA	2	V
Emission wavelength	λ	$I_{op} = 72$ mA	830	nm
Wavelength variation with temperature	$d\lambda/dT$	$I_{op} = 72$ mA	0.25	nm/°K
Beam divergence – parallel	$\Theta \parallel$	$I_{op} = 72$ mA,	6	°
		Full-width half maximum		
Beam divergence – perpendicular	$\Theta \perp$	$I_{op} = 72$ mA,	30	°
		Full-width half maximum		
Slope efficiency	η	$I_{op} = 72$ mA	0.95	W/A

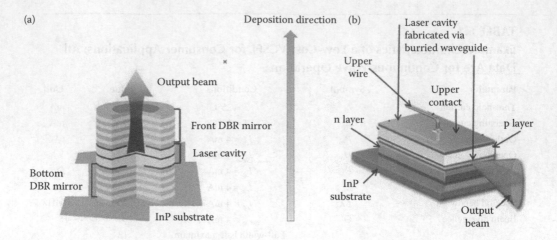

FIGURE 6.3 Principle schemes of semiconductors IR lasers: VCSEL structure (a) and edge-emitting structure (b).

If an edge-emitting laser is used instead [17], laser emission occurs from a cavity realized adding integrated mirrors to an active planar waveguide buried in the laser structure (see Figure 6.3b). The adaptation structure on the silica-on-silicon chip has to be realized so as to accommodate coupling between the silica waveguide surface and the beam emitted by the laser active waveguide, as schematically represented in Figure 6.4b. The structure seems simpler than that required by the VCSEL, but the fact that the laser is essentially inserted inside silicon or silica walls can create thermal control problems, especially if a high-power laser is required.

In both the considered integration cases, the waveguide facets have to be tapered to ease the coupling of the laser-emitted light into the guide, as detailed in Section 6.4.2. The placing and fixing of the upper chip into the adaptation structure in the lower chip is a delicate back-end

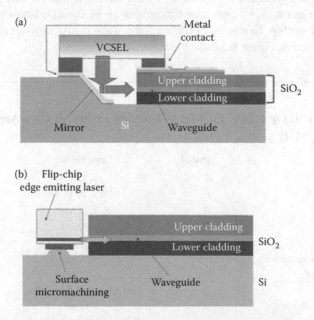

FIGURE 6.4 Scheme of chip-on-chip mounting of a semiconductor IR laser on top of a Si-SiO₂ passive optical integrated structure: mounting of a VCSEL laser (a) and mounting of an edge-emitting laser (b).

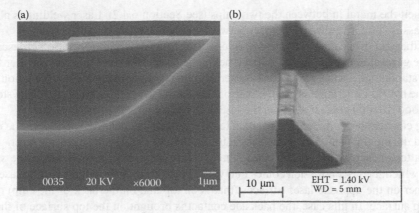

FIGURE 6.5 Realization of a deflection mirror for mounting of a VCSEL laser on a passive Si-SiO$_2$ optical integrated structure (SEM photographs of the structure before resist stripping and the inclined surface metallization): wet etching mirror (a): over-etching can be noted below the resist layer and grey tone lithography mirror (b) realized by several partial exposures to different doses of an electron beam from an E-beam lithography equipment. (Reproduced under permission from Cyoptics Inc.)

operation, which is generally performed by a flip-chip bonder. Different techniques can be used to fix the chips, but the most commonly used are welding and gluing, while soldering also can be used in selected circumstances.

Flip-chip bonders were introduced for microelectronics, where flip-chip is used to avoid too many wire bonding between a chip and the hosting board [19]. Such machines are able to place one chip on the other with a great precision and fixing them. They exist both in semiautomatic versions suited for research and development and in fully automated implementations allowing mass manufacturing. A possible scheme of a semiautomatic flip-chip-bonder is reported in Figure 6.6. The lower chip is fixed to a support while the upper one is placed on a movable arm where the fixing system is incorporated. The whole operation is controlled via an optical system and suitable lighting by a microscope.

Depending on the type of contact that has to be created between the substrate and the integrated chip, it is soldered or glued on the substrate. Welding is generally performed using a strong laser

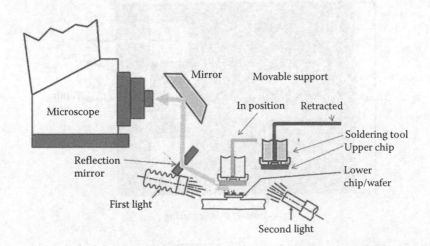

FIGURE 6.6 Flip-chip bonder principle scheme in the case of a semiautomatic machine.

source to melt the metal in between the two chips (see Section 6.4.2). Laser welding is also a good method to assure effective thermal contact between the bonded chip and the substrate.

A good thermal dissipation is a mandatory characteristic of hybrid integration of lasers, since a laser source generates a good amount of heat, being the laser quantum efficiency smaller than 30%. While in a standalone package the laser is generally cooled either using a Peltier junction or a local cooler, if the hybrid integration is used, it has to relay on the general package cooling system so that there is a good thermal contact between the laser and the substrate.

Welding can also be an interesting solution to create electrical continuity between the metallization created during the front end on the substrate and the electrical contacts of the laser.

As a matter of fact, in the VCSEL case, the contacts are normally realized on the same laser facet from which the laser emission comes out, while in the case of the edge-emitting laser they are present either on the opposite laser surfaces (that is on top and on the back of the chip) or both on the top chip surface. In this case, the backside contact is brought on the top surface of the chip via an opportune in the InP wafer.

In both cases, the original laser contacts have to be fixed via an opportune metallization on the substrate to allow wire bonding, as shown in Figure 6.4.

The final structure for the integration of a VCSEL laser and its interfacing with an output optical fiber before the laser mounting is shown in Figure 6.7. The turning mirror, realized in this case by wet etching and metalized to assure the wanted reflection, can be evidenced due to its reflectivity; the great dimension of the V-groove realized to place the output fiber with respect to the other structures on the chip is also evident.

The performances attainable with this kind of hybrid integration in terms of coupling loss between the laser and a square integrated waveguide are reported in Figure 6.8, in the case of an edge-emitting DFB laser [17] emitting at a wavelength of 1300 nm in the near infrared as a function of the vertical misalignment between the laser and the fiber, while the effect of horizontal misalignment and distance fluctuations are reported in Figure 6.9.

From Figures 6.8 and 6.9, the typical precisions that are needed in such alignments results to be 1–3 μm and this is also the limit of a good flip-chip bonder when it refers to lithographic surface micromachining structures like a V-groove [20] or a laser placing site.

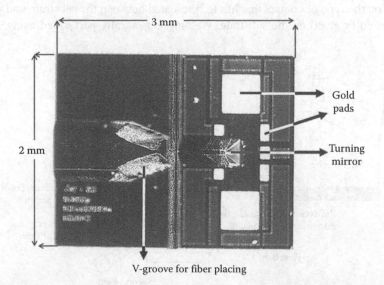

FIGURE 6.7 The final structure for the integration of a VCSEL laser and its interfacing with an output optical fiber before the laser mounting. (Reproduced under permission from Cyoptics Inc.)

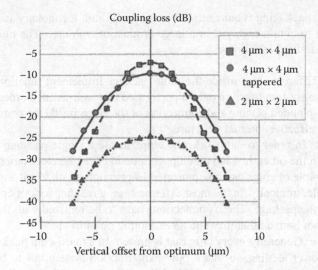

FIGURE 6.8 Coupling loss and effect of vertical offset in the coupling of an edge-emitting DFB laser with a squared SiO_2 waveguide different: squared waveguides are considered with and without a tapered end.

6.3.2 MULTI-CHIP PACKAGING

Multi-chip packaging [21,13] consists of placing several integrated circuits in a single package, either one after the other or in 3D structures that are generally constituted by different layers of superimposed chips [22]. This technology is used in the field of microelectronics, both in order to further reduce costs related to packaging and to shorten the chip-to-chip electrical connections when high-speed signals are considered [22]. When integrated optics and labs on chip technologies were developed, back-end process cost becomes even more relevant (see Section 4.4) so that multi-chip packaging gained importance, besides all solutions designed to alleviate the problem.

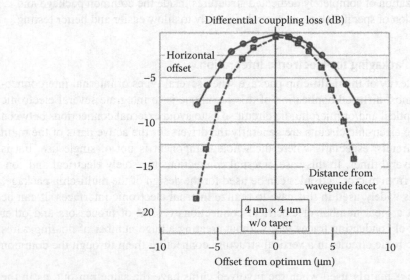

FIGURE 6.9 Coupling losses increase due to offset in distance from the guide facet and in horizontal position for the same alignment considered in Figure 6.8.

Even if multi-chip packaging is quite attractive, it is a difficult technology and requires a careful process development to obtain high yield on large production volumes. The main elements of this technology can be classified as follows:

Chip hierarchy: Different chips inside the same package implement functionalities that produce the final subsystem function only if performed in a well-defined order. This hierarchy calls for a well-planned placing and connection of the chips inside the common package so as to create an effective internal structure.

Chip connections: In order to interwork, the chips inside a single package have to be connected one with the other. In a lab on chip, connections can be electronics, optical, and/or fluidics and couple of chips can be connected in principle in different ways, for example, optically and electronically. In the most extreme case, a real network of connections has to be realized in the package. These connections have to be realized with the most effective technology, from both a reliability and an economic point of view.

Power distribution: Generally, every chip that is present in a multi-chip package has the need of receiving power feeding, so that a power distribution system has to be present inside the package that is able to feed every chip following its own power-feeding requirements.

Heat removal: All active chips, like micro-pumps, lasers, and electronic processors, dissipate power and have to be cooled to assure their correct working. While individual chip cooling can be realized if each chip is individually packaged, this is generally not possible in a multi-chip package design so that heat removal can be a key design point.

Multi-chip module external interfaces: The subsystem constituted by all the chips inside a single package has to communicate with the external environment through a set of different interfaces that have to be connected with the chips inside the package. This is a critical design point, due to the fact that the cost of the back-end process greatly depends on the interface design.

Multi-chip module testability: When different chips are placed inside the same package and connected together they represent a real subsystem that has to be tested both during production and during operation. Improving integration makes testing increasingly difficult, due to the strict relation between the subsystem parts and the difficult accessibility to their internal interfaces. Thus, design for testing is a key point for multi-chip packages and it implies the realization of completely dedicated structures inside the common package and even the integration of specific chips whose role is solely to allow easier and better testing of the component.

6.3.2.1 Multi-Chip Packaging for Electronic Integration

Due to the great complexity of the multi-chip package when several types of internal interconnections are present, the most diffused application of this technique is to integrate several electronic circuits with a single optical and/or microfluidic circuit so as to avoid external connections between different packages. The electronic circuits are generally the drivers for the active parts of the main chip or even digital circuits, especially where the whole component is not of single use, but is designed to be used several times. In this case, internal connections are solely electrical and consolidated technologies from microelectronics can be used for the design of the multi-chip package.

Flip-chip bonding is widely used in this case to realize internal electronic interfaces. It can be used either to connect a great number of electrical connections typical of processors and other digital circuits to a set of conducting traces [23] without creating a huge number of floating wires or to pile different electronic circuits in a vertical structure connecting them through the common surfaces [24].

This last technique is mainly used when the involved chips have the same pin-out, as in the case of use of multiple identical memories or external interface chips inside the same package. An example is the realization of very small memory elements, like those inserted into the micro

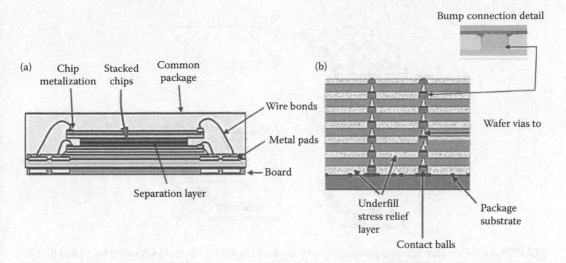

FIGURE 6.10 Schematic representation of chip stacking using wire bonding (a) and using flip-chip bonding (b).

SD cards, by thinning the back of a set of RAM memory chips and superimposing them in a stack. In more sophisticated cases, also connections between chips in different layers can be realized in the stack by suitable vias in the intermediate chips [25]. A stack of electronic circuits is represented in Figure 6.10, when realized both with standard wire bonding and with flip-chip bonding.

6.3.2.2 Flip-Chip Electronic Connection between Chips

Flip-chip, also known as controlled collapse chip connection or its acronym, C4, is a method for interconnecting IC or MEMs chips to external circuitry with solder bumps that are deposited on the chip pads [25]. The solder bumps are deposited on the chip pads on the top side of the wafer during the final wafer processing step. In order to mount the chip onto external circuitry or onto another chip, it is flipped over so that its top side faces down, and aligned so that its pads align with matching pads on the external circuit, and then fixed, generally by soldering to the substrate metal pads. The most common flip-chip bonding process flow is articulated in the following steps (compare Figure 6.11, where the different process steps are listed with the same letters found in the list below):

a. Solder balls are realized in contact with chips metal pads before dicing.
b. Chips are diced and flipped so as to present solder balls on the lower surface.
c. Flipped chips are aligned with the metal pattern on the substrate and the solder balls are put in contact with metal pads.
d. Soldering is realized so as to create conductive contact between the chip and the substrate metal pads; hot air reflow soldering is generally used in this process.
e. An interstitial filling polymer is injected between the chips so as to improve adhesion and release stresses created by the soldering process.
f. After polymer curing, the flip-chip bonding process is ended.

Besides its many advantages, the main disadvantage of flip-chip bonding resides in the very strict bond between the chip and the substrate, which generally has different thermal expansion coefficients. Especially in cases in which a great amount of power has to be dissipated or when thermal management is difficult, as in multi-chip packaging, different thermal expansion can introduce further stress on the contacts, eventually breaking them. In this case, the under-fill polymer has to be chosen so as to mediate between the different chip and substrate materials to protect contacts.

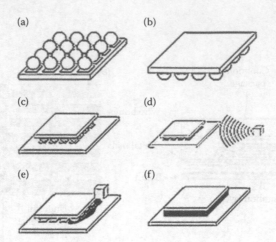

FIGURE 6.11 Flip-chip bonding process steps: (a) Solder balls are realized. (b) Chips are diced and flipped. (c) Flipped chips are aligned with the metal pattern and the solder balls are put in contact with metal pads. (d) Soldering is realized to create conductive contact. (e) An interstitial filling polymer is injected between the chips improve adhesion and release stresses. (f) After polymer curing, the flip-chip bonding process is ended.

6.4 BONDING TECHNIQUES IN MICRO-FABRICATION

Whatever be the hybrid integration method used, fixing a chip on another chip or on a substrate is a key process step. Moreover, bonding technologies are important almost in all back-end processes. Dices have to be fixed on a substrate, wires have to be bonded to metal pads, the package cap has to be fixed to the base, and so on. Different techniques, sometimes used in other technologies fields, are used to produce effective bonding. We will briefly review them in this section, taking into account that the wide array of different materials and techniques used renders almost impossible a general synthesis.

6.4.1 GLUING

In general, an adhesive substance, a glue, is a polymeric or a mixed polymeric material that can be flowed in between two surfaces to be fixed and after curing develops a thin film with a great adhesion to both the surfaces so as to fix them together [26]. A wide variety of adhesives exist, different due to their adhesion characteristics to different materials, curing methods, and physical properties.

Thermal and electrical conductive adhesives are of particular interest since they can be used both to preserve electrical contact between metal pads after gluing and to assure a good thermal contact between the chip and the substrate, especially when they are used to bond a dice to a dissipating package base [27,28]. Also, optical transparent adhesives exist, which are used to preserve optical connection when gluing optical integrated systems.

Conductive adhesives can be either isotropic or anisotropic from an electrical point of view. The mechanism of conduction in these substances is the dispersion of conductive particles in the resin solution. Depending on the type, density, and dimensions of these particles, the conduction results in directional or isotropic. In the isotropic case, small particles with a relatively high concentration are used so that a set of conducting paths are created almost in all directions when the adhesive is cured [29,30], as shown in Figure 6.12. In the anisotropic case, greater particles are dispersed in a small concentration in the resin to be cured [30], as shown in Figure 6.13a. When the substrates to be bonded are put in contact under moderate pressure, the metalized parts are connected by a set of single particles as shown in Figure 6.13b, so as to cause an essentially anisotropic current flow.

From a thermal conductivity point of view, generally isotropic adhesives are used that assure lower thermal resistance [31].

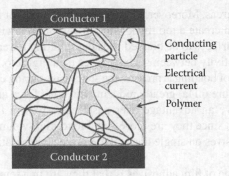

FIGURE 6.12 Working principle of an isotropic conductive adhesive.

The adhesion process through adhesive resins is generally constituted by several stages, which are almost the same if a fluid resin paste or a film adhesive is used.

- *Alignment:* During this step the pieces to be bond are aligned with the bonding tool and superimposed at a distance suitable to operate the second process step;
- *Dispensing:* During this step the fluid resin is dispensed in between the pieces to be bonded.

Paste adhesives generally require sequential dispensing, in which a substrate containing multiple bond locations is indexed under the dispensing head. Despite improvements in dispensing technology, this process remains a significant bottleneck of the whole back-end process flow due to its sequential nature. Printing (see Section 5.3.3) is a cost-effective alternative method of applying paste adhesives that can provide significant increase in throughput. In both cases, the quantity of dispensed resin has to be controlled with accuracy due to various problems that can arise if too much or not enough resin is present.

The presence of too much resin can create resin dispersion out of the area occupied by the surface to be bonded. This can contaminate nearby surfaces and seriously compromise sequent

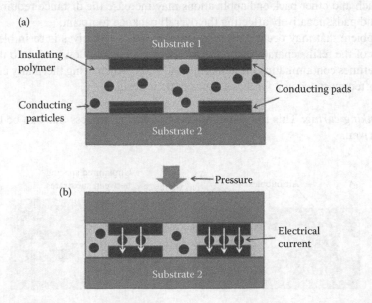

FIGURE 6.13 Working principle of an anisotropic conductive adhesive; the metalized substrate to be bonded before contact (a) and after contact under pressure (b).

bonding processes in those areas. Moreover, if an excessive quantity of resin remains in between the surfaces to be bonded, it can create a too thick film during the following curing processes so as to avoid contact between the surfaces to be bonded. Besides creating a weaker bond, this inhibits good thermal or electrical conductivity between such surfaces (see Figure 6.14b).

If an insufficient quantity of bonding is present, the successive curing can create void volumes under the adhesive surface (see Figure 6.14a) greatly reducing the bond force and damaging conductivity.

Some film adhesives have an advantage over paste adhesives in that they may be applied in batch- or roll-type processes since they are more suitable to high-volume manufacturing. However, the application of film adhesives on single dies can be more problematic. Moreover, film adhesives have their own problems.

One inherent characteristic of film adhesives is that they are in a semi-solid state when applied to a substrate. Since they are preformed, film adhesives tend to flow less than paste during the bonding process, and this can result in a lack of conformability. If not carefully executed, bonds formed with film adhesives may exhibit voiding where they are unable to fully wet the substrate surface.

Due to the rapid development of the adhesive solutions, the subsequent process steps have to be performed immediately after dispensing, requiring either an immediate passing from the dispensing to the curing station or an integrated dispensing and curing equipment.

If this is a problem, the so-called B-staged adhesives can be used [32]. B-staged adhesives are much less instable after being dispensed so that the substrate can be stored for months without sensible degradation of the adhesive film after dispensing. This kind of adhesives also allow substrate manufacturer to supply substrates with a pre-applied adhesive.

- *Thermal curing:* Thermal curing is generally used to evaporate the greater part of the solvent from the resin solution before the final curing process that creates inter-chain bonds in the polymer by hardening the adhesive and creating a good adhesion of the surfaces to be bonded.

This curing step is not always needed, and several adhesives require a single curing where the solvent is eliminated contemporary to the polymer cross-linking.

Resin flow may also be induced during the thermal curing process. Compensating for adhesive flow in die attach and other back-end applications may increase the distance required between the die and the bond pads, negatively affecting the overall package footprint.

Another problem that may occur with thermosetting paste adhesives is resin bleed-out. In this case, a portion of the resin separates from the adhesive matrix and flows out onto the surrounding substrate, sometimes contaminating the adjacent bond pads. When using thermally cured adhesives, IC packagers often must account for these issues in their designs.

- *Cross-linking curing:* This is a standard polymer curing process that can be thermal, IR, or UV driven.

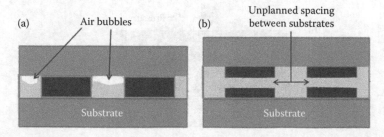

FIGURE 6.14 Problems related to an incorrect adhesive dispensing: insufficient adhesive quantity (a) and excessive adhesive quantity (b).

TABLE 6.3

Example Characteristics of Three Different Adhesives Used in Binding Operation During Back-End Processes

Adhesive Type		Flowable; Self-Priming	Elastomeric; Self-Priming	Self-Priming
Optical characteristics	—	Opaque (black in color)	Translucent	Opaque (grey in color)
Electrical and thermal characteristics	—	Insulating	Thermally conductive	Electrically conductive
Number of components	—	1	1	1
Viscosity	Pa s	210.2	7.3	28
Heat cure temperature	°C	150	180	150
Heat cure time	S	1800 (30 min)	15	3600 (1 h)
Tensile strength	Mpa	—	0.8	—
Elongation	%	—	240	—
Young module	MPa	—	0.9	—
Unprimed adhesion-Lap shear	MPa	6.6	0.6	1.7
Dielectric strength	kV/mm	—	25	—
Dielectric constant A		$-2.82@100$ Hz	$2.8@1$ MHz	—
Dielectric constant B		$-2.81@100$ kHz	—	—
Volume resistivity	Ω cm	2.1×10^{15}	2.7×10^{16}	3.0×10^{-3}
Dissipation factor A	—	1.1×10^{-3} @100 Hz	8×10^{-4} @1 MHz	—
Dissipation factor B	—	2.0×10^{-4} @100 kHz	—	—
Thermal conductivity	W/°K	—	160	—

Two elements are particularly important when using adhesives in packaging labs on chip: the effect of adhesive curing on the glued substrates alignment and the long-term stability of the adhesion.

Crosslinking a polymer generally causes a shrink of the polymer matrix (see Section 5.2) so that the alignment of the bonded parts can change during this process. This effect is taken into account by calibration of the alignment process, especially when well-known adhesives are used to have a large amount of statistical data on the process, and strict alignment requirements have to be satisfied. An alignment accuracy of 100 μm is often considered a lower limit in industrial processes, even if still lower values are reported in the literature. The characteristics of three selected adhesives used for bonding during different back-end processes are reported in Table 6.3: an opaque, insulating adhesive, a thermally conducting, and electrically conducting adhesives are considered.

All the considered adhesives are single phase, that is, there is no need to mix different components before dispensing them. Moreover, they do not require a specific primer for application either on silica or on various polymers like PMI, PMMA, or SU8.

6.4.2 Laser Welding

Welding is a fabrication process that joins materials, usually metals or thermoplastics materials, by causing coalescence. This is generally done by melting the work-pieces and adding a filler material to form a pool of molten material, the weld pool [33,34]. The weld pool cools to become a strong joint, either due to application of pressure, sometimes used in conjunction with heat, or by itself. This is in contrast with soldering and brazing, which involve melting a lower-melting-point material between the work-pieces to form a bond between them, without melting the work-pieces.

Many different energy sources can be used for traditional welding, but in micro-fabrication almost only laser sources are used. Moreover, in order to convey on the welding surface a high laser energy without accumulating a great quantity of heat in the welding zone, pulse lasers are used. Due to this particularity, the welding processes are used in micro-fabrication also to join non-metallic pieces, by depositing a metallic film on the two surfaces. This need not be very thick, since it melts for a very small depth. When a suitable metal is deposited on one of the work pieces, welding can be performed without another filling material, so eliminating a process step is difficult to control.

In laser welding processes, it is also common to perform welding in an atmosphere of inert gas in order to avoid unwanted chemical reaction due to the presence of normal air and various kinds of contaminants with the particles of evaporated welding material. To avoid the enclosure of the whole equipment in an inert atmosphere chamber, this is often realized by injecting continuously in an inert gas welding zone so that it substitutes locally the surrounding atmosphere.

When welding macroscopic pieces, the laser beam is generally focused on the piece either through discrete optics or coupling it with an optical fiber. The mechanic arm of a robot moves the focusing system extreme so that the laser beam follows the form of the pieces to be welded by melt-ing them at any point of the contact surface. A scheme of a possible structure of such an equipment is shown in Figure 6.15, where both the filling dispenser, dispensing the filling material by propel-ling small particles in a suitable gas jet, and the monitoring systems are evidenced.

This method is used in micro-fabrication only when high-accuracy welding is not required, like for closing the top cap of packages. Much better welding accuracy is obtained by avoiding the movement of macroscopic equipment parts and focusing the laser beam at different points by small adjustments of the focusing system. A scheme of such a welding equipment is reported in Figure 6.16. In this case, a welding filler dispenser is not present, assuming to perform filler-less welding, as typical for many back-end processes.

Where superficial bonding of small surfaces is needed and the metal is not to be excavated in deep, generally pulse Nd-Yag or Nd-glass lasers are used. This allows both to minimize the heated area and the stresses accumulated into the bonding and to realize a very precise welding. The selected characteristics of this kind of pulsed lasers are reported in Section 5.7.2.

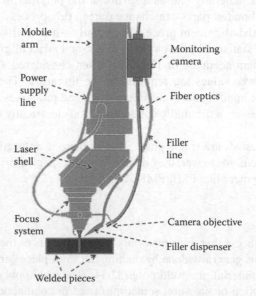

FIGURE 6.15 Scheme of a possible architecture of a laser welding robotized equipment. The filling dis-penser using gas phase dispensing and the monitoring systems are evidenced.

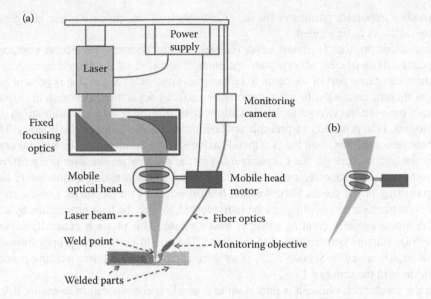

FIGURE 6.16 Scheme of a possible architecture of an optical focus laser welding equipment: equipment scheme (a) and laser beam focus mechanism particular (b).

The interaction of a laser pulse with the surfaces to be bonded can be divided into three phases, even if there is a smooth and seamless separation between them so that the limit where one phase ends and the other begins is not easy to be determined [35,36]. A typical metal surface absorbed power versus times in the three welding phases is represented in Figure 6.17, for a train of high peak power, low repetition rate pulses in Figure 6.17a and for a higher repetition rate, lower peak power pulses train in Figure 6.17b.

In the so-called coupling phase, the pulse hits the surface of the elements to be bonded. Incoming photons are either absorbed or reflected: the absorbed photons generate heating and eventually melting of the material, and the reflected ones are lost for the welding process. Although most metals have high reflectivity, it is important to minimize the reflection so as to optimize the use of laser

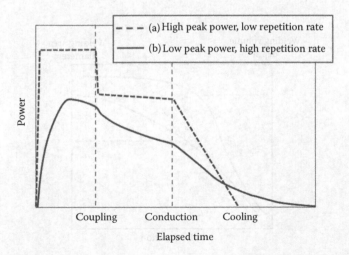

FIGURE 6.17 Typical metal surface absorbed power due to the incident laser pulse versus time in the three welding phases; high peak power, low repetition rate pulses (a) and high repetition rate, low peak power pulses (b).

energy. Another important parameter for the effectiveness of this process phase is a good contact between the surfaces to be welded.

The ideal situation, that is almost never realized, would be a real molecular contact between two completely flat surfaces, allowing an optimum absorption of the laser beam. Any distance between them can cause part of the beam to be lost or even to heat the gas that is present in between the surfaces thereby causing dilatation and further surfaces separation. A common way to favor a good contact between the two surfaces, also allowing to minimize stress accumulation during the welding process, is to proceed to a preliminary heating of the two pieces to be bonded. This facilitates successive contact between the two metal surfaces and elimination of interstitial gas, besides decreasing the temperature gradient experimented by the piece when the laser pulse arrives.

Since laser welding processes used in integrated chips manufacturing almost never has to provoke deep melting of the pieces to be welded, heating happens on the surface of the metal films. Thus, a second phase after coupling can be individuated, where the heat propagates by conduction through the film eventually creating a deeper melting zone. This phase is generally superimposed to the coupling, starting before the end of the pulse. The condition for heat propagation during the pulse duration, discussed in Section 5.7.2, is satisfied in almost every laser welding process where pulse duration is in the order of 1 ms.

During the conduction phase, it is important to control weld temperature to ensure that the weld is well supplied with energy, at the same time ensuring that the weld is not getting overheated. Excessive heating rate can cause weld metal being thrown out of the fusion zone in the form of weld spatter.

The control of weld temperature is easier for high melting alloys, such as stainless steels that are reasonably good absorbers of Nd:YAG laser photons at 1.064 nm wavelength. On the contrary, this is difficult for alloys of aluminum, which are good reflectors, have low melting point, and melt in a narrow temperature range.

The molten metal volume created during the conduction phase is surrounded by a large mass of solid metal. If the laser pulse is terminated abruptly after establishing fusion, the weld will cool very rapidly. Such fast cooling rates can cause many issues, including trapped porosity, high residual stress, cracks, and excessive weld metal hardness. Some of these issues can be alleviated by controlling the cooling rate.

Several potential welding problems can be controlled by controlling the shape of the used laser pulse. As a matter of fact, both the welding area and the welding depth critically depend on the ratio between the pulse peak power and the pulse duration. In Figure 6.18, the behavior of the welding

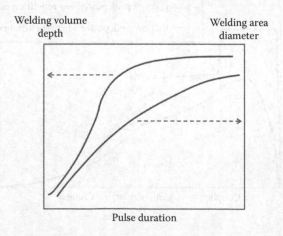

FIGURE 6.18 Qualitative behavior of welding depth and welding area diameter versus the laser pulse duration maintaining constant the pulse peak power.

depth, that is, the depth of the melted metal area and of the welding area versus the pulse duration maintaining constant the pulse peak power, is shown.

The molten metal droplets that are thrown out from the fusion zone are often called welds spatters. Spatter can be controlled by reducing the peak power and reducing the weld temperature. This is particularly an effective way in our case, since a great weld penetration also has to be avoided.

Porosity can form in a laser weld due to multiple reasons. One reason is the rapid closing of the keyhole at the end of the weld pulse. A longer cooling segment can be utilized that encourages the porosity to rise to the top, where it is expelled from the welding volume. Porosity can also be formed due to gases released when contaminants are vaporized. To avoid such porosity, a longer upslope should be utilized to assist in burning away the contaminants before fusion is established. A low-energy pre-pulse can also be used, if required.

Pores can form in the presence of gases that have high solubility in molten metal but poor solubility in solid metal. An example is pore formation due to release of hydrogen as molten aluminum solidifies. Hydrogen is often accidentally introduced in the form of moisture absorbed in the surface of oxide layer or due to water vapor present in the shielding gas.

Another typical problem related to laser welding is cracks insurgence. There are three main criteria for cracks to form in welds, including presence of a defect, high stress state, and brittle material. Microscopic defects are present in practically all welds and are difficult to avoid. Additionally, the weld configuration often introduces geometry defects that provide locations of high stress concentration that can start a crack. It is sufficient to consider what happens when a curve surface like a metalized fiber optic surface is fixed to a plane-shaped V-groove.

A high state of stress is often present in welds, especially spot laser welds that have one of the highest cooling rates of all welding processes. Rapid multi-axial cooling in a three-dimensional molten metal can often lead to very high stresses and cause cooling cracks even in apparently ductile metals such as aluminum. Cooling stresses can be effectively reduced by introducing a relatively long cooling time after the fusion pulse.

A last detrimental effect that can arise from laser welding is the alignment lost between the welded pieces [37]. This is due to the rearrangement of the metal film when cooling after its flow while melting. In order to reduce this effect, the welding temperature has to be optimized, but since melting is needed to fix the involved pieces, the misalignment cannot be completely avoided. When a very good alignment is obtained after the welding process, like when mounting optical interfaces, the process has to be calibrated by a statistical characterization of the welding misalignment and its average compensation by opportune placing of the pieces before the welding. Qualitative characteristic of different metals and alloys when used as weld materials are reported in Table 6.4.

A type of laser welding process can also be used to join the polymer elements by softening the interface to cause permanent bonding. This technique requires one part to transmit the laser beam and either the other part or a coating at the interface to absorb it. The two parts are put under pressure while the laser beam moves along the joining line. The beam passes through the first part and is absorbed by the other one or the coating so as to generate enough heat to soften the interface creating a permanent weld [37,38].

Semiconductor diode lasers are typically used in plastic welding. Wavelengths in the range from 808 to 980 nm can be used to join various plastic material combinations. Power levels from less than 1 to 100 W are needed depending on the materials, thickness, and desired process speed.

In order to obtain a good welding, it is naturally needed that the transparent polymer has a very low absorption at the welding wavelength, whereas the polymer that absorbs the wave has a high absorption coefficient. Since welding happens only if the melted polymer wets the other polymer surface, not all the polymer couples can be welded together. Thus, if this welding technique has to be used, compatible polymers have to be used. A cross compatibility table for selected materials is reported in Figure 6.19 [38]. The meaning of the polymers acronyms is reported in Table 6.5.

Another important condition for a good plastic laser welding is that the two surfaces are in a very good contact so that heat developed on the opaque surface is transferred to the transparent one and

TABLE 6.4

Welding Characteristics of Selected Metals and Alloys

Material	Comments
Aluminum 1100	Welds well; no cracking problem or transformation
Aluminum 2219	No cracks; no filler metal required
Aluminum 2024/5052/6061	Requires filler metal of 4047 Al to make hermetic, crack-free welds
Beryllium copper	Alloys containing higher percentages of alloying agents weld better due to lower reflectivity
Copper	High reflectivity may crease uneven welds; for material less than 0.01" thick, coating may enhance weldability
Hastelloy-X	Requires high pulse rates to prevent hot-short cracking
Nickel	Must be cleaned; good ductile welds and penetration
Steel, Carbon	Good welds with carbon content under 0.25%; for greater carbon content, may be brittle and crack
Steel, 400 Stainless	Generally welds somewhat brittle; may require pre- and post-weld heat treating
Tantalum	Ductile welds; special precautions against oxidation required
Titanium	Ductile welds; special precautions against oxidation required
Tungsten	Brittle welds; requires high energy
Zirconium	Ductile welds; special precautions against oxidation required.

generates melting on both sides. From this point of view, better results are generally obtained when high planarity surfaces are welded, that is the case of polymer labs on chip. The contact is generally improved by applying a moderate pressure on the parts to be welded before starting the process.

A last requirement to obtain a good plastic bond by plastic laser welding is to carefully control the welding power. An excessive welding power can cause permanent distortions in the pieces to be welded while an insufficient power generates a weak weld.

	PS	SAN	ABS	PA	PC	PMMA	POM	PVC	PP	PE-LD	PE-HD	PBT	PET
PS	OK												
SAN		OK	OK		OK	OK		OK					
ABS		OK	OK		OK	OK							
PA				OK									
PC		Ok	OK		OK	OK						OK	OK
PMMA		OK	OK		OK	OK		OK					
POM							OK						
PVC		OK				OK		OK					
PP									OK				
PE-LD										OK	OK		
PE-HD										OK	OK		
PBT					OK							OK	
PET					OK								OK

FIGURE 6.19 Table of compatibility of selected polymers couples with polymers laser welding. Meaning of the polymers acronyms is reported in Table 6.5.

TABLE 6.5

Polymers Acronyms of Figure 1.18

Acronym	Polymer Name	More Informations
PS	Polystyrene	Table 1.11
SAN	Styrene acrylonitrile	—
ABS	Acrylonitrile butadiene styrene	—
PA	Polyamide	Table 1.12
PC	Polycarbonate	Table 1.12, Table 1.15
PMMA	Poly(methyl methacrylate)	Table 1.11, Table 1.15
POM	Polyoxymethylene	—
PVC	Polyvinyl chloride	Table 1.11
PE-LD	Low-density polyethylene	Table 1.11, Table 1.15
PE-HD	High-density polyethylene	Table 1.11
PBT	Polybutylene terephthalate	—
PET	Polyethylene terephthalate	—

Note: If the polymer is considered in more detail in Chapter 1, the table where selected polymer properties or its chemical formula are reported is also indicated

6.4.3 SOLDERING

Soldering is a process in which two or more items, generally metals or alloy parts, are joined together by melting and flowing a filler metal, called solder, into the joint, the filler metal having a lower melting point than the work-pieces [39–41]. Soldering differs from welding in that soldering does not involve melting the work-pieces.

Depending on the type of parts to be soldered and on the soldering material, there is a wide variety of soldering processes for a huge number of applications, from metallurgic industry to plumbing, and so on. In the field of micro-fabrication, soldering is generally used in the last step of the back-end process, where multi-chip packages have to be built or when packaged chips have to be fixed onto a board to connect one to the other. Mostly, wave-soldered or reflow-soldered are used for these applications, though hand soldering is also used especially for prototypes production and research.

In wave soldering, the parts are temporarily kept in place with small dabs of adhesive, then the assembly is passed over flowing solder in a bulk container. This solder is shaken into waves so the whole system is not submerged in solder, but rather touched by these waves. The end result is that solder stays on pins and pads, but not on the substrate itself. The scheme of a wave solder machine with a particular illustrating the soldering principle is reported in Figure 6.20.

Reflow soldering is a process in which a solder paste, a mixture of pre-alloyed solder powder and a flux-vehicle that has a peanut butter-like consistency, is used to stick the components to their attachment pads, after which the assembly is heated by an infrared lamp; a hot air pencil; or, more commonly, by passing it through a carefully controlled oven. The scheme of an oven-like reflow solder machine is reported in Figure 6.21. The oven in divided into different zones having different roles in the soldering process.

The first soldering step involves a rapid rise in temperature of the parts to be soldered, which evaporates the solvent from the paste and burns off the largest amount of contaminants. This generally occurs in the first heated zone of the oven (Zone 1 in the figure). The next heated zones (Zones 2, 3, and 4) are programmed to provide a uniform temperature, with the goal of fully preheating the assembly to a temperature generally between 100 and 150°C. The most critical parameter is the rate of rise of temperature, which should be less than 2°C/s, to avoid solder paste spatter and minimize thermal shock on the components.

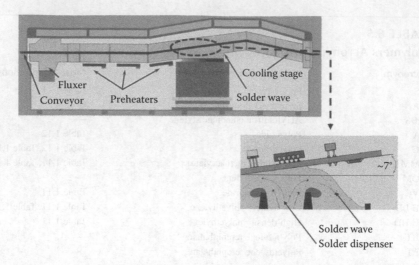

FIGURE 6.20   Scheme of a wave solder machine with a particular illustrating the soldering principle.

The preheating solder section, also referred to as the dry-out, soak, preflow, or activation zone, ensures also that the solder paste is fully dried before hitting reflow temperatures, and acts as a flux activation zone for many solder pastes. Preheating may also cause some slumping of the paste, depending on the specification and quality of the solder paste used. Reflow happens in the last heated zone (Zone 4 in the figure). Here, a rapid rise in temperature causes the solder paste to reflow and wet the surfaces of both pieces to be soldered. Surface tension will determine the shape of the joints, and in some cases the surface tension forces during wetting can generate component movement. Solder reflow starts happening when the paste is taken to a temperature above the melting point of the solder, but this temperature must be exceeded by approximately 20°C to ensure quality reflow. The length of time the solder joint becomes liquid is referred to as the wetting time. This is normally 30–60 s for most pastes. If the wetting time is excessive, intermetallic reactions may occur at the joint, which result in brittle solder joints.

Once the product has reached the end of the heated zones, the process involves slowly cooling, until the assembly reaches a suitable temperature (happening in Zone 5 in the figure). The first stage down to the melting temperature of the solder is critical. Final cooling is both to reduce possible oxidation and make handling safe.

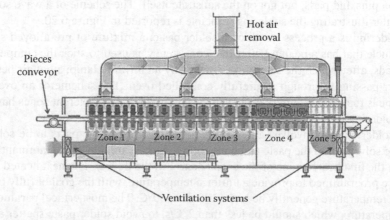

FIGURE 6.21   Scheme of a reflow soldering oven.

Since different components can be best assembled by different techniques, it is common to use two or more processes to fabricate a given subsystem like a board. For example, surface mounted parts may be reflow-soldered first, with a wave-soldering process for the through-hole mounted components coming next, and bulkier parts hand-soldered last.

The soldering temperature is a critical process parameter, due to the damages that can be created both by a too hot process and by a too prolonged not sufficiently hot process. In the first case, the high local temperature can damage sensible components, especially when polymer parts are present, moreover the melted solder can assume a too low viscosity and flow out of the soldering area causing contamination of nearby components. If the soldering process lasts for a too long time due to the too low temperature, heat can diffuse in larger areas of the substrate causing extended heat damages on areas not designed to be soldered.

For the attachment of components to a board, proper selection and use of flux help prevent oxidation during soldering, which is essential for good wetting and heat transfer. The soldering iron tip must be clean and pre-tinned with solder to ensure rapid heat transfer. Components that dissipate large amounts of heat during operation are sometimes elevated above the board to avoid board overheating. After inserting a through-hole mounted component, the excess lead is cut off, leaving a length of about the radius of the pad. Plastic or metal mounting clips or holders may be used with large devices to aid heat dissipation and reduce joint stresses. A heat sink may be used on the leads of heat-sensitive components to reduce heat transfer to the component. This is especially applicable to germanium parts. If all metal surfaces are not properly fluxed and brought above the melting temperature of the solder in use, the result will be an unreliable *cold solder joint*.

Since non-eutectic solder alloys have a small plastic range, the joint must not be moved until the solder has cooled down both through the liquid and solid temperatures. When visually inspected, a good solder joint will appear smooth and shiny, with the outline of the soldered wire clearly visible. A matte gray surface is a good indicator of a joint that was moved during soldering. Other solder defects can be detected visually as well. Too little solder will result in a dry and unreliable joint; too much solder tends to create poor wetting. With some fluxes, flux residue remaining on the joint may need to be removed, using water, alcohol, or other solvents compatible with the parts in question.

A particular reflow process that is frequently used in this field is hot-bar reflow. It is a selective soldering process where two pre-fluxed, solder-coated parts are heated with heating element, called a thermode, to a sufficient temperature to melt the solder. Pressure is applied through the whole process, that lasts usually around 10–20 s, to ensure that the components stay in place during cooling. The heating element is heated and cooled for each connection. Up to 4000 W can be used in the heating element, allowing fast soldering and good results with connections requiring high energy.

When small soldering connections have to be realized laser soldering can also be used. This is a technique where an IR laser emitting a power around 30 W is used to melt the solder. Diode laser systems based on semiconductor junctions are used for this purpose with wavelengths from 808 to 980 nm. The beam is delivered via a large core, multi-mode optical fiber to the work-piece. Since the beam out of the end of the fiber diverges rapidly, lenses are used to create a suitable spot size on the work-piece at a suitable working distance. A wire feeder is generally used to supply solder. Sometimes, not to use a single powerful laser source, several different sources are focused on the solder through a fiber array; in this case the process is frequently called fiber focus infrared soldering.

6.4.4 EUTECTIC BONDING

Eutectic bonding is another bonding technique that is quite extensively used especially for die attach and other chip-to-chip fixing. A gold preform is placed on the substrate while it is heated. When the die is mounted over this gold preform, Si from the die backside diffuses into the gold preform, forming Au–Si alloy. As more Si diffuses into the gold preform, the Si-to-Au ratio of the alloy increases, to achieve the eutectic ratio. The Au–Si eutectic alloy has 2.85% of Si and melts at about

TABLE 6.6
Selected Alloys Used in Eutectic Die Attach Preforms

Composition	Melting Temperature (°C)
80% Au, 20% Sn	280
92.5% Pb, 2.5% Ag, 5% In	300
97.5% Pb, 1.5% Ag, 1% Sn	309
95% Pb, 5% Sn	314
88% Au, 12% Ge	356
100% Au	1063

363°C. Thus, the die attach temperature must be reasonably higher than this temperature to achieve the eutectic melting point. At this point, the alloy melts, attaching the die to the cavity. To optimize the die attachment, the die is scrubbed into the eutectic alloy for even distribution of the die attach alloy. This operation can be performed either manually from an operator or automatically by the die bonder.

Eventually, the diffusion of silicon atoms into the gold preform exceeds the eutectic limit, and the die attach alloy begins to solidify once again. The substrate is then allowed to cool down to completely solidify the eutectic alloy and complete the attach process.

Aside from the Au–Si alloy, semiconductor assembly may employ other metal alloys for eutectic bond. Table 6.6 lists some of the other alloys used for this bonding technique.

6.5 BACK-END PROCESSES

In this section, we will review a set of process that are typically back-end processes and mainly consists in preparing the interfaces needed to the lab on chip to communicate with the environment exchanging matter and signals. Before this step, if the chips have been fabricated using wafer technology, they have to be divided one from the other, since interfacing has to be performed chip by chip. Using several polymer technologies, like micro-molding or hot embossing, this step is not needed.

A lab on chip has several interfaces, so that interfacing processes are, in general, more long and complex with respect to other types of integrated chips. From an electrical point of view, we have electrical signal interfaces that are used to transmit configuration and calibration signal to the chip and to read the results of the performed assay, and power interfaces needed to create power feeds for the onboard active elements, like active valves, micro-pumps, onboard lasers, and optical detectors.

From a microfluidics point of view, we have microfluidics inlets that are needed to insert fluid solutions inside the chip, both in factory and in the field, and sometimes there are also outlet interfaces that could be needed to recover part of the product of the inner microfluidic processing to be fed into other analysis systems or to verify the correct working of the chip.

Finally, if the optical detection is used, we have input and output optical interfaces. Depending on the application, this can be designed to directly interface optical sources or detectors or to provide an output fiber pigtail to be externally connected with the system where the chip is integrated.

6.5.1 WAFER DICING AND DIE ATTACH

Wafer dicing is the process by which single chips (dies) are separated from the wafer that is built during the front-end operation. Dicing has to assure good chips separation without damaging them and creating a sufficient mechanical resistance to allow further process steps.

The most common method used for wafer dicing is by means of a dicing saw, even if also laser dicing is frequently used [42–44]. When a dicing saw is used, the first process step is to thin the wafer by mechanical ablation contemporarily assuring a good planarity of both front and rear

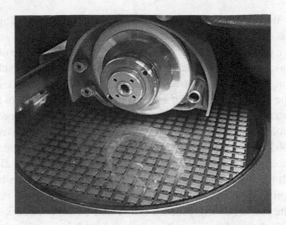

FIGURE 6.22 Example of dicing station evidencing the dicing saw. (Reproduced under permission from Majelac Technologies Inc. from http://www.majelac.com/Wafer_Dicing.html. Accessed on June 2013.)

surfaces [42]. This is very similar to planarization needed before wafer bonding and frequently also before high definition photolithography (see Section 4.10.1).

After thinning, the wafer is fixed to the dicing tape, which has a sticky backing that holds the wafer on a thin sheet metal frame and avoids the dispersion of dies after the cutting operation. The dicing tape is put in position under a dicing saw (see Figure 6.22) that cuts the chips using the guard area left among them during the front-end fabrication. During cut a flux of purified water or another suitable water solution continuously flows on the wafer both to remove small dust created by the saw and to avoid high local heating of the wafer. After cutting, the chips attached to the dicing tape are delivered to the test station. Generally, diamond saws are used for dicing, whose blade is realized by incorporating small artificial diamonds on the metal blade as shown schematically in Figure 6.23.

Diamonds saw dicing is a well-known and effective process, but it has a great disadvantage while dealing with lab on chip applications: whenever an open microfluidic inlet is present on the chip, the continuous washing of the wafer with the dicing liquid can irreversibly damage the chip due to liquid entry into the inlet [45]. Thus, in order to use these methods, the microfluidic inlets have to be protected, adding complexity to the process.

An effective alternative is to use a laser-based technique, the so-called stealth dicing process. It works as a two-stage process in which defect regions are first introduced into the wafer by scanning the beam along intended cutting lines, and second an underlying carrier membrane is expanded to induce fracture [46]. The first step operates with a pulsed Nd:YAG laser, the wavelength of which (1064 nm) is well adapted to the electronic band gap of silicon (1.11 eV, i.e., 1117 nm), so that a very high absorption can be obtained by suitable optical focusing [47]. The defect regions of about 10 μm

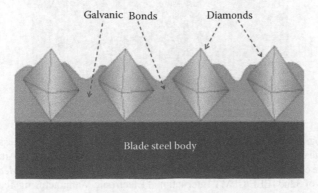

FIGURE 6.23 Schematic structure of the blade of a diamond-based dicing saw.

width are inscribed by multiple scans of the laser along the intended dicing directions, where the beam is focused at different depths of the wafer.

Figure 6.24 displays a photograph of a cleavage plane of a separated chip of 150 μm thickness that was subjected to four laser scans [46]. The topmost defects are the best resolved; from the image it can be deduced that a single laser pulse causes a defected crystal region that resembles the shape of a candle flame. This shape is caused by the rapid melting and solidification of the irradiated region in the laser beam focus, where the temperature of only some μm^3 small volumes suddenly rise to some 1000 K within nanoseconds and fell to ambient temperature again. The laser is typically pulsed by a frequency of about 100 kHz, while the wafer is moved with a velocity of about 1 m/s. The fracture along each defected line is performed in the second step and operates by radially expanding the carrier membrane to which the wafer is attached. The cleavage initiates at the bottom and advances to the surface, so that to optimize the process a high distortion density must be introduced at the bottom.

The advantage of the stealth dicing process is that it does not require a cooling liquid, being particularly suitable to all the applications where open microfluidics inlets are present in the chip so that a dicing liquid bath cannot be used to avoid the liquid entrance into the chip.

After dicing, the dies are detached from the dicing tape and have to be attached on the die support that will render it sufficiently mechanically sturdy to undergo subsequent back-end processes [42]. There are two common die attach processes: adhesive die attach and eutectic die attach. Both of these processes use special die attach equipment and die attach tools to mount the die.

Adhesive die attach uses adhesives such as polyimide, epoxy, and silver-filled glass as die attach material to mount the die on the die pad or cavity. The adhesive is first dispensed in controlled amounts on the die pad or cavity. The die for mounting is then ejected from dicing tape where the wafer is bonded after dicing by one or more ejector needles. While being ejected, a pick-and-place tool commonly known as a *collet* retrieves the die from the wafer tape and positions it on the adhesive. All of the above steps are done by special die attach equipments that are named die bonders. Two different techniques are used in wire bonders to apply pressure on the chip during bonding in order to improve its quality, as shown in Figure 6.25. In the first case, the pressure is applied through a spring, operating on a pad that avoids damage on the chip; in the second case, it is a metal lid to operate the necessary pressure.

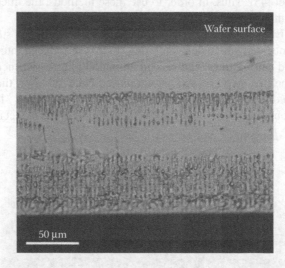

Wafer surface

50 μm

FIGURE 6.24 Photograph of a cleavage plane of a separated chip of 150 μm thickness that was subjected to four laser scans in a stealth dicing process. (Reproduced under Creative Commons Attribution 3.0 Unported license accorded by the copyright owner M. Birkholz; From Teng A., Wilhelmsen F., *Medical device wafer singulation*, Proceedings of 32nd IEEE/CPMT International Electronic Manufacturing Technology Symposium, pp. 108–113, 2007.)

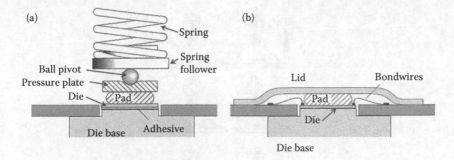

FIGURE 6.25 Methods to press a dice against the die support during die bonding: string method (a) and lid method (b).

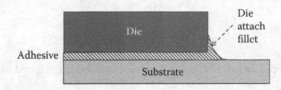

FIGURE 6.26 Die attach fillet.

The mass of epoxy climbing the edges of the die is known as the die attach fillet, and its normal structure is shown in the scheme of Figure 6.26. Excessive die attach fillet may lead to die attach contamination of the die surface. Too little of it may lead to die lifting or die cracking.

Another critical aspect of adhesive die attach is the ejection of the die from the wafer tape during the pick-and-place system's retrieval operation. The use of inappropriate or worn-out ejector needle and improper ejection parameter settings can cause die backside tool marks or micro-cracks that can eventually lead to die cracking.

Eutectic die attach, which is commonly employed in hermetic packages, uses a eutectic alloy to attach the die to the cavity. A eutectic alloy is an alloy with the lowest melting point possible for the metals combined in the alloy. The Au–Si eutectic alloy is the most commonly used die attach alloy in semiconductor packaging [48–50].

6.5.2 ELECTRONIC INTERFACE FABRICATION

Several types of electronics interfaces exist in semiconductor industry, requiring different processes depending on their characteristics. The most complex processes are associated with very high frequency and high power interfaces. In the first case, adaptation and filtering characteristics have to be controlled, whereas in the second case the electronic contact has to be realized to resist the high dissipated power.

Generally, both these types of interfaces are not present in labs on chip components, due to the nature of the application. Signals in the RF and microwave range are generally not used since so fast actuators movement is not needed, if at all possible, and measures are not performed in so short times. Active components like valves or micro-pumps in the microfluidic area and lasers in the optics area are not required to absorb a great power. Thus, standard wire bonding is generally sufficient for labs on chip applications both for signal and for power-feeding interfaces.

6.5.2.1 Wire Bonding

Wire bonding is the method to join the metal pads on chips to electrical contacts on the chip package using electrically conducting wires. Such contacts then pass through the package case and are attached on the electrical contacts on the board that will host the components [51,52].

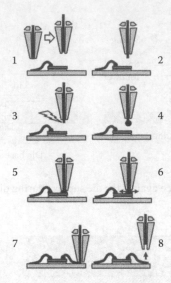

FIGURE 6.27   Process steps in a ball wire bond. The steps numbers are referred to the text where the single steps are described.

Two wire bonding techniques exist: ball wire bonding and wedge wire bonding. The main tool of ball wire bonding is constituted by a needle-like dispose tool called the capillary, through which the wire is fed. The process steps involved in ball wire bonding are schematically represented in Figure 6.27.

1. At the end of a bond, the capillary is lifted and reaches the next bonding position. The inner capillary duct is filled with the bonding wire and a new bond process begins.
2. A small and controlled amount of bonding wire is pushed out of the capillary to form the bonding ball.
3. An electrical discharge is applied at the tip of the capillary through an embedded discharge system.
4. The discharge causes the wire out of the capillary point to melt and to form a melted metal ball that does not leave the capillary point due to the surface tension.
5. The ball quickly solidifies, and the capillary is lowered to the surface of the chip, which is typically heated to at least 125°C.
6. The machine then pushes down on the capillary and applies ultrasonic energy with an attached transducer. The combined heat, pressure, and ultrasonic energy create a weld between the metal ball and the surface of the metal pad on the chip.
7. The wire is passed out through the capillary and the machine moves over a few millimeters to the location of the contact on the package.
8. The machine again descends to the surface, this time without making a ball so that the wire is crushed between the metal pad on the substrate and the tip of the capillary. The resulting weld is quite different in appearance from the ball bond, and is referred to as tail bond, or simply as the second bond.
9. In the final step, the machine pays out a small length of wire and tears the wire from the surface using a set of clamps. This leaves a small tail of wire hanging from the end of the capillary.

An example of ball wire bonding on a set of nearby metal pads is shown in Figure 6.28 [53], while typical performances of ball bonding in terms of adhesion are reported in Table 6.7. In the table, Al wire bonding is considered using a consolidated volume process.

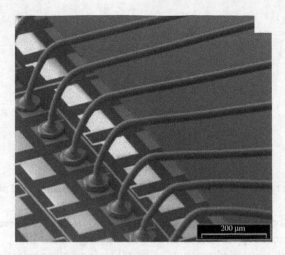

FIGURE 6.28 SEM photograph of ball wire bonds. (Reprinted from *Proceedings of 18th European Microelectronics and Packaging Conference (EMPC)*, Oezkoek M., White N., Clauberg H., Copper wire bond investigation on multiple surface finishes—enabling wire bond packages without gold, 1–6, Copyright 2011, with permission from Elsevier.)

Wedge bonding is a simpler process, which is effective when a large metal pad is available for the bond. It consists of pressing the wire against the metal pad with a tool in order to obtain a deformation of the wire that creates a good contact surface with the metal pad. At this point, ultrasonic energy combined with the heating of the whole bonding surface creates a welding between the metal pad and the wire.

Generally, the material that has to be bonded determines both the bonding tool foot configuration and its material constitution. As far as configurations are concerned, there are several possibilities: the most used are a concave foot and a plain foot (see Figure 6.29). The main difference between the two configurations is given by the type of force that the tool exerts on the wire to be bonded during the pressure phase, as evidenced in Figure 6.29.

The most frequently used materials in wire bonding wires are aluminum, copper, or gold. Wire diameters start at 15 μm and can be up to several hundred microns for high-powered applications. Copper wire has become one of the preferred materials for wire bonding interconnects in many applications; it is used for fine wire ball bonding on pads up to 75 μm. Copper wire has the ability of being used at smaller diameters, providing the same performance as gold without the high material cost [54,55]. However, copper wire poses some challenges, like it is harder than both gold and aluminum, so bonding parameters must be kept under tight control. The formation of oxides is inherent

TABLE 6.7

Wire Ball Bonding Resistance Characteristics (Aluminum Wire Bonding with Standard Process is Considered)

		Ball bond	
Ball diameter in free air	43	μm	
Ball adhesion (shear)	20	MPa	
		Second Bond	
Adhesion	8	MPa	On package standard metal patch
	5	MPa	On leadframe

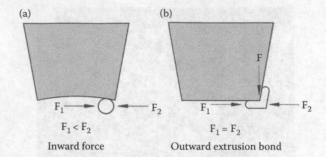

FIGURE 6.29 Different types of tools for wedge bond: concave foot tool (a) and plain foot tool (b).

with this material, so storage and shelf life are issues that must be considered. Special packaging is required in order to protect copper wire and to achieve a longer shelf life.

Gold wire doped with controlled amounts of beryllium and other elements is normally used for ball bonding. Junction size, bond strength, and conductivity requirements typically determine the most suitable wire size for a specific wire bonding application. Typical manufacturers make gold wire in diameters from 12.5 μm with a production tolerance on diameter of $+/-3\%$ [51]. Alloyed aluminum wires are generally preferred to pure aluminum wire except in high-current devices because of greater drawing ease to fine sizes and higher pull-test strengths in finished devices. Pure aluminum and 0.5% magnesium–aluminum are most commonly used in sizes larger than 120 μm.

6.5.3 MICROFLUIDIC INTERFACE FABRICATION

While electronic interfaces fabrication is a well-known technology, proved for huge volumes of IC fabrication and is widely diffused in the market, the situation is quite different for microfluidics interfaces. There is even a diffused idea that one of the main problems in market diffusion of microfluidics-based technologies is the lack of a reliable and cheap interconnection technology.

In fact, a huge research and industrial effort is in act to overcome this limitation, and industrial solutions are emerging after the first laboratory steps so that from the fundamental point of view this is an essentially solved problem [56,57]. The processes, however, have to be still refined up to an industrial level so as to allow very large volume manufacturing with an acceptable yield. This is an important step involving automatic equipment design and testing and metrology methods definition.

Depending on the type of labs on chip application, the chip fabrication materials, and the structure of the system that is designed to host the lab on chip, the microfluidics interconnections have to be designed in a different way.

From the application point of view, we can distinguish

- Cell labs on chip
- Raw biological fluid (like blood, urine, milk, …) labs on chip
- Macro-molecule labs on chip.

In the first case, the lab on chip is designed to perform assays on cells populations. In this case the inner ducts have to be sufficiently wide to host a cell solution, which is hundreds of microns or even a millimeter. With such ducts chips cannot be very small (dimensions of the order of several centimeters are common) and the selected materials are polymers. Under this condition fitting a fluidics interconnection to the labs on chip is easier, due to the fact that there is not so huge difference between the chip internal ducts and the capillaries that can be used as inlets and outlets.

However, the particular characteristics of cells' solutions have to be considered in designing the interconnection since cells lysis and stitching have to be avoided. For example, if sharp points or strong discontinuities are present at the contact between the inner duct and the interconnection capillary, cells lysis can happen. Since cell membranes are essentially composed of water insoluble lipids (see Section 2.6.3), a great number of broken cells can create lipids deposition on the interface up to an interface block. Moreover, cell internal volume hosts a great number of proteins and other macromolecules that in free solution could create a false result of the final assay.

Raw liquid labs on chip are systems designed to perform a macromolecule assay-like proteins or nucleic acids detection starting from a biological fluid-like blood. In the case of blood, for example, it has to be purified in the chip to obtain plasma or even serum. Nevertheless, raw blood has to pass through the interface. If anticoagulation is not performed before the injection into the lab on chip, since it is performed on chip, coagulation has to be avoided during the transit of blood through the interface. Strong hemolysis has to be avoided also, risking both interface blocking and the injection of a great number of spurious cells proteins and membrane fragments into the lab on chip. In case of blood, another problem is not to activate immune system cells during the transit of blood through the interface. As a matter of fact, microphagous or killer cells activation produces a large amount of chemically aggressive enzymes that probably completely spoil the subsequent assay. These problems have to be faced by suitable choice of the material that is in contact with blood and by protecting the interface by contamination not only during fabrication, but also during storage, not to generate contamination-driven immune-system activation.

Finally, if the lab on chip is designed to perform macro-molecules or ion assays, the inner ducts will be smaller than those used for cells, probably in the order of 10–50 μm. In this case, interface blocking is not a problem, due to the nature of the solution under test, but the adaptation of an external capillary to the inner duct is much more difficult, due to the difference in dimension. Generally, an adaptation structure has to be constructed during the front-end fabrication of the chip and insertion of the external interface will be more difficult.

Other application-dependent elements of a microfluidics interconnection are its position and the external interface it has to be connected to. In multi-chip systems, chip-to-chip interfaces have to be built, which should be fabricated on the chip side to allow simpler multi-chip packaging. This can be easier in polymer-based chips, where the chip side is thicker and side working is easier. In the case of small, silica-based chips, it can be a real challenge, since it is almost impossible because of cost. Side fluidics interconnections would be also useful in case of plug-and-play disposable chips, being more suitable to be inserted in a plug-and-play external package.

In other situations on the contrary, for example, when the solution under analysis is inserted via a pipette or a syringe, an interconnection on the upper surface of the chip is well suited for the application. This is also generally true if the chip has to be inserted permanently or quasi-permanently in an external equipment and connected with flexible tubes. In the first case the connection has to be done using an aperture of pipette or syringe size, where the pipette or syringe can be inserted without the risk of breaking it or to force the organic material out of the intended chip interface. In the second case, the interfaces have to be connected with an external flexible tube; thus a suitable fluidics connector has to be used between the interconnect and the external tube.

Another important element is the ability to obtain a good filling of the chip internal chamber and to control the excess test solution that is not inserted into the chip. It can be even dangerous to have a loss of the injected solution toward the external surface of the package, for example in the case of blood of potentially diseased persons or test solutions containing pathogens. This problem can be faced by providing suitable disposal system into the chip for the management of the excess fluid that is not needed by the system during the function.

The death space in a microfluidic interconnect is the space that is filled with liquid at the rear of the interconnection point and that is generally constituted by a liquid quantity that is lost for the interconnection functionality (see Figure 6.30 for an example). The death space has to be minimized, or if possible completely eliminated, in the interconnection. This allows both a better exploitation of the available sample and the avoidance of further risk in case of dangerous samples.

A last, but very important, observation regarding microfluidics interconnections standards. As a matter of fact, in a well-developed market, system vendors and chip producers are generally

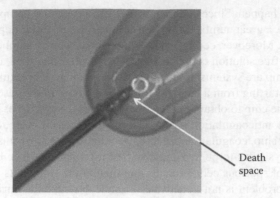

Death
space

FIGURE 6.30 Example of death space location in a simple fluidic interconnection.

different, mainly due to the different technologies needed to produce components and systems and to the quite different ways in which marketing and sales are performed in the two areas. In this situation, system vendors have the need of realizing well-defined fluidics interfaces that are able to accommodate components from a plurality of different component vendors.

This allows both the system design to be decoupled from the component design, with a focalization on the core business of all the market players, and the availability of multiple interchangeable suppliers for the same part of a complex system. A wide discussion is going on about microfluidics standards both for single interfaces and for more complex connectors [58] and it will probably be one of the enabling evolutions for the wide adoption of microfluidics-based assay systems.

6.5.3.1 Microfluidic Vertical Inlet

Greater interconnections can be simply mounted on the top of polymers microfluidic chips by gluing small tubes inside the chip input hole, as schematically represented in Figure 6.31. The gluing process is not difficult to set up, but a few critical aspects have to be considered with care [57]. A tube constituting the interconnect has to face the external system with a specialized end depending on the input tool used: another tube coming from another system, a pipette or a pump syringe. In any case, a good microfluidic model has to be realized of the interconnection to dimension and not to insert fluid with too much high pressure that could influence the working of the microfluidic system in unwanted ways.

Besides the need of reducing as much as possible the dead volume, the adhesive choice is a key step in the process setup. A completely hermetic seal has to be assured, having high chemical resistance if the conveyed fluid is chemically active or suitable not to activate immune cells if raw blood

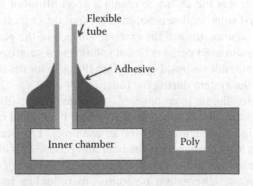

Flexible
tube

Adhesive

Inner chamber   Poly

FIGURE 6.31 Possible scheme of a flexible tube interconnection in a polymer labs on chip.

is used. Moreover, a long duration of the seal with unaltered characteristics is generally needed. In order to evaluate the last requirement, it has to be taken into account that the connection of the chip through a flexible polymer tube to a host system could introduce a permanent stress in the glued part of the interconnection.

If suitable gluing cannot be individuated, laser welding can be used to seal the interconnect, either by depositing a metal film on the tube and on the chip surface in the interconnect area or using plastic welding if compatible materials are used (see Section 6.4.2).

The tube gluing technology is suitable for automation using a simple pick-and-place machine with an embedded gluing station, but it requires apertures of the order of few hundreds microns and with a comparable depth. These dimensions are very common in polymer-based labs on chip and quite standard in labs on chip for cells assays.

The situation is completely different if a macromolecule assay silicon-based chip is used. In this case, the internal ducts can be of the order of magnitude of a few tens of microns and the cover roof of the circuit, obtained by wafer bonding and successive upper wafer thinning can be few hundreds of microns of SiO_2 or polymer. Entering directly with an external micro-tube into such a duct is virtually impossible, thus an adaptation structure has to be built at the front end level to prepare fluidic interconnection.

This structure can be a sort of embedded micro-funnel excavated by lithography and etching in the upper wafer back, as shown in Figure 6.32a. Due to the strong 3D nature of this structure, besides the fact that it is not a very small critical dimension, gray tone lithography used via an optical lithographic process followed by RIE to obtain the required aspect ratio could be a suitable process flow (see Sections 4.5.3 and 4.8.3).

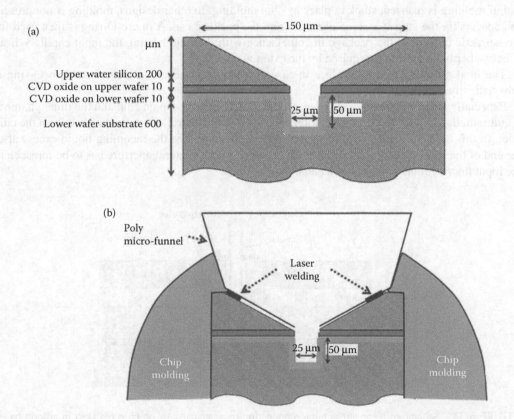

FIGURE 6.32 Possible scheme of a micro-funnel interconnection in a silicon-based lab on chip: front-end fabricated adaptation structure (a) and micro-funnel positioning after chip molding on the carrier (b).

The access fabricated by front-end technologies has to be put in contact with the external system by some sort of adapter, taking into account that, different from polymeric chips, silicon-based chips have to be enclosed in some sort of package, either obtained by simple molding or constituted by a true packaging box.

The adapter is also dependent on the external element that has to be interconnected. If the external element is a pipette, a suitable pipette inlet has to be realized. In this case another micro-funnel can be realized, generally using micro-polymers technologies like micro-molding or hot embossing. This is fixed to the lithographic structure as in Figure 6.32b by gluing or laser welding and stuck at its place when the chip is molded. In case an upper cup is put on the chip, it has to be shaped so as to allow the access to the microfluidic inlet.

In this last case, the micro-funnel once put in place and stuck by molding is allowed to exit from the upper cap using a suitable via, and at the end all is closed using a micro-O-ring that is welded both to the funnel and to the external package cap. The process to place the micro-funnel is not very complex from a technology point of view, resembling in the positioning method, the welding of optical fiber on the V-groove for passive alignment, but it is composed of several steps during which the positioning of the micro-funnel has to be accurately controlled and maintained.

A similar alignment is needed if a flexible tube is to be brought outside instead of a pipette placing site. In this case the front-end adaptation structure has to be fabricated so as to host a ferule that is fixed to the chip by laser welding. The ferule can be either metallic or polymeric, even if the second solution is generally cheaper in case of mass production, and also considering the fact that metallization of the polymer and of the underlying substrate is needed for laser welding. The ferule constitutes the guide for insertion of the flexible tube that is taken into position by the ferule itself and, if molding is realized, stuck in place by chip molding. In other designs, molding is not present and spacers fix the chip at a given distance from the package cap. A micro-O-ring is then used for the hermetic closure of the package in coincidence with the hole hosting the input capillary if an effective hermetic closure is required by the external package.

The final assembly of the interface in case of molding absence and use of a micro-O-ring is schematically reported in Figure 6.33.

Especially when a pipette is used to insert the sample into the lab on chip and the inner chamber is quite small, it is possible that the solution excess has to be controlled to avoid its exit from the chip inlet. In this case a secondary chamber has to be realized to host the incoming liquid excess after the end of the space in the inlet chamber. Moreover, a suitable lateral aperture has to be foreseen in the input micro-funnel to regulate the flux.

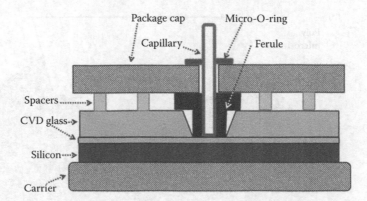

FIGURE 6.33 Scheme of a top surface interconnection to a typical labs on chip realized in silicon-based technology using a flexible micro-tube that is held by a ferule inserted in the chip package. In the figure the chip package is realized via a rigid box and without chip molding.

TABLE 6.8

Adhesion (Pull Resistance) of Different Types of Vertical Microfluidics Interfaces

Interface Type	Bonding Process	Adhesion (Pulling Resistance, N)
Glued interface	Polymer adhesive	10
Micro-funnel interface	Polymer adhesive plus package molding	20
Micro-funnel interface	Laser welding	22
Micro-funnel interface	Laser welding + package molding	30
Ferule + O-ring interface	Laser welding	20

The resistance of a vertical microfluidics interconnections can be measured by standard pull tests to verify the adhesion between the interconnect and the chip. Example values of the pull resistance for different kinds of microfluidics interfaces are reported in Table 6.8.

Testing fluidic interfaces against in–out fluid pressure is also important. The pressure test [1,57] is realized by pumping a fluid (typically water) into the interconnect at a fixed flow rate and measuring the internal pressure in the integrated duct at the output of the interconnect as a function of the input flow rate. If the internal duct is sufficiently long so as to establish stationary Poiseuille flow (see Section 7.3.4), the internal flow rate is easily determined by the measure of the internal pressure. Under this condition, the difference between the internal and the input flow rate is the leakage flow rate, which is the quantity of liquid that the interconnect cannot convey into the chip in the considered conditions. At a determined value of the input pressure, the interconnect will start to be damaged due to the force exerted by the incoming fluid on the interconnect input surface and the internal walls. This threshold input pressure is the interconnect maximum input pressure and fixes the interconnect maximum input flow rate.

A typical behavior of the internal pressure in the integrated duct as a function of the input flow rate is shown in Figure 6.34 [1,57] for a glued interconnection realized in a PDMS lab on chip (see Figure 6.31), and for an interconnect realized for the same lab on chip using the ferule and O-ring technique (see Figure 6.33). The input duct is made of silicon rubber and has a diameter of 1 mm in the case of glued interconnection and of 1.4 mm in the case of the interconnection using a ferule. Different channel dimensions are used in the chip to obtain different internal flow capacities.

Considering the glued interconnect, in the first part of the plot, that is, for low input flow rates, the pressure is approximately linear with the flow rate. This means that in a very first approximation the hydraulic resistance of the interconnect does not depend on pressure and the interconnects

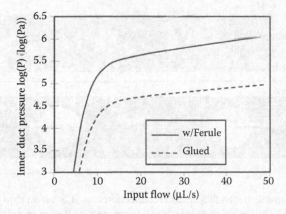

FIGURE 6.34 Typical behavior of the internal pressure in the integrated duct as a function of the input flow rate for a glued interconnection realized in a PDMS lab on chip and for an interconnection realized for the same lab on chip using the ferule and O-ring technique.

behave almost ideally. Increasing the pressure the flow rate starts to saturate, while the hydraulic resistance get higher and higher with pressure, up to the maximum input pressure where the interconnect is damaged by the input flux.

A similar behavior is observed for the ferule plus O-ring interconnect that results to have a lower hydraulic resistance, mainly due to its much better stability. From the results reported in Figure 6.34, it is evident that the considered interconnects behave very well in an extended flow range, covering almost all the practical values considered in labs on chip applications.

6.5.3.2 Microfluidic Horizontal Inlet/Outlet

Vertical interfaces are suitable to connect microfluidic circuits with external elements from the upper surface, but also have a number of disadvantages. The first evident disadvantage is present when the solution enters directly in a chip duct. This causes the fluid to experiment a square angle duct curve passing from the inlet to the embedded duct, which is not the better way to enter the duct.

This is mainly due to the death space that creates near the angle, where the fluid velocity is very small (see Section 7.3.4.4). A very small fluid velocity can provoke stagnant fluid with the possibility of deposition of macro-molecules, on the angle walls, especially for solution containing lipids that are almost insoluble in water and tends to deposit on the ducts. The angle can be avoided by creating a smoother duct end via gray tone lithography, for example, but this complicates the front-end process, especially if such inclined surfaces are to be built only for this reason in the chip.

In addition, vertical connections are usable to insert a liquid into the chip, but are difficult to use to extract it. Thus, when something is to be extracted or when a connection is to be realized to pass from one chip to the other, horizontal connections are very useful. A few techniques do exist to design lateral connections for polymer-based chips.

A technique that is capable to realize both permanent and temporary connections is described in Reference [59]. Here, an SU8 lab on chip is considered, where an input socket is realized near the chip border. This input socket is simply a hole in the SU8 structure that opens from the outside on the chip border that is filled with PDMS after fabrication (see Figure 6.35b). PDMS assures sufficient insulation and adhesion to SU8 to completely insulate the internal microfluidic structure, but it is also possible to penetrate it with a micro-needle without the need of applying a big force due to its viscoelastic nature. During penetration the PDMS mass surrounds the needle and creates a good adhesion, generating a good hermetic sealing of the inside volume. However, this adhesion is not so strong to avoid needle extraction with a simple back-traction without that the PDMS septum is damaged, so that the connection can be created and eliminated several times.

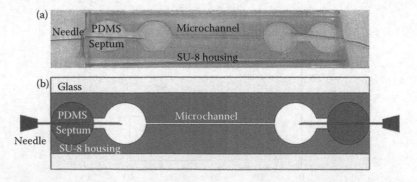

FIGURE 6.35 Lateral reusable micro-fluidics interconnection to a SU8 lab on chip via insertion of a micro-needle in a PDMS socket, Experimental sample (a) and interconnection design principle (b). (Reproduced from *IEEE Transactions On Biomedical Engineering*, vol. 58, no. 4, Johnson D. G., Frisina R. G., Borkholder D. A., In-plane biocompatible microfluidic interconnects for implantable microsystems, pp. 943–948, Copyright 2011, with permission from Elsevier.)

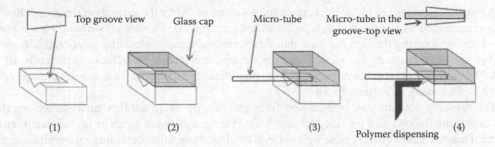

FIGURE 6.36 A possible architecture of a lateral microfluidics connection for a silicon technology lab on chip: interface creation processes macro-steps.

In practical applications, the SU8 chip can be about 0.5 mm thick, while the external diameter of a typical standard micro-needle is about 0.2 mm, so that insertion is not very difficult and is also compatible with automatic machines if mass production is realized.

Lateral connections have also been proposed for silicon-based chips, not only related to labs on chip, but also for implantable micro-pumps that could be used in several medical applications. A possible architecture [60] is represented in Figure 6.36. The process needed to realize the interface is represented by macro-steps in Figure 6.36 and it can be described as follows:

1. A V-groove (or alternatively a U-groove depending on the situation) is realized in the lower wafer; it is opened on one side from the chamber of the microfluidic circuit that the interface has to fill, and on the other side from the chip border.
   The groove width is reduced in the horizontal plane, as indicated in Figure 6.36, to avoid the fixing polymer to enter the microfluidic chamber in the chip and to improve adhesion; Parylene-C is used in [60] to fix a Polyimide micro-tube.
2. The chip roof is created by wafer bonding so that the groove is covered by a silica substrate.
3. A micro-tube is put into the groove from the chip side and maintained in position by the mounting machine; this step is somehow similar to the positioning of an optical fiber in a V-groove, but from the fact that the micro-tube is made of flexible polymer while the fiber being made of glass is much more rigid and fragile.
4. The space between the groove walls and roof is filled with a suitable bonding polymer that is cured after the insertion to be hardened and assure both the hermetic closure of the space and the fixing of the micro-tube.

6.5.3.3 Chip Charging with Reactants

A further step that can be present in the back-end process flow of a lab on chip is the filling of repositories or reaction chambers with test solutions, for example, containing recombining proteins or antibodies that will be used during the assay performed in the chip. If filling of a reservoir is required, it can be realized either connecting a fab fluidic interface with an external pump or exploiting capillary effect to convey the solution into the chip. In both cases, suitable air vents have to be realized, that are closed at the end of the dispensing operation. In other cases, a biochemical solution is charged into the chip to obtain a more complex effect, like the activation of a chip surface.

In the first case, the most suitable interface is a removable one, like that made by PDMS we described in the previous section. If a fixed interface is used, it is to be sealed after the reservoir charging, by adding a further process step. Complex interfaces comprising ferules or similar structures are generally not used and the micro-tubes constituting the fluidic interface can be maintained by the tool of a pick-and-place machine during the filling. After the filling, the interface can be closed by a suitable polymer cap, which is fixed to the chip so as to assure hermetic seal.

If saturation of an activated surface has to be achieved, that is, occupation of all active sites with a molecule, after charging solution into the reaction room through a suitable interface, a sufficiently long time has to elapse to allow the surface to be saturated. After the saturation time, the chamber has to be cleaned by the remaining solution so as to leave a clean saturated surface. This is generally done by injecting through the microfluidic interface a suitable alcoholic solution that does not disrupt the bond between the surface and the trapped molecules, but removes efficiently all the biological molecules from the remaining of the microfluidic circuit (see the macroscopic equivalent in the ELISA assay in Section 3.7.5).

The washing solution can be removed from the chip by using another microfluidic interface and exploiting the pressure provided by an external pump, otherwise it can be accumulated into an internal waste chamber that is close by a valve to insulate it from the remaining microfluidic circuit.

6.5.4 OPTICAL INTERFACE FABRICATION

While microfluidic interfaces are used to inject, and in a few cases also to remove, liquids from the lab on chip, optical interfaces are used to transmit optical signals from and to the lab on chip by interfacing it with suitable sources/detectors. This is required every time an optical detection method is used to detect the assay results and the transmitter/receiver is out of the chip [61]. The simpler way to obtain input/output of optical signal is design the chip so to have a transparent surface. This method is used, for example, to collect fluorescence radiation. In other cases however, optical connections require more complex fabrication techniques, for example to limit optical losses or to interface the chip with a signal coming from an optical fiber. In these cases, an integrated optical waveguide is frequently used.

There are different possible integrated optical interfaces, depending on the external optical system with which the chip has to be connected and to the type of integrated waveguide that is present on the chip. By far the most common waveguides used in labs on chip optical sensors are silica on silicon waveguides designed to be single mode in the near IR frequency region. A photograph of a section of a buried silica-on-silicon waveguide with typical dimensions is reported in Figure 6.37 [62]. Much smaller waveguides can be built if silicon is used for the waveguides core instead of silica, but due to interface and the front-end fabrication difficulties (need of lithography sensitivity around 5–10 nm that call for either electron beam lithography or high definitions stepper with 2D phase masks, see Section 4.3), their use in labs on chip at the state- of- the art is very difficult [63].

A very common optical interface connects an optical fiber with an integrated waveguide. While the optical connection is inside the chip, the fiber exits from the chip package for a certain length and ends with a suitable optical connectors to be interfaced with other optical fibers. This arrangement is generally called, for its shape, a fiber pigtail. Single-mode, low-loss connectors used in single-mode fiber communication systems are too expensive to be adopted in this kind of applications. Very low-cost connectors are designed mainly for multi-mode fibers so that low-cost connector/multi-mode fiber/waveguide is the most suitable arrangement for our application [64,65].

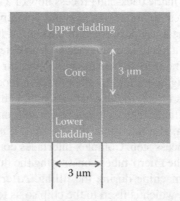

FIGURE 6.37 SEM photograph of the section of a typical silica-on-silicon integrated waveguide that is single mode in the near IR region. (Reproduced under permission from Cyoptics Inc.)

The use of multi-mode fibers is diffused in labs on chip applications also because they are much easier to interface with other optical elements and to manage during manufacturing and field use. Plastic optical fibers are considered too. Their intrinsic advantages are increased by the availability of high-volume connectors developed for application in consumer electronics, especially in high-fidelity systems [66]. Low-cost connectors, both for glass or plastic fibers, do not have very low loss than high-performance connectors, but this is generally not required for the labs on chip, where the optical power budget is not a critical point due to the long duration of the optical measurement.

Another mode of connecting a fiber to another external fiber is to create a splice, that is, to fuse together in a controlled way the two fiber extremes. This is a permanent technique that is useful for permanent mounting of the lab on chip on an external system [67].

If a plug-and-play external package has to be realized, a connector plug can be directly integrated into the package, in order to be inserted into the complementary plug that is present in the equipment. In this case, depending on the internal package structure, the connector plug can be either coupled with the integrated waveguide through a lens or through a very short piece of fiber.

Another possible optical interfacing technique is to directly focalize the optical wave coming out from the integrated waveguide onto the external coupling element via a lens or a set of lenses through a transparent window in the package that can also coincide with the lens itself.

6.5.4.1 Chip Multi-Mode Fiber Interface

An integrated single-mode waveguide in the near IR region has a core linear dimension of the order of a few microns while a glass multi-mode standard fiber has a core diameter of the order of 50 or 62.5 μm, or even 100 μm for low-performance fibers [68]. Similarly, polymeric multi-mode fibers have a core diameter of the order of 60 μm or bigger. Thus, if the waveguide facet is accurately cleaved not to cause light scattering and the fiber is near enough, a good coupling has to be expected.

The difficult aspect of the process is that ideally the axis of the waveguide has to coincide with the axis of the fiber to optimize coupling and this is not trivial with standard back-end methods, especially when a set of nearby waveguides have to be aligned with the corresponding fibers. Two methods can be used to achieve a good alignment: passive and active alignment.

In the case of passive alignment, a front-end fabricated structure is used to accommodate the fiber placing with a pick-and-place machine. Precision is expected from the accuracy of the fabricated hosting structure and of the pick-and-place process. In active alignment, light is coupled into the integrated waveguide during the alignment procedure. This light arrives to the interface and is captured by the output fiber so as to be detected at the fiber pigtails end by a suitable detector. The alignment is realized in the first moment as in the passive case, after that it is optimized by maximizing the light detected at the fiber output. Active alignment is used when a low-loss coupling is needed and it is the characteristics of coupling of single-mode fibers with waveguides. It is rarely used in the case of multi-mode fibers.

Different structures can be realized to host a fiber on the chip: the most used are V-groove and U-groove. The U-groove, as the name says, is similar to the V-groove, but for the fact that the groove bottom is quite rounded due to the lesser anisotropy of the etching process used to fabricate it. Due to the curve shape of the walls, the exact shape of the U-groove is more difficult to control and generally alignment is less precise than the alignment obtained by a V-groove.

In case of multi-mode optical fiber, very large grooves have to be realized and a small distance between the waveguide facet and the multi-mode fiber facet has to be achieved (in the order of few microns). Due to the required dimensions of the groove, the U-groove is sometimes preferred in this case even if the accuracy of passive alignment is inferior, due to the easier required micromachining process (see Section 4.8).

Typical geometric characteristics of a multi-mode fiber passive alignment via a V-groove are reported in Figure 6.38, where typical groove dimensions are also indicated. Typical coupling loss and its dependence on the vertical alignment between the fiber and the waveguide axes are shown in Figure 6.39.

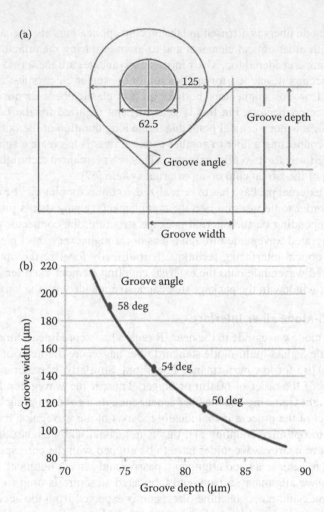

FIGURE 6.38 Geometry of the alignment of a multi-mode fiber in a V-groove considering a 62.5/125 fiber (a) and relationship between the groove depth and width assuming that the nominal position of the fiber axis is on the chip surface (b). All dimensions are in μm.

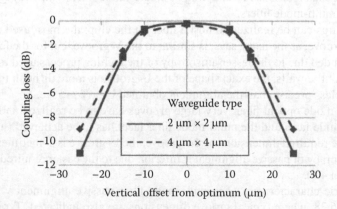

FIGURE 6.39 Coupling loss versus the vertical misalignment of the fiber axis to the waveguide axis for the alignment in Figure 6.38 assuming a groove angle of 54°.

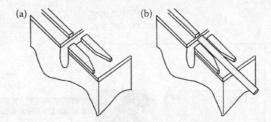

FIGURE 6.40 Multi-mode fiber alignment technique that does not use a groove: front-end hosting structure (a) and positioning of the multi-mode fiber (b).

The great dimension of the V-groove is evident from Figure 6.38: for a groove angle of 54°, that is typical of several etching processes, the groove width is as big as 146.5 μm. The vertical and horizontal placing of the fiber is quite tolerant, allowing a high-accuracy pick-and-play machine to realize it with a very high yield and good performance. The distance between the fiber facets, that is assumed to be cleaved to be a plane as much as possible, is a bit more critical. However, an error in the order of 2–3 μm is not so significant if it is done so as to increase the distance, since it simply implies a greater coupling loss of the order of 0.3–0.5 dB.

Different is the case in which the fiber facet touches the waveguide surface: in this case the probability that the waveguide or the fiber terminations are damaged is very high. For these reasons, if relaxed requirements are to be fulfilled, the fiber is located few microns apart with respect to the optimum distance preferring to improve the process yield with respect to a small difference in coupling loss.

In order to avoid too big grooves on the chip surface, different hosting structures have also been conceived, like that presented in [69] and sketched in Figure 6.40. In this case, two vertical structures are prepared by a suitable front-end processing, and at the back-end stage the fiber is inserted by a pick-and-place machine in between them, either attached by a suitable adhesive or laser welded. The advantage of this technique is that a very wide space can be created between the two vertical structures without making a deep incision into the chip, thus multi-mode fiber can be easily accommodated. On the other hand, the smaller accuracy of placing due to the presence of two independent structures is not so important in the greater part of multi-mode alignments. Losses smaller than 0.5 dB have been measured over a wide near IR bandwidth in Reference [69] using this alignment method; so that it results to have almost the same performances of the traditional V-groove technique without requiring surface micromachining, that is simply substituted with a traditional film deposition plus optical lithography and deep RIE (see Section 4.8).

The above techniques can be used both for glass and for plastic optical fibers that have similar dimensions of the core and cladding. The fixing method, however, can be different in the two cases. If laser welding is used, metallization is needed in both cases. Due to alignment tolerance, adhesive bonding is frequently adopted to couple multi-mode optical fiber, and in this case different adhesives, having also different performances, are needed in the two cases.

In the case of plastic fibers, when the coupling attenuation is not critical and strong cost issues are present, another coupling method has also been proposed, that is much simpler to implement. This consists in realizing a separated silicon holder for the fiber that is placed by welding or gluing in front of the chip, while a spherical micro-lens is either realized by micromachining the waveguide end or integrated into a suitable integration holder during the back-end stage [70]. This is an effective coupling system when the optical beam comes from a large and quite divergent source, like a VCSEL, but it can be used also in coupling with optical waveguides, when a very rough taper is created at the end of the waveguide to form the output beam.

The better coupling loss that can be obtained by this method seems to be around 5 dB in the case of a VCSEL, and greater losses are expected in the case of coupling with a waveguide. However, this system has the great advantage not to require a very small distance between the fiber and the waveguide facet so as to greatly relax the requirements of the process. Moreover, if the coupling

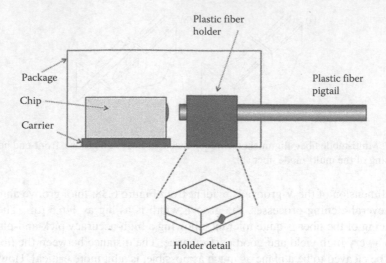

Plastic fiber
holder

Package

Chip

Carrier

Plastic fiber
pigtail

Holder detail

FIGURE 6.41 Scheme of the plastic optical fiber to integrated optical chip proposed in [10] and detail of the fiber holder.

fails, the chip is unaffected, thus reworking during back-end fabrication can be conceived. This is much more difficult in more traditional coupling systems, where the fiber is attached to a hosting structure directly on the chip. Tolerances are even a bit more relaxed in horizontal and vertical alignment with respect to V-groove or other on-chip alignment methods, while naturally they are much more relaxed in terms of distance from the chip lateral surface. In particular, passing from 20 to 40 μm distance from the interface optics of a VCSEL the coupling loss gets worst of only 0.5 dB that has to be added to an optimum value of about 5.5 dB.

The fiber holder that is used in this mounting technique can be a simple silicon element realized by wafer bonding of two silicon wafers and can be produced with simple optical lithography and RIE etching. A polymer holder fabricated by hot embossing or micro-molding can be used too. The scheme of this coupling method is reported in Figure 6.41.

Another way that has been proposed to interface multi-mode fibers to chips, that could be particularly effective in the case of polymer-based labs on chip or for chips having a polymer external package, is to directly realize a plastic ferule on the chip by molding [71]. The plastic optical fiber can then be inserted into the ferule and fixed, for example, by a suitable adhesive. The principle is somehow the same for the system relying on a fiber support: it simplifies the fiber mounting avoiding very short distances from the waveguide of laser surface by paying in terms of coupling losses. In this case, the mounting of the fiber is even simpler, and higher coupling losses are to be expected.

6.5.4.2 Si-SiO$_2$ Chip: Single-Mode Fiber Interface

Coupling an integrated waveguide to a single-mode fiber is completely a different process with respect to the coupling with a multi-mode fiber. As a matter of fact, multi-mode fibers are able to guide a wide variety of optical fields by suitably combining the guided modes so that the coupling is almost only determined by the fiber numerical aperture [62] so that a point surface very near to the fiber facet couple almost all the radiation into the fiber.

In the case of single-mode fibers, all modes are dissipated but one, that is degenerate in polarization, and in order to study how much of the power of the incident field is coupled with the fiber it has to be decomposed in all the fiber modes (radiation, evanescent, and guided modes), so as to determine how much field intensity is related to the only mode that is guided by the fiber. The shape of the incident field is thus a key factor and has to be controlled in order to guarantee a good coupling between the integrated waveguide and the optical fiber. Since this cannot be effectively done by only shaping the end of the integrated waveguide, it is done by simultaneously shaping both the waveguide and the fiber.

The electromagnetic study of the shapes allowing coupling optimization is quite complex [62,64]. Moreover, realistic shapes that can be attained also depend on the technology processes that are needed to fabricate them, so that in general what is done is a compromise between a theoretical optimum and what a realistic process for the considered application can achieve.

Qualitatively, what is done is to try to create both on the fiber and on the waveguide a taper, that is a sort of adiabatic decrease of the guide section up to ideally arrive to an infinitesimal section. If the two "point" terminations are brought to strict contact, the emitting termination emits like a point source, thus it is perfectly adapted to the other termination for the reciprocal nature of Maxwell equations. Once all the radiation is captured by the fiber point termination, it is adiabatically adapted to the fiber-guided mode with a very low loss, which is essentially the fiber loss modulated by the very slow section increase to arrive at the section of the full single-mode fiber core.

From this simple explanation, not only the principle of the coupling between a tapered waveguide and a tapered fiber emerges, but several elements that cannot be realized in a practical system are also evident, so that all practical interfaces have a finite loss due to the fact that the real fabricated coupling system differs from the ideal one. Both the fiber and the waveguides cannot be tapered up to arrive to an infinitesimal section, but the final taper section will always be finite, being generally determined in the case of the fiber by the mechanical resistance of the taper and in the case of the waveguide by the resolution of the process used to attain the tapering.

The two interfaces cannot be brought to perfect contact, not to scrap and ruin them so that good optical coupling will result impossible. Moreover, the tapers cannot be perfectly adiabatic due to their finite length. Finally, the waveguide should be tapered both in the vertical and in the horizontal direction. While tapering in the horizontal direction can be performed with great accuracy using standard planar processes, tapering in the vertical direction would require 3D processing, that is not needed in other parts of the chip. For this reason, very frequently the integrated optical waveguide is tapered only in the horizontal direction, introducing a further element of non-ideality in the coupling design.

After tapering a V-groove is generally realized on the chip and used to accommodate the single-mode fiber in front of the waveguide termination, as schematically shown in Figure 6.42. The V-groove in this case is much smaller than that needed for single-mode fibers, due to the smaller dimension of the single-mode fiber. Typical V-groove dimensions are a width of the order of 25 μm and a depth of the order of 12–15 μm.

Active and passive alignments can be used, with very different results in terms of coupling losses. Characteristic coupling loss in case of active alignment and its dependence on the vertical alignment and in the presence of a taper on the waveguide (the fiber is always assumed tapered) are presented in Figure 6.43. Small coupling losses can be obtained, as expected, paying them with a complex alignment process.

Since fiber positioning has to be very accurate, the fiber is fixed by laser welding, after metallization and the process is accurately calibrated to compensate the welding material rearrangement due to the laser-induced heating.

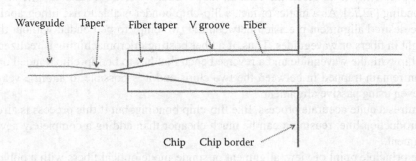

FIGURE 6.42 Schematics of the coupling between a waveguide with horizontal tapering and a tapered fiber via a V-groove on the chip.

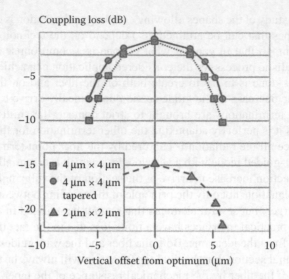

FIGURE 6.43 Coupling loss in the case of active alignment of the system represented in Figure 6.39 and laser welding of the fiber over the V-groove. The loss is measured for different types of tapered and un-tapered waveguides and the sensitivity to the vertical placing accuracy is also represented.

The effect of horizontal tapering of the waveguide and of the waveguide dimension is also represented in Figure 6.43. Horizontal tapering does not change clearly the optimum loss, but gives a great help in relaxing placing tolerances, an effect that would be evident also measuring tolerances with respect to the distance between the fiber and the waveguide termination.

As far as the waveguide dimension is concerned, smaller the waveguide greater the loss if the other parameters are not changed. As a matter of fact, a smaller waveguide has a more divergent mode at the output if no taper is realized, as assumed in the figure. Thus, it should be brought much nearer to the fiber end to optimize coupling. The situation completely changes if tapering is realized. In this case adiabatic mode adaptation is better while the waveguide dimension decreases, at least while silica waveguides are considered, so allowing better alignment.

If passive alignment is simply performed as in the multi-mode fiber case, losses of the order of several dBs are obtained (up to 8–9 dBs) that are generally unacceptable even when the optical power budget is not very critical as in many labs on chip applications. This is clear from observing the results in Figure 6.43 that to obtain a small coupling loss, an alignment precision of the order of 1 μm is needed. Thus, passive alignment has to be performed by using a different process to compensate the impossibility to monitor the effective alignment loss during the process.

The first possibility is to block the fiber in its position by using a suitable silicon bench and flip-chip bonding [72,73]. As a matter of fact, a flip-chip bonder is able to use lithographic markers to attain the desired alignment precision between the two chips to be bonded without the need of injecting light in fibers or waveguides. Thus, if a fiber hosting micromachining is realized onto two chips, the chip with the waveguide and a reverse bench that has to be flip-chip bonded on top of it, the fiber can remain trapped in between the two chips and it is possible to attain a very accurate alignment even using passive alignment.

This requires a quite accurate process, like flip-chip bonding, but if this process is already present in the production line, reusing it can be much cheaper than adding a completely new step like active alignment.

From the principle point of view, alignment of single-mode optical fibers with a polymer waveguide is not different from the same operation if the waveguide is glass based. Since the main polymers used in optical applications have refraction indexes near the glass one, the waveguides dimensions are of the same order of magnitude so that the optical problem is similar. What is completely different is the set of available processes and their cost, so that several processes have been specifically developed for polymeric waveguides alignment.

Hot embossing using LIGA created molds (see Section 5.5) allow, for example, to realize quite precise squared U-grooves to plug single-mode fibers for a precise passive alignment without resorting to high-definition optical lithography [74]. Flip-chip bonding can be used also in the polymer case to attain very precise passive alignment of single-mode optical fibers. In this case, the lower chip simply contains the grooves for fiber placing while the flip-chip bonded element contains the waveguides [75]. These techniques can reach coupling losses between 3.5 and 4 dBs, but they are much simpler than corresponding alignment techniques with silica fiber and silica-on-silicon waveguides and they can be quite suitable for labs on chip applications.

6.5.4.3 Optical Interfaces without Fiber Optics

Even if in transmission systems the connection of a device with an external transmitter/receiver is realized by splicing or joining connectors of two fiber pigtails, this technique is too costly for labs on chip.

A much simple external interface can be obtained by directly inserting a lens in front of a plane waveguide termination that focuses on the beam incoming from a package window at the center of the waveguide facet. The external source or detector has to be put in front of the chip. The beam at the source output has to be rectified by an external lens so as to be approximately transformed into a plane wave so that it is then focused on the waveguide facet by the lens internal to the package. The same architecture has to be used for a detector, where the beam comes from the waveguide and has to be focused on the external detector facet [64]. A scheme of this type of coupling is reported in Figure 6.44. This structure, also called butt coupling, is particularly suitable if low-cost transmitters and detectors are used, and generally contain in standard TO can packages (see Figure 6.45).

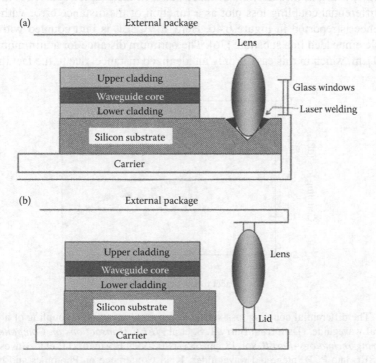

FIGURE 6.44 Waveguide interface with an external source/receiver via a simple hybrid integrated lens: the lens is placed in a micro-machined hosting structure on the chip (a) or supported by a lid and directly fixed to the external package (b). The second mounting is similar to that used in a standard optical TO cans.

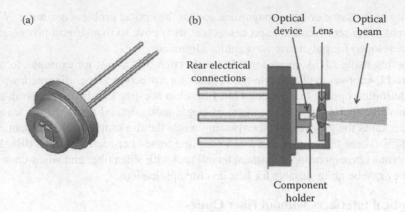

FIGURE 6.45 Scheme of a standard optical TO can: three-dimensional picture (a) and internal mounting scheme (b).

The lens can be mounted in different ways depending on the type of chip and package; common mounting techniques use a hosting surface micromachining on the chip itself or fix the lens to a lid and to the external package, analogously to what is done in TO can packages. Different kinds of lenses are also used besides standard plane lenses, for example, cylindrical lenses are used to couple edge-emitting diodes whose emission pattern tends to be more divergent in the direction perpendicular to the slit.

Butt coupling allows attenuations of the order of 5–6 dBs to be obtained if the optimum coupling is attained and have the advantage of a very good robustness with respect to horizontal and vertical displacements, while, as intuitive, the distance between the coupled sources is more important.

A typical differential coupling loss plot as a function of the distance error with respect to the optimum distance is reported in Figure 6.46. Here, a VCSEL is butt coupled with an integrated glass waveguide embedded in a substrate [76]. The optimum distance for a minimum coupling loss of 0.5 dB is 30 μm, which in this case is only an idealized distance, due to the fact that it cannot be

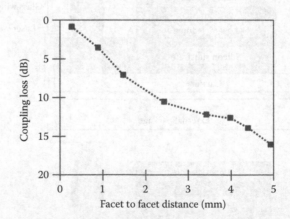

FIGURE 6.46 The differential coupling loss versus distance in case of butt coupling of a VCSEL with an integrated optical waveguide. (Data from Barry T. S. et al., *IEEE Transactions on Components, Packaging, And Manufacturing Technology-Part B*, vol. 18, pp. 685–690, 1995; Hormanski P. et al., Investigation on butt-coupling of VCSEL into PCB integrated waveguides, KNS Conference on Photonics and Nanotechnology, 2004, available at http://www.kns.b2me.pl/art-investigation-on-butt-coupling-of-vcsel-into-pcb-integrated-,57,0.html, last accessed on June 21, 2012.)

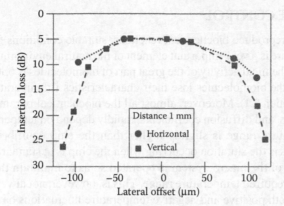

FIGURE 6.47 Coupling loss sensitivity to horizontal and vertical offset from optimum position in case of butt coupling of a VCSEL with an integrated optical waveguide. (Data from Barry T. S. et al., *IEEE Transactions on Components, Packaging, And Manufacturing Technology-Part B*, vol. 18, pp. 685–690, 1995; Hormanski P. et al., Investigation on butt-boupling of VCSEL into PCB integrated waveguides, KNS Conference on Photonics and Nanotechnology, 2004, available at http://www.kns.b2me.pl/art-investigation-on-butt-coupling-of-vcsel-into-pcb-integrated-,57,0.html, last accessed on June 21, 2012.)

attained by such a simple connection for the presence of lenses and relative hosting structures. The nominal distance assumed in Figure 6.43 for the facet-to-facet distance is 1 mm, with a nominal loss of 5.7 dB.

A distance of the order of 1 mm can be guaranteed with a good approximation also by a plug socket, thus this type of interface is suitable for all the cases in which a simple coupling is needed without stringent requirements in terms of coupling losses. This flexibility is confirmed by Figure 6.47, where the coupling loss at the nominal distance is plotted versus horizontal and vertical displacement. A good plug with a simple insertion is able to maintain a good alignment so as to maintain the loss penalty within the acceptable values.

In several cases, a pluggable package has to be fabricated. In this case, the chip package is also inserted into an external package to allow better handling and greater mechanical resistance. The system is then plugged into a socket so that all interfaces have to be created during the plug operation. While electronic pluggable interfaces are quite common and microfluidics interfaces are generally not required in the plug, pluggable optical interfaces are frequently required and not easy to design.

In the case of labs on chip, the problem is generally simplified by relaxed requirements on the interface loss with respect to other applications like telecom or datacom. The first method to design a pluggable optical interface is simply to use a lens interface, as those represented in Figure 6.44, with suitable slides that contemporarily guides the chip inside the socket and protects the interface. A system used to protect the interface is to insert in the external package a sliding plastic window that is closed in front of the interface when the chip is standing alone and is automatically opened when it is inserted into the socket.

Another possibility to create a pluggable interface is to incorporate directly in the external package an optical connector socket whose complementary part is inserted in the external equipment. The optical field is then coupled with the socket inside the package either using a very short pigtail or by a simple optical system in free space like a lens. Many low-loss connectors accommodate glass multi-mode fibers into small ferrules and have to be mounted with great care not to ruin the ferule or even the glass fiber termination. This may not be suitable for a system used even in emergency situations, if it is adopted in medical applications. If plastic fibers are used the connection is less critical and the socket system can be inserted into the external package connection area besides electrical connections and mechanical slides.

6.6 TEMPERATURE CONTROL

As a lab on chip has to reproduce biochemical reactions, suitable conditions for such reactions have to be created. Temperature is a very important element of the natural environment where biochemical reactions happen since chemical activity of the great part of biomolecules is optimized in a very small temperature range and the biomolecules lose their characteristics if temperature deviates too much from this range (see Section 2.1). Moreover, almost all the biochemical parameters, like equilibrium coefficients, kinetic rates, and diffusion coefficients, rapidly depend on temperature (see Section 1.3).

The correct temperature range is slightly higher than the chip equilibrium temperature, thus heating is required. This is the situation occurring when the chip is at standard room temperature or when a general cooling of the macro-system is operated so as to maintain the base temperature of the chip a bit below the required temperature range. This is, however, not always possible and several situations exist where both positive and negative temperature fluctuations have to be compensated.

Temperature stabilization requires a mix of front-end and back-end fabrication processes: we have decided to collect all temperature stabilization techniques together, even if a few of them, like construction of micro-heaters, are more correctly classified as front-end techniques.

6.6.1 HEATERS AND THERMISTORS

If the target temperature range has to be maintained by simply heating the chip, the easier way to do it is to mount a discrete heater below the carrier on the package floor. Heater is essentially a distributed resistance generating heat by Joule effect when current is let to flow through it [77–79]. A uniform temperature is generally desired so that, if temperature gradients are present on the chip, heat generation has to be suitably distributed even if a single heater is used [80]. This happens when heating is needed to compensate an external low temperature, but heat is also locally generated or absorbed on the chip due to chemical reactions. The situation is simpler if no temperature gradients are generated in the chip so that in order to compensate environmental cooling, a simple uniform heater is sufficient.

If the heating principle is simple, practical implementation requires the ability to measure temperature with a good accuracy in the lab on chip so as to provide a feedback to the heating element and stabilize temperature to the wanted value. As a matter of fact, even if the heater resistance is temperature-dependent, the accuracy obtained by using the heater itself to measure temperature is generally not sufficient to obtain a good stabilization. Thus, specific components are used to monitor the temperature, called thermistors [81,82].

Thermistor is an electronic component that exhibits a large change in resistance with a change in its body temperature. The thermistors most used in labs on chip applications are fabricated using ceramic semiconductors so as to obtain a small aspect ratio and a high sensitivity. Such thermistors have either large positive temperature resistance coefficient (PTC devices) or large negative temperature resistance coefficient (NTC devices).

In particular, PCT thermistors are very sensitive and work at higher temperatures, but they are much less stable of NTC components. PCT thermistors are generally used as protection elements against current overshoots and as temperature sensors in high power systems, while NTC devices are more suitable to application in monitoring small temperature changes in very compact system. Thus, we will analyze here only NTC thermistors. The oxides most commonly used as thermistor materials are from manganese, nickel, cobalt, iron, copper, and titanium. In the basic thermistor fabrication process, a mixture of two or more metal oxide powders are combined with suitable binders, formed to a desired geometry, dried, and sintered at an elevated temperature. By varying the types of oxides, their relative proportions, the process atmosphere, and temperature, a wide range of resistivity and temperature coefficient characteristics can be obtained.

After the fabrication the thermistor is enclosed in a protective shell suitable to provide mechanical and chemical insulation and to assure good thermal contact of the active material with the body

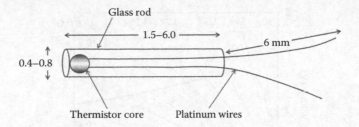

FIGURE 6.48 Scheme of a typical NTC thermistor shielded into a glass road for application in microsystem temperature monitoring with a range of typical dimensions of its parts (all dimensions are in mm).

whose temperature has to be measured. In the labs on chip case, glass shielded thermistors are very useful, due to good chemical characteristics of glass, that allows even the immersion of the thermistor in reaction chambers and other places where biological solutions are present or even when biochemical reactions happen.

Such thermistors have a form of small nail, which is particularly suitable for insertion in several types of systems. The scheme of such a thermistor is reported as an example in Figure 6.48 with a range of typical dimensions of its parts. Besides glass, several other shielding materials are used, and several different thermistor forms exist, adapted to different applications.

Typical resistance–temperature characteristics of NTC thermistors are represented in Figure 6.49 and are compared with the same characteristic of a pure high-resistance platinum thermistor. The tenfold increase in temperature sensitivity with respect to pure resistance sensors explain the advantage that NTC sensors have in applications, where a very good degree of temperature stabilization has to be attained by measuring small temperature changes. Moreover, the difference between curves relative to different kinds of sensors shows a good flexibility of this technology, allowing to adapt the thermistor to different exigencies.

However, the high nonlinearity in the resistance–temperature characteristics calls for a careful calibration of the measurement system and, at the end, poses a limit to the absolute range of temperatures that can be measured with such sensors. In any case, while this is a great disadvantage for pure temperature sensing in systems that undergo wide temperature excursions, this is not so important if the thermistor has to be inserted in a temperature stabilization system.

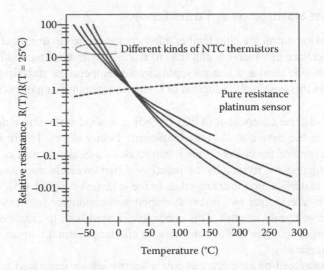

FIGURE 6.49 Resistance–temperature characteristics of NTC thermistors compared with the same characteristic of a pure high resistance platinum thermistor.

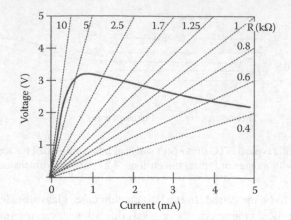

FIGURE 6.50 Typical current–voltage characteristics of a NTC thermistor; equal-resistance curves are also represented in the plot.

The current–voltage characteristic comprising a zone with negative resistance is also the characteristic of this kind of thermistors and has to be taken carefully into account when the temperature has to be estimated by a resistance estimation. A typical current–voltage temperature of an NTC thermistor is reported in Figure 6.50.

When the amount of power dissipated in the thermistor is negligible, the voltage–current characteristic will be tangential to a line of constant resistance that is equal to the zero-power resistance of the device at the specified ambient temperature. As the current continues to be increased, the effects of self-heating become more evident and the temperature of the thermistor rises with a resultant decrease in its resistance. For each subsequent incremental increase in current, there is a corresponding decrease in resistance. Hence, the slope of the voltage–current characteristic decreases with increasing current. This continues until a threshold current value is reached for which the slope becomes zero and the voltage reaches a maximum value. As the current is increased above the threshold value, the slope of the characteristic continues to decrease and the thermistor exhibits a negative resistance characteristic.

6.6.2 Temperature Stabilization by Peltier Elements

Cooling can be used to control the chip temperature whenever the environment temperature is stably below the temperature at which the chip has to work. If both cooling and heating are needed, a simple heater cannot be used and a more sophisticated temperature stabilization is needed. The most used solution in this case is the adoption of temperature stabilizing elements based on Peltier effect [83].

A Peltier thermoelectric component (TEC) [84,85] is a solid-state active device that transfers heat from one side of the device to the other exploiting Peltier effect. The heat transfer direction depends on the direction of the current, thus it can work as a heater or as a cooler. The basic element of a Peltier component is formed by the junction of two inversely-doped semiconductors, that are mostly ceramic materials, and is arranged as in the scheme of Figure 6.51. The thermoelectric junction is created by connecting two inversely-doped semiconductor substrates by a thermal and electrical conductor, generally a metal. This conductor is used both to create electrical continuity between the two semiconductors and to constitute an efficient thermal contact with the element to be stabilized in temperature.

The system is completed by an electrical power supply whose generated voltage intensity and direction can be changed and by a heat sink/source that is used both to dissipate power in case of cooling and to provide heat power in case of heating. The heat sink/source is generally provided by

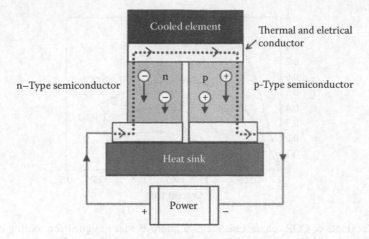

FIGURE 6.51   Principle scheme of a single Peltier element based on a semiconductor thermoelectric junction.

the external environment, which is put in thermal contact with the component by a suitable thermal conductor in contact with the external package.

The current flows through the system in one direction or in the other, so causing heating or cooling and the system is controlled by a temperature sensor so as to provide the control signal to the stabilization system. A practical Peltier element that can be used to stabilize temperature of a lab on chip is composed of several elements that are put in series from an electrical point of view and in parallel from a thermal point of view, as represented in Figure 6.52. The most used semiconductor in micro-Peltier elements is bismuth telluride (Bi_2Te_3) alloyed with antimony or selenium.

The overall efficiency of a Peltier junction if considered as a cooling thermal machine is quite lower than that of a standard cooling machine based on the Rankin cycle: it is generally lower than 10% of the ideal Carnot efficiency and about 25% of a practical Rankin cycle–based cooler.

Typical performances of a Peltier micro-cooler are shown in Figure 6.53, where the coefficient of cooling performance (COP_C) is shown versus the current flowing through the thermoelectric junction for different temperature gradients that are maintained by the cooler between the cooled surface and the heat sink. The coefficient of performance (COP) is a common parameter used to evaluate the performance of thermic machines designed to work as heat pumps and it is defined as [86]

$$COP = \frac{Q_H}{W} \tag{6.1}$$

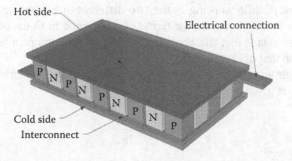

FIGURE 6.52   Arrangement of a set of single Peltier elements in a Peltier component. (Image put in public domain for any use by its author under Creative Commons Attribution 3.0 Unported license, see http://en.wikipedia.org/wiki/File:Peltierelement.png).

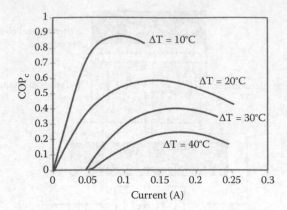

FIGURE 6.53 Example of COP_C characteristics of a micro-Peltier designed for cooling micro-fabricated systems like labs on chip. The Peltier dimension is 2 mm × 2 mm and the operating temperature is 85°C. The COP_C characterization is performed in atmosphere for different required temperature differences maintained by the Peltier element.

where Q_H is the heat supplied by the heat pump to the heat reservoir and W is the work consumed in the process.

The COP for heating and cooling are thus different, because the heat reservoir of interest is different. To represent how well a machine cools, the ratio of the heat removed from the cold reservoir to input work has to be considered, while if heating is considered, the COP is the ratio between the heat removed from the cold reservoir and the heat added to the hot reservoir by the input work:

Thus, if we call Q_C the heat removed from the cold extreme of the heat pump, we can define a coefficient of cooling performance (COP_C) and a coefficient of heating performance (COP_H) that are given by

$$COP_C = \frac{|Q_C|}{W} \tag{6.2}$$

$$COP_H = \frac{|Q_C| + W}{W} \tag{6.3}$$

When the same system is designed to work both as a cooler and as a heater, as a Peltier junction, it is quite intuitive that the two COP values have to be related. In particular, if no effect causes a difference from efficiency while working in the two different directions, as happens with a very good approximation for Peltier junctions, the term Q_C is the same in Equations 6.2 and in 6.3, thus $COP_H = COP_C + 1$. This means that the performance of the heat pump in both directions is well represented by plots like that of Figure 6.53.

Finally, from a straightforward thermodynamic calculation, it can be derived that the maximum possible value of COP_H is given by

$$COP_{H,max} = \frac{1}{\eta_{Carnot}} \tag{6.4}$$

where η_{Carnot} is the efficiency of the Carnot cycle working between the same temperatures. This equation is also intuitive, since in the ideal case the heat pump is an ideal cycle working inversely, that is absorbing work to move heat.

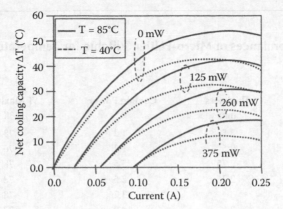

FIGURE 6.54 Net cooling capacity in terms of temperature difference between the cold and the hot extremes of a micro-Peltier component versus the applied current for different heat loads (expressed in mW and represented near the curves) and working temperatures of the cooled extreme.

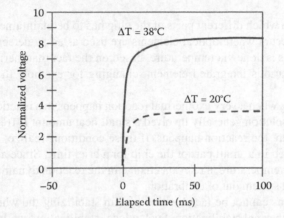

FIGURE 6.55 Typical time response of a fast Peltier cooler versus time for two different effective cooling capacities (in terms of temperature gradient) at a temperature of 85°C.

Although the COP provides indication of the thermodynamic efficiency of the TEC, the design of the temperature stabilization is typically done starting from plots like that of Figure 6.54, where the effective cooling power is provided for a given heat load versus the current for a fixed operating temperature of the cooled element. Increasing the cooling element temperature increases the effective cooling power, as intuitive, while it decreases increasing the heat load.

In several applications, where the activation of different parts of a lab on chip happens in different instants of time, also the reaction time of a Peltier stabilizer can be important, due to the need of following the pace of heat generation by the controlled circuit. In Figure 6.55, the time response of a fast Peltier cooler is represented versus time for two different effective cooling capacities (in terms of temperature gradient) at a temperature of 85°C. The response time is of the order of 35 ms and it is generally quite sufficient to take under control the thermal processes that can happen in biological microsystems. Examples of the performances of micro-Peltier are reported in Table 6.9.

6.6.3 HEATING MICRO-SYSTEMS

Micro-cooler and micro-Peltier elements allow an entire lab on chip to be temperature stabilized in various circumstances so as to render the performed assay independent from external temperature.

TABLE 6.9

Examples of the Performances of Micro-Peltier Suitable for Temperature Stabilization of Labs On Chip

Width mm	Length mm	Thickness mm	Cooling Power W	ΔT Maximum °K	Maximum Operating T °K
4.5	4.5	2.5	1.2	78	80
5.0	5.0	2.5	1.2	76	120
6.0	12.0	2.75	5.5	78	120
6.5	6.5	2.75	2.5	78	120
8.0	8.0	3	3.2	78	80
8.0	8.0	3	10.0	77	225
9.0	9.5	3	4.5	76	120
9.0	9.5	3	4.5	76	225
12.0	13.0	3.5	12.0	77	80

Cases exist, however, in which different parts of the chip has to be maintained at different temperatures. A typical case occurs where optical elements are used as assay detection element. The calibration of such elements is done via temperature, based on the fact that thermal expansion changes the optical length of various integrated element, changing for example the central resonance of interferometers.

A similar need arises when a very exothermal reaction happens in a reaction chamber. Due to the very small quantity of solution generally involved a small heat amount is freed in this way, but this is highly localized where the reaction happens. If these conditions realize, a relevant temperature gradient can be generated in a small part of the chip for a brief time. Since all the chemical parameters depend locally on temperature, a relevant change in the reaction dynamic can happen bringing the whole measurement system out of calibration.

This kind of problems cannot be faced with a system stabilizing the whole chip, but they have to be solved by a local thermal stabilization. Such a local stabilization can be attained by realizing micro-heater or micro-Peltier directly using front-end methods on the chip.

The most frequent structure used when an optical system has to be tuned or calibrated is to stabilize the entire chip a bit below the lower calibration temperature by using a discrete Peltier system and realizing directly on top of the optical system a metal deposition with a controlled resistance that works as a heater when a controlled amount of current is driven through it. The feedback system is generally attained by directly observing the obtained optical signal to verify if it is centered on the correct frequency.

An example of such a structure is shown in Figures 6.56 and 6.57. Here, the problem was to tune a micro-ring-based optical filter for the observation of the spectrum of the transit light. The filter was constructed by two superimposed rings and the tuning was obtained by heating the waveguides constituting the filter.

In Figure 6.56a, the shape of the ring local heater that was designed to heat a single ring is shown, and the thermal distribution over the heater metallization is shown in Figure 6.56b. The heater was realized on top of the filter structure after deposition of the upper cladding and planarization of the obtained structure (see Sections 4.9 and Section 4.10.1). The photograph of the heater after fabrication is shown in Figure 6.57.

In case in which direct observation of the temperature setting effect is not observable, the local temperature can be detected by directly integrating a micro-Peltier on the chip by deposition of the needed junction layers. Micro-Peltier has been directly integrated both on a polymer substrate [87] and on a semiconductor substrate [88] and depending on their dimensions and

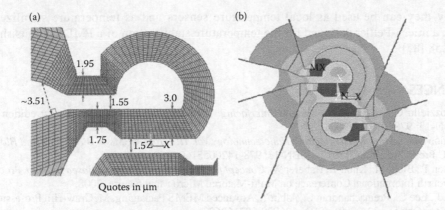

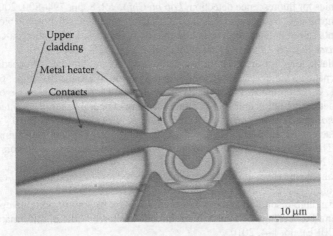

FIGURE 6.56 Design shape (a) and calculated local temperature distribution (b) of the monolithically integrated micro-heater designed to tune a double-ring optical resonator. (Reproduced under permission of Cyoptics Inc.)

FIGURE 6.57 Optical photograph of the chip where the micro-heater considered in Figure 6.56 was fabricated. (Reproduced under permission of Cyoptics Inc.)

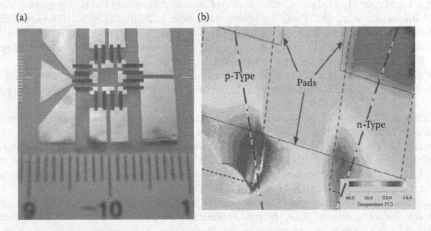

FIGURE 6.58 Photograph (a) and induced local temperature distribution (b) for a micro-Peltier realized monolithically on top of a PMDS substrate. (Reprinted from *Sensors and Actuators*, vol. 145–146, Goncalves L. M. et al., On-chip array of thermoelectric Peltier microcoolers, pp. 75–80, Copyright 2008, with permission from Elsevier.)

capability they can be used as local temperature sensors and as temperature stabilizers. For example, a micro-Peltier designed for the temperature stabilization of a PMDS chip is shown in Figure 6.58 [87].

REFERENCES

1. Perozziello G., *Microfluidics Systems Interfacing*, Lambert Academic Publishing, 1st edition (2011), ISBN-13: 978-3844327700.
2. Madou M. J., *Microfabrication and Nanotechnology Vol. III, From MEMs to Bio-MEMs and Bio-NEMS*, CRC Press, 3rd edition (2012), ISBN-13: 978-1420055160.
3. Velten T., Biehl M., Knoll T., Haberer W., *Concept for Packaging of a Silicon-Based Biochip*, Proceedings of Fourth International Conference on Multi-Material Micro Manufacture, 2008.
4. Lau J., Lee C., Premachandran C., Albin Y., Advanced MEMS Packaging, McGraw-Hill Professional, 1st edition (October 22, 2009), ISBN-13: 978-0071626231.
5. Ahn C. H. et al., Disposable smart lab on a chip for point-of-care clinical diagnostics, *Proceedings of the IEEE*, vol. 92, pp. 154–173, 2004.
6. Pais A., Banerjee A., Klotzkin D., Papautsky I., High-sensitivity, disposable lab-on-a-chip with thin-film organic electronics for fluorescence detection, *Lab on Chip*, vol. 8, pp. 794–800, 2008.
7. Xie L., Premachandran C. S., Chew M. Chong S. C., Development of a disposable bio-microfluidic package with reagents self-contained reservoirs and micro-valves for a DNA lab-on-a-chip (LOC) application, *IEEE Transactions on Advanced Packaging*, vol. 32, pp. 528–535, 2009.
8. Blionas S., Scalable low cost architecture for analysis of lab-an-chip data, Proceedings of Electronics, 17th IEEE International Conference on Circuits, and Systems (ICECS), 2010, pp. 563–566.
9. Constandinou T. G., Georgiou P., Prodromakis T., Toumazou C., A cmos-based lab on chip array for the combined magnetic stimulation and opto-chemical sensing of neural tissue, *12th International Workshop on Cellular Nanoscale Networks and their Applications (CNNA)*, pp. 10–16, 2010.
10. Ucok A. B., Giachino M. B., Najafi K., Compact, modular assembly and packaging of multi-substrate microsystems, The 12th International Conference on Solid Stale Sensors, Actuators and Microsystems, pp. 1877–1878, 2003.
11. Kigala C. V. et al., Inexpensive, universal serial bus-powered and fully portable lab-on-a-chip-based capillary electrophoresis instrument, *IET Nanobiotechnology*, vol. 3, pp. 1–7, 2009.
12. Jin X.-L., A novel high resolution and low noise cmos vision sensor for portable optical analytical lab-on-a-chip system, Proceedings of Fourth International Conference on Bioinformatics and Biomedical Engineering (iCBBE), pp. 1–4, 2010.
13. Ghafar-Zadeh E., Sawan M., Therriault D., A microfluidic packaging technique for lab on chip applications, *IEEE Transactions on Advanced Packaging*, vol. 32, pp. 410–416, 2009.
14. Tingkai L., Mastro M., Dadgar A., editors, *III-V Compound Semiconductors: Integration with Silicon-Based Microelectronics*, CRC Press, 1st edition (December 2, 2010), ISBN-13: 978-1439815229.
15. Noriki A., Kiyoyama K., Fukushima T., Tanaka T., Koyanagi M., Three-dimensional hybrid integration technology of CMOS, MEMS, and photonics circuits for optoelectronic heterogeneous integrated systems, *IEEE Transactions on Electron Devices*, vol. 58, pp. 748–757, 2011.
16. Kaler K. V. I. S., Yadid-Pecht O., Hybrid integration of an active pixel sensor and microfluidics for cytometry on a chip, *IEEE Transactions on Circuits and Systems I: Regular Papers*, vol. 54, pp. 99–110, 2007.
17. Coldren A. L.,Corzine S. W., Mashanovitch M. L., *Diode Lasers and Photonic Integrated Circuits*, Wiley, 2nd edition (20 March 2012), ISBN-13: 978-0470484128.
18. Michalzik L. editor, *VCSELs: Fundamentals, Technology and Applications of Vertical-Cavity Surface-Emitting Lasers*, Springer, 2012 edition (June 30, 2012), ISBN-13: 978-3642249853.
19. Chen A., Lo R. H.-Y., *Semiconductor Packaging: Materials Interaction and Reliability*, CRC Press, 1st edition (October 10, 2011), ISBN-13: 978-1439862056.
20. Oh K., Paek U.-C., *Silica Optical Fiber Technology for Device and Components: Design, Fabrication, and International Standards*, Wiley, 1st edition (February 28, 2012), ISBN-13: 978-0471455585.
21. Perozziello G., Packaging of microsystems, in *Microsystem Engineering of Lab-on-a-Chip Devices*, Geschke O., Klank H., Tellerman P., editors, Wiley-VCH, 2nd edition (June 17, 2008), ISBN-13: 978-3527319428.
22. Tummala R. R., Multichip packaging: A tutorial, *Proceedings of the IEEE*, vol. 80, pp. 1924–1940, 1992.

23. Abdel-Majeed M., Chen M., Annavaram M., A case for 3d stacked analog circuits in high-speed sensing systems, Proceedings of 13th International Symposium on Quality Electronic Design (ISQED), pp. 412–417, 2012.

24. Vempati S. R. et al., Development of 3-d silicon die stacked package using flip chip technology with micro bump interconnects, Proceedings of 59th Electronic Components and Technology Conference, pp. 980–987, 2009.

25. Canumalla S., Viswanadham P., *Portable Consumer Electronics: Packaging, Materials, and Reliability*, PennWell Corporation (May 15, 2010), ISBN-13: 978-1593701253.

26. Ebnesajjad S., *Adhesives Technology Handbook*, William Andrew, 2nd edition (August 21, 2008), ISBN-13: 978-0815515333.

27. Lu D., Wong C. P., High performance conductive adhesives. *IEEE Transactions on Electronics Packaging Manufacturing*, vol. 22, pp. 324–330, 1999.

28. Kang S. K. et al., Development of conductive adhesive materials for via fill applications. *IEEE Transactions on Components and Packaging Technologies*, vol. 24, pp. 431–435, 2001.

29. Windlein M., Nicolics J., Modeling of particle arrangement in an isotropically conductive adhesive joint, Proceedings of Fourth IEEE International Conference on Polymers and Adhesives in Microelectronics and Photonics, pp. 251–256, 2004.

30. Lyons A. M., Dahring D. W., Electrically conductive adhesives, in *Handbook of Adhesive Technology*, Revised and Expanded, Pizzi A., Mittal K. L. editors, CRC Press, 2nd edition (August 1, 2003), ISBN-13: 978-0824709860.

31. Inoue M., Muta H., Maekawa T., Yamanaka S., Suganuma K., Thermal conductivity of isotropic conductive adhesives composed of an epoxy-based binder, Conference on High Density Microsystem Design and Packaging and Component Failure Analysis, pp. 236–241, 2006.

32. Schildgen W. R., Murray C. T., Material set comparison in moisture sensitivity classification of nonhermetic organic packages, Proceedings of 35th International Symposium on Microelectronic, pp. 679–684, 2002.

33. Steen W. M., Mazumder J., Watkins K. G. *Laser Material Processing*, Springer, 4th edition (September 7, 2010), ISBN-13: 978-1849960618.

34. Duley W. W., *Laser Welding*, Wiley-Interscience, 1st edition (October 9, 1998), ISBN-13: 978-0471246794.

35. Chander D., Mazumder J., Estimating effects of processing conditions and variable properties upon pool shape, cooling rates, and absorption coefficient in laser welding, *Journal of Applied Physics*, vol. 56, pp. 1981–1986, 1984.

35. Zhigang X., Le H., Hongyan G., The effect of processing parameters on performance of laser welding tailored blanks of different thickness, Proceedings of Second International Conference on Digital Manufacturing and Automation, pp. 1279–1283, 2011.

36. Yaomin L.; Eichele C., Shi F.-G., Effect of welding sequence on welding-induced-alignment-distortion in packaging of butterfly laser diode modules: Simulation and experiment, *IEEE Journal of Lightwave Technology*, vol. 23, pp. 615–623, 2005.

37. Troughton M. J., *Handbook of Plastics Joining, A Practical Guide*, William Andrew, 2nd edition (September 18, 2008), ISBN-13: 978081551581-4.

38. Brown J., *Laser Plastic Welding Design Guidelines Manual*, LPKF Laser and Electronics, freely downloadable from http://www.laserplasticwelding.com/, last accessed on June 6, 2012.

39. Lau J. H., *Solder Joint Reliability: Theory and Applications*, Springer, 1st edition (January 15, 1991), ISBN-13: 978-0442002602.

40. Frear D. R., Burchett S. N., Morgan H. S., Lau J. H., *Mechanics of Solder Alloy Interconnects*, Springer, 1st edition (January 1, 1993), ISBN-13: 978-0442015053.

41. Tu K.-N., *Solder Joint Technology: Materials, Properties, and Reliability*, Springer, 1st edition (August 22, 2007) ISBN-13: 978-0387388908.

42. Harper C., *Electronic Assembly Fabrication*, McGraw-Hill Professional, 1st edition (March 22, 2002), ISBN-13: 978-0071378826.

43. Efrat U., Optimizing the wafer dicing process, Proceedings of Fifteenth IEEE/CHMT International Electronic Manufacturing Technology Symposium, pp. 245–253, 1993.

44. Chen S., Tsai C. Z., Wu E., Shih I. G., Chen Y. N., Study on the effects of wafer thinning and dicing on chip strength, *IEEE Transactions on Advanced Packaging*, vol. 29, pp. 149–157, 2006.

45. Teng A., Wilhelmsen F., Medical device wafer singulation, Proceedings of 32nd IEEE/CPMT International Electronic Manufacturing Technology Symposium, pp. 108–113, 2007.

46. Birkholz M., Ehwald K.-E., Kaynak M., Semperowitsch T., Holz B., Nordhoff S., Separation of extremely miniaturized medical sensors by IR laser dicing. *Journal of Optoelectronics Advanced Materials*, vol. 12, pp. 479–483, 2010.

47. Ohmura E., Fukuyo F., Fukumitsu K., Morita H. Internal modified layer formation mechanism into silicon with nanosecond laser. *Journal of Achievements in Material Manufacturing Engineering* vol. 17, pp. 381–384, 2006.

48. Lani S., Bosseboeuf A., Belier B., Clerc C., Gousset, C., Aubert J., Gold metallizations for eutectic bonding of silicon wafers. *Microsystem Technologies*, vol. 12, pp. 1021–1025, 2006.

49. Matijasevic G. S., Lee C. C., Wang C. Y., Au-sn alloy phase diagram and properties related to its use as a bonding medium. *Thin Solid Films*, vol. 223, pp. 276–287, 1993.

50. Sood, S., Farrens, S., Pinker, R., Xie, J., Cataby, W., Al-ge eutectic wafer bonding and bond characterization for cmos compatible wafer packaging. *ECS Transactions*, vol. 33, pp. 93–101, 2010.

51. Harman G. G., *Wire Bonding In Microelectronics*, McGraw-Hill Professional, 3rd edition (January 20, 2010), ISBN-13: 978-0071476232.

52. Prasad S. K., *Advanced Wirebond Interconnection Technology*, Springer, 1st edition (April 30, 2004), ISBN-13: 978-1402077623.

53. Ho H. M. et al., Direct gold and copper wires bonding on copper, *Microelectronics Reliability*, vol. 43, pp. 913–923, 2003.

54. Oezkoek M., White N., Clauberg H., Copper wire bond investigation on multiple surface finishes—enabling wire bond packages without gold, Proceedings of 18th European Microelectronics and Packaging Conference (EMPC), pp. 1–6, 2011.

55. Ho H. M., Advanced copper wire bonding technology, Proceedings of 34th IEEE/CPMT International Electronic Manufacturing Technology Symposium (IEMT), pp. 1–2, 2010.

56. Haeberle S., Zengerle R., Microfluidic platforms for lab-on-a-chip applications, *Lab on a Chip*, vol. 7, pp. 1094–1110, 2007.

57. Fredrickson C. K., Fan Z. H., Macro-to-micro interfaces for microfluidic devices, *Lab on a Chip*, vol. 4, pp. 526–533, 2004.

58. van Heeren H., Standards for connecting microfluidic devices?, *Lab on a Chip*, vol. 12, pp. 1022–1025, 2012.

59. Lo R., Meng E., Integrated and reusable in-plane microfluidic interconnects, *Sensors and Actuators* B vol. 132, pp. 531–539, 2008.

60. Johnson D. G., Frisina R. G., Borkholder D. A., In-plane biocompatible microfluidic interconnects for implantable microsystems, *IEEE Transactions on Biomedical Engineering*, vol. 58, no. 4, pp. 943–948, 2011.

61. Zourob M., Lachtakia A., editors, *Optical Guided-wave Chemical and Biosensors Volume I and Volume II*, Springer, 1st edition (26 March 2010), ISBN-13: 978-3540882411, for volume I and ISBN-13: 978-3642028267 for volume II.

62. Hunsperger R. G., *Integrated Optics: Theory and Technology*, Springer, Reprint of 2009 edition (October 29, 2010), ISBN-13: 978-1441928023.

63. Deen M. J., Basu D. K., *Silicon Photonics: Fundamentals and Devices*, Wiley, 1st edition (May 8, 2012), ISBN-13: 978-0470517505.

64. Keiser G., *Optical Communications Essentials*, McGraw-Hill, Networking Professional Series, 1st edition (August 2003), ISBN-13 978-0071412042.

65. *Fiber Optic Connectors Reference*, http://www.ertyu.org/steven_nikkel/fiberconnect.html, last accessed on June 16, 2012.

66. Kuzik M. G., *Polymer Fiber Optics: Materials, Physics, and Applications*, CRC Press, 1st edition (September 11, 2006), ISBN-13: 978-1574447064.

67. *Fiber Optics Slicing*, TPUB integrated Publisher, http://www.tpub.com/neets/tm/108-7.htm, last retrieved on June 6, 2012.

68. Weik M., *Fiber Optics Standard Dictionary*, Springer, 3rd edition (January 15, 1997), ISBN-13: 978-0412122415.

69. Barry T. S. et al., Efficient multimode optical fiber-to-waveguide coupling for passive alignment applications in multichip modules, *IEEE Transactions on Components, Packaging, And Manufacturing Technology-Part B*, vol. 18, pp. 685–690, 1995.

70. Jing Z. et al., Development of optical subassembly for plastic optical fiber in high speed applications, Proceedings of the 10th IEEE Electronics Packaging Technology Conference, pp. 1220–1225, 2008.

71. Mori H., Tamura S., Suga S., Iwase M., Plastic optical module having a pre-insert molded sc ferule and a laser diode with mode-field converter, Proceedings of 1998 Optical Fiber Conference, paper ThS2, pp. 347–348, 1998.

72. Lecarpentier G., Mottet J.-S., Dumas J., Cooper K., High accuracy machine automated assembly for opto electronics, Proceedings of 2000 IEEE Electronic Components and Technology Conference, pp. 1–4, 2000.

73. Hauffe R., Siebel U., Petermann K., Moosburger R., Kropp J.-R., Arndt F., Methods for passive fiber chip coupling of integrated optical devices, *IEEE Transactions On Advanced Packaging*, vol. 24, pp. 450–455, 2001.

74. Henzi P., Rabus D. G., Bade K., Wallrabe U., Mohr J., Low cost single mode waveguide fabrication allowing passive fiber coupling using LIGA and UV flood exposure, In Micro-Optics: Fabrication, PaCkaging, and Integration, Van Daele P., Mohr J., editors, *Proceedings of SPIE*, vol. 5454, pp. 64–73, 2004, ISBN-13: 978-0819453778.

75. Kim J. T., Yooh K. B., Choi C.-G., Passive alignment method of polymer PLC devices by using a hot embossing technique, *IEEE Photonics Technology Letters*, vol. 16, pp. 1664–1666, 2004.

76. Hormanski P., Nieweglowski K., Wolterk.-J., Patela S., *Investigation on Butt-Coupling of VCSEL into PCB Integrated Waveguides*, KNS Conference on Photonics and Nanotechnology, 2004, available at http://www.kns.b2me.pl/art-investigation-on-butt-coupling-of-vcsel-into-pcb-integrated-,57,0.html, last accessed on June 21, 2012.

77. Laconte J., Flandre D., Raskin J.-P., *Micromachined thin-film sensors for SOI-CMOS co-integration*, Springer, Reprint 2006 edition (October 29, 2010), ISBN-13: 978-1441939579.

78. Cobianu O. M., Cobianu C., Comparison of microheaters efficiency for sensing applications, Proceedings of International Semiconductor Conference, *CAS 2004*, vol. 1, pp. 1–5, 2004.

79. Liu L., Peng S., Niu X., Wen W., Microheaters fabricated from a conducting composite, *Applied Physics Letters*, vol. 89, pp. 223521- 223521-3, 2006.

80. Sebastian A., Weissman D., Modeling and experimental identification of silicon microheater dynamics: A systems approach, *IEEE Journal of Micromechanical Systems*, vol. 17, 2011–2020, 2008.

81. Michalski L., Eckersdorf K., Kucharski J., McGhee J., *Temperature Measurement*, Wiley, 2nd edition (December 15, 2001), ISBN-13: 978-0471867791.

82. Boyes W., *Instrumentation Reference Book*, Butterworth-Heinemann, 3rd edition (December 3, 2002), ISBN-13: 978-0750671231.

83. MacDonald D. K. C., *Thermoelectricity: An Introduction to the Principles*, Dover Publications (October 27, 2006), ISBN-13: 978-0486453040.

84. Hwang G. S., Micro thermoelectric cooler: Planar multistage, *International Journal of Heat and Mass Transfer*, vol. 52, pp. 1843–1852, 2009.

85. Bottner H., Nurnus J., Shubert N., Volkert F., New high density thermogenerators for stand-alone sensor systems, *IEEE Journal of Micromechanical Systems*, vol. 13, pp. 414–420, 2004.

86. Kandasamy S., Kalantar-zadeh K., Rosengarten G., Wlodarski W., Modelling of a thin film thermoelectric micro-peltier module, *2004 IEEE Region 10 Conference TENCON*, vol. D (vol. 4), pp. 310–313, 2004.

87. Goncalves L. M., Rocha J.G., Couto C., Alpuim P., Correia J.H., On-chip array of thermoelectric peltier microcoolers, *Sensors and Actuators A*, vol. 145–146, pp. 75–80, 2008.

88. Dilhaire S., Ezzahri Y., Grauby S., and Claeys W., Thermal and thermomechanical study of micro-refrigerators on a chip based on semiconductor heterostructures, Proceedings of IEEE International Conference on Thermoelectrics, pp. 519–523, 2003.

Section III

Lab on Chip Design

7 Fluid Dynamics in Microfluidic Circuits

7.1 INTRODUCTION

This is the first chapter of the third part; the part devoted to labs on chip design methods. Several different techniques have to converge in the design of such systems that are characterized by their multidisciplinary nature. Synthesis between exigencies of different technologies in order to optimize the whole system is perhaps the most difficult part of the design.

In this chapter, we will deal with the design of the microfluidic circuit embedded in the lab on chip. This is somehow the core of the chip, where the solutions containing reactants are purified and concentrated and the key assays are performed. Design of microfluidic circuits involves a wide set of methods typical of fluid dynamics, moreover technological aspects of fabrication of the structures under design have always to be taken into account. As a matter of fact, technology constraints are never negligible and a purely theoretical design frequently brings to structures that are difficult to fabricate, completely cancelling the design advantages.

Fluid dynamics have to consider quite often the presence of electrical and magnetic fields besides traditional pressure and diffusion forces, and chemistry in systems out of mechanical equilibrium. These elements render the theoretical analysis of system dynamics quite difficult and calls for the use of complex mathematical methods to correctly catch the main elements of the design. However, turbulence phenomena are almost absent in microfluidic circuits, while they are fundamental in many macroscopic fluid dynamics.

Situations are present in specific cases where more complex mechanical evolution happens, for example, involving multiphase fluxes. In this cases, an even more complex representation of the set of moving fluids is needed, where modeling and mathematical equation treatment intersect creating very interesting situations under the point of view of the theoretical fluid-dynamics [1–3].

In the first part of the chapter, we will review fluid dynamics fundamentals, with particular attention to those conditions typical of microfluidic circuits. A coherent description of fluid kinematics will allow us to clarify concepts like flow lines and material coordinates. On the ground of this basic concept we will introduce the main fluid dynamics equations for different types of liquids. In doing that we are not to forget that often we will deal with biological liquids like blood serum, that are not completely compliant with more intuitive liquid properties modeled on water.

We will consider in some detail a set of basic solution techniques for our dynamic equations that in the next chapters will allow us to set up a correct theoretical modeling for the key microfluidic building blocks, like mechanical filters, micro-valves, and so on.

In microfluidic problems, due to the planar technology used to realize the circuits, it is quite uncommon to face fluid motion along curve surfaces, thus we can get rid of the difficulty of considering motion on non-Euclidean Riemann varieties and the consequent use of non-Euclidean complex tensor calculus. The interested reader is encouraged to access the rich and detailed technical literature on these methodologies that are on the contrary very important, for example, in aerodynamics [4,5].

After the review of fluid dynamics tailored to its application to microfluidic, we will face diffusion processes that are very common when a solution is injected by diffusion in the reaction chamber of a microfluidic circuit. In these cases, diffusion is often accompanied by chemical reactions so that we will face the problem to derive and solve chemical–diffusion models and convection–diffusion models that are needed where a solution is put in motion by an external pressure while diffusion reshapes the solutes concentration.

In reviewing this large set of mathematical design methods, we will face the need of frequently using Euclidean tensor algebra and calculus. Different notations have been used in various fluid-dynamics applications: we will use both formal notation for vector and tensors equations and the Einstein notation when the equations are expressed through the coordinates [6]. A detailed description of the conventions used for tensor and vector equations in this book is reported in Appendix 2.

7.2   KINEMATIC OF FLUID MOTION

7.2.1   The Continuous Fluid Model

The kinematic is the part of mechanic describing the motion. In this sense, no hypothesis is done on forces causing the motion or on the nature of the moving fluid, but for the fact that it is considered a continuum medium. This means that all the derivations are carried out starting from the concept that an infinitesimal volume of the fluid, that is a volume whose linear dimensions are much smaller than the critical dimension of the structure guiding the fluid motion, can still be considered a continuous medium.

In classical fluid dynamics, this infinitesimal volume is, in general, called fluid particle, that has naturally no relation to the real fluid particles that are the molecules composing the fluid. While the real molecules of the fluid are animated by a random motion, whose average is the macroscopic fluid flow, the classic fluid particle is a small part of a continuous system, moving with a deterministic velocity along a trajectory that is part of the overall fluid flow. The first step of a micro-fluidics theory is to verify whether the hypothesis is still true in small structures like labs on chip.

To refer to a specific case, let us consider a microfluidic duct that has a section 10×10 μm wide filled with water. A stereographic model of the water molecule is represented in Figure 7.1. From the figure it can be deduced that we do not make a great error by considering the space occupied by a water molecule external orbital equal to a sphere of diameter of 3 Å. Thus, we can divide our microfluidic duct in elementary volumes of 3×10^3 nm^3 that we can fill with more than 10^6 water molecules.

On the other end, we have as much as 3×10^6 of such elements in 10 μm^3 of our duct, so that we can conclude that the elementary volume of 3×10^3 nm^3 is sufficiently small with respect to the duct dimension and contains a sufficiently high number of water molecules to allow the continuous approximation.

Frequently, the organic fluids we will consider are diluted solutions, where biological macromolecules are present in very small amount in water solution, generally in the presence of small ions such as Na$^+$ or Cl$^-$ and sometimes of alcohols such as glycerol, that are added to the solution in small quantity, for example, to avoid jellification. The stereographic model of a glycerol molecule in represented Figure 7.2. Macromolecules are sufficiently diluted so that fluid dynamics properties almost only depends on the solute, that is a saline water solution, but for diffusion-driven phenomena that are in any case dealt with using specific models.

Thus, in almost all practical cases, where dimensions of the microns order of magnitude are considered, a continuous liquid approximation is allowed. Care has to be taken if concentrated solution of macromolecules appears, or if separation phenomena, like fatty acids precipitation, are present. In this case however, it is not the continuous model that loses its validity, but the single phase approximation and frequently a more complex multi-phase continuous model has to be adopted.

The situation would be quite different if we would like to consider nano-fluidics, which are ducts of the order of 100 nm. In this case, careful consideration of the continuous model has to be done since it loses its validity in several cases. However, such systems are used for different applications and hardly can be classified as labs on chip, thus we will not take them into consideration in this book.

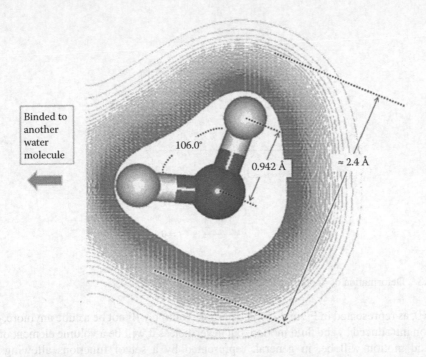

FIGURE 7.1 Stereographic model of the water, the two hydrogen atoms and the oxygen atom are represented through the internal electrons energy levels, while equal density curves of the shared electrons molecular orbital in the binding plane are represented with lines besides a point density that qualitatively suggest the electron density for c certain equal density line.

7.2.2 FLUID MOTION DESCRIPTION

If we fix the fluid state in an instant, call it the initial instant $t = 0$, and we divide the fluid mass in "particles" in the sense considered in the above section, each fluid particle has a position whose coordinate will be called ξ_j ($j = 1, 2, 3$).

Since the fluid motion is continuous, following the motion of all the points belonging to an elementary particle in the instant $t = 0$ (let image it is a cube) we will always find that those points will define a three-dimensional volume in the vicinity of the point that was the cube center at the

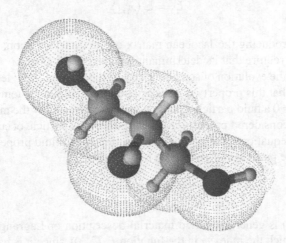

FIGURE 7.2 Stereographic model of a glycerol molecule.

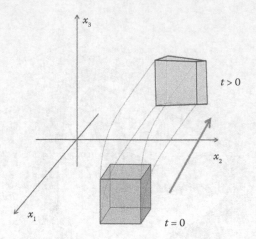

FIGURE 7.3 Deformation of the fluid particle during motion.

instant $t = 0$, as represented in Figure 7.3. The particle volume will not be a cube anymore, due to the deformation introduced by the fluid motion, but nevertheless it will be a volume element of the fluid.

The fluid motion will be, in general, represented by a set of functions allowing to calculate the position of the points belonging to a fluid particle in an instant t if the particle occupied at $t = 0$ the point of coordinates ξ_j. Thus, the generic description of the fluid motion can be represented by the following set of three functions of four variables:

$$x_j = x_j(\xi_i, t) \tag{7.1}$$

For the indexes convention (see Appendix 2), the fact that the second member of Equation 7.1 depends on ξ_i and the index i is not repeated anywhere does mean that it depends on all the ξ_i, that is from all the coordinates of the vector $\xi = (\xi_1, \xi_2, \xi_3)$.

Since the motion has to be continuous we have to require that Equation 7.1 is invertible so that the initial position of each fluid particle identified at the instant t by the coordinates x_i can be derived univocally from the equations

$$\xi_j = \xi_j(x_i, t) \tag{7.2}$$

This means that, introducing the Jacobean matrix of the transformation, (7.1) that is defined as $J_{i,j} = \partial x_i / \partial \xi_j$, we have to require that its determinant is different from zero.

Let us now imagine the evolution of some property of the flowing fluid; let us call it F, and let us imagine for simplicity that this property is a scalar one, for example, the temperature. We can individuate at the instant $t = 0$ a fluid particle via its coordinates and follow the motion of the particle in time by evaluating the considered property in all the points this particle occupies.

This means that the equation representing the evolution of our fluid property will depend on the initial coordinates of the particle and on time so to be

$$F = F_m(\xi_j, t) \tag{7.3}$$

The description (7.3) is generally called material description or Lagrangian description of the fluid evolution (from which the index m in the function $F_m(\xi_j, t)$), since it is based on the idea of following a well-identified portion of the fluid during its time evolution.

An alternative way of describing a fluid property is to fix a position in the domain occupied by the fluid and look at the evolution of the considered property in that point, while continuously different fluid particles travels through it. This description is related with the material description by the fact that the transformation relating initial coordinates of a particle with its position in time are invertible and can be obtained by Equation 7.3 substituting to the initial coordinates their expressions as a function of time and of the coordinates of the observation point.

In this way, the initial coordinates assume in each instant the value of the starting point of the particular fluid particle travelling through the observation point at the considered instant and Equation 7.3 writes

$$F = F_l(x_j, t) \tag{7.4}$$

The corresponding description of the fluid property is called Eulerian or local description (from which the index l in the function $F_l(\xi_j, t)$).

Both Equations 7.3 and 7.4 will be derivable with respect to t, and both the derivative can be called derivate of the property F of the fluid with respect to time. Nevertheless they are different functions, due to the different ways in which the evolution of the considered property is described. Thus, it is necessary to mark their difference and find a relationship between them, since they describe in different ways the same evolution.

Following the name we gave to the representation provided by Equation 7.3, the derivative of $F_m(\xi, t)$ with respect to time is generally called material or substantial derivative and it is indicated with D/Dt, while the derivative of $F_l(x_j, t)$, defined in Equation 7.4 is called local derivative and it is indicated with the usual formalism used for partial derivatives.

The relationship between the two kinds of derivatives can be easily found substituting in Equation 7.4 the dependence of the observation point coordinates on the initial particle coordinates and observing that the velocity of the particle passing from the observation point at the instant t (i.e., the velocity in the local description) is given simply by

$$v_j = \frac{\partial x_j(\xi_i, t)}{\partial t} \tag{7.5}$$

At the end of the computation the following expression is found, which we report both in the abstract and in the index notation

$$\frac{DF}{Dt} = v_j \frac{\partial F}{\partial x_j} + \frac{\partial F}{\partial t} \tag{7.6a}$$

$$\frac{DF}{Dt} = (v \cdot \nabla)F + \frac{\partial F}{\partial t} \tag{7.6b}$$

From the local expression of the velocity we can deduce a set of curves, called the streamlines, whose parametric equations $\vartheta_j(\xi_i, \tau)$ where τ is the curve parameter, are solution of the following differential equations:

$$\frac{\partial \vartheta_j}{\partial \tau} = v_j(\vartheta_i, \tau) \tag{7.7}$$

We cannot confuse the streamlines with the fluid particles trajectories, since in Equation 7.7 the time coordinate is maintained constant so that, in general, the streamline will vary with varying time. However, at any time, a streamline is tangent to the real trajectory of the particle traveling by the observation point in the considered instant. As a matter of fact, trajectories are the solutions of the equation

$$\frac{\partial x_j}{\partial t} = v_j(x_i, t) \tag{7.8}$$

subject to the given initial conditions. It is clear from Equation 7.8 that, if t is taken as curve coordinate on the trajectories, in a given instant the derivative with respect to the curve coordinate of the streamline and of the trajectory in the same point are the same. This effect is shown in Figure 7.4a, where the evolution of a set of streamlines during a nonstationary fluid flow is shown evidencing the real fluid particles trajectories.

In the case of stationary flux, that is when the local velocity does not depend on time, the streamlines identify with particles trajectories. This is shown in Figure 7.4b, where the streamlines and the trajectories of a stationary motion are considered. As a matter of fact, since the velocity of the particle travelling through a point does not change, this means that all the particles travelling through that points share the same trajectory that is exactly the streamline.

The stationary motion is not the only particular case where streamlines coincide with trajectories [4], but we will not go deeply into this issue, as it is not very important for our application.

A striking idea of realistic streamlines of fluid motion is given in Figure 7.5, where the streamlines of air around a moving sphere are shown in a particular instant. In this case, it is to be noted that if the sphere motion is linear and uniform, the fluid motion in the reference frame in which the sphere is still is also stationary, thus the streamlines are also the particles trajectories in this particular reference frame.

A concept that helps many times in visualization of the characteristics of the fluid flow it that of streamtube, that is the surface constituted by all the streamlines travelling through the points of a closed line in space. An example of streamtube is given in Figure 7.6. Due to the continuity of the motion, this constitutes a regular surface if the closed curve is regular. However, as the streamlines, the streamtube also changes in time. Streamtubes have an important property, deriving from the fact that during any kind of fluid motion they evolve in such a way that real particles trajectories are

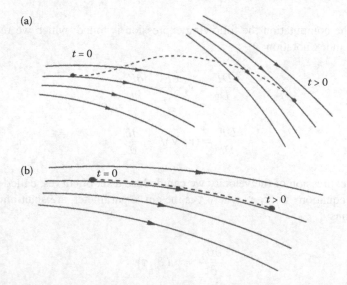

FIGURE 7.4 Streamlines variation with time in a generic fluid motion (a) where the fact that the stream lines are always tangent to the fluid particles trajectories is evidenced; coincidence of streamlines with trajectories in a stationary fluid motion (b).

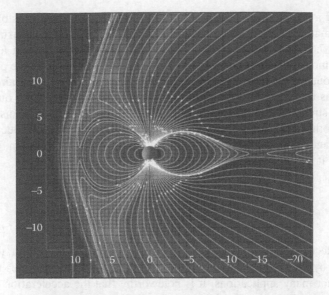

FIGURE 7.5 Streamlines of air flux around a moving balls: gray tones represents qualitatively the local air pressure.

always tangent to the streamlines constituting the streamtube surface. Particles inside the streamtube will remain inside and never exits from the tube during motion and particles outside the tube remains outside during all the motion. Thus, even if the streamtube evolves during motions, we can define a streamtube rate of flow, that is, the fluid mass flowing through the streamtube.

Let us call S a regular open surface whose border is one of the closed lines defining the streamtube and let us define a parametric equation of S that is function of the two parameters σ_1 and σ_2 so that the surface can be described by the three equations

$$x_j = x_j(\sigma_1, \sigma_2) \tag{7.9}$$

The fluid mass flowing through this surface in a unit time, that is the same in any streamtube section, is the streamtube flow rate Q and it is given by

$$Q = \iint_S \rho(\sigma_1, \sigma_2) v_j(\sigma_1, \sigma_2) n_j(\sigma_1, \sigma_2) dS \tag{7.10}$$

where $v_j \, n_j$ is the scalar product between the fluid velocity in a point of the surface and the normal unit vector to the surface in that point.

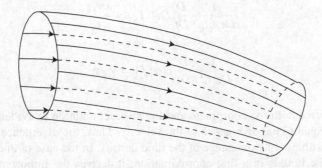

FIGURE 7.6 Example of streamtube where the streamlines on the limit surface are evidenced.

The property of a streamtube to catch a fluid flow inside it is also a possible definition of the streamtube. As a matter of fact, if we consider a generalized cylindrical surface like those represented in Figure 7.6, the fact that the fluid local velocity is always tangent to the external tube surface is easily demonstrated to be a necessary and sufficient condition for the permanency of fluid particles inside or outside the tube. This implies that if a physical duct constrains the fluid motion, so that the fluid has to remain into the duct from the duct input to the duct output, its surface is necessarily also a streamtube. This is true in any case, even if the motion inside the duct is not stationary and the other stream tubes vary with time, due to the fact that the duct is physically still.

Another important kinematic variable of the fluid motion is the acceleration, which is the rate of change of velocity. It is generally defined in the material representation as

$$a_j = \frac{Dv_j}{Dt} = \frac{\partial v_j}{\partial t} + v_i \frac{\partial v_j}{\partial x_i} \tag{7.11}$$

Even if a local acceleration could also be defined as $a_j = \partial v_j/\partial t$ this concept, that is the acceleration experimented by the different fluid particles travelling in different times through the observation point, has not many applications. It is noteworthy that the acceleration does not vanish if the velocity is constant. This property is due to the fact that the velocity v_i is defined in the local representation while the acceleration in the material one. Thus, if the velocity is constant we are not saying that a single particle is travelling of linear uniform motion (case in which the acceleration is zero), but that the particles passing from the observation point at different instants have all the same velocity, condition that for sure does not assure that the particle acceleration while travelling from that point is zero.

Finally, we can consider the compression (or dilation) of a fluid during motion. This property is directly linked to the transformation bringing from the material to the local representation, since the Jacobean of that transformation is exactly the ratio between the volume of the fluid particle before and after the transformation, that in our case coincides with the volume of the particle at $t = 0$ and at a successive instant. Thus, since the mass of a fluid particle has to maintain during motion for the continuity of the motion itself, we can write

$$Det(J_{ij}) = \frac{dV}{dV_0} = \frac{\rho_0}{\rho} \tag{7.12}$$

where ρ is the fluid density. Thus, the Jacobean represents the dilation (or compression) of the fluid during motion.

It is possible to demonstrate with a trivial but cumbersome computation that the material derivative of the Jacobean determinant with respect to the time can be expressed as follows [4]:

$$\frac{1}{Det(J_{ij})} \frac{D}{Dt} Det(J_{ij}) = \frac{\partial v_j}{\partial x_j} \tag{7.13a}$$

$$\frac{1}{Det(\underline{J})} \frac{D}{Dt} Det(\underline{J}) = \nabla \cdot v \tag{7.13b}$$

where we have reported both the coordinate and the abstract notation to evidence the fact that the second member is equal to the divergence of the velocity. Thus, the divergence of the velocity has the meaning of logarithmic rate of change of the fluid density. In the case of uncompressible fluids, that is, almost all the liquids in a first approximation, it derives the important property that the velocity field is conservative, that is it admits a scalar potential [2].

7.2.3 Continuity Equation

The continuity equation is one of the most important elements of the description of fluid motion.

Even if this equation regards essentially mass conservation in the absence of sinks and sources, it finds its place in the kinematic part of fluid dynamics due to the fact that it is a purely descriptive property of the motion.

We will also derive the mass continuity equation from a more general continuity equation for a motion invariant. This general equation will be useful several times like evaluating the momentum, the electrical charge and the energy flow. Let us image that $h_i(r_j, t)$ is the density of an intensive vector quantity that is conserved during fluid motion, so that the conserved quantity in a volume V can be written as

$$H_i = \int_V h_i(r_j, t)dV \tag{7.14}$$

If we define the normal unit vector n_k to every point of the surface ∂V of the volume V as positive, if directed out of the volume as shown in Figure 7.7a, the flux Φ_{ij} (quantity per unit surface area and unit time) of H_i through the infinitesimal element $d\sigma$ of the surface is given by $\Phi_{ij} = h_i v_j$, where v_j is the local velocity and the flux is in this case a matrix since it is in reality the joint representation of the three fluxes of the components of H_i. Since h_i transforms as a vector we can conclude that the flux Φ_{ij} is a tensor of order two.

The local time derivative of H_i can be written both as integral of the time derivative of its density $h_i(r_j, t)$ and in terms of the flux of the quantity H_i. This second expression gives

$$\frac{\partial H_i}{\partial t} = -\int_{\partial V} n_k h_i v_k \, d\sigma = -\int_V \frac{\partial}{\partial x_j}(h_i v_j) dV \tag{7.15}$$

where the last expression is obtained by using three times, one for each component of h_i, the Gauss theorem on the vector $h_i v_j$ (applying the Gauss theorem the vector index is j, while i simply indicates one of three vectors with $i = 1, 2, 3$).

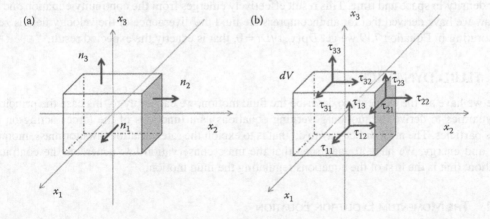

FIGURE 7.7 Graphical illustration of the convention on the direction of the unit vector perpendicular to the boundary surface of a given volume (a) and of the physical meaning of the components of the stress tensor $\underline{\tau}$ (b).

Equating the integral of the time derivative of the density to the last expression comparing in Equation 7.15 we get

$$\int_V \frac{\partial}{\partial x_j}(h_i v_j)\, dV = -\int_V \frac{\partial h_i}{\partial t}\, dV \tag{7.16}$$

Since Equation 7.17 has to hold for all possible choices of the volume V, it derives that the functions under the integral sign have to be equal. From this observation we obtain the continuity equation for H_i

$$\frac{\partial h_i}{\partial t} + \frac{\partial}{\partial x_j}\Phi_{ij} = \frac{\partial h_i}{\partial t} + \frac{\partial}{\partial x_j}(h_i v_j) = 0 \tag{7.17}$$

If the conserved quantity is the mass, h_i is a scalar, that is the mass density of the fluid, and we obtain the mass continuity equation:

$$\frac{\partial \rho}{\partial t} + \frac{\partial}{\partial x_j}(\rho v_j) = 0 \tag{7.18}$$

Observing that the local derivative can be expressed as a function of the material derivative by Equation 7.6, the continuity equation can be also expressed using the material derivative of the density as

$$\frac{D\rho(x_i,t)}{Dt} + \rho(x_i,t)\frac{\partial v_j}{\partial x_j} = 0 \tag{7.19a}$$

$$\frac{D\rho(\mathbf{x},t)}{Dt} + \rho(\mathbf{x},t)\nabla \cdot \mathbf{v} = 0 \tag{7.19b}$$

It is to be noted that for many fluids the incompressible model applies, that should imply a constant density in space and time. This result effectively emerges from the continuity equation and for the law we have derived that for an incompressible fluid the divergence of the velocity field is zero. Substituting in Equation 7.19 we get $D\rho(x_i, t)/Dt = 0$, that is exactly the expected result.

7.3   FLUID DYNAMICS

Once we have all the elements to describe the fluid motion, we can apply to this case the principles of dynamics to derive the motion governing equations as a functions of the forces acting on the fluids particles. The most direct way to do that is to exploit the rate variation laws for mass, momentum, and energy. We have already seen that the mass conservation law generates the continuity equation, that is the first of the equations regulating the fluid motion.

7.3.1   THE MOMENTUM EVOLUTION EQUATION

The basic law of classical mechanics is the Newton's second law which is written essentially as a rule giving the momentum rate of change of a particle versus the applied force. Let us fix, in the local fluid description, a fixed volume V around the observation point.

The local derivative of the momentum density $q_i = \rho v_i$ in the volume V can be written as follows:

$$\frac{\partial q_i}{\partial t} = \frac{\partial}{\partial t} \iiint_V \rho v_i \, dV = \iiint_V \left[\frac{\partial \rho}{\partial t} v_i + \rho \frac{\partial v_i}{\partial t} \right] dV \qquad (7.20)$$

where the local derivative can be moved inside the integral since in the local description the volume V is constant in time.

The momentum can change due to two possible causes: either the mass of the fluid in the volume changes, entering in the infinitesimal time a mass with a momentum different from the mass that is exiting in the same time interval, or for the action of forces acting on the fluid.

Different kinds of forces can act on the fluid, both acting on the overall momentum due to the Newton's second law:

- External forces acting on the fluid body as, for example, gravity or an electromagnetic field if the fluid is charged
- The effect of the fluid pressure acting on the surface of the volume V
- The inner resistance to motion due to the attrition between the fluid particles, that is called viscous force

Thus, we can decompose the expression of the momentum variation as follows:

$$\left.\frac{\partial q_i}{\partial t}\right)_{motion} + \left.\frac{\partial q_i}{\partial t}\right)_{pressure} + \left.\frac{\partial q_i}{\partial t}\right)_{viscous} + \left.\frac{\partial q_i}{\partial t}\right)_{body\ forces} = \iiint_V \left[\frac{\partial \rho}{\partial t} v_i + \rho \frac{\partial v_i}{\partial t} \right] dV \qquad (7.21)$$

Expression (7.21) is essentially the momentum rate equation, that is the equivalent of the second law of dynamics for fluids. Now all the terms at the first member has to be evaluated as functions of the fluid motion variables.

7.3.1.1 Change of Momentum Due to Fluid Motion

In order to evaluate the momentum flux through the volume surface we have to define, for each momentum component, a relative flux, as we have done in general in Section 7.2.3. The flux of the jth momentum component is equal to the mass current through the surface multiplied by the corresponding velocity component, thus we have that the jth flux vector is given by

$$\Phi_{j,i} = \rho v_j v_i \qquad (7.22)$$

As in the general case the flux of the momentum vector is a tensor of order two, whose expression is given by Equation 7.22. Indicating with Ω the surface of the volume V, the expression of the momentum change due to mass flux through the volume surface can be written specializing to this case Equation 7.15 as

$$\left.\frac{\partial q_j}{\partial t}\right)_{motion} = -\iint_\Omega \rho v_j v_i n_i \, d\Omega \qquad (7.23)$$

where the minus sign comes from the usual convention to point outside the volume the unit vector normal to a volume boundary surface (see Figure 7.7a).

7.3.1.2 Stress Tensor in the Fluid, Pressure and Viscosity

In all the branches of continuum mechanics the internal forces acting of the surface of an infinitesimal volume of the continuous body due to interactions with the nearby body parts are represented by the so-called stress tensor τ_{ij}. Quantitatively, the stress tensor elements are a measure of the average force per unit area of a surface within the body on which internal forces act. Considering an elementary body volume shaped like a cube the different tensor components can be easily identified as the forces acting on the cube faces in the different directions, as it is represented in Figure 7.7b.

If the fluid mass is still, tangent forces cannot exist between nearby parts of the fluid, since they would cause fluid motion. Thus, the stress tensor reduces to a diagonal tensor in mechanical equilibrium. Moreover, the three component of the equilibrium stress tensor have to be equal, due to the fact that otherwise a deformation of the fluid would happen. Thus, in mechanical equilibrium the stress tensor depends simply by a scalar parameter, that we call p. The parameter p can be identified with the pressure as defined in thermodynamic transformations.

This property can be shown if we consider the basic thermodynamic experiment where a fluid is put into a cylinder with a piston parallel to the $(x_1 \, x_2)$ plan, as shown in Figure 7.8. When the piston is pushed against the fluid surface by applying a constant pressure on the piston surface equal to Δp and equilibrium is reached, the stress tensor remains diagonal since no fluid motion happens. Since the only applied force is uniform and perpendicular to the $(x_1 \, x_2)$ plane the stress tensor components, due to the isotropy of the fluid properties, changes all by an amount equal to Δp. Thus, p scales exactly as the thermodynamic pressure so that it can be identified with it.

In a dynamic situation, where the fluid moves, the stress tensor is generally not diagonal, so that, calling p the pressure, it can be written as

$$\tau_{ij} = p\delta_{ij} + \gamma'_{i,j} \qquad (7.24)$$

Since τ_{ij} is a tensor also $\gamma'_{i,j}$ has to transform as a tensor and, since it is different from zero only during motion, it has to depend on the forces generated between nearby portions of the fluids due to their relative change of position. These forces are called viscous forces, and $\gamma'_{i,j}$ is generally called the viscous tensor.

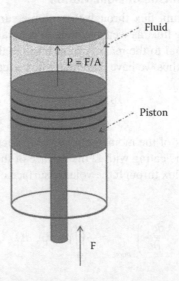

FIGURE 7.8 Example of uniform compression of a fluid in a piston used to show the equivalence between thermodynamic and fluid-mechanical definitions of pressure.

7.3.1.3 Change of Momentum Due to Pressure and Viscous Forces

The presence of internal forces generates a change of local momentum during motion. Starting from the term depending on pressure, we can write the related change of momentum density as

$$\left. \frac{\partial q_i}{\partial t} \right)_{pressure} = -\iint_\Omega p \delta_{i,j} n_j \, d\Omega \tag{7.25}$$

where $\delta_{i,j}$ is the Kronecker symbol and $p_i \delta_{i,j}$ represents the stress tensor pressure component. Sometimes Equations 7.25 and 7.23 get together by defining a generalized momentum flux tensor given by

$$\Pi_{i,j} = p \delta_{i,j} + \rho v_j v_i \tag{7.26}$$

so that the overall momentum flux due to the combined action of motion and pressure is given by

$$\left. \frac{\partial q_i}{\partial t} \right)_{motion} + \left. \frac{\partial q_i}{\partial t} \right)_{pressure} = -\iint_\Omega \Pi_{i,j} n_i \, d\Omega \tag{7.27}$$

The expression of the momentum change due to the viscous stress tensor $\gamma'_{i,j}$ is completely analogous, so that we can write

$$\left. \frac{\partial q_i}{\partial t} \right)_{viscous} = -\iint_\Omega \gamma'_{i,j} n_j \, d\Omega \tag{7.28}$$

It is possible to obtain a more specific expression of the viscous stress tensor by considering a set of properties that the relative attrition between fluid particles must have. First of all, attrition happens only when fluid particles move one with respect to the other. Thus, the stress tensor coordinates have not to depend on the absolute value of the velocity, but only on the velocity derivatives with respect to spatial coordinates. This reflects the fact that, when the fluid moves as a whole, with a rigid movement, there is no viscous force. If very fast motion is involved, as it is possible in some macroscopic fluid mechanics, the dependence of the stress tensor from the second-order derivative of the fluid velocity can have some impact, but in microfluidic circuits the fluid speeds are always quite low, so that we can assume that the viscous tensor elements depend only on the velocity gradient $\partial v_i/\partial x_j$.

No viscous force is also present if the fluid rotates as a rigid body, since also in this case there is no change in the reciprocal positions of the fluid particles. A rigid rotation is usually described in terms of the angular velocity vector ω defined in such a way that the velocity of each point of the body is given by the vector product of the point position vector r and ω.

To adapt this description to our tensor formalism we have to use the Levi Civita symbol as described in Appendix 2. Thus, the rigid rotation velocity field can be written as

$$v_i = \epsilon_{i,j,k} \omega_j x_k = \epsilon_{i,j,k} b_{j,k} \tag{7.29}$$

where the order two tensor $b_{j,k} = \omega_j x_k$ is called the rotation tensor. If we derive the expression of the rigid rotation velocity field we obtain, due to the properties of the Levi Civita symbol, the following remarkable property:

$$\frac{\partial v_i}{\partial x_j} = -\frac{\partial v_j}{\partial x_i} \tag{7.30}$$

On the contrary, if we suppose that a particular velocity field obeys the relation (7.30) we obtain that the velocity field has necessarily to be obtained as in Equation 7.30 where $b_{j,k}$ is a nonnull tensor. Thus, we can conclude that Equation 7.30 univocally identifies a rigid rotation induced velocity field so that we can state that the viscous stress tensor has to be null for every velocity field characterized by the Equation 7.30.

The conditions that the viscous tensor depends only on the first derivative of the velocity and that it is zero if the velocity field is characterized by Equation 7.30 can be achieved simultaneously only if the viscous stress tensor contains only symmetrical combinations of terms in the form $(\partial v_i/\partial x_j + \partial v_j/\partial x_i)$ and $\partial v_k/\partial x_k$, that are all zero if Equation 7.30 holds. Moreover, in order to be a correctly defined tensor, the dependence of the viscous stress tensor on these terms has to be linear.

The most general tensor of this kind can be written as a function of only two constants η and ζ or the related constants η and $\beta = (\zeta/\eta + 1/3)$ as follows:

$$\gamma'_{i,j} = \eta\left(\frac{\partial v_i}{\partial x_j} + \frac{\partial v_j}{\partial x_i} - \frac{2}{3}\frac{\partial v_k}{\partial x_k}\right) + \zeta\delta_{ij}\frac{\partial v_k}{\partial x_k}\ (\Sigma\,i,j) =$$

$$= \eta\left(\frac{\partial v_i}{\partial x_j} + \frac{\partial v_j}{\partial x_i}\right) + (\beta - 1)\eta\delta_{ij}\frac{\partial v_k}{\partial x_k}\ (\Sigma\,i,j) \tag{7.31}$$

where, as explicitly indicated, the summation convention has not to be applied on the index i and j, even if they are repeated in the equation, as it is evident from the fact that the result is a rank two tensor and not a scalar also in the case $\zeta = 0$.

The parameters that characterize the material response appearing in Equation 7.31 are generally named as follows:

- Dynamic viscosity (η)
- Second viscosity (ζ)
- Dimensionless viscosity ratio (β)

Values of the dynamic viscosity for different fluids at room temperature (25°C) are reported in Table 7.1, while the dependence of the dynamic viscosity from temperature for a few liquids is represented in Figure 7.9. From the table we can see that viscosity ranges from very low values (in the order of 10^{-5}) to high values (in the order of 10^{12}), thereby spanning a range of more than 17 orders of magnitude. Thus, the behavior of viscous forces is very different from fluid to fluid.

The first of the two expressions of the viscous coefficients given by Equation 7.31 is normalized to insulate, analogously to what is done defining the stress tensor in the elasticity theory, the shear stress from the compressive stress. Under this point of view, the dynamic viscosity represents the shear module of the fluid and the second viscosity the compression module.

This interpretation of Equation 7.31 also allows an important simplification of the expression of the viscosity tensor to be obtained in case of uncompressible fluids, as almost all liquids used in microfluidic circuits are. In this case, the compression module has to be set to zero and the viscosity tensor expression simplifies as

$$\gamma'_{i,j} = \eta\left(\frac{\partial v_i}{\partial x_j} + \frac{\partial v_j}{\partial x_i}\right)\ (\Sigma\,i,j) \tag{7.32}$$

In order to evaluate theoretically the value of viscosity in liquids a microscopic theory of the interaction between liquid particles is needed. A quite complete review of classical theories is reported in [9], while more articulated theories based on statistical mechanical models are summarized in [10].

TABLE 7.1
Viscosity of Selected Fluids

Fluid	Viscosity (Pa s)
Air	1.8×10^{-5}
Helium	1.9×10^{-5}
Methane	2.0×10^{-5}
Oxygen	2.0×10^{-5}
Gasoline	6×10^{-4}
Water	10^{-3}
Ethyl alcohol	1.2×10^{-3}
Blood plasma*	1.5×10^{-3}
Mercury	1.6×10^{-3}
Blood (whole)*	4.0×10^{-3}
Ethylene glycol	20×10^{-3}
Olive oil	0.1
Lubrication oil	0.66
100% Glycerol	1.5
Honey	10
Corn syrup	100
Bitumen	10^{8}
Molten glass	10^{12}

Note: A temperature of 25°C is assumed but for blood and blood plasma* that are considered at physiological temperature of 37°C.

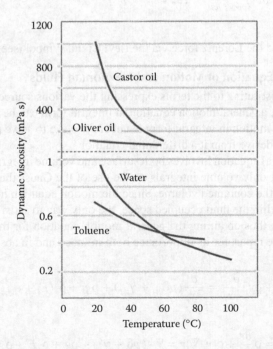

FIGURE 7.9 Dependence of the viscosity on temperature in selected Newtonian fluids.

The final equation for the momentum rate of change due to the attrition between fluids particles is

$$\left.\frac{\partial q_i}{\partial t}\right)_{viscous} = -\iint_{\Omega} \left[\eta\left(\frac{\partial v_i}{\partial x_j} + \frac{\partial v_j}{\partial x_i} - \frac{2}{3}\frac{\partial v_k}{\partial x_k}\right) + \zeta\delta_{ij}\frac{\partial v_k}{\partial x_k}\right]_{\Sigma ij} n_j \, d\Omega \tag{7.33}$$

7.3.1.4 Change of Momentum Due to Body Forces

Body forces are forces that act on each fluid particle due to some particular characteristic of the fluid.

We will take apart the problem of dealing with electromagnetic forces acting on charged fluids in such conditions that a static approximation cannot be done. On one side this is a very difficult subject, requiring relativistic fluid motion theory to be dealt correctly, on the other side this situation never occurs in microfluidic circuits, where the fluid velocity is always sufficiently small to neglect the fluid particles generated field and assume electrostatic or magneto-static approximation.

Thus, we will imagine a moving charged fluid undergoing gravity due to its mass and electrostatic and magneto-static forces due to its intrinsic charge. Beside the mass density of the fluid, we have to introduce the charge density ρ_e, driving electrostatic and magneto-static phenomena. Since the electrical charge is a quantity that is conserved during fluid motion, the charge density obeys a continuity equation completely analogous to Equation 7.18. In this approximation, not only will the gravitational field be unperturbed by the fluid motion and represented with a constant field through the gravity acceleration, but also the electrical and the magnetic fields can be considered constant external fields, not influenced by the motion of the charged fluid.

In this case, Newton second law can be applied directly so as to write the momentum rate of change as

$$\left.\frac{\partial q_i}{\partial t}\right)_{body\ forces} = \iiint_V \left[\rho g_i + \rho_e\ (E_i + \epsilon_{i,j,k}\ v_j B_k)\right] dV \tag{7.34}$$

where we have expressed the Lorentz force via the Levi Civita symbol (see Appendix 2).

7.3.1.5 The General Equation of Motion and Newtonian Fluids

From Equation 7.21, substituting to the terms expressing the various sources of momentum change their explicit expression, a general motion equation in integral form can be obtained. As frequently happens, an equation of motion in integral form is not easy to use to solve practical problems, thus it is customary to try to derive from it a differential equation.

In our case, the integral equation involves both surface and volume integrals and it can be reduced to an equation involving only volume integrals by the use of the Gauss theorem to rewrite surface integrals as integrals to the contained volume. Since the motion equation holds for every finite and infinitesimal volume within the fluid occupied space, the only way to satisfy it is to equal the functions under the integral; thus obtaining the general motion equation for the fluid local velocity in differential form, that we report for its importance both in index and in abstract notation:

$$\rho\frac{\partial v_i}{\partial t} + \rho v_j\frac{\partial v_i}{\partial x_j} = \frac{\partial}{\partial x_j}(p\delta_{i,j} + \gamma'_{i,j}) + \rho g_i + \rho_e(E_i + \epsilon_{i,j,k}v_j B_k) \tag{7.35a}$$

$$\rho\frac{Dv}{Dt} = \rho\frac{\partial v}{\partial t} + \rho(v\cdot\nabla)v = \nabla\cdot(p\underline{\delta} + \gamma') + \rho g + \rho_e E + \rho_e v \times B \tag{7.35b}$$

In the abstract expression of the general motion equation also Equation 7.6 for the material derivative has been used, so as to simplify the equation. The form (7.35b) of the motion equation is also quite intuitive, since it has essentially the same form of the Newton's second law, where the product of mass by acceleration (see Equation 7.11) equates the sum of the local applied forces. In general, Equations 7.35 makes no assumption of the viscosity parameters, so that they can depend, for example, on the shear stress or on other fluid motion variables, but for the fluid velocity.

In the case of several practical fluids, the dependence of the viscosity parameters on the stress terms, is very slow and in normal condition it can be completely neglected. The most important of these fluids, called Newtonian fluids, is water so that quite frequently diluted solutions of molecules in water behave as Newtonian fluids. However, remarkable exceptions exist (see Section 7.3.6), that are quite important in labs on chip design since they involve polymers chains and solutions where cells are diluted.

If a Newtonian fluid is considered, the constant nature of the coefficients η and β can be exploited to simplify the equation of motion. The computation is straightforward but cumbersome, and we encourage the interested reader to find it on standard books of fluid dynamics as in References [1–3]. The final result is the so-called Navier–Stokes equation, that is the general motion equation for Newtonian fluids, and writes

$$\rho \frac{\partial v_i}{\partial t} + \rho v_j \frac{\partial v_i}{\partial x_j} = -\frac{\partial p}{\partial x_i} + \eta \frac{\partial^2 v_i}{\partial x_i^2} + \beta\eta \frac{\partial}{\partial x_i} \frac{\partial v_j}{\partial x_j} + \rho g_i + \rho_e(E_i + \epsilon_{i,j,k} v_j B_k) \qquad (7.36a)$$

$$\rho \frac{\partial v}{\partial t} + \rho(v \cdot \nabla)v = -\nabla p + \eta \nabla^2 v + \beta\eta \nabla(\nabla \cdot v) + \rho g + \rho_e E + \rho_e v \times B \qquad (7.36b)$$

While dealing with microfluidics circuits, the fluid that is considered is quite frequently a liquid and the considered velocities are quite low with respect to the sound velocity in the fluid. The compressibility of various liquids at room temperature (25°C) and assuming a local velocity field much smaller than the sound speed in the liquid is shown in Table 7.2. From the table it results that neglecting the fluid compressibility to consider the fluid uncompressible is a well-verified approximation. Thus, in this case we can set $\beta = 0$ and the Navier–Stokes equations further simplifies as

$$\rho \frac{\partial v_i}{\partial t} + \rho v_j \frac{\partial v_i}{\partial x_j} = -\frac{\partial p}{\partial x_i} + \eta \frac{\partial^2 v_i}{\partial x_i^2} + \rho g_i + \rho_e(E_i + \epsilon_{i,j,k} v_j B_k) \qquad (7.37a)$$

$$\rho \frac{\partial v}{\partial t} + \rho(v \cdot \nabla)v = -\nabla p + \eta \nabla^2 v + \rho g + \rho_e E + \rho_e v \times B \qquad (7.37b)$$

Although quite simplified with respect to the general equation of motion (7.35) the Navier–Stokes equation for incompressible fluids is still very complex under a mathematical point of view,

TABLE 7.2

Compressibility (Change in Volume for a Change of 1 Pa in Pressure) for Selected Liquids at 25°C

Liquid	Compressibility (10^{-11}/Pa)
Carbon disulfide	93
Ethyl alcohol	110
Glycerine	21
Mercury	3.7
Water	45.8

mainly due to the nonlinear term $\rho(v \cdot \nabla)v$ that makes it very difficult to deal using analytical solution techniques.

In order to further simply the motion equations by maintaining a good accuracy in the microfluidic case, it can be noted that in a lab on chip the fluid velocity is generally quite small, due both to the small pressure and to the small dimensions of the microfluidics ducts that increase the effect due to attrition between the duct walls and the fluid. In order to exploit approximations that hold when a certain variable is small or great, we have to introduce a scale factor with which the considered variable can be compared, to quantitatively define what small and great means.

In our case, let us introduce scale factors for length and time, that we will indicate with ℓ_0 and t_0, respectively. The length scale factor is generally assumed as the typical length scale of the system under consideration while the time scale factor as the typical time characterizing the considered phenomena. Using the scale factors, the time and the coordinates can be substituted by dimensionless variables defined as

$$\bar{x}_i = \frac{x_i}{\ell_0} \tag{7.38}$$

$$\bar{t} = \frac{t}{t_0} \tag{7.39}$$

while scale factors for velocity and pressure immediately derive from the above assumptions allowing to define dimensionless velocity and pressure as

$$\bar{v}_i = \frac{t_0}{\ell_0} v_i = \frac{v_i}{v_0} \tag{7.40}$$

$$\bar{p} = \frac{t_0}{\eta} p = \frac{p}{P_0} \tag{7.41}$$

Substituting the dimensionless variables into the Equation 7.37, eliminating the term relative to body forces, that is naturally unaffected by the scaling and by the velocity regime of the fluid, and scaling the derivatives, the following result is obtained:

$$\mathcal{R}_e \left(\frac{\partial \bar{v}_i}{\partial \bar{t}} + \bar{v}_j \frac{\partial \bar{v}_i}{\partial \bar{x}_j} \right) = -\frac{\partial \bar{p}}{\partial \bar{x}_i} + \frac{\partial^2 \bar{v}_i}{\partial \bar{x}_i^2} \tag{7.42}$$

The dimensionless number $\mathcal{R}_e$ is defined as

$$\mathcal{R}_e = \frac{\rho v_0 \ell_0}{\eta} = \frac{\rho \ell_0^2}{\eta t_0} \tag{7.43}$$

and it is called the Reynolds number. The Reynolds number multiplies the term related to the inertia of the fluid and it allows to individuate two distinct regimes in the Newtonian fluid motion, corresponding to the conditions $\mathcal{R}_e \ll 1$ and $\mathcal{R}_e \gg 1$. In the first regime, the viscous term, represented by the second member of Equation 7.42, prevails on the inertia term, the motion is called viscous and the nonlinear term in Equation 7.43 can be neglected.

In the second regime, the motion is called inertial; in this case it is the viscous term that can be neglected and the motion equation is essentially nonlinear.

In a typical microfluidic circuit, the characteristic dimensions of ducts and reaction chambers are under the millimeter, and we do not make a great error fixing $\ell_0 = 0.1$ mm $= 10^{-4}$ m. As far as characteristics times they are of the order of 10 s so that velocities are of the order of 10 μm/s; thus, we can set $v_0 = 10^{-5}$ m/s. Assuming to deal with a diluted water solution at standard conditions we can also assume $\rho = 10^3$ Kg/m^3 and $\eta = 10^{-3}$ Pa s.

Substituting the above values in the expression of the Reynolds number we obtain $\mathcal{R}_e = 10^{-3}$. This is a really small value, so that, dealing with labs on chip, when the Newtonian approximation holds, generally also the so-called Stokes approximation can be performed, consisting in setting $\mathcal{R}_e \approx 0$.

Returning to dimensional variables and inserting the Stokes approximation into the motion equation in the absence of volume forces, we get the so-called Stokes equation, regulating the motion of Newtonian fluids in the viscous regime. If the Stokes approximation is applied rigorously, not only the inertial term $\bar{v}_j(\partial \bar{v}_i / \partial \bar{x}_j)$, but also the time derivative of the velocity can be neglected in Equation 7.42. However, in some problems it happens that the time reference scale is not related to the length and velocity scale, that is, to a characteristic time of the fluid motion, but it is imposed separately by the problem. As an example we can consider a rapidly opening and closing valve. The valve characteristic closing time can be of the order of 10^{-2} s, but this is not the correct time scale for the fluid motion, since the time scale has to be related correctly with the velocity scale. Other similar cases happen when fast time varying volume forces are considered like a fast varying electrical field. In these cases the velocity time derivative cannot be neglected even if the Reynolds number is very low.

Thus, a more general version of the Stokes equation is obtained by also including the time derivative of the speed so as to obtain

$$\rho \frac{\partial v_i}{\partial t} = -\frac{\partial p}{\partial x_i} + \eta \frac{\partial^2 v_i}{\partial x_i^2} \tag{7.44a}$$

$$\rho \frac{\partial v}{\partial t} = -\nabla p + \eta \nabla^2 v \tag{7.44b}$$

7.3.2 THE ENERGY EVOLUTION EQUATION

The general fluid dynamic phenomenon cannot be studied on the ground of the two basic governing equations we have deduced up to now, that is the continuity Equation 7.19 and the motion Equation 7.35 due to the fact that viscosity and other dissipative forces generates conversion of mechanical energy in heat during fluid motion. The generated heat is transported by the moving fluid and transmitted by one part of the fluid to the other by conduction, to generate a phenomenon of energy transportation during fluid motion. In labs on chip the heat generation or absorption can be also related to chemical reactions happening during motion, so that energy is also added or subtracted to the fluid.

It is thus clear that the study of energy dynamics is needed to derive a self-consistent model allowing a complete study of fluid-dynamics phenomena. Energy-related phenomena during fluid motion are better described by considering, besides thermodynamic intensive variables like pressure and temperature, extensive variables per unit mass so that the real value can be simply obtained by multiplying the result by the real fluid mass M.

Thus, we will introduce three intensive variables per unit mass: the internal fluid energy $u = U/M$, the entropy per unit mass $s = S/M$, and the volume per unit mass $v = V/M = 1/\rho$. The spatial densities related to the considered variables are obtained by multiplying the variables per unit mass by the mass density ρ so that, for example, the internal energy density μ is given by $\mu = U/V = \rho u$. Using these variables, the first thermodynamic principle writes

$$du = Tds - pd\left(\frac{1}{\rho}\right) = Tds + \frac{p}{\rho^2}d\rho \tag{7.45a}$$

The energy transport equation can be obtained with the same method already used for the motion equation: evaluating the internal energy variation rate taking into account all the energy conversion and transport phenomena and substituting its overall expression in the first thermodynamic principle.

Thus, let us fix a volume V of the fluid around a well-defined observation point. The overall fluid energy $\mathcal{E}$ is provided by the sum of the kinetic and the internal energy so that we can write

$$\frac{\partial \mathcal{E}}{\partial t} = \frac{\partial}{\partial t} \iiint_V \left(\frac{1}{2}\rho v^2 + \rho u \right) dV = \iiint_V \frac{\partial}{\partial t} \left(\frac{1}{2}\rho v^2 + \rho u \right) dV \tag{7.46}$$

where $v^2 = v \cdot v = v_i v_i$.

Possible causes of energy change are convection of mass through the surface Ω of the volume V, work done by pressure and by the viscous forces from the surrounding on the volume surface and by heat conduction due to the thermal gradient created at the volume surface.

Thus, we can write

$$\left. \frac{\partial \mathcal{E}}{\partial t} \right)_{conv} + \left. \frac{\partial \mathcal{E}}{\partial t} \right)_{press} + \left. \frac{\partial \mathcal{E}}{\partial t} \right)_{visc} + \left. \frac{\partial \mathcal{E}}{\partial t} \right)_{cond} = \iiint_V \frac{\partial}{\partial t} \left(\frac{1}{2}\rho v^2 + \rho u \right) dV \tag{7.47}$$

The computation of the four terms directly derives from the general description of the fluid motion we have done in the previous Section [3], but for the conduction term, that has to be evaluated by introducing a specific law for heat conduction, that is not included in the fluid motion analysis we have done up to now.

In particular, if we indicate with Φ_i^{conv} the energy flux by convection through the surface of the volume V we can write

$$\left. \frac{\partial \mathcal{E}}{\partial t} \right)_{conv} = -\iint_\Omega n_i \Phi_i^{conv} \, d\Omega = -\iint_\Omega \left(\frac{1}{2}\rho v^2 + \rho u \right) n_i v_i \, d\Omega \tag{7.48}$$

where the energy flux by convection is defined as (see Section 7.2.3):

$$\Phi_i^{conv} = \left(\frac{1}{2}\rho v^2 + \rho u \right) v_i \tag{7.49}$$

Regarding the contribution due to the work of the forces represented by the stress tensor we can write

$$\left. \frac{\partial \mathcal{E}}{\partial t} \right)_{press} + \left. \frac{\partial \mathcal{E}}{\partial t} \right)_{visc} = \iint_\Omega v_i (p\delta_{i,j} + \gamma'_{i,j}) n_j \, d\Omega \tag{7.50}$$

being $v_i(p\delta_{i,j} + \gamma'_{i,j})n_j$ the work of the stress forces acting on a unit surface.

As far as the heat conduction term is concerned, heat is transmitted when a temperature gradient is present, while when two bodies at the same temperature are put statically in contact no heat transfer happens. This means that the heat flux depends on the temperature difference. Transporting this observation in a continuous medium we can say that the local heat flux will depend on the derivatives of the scalar temperature field. Considering nearby points linear dependence can be assumed since higher degree terms nullify in the limit of zero distance more rapidly.

Thus, we can assume, in general, that in a continuous medium a local heat flux Φ_i^{heat} is present, whose components are a linear combination of the components of the temperature gradient. Defining a thermal conductivity tensor $\kappa_{i,j}$, that is independent from temperature and is a characteristic parameter of the considered material we have

$$\Phi_i^{heat} = -\kappa_{i,j}\frac{\partial T}{\partial x_j} \tag{7.51}$$

where the minus sign comes from the usual thermodynamic convention indicating as positive the acquired heat that corresponds to a negative temperature gradient.

Dealing with fluid dynamics, generally, the fluid medium can be considered isotropic, so that the thermal conductivity tensor depends on one parameter only being $\kappa_{i,j} = \kappa\delta_{i,j}$. In this case, the heat flux is simply proportional to the temperature gradient, being

$$\Phi_i^{heat} = -\kappa\frac{\partial T}{\partial x_i} \tag{7.52}$$

However, particular cases can occur also in fluid dynamics when anisotropy plays a role, for example, when long polymeric chains are diluted into a solution and are oriented in a well-defined direction. Using Equation 7.48 and recalling the convention on the orientation of the unit vector normal to a given surface (see Figure 7.8a) it is obtained

$$\left.\frac{\partial \mathcal{E}}{\partial t}\right)_{cond} = \iint_\Omega n_j \kappa\frac{\partial T}{\partial x_j}\, d\Omega \tag{7.53}$$

Substituting the energy rate expressions in Equation 7.47 we have an integral equation involving both volume integrals and integrals to the volume boundary surfaces. As in all the similar cases we can use the Gauss's theorem to reduce it to an equation involving only volume integrals and, by noting that such an equation have to hold for every volume inside the fluid occupied zone, we can equate the integrands. From this procedure the first form of the energy transport equation is obtained:

$$\frac{\partial}{\partial t}\left(\frac{1}{2}\rho v^2 + \rho u\right) = -\frac{\partial}{\partial x_i}\left[\left(\frac{1}{2}\rho v^2 + \rho u + p\right)v_i - \gamma_{ij}'v_j - \kappa\frac{\partial T}{\partial x_i}\right] \tag{7.54}$$

This form of the energy transport equation is useful due to its easy physical interpretation as an energy flux continuity equation. Looking at the term under parenthesis at the second member, it is possible to recognize it as the overall energy flux density

$$\Phi_i^{energy} = \left(\frac{1}{2}\rho v^2 + \rho u + p\right)v_i - \gamma_{ij}'v_j - \kappa\frac{\partial T}{\partial x_i} \tag{7.55}$$

so that Equation 7.54 can be rewritten in abstract notation as a continuity equation for the energy, that is intuitive since energy is a conserved quantity

$$\frac{\partial \mathcal{E}}{\partial t} = -\nabla \cdot \Phi^{energy} \tag{7.56}$$

The energy continuity equation is effectively a heat transfer equation, since the energy flux through the moving fluid is generated, in the Euler representation, by heat transmission causing the temperature of the fluid particles to change in time.

In order to render more explicit this nature of Equation 7.54 it is customary to express it as a function of the product $\xi = s\rho T$ where s is the entropy per unit mass.

By using the continuity equation and the Navier–Stokes equation to express differently the left-hand side of Equation 7.54 and exploiting the first principle of thermodynamic [2,3], the second form of the energy conservation equation is obtained:

$$\rho T\left[\frac{\partial s}{\partial t} + \left(v_j \frac{\partial}{\partial x_j}\right)s\right] = \gamma'_{ij} \frac{\partial v_i}{\partial x_j} + \frac{\partial}{\partial x_j}\left(\kappa \frac{\partial T}{\partial x_j}\right) \tag{7.57a}$$

$$\rho T\left[\frac{\partial s}{\partial t} + (v \cdot \nabla)s\right] = (\gamma'\nabla)v + \nabla(\kappa\nabla T) \tag{7.57b}$$

Due to its importance, Equation 7.57 is written both in index and in abstract notation and, as intuitive, the tensor product $(\gamma'\nabla)$ in Equation 7.57b has to be interpreted as a matrix product between the matrix representations of the tensors in the given reference frame.

Equation 7.57 can be easily interpreted by observing that the first member is the total time derivative of the entropy per unit mass times the density and the temperature, thus representing the overall heat density change of a moving fluid particle. At the second member we have the terms causing the heat density change: the friction due to viscosity and the heat conduction through the fluid.

Equation 7.57 is valid whatever fluid motion regime we are considering and it has a very wide application range. In microfluidics systems however, generally a set of approximations can be used to simplify the fluid-dynamics part of the problem. Pressure deviations are quite small in microfluidic problems and they can be neglected. Due to the fact that fluid speed is much smaller that sound speed in the fluid, this condition is also compliant with the fact that biochemical reactions are generally better performed under a constant pressure regime.

The entropy per unit mass is function of temperature and pressure, if pressure is almost constant it depends only on temperature. Using the thermodynamic relation $c_p = T\left.\frac{\partial s}{\partial T}\right)_p$, that gives the expression of the specific heat when the pressure is maintained constant, Equation 7.57 simplifies as

$$\rho c_p\left[\frac{\partial T}{\partial t} + \left(v_j \frac{\partial}{\partial x_j}\right)T\right] = \gamma_{ij} \frac{\partial v_i}{\partial x_j} + \frac{\partial}{\partial x_j}\left(\kappa \frac{\partial T}{\partial x_j}\right) \tag{7.58}$$

Equation 7.58 has the form of an equation for the temperature field in the fluid, once the fluid velocity field is known. Quite frequently, the system main parameters (i.e., $c_p, \gamma'_{ij}, \kappa$) can be assumed almost constant with respect to temperature, since temperature fluctuations are small with respect to their scale of variation. Moreover, considering a single phase incompressible liquid, the density is also constant.

Introducing the temperature diffusion coefficient $D_T = (\kappa/\rho c_p)$, Equation 7.58 further simplifies as

$$\frac{\partial T}{\partial t} = D_T \nabla^2 T \tag{7.59}$$

This is the so-called Fourier equation that is the simplest possible form of heat transmission equation in microfluidics and coincides with the heat transmission equation in isotropic solids.

7.3.3 NEWTONIAN LIQUIDS FLOW IN LAB-ON-CHIP DUCTS: SIMPLIFIED MODEL

At this point we can try to formulate a general form of the fluid dynamic problem. Once external forces, boundary conditions, and initial conditions are given, the problem is solved if the velocity vector field and three other scalar fields, the fluid temperature, density, and pressure, are determined. In order to do that, fluid dynamics provides a system of five partial differential equations: the three components of the vector Navier–Stokes equation (7.37), the mass continuity equation (7.19), and the energy transport equation (7.54). In order to have a well-conditioned problem we have to add a further equation relating the unknown fields. This is provided by the fluid state equation that describes the fluid material properties via a further relation among the fluid pressure, density, and temperature. The characteristic equation can be very simple, as in the case of ideal gasses, or quite complex, involving dependence of the fluid characteristics in a point from other characteristics in nearby points (see e.g., Section 7.3.6).

If no simplification is possible, the fluid dynamics problem is thus very complex; in several cases, however, it can be considerably simplified by exploiting either specific fluid characteristics or specific features of the system under analysis. In this section we will exploit general approximations that are almost always valid in microfluidics systems to simplify the fluid dynamic problem in a way suitable for the analysis of labs on chip circuits. As a first application we will analyze the flow of a Newtonian liquid through microfluidic ducts.

7.3.3.1 State Equation: Incompressibility Hypothesis

We will assume that the state equation of our liquid will reduce simply to the uncompressible property, that is, $\rho = \rho_0$, where ρ_0 is a given constant. The incompressibility hypothesis eliminates from the fluid-dynamic system the mass continuity equation and considerably simplifies the Navier–Stokes equation (see Section 7.3.1.5). Since electrical charges are transported by molecules and atoms, if the incompressibility approximation holds, generally also the electrical charge density, if present, can be considered constant.

Frequently, in microfluidic circuits the flowing liquids are diluted water solutions of macromolecules. In general, the density of a solution can be calculated by dividing the mass contribution m_j of each solution component by the overall volume V of the solution, that is, if we have h-1 solutes and indicate with the h component the solvent, we have

$$\rho = \frac{1}{V} \sum_{j=1}^{h} m_j = \frac{1}{V} \sum_{j=1}^{h} \rho_j V_i \tag{7.60}$$

being the overall volume not equal to the sum of volume V_i of the components of the solution. This is due to the hydration phenomenon (see Section 1.3), so that the overall volume is equal to the volume of the solvent part that is not involved in the hydration of the solutes plus the volume of the hydrates solutes that is quite different from the volume of the nonhydrate substances. From Equation 7.60, it is clear that, in case we deal with diluted solutions, the contribution of the solute is dominant, so that frequently no great error is done by considering the solution density equal to the solvent density.

Even in cases in which dilution is not sufficient to neglect the solute contribution, Equation 7.60 assures that, unless some element exists that changes the molar volume of the hydrated solute (like chemical reactions) the hypothesis of constant density holds for the solution very well if it holds for the solvent and for the dispersed molecules of hydrated solute.

The compressibility of water, defined as derivative of volume with respect to pressure divided by the volume, is very small and varies with temperature [11]. At $0°C$, at the limit of zero pressure, the compressibility is 5.1×10^{-10} Pa^{-10}. As the pressure is increased, the compressibility decreases,

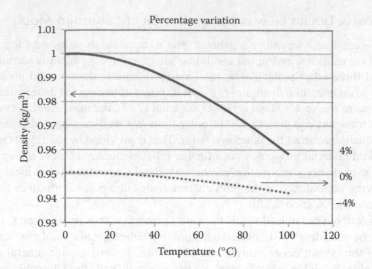

FIGURE 7.10 Absolute value and variation with respect to standard conditions of liquid water density versus temperature.

being 3.9×10^{-10} Pa^{-1} at 0°C and 100 MPa. Thus, in all microfluidics applications, water and diluted water solution can be considered incompressible.

Considering density of water in liquid state, its values are shown in Figure 7.10 versus temperature [11]. Also, the percentage density change with respect to normal conditions (25°C and pressure of one atmosphere) is shown in the figure. From Figure 7.10 it is evident that in a very wide range of temperature (from 0°C to about 40°C) the water density variation with temperature is smaller than 0.5% with respect to the density at standard conditions. Since almost all biological reaction happens well within this temperature range, diluted water solutions can be considered not only uncompressible, but also characterized by a temperature independent density when considering labs on chip.

7.3.3.2 Low Reynolds Number and Temperature Fluctuations

In Section 7.3.1.5 we have seen that some general characteristics of the motion of a fluid is determined by the value of a characteristic parameter of the motion, called Reynolds number ($\mathcal{R}_e$) . In particular, this parameter is related to the ration between the inertial contribution and the viscous contribution to the motion. In microfluidic circuits, due to the small linear dimensions involved and to the small fluid speeds, the Reynolds number is always much smaller than one, causing the inertial term to be negligible in the motion equation. This also implies (see Section 7.3.1.5) that using constant density, the Navier–Stokes equation can be used in the simplified Stokes form.

Due to temperature sensitivity of biochemical reactions, great temperature fluctuations cannot happen in labs on chip. On this ground, we can assume that the liquid dynamic viscosity and specific heat at constant pressure are independent from temperature. The validity and limits of this approximation in case of water can be understood by looking at Figures 7.10 and 7.11, where the dynamic viscosity at 100 kPa and the constant pressure heat capacity of liquid water are shown versus temperature [11].

The only appreciable variation with temperature within the relevant temperature range for biochemical reactions is the dynamic viscosity that however changes only 20% in between 20°C and 30°C. Thus, the constant parameters approximation can be assumed without great errors, taking under consideration that, if temperature fluctuations in the order of 10°C can be

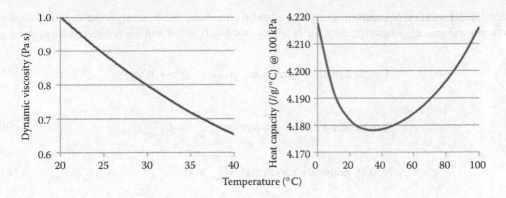

FIGURE 7.11 Dynamic viscosity and heat capacity of liquid water versus temperature.

forecasted and an accurate analysis of fluid motion has to be carried out, viscosity variations have to be considered.

Assuming the constant parameters approximation the temperature evolution equation can be approximated as a diffusion equation (see Section 7.3.2).

7.3.3.3 No-Slip Boundary Condition

Once the overall equation system regulating the fluid motion and energy exchange has been suitably simplified, it is important to state the form of the problem boundary conditions. The simpler situation under this point of view is fluid flow in a duct.

Such conditions summarize at a macroscopic level the interaction of the liquid molecules with the molecules of the duct walls. It is reasonable to assume that, in the absence of a particular interaction between the fluid and the walls (like the presence of an hydrophobic walls material or a chemical reaction between the fluid and the walls material) the loss of energy for attrition between the walls and the liquid is greater than that between adjacent liquid layers. Assuming that complete momentum relaxation happens when a fluid molecule hits the duct walls, it is possible to assume that the speed of fluid molecules adjacent to the duct walls is equal to the speed of the walls themselves. Thus, it is zero in a reference in which all the duct walls are still. This approximation is called no-slip boundary condition, since it assumes that the fluid does not slip when in contact with the duct walls.

The no-slip condition has been extensively studied both theoretically and experimentally in order to verify the validity and limits of the underlying approximation [12,13]. In Reference [12], in particular, an extended set of experimental measurements of the real slip degree of different liquids in contact with different solid materials during liquid flow is presented in order to allow a detailed evaluation of the accuracy of the no-slip approximation if needed.

Even if frequently quite accurate, practical cases exist where the no-slip assumption causes relevant errors due to a sensible slip on the walls. Besides the case of use of hydrophobic materials to fabricate the duct walls [14] slippage can occur on patterned surfaces or on surfaces [15] incorporating microstructures [16]. A very good review of more complex and accurate boundary conditions for Newton liquid flow that takes into account the slip of the liquid in contact with a solid surface is reported in Reference [17].

7.3.4 The Liquid Flow in a Microfluidic Duct: Poiseuille Flow

Summarizing all the assumptions we have detailed in Section 7.3.3, the flow of a Newtonian fluid in a microfluidic duct in the absence of electromagnetic phenomena, for example, the flow of a water diluted solution of macromolecules in a lab on chip duct, can be analyzed using the following mathematical model, where the duct walls are assumed still in the considered reference system:

$$\text{Stokes equation of motion} \quad \rho \frac{\partial v}{\partial t} = -\nabla p + \eta \nabla^2 v \quad (7.61\text{a})$$

$$\text{Temperature diffusion equation} \quad \frac{\partial T}{\partial t} = D_T \nabla^2 T \quad (7.61\text{b})$$

$$\text{No-slip boundary condition} \quad v\big|_{wall} = 0 \quad (7.61\text{c})$$

In this simplified form, the temperature-related problem is independent of the fluid motion problem, but for the case in which the fluid speed appears in the boundary conditions or in the initial conditions of the temperature equation.

Even with the great number of approximations we have done, the problem constituted by Equations 7.61 is in general a very complex problem, and a classification of the possible kind of motion helps in the analysis of practical cases.

A class of motions whose analysis is much simpler with respect to the general case is that of stationary motions, where the speed field does not depend on time. In this case, the first term of Equation 7.61a is zero and all the dynamic variables do not depend on time. In particular, the motion equation becomes simply

$$\nabla^2 v = \frac{1}{\eta} \nabla p \quad (7.62)$$

In stationary motions, the pressure is time independent and can be deduced from the problem conditions, so that Equation 7.62 simply states that the fluid velocity is a solution of the Laplace equation with the condition that v has to be zero on the duct border. In stationary problems, the local temperature has to remain constant in time. Generally, it is also assumed to be constant in space in the absence of external heat sources or sinks, neglecting heat generation due to viscosity.

External heat sources and sinks, like external heater or ongoing chemical reactions, can be present in stationary problems. In order to produce a constant local temperature, no net heat has to be added to the fluid and heat from sources has only to be transmitted by the fluid to the sinks where it is absorbed. In this case also the temperature equation becomes the Laplace equation, reducing to

$$D_T \nabla^2 T = 0 \quad (7.63)$$

Stationary motion through a microfluidic duct under the above conditions is generally called Poiseuille flow.

The simpler fluid dynamic problem that is practically relevant for labs on chip is pressure-driven fluid flow in a straight duct obtained by translation of its section $\mathcal{B}$ along the x-axis. In a realistic case a transition region is present near the input and the output sections of the duct, where the velocity profile is different from the stable profile existing well inside the duct. We will assume that our duct is so long that the transition region at the input and at the output are very small with respect to the duct length assuming that the input and the output velocity distributions are the same for the distribution inside the duct, so preserving the duct translational symmetry.

Let us assume a coordinate system where the x-axis coincides with the duct axis. In this way the duct profile is a closed regular curve on the (y, z) plane. To model this problem under a fluid dynamic point of view we have to solve Equation 7.62 with the no-slip condition all over the duct boundary. A first observation is that the volume forces acting on the fluid reduce to gravity, whose contribution is always orthogonal to the duct axis. It is thus completely compensated by the duct wall reaction and has no role in determining the characteristics of motion. Thus, the only element relevant to determine the motion characteristics is the pressure difference along the duct and, due to the duct symmetry and the uniformity of the boundary conditions, we derive that the pressure along the duct does not depend on the transversal coordinates (y, z), but only on the longitudinal coordinate x. Thus, the pressure along the duct can be written as $p(x)$.

The same problem symmetry forces the velocity field to be composed by vectors parallel to the x-axis and depending only on y and z, since no translational symmetry can be fulfilled if the y or z components are different from zero and if the velocity varies in different duct sections. Thus, the velocity field has to be written as

$$v = v(y,z)x \tag{7.64}$$

where x is the unit vector parallel to the x axis.

If the velocity field has the expression (7.64) we have $(v \cdot \nabla)v = 0$ so that in this case the nonlinear term can be eliminated from the Navier–Stokes equation without any approximation. Substituting the expression of the pressure and of the velocity field in the Stokes equation (7.62) we obtain the expression of the motion equation in this case

$$\eta\left(\frac{\partial^2 v}{\partial y^2} + \frac{\partial^2 v}{\partial z^2}\right) = \frac{\partial p}{\partial x} \tag{7.65}$$

Since the first member of Equation 7.65 depends only on y and z while the second depends only on x, the only possibility to fulfill the equation is that both are constant. From this condition we obtain the equation for the pressure along the duct that results simply to be

$$\frac{\partial p}{\partial x} = const \tag{7.66}$$

Setting $p(0) = p_0 + \Delta p$, where, $x = 0$ represents the duct input section, and $p(L) = p_0$ where $x = L$, is the duct output section, we get

$$p(x) = \frac{\Delta p}{L}(L - x) + p_0 \tag{7.67}$$

Thus, the motion equation reduces to a second-order linear differential equation for the speed field that writes

$$\frac{\partial^2 v}{\partial y^2} + \frac{\partial^2 v}{\partial z^2} = \frac{\Delta p}{L\eta} \tag{7.68}$$

that has to be solved imposing the no-slip boundary condition on the duct walls. Once the velocity field is determined, the volumetric flow rate Q, that is the fluid volume traversing the generic duct section in the unit time, can be evaluated from the simple flow rate definition

$$Q = \iint v(y,z)\,dydz \tag{7.69}$$

The flow rate depends naturally on the applied pressure difference Δp and it is quite interesting to deduce a relation between Q and Δp.

Let us consider the velocity field $v(y,z)$: it is surely a nonnegative limited and continuous function in a limited bi-dimensional domain, the duct section $\mathcal{B}$.

This means that it is a member of a suitably defined Hilbert functional space over $\mathcal{B}$ and the transversal operator $\nabla_t = (\partial^2/\partial y^2) + (\partial^2/\partial z^2)$ is a linear operator acting in this space. We can use the formal solution (A2.30) from Appendix 2 to express the solution of Equation 7.68 as a function of the eigen-functions $\varphi_n(y,z)$ of the transverse Laplace operator and, adopting the Dirac notation (see Appendix 2), we can express the velocity field as

$$| v \rangle = \frac{\Delta p}{L\eta} \sum_n \frac{\langle \varphi_n | 1 \rangle}{k_n} | \varphi_n \rangle \tag{7.70}$$

Where $|1\rangle$ is equal to one over all the duct section. Integrating to obtain the volumetric flow rate and remembering the definition (A2.21), we have

$$Q = \iint v(y,z)\,dy\,dz = \langle 1 | v \rangle = \frac{\Delta p}{L\eta} \mathcal{R}^2 B \sum_n \frac{1}{k_n \mathcal{R}^2} \frac{B_n}{B} \tag{7.71}$$

where the so-called hydrodynamic radius of the duct is defined as a function of the duct section area B and the duct perimeter as

$$\mathcal{R} = \frac{2B}{\mathcal{P}} \tag{7.72}$$

and the effective area covered by each eigenfuction of the transversal Laplace operator is defined as

$$B_n = \langle \varphi_n | 1 \rangle \langle 1 | \varphi_n \rangle \tag{7.73}$$

In the case of circular duct section, the volumetric flow rate can be exactly evaluated, obtaining simply

$$Q = \frac{1}{2} \frac{\Delta p}{L\eta} \frac{B^3}{\mathcal{P}^2} = \frac{1}{8} \frac{\Delta p}{L\eta} \mathcal{R}^2 B \tag{7.74}$$

Considering that generally real ducts have frequently a cross section with dimensions of the same order of magnitude in the y and z directions, let us rewrite Equation 7.71 as

$$Q = \frac{1}{2\vartheta} \frac{\Delta p}{L\eta} \frac{B^3}{\mathcal{P}^2} \tag{7.75}$$

where the form factor ϑ is provided by the expression

$$\frac{1}{\vartheta} = \sum_n \frac{8}{k_n \mathcal{R}^2} \frac{B_n}{B} \tag{7.76}$$

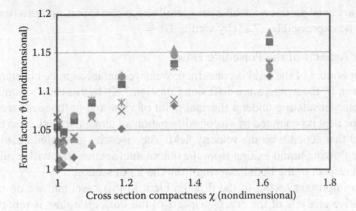

FIGURE 7.12 Form factor appearing in the expression of the volumetric flow rate versus the cross section dimensional compactness χ for various channels with regular cross section.

For ducts of different cross sections, the form factor can be evaluated numerically with great precision and a few results of such evaluations are synthesized in Figure 7.12. Form factors for various channels with regular cross sections are shown versus the cross section compactness χ, that is defined as

$$\chi = \frac{\mathcal{P}^2}{4\pi B} \tag{7.77}$$

where the factor 4π is added at the denominator to have unitary compactness in the case of the circle. To evidence the meaning of the compactness, it is put in relation with the eccentricity in the case of an ellipse in Figure 7.13. Here the eccentricity is defined as the ratio between the major and the minor ellipse axis, so that the eccentricity of a circle is one instead that zero resulting for the traditional definition. A compactness of 1.5 corresponds in this case to an eccentricity around 3.2, that is, to a section with the major axis about three times longer than the minor one.

From Figure 7.12 it is evident that $1/\vartheta$ is of the order of unit and it is really almost equal to one for the great majority of realistic ducts that are rarely characterized by a compactness greater than 1.5. Thus, quite surprisingly, almost all the geometrical dependence of the flow rate is captured by

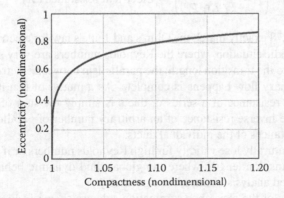

FIGURE 7.13 Compactness of an ellipse versus the ellipse eccentricity.

the cross section area and perimeter, with a very small shape correction, and in a first approximation the flow rate can be expressed by (7.85) by setting $1/\vartheta = 1$.

7.3.4.1 Energy Aspects of the Poiseuille Flow

As far as the temperature of the fluid is concerned, we have that it has to be constant in time and its distribution is given by the temperature diffusion Equation 7.63. In this case, assuming that the duct walls are completely insulating under a thermal point of view and at the same temperature of the incoming fluid, the heat is generated by viscous dissipation all along the motion, so that a distributed heat source exists that depends on the velocity field. The viscosity generated heat is removed from the system by the flowing liquid exiting from the output duct section that will result to be at higher temperature with respect to the liquid entering from the input section.

This is not an important aspect of the flow problem in this case, and we do not analyze it in detail, a quantitative analysis of the energy aspects of the Poiseuille flow is reported for example in References [2,3].

The final result is in any case quite interesting: the power dissipated by the viscous forces during the flow (W_d), that is exactly the energy per unit time exerted on the fluid by the external source creating the pressure difference, has a very simple and intuitive expression

$$W_d = Q \, \Delta p \tag{7.78}$$

The heat transport problem is the main part of the problem in cases in which the duct walls are at higher temperature with respect to the flowing fluid and the fluid is used to carry out heat from the duct walls and transport it out of the system through the output section: in this case the duct acts like a heat exchanger. This is an important application of microfluidic ducts, when they are used to create cooling of microsystems like very high performance electronic processors [18,19].

7.3.4.2 Hydrodynamic Circuit Theory

Equations 7.75 and 7.78 suggest an interesting parallel between the fluid dynamics of ducts circuits and electrical circuits.

In particular, setting the parallelism

- Flow rate (Q) $\rightarrow$ Electrical voltage (V)
- Pressure difference (Δp) $\rightarrow$ Electrical current (i)
- Hydraulic resistance

$$\left(r = \frac{1}{2\gamma} \frac{1}{L\eta} \frac{B^3}{\mathcal{P}^2} \right) \rightarrow \text{Electrical resistance } (\mathfrak{R})$$

Equations 7.75 and 7.78 exactly match the Ohm's and Joule's law for electrical resistive elements.

In a typical microfluidic situation, where the Reynolds numbers are very small and the ducts are quite long with respect to the transition length, the parallelism between electrical and fluidic circuits where Poiseuille stationary flow happens is complete. As a matter of fact it can be demonstrated [2,3] that the hydraulic resistance of a series of ducts is simply the sum of the resistances of the individual ducts and the inverse resistance of an arbitrary number of parallel ducts is equal to the sum of the inverse resistances of the individual ducts.

These simple rules naturally lose validity for high Reynolds numbers or if the duct is of the order of magnitude of the transition length, where the global fluid dynamic behavior have to be determined by a more detailed analysis of the system geometry.

The limits of validity of the resistance summation rule are shown in Figure 7.14. In this figure an example of a cascade of two rectangular microfluidic ducts where Poiseuille flow takes place is represented. The width of the two ducts (100 μm) is the same, while the height changes continuously

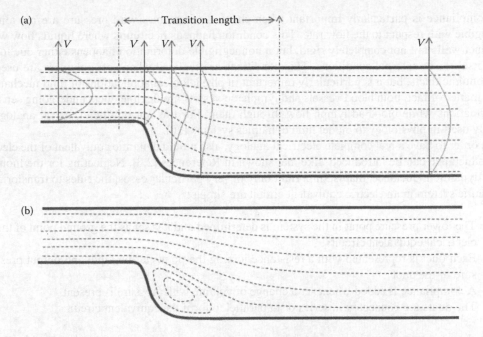

FIGURE 7.14 Example of two series of rectangular microfluidic ducts where Poiseuille flow takes place. The width of the two ducts is the same, while the height changes continuously as shown in Figure. In case (a), the Reynolds number is 0.001; in this condition the summation rule for series hydraulic resistances holds. In case (b), the Reynolds number is 100; vortices appears in the velocity field and the resistance summation rule does not hold.

as shown in the figure from 30 to 60 μm; the velocity field is obtained by numeric finite element simulation of the complete Navier-Stokes equation. The velocity field is represented in the figure through the flow line and the velocity dependence on z in selected duct sections.

In Figure 7.14a, the pressure difference is selected so as to obtain a Reynolds number of 0.001 so that the nonlinear term in the Navier–Stokes equation can be neglected and the velocity field has a null curl. In this condition, the summation rule for hydraulic resistances in series holds. In Figure 7.14b, the Reynolds number is 100 by setting a very high pressure difference. Here, the nonlinear term in the velocity equation cannot be neglected, vortices appear in the field and the resistance summation rule does not hold.

If the electrical analogy holds for the hydraulic resistance, it is possible to further develop it by introducing the hydraulic capacitance, generally called compliance. The electrical capacity is the derivative of the charge with respect to the applied voltage, thus following the hydrodynamic-electrical analogy we can introduce the compliance (C_{Hy}) as

$$C_{Hy} = \frac{dV}{dp} = \frac{Q}{(\partial p/\partial t)} \tag{7.79}$$

where V represents the volume of the fluid, so that C_{Hy} is the volume variation due to a pressure variation or, that is the same, the flow rate variation corresponding to a pressure variation in the unit time. Even if the fluid flowing through the ducts is assumed uncompressible, a very small variation of volume always happens if the pressure varies, so causing nonzero compliance. Within the same ranges of validity of the resistance summing rule, the hydraulic compliance of different ducts constituting a cascade or a parallel is summed exactly as electrical capacitance, completely extending the electrical-hydrodynamic parallel.

Compliance is particularly important when changes of volumes with pressure are not almost negligible with respect to the flow rate. This condition happens in circuits where liquids flow when the duct walls are not completely rigid, but a nonnegligible deformation happens either due to the flow itself or to external conditions. This conditions are realized when soft polymers are used in microfluidic ducts, but it is particularly important in physiological applications of fluid mechanics. As a matter of fact, both blood vessels and lymphatic vessels are flexible ducts undergoing sensible deformations while blood ad lymph flow through them. For this reason, the electrical analogy is widely used in physiology to model fluid dynamics systems [20].

In order to have a real complete electrical analogy, also a fluid dynamic equivalent of the electrical inductance can be introduced, like that shown in References [2,3]. Neglecting for the moment fluid dynamic inductance, that is, important only in very particular cases, the rules to transform an hydraulic system in an electric equivalent circuit are simple:

1. The lower pressure point in the system is determined and it is set as the ground point of the electrical equivalent circuit
2. Each duct is represented with a resistance joining the points at the input and output pressure of the duct
3. A compliance is added whenever a change of volume with pressure is present
4. The ducts are connected in series or in parallel to form the equivalent circuit

To show an example of application of this principle, let us analyze the bifurcation of a blood vessel in a main vessel and a side one, as it is shown in Figure 7.15. The scheme of the system is shown in Figure 7.15a besides the main fluid dynamic variables. The equivalent electrical circuit is shown in Figure 7.15b. In the limits of validity of the equivalence, the electrical circuits theory allows us to evaluate all the parameters in the circuits, like the flow rate in every branch and the response to the addition of a fluctuating part to one of the generators and so on.

7.3.4.3 Poiseuille Flow in Ducts with a Simple Geometry

In real microfluidic systems the ducts shape depends on the processes that are used to fabricate them. A summary of common fabrication techniques for microfluidic duct used in silica on silicon and polymers labs on chip is reported in Table 7.3. Besides the fact that practical ducts have

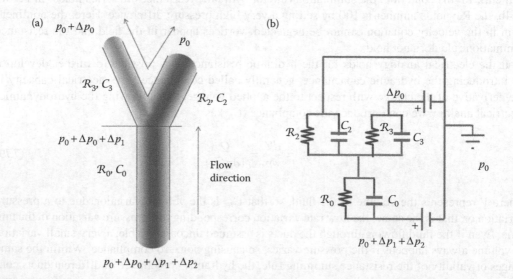

FIGURE 7.15 Simplified scheme of an arterial bifurcation (a) and the relative equivalent electrical circuit (b).

TABLE 7.3

Shapes of Practical Microfluidic Ducts versus the Used Material and the Fabrication Process

Application	Material	Fabrication Process	Shape	Compact-ness	Notes	Applicable Section of This Book
Chip inlet	Polymers	—	Circular	1		Section 6.5.3
On-chip duct	Silica on silicon	Anisotropic wet etching	Equilater triangle	1.65		Section 4.7.1
On-chip duct	Silica on silicon	Isotropic wet etching/RIE	Semi-circular	1.34	No fabrication on the upper wafer	Section 4.7
On-chip duct	Silica on silicon	Isotropic wet etching/RIE	Circular	1	Symmetric fabrication on the upper wafer	Section 4.7
On-chip duct	Silica on silicon	Anisotropic RIE	Rectangular	≥1.27	Minimum compactness for square duct	Section 4.7.3
On-chip duct	Polymers	Micro-molding/ hot embossing	Any	≥1	Fabrication on the upper wafer	Section 5.4
On-chip duct	Polymer	Laser ablation	Plane upper wall	≥1.34	No fabrication on the upper wafer	Section 5.7

Note: The duct application and the compactness are also reported.

generally small compactness, the recurrence of some particularly symmetrical shapes like rectangular, circular, and elliptical ducts can be observed. The velocity field in a few of such ducts can be calculated analytically under the hypothesis of Poiseuille flow, allowing to get rid of the approximations used up to now in this section (like $\vartheta = 1$). Here, we will review a few exact solutions for Poiseuille flow in particular ducts.

7.3.4.3.1 Elliptical and Circular Sections

Equation 7.68 can be exactly solved in a duct with an elliptical section by passing in elliptical coordinates in the (y, z) plane [2,3]. The problem solution is analytically trivial and the results in terms of velocity field and volume flow rate, assuming the ellipse main axis parallel to the y reference axis, can be written as

$$v(y,z) = \frac{\Delta p}{2L\eta a^2} \frac{\varepsilon^2}{1 + \varepsilon^2}\left(a^2 - y^2 - \frac{z^2}{\varepsilon^2}\right)$$

(7.80)

$$Q = \frac{\pi}{4}\frac{\Delta p}{L\eta}a\frac{\varepsilon^3}{1 + \varepsilon^2}$$

(7.81)

where a is the ellipse main semi-axis and ε the eccentricity (i.e., the ratio between the minor and the main axes). Setting in Equations 7.80 and 7.81 $\varepsilon = 1$ and $a = R$ we obtain the velocity field and the flow rate for a circular duct:

$$v(y,z) = \frac{\Delta p R^2}{4L\eta}\left(1 - \frac{y^2 + z^2}{R^2}\right)$$

(7.82)

$$Q = \frac{\pi}{8}\frac{\Delta p}{L\eta}R$$

(7.83)

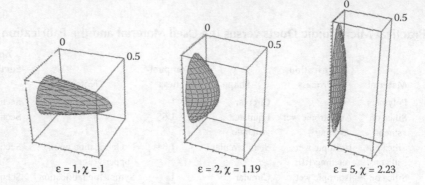

$\varepsilon = 1, \chi = 1$ $\varepsilon = 2, \chi = 1.19$ $\varepsilon = 5, \chi = 2.23$

FIGURE 7.16 Velocity field profile for elliptic ducts with different eccentricity, the same area and duct length and the same pressure difference on the terminal facets. The section compactness is also shown.

As anticipated, Equation 7.83 can also be written in the form (7.74) with the correct definition of the circle hydrodynamic radius. The shapes of the velocity field for elliptic ducts with different eccentricity, the same area and duct length and the same pressure difference on the terminal facets are shown in Figure 7.16, while the flow rate of the same family of ducts is shown in Figure 7.17. As intuitive, if ducts with the same length, area, and pressure difference are considered, the flow rate and the maximum of the velocity field decreases with the eccentricity and with compactness.

7.3.4.3.2 Equilateral Triangle Section

The equilateral triangle section is interesting for microfluidics since it can be obtained in practice by wet anisotropic etching in silicon (see Table 7.3). Let us consider a triangle section like that presented in Figure 7.18a, with the lower side parallel to the y-axis and the opposite vertex in the origin. Let us call a the triangle side.

The velocity field can be determined exactly in this kind of duct by assuming as trial solution of the motion equation the product of the equations of the three lines constituting the borders of the triangular cross section. Substituting the trial solution into the motion equation it is possible to determine the unknown constant, thus obtaining the following exact expression of the velocity field:

$$v(y,z) = \frac{1}{2\sqrt{3}} \frac{\Delta p}{\eta L} \left(\frac{\sqrt{3}}{2} - \frac{z}{a} \right) (z^2 - 3y^2) \tag{7.84}$$

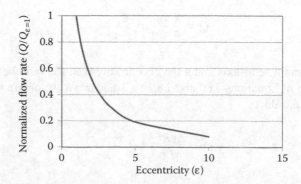

FIGURE 7.17 Relative flow rate versus ellipse eccentricity for the family of ducts considered in Figure 7.16. The flow rate is normalized to its value for a circular cross section.

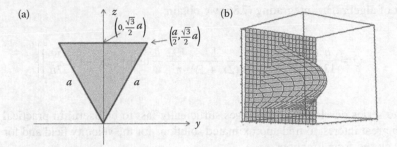

FIGURE 7.18 The triangular cross-section considered in the evaluation of the Poiseuille velocity field and flow rate (a) and the velocity field profile (b).

The profile of the velocity field is reported in Figure 7.18b. The flow rate can be simply obtained by integration as

$$Q = \frac{\sqrt{3}}{320} \frac{a^4}{\eta L} \Delta p \tag{7.85}$$

7.3.4.3.3 Rectangular Section

In microfluidic applications, the rectangular section is perhaps the most important, being possible to fabricate rectangular ducts both for silica on silicon and polymer labs on chip. In this case however, in spite of the simple and symmetry rich cross-section shape, a close form exact solution for the velocity field does not exist. A series expansion of the solution can be found that converges with reasonable rapidity, increasing the number of considered terms, so as to be useful for practical applications.

This solution can be found by considering the cross section placed as in Figure 7.19 with respect to the reference system and considering every function as periodical with period $(-w, w)$ along the y-axis and $(-h, h)$ along the z-axis. Applying the Fourier development to both terms of the motion equation and solving for the coefficients we obtain

$$v(y, z) = \frac{4h^2}{\pi^3} \frac{\Delta p}{\eta L} \sum_{n=0}^{\infty} \frac{1}{(2n+1)^3} \left[1 - \frac{\cosh((2n+1)\pi y/h)}{\cosh((2n+1)\pi w/2h)} \right] \sin\left[(2n+1)\pi \frac{z}{h} \right] \tag{7.86}$$

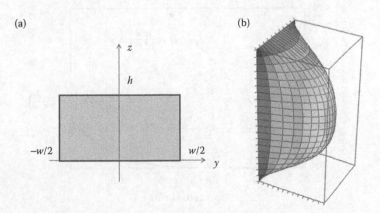

FIGURE 7.19 The rectangular cross-section considered in the evaluation of the Poiseuille velocity field and flow rate (a) and the velocity field profile (b).

With a bit of algebra, by integrating (7.86) we obtain

$$Q = \frac{h^2 w}{12\eta L}\Delta p\left\{1 - \sum_{n=0}^{\infty}\frac{1}{(2n+1)^5}\frac{192}{\pi^5}\frac{h}{w}\tanh\left[(2n-1)\pi\frac{w}{2h}\right]\right\} \tag{7.87}$$

Even if the series development converges sufficiently fast to be useful in practical problems, it has anyway a great interest to find approximated solutions for the velocity field and for the flow rate expressed by closed form functions.

A first approximation attempt, that is useful in many cases in planar microfluidics is to consider the rectangular duct like a slab. This happens when $w \gg h$. In this approximation the effect on the flow of the smallest duct walls can be neglected considering the duct as infinitely wide in the y direction. In this case the equation for the stationary flow becomes an ordinary differential equation whose solution is

$$v(z) = \frac{1}{2}\frac{\Delta p}{\eta L}(h - z)z \tag{7.88}$$

The corresponding flow rate is easily found to be

$$Q = \frac{h^3 w}{12\eta L}\Delta p \tag{7.89}$$

The accuracy of such an approximation in the case of a rectangular duct in terms of error in the flow rate estimation is reported in Figure 7.20 versus the aspect ratio w/h of the duct. The error is still as high as 23% for an aspect ratio of 3 and becomes 7% for an aspect ratio of 10. The slab approximation thus is usable only if the duct is a real slab, with an aspect ratio greater than 10. Considering the flow rate only, a much better approximation can be attained starting from (7.87) and noting that if $w > h$ the hyperbolic tangent can be approximated with its limit value equal to one. Using this approximation and exploiting the properties of the Riemann zeta function [3] we get to the following approximation for the flow rate in a rectangular duct:

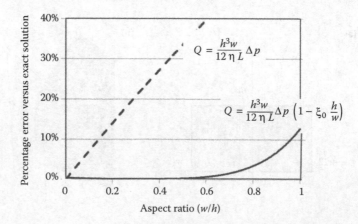

FIGURE 7.20 Error for different approximations of the Poiseuille flow rate through a rectangular duct versus the duct aspect ratio.

$$Q = \frac{h^3 w}{12\eta L} \Delta p \left(1 - \xi_0 \frac{h}{w}\right) \tag{7.90}$$

where the approximation parameter ξ_0 can be expressed as

$$\xi_0 = \frac{192}{\pi^5} \frac{31}{32} Z(5) \approx 0.630 \tag{7.91}$$

where $Z(s)$ is the Riemann zeta function of the complex number s. The error due to approximation (7.90) is also reported in Figure 7.20. This is a much better approximation of the flow rate: in the most unfavorable case, that is $w = h$, the error is only 13% and it is below 0.2% for an aspect ratio smaller than 0.5.

7.3.4.4 Transition Region at the Duct Input/Output

The solutions for the viscous flow problem in microfluidics ducts we have found in this section assume that the duct is very long and that the transition between the external fluid velocity and the spatially stationary velocity at the input and output of the duct is negligible.

This condition is not always fulfilled in real ducts, thus it is interesting to estimate the width of such a transition region. This problem is very hard to be solved in general, whatever is the duct section; however, it is easy to imagine that the order of magnitude of the transition length does not critically depend on the duct section. We will consider the flow in a semi-infinite circular duct starting from a uniform speed distribution v_0 at the duct input; the situation is represented schematically in Figure 7.21. The pressure difference for unit length is given through the constant pressure derivative along the duct axis $\partial p / \partial x$.

The input pressure and the input flow velocity are naturally related by the fact that we are assuming that all the fluid at the input section enters the duct and that, far from the duct input, a Poiseuille flow is established. This relation can be found by noting that the flow is constant in every duct section.

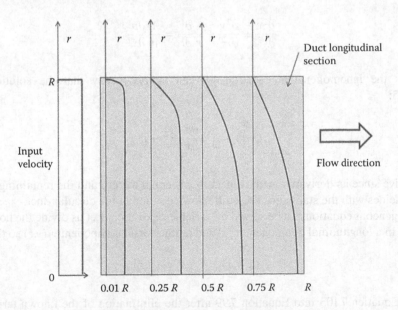

FIGURE 7.21 Flow velocity profile in different sections of a duct fed with a constant velocity flow. Half the longitudinal section of the duct is represented.

The offered flow rate is equal to $Q_{off} = \pi R^2 v_0$ while the maximum duct flow rate with the a given pressure is $Q_{in} = (\pi R^4/8\eta)(\partial p/\partial x)$. Setting $Q_{in} = Q_{off}$, we find

$$\frac{\partial p}{\partial x} = \frac{8\eta v_0}{R^2} \tag{7.92}$$

so that the pressure drop along the duct is determined by the input flow velocity. The motion equation is the Stokes equation that writes

$$\frac{\partial^2 v}{\partial x^2} + \frac{\partial^2 v}{\partial y^2} + \frac{\partial^2 v}{\partial z^2} = \frac{1}{\eta}\frac{\partial p}{\partial x} \tag{7.93}$$

The boundary conditions, taking into account the prescribed input velocity distribution, the fact that in the case of infinitely long duct the speed distribution has to reduce to a Poiseuille stationary distribution and the no-slip condition on the duct walls, write

$$v(x,R) = 0 \tag{7.94a}$$

$$v(0,r) = v_0 \tag{7.94b}$$

$$\lim_{x \to \infty} v(x,r) = \frac{1}{4\eta}\frac{\partial p}{\partial x}(R^2 - r^2) \tag{7.94c}$$

where v_0 is the input velocity and R is the duct radius.

Equation 7.93 is an inhomogeneous linear differential equation, thus we can write its solution as the sum of a solution of the inhomogeneous equation plus the general solution of the homogeneous one.

Considering polar coordinates on the duct transverse plane and assuming the velocity field independent from the azimuthal angle due to the circular symmetry of the problem 7.93 writes

$$\frac{\partial^2 v}{\partial x^2} + \frac{\partial^2 v}{\partial r^2} + \frac{1}{r}\frac{\partial v}{\partial r} = \frac{1}{\eta}\frac{\partial p}{\partial x} \tag{7.95}$$

As far as the inhomogeneous equation we can simply verify that the solution satisfies Equation 7.95:

$$v_{in}(x,r) = \frac{1}{4\eta}\frac{\partial p}{\partial x}(R^2 - r^2) \tag{7.96}$$

This is intuitive since its derivative with respect to x is equal to zero and the remaining part of the equation coincides with the stationary Poiseuille flow equation in the circular duct.

The homogeneous equation can be solved by variable separation. Let us divide the homogeneous velocity field in a longitudinal component $v_L(x)$ and a transversal component $v_T(y,z)$ so that

$$v_{ho}(x,y,z) = v_L(x)\,v_T(y,z) \tag{7.97}$$

Inserting Equation 7.103 into Equation 7.99 after the elimination of the known term, dividing the variables through the introduction of the parameter K^2 and passing in polar coordinates in the transverse equation we get

$$\frac{\partial^2 v_L}{\partial x^2} - K^2 v_L = 0 \tag{7.98a}$$

$$\frac{\partial^2 v_T}{\partial r^2} + \frac{1}{r}\frac{\partial v_T}{\partial r} = -K^2 v_T \tag{7.98b}$$

Both this equations can be solved analytically. The first equation, after eliminating the divergent solution that has no physical meaning has the solution

$$v_L(x) = v^* e^{-Kx} \tag{7.99}$$

While the second equation is well known in the theory of Bessel functions, since its general solution is a linear combination of the zeroth order Bessel functions of the first and second kind, $J_0(x)$ and $Y_0(x)$, respectively [21]. Since $Y_0(x)$ diverges for $x = 0$ we can eliminate this part of the solution and write

$$v_T(r) = c_n J_0(Kr) \tag{7.100}$$

The plot of the function $J_0(r)$ is provided for reference in Figure 7.22. Using the set of base solutions we have found we can express the velocity field as

$$v(x,r) = \frac{1}{4\eta}\frac{\partial p}{\partial x}(R^2 - r^2) + \sum_{n=1}^{\infty} c_n J_0(K_n r) e^{-K_n x} \tag{7.101}$$

where the constant v^* has been inserted into the coefficients c_n.

The parameters that are still present in the solution have to be determined by imposing the boundary conditions. We found easily that the no-slip condition is satisfied automatically by the first term of the solution, while to satisfy it also for the second term we have to write

$$K_n = \frac{\varphi_n}{R} \tag{7.102}$$

where φ_n is the set of zeros of the function $J_0(r)$. This sets the values of the variable separation parameter K_n. The parameters c_n has to be determined with the condition that $v(0, r) = v_0$.

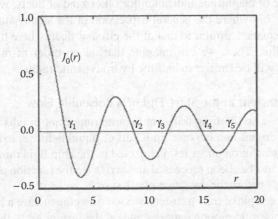

FIGURE 7.22 Plot of the zeroth-order Bessel function with its zeros put in evidence.

This brings to set the following equality

$$\sum_{n=1}^{\infty} c_n J_0\left(\frac{\varphi_n}{R} r\right) = v_0 - \frac{1}{4\eta} \frac{\partial p}{\partial x}(R^2 - r^2) = -\frac{1}{4\eta} \frac{\partial p}{\partial x}(D^2 - r^2) \tag{7.103}$$

being

$$D = \sqrt{R^2 - \frac{4\eta v_0}{\dfrac{\partial p}{\partial x}}} = \frac{R}{\sqrt{2}} \tag{7.104}$$

With this assumption 7.103 can be explicitly solved by multiplying both the members by $J_0((\varphi_m/R)r)$ and integrating. Using the orthogonal property of $J_0((\varphi_m/R)r)$ [21] and the property of the first type Bessel function

$$\int J_0(\omega)\omega\, d\omega = J_1(\omega)\omega \tag{7.105}$$

we obtain

$$c_n = -\frac{R^2}{8\eta} \frac{\partial p}{\partial x} \frac{8 - \varphi_n^3}{\varphi_n^3 J_1(\varphi_n)} \tag{7.106}$$

being $J_1()$ the order one Bessel function and Equation 7.105 has been used.

The final result for the velocity field is thus

$$v(x,r) = \frac{1}{4\eta} \frac{\partial p}{\partial x}(R^2 - r^2) - \frac{R^2}{4\eta} \frac{\partial p}{\partial x} \sum_{n=1}^{\infty} \frac{8 - \varphi_n^3}{\varphi_n^3 J_1(\varphi_n)^2} J_0\left(\frac{\varphi_n}{R} r\right) e^{-\frac{\varphi_n}{R} x} \tag{7.107}$$

This is a rapidly converging series and the plots in Figure 7.21 are obtained evaluating the shape of the velocity field for different abscissas along the duct axis. From Equation 7.107 it is evident that the main length scale determining the length of the transient region is R/φ and since $\varphi_1 \approx 2.405$ it is near the half of the duct radius.

If we search an order of magnitude indication for other kind of ducts, we have to remember the approximated Equation 7.74 where the general expression of the steady state flow rate in a duct is approximated with an equation similar to that of the circular duct, where the hydrodynamic radius substitutes the duct radius. Thus, we can imagine that, as an order of magnitude, the transition region in a general duct will be similar to half the hydrodynamic radius.

7.3.4.5 Temporal Transient at the Start/End of a Poiseuille Flow

Besides space transition, also the time transient is quite important in labs on chip. As a matter of fact, the hydrodynamic circuit in a lab on chip is full of liquid before starting the operation and at the moment in which the solution under test is injected in the chip fluid motion begins. Conversely, when the solution under test has been processed and arrives in the reaction chamber it is not unusual that the fluid motion ends before the detection phase starts.

In order to study an example of time transient, we will imagine to have a long section of a circular duct when stationary Poiseuille motion happens and, at the instant $t = 0$, the pressure difference is instantaneously dropped so that, after a time transient, the fluid comes to a stop.

Even if the pressure source, a pump for example, is instantaneously switched off, the pressure difference does not decay instantaneously through the duct, but a pressure wave propagates along the duct at the speed of sound in the fluid. This means not only that the perturbation arrives with a certain delay to a generic duct section, but also that the pressure transition at the generic duct section is not abrupt, but has a duration that depends on the fluid elastic time constant.

In microfluidic circuits the fluid speed is generally much smaller than the sound speed in the considered liquid (sound speed in water is for example 1484 m/s at standard conditions). Thus, the dynamics of the pressure wave propagating through the duct can be neglected if the fluid motion is under analysis. Under this hypothesis we can assume that an instantaneous pressure transition happens at each duct section so that the motion equation for $t > 0$ writes

$$\rho \frac{\partial v}{\partial t} = \eta \left(\frac{\partial^2 v}{\partial y^2} + \frac{\partial^2 v}{\partial z^2} \right) \tag{7.108}$$

This time we have an homogeneous problem that has to be solved under the following conditions:

$$v(R,t) = 0 \tag{7.109a}$$

$$v(r,0) = \frac{1}{4\eta} \frac{\partial p}{\partial x} (R^2 - r^2) \tag{7.109b}$$

$$\lim_{t \to \infty} v(r,t) = 0 \tag{7.109c}$$

where r is the radial coordinates on the transversal duct section and, due to the infinite sound speed hypothesis, the velocity field is the same in every transversal section.

Equation 7.108 can be solved by variable separation using a procedure quite similar to those adopted in the previous section. The final result writes

$$v(r,t) = \frac{R^2}{4\eta} \frac{\partial p}{\partial x} \sum_{n=1}^{\infty} \frac{8}{\varphi_n^3 J_1(\varphi_n)^2} J_0\left(\frac{\varphi_n}{R} r\right) e^{-\frac{\varphi_n^2}{R^2} \frac{\eta}{\rho} t} \tag{7.110}$$

Here, the first series term contains the exponential factor that regulates the decay in time of the velocity field. Thus, the main time constant of the velocity decay is given by

$$= \frac{R^2}{\varphi_1^2} \frac{\rho}{\eta} \tag{7.111}$$

In the case of a typical microfluidic duct, with a radius of 30 μm, using data from water and remembering that $\varphi_n 1 \approx 2.405$ we get $\tau \approx 180$ μs. The velocity profiles for different instants during the velocity field relaxation are shown in Figure 7.23.

7.3.5 INTERFACES PHENOMENA AND DROPLETS

Up to now we have considered the flow of a fluid, mainly a liquid, into a duct. The contact between the duct walls and the liquid has been described using the no-slip condition, assuming that the fact that two surfaces are at contact produces a force opposing the fluid motion so strong that it completely stops the motion of the fluid particles in contact with the solid wall.

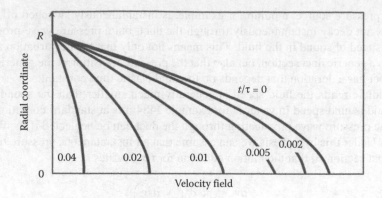

FIGURE 7.23 Flow velocity profile at different times during the relaxation of a Poiseuille velocity field in a circular duct due to pressure difference elimination.

In this section, we will go more in deep into the mechanisms causing this force and we will review a few related effects.

If we consider a particle inside a fluid that is not a perfect gas, they interact one with the other up to reach a minimum energy state that determines the properties of the fluid in thermodynamic equilibrium. For example, water molecules in liquid water interacts via hydrogen bonds as shown in Figure 7.24 (see Section 1.2.6). The presence of the intermolecular bonds decreases the Gibbs free energy per unit fluid volume allowing it to remain in a minimum energy state.

Molecules that are present on the contact surface between the fluid and another material (both another fluid or a solid) lack interaction with similar molecules all around them and, even if they can create weak bonds with the molecules of the other material, they have generally a greater energy with respect to the inner molecules of the fluid. This effect creates a specific amount of free energy G for unit area A that is called surface tension and mathematically is defined as

$$\gamma = \left(\frac{\partial G}{\partial A} \right)_{p,T,M} \tag{7.112}$$

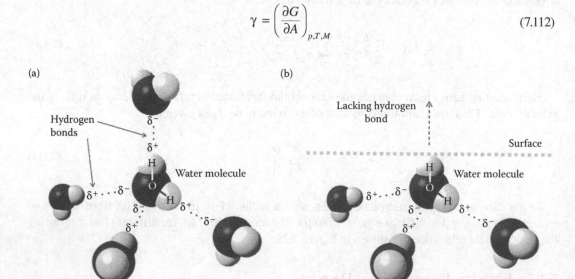

FIGURE 7.24 Hydrogen bonds among molecules in liquid water. Molecules in the water volume, (a) are bonded with four other molecules: two bonds are formed by the two hydrogen toward oxygen atoms and two bonds are created by the oxygen toward other molecules hydroges. Molecules on a surface (b) lack at least one bond, so having an higher energy.

Since, the temperature, the pressure, and the overall mass (or number of moles) of the fluid changes the free energy, these thermodynamic quantities have to be maintained constant in order to determine the effect of the presence of the surface on G; the surface tension is measured in $J/m^2 = N/m = Pam$ from which its name.

The existence of a surface tension means that in order to create a surface, for example, dividing a fluid mass in two parts, it is needed to spend energy and the quantity of spent energy depends essentially on the fluid and on the extension of the surface. It also means that a force is generated at the surface between a fluid and another material when the equilibrium situation is changed, that tends to restore the minimum energy situation.

The value of the surface tension depends mainly on the materials in contact and on temperature. An example of the dependence on temperature is shown in Figure 7.25, where surface tension data for pure water and benzene at equilibrium pressure with air are shown at different temperatures.

The study of the dependence of the surface tension on temperature starting from prime principles is quite complex and generally has to be carried out specifically for a given couple of substances [22–24]. In order to use a general model, empirical formulas are generally used [25]. The most known of such empirical models is the Eötvös model based on the following relation:

$$\gamma V^{2/3} = K_\gamma (T_c - T - T_{corr}) \tag{7.113}$$

where

- T_c is the vapor-liquid critical temperature at which no phase boundary exists between the vapor and liquid phases of the material; for water the critical temperature is about $374°C$.
- V is the molar volume of the considered substance; for water it is equal to 1.8×10^{-2} L/mole.
- K_γ is a constant independent of the specific substance; a typically used value is 2.1×10^{-7} $[JK^{-1} \, mol^{-2/3}]$.
- T_{corr} is a substance independent correction factor that has to be determined to optimize the fit of the equation; its most used value is 6 K at low temperatures, well below $0°C$, and 0 K at standard conditions.

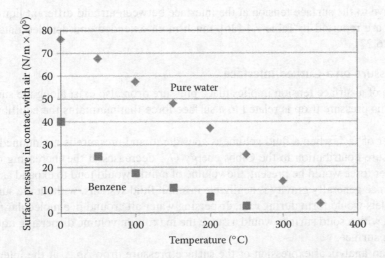

FIGURE 7.25 Surface tension data for pure water and benzene at equilibrium pressure with air are shown at different temperatures. (Data from Speight J., *Lange's Handbook of Chemistry, McGraw-Hill Professional*; 16th edition (December 20, 2004), ISBN-13, 978-0071432207; Jasper J. J., The surface tension of pure liquids compounds, *Journal of Physical Chemistry Reference Data*, vol. 1, pp. 841–1009, 1972.)

TABLE 7.4

Surface Tension of Different Liquids in Contact with Air at Selected Temperatures

Liquid	Surface Tension, $\gamma(N/m \times 10^{-3})$	Temperature (°C)
Acetic acid	27.6	20
Acetic acid (40.1%) + water	40.68	30
Acetic acid (10.0%) + water	54.56	30
Acetone	23.7	20
Diethylether	17.0	20
Ethanol	22.27	20
Ethanol (40%) + water	29.63	25
Ethanol (11.1%) + water	46.03	25
Glycerol	63	20
n-Hexane	18.4	20
Isopropanol	21.7	20
Liquid helium II	0.37	−273
Liquid nitrogen	8.85	−196
Mercury	487	15
Methanol	22.6	20
n-Octane	21.8	20
Sucrose (55%) + water	76.45	20
Water	75.64	0
Water	71.97	25
Water	67.91	50
Water	58.85	100
Toluene	27.73	25

Data relative to the surface tension at the interface between air and different liquids at selected temperatures are reported in Table 7.4 [26], much more extended and detailed data are found in References [26,27].

7.3.5.1 Pressure on a Curved Interface

The existence of a surface tension implies that a pressure drop also exist along the surface between two fluids. This pressure drop is related to a surface force that maintains the equilibrium shape of the interface.

As a matter of fact, when a fluid volume is considered and pressure is maintained constant, the volume–pressure contribution to the Gibbs energy G_{VP} decreases at the increasing of the volume and, if no other force would be present, the volume of a fluid would tend to expand as much as possible. Thus, since generally gravity is negligible in small fluid systems, without the surface pressure drop, no droplets would form during rain, dispersing water all around in a molecular mist and a liquid in contact with a solid surface would assume the maximum volume dispersing liquid molecules all around the surface.

To derive an analytical expression of the surface pressure drop Δp_{surf} at the interface between two fluids, let us consider a very small part of the equilibrium surface, whose lateral dimensions are δx and δy and let us assume that the areas of the surface δA can be well approximated with

$$\delta A = \delta x \delta y \tag{7.114}$$

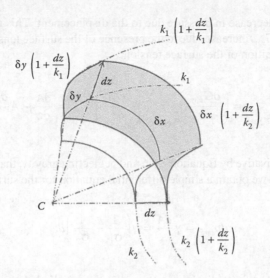

FIGURE 7.26 Graphical definition of the parameters used in the evaluation of the surface pressure on a curve surface where the surface undergo an infinitesimal displacement.

Let us also imagine a surface perturbation that moves the surface of an infinitesimal displacement dz as it is depicted in Figure 7.26. If the displacement dz is operated on every point of the surface by connecting that point to a displacement center C (see Figure 7.26) and moving all the points either toward or on the opposite side of that center, the surface element not only varies its area, but it is also deformed.

The two local main curvature radii (σ_1 and σ_2) in the hypothesis of very small surface element are at first-order constant over the whole surface element both before and under the displacement. These radii changes from σ_j to σ'_j due to the displacement and their first-order variation be written as

$$\sigma'_j = (\sigma_j + dz) = \left(1 + \frac{dz}{\sigma_j}\right)\sigma_j(\Sigma j) \quad (j = 1,2) \tag{7.115}$$

where the implicit summation rule has not to be used. The surface element area variation can also be expressed as a function of the displacement as

$$dA = \left(1 + \frac{dz}{\sigma_1}\right)\left(1 + \frac{dz}{\sigma_2}\right)\delta x \, \delta y - \delta x \, \delta y = \left(\frac{1}{\sigma_1} + \frac{1}{\sigma_2}\right)A \, dz \tag{7.116}$$

where the second-order term in the displacement has been neglected.

Since we started from a portion of the equilibrium surface, this was a minimum free energy surface and the following condition has to be verified:

$$\left(\frac{\partial G}{\partial z}\right)_{T,p,M} = 0 \tag{7.117}$$

The variation of the free energy related to an equilibrium surface displacement is essentially composed of two terms: the first is the decrease of the volume–pressure free energy G_{pV}, as anticipated previously, that can be written as the product of the incremental volume and of the pressure surface drop, that is the decrease in pressure due to the displacement. This term has to be balanced by a surface free energy G_{surf} increase, due to the presence of the surface tension. Thus we can write, on the ground of the definition of the surface tension:

$$\left(\frac{\partial G}{\partial z}\right)_{T,p,M} = \left(\frac{\partial G_{surf}}{\partial z}\right)_{T,p,M} + \left(\frac{\partial G_{pV}}{\partial z}\right)_{T,p,M} = \frac{\partial A}{\partial z} - A\frac{\partial p_{surf}}{\partial z} \tag{7.118}$$

evaluating the surface derivative by Equation 7.116 and neglecting gravity, that is generally very small for microfluidics systems, we obtain a simple differential equation for the surface pressure drop:

$$dp_{surf} = \gamma\frac{dA}{A} = \gamma\left(\frac{1}{\sigma_1} + \frac{1}{\sigma_2}\right)dz \tag{7.119}$$

Integrating to a small but finite displacement we get the so-called Young–Laplace equation that relates the surface tension to the pressure drop along the surface and to the equilibrium surface shape:

$$\Delta p_{surf} = \left(\frac{1}{\sigma_1} + \frac{1}{\sigma_2}\right)\gamma \tag{7.120}$$

As intuitive, the pressure drop increases with the surface tension.

Equation 7.120 clearly shows the effect of the surface shape on the surface pressure, but it is frequently difficult to be used in practice. The term $((1/\sigma_1) + (1/\sigma_2))$ is defined in an operative way and it generally depends on the reference system. A more rigorous definition is required to apply the Young–Laplace equation to a completely generic situation. To obtain such definition the contact surface has to be described in terms of its curvature tensor [28] and the derivation has to be carried out using generic coordinates. Defining the curvature κ in a point and along a given direction as the inverse of the curvature radius σ along the same direction, it is obtained that the term $((1/\sigma_1) + (1/\sigma_2))$ has to be substituted in Equation 7.120 by $2\bar{\kappa}$ where $\bar{\kappa}$ is the so-called mean curvature of the surface in the considered point.

Let us assume that our surface is derivable up to second order and all second derivatives are limited in the points where we want to evaluate the mean curvature. Consider all the curves having the following properties:

- They belongs to the surface
- They pass through the considered point
- They have here a definite curvature

We can individuate the set $\{\kappa\}$ of the curvatures of those curves; since $\{\kappa\}$ is a set of positive or null numbers, a minimum curvature always exist, called κ_m. It can be demonstrated that a maximum curvature κ_M also exist, due to the assumed hypothesis on the second derivatives of the curve. The values κ_m and κ_M are called principal curvatures of the surface. The mean curvature is defined as [4–30]:

$$\bar{\kappa} = \frac{\kappa_m + \kappa_M}{2} \tag{7.121}$$

Once the mean curvature is correctly evaluated, a more mathematically rigorous form of the Young–Laplace equation can be written as [4–30]

$$\Delta p_{surf} = 2\bar{\kappa}\gamma \tag{7.122}$$

7.3.5.2 Contact Angle and Wetting Capacity of a Liquid

A first important application of the concept of surface tension and surface pressure is the evaluation of the contact angle of a fluid in a point where three phases comes in contact. A first example of this contact happens along the line where a droplet of fluid deposited on a flat solid surface touches both the solid and the air or some other environmental fluid (see Figure 7.27a). A similar case happens when a fluid is contained in a container with the upper surface in contact with another fluid (see Figure 7.26b). In this case, the fact that the contact angle can be either smaller or greater than $\pi/2$ determines the possibility to form both concave and convex meniscuses on top of the liquid volume depending on the types of fluids in contact and on the container material characteristics.

To analyze quantitatively the phenomenon we start from the fact that the equilibrium contact angle corresponds to the minimum free energy situation. To exploit this property let us imagine to decrease the drop height so as to change the contact surface enlarging it by maintaining the same contact angle. Air is assumed as an example, but naturally the situation is identical in whatever environmental fluid the droplet is immerged. Three effects are related to this change: at the air–liquid and at the liquid–solid interface a surface pressure arises, that tends to restore the equilibrium surface. Around the contact line interfacing the three materials, however, a net change in the contact areas happens due to the displacement. Since contact areas between different materials have different surface energies, this also introduces a change in the overall free energy; a graphical detail of this phenomenon is reported in Figure 7.28. Let us indicate with dA_{al}, d_{Aas}, and d_{Asl}, the changes in contact areas between air and liquid, between air and solid, and between solid and liquid, respectively. Since rotational symmetry around the vertical axis of the droplet can be assumed due to free energy minimization, calling r the liquid–solid surface radius before the displacement and dl the displacement itself (see Figure 7.28) we can write

$$dA_{al} = \pi[(r + \cos(\theta)\,dl)^2 - r^2] \tag{7.123a}$$

$$dA_{sl} = \pi[(r + dl)^2 - r^2] \tag{7.123b}$$

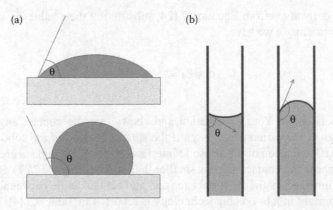

(a)   (b)

FIGURE 7.27 Scheme of positive and negative contact angles θ at the edge of a liquid drop put on a solid surface and in contact with air (a) and at the border of the free surface of a liquid in a container (b). In the last case, due to the different sign of the contact angle convex and concave meniscuses are formed on top of the liquid volume.

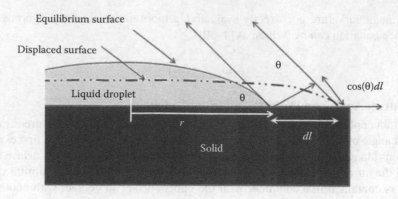

FIGURE 7.28 Geometry of the triple contact curve between air–liquid and a solid surface before and after a displacement from the equilibrium situation.

$$dA_{as} = -\pi[(r + dl)^2 - r^2]$$ (7.123c)

The changes in the related free energies are given by

$$dG_{sl} = \pi[(r + dl)^2 - r^2]\gamma_{sl} = 2\pi r \, dl \, \gamma_{sl}$$ (7.124a)

$$dG_{as} = -\pi[(r + dl)^2 - r^2]\gamma_{as} = -2\pi r \, dl \gamma_{as}$$ (7.124b)

$$dG_{al} = \pi[(r + \cos(\theta)dl)^2 - r^2]\gamma_{al} = 2\pi r \cos(\theta) dl \, \gamma_{al}$$ (7.124c)

The minimum free energy condition is imposed by imposing that the derivative of the free energy with respect to the displacement is zero, that is,

$$\left(\frac{dG}{dl}\right)_{T,p,M} = \left(\frac{dG_{sl}}{dl}\right)_{T,p,M} + \left(\frac{dG_{as}}{dl}\right)_{T,p,M} + \left(\frac{dG_{al}}{dl}\right)_{T,p,M} = 0$$ (7.125)

Evaluating the derivatives from Equation 7.124, substituting their values in Equation 7.125, and solving for the contact angle we have

$$\cos(\theta) = \frac{\gamma_{as} - \gamma_{sl}}{\gamma_{al}}$$ (7.126)

Equation 7.126 is called Young's equation and shows that the contact angle sign essentially depends on the sign of the difference $\gamma_{as} - \gamma_{sl}$: if the surface tension of the solid–liquid interface is greater than the surface tension of the air–solid interface, the contact angle is greater than $\pi/2$ while if the contrary happens the contact angle is smaller than $\pi/2$ (see Figure 7.27). Referring to a situation where all is immersed in air, the surface tension and contact angle between a set of liquids and solids that are important in labs on chip technology is reported in Table 7.5 [4].

The fact that the contact angle is smaller or greater than $\pi/2$ has an important physical meaning. We have to remember that the origin of the surface tension is the anisotropy that the surface liquid particles see between the part exposed to the same material and the part exposed to the other material, as shown in Figure 7.24. In the bulk of the liquid a molecule forms weak bonds with all the

TABLE 7.5

Surface Tension and Contact Angle between Liquid–Solid Couples Immersed in Air at 20°C and Atmospheric Pressure

Liquid	Solid	Contact Angle (deg)
Water	Glass	0
Water	Gold	0
Water	Crystalline Si	22
Water	PMMA	72
Water	Teflon	115
Ethanol	Glass	0
Mercury	Glass	140

Source: Data from Aris R., *Vectors, Tensors and the Basic Equations of Fluid Mechanics*, Dover Publications (January 1, 1990), ISBN-13: 978-0486661100.

other liquid molecules, like hydrogen bonds in liquid water, while on the surface generally similar bonds cannot be constituted and a surface molecule has a higher energy with respect to the bulk molecule. At the interface, however, bonds could be formed between molecules of different materials if this is effective in decreasing the surface free energy. Stronger the bonds, smaller the surface free energy and smaller the surface tension. This means that, if $\gamma_{as} - \gamma_{sl} > 0$ the liquid forms stronger bonds with the solid surface with respect to the environmental fluid. If the surrounding fluid is air, this is generally expressed saying that the liquid wet the solid surface. However, it is clear that the fact that a liquid wets or not a surface depends also on the fluid where both are immersed. Smaller the angle, stronger the surface bonds, so that the liquids forming small contact angles with solid surfaces exhibits a very good adhesion to the surface, that is, a strong force is needed to divide the unit area of contact surface. In the extreme limit, if the surface bonds have greater energy with respect to the bulk bonds no droplet forms on the surface and the liquid disperses on the surface.

On the contrary, if $\gamma_{as} - \gamma_{sl} < 0$ the liquid forms weaker bonds with the solid surface with respect to the environmental fluid. If the surrounding fluid is air, this is generally expressed saying that the liquid does not wet the solid surface. In the extreme case of very high surface energy, a spherical droplet forms so as to minimize the contact surface up to a single point.

The above considerations can be expressed in a quantitative form by observing that the surface tension is the energy per unit area that is accumulated at the surface so that, the energy per unit area W needed to divide a droplet from the solid surface where it adhere is given by

$$W = \left(\frac{dG_{sl}}{dl} \right)_{T,p,M} - \left(\frac{dG_{as}}{dl} \right)_{T,p,M} + \left(\frac{dG_{al}}{dl} \right)_{T,p,M} \tag{7.127}$$

Equation 7.127 is simply justified by the fact that the interface solid–liquid and liquid–air are removed while a new interface solid–air is created. Substituting the expressions of the derivatives and the definition of the contact angle in Equation 7.127 we obtain the so-called Young–Duprè equation:

$$W = \gamma_{sl} \left(1 + \cos(\theta) \right) \tag{7.128}$$

This equation reflects the qualitative link between the liquid–solid adhesion, the wetting and the contact angle.

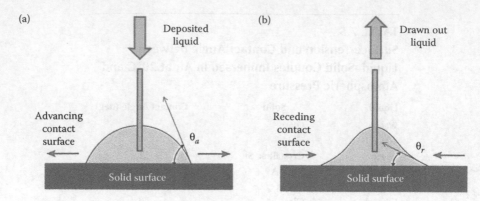

FIGURE 7.29 Illustration of the contact angle hysteresis in rough surfaces. The advancing contact angle θ_a is shown in part (a) while the receding contact angle θ_r in part (b).

On a surface that is rough or contaminated, Young's equation is still locally valid, but the equilibrium contact angle may vary from place to place on the surface [31]. According to the Young–Dupré equation, this means that the adhesion energy varies locally—thus, the liquid has to overcome local energy barriers in order to wet the surface. One consequence of these barriers is contact angle hysteresis: the extent of wetting, and therefore the observed contact angle, averaged along the contact line, depends on whether the liquid is advancing or receding, that is deposited on or drawn out of the surface, as represented in Figure 7.29. Since liquid advances over previously dry surface but recedes from previously wet surface, contact angle hysteresis can also arise if the solid has been altered due to its previous contact with the liquid, for example, by a chemical reaction, or absorption.

In several applications it is needed to have a combination of a strong hydrophobic surface, so that the liquid droplets do not wet the surface, and of a good surface adhesion so as to avoid the droplet to move along the surface too easily. In this case, the most used technique is to alter the surface mechanically so as to create a complex surface texture composed by a steep surface periodic undulation (see Figure 7.30) and, on top of it, a nanostructured set of needles that depart from the surface, as shown in Figure 7.31. The steep undulation causes the fluid not to penetrate into the structure, thereby reducing greatly the contact area and the contact energy. As a matter of fact, entering into the steep oscillations of the surface would require the contact surface to have a huge curvature; thus, increasing the surface pressure greatly. Moreover, during liquid deposition on the surface, air remains trapped within the periodic perturbation of the surface, rendering still more difficult for the liquid to penetrate [32,33].

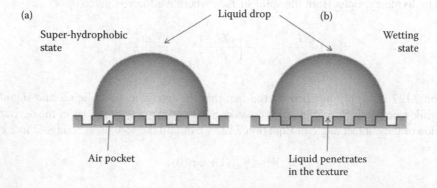

FIGURE 7.30 A textured super-hydrophobic surface in contact with a liquid droplet is shown in part (a), while the effect of air pockets elimination and the consequent wetting transition is shown in part (b).

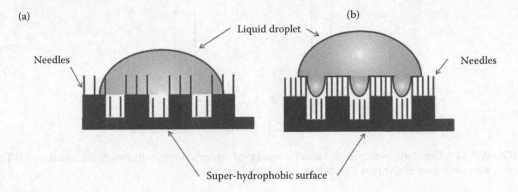

FIGURE 7.31 The Petal effect: different effect of nanometric needles on a textured super-hydrophobic surface due to the different distance between adjacent needles: (a) droplet movement along the surface elimination, (b) further decrease of the contact surface area.

Depending on the structure of the surface, it is possible that while time passes, or when temperature is raised, the air pocket trapped below the liquid drop either evaporate or are diluted into the liquid drop. In this case, the hydrophilic property of the surface decreases greatly and it is possible that the liquid starts to enter within the oscillations of the surface by wetting it, as shown in Figure 7.30b [32]. Surfaces that have this structure are called super-hydrophobic and exhibit a contact angle very near to π. If no other structure is realized on the surface, the liquid droplet moves almost freely on the surface, by almost maintaining its shape unchanged. If nanometric section needles are realized with a suitable periodic repetition, they are sufficiently small to penetrate into the liquid and form bonds with liquid particles. This bond gives a contribution to the adhesion energy thwarting the droplet movement along the surface [34,35]. This is frequently called "petal effect."

7.3.5.3 Capillary Effect

Up to now we have neglected the effect of gravity assuming to work with a microfluidic system. Assuming the fluid immersed in a gas such as air and indicating with γ the surface tension of the fluid with respect to this gas, booth γ/l^2 and the volume force related to gravity, $\rho\,g$ have the dimensions of (N/m^3). Thus, we can assume that the length l_{cap} for which these two quantities are equal is the typical length scale on which surface tension and gravitational effects are of the same order of magnitude. This length scale is called capillary length of the fluid. From the equation $\gamma/l_{cap} = \rho g$ we get

$$l_{cap} = \sqrt{\frac{\gamma}{\rho g}} \tag{7.129}$$

If we substitute data relative to water in contact with air on the earth surface in Equation 7.129 we obtain $l_{cap} = 2.7$ mm. This is a length much greater than the typical lengths of a lab on chip microfluidic circuit that are generally comprised between 10 and 100 μm; thus, the approximation of neglecting gravity in these systems generally causes very small errors.

However, there are gravity-driven phenomena, where obviously the gravity cannot be neglected. The most evident of these phenomena are probably the so-called capillarity effect.

The capillarity effect can be easily observed when a small tube with section width much smaller than the capillary length is immersed into a liquid container, as shown in Figure 7.32. When the liquid wets the tube walls (the upper meniscus is convex) it rises into the tube with respect to the container; conversely, when the liquid does not wet the tube walls (the meniscus is concave), it goes down into the tube with respect to the surface of the liquid in the container. To evaluate the capillary

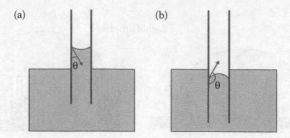

FIGURE 7.32   Capillarity effect in the case of a small tube immersed vertically in a liquid container. (a) The liquid wets the tube walls, (b) the liquid does not wet the tube walls.

rise length, let us assume that the capillary has a circular section, so that, due to the global rotational symmetry of the system, the capillary meniscus is always a sphere segment.

The two principal curvature of a sphere are identical since all the lines passing through a point have there the same curvature radius. Moreover, as it is evident from the geometry of Figure 7.32, calling R the tube section radius, we have

$$\bar{\kappa} = \frac{\cos(\theta)}{R} \tag{7.130}$$

Considering the Young–Laplace expression 7.120 of the interface pressure and noting that it is positive crossing the interface toward the liquid if the meniscus is convex, we can write the pressure difference between the liquid just below the surface (at a level h with respect to the container surface) and the air just above the surface as

$$p_{liq}(h) = p_0 - 2\frac{\gamma}{R}\cos(\theta) \tag{7.131}$$

where p_0 is the air pressure. The pressure at a point just below the tube end into the contained has to be equal to the atmospheric pressure, due to the liquid characteristics to distribute pressure uniformly in each direction that is to the fact that the pressure tensor is diagonal with all the trace elements equal to the scalar pressure p.

In order to be at equilibrium at a height h above the liquid surface of the contained, the pressure difference has to be balanced by the weight of the liquid column above this surface. Thus, we can write

$$p_{liq}(h) = p_0 - 2\frac{\gamma}{R}\cos(\theta) = \rho g h \tag{7.132}$$

It is to observe that in case of a noncircular duct, the duct radius in Equation 7.132 can be substituted by the capillary radius $R_{cap} = \mathcal{P}_W/(2\pi)$ where $\mathcal{P}_W$ is the wetted perimeter of the duct, generally corresponding to the duct section perimeter. This is due to the fact that the capillary pressure originates from a force acting on the contact curve between the duct, the liquid and the environmental fluid.

Equation 7.132 also holds if the value of h is negative due to a negative surface pressure, thus in any case we can write, solving (7.132) for h

$$h = \frac{2\gamma}{\rho g R}\cos(\theta) = 2\frac{l_{cap}^2}{R}\cos(\theta) \tag{7.133}$$

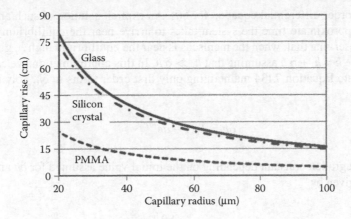

FIGURE 7.33 Capillary rise for capillaries of different solids used in microfluidics labs on chip when used with water in air. Data evaluated at 20°C and atmospheric pressure.

confirming the fact that l_{cap} is the characteristic length at which gravity and surface tension balances.

The capillary rise can be sensible if microfluidic ducts are considered. As an example, in Figure 7.33 the capillary rise of water is shown for different tubes radii and for different solid materials used in microfluidic devices.

Due to the possibility to use the capillary effect in different ways in labs on chip, it is relevant to assess the speed of the effect, that is the speed of the meniscus rise or descend after the entering of the capillary in the liquid container.

We will consider a circular capillary that is vertically inserted into the container and we also assume that the liquid flux into the capillary during the meniscus rise or descend is a fully developed Poiseuille flow, so as to be able to use the results we obtained for this kind of flow. In order for this approximation to be valid, we must have that the capillary rise time is much longer than that the Poiseuille flow stabilization time, that as we have seen is in the order of milliseconds for the water-fluxes. Thus, we will be able to verify a posteriori the correctness of this hypothesis.

The average velocity v of the flow in a tube can be written as a function of the flow rate as

$$v = \frac{Q}{\pi r^2} \tag{7.134}$$

Due to the definition of the flow rate, the average speed at which the liquid goes up into the capillary can also be written as dh/dt, so that, exploiting Equation 7.83 for the flow rate, we get

$$\frac{dh}{dt} = \frac{Q}{\pi r^2} = \frac{r^2 \Delta p}{8\eta} \frac{1}{h} \tag{7.135}$$

The overall pressure causing the liquid motion through the capillary is caused by the surface tension pressure minus the gravity pressure induced by the liquid column into the capillary. Using the fact that the meniscus can be assumed a segment of sphere to express the meniscus mean curvature and substituting the expression of the surface pressure in Equation 7.135 we can write

$$\frac{dh}{dt} = \frac{\gamma}{8\eta} \left[\frac{2r\cos(\theta)}{h} - \frac{r^2}{l_{cap}^2} \right] \tag{7.136}$$

This is a first-order differential equation for $h(t)$. An explicit solution of such an equation is not known, but the approximate time the system takes to arrive near the equilibrium position can be determined by observing that, when the meniscus is near the equilibrium high h_e given by Equation 7.133 we can write $h = h_e + \delta h$ assuming that $h_e \gg \delta h$. In this approximation, we can substitute the expression of h into Equation 7.134 maintaining only first order terms in δh. Solving this equation we have

$$\delta h = h_e (1 - a e^{-t/\tau_{cap}}) \qquad (7.137)$$

where a is the integration constant depending on the initial value assumed for δh and the characteristic rise time is given by

$$\tau_{cap} = \frac{8 \eta h_e}{\rho g r^2} \qquad (7.138)$$

This is the characteristic time needed to the capillary to get hydrostatic equilibrium. In case of water, in a 100 μm radius tube made of PMMA in contact with air we get, using the value from Figure 7.33 for the equilibrium value of the capillary rise, $\tau_{cap} = 3.4\ s$ while in the case of a glass tube of the same diameter we obtain in the same way $\tau_{cap} = 11.9s$. These values are much higher than the characteristic times needed to establish a fully developed Poiseuille flow in the same duct; thus, confirming the approximation we put at the ground of the calculation of τ_{cap}.

The capillary effect has an important application in labs on chip if the duct where the liquid flows is horizontal instead of vertical. In this case, the analysis we have done holds if we drop the effect of gravity from equations. Thus, no pressure is present to balance the surface pressure and equilibrium is never reached. The liquid simply flows through the tube up to the tube end, where capillary effect is no more present. Since all ducts in a microfluidic circuit can be considered capillaries, the capillary effect can be used to create passive pumps, that have no need of moving parts and power feed. This point will be better developed by considering labs on chip building blocks in Chapter 8.

7.3.5.4 Droplet Generation

Another important phenomenon related to the presence of surface pressure and having a wide application in labs on chip is droplet generation. The most common way droplets forms is the so-called pendant drop. In this case we have a small circular tube vertically placed and the liquid is left to get out of the tube, subject both to surface tension and gravity as shown in Figure 7.33.

Surface tension tends to maintain the mass of the liquid compact maintaining continuity between the liquid out of the tube and the liquid into the tube, while the gravity tends to get the liquid out of the tube. This effect can be represented by a couple of forces: the gravity force $\boldsymbol{F}_g$ and the surface tension force $\boldsymbol{F}_s$. The gravity force is a volume force while the surface tension gives rise to a force acting on the tube-liquid contact along the tube wall lower border. The nature of the surface tension force can be understood noting that the surface tension can be also measured in $N\ m$, so suggesting it can give rise to forces acting on contact curves between different materials. This force is tangent to the liquid surface, so as to obtain the better possible liquid adhesion to the tube border.

A first idea of the droplet formation phenomenon can be obtained by imagining in a very first approximation that the gravity force acts on the droplet center of mass. Setting a reference system as shown in Figure 7.34, the relevant forces write

$$\boldsymbol{F}_g = V \rho g \boldsymbol{u}_z \qquad (7.139a)$$

$$\boldsymbol{F}_s = \pi r \gamma [\cos(\theta) \boldsymbol{u}_y - \sin(\theta) \boldsymbol{u}_z] \qquad (7.139b)$$

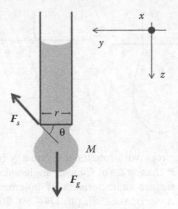

FIGURE 7.34 Droplets formation at the lower output of a vertical tube: simplified scheme of the playing forces.

where u_x, u_y, and u_z are the coordinate axes unit vectors, V is the liquid volume out of the tube, γ the surface tension between the tube material and the liquid, r the tube radius, and (x, y, z) the coordinate axes unit vectors. While on the y direction the surface tension force is balanced by the reaction of the tube wall, in the vertical direction the overall force acting on the droplet is

$$F_z = V\rho g - \pi r\gamma\sin(\theta) \quad (7.140)$$

The drop detaches from the tube when the surface tension is overcome by the drop weight so that an estimate of the drop volume can be attained by equating gravity and surface tension obtaining

$$V = \frac{\pi r\gamma\sin(\theta)}{\rho g} = \pi r l_{cap}^2 \sin(\theta) \quad (7.141)$$

In order to evaluate the droplet shape and the dynamics of the droplet formation process, the simple approximation (7.139) is not sufficient and a more complex model has to be carried out by taking into account the distributed forces on the tube border, on the droplet boundary surface and on the droplet volume and minimizing the overall free energy [36,37]. Precise numerical calculations can be done regarding the drop surface both in hydrodynamic equilibrium, when the droplet remains attached to the tube end, and during the droplet detach process [38]. The shape depends strongly on the contact angle between the tube walls and the liquid, as shown in Figure 7.35, where real shapes of pendant drops with rotational symmetry are shown in correspondence to different contact angles [39,40].

In order to correctly study the process of drop formation and detachment from the liquid inside the tube the Navier-Stokes Equation 7.36 has to be solved for the liquid taking into account the correct boundary conditions both for the liquid–solid contact and for the liquid–gas contact and imposing in each phase of the process the correct shape of the drop surface [38,41]. The resulting mathematical problem is very complex and it can be solved in specific cases only by simulation. The result of a simulation showing the droplet detachment of a water droplet from a PMMA circular tube having 300 μm of diameter is shown in Figure 7.36.

From this figure it results that the drop formation process can be divided into different phases. At first the droplet starts to form while maintained in contact with the originating tube (part (a) of the figure), in the case of the figure the 72° contact angle between the droplet upper section and the PMMA constituting the tube is evident. The neck of the droplet, dividing the main part of the droplet from the section in contact with the tube slowly is elongated while its section decreases, always

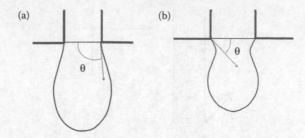

FIGURE 7.35 Shapes of pendant drops with rotational symmetry in correspondence to different contact angles; (a) contact angle greater than $\pi/2$. (b) Contact angle smaller than $\pi/2$. (Data from Yang D. et al. Experimental study on the surface characteristics of polymer melts, *Colloids and Surfaces A: Physicochemical and Engineering Aspects*, vol. 367, pp. 174–180, 2010; Gardas R. L. et al. Interfacial tensions of imidazolium-based ionic liquids with water and n-alkanes, *Fluid Phase Equilibria*, vol. 294, pp. 139–147, 2010.)

maintaining a constant contact angle with the tube (part (b) of the figure) up to a moment in which the neck central part arrives at a critical width, being reduced to a very thin liquid fillet (part (c) of the figure). After this point, the fillet maintaining the contact between the liquid contained in the tube and the droplet breaks contemporary both at the level of the droplet surface and at the contact with the bulk of the liquid (part (d) of the figure). The two liquid masses that are now detached from the tube fall while adjusting their shape to reach a minimum free energy contact with the surrounding gas up to reach the final shape while falling down (part (e) of the figure). In the presence of very small perturbations that do not alter the main drop shape, but influences the detachment process, the fillet breaks also in other intermediate points, for example, in correspondence with minimum width points generated by a perturbation.

This process creates two or more droplets of a very different shape: a main droplet and a set of secondary droplets, created by the simultaneous breakage of the pendant droplet neck. The creation of secondary droplets is practically unavoidable and it frequently happens when droplets are formed inside a lab on chip by mechanical methods [43,44].

Another phenomenon creating droplets at the lower output of a tube is the so-called Plateau–Rayleigh instability [41,45] generated in the continuous flux out of the tube. This phenomenon is graphically shown in Figure 7.37a. The instability is generated by small perturbations in the stream due to various reasons. By writing the Navier–Stokes equation for the steam in steady state with the

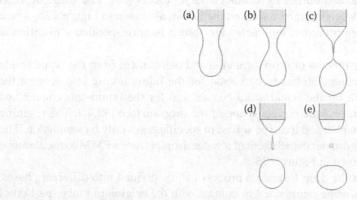

FIGURE 7.36 Phases of the drop formation and detachment: a water drop forming out of a PMMA circular tube having 300 μm of diameter is considered. The correct drop shapes, having rotational symmetry, are obtained by simulation.

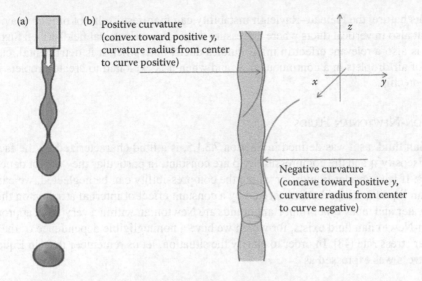

FIGURE 7.37 Droplets generation by Plateau–Rayleigh instability: pictorial scheme of the phenomenon (a) and geometry of the liquid flux under a single frequency perturbation (b).

correct boundary conditions and adding a very small perturbation, it is possible to see that whatever the perturbation initial shape, after a certain time a clear harmonic undulation appears on the surface of the stream, as shown in Figure 7.37b. This behavior can be clarified by expressing the perturbation using the Fourier integral and linearizing the equation for the perturbed fluid surface. It is found that, while propagating along the liquid surface at the sound speed, the perturbation is also filtered in the frequency domain by a function depending essentially on the radius of the tube generating the stream. In particular, the frequency filter has a positive amplitude (i.e., implies an amplification of the perturbation) if the following equation is satisfied:

$$2\pi \frac{f}{v_s} r = k(f) r < 1 \qquad (7.142)$$

being

- the frequency of the harmonic perturbation component
- v_s the sound speed in the liquid
- r the radius of the stream originating tube
- $k(f)$ the wave number of the considered frequency components

The amplifying part of the frequency response has a clearly defined maximum, generating the amplification of a very sharp frequency packet at the expenses of all other frequencies of the original perturbation, in such a way that rapidly the alteration of the stream surface becomes almost monochromatic. The presence of this amplifying region of the frequency response can be justified by observing the behavior of the surface pressure when the stream surface is perturbed by a "long frequency" perturbation (compare Figure 7.37b). The perturbed fluid stream has areas with positive curvature and other areas with negative curvature. Applying the Young–Laplace equation we can see that the pinched sections have higher pressure ($\bar{\kappa}$) and the bulging sections have lower pressure ($\bar{\kappa}$ is smaller), thereby producing a fluid flow internal to the flowing stream due to pressure gradient. This internal flux causes the growth of displacement amplitude which eventually initiates droplet formation.

Due to its nature, the Plateau–Rayleigh instability can manifest itself not only in gravity caused streams, but also in vertical ducts where a pressure driven or an electrical field-driven flux happens. Thus, this is also a relevant effect in microfluidics ducts, both when it is detrimental, causing the formation of air droplets in a continuous flow and when it is exploited to create droplets in droplet based labs on chip.

7.3.6 NON-NEWTONIAN FLUIDS

A Newtonian fluid, as it was defined in Section 7.3.1.5, is a fluid characterized by the fact that the dynamic viscosity η and the compressibility β are constant, in particular they do not depend on the shear stress. If we consider liquids for which the compressibility can be neglected, we can say that a Newtonian liquid is a liquid characterized by a constant effect of internal attrition on the motion.

While water and many other important liquids are Newtonian within a very good approximation, several non-Newtonian fluid exists, for which we have a nonnegligible dependence of the viscosity on the shear stress rate [48]. In order to clarify the situation, let us remember that, in Equation 7.32 the shear stress was expressed as

$$\gamma'_{i,j} = \eta\left(\frac{\partial v_i}{\partial x_j} + \frac{\partial v_j}{\partial x_i}\right) = \eta\dot{\gamma}_{ij} \tag{7.143}$$

where $\dot{\gamma}_{ij}$ is a symmetric tensor called, for its physical meaning, shear stress rate. Thus, the components of the shear tensor are proportional to the shear stress rate via a single constant that is called viscosity. In the general case of non-Newtonian fluid, Equation 7.140 has to be rewritten as [49]

$$\gamma'_{i,j}(t) = \int_{-\infty}^{t} \eta_{i,k}(\dot{\gamma}_{m,h}(\tau),t)\,\dot{\gamma}_{kj}(\tau)d\tau \tag{7.144}$$

where, in principle, since the viscosity changes during motions, values of the shear rate at different instants can be involved in the evaluation of the instantaneous value of the viscosity and, due to the causality principle, we must have $\tau \le t$.

In many practical cases the dependence of the viscosity from the shear rate is simpler than the generic expression 7.144. Let us introduce two scalar invariant of the shear rate tensor: the trace $Tr(\dot{\gamma}_{kj}(t))$ and the magnitude $\left|\dot{\gamma}_{kj}\right|$ that are defined as

$$Tr(\underline{\dot{\gamma}}) = \dot{\gamma}_{kj}(t)\delta_{kj} = 2\nabla \cdot v \tag{7.145a}$$

$$\left|\underline{\dot{\gamma}}\right| = \sqrt{\frac{\dot{\gamma}_{kj}(t)\dot{\gamma}_{jk}(t)}{2}} \tag{7.145b}$$

The viscosity can be frequently expressed as a scalar function of the scalar invariants of the shear rate. Moreover, for incompressible fluids, $Tr(\underline{\dot{\gamma}}) = 0$ (see Section 7.3.3) so that Equation 7.144 simplifies as [48,4]

$$\gamma'_{i,j}(t) = \int_{-\infty}^{t} \eta\left(\left|\dot{\gamma}_{m,h}(\tau)\right|,t\right)\dot{\gamma}_{ij}(\tau)d\tau \tag{7.146}$$

In any case, this is a very complex situation. Since the behavior of non-Newtonian fluids depends on the microscopic structure of the material, it is not completely generic and an approximated classification of possible behaviors is possible. Roughly non-Newtonian fluids can be classified into three classes:

- Time independent or generalized Newtonian
- Time dependent
- Visco-elastic

It is to be noted that this is a rough classification of possible behaviors, not a materials classifications. Specific fluids often exhibit two or even all three behaviors depending on the observation conditions. For instance, it is not uncommon for a melted polymer to show time-independent or visco-elastic behavior depending on the values of the shear stress and for a china clay suspension to exhibit a combination of time-independent and time-dependent features at certain concentrations and/or at appropriate shear rates.

To illustrate the physical characteristics of the viscosity it is useful to consider a simple method for viscosity measurement. The experimental equipment is schematically constituted by two parallel plates, put at a distance d much smaller than their linear dimensions, containing in between the considered liquid. The upper plate is moved at a constant velocity, while the lower plate is maintained still in the considered reference system. The scheme of the equipment with the adopted reference system is shown in Figure 7.38.

Since the pressure difference is zero, the fluid moves only due to the movement of the upper plate and the viscosity no more appears in the stationary Stokes equation (7.62), whose solution is for any kind of liquid (if the no-slip boundary condition can be applied):

$$v(z) = v_0 \frac{z}{d} \tag{7.147}$$

This kind of motion is called Couette flow. The force needed to pull the upper plate at the desired speed can be directly deduced by the definition of the stress tensor $\gamma'_{i,j}$ obtaining

$$F = F u_y = \gamma'_{2,3} A u_y = \eta \frac{v_0 A}{d} y = \eta \dot{\gamma}_{2,3} A u_y \tag{7.148}$$

where u_y is the y axis unit vector, A is the transversal area of the system and the other variables are defined in Figure 7.38. Thus, by measuring the force needed to pull the upper plate, the viscosity for different shear rates can be directly evaluated. We will use in the following this type of measurement equipment to illustrate a few key features of non-Newtonian fluids.

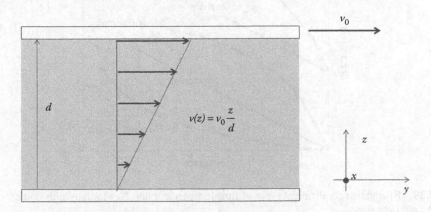

FIGURE 7.38 Flow of a liquid between a still and a moving plate.

7.3.6.1 Time-Independent Non-Newtonian Fluids

This type of non-Newtonian behavior is characterized by an instantaneous relation between the viscosity and the shear rate trace, so that we can write

$$\gamma'_{i,j} = \eta(|\underline{\dot{\gamma}}|)\dot{\gamma}_{ij} \tag{7.149}$$

If we assume an instantaneous relation between the shear stress and the shear rate, we can individuate three possible behaviors of the fluid:

1. Shear-thinning or pseudoplastic behavior
2. Visco-plastic behavior with or without shear-thinning behavior
3. Shear-thickening or dilatant behavior

These behaviors can be observed easily by the viscometer sketched in Figure 3.38 by observing as the force changes by increasing the velocity of the upper plate. Figure 7.39 shows qualitatively the curves representing the dependence of the shear stress from the shear rate, also called flow curves or rheograms, characteristics of these categories of fluid behavior as detected by the viscometer. In this case, both the shear stress and the shear rate have only one component different from zero and their intensity reduces to the square of this component.

The shear thinning behaviors is perhaps the most common among melted polymeric materials. In this case, a particular shear thinning effect is observed, that is qualitatively shown in Figure 7.40. At low shear rate the viscosity is almost constant and the polymer behaves as an almost Newtonian fluid. Increasing the shear rate beyond a critical value the viscosity starts to decrease up to a second critical value where it returns to be almost constant [50,51]. Qualitatively, the transition region can be interpreted as the shear stress rate region where the polymeric chains loose, due to the motion, their chaotic configuration and starts to align along the motion direction. Thus, a transition between two regions with different polymeric chains average configuration is also characterized by the transition between two different viscosity regimes.

The visco-plastic behavior is characterized by the existence of a threshold stress γ'_0, called yield stress or apparent yield stress, which must be exceeded for the fluid to deform or flow. Conversely, such a substance will behave like an elastic solid or moves like a rigid body when the externally applied stress is less than the yield stress. Once the magnitude of the external yield stress exceeds

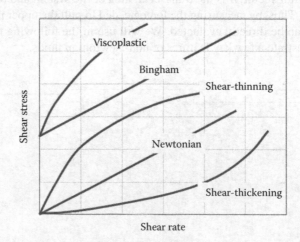

FIGURE 7.39 Rheograms for different types of time independent non-Newtonian fluids compared with the Newtonian fluid behavior.

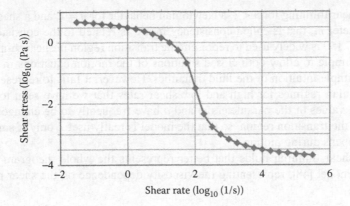

FIGURE 7.40 Example of non-Newtonian shear thinning behavior of a melted polymer showing limit Newtonian behaviors for high and low shear rates.

the value of γ'_0, the fluid may exhibit Newtonian behavior or shear-thinning characteristics. Moreover, in the absence of surface tension effects, such a material will not level out under gravity to form an absolutely flat free surface. Perhaps, the most known among visco-plastic substances is PDMS, introduced in Section 1.4.3 and used in several applications in labs on chip technology (see, e.g., soft lithography described in Section 5.2 and the fluidic interfaces described in Section 6.5.3.2).

Quantitatively, this type of behavior can be explained assuming that, at rest, the substance consists of three-dimensional structures of sufficient rigidity to resist any external stress less than γ'_0 and therefore offers an enormous resistance to flow, albeit it still might deform elastically. For stress levels above γ'_0, however, the structure breaks down and the substance behaves like a viscous material. In some cases, the build-up and breakdown of structure has been found to be reversible, so that the substance may regain its initial value of the viscosity at the end of the stress. Other times the value of the viscosity after the end of the stress is lower than the initial one. In this case, the behavior can be interpreted assuming a few macrostructures being definitively broken by the insurgence of the stress, while the great number of them are able to return at their initial ordered state.

Finally, shear thickening systems are similar to shear thinning once in that they show no yield stress, but their apparent viscosity increases with the increasing shear rate and hence the name shear-thickening. Originally, this type of behavior was observed in concentrated suspensions, and one can qualitatively explain it as follows: at rest, the void spaces among suspension particles is minimum and the liquid present in the sample is sufficient to fill the voids completely. At low shearing levels, the liquid lubricates the motion of each particle past another thereby minimizing solid–solid friction. Consequently, the resulting stresses are small. At high shear rates, however, the mixture expands so that the available liquid is no longer sufficient to fill the increased void space and to prevent direct solid–solid contacts and friction. This leads to the development of much larger shear stresses. This mechanism causes the viscosity to rise rapidly with the increasing rate of shear.

One elementary model for viscosity in both shear thinning and shear thickening fluids is the so-called Power model, that consists in a simple relation between the shear rate intensity and the viscosity:

$$\eta(|\dot{\underline{\gamma}}|) = m(|\dot{\underline{\gamma}}|)^{n-1} \qquad (7.150)$$

where we have shear thinning for $n < 1$, a Newtonian behavior for $n = 1$, and a shear thickening for $n > 1$. The parameter m, that is called consistency index, is related to the consistency of the substance. Equation 7.150 is widely used to represent the transition region in shear thinning fluids since it is sufficiently simple to allow both closed solutions of the motion equations in several interesting cases and a simple intuition of the fluid dynamics. However, it fails to represents the presence of pseudo-Newtonian regimes for high and low shear rates that we have seen to exist in melted polymers and the values of the parameters m and n have frequently to be changed to correctly fit different parts of the transition region, so that the model is really useful only if small variations of the shear rate happens during motion.

A model for shear thinning fluids that better represents the whole rheogram is the so-called Carreau–Yasuda model [48], representing the viscosity dependence on the shear rate with a more complex equation

$$\eta(|\underline{\dot{\gamma}}|) = \eta_\infty + (\eta_0 - \eta_\infty)[1 + (\lambda|\underline{\dot{\gamma}}|)^a]^{\frac{n-1}{a}} \tag{7.151}$$

Equation 7.151 depends on four parameters:

- η_∞ represents the infinite limit viscosity
- η_0 represents the zero limit viscosity
- λ represents the typical time scale of viscosity changes
- a controls the curvature in the middle of the transition region
- n the slope of the curvature in the middle of the transition region.

Many other models have been adopted both on a purely empiric base and starting from microscopic elements to improve the empiric interpolation of experimental data. It is out of the scope of this brief section on non-Newtonian fluids to list and compare such models and the interested reader is encouraged to analyze the rich technical literature for such a study [48,50,51].

7.3.6.2 Time-Dependent Non-Newtonian Fluids

In the case of time-dependent fluids, the viscosity cannot be expressed as an instantaneous function of the shear rate, since the fluid behavior depends on its time behavior. For example, fluids like cement paste, waxy crude oil, hand lotions, and creams slowly create internal weak bonds among molecules when at rest. These bonds generate an increase in viscosity so that the fluid has a high viscosity when motion starts. When subject to a shear rate, the weak bonds among molecules are progressively broken at a rate greater than the creation rate and the viscosity decreases up to the moment in which the number of internal bonds gets at equilibrium and the viscosity assumes a minimum stationary value. This behavior is represented, for example, in Figure 7.41, where experimental data showing time-dependent behavior in a red mud suspension are shown [52].

Depending upon the response of a material to shear over a period of time, it is customary to subdivide time-dependent fluid behavior into two types, namely, thixotropy and rheopexy (also called negative thixotropy).

If the rheogram of such a fluid is measured into a viscometer increasing the shear rate after a long period of rest and then decreasing it again up to restoring a rest situation, an hysteresis loop of the form shown schematically in Figure 7.42 is obtained. Thixotropic and rheopexic fluids are distinguished from the form of the hysteresis, as shown in Figure 7.42. In both cases the height, shape, and area enclosed by the loop depend on the experimental conditions like the rate of increase/decrease of shear rate, the maximum value of shear rate, and the past kinematic history of the sample. Generally, the larger the enclosed area, more severe is the time-dependent behavior of the material under discussion.

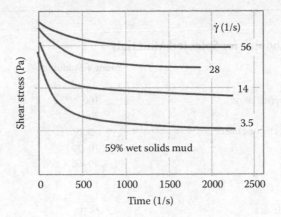

FIGURE 7.41 Example of time dependent viscosity behavior in a trixotropic fluid. (Data from Nguyen Q. D., Uhlherr P. H. T., *Thixotropic Behaviour of Concentrated Real Mud Suspensions.* Proceedings of the 3rd National Conference on Rheology, Melbourne, pp. 63–67, 1983.)

7.3.6.3 Visco-Elastic Non-Newtonian Fluids

For an ideal elastic solid, stress in a sheared state is directly proportional to strain. However, in a real solid, when a yield stress is overcome, the deformation becomes permanent and the solid creeps. In the case of some solids this phenomenon is so evident that the material starts to flow, like it was a high viscosity liquid. Here it is possible that, after flowing, the material does not recover the solid behavior, being unable to restore the broken bonds. Conversely, in other cases the bonds between nearby molecules are completely or partially recovered after flowing, thus restoring a solid-like behavior.

Table 7.6 presents typical values of the Young's modulus $\mathcal{E}$ for a range of materials including metals, plastics, polymer, and colloidal solutions. These values provide a basis to label some of the substances as *soft solids:* these could be, for example, defined as solids with a Young module smaller than 0.1 MPa. Soft solids generally exhibit visco-elastic characteristics if subject to a sufficiently high shear stress.

Time dependence can exist for visco-elastic materials, generally however it is not so relevant allowing to use an instantaneous model for the viscosity for many practical purposes. A characteristic of visco-elastic materials is that if solicited with unidirectional shear rate (as in the viscometer of Figure 7.38, they generate a shear stress in the direction orthogonal to the shear rate). This means

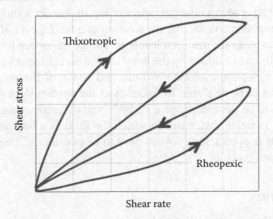

FIGURE 7.42 Schematic plot of the hysteresis cycle in the rheogram of a thixotropic and a rheopexic fluid.

TABLE 7.6
Young's Modulus for Selected Materials

Material	Young's Modulus	Unit
Glass	70	GPa
Aluminum, copper, alloys	100	GPa
Steel	200	GPa
High modulus oriented fibers	>300	GPa
Concrete	10–20	GPa
Stones	40–60	GPa
Wood	1–10	GPa
Ice	10	GPa
Engineering plastics	5–20	GPa
Leather	1–100	MPa
Rubber	0.1–5	MPa
Polymer and colloidal solutions	1–100	Pa

Note: Materials with low Young's modulus (as a Reference <50 MPa) can be generally considered as "soft materials."

that the viscosity cannot be considered a scalar, but has to be described as a tensor so that Equation 7.149 has to be substituted by

$$\gamma'_{i,j} = \eta_{i,k}(|\underline{\dot{\gamma}}|)\dot{\gamma}_{kj} \tag{7.152}$$

Assuming the viscometer configuration of Figure 7.38, the only share rate component that is different from zero is $\dot{\gamma}_{2,3}$ while, if visco-elastic behavior is present, $\dot{\gamma}'_{2,3}, \dot{\gamma}'_{2,1}$, and $\dot{\gamma}'_{2,2}$ are all different from zero.

7.4 SOLUTIONS DYNAMICS: DIFFUSION

Up to now we have introduced a few key concepts of fluid dynamics that are widely used in the analysis and design of labs on chip. By far the greatest number of fluids flowing in labs on chip microfluidics structures analyzed are diluted solutions of macromolecules and other particles, such as ions and sometimes cells. We have seen in the previous section that under a fluid-dynamic point of view it is possible to study the motion considering the solution as a whole, even if in the case in which the concentration is so high to make the macromolecules presence important for the fluid flow characteristics, many complications can be added by the non-Newtonian characteristics of the resulting fluid.

However, in several cases the evolution in time and space of the solute concentration is the relevant quantity that has to be analyzed to understand the system dynamics. In these cases, the solute concentration has to be the independent variable and dynamic equations have to be found to determine its evolution. In doing that, cases in which the fluid as a bulk is in motion and cases in which chemical reactions happen among solutes have to be considered, due to the fact that they are relevant phenomena in labs on chip.

7.4.1 DIFFUSION MODELS

In Section 1.6, we have derived a few key points regarding the microscopic dynamics of macromolecules diluted solutions. In particular, we have pointed out the following elements:

- Since macromolecules are much greater than the solvent molecule a diluted solution dynamics can be suitably represented as the evolution of a population of macromolecules in a continuum constituted by the solvent molecules.
- The above model does not change if other small molecules (such as ions or light alcohols) are present, as usual in biological solutions. They enter as a part of the continuous background.
- If different macromolecules are considered, they can be described as different populations all immersed in the same background.
- Due to the phenomenon of hydration, if this model is used to derive results from a system microscopic model, a sort of virtual macromolecule has to be considered, whose parameters takes into account hydration.
- The average distance among macromolecules in a diluted solution is sufficiently high that the only relevant interaction is constituted by rare collisions between couple of molecules: thus, the molecule population can be considered a perfect gas.
- The dynamic of this perfect gas has to take into account that the viscous background causes almost all the motion of a macromolecule to happen at the limit velocity determined by the background viscosity.

We will use these elements to derive a macroscopic dynamical model of the macromolecules concentration evolution [53].

Since the solute particles move and we can assume in a first moment that their number is conserved, for example, no chemical reaction happens, we can introduce a particles flux $\Phi_p(r,t)$ representing with its intensity the variation in the unit time of the number of particles in the space element, that is, of the particles concentration. Thus, we can write the continuity for the solute concentration by specializing Equation 7.17 as

$$\frac{\partial c(r,t)}{\partial t} + \nabla \cdot \Phi_p(r,t) = 0 \tag{7.153}$$

In many practical cases however, the hypothesis that the number of particles is constant is not true, but sources/sinks can be present for solute particles. This can happen, for example, when a chemical reaction transforms particles of selected solutes in particles of other solutes or when particles are subtracted from the solution by selective filters. In a lab on chip it is possible that two reagents, A and B, diffuse from two inlets in a reaction chamber where they react to generate the product C while diffusing into the solvent. Let us imagine that the reaction generating C writes

$$A + B \rightleftharpoons C \tag{7.154}$$

If the diffusion coefficient is correctly evaluated in order to represent the situation, the diffusion terms are independent so that the time evolution of the three concentrations due to the molecule motion can be represented with standard diffusion equations. However, when a reaction happens, either two molecules of A and B are destroyed to create a molecule of C or, inversely, a molecule of C decades into a molecule of A and a molecule of B. This mechanism generates a source/sink term in the diffusion equation.

In these cases, Equation 7.153 can be generalized by adding a source/sink term as

$$\frac{\partial c(r,t)}{\partial t} + \nabla \cdot \Phi_p(r,t) = S(r,t) \tag{7.155}$$

The flux can be written as in Equation 7.17 as a function of the concentration of the solute (number of solute molecules in the unit volume) and the average molecules velocity (number of molecule transiting through the unit surface in the unit time) as

$$\Phi_p(\boldsymbol{r},t) = c(\boldsymbol{r},t)\boldsymbol{v}(\boldsymbol{r},t) \tag{7.156}$$

Since we have assumed that molecules moves in a high viscosity environment, the average molecule velocity module v is given by

$$v = \sigma F \tag{7.157}$$

where F is the average active force that is exactly counterbalanced by the viscous attrition and σ, called molecules mobility, is the parameter relating the limit velocity in the viscous fluid and the active force that depends on both the viscosity and the molecule shape once hydrated. To determine the average active force, let us consider the chemical potential that in this case is exactly the potential of the average active force, since it determines the tendency of the molecule population to arrive at a status of minimum free energy.

At thermal equilibrium, the local chemical potential (see Section 1.2.3) can be written as

$$\mu = \mu_0 + \kappa T \log\left(\frac{c}{c_0}\right) \tag{7.158}$$

where κ is the Boltzmann constant. Thus,

$$F = -\nabla\mu = -\frac{\kappa T}{c}\nabla c \tag{7.159}$$

Substituting the expression of the force into the velocity and the velocity expression in the flux we get the so-called Fick law:

$$\Phi_p(\boldsymbol{r},t) = -\sigma\kappa T\nabla c \tag{7.160}$$

Returning to the continuity Equation 7.155 and defining the diffusion coefficient as $D = \sigma\,\kappa\,T$ we obtain the general form of the diffusion equation

$$\frac{\partial c(\boldsymbol{r},t)}{\partial t} = \nabla \cdot (D\nabla c) + S(\boldsymbol{r},t) \tag{7.161}$$

There are several reasons causing the diffusion coefficient to depend on the space variables: a thermal gradient can be present, for example, or the solution is not so diluted to neglect interaction between solute particles, in which case we will see that D will depend on $c(\boldsymbol{r},t)$. If the diffusion coefficient is constant, we obtain

$$\frac{\partial c(\boldsymbol{r},t)}{\partial t} = D\nabla^2 c + S(\boldsymbol{r},t) \tag{7.162}$$

The first interesting notation is that diffusion equation, which we have derived in correspondence with solute particle diffusion, is similar to the simpler form of the thermal diffusion equation we obtained in Section 7.3.2. This is not completely casual, but is more a hint that somehow heat is carried around by virtual particles that diffuses into solids and fluids. This hint is completely confirmed by the phonons theory both in solids [54], where full phonons exists, and in systems with a partial local order, where phonons are defined locally and are continuously absorbed and emitted due to the limited range of order of the material [55].

The diffusion coefficient has the dimensions of m^2/s, thus we can assume that the diffusion characteristic time is given by

$$\tau = \ell^2/D \tag{7.163}$$

where l is the characteristic length of the system. Assuming $D = 10^{-11} \; m^2/s$ (a typical value in labs on chip) and $l = 100 \; \mu m$ we have a characteristic time $\tau = 100$ s, thus diffusion of macromolecules is generally a slow phenomenon even in labs on chip. In Sections 2.4.2 and 3.3.3 we have seen that the most important protein-related reactions are characterized by characteristic times of the order of 0.1–1 ms. This allows us to consider the chemical reaction almost instantaneously with respect to diffusion and insert thus an instantaneous source/sink term equal to the chemical rate if chemical reactions happen.

Thus, if the chemical reaction 7.154 happens during diffusion, the concentration dynamics is well described by a system of three diffusion-chemical equations that writes

$$\frac{\partial c_\alpha(\boldsymbol{r},t)}{\partial t} = D\nabla^2 c_\alpha - \lambda_\alpha \; v_+ \; c_A \; c_B + \lambda_\alpha \; v_- c_C \tag{7.164}$$

where $\alpha = \{A,B,C\}$, $\lambda_A = \lambda_B = +1$ and $\lambda_C = -1$.

Another important case in which the pure diffusion equation has to be modified adding additional terms is the case of the presence of a pressure causing the movement of both the solute and the solvent as a whole. In this case, we have to come back to the expression of the flux (7.160) and add to the flux due to the variation of the chemical potential caused by concentration gradient another term, due to the whole movement of the solution. This term is identical to the flux considered in the derivation of the continuity equation (see Section 7.2.3) but for the fact that, assuming the solution an uncompressible fluid, it has to be written assuming for the solute $\rho(\boldsymbol{r},t) = c(\boldsymbol{r}, t)$. Thus, the overall flux gets

$$\Phi_p(\boldsymbol{r},t) = -\sigma\kappa T\nabla c - c(\boldsymbol{r},t)v_w(\boldsymbol{r},t) \tag{7.165}$$

where v_w is the fluid velocity as a whole.

Substituting Equation 7.160 into the Equation 7.155 and assuming that there are no sources or sinks, since the divergence of the velocity field of an uncompressible liquid is zero and that the diffusion coefficient is constant, we have

$$\frac{\partial c(\boldsymbol{r},t)}{\partial t} = D\nabla^2 c + v_w \cdot \nabla c \tag{7.166}$$

This is the so-called diffusion-convection equation that regulates the solute concentration in cases in which the solution undergoes an hydrodynamic motion.

7.4.2 THE DIFFUSION COEFFICIENT

To correctly model diffusion phenomena in labs on chip it is very important to determine accurate values for the diffusion coefficients of macromolecules in different situations. The most direct way of calculating the diffusion coefficient is to imagine a rigid spherical particle immersed in a continuous fluid. In this case, we can use for the particle mobility the Stokes relation [4,53] that writes $\sigma = 1/6\,\pi\,\eta\,r$ where η is the solvent dynamic viscosity and r is the particles radius.

Since we can neglect the collision between particles due to the assumption of diluted solution, substituting the Stokes relation into the expression of the diffusion coefficient we have

$$D = \kappa\,T/6\,\pi\,\eta\,r \qquad\qquad (7.167)$$

This relation is often used to evaluate the order of magnitude of a diffusion coefficient. For example, if we consider a protein as a molecule with a radius of the order of 0.05 nm, we get as order of magnitude $D \sim 4\,10^{-12}$. This is a correct forecast regarding the order of magnitude of diffusion coefficient of proteins, that varies from 10^{-10} to 10^{-13}. However, Equation 7.167 cannot provide a more quantitative value, since many important effects influencing the value of the diffusion coefficient are not taken into account.

It is intuitive that the diffusion coefficient has to depend on the configuration of the considered macromolecule once hydrated in the solution. If we consider the configuration phase space introduced in Section 1.6, we should determine all the different configurations corresponding to the minimum configuration energy and determine the value of the diffusion coefficient for each of them. The macroscopic diffusion coefficient will be the average over the configuration space. This is a quite complex task, even if methods to describe and forecast the configuration of macromolecules with the methods of statistical mechanics are effectively available [56,57].

An important part of the dependence on the molecule configuration is the dependence on the molecule hydration that differentiates the insulated molecule configuration from the configuration of the molecule while in the solution.

If the solution is quite diluted, different kinds of macromolecules are effectively independent. However, in the solution processing that happens in a lab on chip to ease the final detection stage, it is frequent that the solution is concentrated so that collision among different types of macromolecules are no more independent. Moreover, in intra-tissue and intracellular environment the macromolecules solution is not always diluted. In all these cases, the diffusion coefficient depends not only on the considered macromolecule, but also on the concentration of all the other macromolecules in the solution [58–60].

A great effort has been carried out to set-up more accurate methods to forecast the diffusion coefficient of macromolecules, both trying to introduce more complexity in the simple Stokes-Einstein model and to develop new models starting from a more accurate description of the macromolecules [61,62]. Measurements of diffusion coefficients in different situations are key to tune and verify different theories on their calculation and different measurement techniques have been developed to measure diffusion coefficients of macromolecules [63–66].

In Table 7.7, the diffusion coefficients of selected diluted solutions of carbohydrates are reported at a temperature of 303 K [59]. Data relative to proteins in diluted water solution are reported in Table 7.8 [77–79]. The data presented in Table 7.8 are also shown on a Dispersion Coefficient versus Molecular Weight plot in Figure 7.43 and interpolated with a function depending on the inverse of the cubic radix of the molecular weight. The interpolation function is suggested by the Stokes-Einstein relation, where the diffusion coefficient depends on the inverse of the solute molecule radius. Imagining the density of the molecule constant and a spherical shape this implies the dependence on the inverse of the cubic radix of the molecular weight.

The interpolating curve catches well the qualitative behavior of the experimental points, but substantial deviations are present, far beyond the experimental errors [77,78] that identify the importance of the configuration of the molecule. Finally, in Table 7.9 [79], diffusion coefficients at 25°C are reported for cells in water solution. These are big particles with respect to molecules and frequently much more compact. The values of the diffusion coefficient are much smaller than those of macromolecules, as intuitive.

TABLE 7.7

**Experimental Values of the Diffusion Coefficients
of Selected Carbohydrates in Diluted Water Solution
at a Temperature of 303 K**

Carbohydrate	Diffusion Coefficient ($m^2/s \times 10^{-11}$)
Lactose	64
Sucrose	61
Glucose	76
Fructose	77

Source: Data form Ribeiro A. C. F. et al., Binary mutual diffusion coefficients of aqueous solutions of sucrose, lactose, glucose, and fructose in the temperature range from (298.15 to 328.15) K, *Journal of Chemical Engineering Data*, vol. 51, pp. 1836–1840, 2006.

Besides diffusion coefficients in water solution, the diffusion coefficient in electrophoretic gel (see Section 2.3.1 and 2.3.5) is relevant for all polar molecules. Motion of polar molecules in gel is not strictly a combination of convection generated by the electrical field and diffusion. The gel acts as a porous material where molecules moves in spaces among gel molecules, frequently widening them. Thus, a complex model based on percolation in a porous medium that is modified by the moving molecule population should be adopted. However, simple convection-diffusion description of the molecules movement is frequently adopted for a rough evaluation of the electrophoresis run length and linewidth. Under this approximation, the width of the electrophoresis line depends on the width of the insertion zone and on the diffusion of particles in gel that randomizes their motion. Since the diffusion coefficient in gel is measured typically to model

TABLE 7.8

Experimental Values of the Diffusion Coefficients of Selected Proteins in Diluted Water Solution

Protein	Source	Diffusion Coefficient ($m^2/s \times 10^{-11}$)	Molecular Mass (kDa)	Reference
Insulin	Porcine	13	5.8	[77]
Ribonuclease	Human	13	13.7	[79]
Lysozyme	Chicken egg white	13	14.5	[78]
Myoglobin	Horse	11.3	16.9	[78]
VEGF 165	—	5.2	19	[77]
Chymotrypsinogen	Bovine	7.1	24	[77]
Insulin	Human	7.7	24.2	[79]
Ovalbumin	Chicken egg	7.76	43.5	[78]
α-Glycoprotein	Human pleural fluid	6.75	45.2	[78]
Albumin monomer	Bovine serum	7.1	66.5	[77]
Hemoglobin	Bovine	8.4	68	[77]
Hemoglobin	Human	7.3	68	[79]
Actin	Human	5.3	130	[79]
IgG	Human	3.88	150	[77]
Apoferritin	Horse	3.6	443	[78]
Tyroglobulin	Bovine	2.61	669	[78]
IgM	Human	1.8	970	[77]

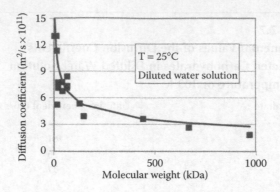

FIGURE 7.43 Data from Table 7.8 on a diffusion coefficient versus molecular weight plot. The solid line represents the best fit with a function depending on the inverse of the cubic radix of the molecular weight.

the electrophoresis process it is customary to consider the presence of ions into the gel besides polar macromolecules such as proteins, peptides, or nucleic acids. Moreover, the diffusivity coefficient is evaluated in a gel membrane, like those used in electrophoresis measurements.

Two reasons tend to make the diffusion coefficient in a membrane smaller than that in the bulk of a solution with the same viscosity of the gel. First, hydrodynamic interactions between the macromolecular solute and fibers that compose the gel membrane reduce the mobility of the solute. As a matter of fact, the continuous approximation is not completely suitable for the gel, composed by a very dense solution of fibers, which results having a high degree of orientation in a thin membrane.

Second, steric and/or electrostatic interactions between macromolecules and the gel fibers tend to reduce the diffusion coefficient further when calculated in a thin slab. To represent macroscopically these effects the diffusion coefficient D_{eff} in a gel membrane is frequently expressed as follows:

$$D_{eff} = \Phi D = \Phi \Gamma D_{\infty} \qquad (7.168)$$

where D_{∞} is the diffusion coefficient in a bulk solution, and the two coefficients Φ and Γ, both smaller than one, represents, respectively, the interaction with the gel fibers and the steric and electrostatic interaction with the gel. In Table 7.10 [80], the diffusion coefficient in agarose gel containing ions is evaluated for selected proteins for different ionic strength at 25°C. The limits of the dilutes approximation are shown in Figure 7.44, where the diffusion coefficient of lactose in water is shown for different temperatures as a function of the lactose concentration in moles per liter [59]. For small concentration, the diffusion coefficient remains unchanged, but by increasing the concentration it starts to decrease as collisions among lactose molecules are more and more important. This can be a relevant effect in the last stages of a lab on chip, where the solution under test has been concentrated to ease the detection.

TABLE 7.9

Diffusion Coefficients and Mass of Selected Cells in Diluted Water Solution

Cell	Cells' Weight	Diffusion Coefficient $(m^2/s \times 10^{-11})$	Reference
Tobacco mosaic virus	31.34 MDa	0.56	[79]
T7 Bacteriophage	37.5 MDa	0.95	[79]
Polyhedral silkworm virus	916.2 MDa	0.23	[79]
Platelet (human)	4 TDa	0.016	[79]
Red blood cell (human)	60 TDa	0.0068	[79]

TABLE 7.10

Diffusion Coefficients in Charged Sulfated Agarose Gel with Different Ionic Strengths for Selected Proteins at 25°C

Protein	Molecular Weight	Ionic Strength (mol/m³)	D_∞ (m²/s × 10⁻¹¹)	D (m²/s × 10⁻¹¹)	D_{eff} (m²/s × 10⁻¹¹)
Bovine serum albumin	66.5	1.01	5.7	2.7	1.809
		0.11	5.8	2.6	1.222
		0.01	5.8	2.6	0.754
Ovalbumin	45	1.01	6.7	3.1	1.984
		0.11	6.8	3.0	1.77
		0.01	6.8	2.8	0.812
Lactalbumin	14.2	1.01	9.2	4.9	3.822
		0.11	9.3	4.5	3.375
		0.01	9.9	3.8	1.672

Source: Data from Johnson E. M. et al., Diffusion and partitioning of proteins in charged agarose gels, *Biophysical Journal*, vol. 68, pp. 1561–1568, 1995.

7.4.3 Diffusion Equation Basic Solutions: Free Diffusion

The first step is to consider a solution of the diffusion equation in a practically unlimited volume. Besides the theoretical importance of such problem, solving it is also practically important when the diffusion happens in a limited volume, but all the interesting dynamics is limited to short times, when the concentration near the far end walls is still almost zero. In this case, the diffusion volume can be considered unlimited.

Such results are also useful when the diffusion volume is half limited (a semi space limited by a plane) and all the diffusion sources/sinks are along the plane. In this case, for the symmetry of the problem, no diffusion can happen through the limiting plane, that is the center of a reflection symmetry. Thus, the unlimited volume approach can be adopted.

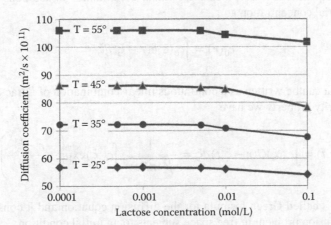

FIGURE 7.44 Diffusion coefficient of lactose in water for different temperatures as a function of the lactose concentration in moles per liter. (Data from Ribeiro A. C. F. et al., Binary mutual diffusion coefficients of aqueous solutions of sucrose, lactose, glucose, and fructose in the temperature range from (298.15 to 328.15) K, *Journal of Chemical Engineering Data*, vol. 51, pp. 1836–1840, 2006.)

7.4.3.1 Green Function and Free Diffusion from an Initial Distribution

The first case to be considered is the diffusion from a point source, that is, a source mathematically represented by a Dirac distribution. Physically, this condition represents the case in which a quantity of solute is inserted in a very small volume at the initial instant and then it diffuses freely into the solvent. The solution of this problem is mathematically called Green function [81] for the free diffusion problem.

In the absence of source/sink terms, the diffusion equation writes

$$\frac{\partial c(r,t)}{\partial t} = D\nabla^2 c \tag{7.169}$$

By Fourier transforming with respect to the three spatial variables and direct integration with respect to the time variable we find a simple Fourier transform of a solution of Equation 7.169. Its inverse transform can be directly evaluated obtaining

$$G(r,t) = \frac{1}{\sqrt{(4\pi Dt)^3}} \exp\left(-\frac{x^2 + y^2 + z^2}{4Dt}\right) \tag{7.170}$$

It is easy to note that the distributional limit of such a function for $t \to 0$ is $G(r, 0) = \delta(r)$ thus it is exactly the solution we were searching.

Equation 7.170 has the properties we intuitively require from free diffusion. By increasing time, the variance of the Gaussian function representing the concentration increases, thus representing the fact that diffusion disperses the solute progressively into the solvent.

The concentration standard deviation increases slowly with time, only with the square root of time, representing the intuitive fact that diffusion is the result of a great number of random events so that their effect accumulates slowly [82]. However, the average of the concentration remains zero, that is, the center of mass of the concentration remains always fixed at the point where the solute was inserted into the solvent. Thus, representing the fact that free diffusion has no preferential directions in isotropic media.

In more practical cases, the initial concentration is not point-like, but it is constituted by a spatial function $c_0(r)$. In order to solve the corresponding free diffusion problem we can use the fact that the diffusion equation is linear, thus every linear combination of solutions is a solution itself. Expressing the initial concentration as

$$c_0(r) = \int c_0(\xi)\delta(r - \xi)d\xi \tag{7.171}$$

we recognize that it can be written as a continuous linear combination of Dirac distributions. Thus applying the linearity property we have

$$c(r,t) = \int c_0(\xi)G(r - \xi,t)d\xi = \frac{1}{\sqrt{(4\pi Dt)^3}} \int c_0(\xi)\exp\left(-\frac{|r - \xi|^2}{4Dt}\right)d\xi \tag{7.172}$$

Equation 7.172 is called Green formula for the diffusion equation and it constitutes the general solution of the diffusion problem in free space subjects to an initial condition.

To provide an example of the use of Equation 7.172 let us imagine that diffusion happens in a very thin slab, so that the concentration along the vertical direction can be always considered constant and the problem reduces to a bidirectional problem. Let us also assume that the initial distribution is constant in the interval $(x,y) \in \left[(-L,-L),(L,L)\right]$.

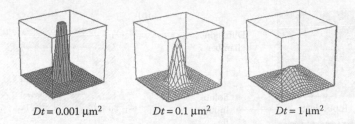

$$Dt = 0.001\ \mu m^2 \qquad Dt = 0.1\ \mu m^2 \qquad Dt = 1\ \mu m^2$$

FIGURE 7.45 Concentrations at different times after two-dimension diffusion from a square initial concentration.

In this case, the integral (7.172) can be solved analytically using the error function erf(*) [83] obtaining

$$c(\boldsymbol{r},t) = c_0(0,0)\left[\mathrm{erf}\left(\frac{x-L}{\sqrt{4\,Dt}}\right) - \mathrm{erf}\left(\frac{x+L}{\sqrt{4\,Dt}}\right)\right]\left[\mathrm{erf}\left(\frac{y-L}{\sqrt{4Dt}}\right) - \mathrm{erf}\left(\frac{y+L}{\sqrt{4\,Dt}}\right)\right] \qquad (7.173)$$

The concentration profiles for different times coming out from Equation 7.173 are shown in Figure 7.45 at different times.

7.4.3.2 Source and Flux-Driven Free Diffusion

Besides initial conditions, we have the presence of a source in the chamber where diffusion appears that, while diffusion disperses the solute into the chamber, adds in time new solute to the solution. The first step to address this problem is to write the overall diffusion equation solution as the super-position of the solution corresponding to the initial condition (see Equation 7.172) and a solution corresponding to the problem with the source and initial condition equal to a zero. This separation is allowed by the linearity of the diffusion equation and allows us to concentrate here on the source problem with zero initial condition.

Let us assume that the source can be expressed with a function of time and position $c_{sou}(\boldsymbol{r}, t)$ providing the quantity of solute added to the diffusion chamber by the source in the unit time. As we have done for the space variables in Equation 7.171 we can decompose the source function in a continuous linear superposition of sources acting in a specific instant. This corresponds to decompose the problem in a continuous set of diffusion problems, each of which starts from a different instant and with a different initial condition corresponding to the value of the source in that instant. Since the diffusion equation is linear, the final solution will be the superposition of the solutions of each individual problem. In particular, the quantity of solute added to the diffusion chamber by a continuous source in a time is simply given by the source function multiplied by dt, using Equation 7.172 to solve the instantaneous problem and adding the obtained functions we find the wanted solution of the diffusion equation as

$$c(\boldsymbol{r},t) = \int_0^t \int_V c_{sou}(\xi,\tau)G(\boldsymbol{r}-\xi,t-\tau)\eta_H(t-\tau)\,d\xi\,d\tau \qquad (7.174)$$

where the integral on V represents the triple spatial integral and $\eta_H(t-\tau)$ is the Heaviside function that is equal to one for $t-\tau \geq 0$ and equal to zero for $t-\tau < 0$. The presence of the Heaviside function remembers that the value of the source at the instant τ influences the solution only in instants greater than τ for the causality principle. It is useful to include it explicitly into the integral, since frequently it is possible to express the concentration source in a simple way using functions that have not the property to be different from zero only for positive times.

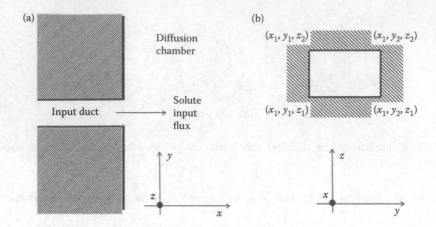

FIGURE 7.46 Reference geometry for the solution of the flux driven free diffusion problem. Section parallel to the (x, y) coordinate plane (a), section parallel to the (y, z) coordinate plane (b).

A particularly interesting case is the flux driven diffusion. In this case, the source is given by the flux of the solute through an input duct opening on the considered chamber. For a reference let us consider the geometry represented in Figure 7.46. Let us assume that in the input duct the concentration depends only on the longitudinal variable x and is constant along y and z. This is the case in which the solution is injected in the input duct when it is divided by a valve from the diffusion chamber, equilibrium is reached and only at the end is the valve opened and the diffusion from the duct to the chamber begins.

The flux of the concentration is given by the concentration gradient changed in sign, thus the incoming flux through the input duct end into the diffusion chamber is

$$\Phi_c(\boldsymbol{r},t) = -\nabla c_d(\boldsymbol{r},t)\big|_{x=0} = -\frac{\partial c_d(\boldsymbol{r},t)}{\partial x}\big|_{x=0} \; \boldsymbol{x} \tag{7.175}$$

where $c_d(\boldsymbol{r}, t)$ is the concentration in the input duct and x is the unitary vector along the x-axis. If we imagine that the valve is instantly opened, at the initial instant the concentration derivative is infinite, being the concentration finite just a step into the duct and zero just a step into the chamber.

This is a consequence of the unphysical hypothesis that the valve opens instantaneously. There are mathematical tricks to cure this problem while maintaining the valve aperture instantaneous [84,85], which are useful especially when this kind of phenomena are found in more complex problems that have to be solved by simulation. Here, we simply prefer to introduce a finite time for the valve opening. Let us assume that the valve opens like a plane shatter in a characteristic time equal to T_{val} so that the area that is open for diffusion at the instant t is given by $A(t) = (y_2 - y_1)(x_2 - x_1)\psi(t,T_{val})$ where the function $\psi(t,T_{val})$ is zero for $t = 0$, one at the limit of very long times and it approaches its asymptotic limit monotonically with a characteristic time equal to T_{val}. Thus, the net flux of solute entering the diffusion chamber is

$$\Phi_c(\boldsymbol{r},t) = -\frac{\partial c_d(\boldsymbol{r},t)}{\partial x}\bigg|_{x=0} A(t)\delta(x)\boldsymbol{x} \tag{7.176}$$

The flux-driven diffusion can be reduced to a source-driven diffusion by observing that, if we introduce a source that exists only on the duct end, it provides a solute quantity to the diffusion chamber equal to the flux in the unit time. Thus we can write the solution as in Equation 7.74 with

$$c_{sou}(\boldsymbol{r},t) = -\left.\frac{\partial c_d(\boldsymbol{r},t)}{\partial x}\right|_{x=0} A(t)\delta(x) \tag{7.177}$$

The integral in the longitudinal direction is immediately solved and the following expression is obtained for the final solution

$$c(\boldsymbol{r},t) = -\int_0^t\int_{y_1}^{y_2}\int_{z_1}^{z_2} \left.\frac{\partial c_d(\xi,\ \theta,\xi,\tau)}{\partial\xi}\right|_{\xi=0} A(\tau)\, G(x,y-\theta,z-\zeta,t-\tau)\,d\theta d\zeta d\tau \tag{7.178}$$

As an example, let us imagine that a duct of length L_d is full of a water solution containing a certain macromolecule in a concentration c_0, constant along the duct. At the instant $t = 0$, the valve is opened in a time much smaller than the diffusion time of the macromolecule along the duct and it starts to diffuse in the diffusion chamber. While the macromolecule diffuses in the diffusion chamber the concentration decreases in the input duct, so that the fluxes changes in time.

As far as the input duct is considered, due to the overall axial symmetry and to the fact that no flux has to happen from the rear duct end, it can be considered a one-dimensional system regulated by the diffusion equation

$$\frac{\partial c_D(x,t)}{\partial t} = D\frac{\partial^2 c_D(x,t)}{\partial x^2} \tag{7.179}$$

In order to force diffusion only from the open to the diffusion chamber, we assume that the solution is periodic with period $2L$, as if two identical ducts were put with the end walls one after the other. Since the dynamic in the two ducts is identical, there is no reason why matter passes from one to the other and generally no unprovoked passage of matter can happen from one duct to the other: that means that no flux happens from the end wall. Under these conditions, the one-dimensional diffusion equation solves easily by the Green formula 7.172 obtaining

$$c_D(x,t) = c_0\left[\operatorname{erf}\left(\frac{x}{\sqrt{2Dt}}\right) - \operatorname{erf}\left(\frac{2L+x}{\sqrt{2Dt}}\right)\right] \tag{7.180}$$

The variation of the concentration in the input duct while it diffuses in the diffusion chamber is represented in Figure 7.47 versus time and longitudinal coordinates using the data in Table 7.11.

The diffusion in the diffusion chamber cannot be described as a one-dimensional process, but due to the very small vertical dimension, it can be approximated with a two-dimensional model. As a matter of fact, as it can also be deduced in Figure 7.47, the typical time scale T of the problem is of the order of 1 s. The considered macromolecule, due to its diffusion coefficient, travels by diffusion more or less $\sqrt{DT} = 26\,\mu m$ that is a distance much longer than the vertical dimension of the diffusion chamber.

Approximating the diffusion chamber as a slab and assuming the valve opening an exponential process with a time scale of the order of 1 ms, we can write the flux in the diffusion chamber as

$$\Phi(x,t) = -\left.\frac{\partial}{\partial x}c_D(x,t)\right]_{x=0} A(t)x = \frac{c_0}{\sqrt{2\pi Dt}} H_{y_1,y_2}(y)\left(1 - e^{-\frac{t}{T_{val}}}\right)x \tag{7.181}$$

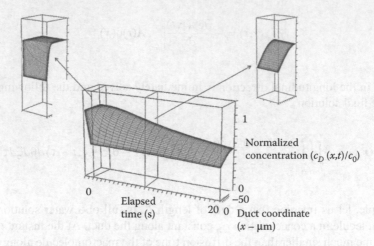

FIGURE 7.47 Diffusion of the macromolecule considered in the example of flux driven diffusion into the incoming duct as a function of the longitudinal coordinate x and of time.

where $H_{a,b}(y)$ is the so-called rectangular function defined as

$$H_{a,b}(y) = \begin{cases} 1 & y \in [a,b] \\ 0 & \text{Otherwise} \end{cases} \tag{7.182}$$

Substituting Equation 7.181 into Equation 7.178 and integrating we get

$$c(x,y,t) = c_0 \int_0^t \left[\text{erf}\left(\frac{1}{4D} \frac{x}{t-\tau} \right) - 1 \right] \left[\text{erf}\left(\frac{1}{4D} \frac{y-L/2}{t-\tau} \right) - \text{erf}\left(\frac{1}{4D} \frac{y-L/2}{t-\tau} \right) \right] \left(1 - e^{-\frac{\tau}{T_{val}}} \right) d\tau$$

$$\approx c_0 \left[\text{erf}\left(\frac{1}{4D} \frac{x}{t} \right) - 1 \right] \left[\text{erf}\left(\frac{1}{4D} \frac{y-L/2}{t} \right) - \text{erf}\left(\frac{1}{4D} \frac{y-L/2}{t} \right) \right] \quad \text{for } t \gg T_{val}$$

$$\tag{7.183}$$

TABLE 7.11

Numerical Data of the System Used for the Examples of Sections 7.4.3.2 and 7.4.4

Free and Limited Volume Diffusion

Incoming duct length	L	50 μm
Duct horizontal width	$y_2 - y_1$	10 μm
Duct vertical width	$z_2 - z_1$	5 μm
Diffusion chamber vertical width	—	5 μm
Initial protein concentration	c_0	0.02 PPM mol, 0.09 mol/L
Protein molecular weight	M	8 kDa
Protein diffusion coefficient	D	7×10^{-10}
Valve opening characteristic time	T_{val}	1 ms

Limited Volume Diffusion Only

Diffusion chamber length	L_1	200 μm
Diffusion chamber width	L_2	100 μm

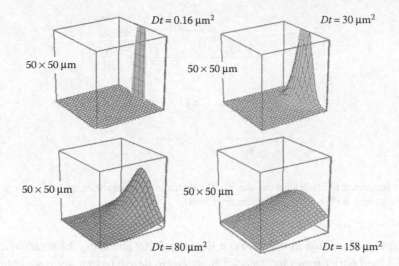

FIGURE 7.48 Diffusion of the macro molecule considered in the example of flux driven diffusion into the diffusion chamber at different instants.

The evolution of the concentration in the diffusion chamber at different instants is shown in Figure 7.48, demonstrating the typical diffusion dynamics, starting from the initial shape reproducing the outlet of the incoming duct.

7.4.4 Diffusion Equation Basic Solutions: Diffusion in Limited Volumes

Diffusion solution in conditions of free diffusion are very useful in several practical cases, however it is also frequently the case in which the fact that diffusion happens in a limited volume cannot be ignored. In this case, boundary conditions are added to the initial condition and the free diffusion Green methods cannot be used. In labs on chip, the ducts and chambers where diffusion happens are generally squared, due to the processes that produce them. Thus, the case of a square domain for diffusion is not only particularly simple, but it is also important in our case.

Let us imagine that diffusion happens in a chamber of dimensions L_i ($i = 1, 2, 3$) whose vertex with smaller coordinates is (x_0, y_0, z_0) as shown in Figure 7.49. The most common boundary conditions for the concentration diffusion equation prescribe a value for the flux on the chamber walls. In particular, the initial conditions problem is generally solved by assuming that the flux on the chamber walls is zero, which means in mathematical terms

$$\left.\frac{\partial c}{\partial x}\right)_{x_0} = \left.\frac{\partial c}{\partial y}\right)_{y_0} = \left.\frac{\partial c}{\partial z}\right)_{z_0} = 0 \tag{7.184}$$

The above boundary conditions can be imposed by developing in Fourier series in the domain of Figure 7.49 the concentration and imposing on the series the condition (7.184) [86]. Since the Fourier functions are orthogonal the boundary condition has to be valid for every term of the series, so obtaining

$$c(x, y, z, t) = \sum_{i,j,k} c_{i,j,k}(t) \cos\left(\pi i \frac{x - x_0}{L_1}\right) \cos\left(\pi j \frac{y - y_0}{L_2}\right) \cos\left(\pi k \frac{z - z_0}{L_3}\right) \tag{7.185}$$

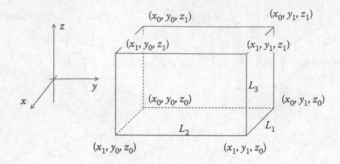

FIGURE 7.49 Reference geometry for the study of the diffusion in a parallelepiped diffusion chamber from an initial condition with no flux through the chamber walls.

Substituting Equation 7.185 in the diffusion Equation 7.169 and using the absolute and uniform convergence of the Fourier series for class $\mathbb{C}^2$ functions to derive term to term we obtain a simple differential equations for the Fourier coefficients

$$\frac{dc_{i,j,k}(t)}{dt} = -D\pi^2 \left(\frac{i^2}{L_1^2} + \frac{j^2}{L_2^2} + \frac{k^2}{L_3^2} \right) c_{i,j,k}(t) \tag{7.186}$$

This equation can be directly solved and the integration coefficients can be determined by imposing that at $t = 0$; the solution coincides with the initial condition $c(x, y, z, 0)$. This is simply obtained by developing the initial condition in Fourier series and equaling the coefficients with the same indices. Calling $c_{i,j,k}(0)$ the Fourier coefficients of the initial condition we get the final expression of the Fourier coefficients appearing in Equation 7.185

$$c_{i,j,k}(t) = c_{i,j,k}(0) e^{-D\pi^2 \left(\frac{i^2}{L_1^2} + \frac{j^2}{L_2^2} + \frac{k^2}{L_3^2} \right) t} \tag{7.187}$$

Equation 7.187 indicates that the diffusion from an initial condition in a limited chamber, differently from the diffusion in free space, tends to a stationary regime with a characteristic time equal to

$$\tau = \frac{L_{max}^2}{D\pi^2} \quad L_{max}^2 = \max(L_1^2, L_2^2, L_3^2) \tag{7.188}$$

The stationary value has to be constant in all the diffusion domains, since by direct inspection of the diffusion equation this is the only condition assuring both null flux out of the domain and zero concentration time derivative. The exact stationary value c_{st} can be derived from the conservation of mass inside the domain, due to the null flux boundary condition, and it is given by

$$c_{st} = \frac{1}{V} \int_V c(\mathbf{r}, 0) \, d\mathbf{r} \quad V = L_1 L_2 L_3 \tag{7.189}$$

It is also interesting to consider the flux-driven diffusion equation solution in the case of a limited diffusion domain. In this case, if imagine to have a diffusion chamber and an incoming duct from which at the instant $t = 0$ the solute starts to diffuse into the diffusion chamber where only the solvent is present; the situation is depicted in Figure 7.50. In this case, the initial condition is zero and the boundary condition on the domain wall at $y = y_0$ writes

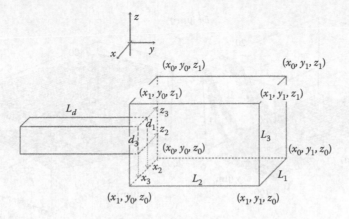

FIGURE 7.50 Reference geometry for the study of the diffusion in a parallelepiped diffusion chamber driven by the solute flux coming from an incoming duct.

$$\left.\frac{\partial c}{\partial y}\right)_{y_0} = H_{x_2,x_3}(x)H_{z_2,z_3}(z)\left.\frac{\partial c_D}{\partial y}\right)_{y_0} \tag{7.190}$$

where the rectangular function $H_{x_2,x_3}(x)$ is defined in Equation 7.182.

In order to solve the problem, let us imagine that the diffusion chamber is replied twice, symmetrized with respect to the $y = y_0$ plane. The solution in the diffusion chamber and in its specular replica is the same, but for a specular symmetry. This assures that no flux will happen through the $y = y_0$ plane, but for the flux from the incoming duct. The flux from the incoming duct, in this extended diffusion chamber appears as a continuous source placed along a part of a plane. This source has to generate a flux that is considered toward positive y when coming near the source from $y > 0$ and toward negative y when coming near the source from $y < 0$ so as to satisfy the mirror symmetry we have constructed.

In order to do that, let constructing a concentration in an imaginary mirrored duct be as follows:

$$c_M(y) = \begin{cases} c_D(y - y_0) & y \geq y_0 \\ c_D(y_0 - y) & y \leq y_0 \end{cases} \tag{7.191}$$

The flux expression is obtained directly by Equation 7.191 as.

$$\Phi(x,y,z,t) = H_{x_2,x_3}(x)H_{z_2,z_3}(z)\left.\frac{\partial c_M}{\partial y}\right)_{y_0}\delta(y - y_0) \tag{7.192}$$

where the derivative of $c_M(y)$ has to be evaluated suitably considering the direction from where we get near $y = y_0$.

The problem of diffusion from a continuous source in a limited volume can be solved using the same procedure we have used in the case of free diffusion. In particular, let us consider the Fourier components of the equivalent source (7.192), which are defined as

$$\xi_{i,k}(t) = \int_{y_0-L_2}^{L_2+y_0}\int_{x_0}^{L_1+x_0}\int_{z_0}^{L_3+z_0} c_{eq}(x,y,z,t)\cos\left(\pi i\frac{x-x_0}{L_1}\right)\cos\left(\pi k\frac{z-z_0}{L_3}\right)\cos\left(\pi j\frac{y-y_0}{L_3}\right)dy\,dz\,dy \tag{7.193}$$

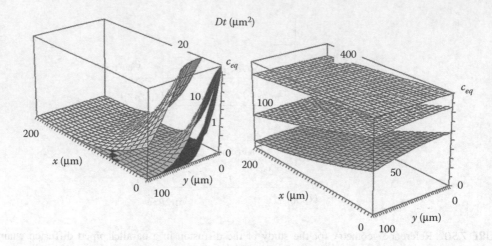

FIGURE 7.51 Diffusion from an incoming duct of a macromolecule in a two-dimensional diffusion chamber of limited length and width. The concentration is shown versus the coordinates in the diffusion chamber for different times after the start of the diffusion.

In order to correctly evaluate $\xi_{i,k}(t)$ we have to split the integral in two parts: one in the interval $[y_0, L_2 + y_0]$ and the other in the interval $[y_0, L_2 - y_0]$ since in the two interval the derivative of the function $_{cM}$ has to be considered different. The two resulting integrals are equal, as it can be seen by changing y in $-y$. Considering also the presence of the rectangular functions we have

$$\xi_{i,k}(t) = 2\int\limits_{x_2}^{x_3}\int\limits_{z_2}^{z_3} \left(\frac{\partial c_D}{\partial y}\right)_{y_0} \cos\left(\pi i \frac{x - x_0}{L_1}\right)\cos\left(\pi k \frac{z - z_0}{L_3}\right) dz\, dy \qquad (7.194)$$

Finally, the Fourier coefficients of the concentration in the diffusion room are given by

$$c_{i,j,k}(t) = \int\limits_0^t \xi_{i,k}(\tau)A(\tau)\, e^{-D\pi^2\left(\frac{i^2}{L_1^2}+\frac{j^2}{L_2^2}+\frac{k^2}{L_3^2}\right)(t-\tau)}\, d\tau \qquad (7.195)$$

where $A(\tau)$ represents the aperture of the duct end valve (see Section 7.3.4.2).

As an example of application of this solution of the diffusion equation let us consider the diffusion in a two-dimensional diffusion room with dimensions equal to that reported in Table 7.11 for times much longer than the valve typical aperture time ($T_{val} = 1$ ms in this case). Results obtained by using Equations 7.194 and 7.195 are reported in Figure 7.51, where c_{eq} indicates the equilibrium concentration. The behavior is quite clear, while the solute passes from the incoming duct to the diffusion chamber the quantity of solute increases in the diffusion chamber and decreases in the incoming duct. Due to diffusion a sort of diffusion wave propagates further from the duct output into the diffusion chamber up to the equilibrium situation where the concentration is constant over the diffusion chamber and the incoming duct and equal to $c_{eq} = c_0(V_d + V_c)/V_d$ being V_c and V_d the volumes of the diffusion chamber and of the incoming duct, respectively.

7.4.5 THE CHEMICAL–DIFFUSION MODEL: EXAMPLES

If we assume a single order neutralization reaction like 7.162 happening in the diffusion chamber and we add the corresponding chemical terms to the diffusion equation we obtain the system

(7.164), that is, in general, much harder to solve with respect to a simple diffusion equation. In this section we will introduce two results that allow to use solutions of the simple diffusion equation to approach the solution of the chemical-diffusion problem.

A first step is to assume that, since we are dealing with an assay in a lab on chip, the reaction is almost unidirectional (see Section 3.3.2), so that the quantities of the reagents that remain not combined in the reaction room is very small. This does not imply that both A and B are not present at equilibrium, due to the fact that the overall molarity of one of them can be larger than that of the other. In this hypothesis, the term representing the decay of C into $A + B$ at the second member of the system (7.164) can be eliminated in a first approximation.

In certain practical cases, the first term of reaction 7.162 is composed by two molecules with very different molecular weights (see Sections 3.3.3 and 3.3.4). A first example is the immunoassay of great bodies, like viruses or great antigenic molecules via reaction with a specific antibody. In this case, the difference in diffusion coefficients between the two reacting species can be more than one order of magnitude. Another example is the detection of a heavy protein via a single segment of a specific antibody (e.g., one of the branches of an IgG).

In these cases, a first-order perturbation theory can be used to approximate the evolution in the reaction chamber, assuming at order zero that the heavy species, for example, the antigen and the neutralized antigen, are still and evaluating its diffusion only at first order.

Let us indicate with the indices B and C the heavy species and with A the light one. Under the above hypotheses the system (7.164) becomes

$$\frac{\partial c_{A1}(r,t)}{\partial t} = D\nabla^2 c_{A1} - v_+ c_{A1} c_{B0} \tag{7.196a}$$

$$\frac{\partial c_{B1}(r,t)}{\partial t} = -v_+ c_{A1} c_{B1} \tag{7.196b}$$

$$\frac{\partial c_{C1}(r,t)}{\partial t} = v_+ c_{A1} c_{B1} \tag{7.196c}$$

where c_{B0} indicates the zeroth order approximation for the concentration of the species B and all the other concentrations are first-order approximations. Moreover, equations b and c come from the reaction stoichiometry and from the hypothesis that at zero-th order the molecules of the species B and C do not move in space.

We can divide the derivatives of the concentrations into two terms: a chemical term that is fast and a diffusion term that is slow. The fast derivatives are related to the stoichiometry of the chemical reaction. Moreover, at the zero-th order both $c_{B0}(r, t)$ and $c_{C0}(r, t)$ do not depend on diffusion, being their fast derivative coincident with the whole time derivative. As a conclusion we can write

$$\left.\frac{\partial c_{A1}(r,t)}{\partial t}\right)_{fast} = \frac{\partial c_{B0}(r,t)}{\partial t} = -\frac{\partial c_{C0}(r,t)}{\partial t} \tag{7.197}$$

A first case in which Equation 7.197 can be solved is in the case in which the overall mass of the substance A that is present in the system at the instant $t = 0$ is much smaller than the overall mass of the substance B. This is a realistic situation if A is the substance to be detected into the lab on chip via an assay and B is the assay reference substance since in many assays the reference substance is present in larger concentration with respect to the substance to be detected. It is also generally verified that in the reaction chamber $c_{A1}|_{t=0} = 0$ since the substance to be detected is injected into the reaction chamber either via diffusion or in other ways starting at the initial assay instant.

Under all these hypotheses the quadratic term of Equation 7.196a becomes

$$\frac{\partial c_{A1}(\boldsymbol{r},t)}{\partial t} = D\nabla^2 c_{A1} - K_+ c_{A1} \qquad (7.198)$$

where $K_+ = v_+ c_{B0}\big|_{t=0}$ being $c_{B0}\big|_{t=0}$ the initial condition for the species B. The physical meaning of K_+ is quite clear, it is a sort of effective reaction speed, depending both on the reaction rate and on the concentration of the abundant regent.

Equation 7.198 can be solved exactly with the method of the integrating factor [87] if a solution of the corresponding diffusion equation under the problem initial and the boundaries conditions is known. Let us assume the following expression of the solution of Equation 7.198:

$$c_{A1}(\boldsymbol{r},t) = e^{-K_+ t} c_D(\boldsymbol{r},t) \qquad (7.199)$$

where $c_D(\boldsymbol{r}, t)$ is a solution of the corresponding diffusion equation.

Substituting into Equation 7.199 and collecting terms the integrating factor $e^{-K_+ t}$ can be eliminated and it is obtained

$$D\nabla^2[c_D(\boldsymbol{r},t)] - K_+ c_D(\boldsymbol{r},t) = \frac{\partial}{\partial t}[c_D(\boldsymbol{r},t)] - K_+ c_D(\boldsymbol{r},t) \qquad (7.200)$$

Since $c_D(\boldsymbol{r}, t)$ is a solution of the corresponding diffusion equation the equality (7.200) is satisfied so that its result demonstrated that expression 7.199 is the solution of Equation 7.198.

The solution 7.199 has a very intuitive meaning. Faster the reaction (higher K_+), faster the concentration of the species A decreases in time and it is not allowed to diffuse beyond its initial position. A simple example is provided if we consider the reaction chamber described in Table 7.11 with its feeding duct and imagine that the reaction chamber is filled with a solution containing the heavy species B, while the species A is injected into the chamber from the incoming duct.

The analysis of the incoming duct is the same as the previous example, but for the fact that here the one-dimensional assumption is not exact due to the asymmetry of its position with respect to the reaction chamber, the approximation is in any case quite small with the given parameters. The concentration of the species A at order one is represented in Figure 7.52 versus the space coordinates if the parameters listed in Table 7.12 are used besides the geometrical parameters of Table 7.11. Also in this case, the approximation of two-dimensions reaction chamber is considered.

The above discussion is based on the approximation that the concentration of the reference substance in the assay is much greater than that of the substance to be detected. Since it is not always true, it is useful to find a method to solve Equation 7.197 even when the quadratic term at the second member cannot be neglected. A useful instrument in this case is the so-called time scales separation method, whose demonstration is reported in Appendix A3 in its main traits [88]. This theorem is based on the fact that the chemical reaction is much faster than diffusion, so that an adiabatic approximation can be used, considering the slow varying diffusion term as an initial condition for the fast varying chemical dynamics.

Using this approach an approximated solution of Equation 7.197 can be constructed by separately solving the diffusion equation and the chemical equation that regulates the chemical reaction dynamics.

If only the fast dynamic is considered, the time derivative of all the concentrations will coincide with the fast derivative term only so that Equation 7.197 in this case can be directly solved.

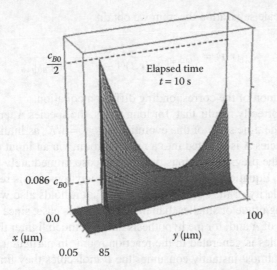

FIGURE 7.52 Diffusion from an incoming duct of a protein in a two-dimensional diffusion chamber of limited length and width while it recombines with a much more concentrated recombining molecule.

Substituting its solution in the general form of the chemical dynamics equations (see Equation 3.5 Section 3.3.3) we get

$$\frac{\partial c_{A1}(\boldsymbol{r},t)}{\partial t} = -v_+ c_{A1}^2 - K_+ c_{A1} \qquad (7.201)$$

It is apparent that the chemical equation can also be obtained by eliminating from Equation 7.197 the diffusion term (i.e., the slow term), contrary to the diffusion equation that is obtained by eliminating the chemical term (i.e., the fast term). From this interpretation the name of time scales separation theorem emerges. In our case, the solution of the associated chemical equation is simply

$$c(\boldsymbol{r},t) = \frac{c_{B0}|_{t-0} c_0 e^{-K_+ t}}{c_0(1 - e^{-K_+ t}) + c_{B0}|_{t=0}} \qquad (7.202)$$

TABLE 7.12

Numerical Data of the Assay Substances Used for the Example of Section 7.4.5

A species molecular weight	M_A	8 kDa
B species molecular weight	M_B	300 kDa
A species initial concentration in the duct	c_{A0}	0.02 PPM mol
B species concentration in the reaction chamber	c_{B0}	0.01 PPM mol
A molarity/B molarity	—	1/40
Direct reaction specific rate	v_+	10^7 1/s/mol
Direct initial reaction rate	$v_+ c_{B0}$	10^5 1/s
Inverse reaction rate	v_-	10^3 1/s

Applying the time scale separation theorem we obtain

$$c_{A1}(\boldsymbol{r},t) = c_{B0}|_{t=0} \frac{c_D(\boldsymbol{r},t)e^{-K_+ t}}{c_D(\boldsymbol{r},t)(1 - e^{-K_+ t}) + c_{B0}|_{t=0}} \tag{7.203}$$

where $c_D(\boldsymbol{r}, t)$ is the solution of the corresponding diffusion equation.

From this solution correctly results that, for long times, the species A tends to disappear in favor of the reaction result. The time scale of this evolution is $t_{chem} = 1/K_+$ as intuitive. However, this does not mean that if the species A is inserted into a reaction room via an input duct, as in the examples we have considered in the previous sections, it is in any case immediately consumed near the duct end. As a matter of fact, Equation 7.203 does not contain any hypothesis regarding the relationship between the overall molarity of the species A and B, so that it holds also when the molarity of B is of the same order of magnitude or smaller than that of A. In this case, since the chemical reaction is faster than the diffusion of A and, for the hypothesis that A is much lighter than B, a sort of diffusion wave of the fast molecules is generated in the reaction room. In particular, while entering into the room, the A molecules almost instantly consumes the B molecules they find on their way, creating zones that are almost free of B molecules, since they are too heavy to be able to replenish them. After freeing a reaction room zone from B molecules, the A molecules diffuses up to encounter a zone where the B molecules are present and repeat the cycle.

This effect is shown in Figure 7.53, where the behavior with time of the concentration of the reagent A in three different points of the reaction chamber is shown versus time. Once an approximated solution of Equation 7.196a is known, the other equations of the system 7.164 provide the concentration of the other reagent and of the reaction product at first order in the diffusion of the slow molecules. Both these equations can be solved with the integrating factor method obtaining the concentrations of the slow molecules with their diffusion taken into account at the first order.

Even if the approximation that one molecule diffuses much slower than the other is true in important cases, it is not always valid in practical cases. In many interesting assays, the molecules involved in the chemical reaction have similar diffusion coefficients, so that the chemical diffusion equation system cannot be solved with the approximations we have presented. In these cases, due to the fact that this is a system of three nonlinear equations, simulation is needed to obtain the concentration dynamic in the reaction chamber.

7.4.6 DIFFUSION–CONVECTION MODEL: EXAMPLES

The diffusion-convection model based on Equation 7.176 is used when a solute is transported by a moving solvent through a microfluidic circuit. In these cases, the fluid dynamic problem involving the motion of the solution as a whole has to be solved so as to determine the velocity field, thus the diffusion-convection equation can be used to determine the evolution of the solute concentration. In doing this procedure, when macromolecules are dissolved in water or another solute a first difficulty is often encountered in the fluid dynamic analysis if the solution is not very diluted. As a matter of fact the presence of a high concentration of macromolecules generates frequently a non-Newtonian behavior of the fluid with all the complications introduced in Section 7.3.6.

Here we will analyze the second part of the problem, the solution of the diffusion-convection equation. Since, in general, this is a formidably difficult problem, we will restrict ourselves to the solution motion through a microfluidic duct that we will imagine to be circular. We know that this is a representative problem and that the obtained results are valid as orders of magnitude also for other types of ducts provided that the correct expression of the hydrodynamic radius is adopted (see Section 7.3.4). The phenomenon we will consider is called Taylor dispersion [1,2,3].

The initial instant situation is shown in Figure 7.54: a solution with Newtonian characteristics is experiencing a fully developed Poiseuille flow through a circular duct and the solute concentration, at the initial instant, is constant for $x < 0$ and null for $x > 0$. The considered system has

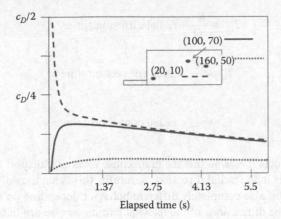

FIGURE 7.53   Concentration of the reagent A in three different points of the reaction chamber versus time.

two characteristic lengths: the duct radius R and the duct length L. Since mass transport happens through both convection and dispersion we can define different characteristic times relative to transport both in the radial and in the axial direction through the duct. The characteristic parameters of the two transport phenomena are the average Poiseuille velocity in the axial direction $\bar{v}$ and the diffusion coefficient D, being

$$\bar{v} = \int_0^R 2\pi r v(r)\, dr = \frac{v(r)}{2\left(1 - \dfrac{r^2}{R^2}\right)} \tag{7.204}$$

where $v(r)$ is the Poiseuille velocity field.

Combining the two characteristic length and the characteristic transport parameters we obtain the four characteristic times defined as

$$T_{ad} = \frac{L^2}{D} \quad \text{axial diffusion time}$$

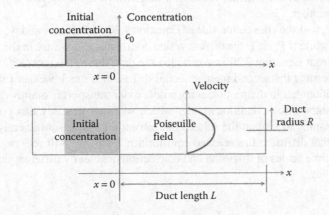

FIGURE 7.54   Initial situation for Taylor dispersion in a circular duct.

$$T_{rd} = \frac{R^2}{D} \quad \text{radial diffusion time}$$

$$T_{ac} = \frac{L}{\bar{v}} \quad \text{axial convection time}$$

$$T_{rc} = \frac{R}{\bar{v}} \quad \text{radial convection time}$$

In practical system, ducts $R \ll L$ so that the main cause of axial transport is the convection while diffusion mainly operates in the radial direction. Naturally, this is not the only possible dynamics of the system that can exhibit also completely different behavior depending on the value of the system parameters. Observing the dimensions of the relevant parameters we are induced to define a nondimensional characteristic number that, like Reynolds number for pure fluid dynamics, can help us to individuate the conditions in which different motion regimes appears.

This is the so-called Pécle number (P_e) that is the ratio between the characteristic time for radial diffusion and the characteristic time for axial convection:

$$P_e = \frac{T_{rd}}{T_{ac}} = \frac{\bar{v} R}{D} \tag{7.205}$$

If we rewrite Equation 7.166 in cylindrical coordinates we obtain

$$\frac{\partial c}{\partial t} + v \frac{\partial c}{\partial x} = D \left(\frac{\partial^2 c}{\partial r^2} + \frac{1}{r} \frac{\partial c}{\partial r} + \frac{\partial^2 c}{\partial x^2} \right) \tag{7.206}$$

where we have grouped at the first member the convection terms that are independent of the diffusion coefficient, and at the second member the diffusion terms.

Rearranging Equation 7.206 in order to put in evidence the Pécle number, we can write

$$P_e \frac{\partial c}{\partial t} + P_e \frac{R}{L} v \frac{\partial c}{\partial x} = \left(\frac{\partial^2 c}{\partial r^2} + \frac{1}{r} \frac{\partial c}{\partial r} \right) + \frac{R^2}{L^2} \frac{\partial^2 c}{\partial x^2} \tag{7.207}$$

The equation now shows clearly its dependence from two characteristic numbers: the ratio between radial and longitudinal dimensions, that determines if the system is a duct ($R/L \ll 1$) or not, and the Pécle number.

In particular, if $P_e \gg 1$ the convection side of Equation 7.206 dominates and we are in the so-called convection regime, while if $P_e \ll 1$, the diffusion side dominates and we are in the so-called diffusion regime. Moreover, from Equation 7.206 we can also see that, due to the term $R^2/L^2 \ll 1$ that multiply the axial diffusion term at the second member, axial diffusion is much weaker than radial diffusion, confirming the intuition that in the motion along a duct axial transport is mainly due to convection.

Let us now fix some basic conditions under which we want to study this convection-diffusion phenomenon. We assume to look at the solute concentration for times sufficiently long with respect to the motion start that diffusion has reached equilibrium. Thus, we will set $t \gg T_{rd}$ We are induced to imagine that the time scales of diffusion and convection are clearly different due to their different length scales by setting

$$T_{rc} \ll T_{rd} \ll T_{ac} \Leftrightarrow 1 \ll P_e \ll \frac{L}{R} \tag{7.208}$$

Let us now rewrite Equation 7.205 in the frame moving along the duct axis with the average Poiseuille velocity $\bar{v}$ Neglecting the axial diffusion term in Equation 7.205 due to the assumption that we are in a duct, we see that the only axial coordinate depending terms are related to convection, thus we can assume that the axial evolution is independent from the radial evolution and the radial dependence of the concentration is the same in all the duct sections. Moreover, since we have stated that we search for a solution for long times, that is, in the limit where diffusion has reached stationary regime, it is also reasonable to neglect the time derivative, assuming that the concentration shape is the same in all the duct sections.

Applying the above approximations and rewriting Equation 7.205 in the frame moving along the duct axis with the average Poiseuille velocity $\bar{v}_3$, we obtain

$$\left(1 - 2\frac{r^2}{L^2}\right)\bar{v}\frac{\partial c}{\partial \zeta} = D\left(\frac{\partial^2 c}{\partial r^2} + \frac{1}{r}\frac{\partial c}{\partial r}\right) \quad \zeta = x - \bar{v}t \tag{7.209}$$

It is to be noted that, since $\partial c/\partial \zeta$ is independent of r due to the assumption that the axial and the radial evolutions of the concentrations are independent, Equation 7.209 is an ordinary differential equation allowing us to determine the dependence of the solute concentration on the radial coordinate. It can be solved starting from a test solution in the form of a polynomial of degree N of the ratio r/R. By direct substitution of the test solution it is obtained

$$c(r,\zeta) = \bar{c}(\zeta) + \frac{\bar{v}R^2}{4D}\frac{\partial c}{\partial \zeta}\left(-\frac{1}{3} + \frac{r^2}{R^2} - \frac{1}{2}\frac{r^4}{R^4}\right) \tag{7.210}$$

where $\bar{c}(\zeta)$ is the radial average concentration. Since we have assumed that the axial gradient has to be independent from the radial coordinate, we must verify that Equation 7.210 fulfills this condition.

Deriving with respect to the radial coordinates and assuming that the radial dependent term is negligible with respect to the radial independent one we get

$$\frac{\bar{v}R^2}{4D}\frac{1}{L} \ll 1 \Leftrightarrow P_e \ll 4\frac{L}{R} \tag{7.211}$$

This condition is coherent with Equation 7.208 confirming the fact that we have got a solution coherent within the considered approximations. At this point a complete solution of the Taylor dispersion problem is obtained by expressing $\bar{c}(\zeta)$ with respect to the problem parameters and coming back to a fixed reference system.

The first operation can be accomplished by averaging Equation 7.210 to determine the average flux through the duct section. We get

$$\Phi(\zeta) = 2\pi \int_0^R r\rho c(r,\zeta)[v(r) - \bar{v}]\,dr = -D_{eff}\rho\frac{\partial \bar{c}}{\partial \zeta} \tag{7.212}$$

where we have collected all the multiplicative constants in the so-called Taylor diffusion coefficient (or effective diffusion coefficient) D_T whose expression is

$$D_T = \frac{R^2\bar{v}^2}{48D} = \frac{P_e^2}{48}D \tag{7.213}$$

Let us now imagine that pure diffusion in the fixed frame due to molecular collisions is negligible with respect to Taylor diffusion happening in the moving system. In order for this approximation to be valid we must have

$$D_{eff} \gg D \Leftrightarrow P_e \gg \sqrt{48} \approx 7 \qquad (7.214)$$

This approximation is coherent with the first part of Equation 7.208, thus we can assume that it is verified in our situation. If pure diffusion is negligible, we can apply the mass continuity equation in the moving frame to the average flux and the average concentration. This results in a one-dimensional equation relating the derivative of the flux to the time derivative of the radial average concentration. Using expression 7.212 for the flux, we finally get, after simplifying the constant density of the fluid

$$\frac{\partial^2 \overline{c}}{\partial t^2} = D_T \frac{\partial \overline{c}}{\partial \zeta} \qquad (7.215)$$

This is a one-dimension diffusion equation that can be solved under the given initial condition $\overline{c}(\zeta, 0) = c_0$ using the Green formula. Coming back to the fixed coordinate system we get

$$c(x, t) = \frac{c(x, 0)}{\sqrt{\pi D_T t}} e^{-\frac{(x - \overline{v}t)^2}{4D_T t}} \qquad (7.216)$$

Equation 7.216 has an immediate physical interpretation: the solute is transported globally by the solution deterministic motion while it diffuses with an equivalent diffusion coefficient equal to D_T. This dispersion effect depends on the system parameters through the Taylor dispersion coefficient. In particular, due to Equation 7.213 the dispersion is highly efficient while increasing both the duct radius and the average velocity of the solution Poiseuille motion.

It is to be observed that Taylor diffusion also happens in rectangular ducts. With a similar derivation Equation 7.213 is proved again under equivalent conditions with the difference that R is now the hydrodynamic radius of the duct and the constant 48 is substituted by 128.

7.5 ELECTRO-HYDRODYNAMICS

As it is evident from the Navier-Stokes Equation 7.36, besides gravity, the electromagnetic forces are very important in determining the fluid motion when electrical charges or dipoles are present. This is a quite common situation in labs on chip, since as we have seen in Section 2.3 that biomolecules are generally polar and, in particular, proteins and nucleic acids acquire a charge in ion charged water solution. Electro-hydrodynamic is also a key technique in protein and nucleic acids detection and purification through the electrophoresis procedure that we have already introduced in Section 3.6. In this section, we will lay a theoretical foundation for the analysis of those electro-hydrodynamic effects more frequently occurring in labs on chip.

When an electromagnetic field is present, besides the material constitutive equation and the Navier-Stokes equation we have to add the Maxwell equation providing the electromagnetic field dynamics to the mathematical system modeling.

If the whole complexity of Maxwell equations is carried in, the analysis of electromagnetic phenomena occurring while an electromagnetic active fluid moves is very difficult. Maxwell equations are not invariant for the Galilean transformations [89,90], thus it is impossible to pass from a still reference to a suitable reference with the average fluid velocity is zero without formulating a relativistic version of fluid mechanics [91]. This is possible, but it is not needed in our case. As a matter of fact, irradiative phenomena are important only when the speed of the moving charges are sufficiently high to make the radiated energy nonnegligible with respect to the other energy terms involved in the problem. High speeds are never reached in microfluidic circuits, thus radiation can be always neglected and the interaction between the moving fluid and the electromagnetic field can be modeled either as an electrostatic or as a magneto-static interaction.

The electrostatic version of the Maxwell equations in a continuous medium can be written as

$$\epsilon_{i,j,k} \frac{\partial E_j}{\partial x_k} = 0 \tag{7.217a}$$

$$\frac{\partial D_j}{\partial x_j} = \rho_e \tag{7.217b}$$

where ρ_e represents the charge density and the electrical displacement vector D can be expressed as a function of the electrical field E and of the medium polarization vector P as

$$D_j = \varepsilon_0 E_j + P_j = \varepsilon_0 (\delta_{j,k} + \chi_{j,k}) E_k \tag{7.218}$$

being ε_0 the void dielectric constant and $\chi_{j,k}$ the dielectric susceptibility tensor. In general, fluids are isotropous, thus the susceptibility reduces to a constant and the polarization vector is parallel to the electrical field, but in the case of labs on chip practical cases exists where this condition is not fulfilled. Typically, this happens when macromolecules in the medium are like chains aligned in a prevalent direction, creating a directional behavior of the medium. This is the case, for example, of a few electrophoresis gels, in which the gel molecules are long chains that align in a prevalent direction when the gel is deposited and, since the gel hardens after deposition, maintain their alignment in time. We have already encountered this phenomenon dealing with diffusion of proteins in electrophoretic gel in Section 7.4.2.

If the electrical field energy is sufficiently low not to perturb the chemical structure of the medium, it is possible to assume the dielectric susceptibility as a constant so that the medium results to be linear. For high electrostatic energies the field presence is not negligible in determining the properties of the fluid and the susceptibility dependence on the electrical field become evident so that the medium becomes nonlinear. This condition is almost never verified in labs on chip, so that in the following section we will assume the electrostatic susceptibility as a scalar constant, assuming our fluid homogeneous and isotropic.

Equation 7.217 implies that the electrical field can be expressed as the divergence of a scalar potential $\psi(r, t)$. Substituting the expression of the electrical displacement vector in the second of the (7.217) and exploiting the expression of the displacement vector we can introduce the medium dielectric constant as $\varepsilon = \varepsilon_0(1 + \chi)$ so that the equation for the potential writes, calling u_i the vector whose coordinates are all equal to unit,

$$\frac{\partial^2 \psi}{\partial x_i^2} u_i = -\frac{1}{\varepsilon} \rho_e(x_j) \tag{7.219a}$$

$$\nabla^2 \psi = -\frac{1}{\varepsilon} \rho_e(r) \tag{7.219b}$$

Equation 7.220, for its importance we have written both in index and in abstract notation, is called Poison equation and it is the basic equation of electrostatics.

It is interesting to consider the force acting on a small volume δV of a continuous medium subject to an electrical field. Calling r_0 the center of mass of δV, exploiting the small dimension of δV to use a second-order Taylor expansion of the electrical field, we can write

$$
\begin{aligned}
F_i &= \int_{\delta V} \rho_e(x_j - x_{0j}) E_i(x_j - x_{0j}) \, dV \\
&= E_i(x_{0j}) \int_{\delta V} \rho_e(x_j - x_{0j}) \, dV + \left. \frac{\partial E_i}{\partial x_k} \right)_{x_{0j}} \int_{\delta V} \rho_e(x_j - x_{0j}) x_k \, dV
\end{aligned}
\tag{7.220}
$$

The first term of Equation 7.221 is evidently the contribution of the net charge of the material while the second term depends on the reciprocal position of the charges that are present through the coordinates inside the integral and represents the dipole moment of the considered piece of material.

If we assume as the volume δV the so-called fluid particle, that is the volume where we average our physical quantities to pass from the real discrete nature of the fluid to a continuous model (see Section 7.1), the charge density $\rho_e(x_j - x_{0j})$ is due to all the charged particles in the volume and the polarization vector can be expressed as dipole moment density, that is as

$$
P_k(x_{0j}) = \frac{1}{\delta V} \int_{\delta V} \rho_e(x_j - x_{0j}) x_k \, dV
\tag{7.221}
$$

Thus, passing from the total force to the force density f_i we can rewrite Equation 7.221 in the continuous model as the sum of a net charge effect and of a dipole effect represented by the polarization vector as

$$
f_i(x_j) = \rho(x_j) E_i(x_j) + P_k(x_j) \frac{\partial E_i}{\partial x_k}
\tag{7.222}
$$

While the second-order approximation in Equation 7.221 is generally sufficient in lab on chip analysis, cases can happen where further terms of the Taylor expansion (7.221) has to be considered, typically when electrostatic effects are nonnegligible but both the net charge and the polarization vector are zero. In these cases further terms of the development give raise to three-pole and other multipolar terms [92].

7.5.1 Ions Electrophoresis

A first and simple example of electro-kinetic effect in labs on chip is ions electrophoresis. This phenomenon happens when an ionic solution fills a reaction chamber where two electrodes are present on opposite sides, as represented in Figure 7.55. The total force acting on the ions is the sum of the electrostatic force and the viscous drag due to the surrounding fluid. As represented in Figure 7.55, let us imagine that the reaction chamber under an electrostatic point of view is a plane plate capacitor and that border effects can be neglected assuming straight electrical field lines. Due to the compact structure of almost all ions, let us approximate the ions shape to be like a rigid sphere so as to apply the expression of the Stokes drag (see Section 7.4.2 [3,53]) to represent the effect of the solvent viscosity. In this condition, calling Z and R the ions charge in terms of multiples of the electron charge q and the ions radius, the dynamic equation for the ions is

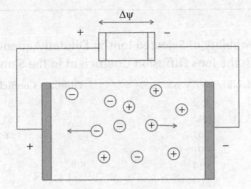

FIGURE 7.55 Scheme of a reaction chamber for ions electrophoresis. Electrodes are indicated in light grey and the ions inside the solution as small circle with the charge sign inside.

$$qZE - 6\pi\eta R v_x = m a_x \tag{7.223}$$

The solution of this dynamic equation is known: it relaxes after a very short time (in the order of one μs in the current example) on a constant velocity motion due to the equilibrium of electrical and viscous forces. The steady-state velocity is then

$$v_x = \frac{qZ}{6\pi\eta R} E = \mu E \tag{7.224}$$

where μ is called ions mobility in the solution. This very simple theoretical model however, does not take into account the phenomenon of hydration (see Section 1.3.3) that impact in an important way on the physical characteristics of diluted particles.

We can calculate the ions mobility from Equation 7.224 by considering the so-called hydrated radius instead of the ionic radius. As a matter of fact, while the ionic radius, evaluated from the density of external occupied orbitals, is about 0.05 nm for small ions, the hydrated radius, evaluated starting from the structure obtained surrounding the ions with polar water molecules, is instead of the order of 0.2 nm for the same ions.

If we use the correct value for the radius of hydrated ions Equation 7.224 produces results in very good agreement with experience, even if it is obtained using a very simple model. Experimental values of the mobility of selected monovalent ions in diluted water solution are reported in Table 7.13 and compared with their diffusion coefficient in the same condition. Since the hydrated radius of monovalent ions is almost the same, Equation 7.224 indicates that their mobility also has to be almost the same. This is verified by inspecting Table 7.13, but for the case of hydrogen and hydroxyl ions, whose mobility is much greater. This is the hint that these ions do not simply move due to the electrical field, but exploit a different transport mechanism. As a matter of fact, a detailed study of the mobility of hydrogen and hydroxyl ions in water [93,94] reveals that they rapidly move among water molecules with the so-called "electron exchange mechanism" instead of exploiting the bare electrostatic force.

7.5.2 STERN AND DEBYE LAYERS

The analysis we have performed in the previous section implicitly assumes that, on reaching the electrophoresis electrodes, ions are removed from the solution so that the potential generated by the electrodes in the electrophoresis chamber is constant all over the process. Frequently, however, this

TABLE 7.13

Experimental Mobility of Selected Ions in Diluted Aqueous Solution Compared with the Ions Diffusion Coefficient in the Same Conditions

Ion	Mobility ($m^2/(V\ s) \times 10^{-8}$)	Diffusion Coefficient ($m^2/s \times 10^{-9}$)
H^+	36.2	9.31
Ag^+	6.42	1.65
K^+	7.62	1.96
Li^+	4.01	1.03
Na^+	5.19	1.33
Br^-	8.09	2.08
Cl^-	7.91	2.03
F^-	5.70	1.46
I^-	7.96	2.05
OH^-	20.6	5.30

Source: Bruus H., *Theoretical Microfluidics*, 2007, by permission of Oxford University Press.
Note: Values are measured at 25°C.

is not the case and ions deposit on the electrode when reaching it. In this situation it is intuitive that a layer of charges of opposite sign starts to deposit on each electrode and to shield it so as to progressively decrease the potential in the electrophoresis chamber. In the absence of thermal motion of the ions, this will eventually shield completely the electrodes nullifying the electrophoresis field and stopping the process. Thermal motion removes now and then an ion from the electrode surface on a random basis, generating a dynamical equilibrium where the field inside the electrophoresis chamber is only partially screened. At equilibrium we can imagine that different zones are formed all around the charged surface [95,96,97]. A first ion layer, known as Stern layer, is formed in direct contact with the charged plane; this is a very thin layer of almost still ions,even a single particle layer in few cases that provides a first screening of the surface-generated field.

When the screening arrives to a critical value the residual field is no more sufficient to capture more ions due to their thermal motion and ions out of the Stern layer are free to move. However, the existence of an electrical field still attract or repel ions depending on their charge, thus creating a thicker layer of mobile ions where the concentration of ion with a certain charge is greater than the concentration of ions with the opposite charge. This layer is called Debye layer or diffusion layer [98,99]. The structure generated by the Stern and the Debye layers is qualitatively shown in Figure 7.56.

A quite similar phenomenon is present also when a plasma discharge is generated in a neutral gas through the application of a continuous voltage, as it was described in Section 4.7.2 dealing with plasma creation. Here we want to review more in detail the effect in ionic solutions.

The Stern layer causes a simple electrical potential drop between the voltage externally applied to the electrodes and the electrophoresis effective voltage, the electric potential on the external boundary of the Stern layer versus the bulk electrolyte is referred to as Stern potential or zeta potential. Electric potential difference between the fluid bulk and the surface is called the electric surface potential. It is interesting to note that, increasing the surface potential from zero, the Stern layer builds progressively so that the effective potential experimented by the solution increases in a nonlinear way up to arrive to the zeta potential. When the effective potential is equal to the zeta potential the Stern layer is completely build and a further increase of the surface potential do not increase the effective potential, but increases the number of ions in the Stern layer up to the moment in which the external potential is so high to cause the dielectric breakdown of the solvent or some other nonlinear phenomenon.

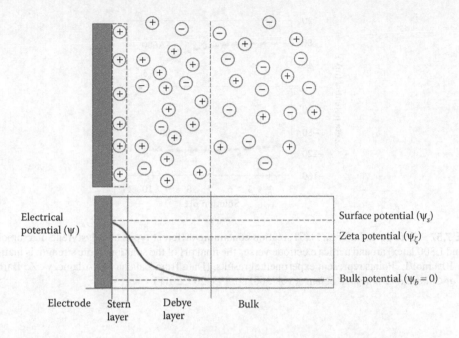

FIGURE 7.56 Structure generated by the Stern and the Debye layers near a charged surface in contact with a ionic solution and qualitative scheme of the corresponding electrical potential behavior.

The Stern potential greatly depends on the kind of solution we are considering [95]. Generally, besides ions other chemical species are present in the solution either in order to stabilize it or for other reasons. For example, a certain ionic concentration is always maintained in proteins solutions, even when they are artificially generated, in order to favor protein solubility in water. When protein electrophoresis is performed, also ion electrophoresis happens and, given enough time, a zeta potential could be generated, even if this situation is in practical assays avoided by limiting the assay time. In this case, the zeta potential depends on the type and concentration of the proteins that are present in the solution.

An example of this dependence is reported in Figure 7.57 [100] where the zeta potential around a mica electrode is reported for a solution of NaCl and two different types of polystyrene macromolecules (A500 and L800 latex) versus the final pH of the solution. In order to change the pH in a controlled situation the overall ionic strength (see Equation 7.178) equals to 10^{-2} mol/L. The strong dependence of the zeta potential both on the ratio between the ions concentrations and on the presence of different macromolecules in the solution is evident from the figure.

The Debye layer constituted by almost free moving ions can be studied by considering the ions of a given charge that are present in the solution as a perfect gas. The equilibrium situation is reached when the overall chemical potential of the system is constant. Assuming that the solvent is completely dielectric so that it does not contribute to the electrostatic phenomena, the chemical potential is due only to the ion concentration and to the electrical potential. The ion concentration contribution is simply obtained deriving Equation 1.15 reporting the free energy of a solution. The electrostatic term is simply equal to the potential energy of the electrostatic field. Collecting the two terms we get, considering the potential per mole of ions,

$$\mu_\beta(\boldsymbol{r}) = \mu_0 + \kappa_B T \log\left(\frac{c_\beta(\boldsymbol{r})}{c_0}\right) + \beta Z q \psi(\boldsymbol{r}) \quad \beta = +,- \tag{7.225}$$

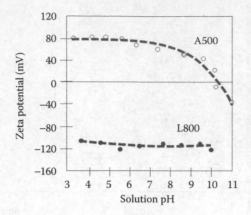

FIGURE 7.57 Zeta potential of an NaCl solution containing different types of polystyrene macromolecules (A500 and L800 latex) around a mica electrode versus the final pH of the solution. Ionic strength is maintained equal to 10^{-2} mol/L. Points represent experimental results. (Data from Zaucha M., Adamczyk Z., Barbasz J., *Journal of Colloid and Interface Science*, vol. 360, pp. 195–203, 2011.)

where

μ_0 is the initial chemical potential that is assumed to be the same for both the ions populations;

c_0 is the initial concentration that is assumed to be the same for both the ions populations;

Z is the ion charge in terms of electron charges that is assumed to be the same for both the ions populations;

q is the module of the electron charge;

κ_B is the Boltzmann constant;

$\beta = +$ represents positive ions while $\beta = -$ represents negative once.

Imposing that the chemical potential has a minimum, so that the system is at equilibrium brings to set to zero its gradient obtaining the following equation:

$$\kappa_B T \nabla \log\left(\frac{c_\beta(r)}{c_0}\right) = -\beta Z q \nabla \psi(r) \quad \beta = +,- \tag{7.226}$$

The potential on the electrode, beyond the Stern layer, is the zeta potential ψ_ζ and if the solution chamber is sufficiently extended we can assume that in the bulk of the solution (mathematically at infinity) the electrical potential is constant and equal to zero and the concentration is coincident with the initial value c_0. Under these conditions Equation 7.226 is easily integrated yielding

$$c_\beta(r) = c_0 e^{-\beta \frac{Zq}{\kappa_B T} \psi(r)} \tag{7.227}$$

The charge density is obtained as $\rho_e(r) = Zq(c_+(r) - c_-(r))$ and expressing $\rho_e(r)$ via the Poisson equation the so-called Poisson–Boltzmann equation for the electrical potential is obtained:

$$\nabla^2 \psi(r) = \frac{2Zqc_0}{\varepsilon} \sinh\left(\frac{Zq}{\kappa_B T} \psi(r)\right) \tag{7.228}$$

It is interesting to observe that the version Equation 7.228 of the Poisson–Boltzmann equation presents the sinh(*) at the second member due to the fact that we have charges of two opposite signs in our solution. In other cases, only a single type of charge is present, so that the Poisson–Boltzmann equation presents a simple exponential instead of the sinh(*). We have already encountered the Poisson–Boltzmann equation dealing with implicit solvent statistical models in Section 1.5.1.

Equation 7.228 is quite difficult to solve and simulation is generally needed, but for specific cases corresponding to particular system geometries. The simpler, but quite significant case in which an analytical solution can be obtained is that of a conductive plane limiting a half space containing the ions solution. The problem becomes one dimensional, since the potential and the concentrations only depend on the x coordinates (see Figure 7.58) and the analytic solution of the Poisson–Boltzmann equation can be obtained by the Gouy–Chapman procedure [3] obtaining

$$\psi(x) = \frac{4\kappa_B T}{Zq} \text{arctanh}\left[\tanh\left(\frac{Zq\psi_\zeta}{4\kappa_B T}\right) e^{-\frac{x}{\lambda_D}} \right] \tag{7.229}$$

where the Debye layer typical width λ_D (called Debye length) is given by

$$\lambda_D = \sqrt{\frac{\varepsilon \kappa_B T}{2(Zq)^2 c_0}} \tag{7.230}$$

A very interesting approximation that allows Equation 7.225 to be solved in several practically interesting cases is the so-called Debye–Hückel approximation. In this case, it is assumed that the thermal energy is much greater than the energy of the electromagnetic field, so that it is possible to write $Zq\psi_\zeta \ll \kappa_B T$.

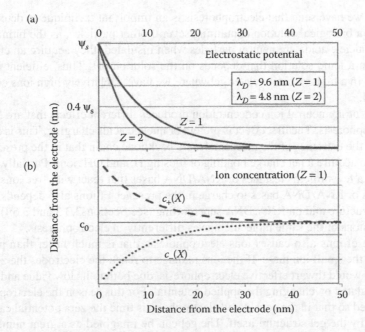

FIGURE 7.58 Electrical potential in the Debye–Hückel approximation for a diluted solution of mono and bivalent ions (a) and ion concentration the case of monovalent ions (b). In both cases, the initial concentration is 1 mol/m³ and the reference temperature is 25°C.

Under the Debye–Hückel approximation we can use the first-order approximation $\sinh(y) \approx y$ so that the Poisson–Boltzmann equation becomes

$$\nabla^2 \psi(r) = \frac{1}{\lambda_D^2} \psi(r) \tag{7.231}$$

confirming the meaning of the Debye length not only in the case of a flat plate, but more, in general, for any configuration. Solving Equation 7.231 in the case of a flat plate, where Equation 7.229 is the exact Poisson–Boltzmann equation solution, provides

$$\psi(r) = \psi_\zeta e^{-e^{\frac{x}{\lambda_D}}} \tag{7.232}$$

that simply coincides with the first-order approximation of Equation 7.231. The charge density can be evaluated by the Poisson equation and the concentrations of the ions from Equation 7.227 that has to be approximated at first-order to take into account coherently the adopted approximation. It is obtained

$$c_\beta(x) = c_0 \left[1 + \beta \frac{Zq\psi_\zeta}{\kappa_B T} e^{-e^{\frac{x}{\lambda_D}}} \right] \tag{7.233}$$

The electrical potential in the Debye–Hückel approximation for a diluted solution of mono and bivalent ions is shown in Figure 7.58. The ion concentration is also shown in the case of monovalent ions. In both cases, the initial concentration is 1 mole/m^3 and the reference temperature is 25°C.

7.5.3 Protein and Nucleic Acids Electrophoresis

In Sections 3.6, we have seen that electrophoresis is an important technique to detect proteins and nucleic acids in a biological solution containing several other particles, as the human blood. Even if proteins and nucleic acids are neutral particles when insulated, they acquire an electrical charge when inserted in a ionic solution that depends on the solution pH. Thus, efficient electrophoresis can be executed in a high viscosity water gel where we have a relatively high ions concentration to set a suitable pH.

The presence of nonneutral ion concentration produces different effects that are fundamental to carry out electrophoresis. The first effect is protein or nucleic acids charging. This is due partially to the reactivity of the extremes of the macromolecule backbone chain that in the presence of charged particles tends to acquire a net charge bonding or loosing H$^+$ and OH$^-$ ions. Partially, it is caused by the reactivity of a few proteins residues or RNA/DNA bases that react with free ions. The ability of reactive residues or RNA/DNA bases to charge in the presence of ions also depends on the tertiary protein/RNA structure and on RNA/DNA supercoiling (see Sections 3.3.3 and 3.6.1), so that differently coiled versions of the same molecule moves differently in electrophoresis.

The presence of ions also causes ions electrophoresis that is much faster than protein electrophoresis, due to the small ion mass. If the ions manage to reach the electrodes the zeta potential is established, that would thwart effective electrophoresis, due both to its low value and to the fact that it cannot be regulated by changing the applied potential. For this reason the electrophoresis system has to be designed so that in the considered electrophoresis time the zeta potential cannot establish. This is allowed by the gel structure itself. The gel can be imagined as a great number of polymer chains entangled one to the other and capturing a great quantity of water. Macromolecules like proteins cannot penetrate into the chains twists so that they open a way in between different chains. Much smaller ions conversely travels through all the twists and hovels, so experiencing a much greater resistance to motion and traveling a much longer way. In standard electrophoresis gels this effect, similar to the principle of size exclusion chromatography (see Section 3.5.3.2), is so relevant that ions displacement from the initial injection point is almost irrelevant.

The charge distribution on the macromolecules surface is generally nonuniform so that rotational motion and excitation of internal degrees of freedom can be generated besides the transport toward the opposite charged electrode. Rotation effect depends on the macromolecule configuration also and for complex molecules it generates a complex viscous motion while internal degrees of freedom excitation subtract energy to the motion toward the electrode. For this reason, protein mobility during electrophoresis cannot be forecasted by Equation 7.224, not even approximately.

We also know that in a macroscopic electrophoresis equipment, a protein or a nucleic acid occupy a wide bandwidth more than a single line (compare Figures 3.32 and 3.33). This is evident also when an artificially prepared solution, containing all molecules in the same configuration, is used for electrophoresis.

This effect is due to two reasons. The first reason is trivial and depends on the fact that the molecules are not injected in the electrophoresis slab in a mathematical point, but the injection area has its own thickness, reflecting in a thickness in the final electrophoresis line. The second cause is the macromolecule diffusion in the gel.

7.5.4 ELECTROOSMOSIS

Electroosmosis is the process involving the movement of a charged fluid in a microfluidic channel due to the action of an electrical field on the Debye layer. In particular, let us consider the situation of Figure 7.59, where two orthogonal potentials are applied on a circular duct where a liquid containing a certain ionic concentration can flow. When the voltage along the radial direction is created, a Debye layer generates along the walls of the duct. If a voltage is applied also to the vertical electrodes, an electrical field is created along the x direction pushing the Debye layer in the x direction. The Debye layer creates a viscosity drag on the whole fluid mass that start to move in the x direction. If charges depositing on the vertical electrodes are not removed the motion lasts only up to the moment where the Stern and Debye layers shield the horizontal field so much that it is no more sufficient to win viscous resistance and the fluid stops. However, charged ions can be removed in different ways when reaching the end of the duct, for example, by chemical recombination or simply fluid extraction, so that the motion can become stationary creating the electroosmosis process.

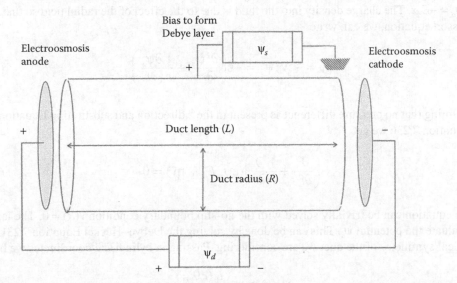

FIGURE 7.59 Scheme of the set-up for electroosmosis in a circular duct.

This process is called electroosmosis due to the fact that it was discovered by applying an electrical potential to a porous osmosis membrane, where a great number of small channels are present where electrical drag happens. To analyze the motion in this case we have to maintain the volume force due to the electrical field in our simplified form of Equation 7.61a of the Navier-Stokes equation so as to obtain the electro-hydrodynamic form of the Stokes equation:

$$\rho \frac{\partial v}{\partial t} = -\nabla p + \eta \nabla^2 v + \rho_e E \tag{7.234}$$

The electrical field is the sum of two components: an equilibrium component due to the voltage applied to the duct walls creating the Debye layer and a dynamic component due to the horizontal field. The pressure can also be decomposed in a hydrostatic pressure, due for example to the presence of gravity, that in an horizontal duct is balanced by the reaction of the walls and by the incompressible fluid internal stress, and by a dynamic pressure that can be applied in the x direction and that can act besides the electroosmosis to create fluid motion.

If we write all the quantities as the sum of a stationary part and of a dynamic part and insert it into the motion Equation 7.234 we see that all the static quantities at the second member simplifies, due to the assumption of hydrostatic equilibrium before the start of electroosmosis. The motion equation involves only dynamic quantities, which we will indicate with an index d, while we will indicate with s the static components. Equation 7.234 thus rewrites

$$\rho \frac{\partial v}{\partial t} = -\nabla p_d + \eta \nabla^2 v - \rho_e \nabla \psi_d \tag{7.235}$$

Due to the orientation of the electrical field and to the round symmetry of the duct, the only component of the velocity to be different from zero is the x component, and assuming steady-state motion, Equation 7.235 can be rewritten as

$$-\frac{\partial p_d}{\partial x} + \eta \frac{\partial^2 v}{\partial r^2} + \frac{1}{r} \frac{\partial v}{\partial r} - \rho_e \frac{\partial \psi_d}{\partial x} = 0 \tag{7.236}$$

Neglecting boundary effects, the field along the x direction can be considered constant so as to write $\psi_d = -E_d x$. The charge density into the fluid is due to the effect of the radial field so that, using the Poisson equation, we can write

$$\rho_e = -\varepsilon \nabla_r^2 \psi_s = -\varepsilon \left(\frac{\partial^2 \psi_s}{\partial r^2} + \frac{1}{r} \frac{\partial \psi_s}{\partial r} \right) \tag{7.237}$$

Assuming that no pressure difference is present in the x direction and substituting Equation 7.237 into Equation 7.236 we get

$$\left(\frac{\partial^2}{\partial r^2} + \frac{1}{r} \frac{\partial}{\partial r} \right)(\varepsilon \psi_s E_d + \eta v) = 0 \tag{7.238}$$

This equation can be trivially solved with the no-slip boundary condition $v(R) = 0$. The last step is to evaluate the potential ψ_s. This can be done by solving the Debye–Hückel Equation 7.231 in the cylindrical symmetry of the duct we are considering. Passing in cylindrical coordinates we have

$$\psi_s(r) = \psi_\zeta \frac{I_0(r/\lambda_D)}{I_0(R/\lambda_D)} \tag{7.239}$$

Using the expression of $\psi_s(r)$ we can write the radial distribution of the velocity as

$$v(r) = v_{EO}\left[1 - \frac{I_0\left(r/\lambda_D\right)}{I_0\left(R/\lambda_D\right)}\right] \tag{7.240}$$

where

$$v_{EO} = \frac{\varepsilon}{\eta}\,\psi_\zeta\,E_d = \mu_{EO}\,E_d \tag{7.241}$$

$\mu_{EO} = \varepsilon\psi_\zeta/\eta$ being the electroosmotic mobility. Using values relative to a diluted water solution and $\psi_\zeta = 100$ mV we obtain $\mu_{EO} = 7 \times 10^{-8}$ m²/V/s and $v_{EO} \sim 10^{-3}$ m/s. The Debye–Hückel approximation is at its limit in this case, since from the above values we see that $\varepsilon\psi_\zeta/\kappa_B T \approx 4$ so that the electrostatic energy is not much smaller than the thermal energy. Nevertheless, results obtained with the above procedure are qualitatively in good agreement with measurements.

The velocity profile due to electroosmosis is shown in Figure 7.60 for different values of the ratio λ_D/R between the duct radius and the Debye length. Largely, the most common situation is that the Debye length, of the order of 10 nm, is much smaller than the duct radius. In this case, the velocity profile is quite different from the Poiseuille profile, being almost constant far from the Debye layer boundary. This means that imagining a duct of radius 50 μm and a Debye layer of 10 nm we have $\lambda_D/R = 0.001$. In this condition, but for a very thin layer near the duct walls of the radial dimension approximately 20 nm, the fluid velocity is almost constant in the duct and the volume flow rate can be easily evaluated as $Q = \pi R^2\,v(0)$.

While the ratio λ_D/R becomes greater, that is, the Debye length gets nearer to the duct radius, the velocity profile gets more rounded, up to the moment in which the Debye length coincides with the radius. In this case, no viscosity drug happens, a volume force is exerted on the whole fluid volume by the field and the velocity profile becomes parabolic, like that obtained by the Stokes equation when a constant volume force pushes the fluid. The same dynamics is also obtained from a different point of view by looking at the maximum attainable velocity in the channel by varying the ratio λ_D/R, as shown in Figure 7.61.

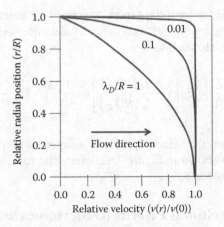

FIGURE 7.60 Radial dependence of the fluid velocity versus the ratio between the fluid radius and the Debye length during electroosmosis in a circular duct.

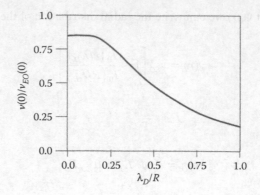

FIGURE 7.61   Dependence of the maximum velocity during electroosmosis in a circular duct versus the ratio between the fluid radius and the Debye length.

Adding an external pressure the motion equation becomes

$$-\frac{\Delta p_d}{L} + \left(\frac{\partial^2}{\partial r^2} + \frac{1}{r}\frac{\partial}{\partial r}\right)(\varepsilon\psi_s E_d + \eta v) = 0 \tag{7.242}$$

This is an interesting case for applications where electroosmosis is used to pump the solution against an external pressure. The problem (7.242) can be solved directly using the linearity of the equation. As a matter of fact we can write the overall velocity as the sum of two components, a Poiseuille component and an electroosmotic component as $v = v_{eo} + v_{poi}$. The equation is satisfied if the following two equations are simultaneously verified:

$$\left(\frac{\partial^2}{\partial r^2} + \frac{1}{r}\frac{\partial}{\partial r}\right)(\varepsilon\psi_s E_d + \eta v_{eo}) = 0 \tag{7.243a}$$

$$-\frac{\Delta p_d}{L} + \eta\left(\frac{\partial^2}{\partial r^2} + \frac{1}{r}\frac{\partial}{\partial r}\right)v_{poi} = 0 \tag{7.243b}$$

where L is the duct length. Since from the general theory of differential equations the solution of (7.242) under the no-slip boundary conditions is unique, the unique solution providing the following expression of velocity profile into the duct is

$$v = \frac{\varepsilon}{\eta}\psi_\zeta E_d\left[1 - \frac{I_0(r/\lambda_D)}{I_0(R/\lambda_D)}\right] + \frac{1}{4\eta}\frac{\Delta p_d}{L}(R^2 - r^2) \tag{7.244}$$

The result is quite intuitive: the velocity profile is a superposition of an electroosmotic profile and of a Poiseuille profile as shown in Figure 7.62, where the case of a pressure opposing to the electroosmosis motion is considered.

7.5.5   Electrophoresis of Neutral Particles (Dielectrophoresis)

The mechanism causing electrophoresis of neutral particles is the fact that the particle, if subject to an electrical field, develops a dipole momentum, so experimenting a dipole force due to the

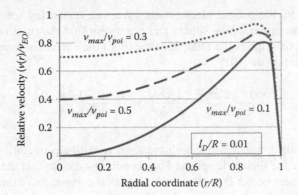

FIGURE 7.62 Velocity profile for different ratios between the maximum electroosmosis velocity v_{max} and the maximum Poiseuille velocity v_{poi} for electroosmosis with counter-pressure. The ratio between the Debye length and the duct radius is set to 0.01.

presence of the electrical field. Let us imagine a parallelepiped electrophoresis chamber where the field is generated by two parallel electrodes that are sufficiently extended so that border effects can be neglected (see Figure 7.63), filled with a solution containing a dielectric particles. If no molecule would be present inside the chamber, the field inside the chamber would depend on the applied voltage and would be uniform in the chamber. The presence of dielectric particles completely changes the situation.

Assuming to have a dielectric spherical particle in solution in a dielectric liquid and subject to a uniform electrical field whose expression is (see Figure 7.63)

$$E = E_0 u_x = -\frac{\psi_0}{L} u_x \qquad (7.245)$$

where u_x is the x axis unit vector, L is the length of the electrophoresis chamber and ψ_0 the applied potential. The Poisson equation can be written setting to zero the charge term becoming

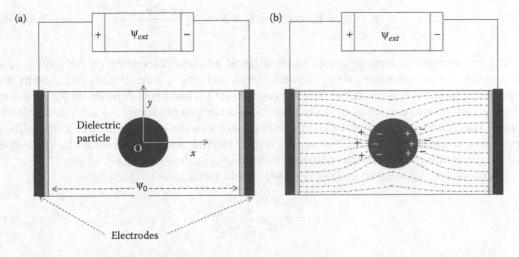

FIGURE 7.63 Scheme of the situation considered in the analysis of electrophoresis of a dielectric sphere (a) and field lines due both to the external potential and to the polarization of the solvent and the sphere (b).

the Laplace equation for the overall electrostatic potential. Assuming spherical coordinates (r, φ, θ) with center in the center of the sphere and observing that the rotational symmetry of the system around the x axis implies the independence of all the variables from the angle ϕ, we can write the Laplace equation as [101]

$$\frac{\partial^2 \psi}{\partial r^2} + \frac{2}{r} \frac{\partial \psi}{\partial r} + \frac{1}{r^2} \frac{\partial^2 \psi}{\partial \theta^2} + \frac{1}{r^2} \frac{\cos(\theta)}{\sin(\theta)} \frac{\partial \psi}{\partial \theta} = 0 \qquad (7.246)$$

This is a deeply studied equation that we have to solve with electrostatic boundary conditions both inside and outside the dielectric sphere. Such conditions dictate that the radial component of the dielectric displacement vector $\boldsymbol{D} = \varepsilon \boldsymbol{E}$ and the tangential component of the electrical field $\boldsymbol{E}$ are both continuous on the dielectric sphere surface. Indicating with ε_s and ε_L the sphere and the surrounding liquid dielecric constant and the potentials inside and outside the sphere with the same indices, we have the following boundary conditions

$$\psi_s(0,\theta) \quad \text{is finite} \qquad (7.247a)$$

$$\psi_s(R,\theta) = \psi_L(R,\theta) \qquad (7.247b)$$

$$\varepsilon_s \left. \frac{\partial \psi_s}{\partial r} \right|_{r=R} = \varepsilon_L \left. \frac{\partial \psi_L}{\partial r} \right|_{r=R} \qquad (7.247c)$$

$$\lim_{r\to\infty} \left[\psi_L(r,\theta) - E_0 r \cos(\theta) \right] = 0 \qquad (7.247d)$$

where R is the dielectric sphere radius, E_0 is the external field that in this case is directed toward the x direction and the last condition assures that very far from the sphere the field reduces to the unperturbed field generated by the electrodes. Equation 7.246 with the conditions 7.247 can be solved using Legendre Polynomial [101] obtaining a simple constant potential inside the sphere and the following expression of the potential outside the sphere:

$$\psi_L(r,\theta) = E_0 r \cos(\theta) + E_0 R^3 K(\varepsilon_s, \varepsilon_L) \frac{\cos(\theta)}{r^2} \qquad (7.248)$$

The first term is the term generated by the external potential, depending on the coordinate x since in the adopted reference $x = r \cos(\theta)$ while the second term is a dipole term, as shown by the dependence from the coordinates in the form $\cos(\theta)/r^2$ [90]. This dipole depends on the dielectric sphere polarization as confirmed by the fact that the constant potential implies a null field inside the sphere. This is a consequence of the distribution of charges on the sphere surface that, due to their orientation, shield the external field preventing it from entering inside the sphere itself. The sphere and the surrounding liquid are thus polarized, for example, as shown in Figure 7.63b.

The factor $K(\varepsilon_s, \varepsilon_L)$ is the so-called Clausius–Mossotti factor whose expression is

$$K(\varepsilon_s, \varepsilon_L) = \frac{\varepsilon_L - \varepsilon_s}{\varepsilon_L + 2\varepsilon_s} \qquad (7.249)$$

The expression of the Clausius–Mossotti factor is important since it allows another important property of dielectrophoresis to be pointed out. This is evidenced by evaluating the dipole moment of the sphere starting from the dipole potential. We know that, in general, the dipole potential can be written as a function of the dipole momentum module p as

$$\psi(r) = \frac{p}{4\pi\varepsilon} \frac{\cos(\theta)}{r^2} \tag{7.250}$$

Comparing Equation 7.249 with the second term of Equation 7.248 we get in our case

$$p = 4\pi\varepsilon_L R^3 K(\varepsilon_s, \varepsilon_L) E_0 \tag{7.251}$$

The direction of the dipole depends on the difference between the dielectric constant of the sphere and that of the surrounding liquid: if the liquid dielectric constant is greater, the dipole is oriented in the same direction of the external electrical field, otherwise it is directed in the opposite direction.

This behavior can be explained considering the fact that the liquid itself is a dielectric so that every liquid portion polarizes due to the field. Naturally, the effect of the polarization of nearby liquid portions neutralizes, but this is not true for the liquid elements in contact with the sphere surface. The fact that the dielectric constant across the sphere surface has a discontinuity creates locally a net charge that induces a global dipole generated by the dielectric sphere and the surrounding liquid. This dipole depends on the dielectric constants that physically represent the ability of a dielectric of creating a dipole distribution to counteract an external field, as demonstrated by Equation 7.219.

We have deduced Equation 7.251 by assuming that our sphere is still in the electrical field. This is not the situation in dielectrophoresis, where polarized particles move through the electrical, simultaneously changing the field while their position changes. In a general situation, where the physical dimension of the moving particles is taken into account, the situation is quite complex and in order to evaluate the force exerted by the field on the particles, higher order multipole components have to be taken into account. In cases in which dielectrophoresis of macromolecules or very small particles is performed, the molecules dimension is very small, in particular much smaller than the typical electrical field variation length. In this case, an adiabatic approximation can be used, that is we can imagine that for a very small time period the particles movement do not change the surrounding electrical field due to the fact that it is almost constant in the volume traversed by the particle.

In this case, the field derived from Equation 7.248 and constituted by the constant electrical field and the sphere induced polarization field acts as if it was an external field E, while the sphere polarization moment can be still expressed by Equation 7.251. In this particular condition, the force acting on the molecules can be expressed with a good approximation using Equation 7.222 and eliminating the term due to the net charge that in this case is zero. Transforming the force density into a force can be performed passing from the polarization vector of a continuous medium to the polarization moment of each molecule and considering a general situation where the field direction can be arbitrary we obtain

$$F_j = 2\pi\varepsilon_s K(\varepsilon_s, \varepsilon_L) R^3 E_k \frac{\partial E_j}{\partial x_k} \tag{7.252}$$

Equation 7.252 is very important in understanding the characteristics of dielectrophoresis. As a matter of fact, if we imagine to perform electrophoresis in a very viscous medium so as to enhance the particles separation, we know that after a very small period in which the particles accelerate, their motion becomes uniform, with the equilibrium speed determined by the balance between the dielectrophoresis force and the viscous drag. Assuming that the dielectrophoresis force and thus the particles is along the x direction and that the particles have all the same density ρ_0, that is an approximation completely acceptable if we assume they are spheres so as to use Equation 7.250, the equilibrium velocity can be expressed as

$$v_x = \frac{3}{2} \frac{\varepsilon_s}{\rho_0} K(\varepsilon_s, \varepsilon_L) M \left[E_x \frac{\partial E_x}{\partial x} + E_y \frac{\partial E_x}{\partial y} + E_z \frac{\partial E_x}{\partial z} \right] \tag{7.253}$$

where the speed sign is essentially given by the Clausius–Mossotti factor since the square of the electrical field is present and M represents the mass of the dielectric particle.

Equation 7.49 justifies qualitatively two important characteristics of dielectrophoresis. First, certain dielectric particles move in a direction while others in the opposite direction: this is due to the Clausius–Mossotti factor having opposite sign in the different cases. Second, the average space that is covered by particles during the dielectrophoresis time is proportional to their volume and thus to their mass if they have all the same density, as it is evident from Equation 7.253.

7.5.6 ELECTROWETTING

Electrowetting is an electrostatic effect due to the contribution of electrostatic energy to the interface tension of a liquid. This effect is particularly relevant when dealing with electrolytes droplets in contact with a partially wetted conductive surface [102]. Let us assume that a droplet of an electrolyte solution is in contact with a conducting surface that is partially wetted from it so that the contact angle is greater than $\pi/2$ as in Figure 7.64a. When applying an electrostatic potential to the surface, a static field is generated in the space occupied by the droplet so that an electrostatic contribution to the free energy of the liquid–solid surface appears.

Since we are considering a mesoscopic dimension droplet, with a height of the order of at least 10 μm, the Debye length is generally much smaller than the droplet dimension (compare Section 7.5.2) and a fully developed double layer forms between the charged electrode and the droplet internal volume.

The droplet internal volume, beyond the Debye layer, is a conducting fluid so that the potential stabilizes inside the droplet to a constant value and the double layer acts as a sort of plane plates capacitor supporting a potential difference equal to $\Delta\psi$. This capacitor stores an energy that depends on its capacitance and that has to be considered among the different contributions to the surface free energy.

If the surrounding environmental fluid does not acquire a charge due to the electrolyte drop, as it is the case of air or water, it is possible to refer all potentials to the constant potential inside the droplet that would be the same as the bulk environmental fluid. In this case, we can assume $\Delta\psi$ equal to the applied potential. Cases exists in which the environmental fluids acquire a charge due to the

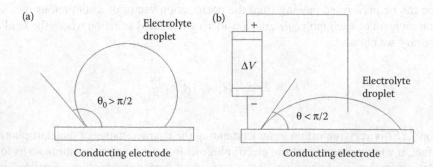

FIGURE 7.64 Electrowetting phenomenon: droplet on the surface before (a) and after (b) the application of the electrowetting potential.

droplet presence, like in the mercury case that was first studied in relation to electrowetting: in this cases, the potential $\Delta\psi$ cannot be assumed to be equal to the applied potential, but the potential drop at the droplet environment interface have to be subtracted to the applied potential to obtain $\Delta\psi$ [102].

We can write the free energy of the droplet surface in this case as

$$G = G_0 - C_{dl}\,\Delta\psi^2 \tag{7.254}$$

Applying the definition of surface tension we gave in Equation 7.112 we obtain

$$\gamma_{ls} = \left.\frac{\partial G}{\partial A}\right)_{p,T,M} = \gamma_{0ls} - \Delta V \left.\frac{\partial C_{dl}}{\partial A}\right)_{p,T,M} = \gamma_{0ls} - \Delta\psi^2\delta C \tag{7.255}$$

where γ_{0ls} is the surface tension in the absence of electrostatic potential and $\delta C = \partial C_{dl}/\partial A)_{p,T,M}$ is the capacity variation achieved by an infinitesimal variation of the contact area between the surface and the droplet, while it is assumed that, due to the double layer formation mechanism, the potential across the double layer does not change if the contact area is changed of an infinitesimal amount.

The explicit evaluation of the term δC requires the solution of the Poison–Boltzmann equation to determine the behavior of the Debye layer and the consequent accumulated charge and capacity. This can be done explicitly in the case of monovalent ions [102] or when the Debye–Hückel approximation can be used. However, the Debye–Hückel approximation has to be used with care in this case since relevant deviations are observed in many cases. A first approximation sufficient for many evaluations can be obtained with a simple approach: that is, assuming the double layer as a plane capacitors. In this way, the dependence of the capacitance on the area of the electrode is linear and a simple expression is obtained for δC

$$\delta C = \varepsilon_0 \frac{\varepsilon_l}{d_H} \tag{7.256}$$

where d_H is the equivalent double layer thickness and ε_l is the dielectric constant of the liquid.

Recalculating the contact angle between the droplet and the surface similar to Equation 7.126 we obtain

$$\cos(\theta) = \frac{\gamma_{as} - \gamma_{0sl} + \Delta\psi^2\delta C}{\gamma_{al}} \tag{7.257}$$

The overall effect is that the contact angle decreases due to the applied tension, and full wetting (i.e., $\theta < \pi/2$) can be obtained for sufficiently high electrical potentials as shown in Figure 7.64b.

Using the approximation Equation 7.256 we can rewrite Equation 7.257 as

$$\cos(\theta) = \cos(\theta_0) + \varepsilon_0 \frac{\varepsilon_l}{d_H} \frac{\Delta\psi^2}{\gamma_{al}} \tag{7.258}$$

For typical values of $d_H = 2$ nm, $\varepsilon_l = 81$, and $\gamma_{al} = 0.072$ mJ/m^2 the contact angle decreases rapidly upon the application of a voltage. It should be noted, however, that Equation 7.258 is only applicable within a voltage range below the onset of electrolytic processes, typically up to a few hundred millivolts. In many applications this problem, that limits the control on the reduction of the contact angle, is circumvented by introducing a thin dielectric film, which insulates the droplet from the electrode [103]. In this ElectroWetting On Dielectric (EWOD) configuration, the electric double layer builds up at the insulator–droplet interface. Since the insulator thickness d is usually much larger than d_H, the total capacitance of the system is greatly reduced.

This system may be described as two capacitors in series, namely the double layer at the dielectric film interface and the dielectric film itself. Since the dielectric film has a much lower capacitance, the series capacitance can be approximated as that of the dielectric layer alone. Thus, neglecting possible charges on the droplet-environmental fluid interface, we can write the contact angle due to electrowetting as

$$\cos(\theta) = \cos(\theta_0) + \varepsilon_0 \frac{\varepsilon_l}{d} \frac{\Delta\psi^2}{\gamma_{al}} \tag{7.259}$$

A problem of the simple electrowetting theory we have presented is that the phenomenon exhibits saturation: after a specific voltage, the saturation voltage, the increase of voltage will not change the contact angle, and with extreme voltages the interface will show instabilities. Qualitatively, this behavior can be ascribed by the fact that surface charge is perhaps the main component of surface energy due to the electrostatic field, but not the only. Other components are negligible at low voltage but becomes important at high voltage, generating the contact angle saturation.

The full behavior of electrowetting, comprising saturation and instabilities, can be only justified quantitatively by taking into account accurately both the charged layer structure and the droplet and surface shape [104]. Within this framework it is predicted that reversed electrowetting is also possible in particular circumstances, causing the contact angle to grow with the applied voltage.

7.6   MAGNETO-HYDRODYNAMICS

In Chapter 3 we have seen that several analytical procedures used in biology use the so-called magnetic beads. They are used, for example, in specific nucleic acids amplification procedures (see Section 3.3), to fix antibodies to their surface in immunoassays (see Section 3.5) and in second- and third-generation DNA sequencing techniques (se Section 3.8).

A magnetic bead is a big solid particle, with a diameter at least of the order of 1 μm, presenting several magnetic dipoles fixed in its body so as to be oriented all in the same direction. The surface of a magnetic bead is activated creating the possibility to capture a target macromolecule. Frequently, the magnetic bead matrix is constituted by a magnetic inert polymer; strongly diamagnetic nanoparticles are inserted in the matrix and surface activation is obtained by coating the bead with a suitable material. The structure of this type of beads is reported in Figure 7.65.

Since the overall magnetic dipole of a magnetic bead is the sum of all internal dipoles, a magnetic field can be used to move it in a microfluidic circuit. In this section, we will study the interaction of a magnetic bead with an external magnetic field.

7.6.1   MAGNETOSTATIC BASICS

The first step to analyze the interaction of magnetic beads with an external magnetic field is to recap the main elements of magnetostatic. As a matter of fact, magnetostatic equations have to be added in this case to fluid dynamics and, in case, diffusion equation. As in the electrostatic case we will consider uniquely stationary currents so as to deal only with constant magnetic field and neglect radiation-related phenomena.

However, several times materials with strong magnetic properties are used in magnetostatic systems, so that magnetization has to be explicitly taken into account in magnetostatic equations. Magnetic materials can be described as a system constituted by a large set of microscopic magnetic dipoles due both to micro-currents flowing internally to the material due to electron motion and to the spins of the involved particles.

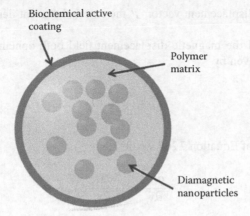

FIGURE 7.65   Structure of a paramagnetic bead.

Once the intensity m and the location r_i, of all magnetic dipoles that are present in the material are known, the overall magnetic dipole of a material volume V can be evaluated. As we have already done for fluid dynamics in Section 7.1, we can adopt a continuous representation of the magnetic material defining a reference volume $\Omega(r)$ whose center is the point r and with measure Ω_V small with respect to the volume scale of the macroscopic problem, but still sufficient to contain a very large number of magnetic dipoles. The macroscopic value of the magnetization $M(r)$ in the continuous model is then provided by

$$M(r) = \frac{1}{\Omega_V} \int\limits_{\Omega(r)} m(r')\delta(r' - r_i)\, dr' \tag{7.260}$$

so that the magnetization results to be a mesoscopic density of magnetic moment.

When the microscopic magnetic moment is due to a micro-current a link exists between the micro-current and the associated magnetic moment. To simplify magnetostatic equations, generally a sort of apparent micro-current is introduced correlated to the spin magnetic moments, so that a mesoscopic material current density J^m can be introduced with a procedure similar to that used for magnetization. Due to the definition of the material internal current density the following equation is immediately derived,

$$J_i^m = -\epsilon_{i,j,k} \frac{\partial M_j}{\partial x_k} \tag{7.261}$$

relating the overall internal current to the magnetic moment curl. Introducing also a macroscopic current flowing in an electrical circuit built into the system, the magnetostatic equations can be obtained by Maxwell equations eliminating the radiation-related terms and taking only the equations for magnetic fields. They write

$$\frac{\partial B_j}{\partial x_j} = 0 \tag{7.262a}$$

$$\epsilon_{i,j,k} \frac{\partial B_j}{\partial x_k} = \mu_0 \left(J_i^e + J_i^m \right) \tag{7.262b}$$

where B is the magnetic displacement vector, J^e the external current density, and μ_0 the magnetic vacuum permeability.

The magnetization and the magnetic displacement field both concurs to the definition of the magnetic field H, that is given by

$$H_j = \frac{B_j}{\mu_0} - M_j \tag{7.263}$$

Taking the divergence of Equation 7.264 we obtain

$$\frac{\partial H_j}{\partial x_j} = -\frac{\partial M_j}{\partial x_j} \tag{7.264}$$

The definition of the magnetic field is useful to simplify, at least formally, Equation 7.262b by eliminating the magnetic current density, that is a microscopic characteristic of the material. As a matter of fact, using Equations 7.263 and 7.264 in Equation 7.262b we get

$$\epsilon_{i,j,k} \frac{\partial H_j}{\partial x_k} = \mu_0 J_i^e \tag{7.265a}$$

$$\nabla \times \mathbf{H} = \mu_0 \mathbf{J}^e \tag{7.265b}$$

that is the most traditional form of the second law of magnetostatics.

From Equation 7.62 we get that the relation between the magnetic field H and the inner material magnetization M is quite complex. Besides the explicit linear dependence, an implicit dependence is contained in the B field. In the more complex case, the case of ferromagnetic materials, this is a noninstantaneous dependence, so that the magnetic displacement depends on values of the magnetization not only in the same instant, but also in a previous time interval, called material memory time. When an external magnetic field is applied to a ferromagnetic material such as iron, the atomic dipoles align themselves with it. Even when the field is removed, part of the alignment will be retained: the material has become magnetized. Once magnetized, the magnet will stay magnetized for a very long time, since the only demagnetization mechanism is thermal energy, which at room temperature has generally little impact on ferromagnetic dipoles. Magnetization can be removed greatly increasing thermal energy, that is heating the material or via a new magnetic field. If we represent magnetization and demagnetization on the H–M plane, since the application of a new magnetic field is done on a magnetized material, the process of demagnetization does not follow the inverse path of the first magnetization process, causing magnetic hysteresis. An example of magnetic hysteresis cycle is shown in Figure 4.66.

In the case of paramagnetic and diamagnetic materials, no memory exists in the dependence of the magnetic field by the magnetization, and the magnetic properties of the material are described by the magnetic susceptibility tensor χ, that is defined as

$$\chi_{i,j} = \left. \frac{\partial M_i}{\partial H_j} \right)_{V,T} \tag{7.266}$$

The tensor nature of χ indicates anisotropy of the material magnetic properties. In isotropic materials the vectors H and M are parallel, having the same direction for paramagnetic material and opposite directions for diamagnetic ones. In this case, the magnetic susceptibility becomes a scalar

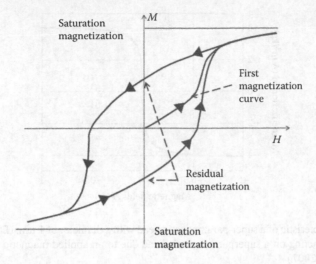

FIGURE 7.66   Example of magnetic hysteresis cycle.

and frequently the magnetic susceptibility does not depend on the magnetic field in wide ranges of magnetic and environmental conditions. In these cases, dependence of the between H and M is linear; in this case we can write

$$M = \chi H \tag{7.267a}$$

$$B = \mu_0(1 + \chi)H = \mu H \tag{7.267b}$$

Here, μ is called magnetic permeability of the medium and the relation between H and B is similar to the relation between E and D.

Among paramagnetic materials, particularly important in the fabrication of magnetic beads are the so-called super-paramagnetic materials. This kind of material shows no hysteresis, but the transition between the two saturation values of the magnetization for positive and negative magnetic fields is quite abrupt, so that for practical purposes they can be considered as having two possible magnetization values and passing from one to the other when the magnetic field changes direction. This characteristics is quite useful in beads since it allows the magnetization of the bead to be fixed practically whatever the magnetic field and the bead behavior in the system to be easier to forecast and more reproducible. An example of magnetization characteristics of a super-paramagnetic bead with a diameter of 1 µm is reported in Figure 7.67 [105].

7.6.2   MAGNETOPHORESIS

The name magnetophoresis characterizes all the systems where magnetic beads with absorbed macromolecules are moved through a macroscopic assay system or through a lab on chip by magnetic forces. This technique has several applications, as we have seen in Chapter 3.

The first step to face the problem is to determine the magnetic force acting on a magnetic bead. The evaluation of such a forces is not trivial [90,105], and the most direct way of doing it is to evaluate the magnetic contribution to the free energy starting from the equation giving the energy ϵ_M of the magnetic field that writes

$$\epsilon_M = -B_j H_j = -\frac{B_j B_j}{\mu_0} - M_j B_j \tag{7.268}$$

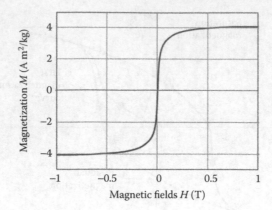

FIGURE 7.67 Characteristic of a super-paramagnetic bead with a diameter of 1 μm. (Data from Shevkoplyas S. S. et al., The force acting on a superparamagnetic bead due to an applied magnetic field, *Lab on a Chip*, vol. 7, pp. 1294–1302, 2007.)

Starting from this expression the virtual works theorem can be used to estimate the force acting on the bead as a whole. Assuming a nonconductive homogeneous bead occupying the volume V, the resulting force on the bead center of mass results

$$F_j = \mu_0 \int_V M_k \frac{dH_j}{dx_k} dV \qquad (7.269)$$

In the magnetostatic case, considering linear diamagnetic or paramagnetic materials, the fact that the magnetic field has a null curl can be used to introduce a scalar magnetic potential $\phi(r)$, in strict analogy to the electrostatic potential, so that $H_j = \partial\phi/\partial x_j$. Proceeding in analogy to dielectrophoresis, the following expressions are found for magnetization of the bead and for the force acting on it:

$$M_j = \frac{3\mu - \mu_0}{\mu + 2\mu_0} H_j^e \qquad (7.270)$$

$$F_j = 2\pi\mu_0 K(\mu, \mu_0) R^3 \frac{\partial}{\partial x_j} (H_k H_k) \qquad (7.271)$$

where μ and R are the bead radius and magnetic permeability, respectively, $K(\mu, \mu_0)$ is the Clausius–Mossotti factor (see Equation 7.249) and H^e is the externally applied magnetic field.

Equation 7.272 is essentially identical to the expression of the dielectrophoresis force. However, magnetic materials frequently show substantial deviations from the simple linear behavior, so that experimental results deviate frequently from results from Equation 7.272. In these cases, a more accurate, and frequently numeric, approach has to be considered.

Magnetophoresis can be used to selectively separate a biochemical species due to the fact that almost all biomolecules are not magnetically active. The device implementing magnetophoresis is represented schematically in Figure 7.68. In a first step the solution containing the target macromolecule besides nonspecific species is mixed with a certain concentration of magnetic beads. The target macromolecule is absorbed on the surface of the beads, in case through an intermediate antibody previously attached to the bead surface. If the number of used beads is sufficient, almost all

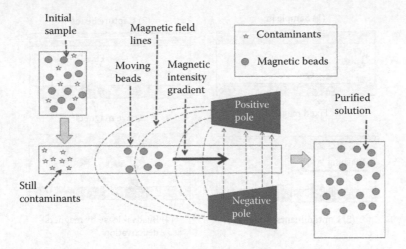

FIGURE 7.68   Principle scheme of a magnetophoresis system based on bead motion in a duct.

the target molecules are absorbed. After this step, the bead enriched solution is put in a duct where a magnetic field is created. The magnetic field operates only on the beads, causing their movement through the duct toward the final chamber, while the other macromolecules are not affected by the field. At the end the target molecules attached to the beads are assayed to determine their concentration. The bead movement depends on the gradient of the magnetic field intensity so that better performances are attained by increasing the magnetic gradient.

Magnetophoresis beads on beads motion is a powerful technique, but has a problem if the required bead concentration is high. As a matter of fact, bead movement can cause hydrodynamic drag of the solvent and of part of the contaminating species that exist in the original solution. Thus, a threshold bead concentration cannot be overcome if the purification has to be efficient.

Another possible technique relies on the use of switchable magnets to capture the beads: the scheme of this arrangement is reported in Figure 7.69. In this case also, the sample is enriched with magnetic beads and sent to a duct. Switchable magnets on the duct walls are activated so as to capture the beads and the solution in the duct is washed with a suitable washing solution. The target molecule remains attached to the beads while all the contaminants are washed away. At the end of the washing a suitable solvent is sent to the duct and the magnets are switched off so as to release the beads. In this case, the type of washing solution and the washing pressure has to be carefully chosen not to provoke target molecules detachment during washing.

7.6.3   Bead Concentration Evolution

In every case in which bead motion happens, a detailed prediction of it is needed to design the magnetophoretic system. Beads motion is essentially determined by the bead density, since this factor influences the interaction between the beads and the fluids where they are suspended [106].

In the extreme case of very small bead density, not only collision among beads can be neglected in studying the motion, but also hydrodynamic drags of the surrounding fluid due to interaction between with bead surfaces is negligible. In this case, the problem reduces to analyze the beads concentration in a surrounding fluid whose motion state is not influenced by the beads presence [107].

The forces acting on the single bead are essentially three: drag from the surrounding fluid, magnetic force, and a random walk caused by thermal motion. The correct approach in this extreme case is to insert in the diffusion-convection Equation 7.166, a term representing a force acting only on the beads. This term can be easily evaluated taking into account that a particle that is subject to a force

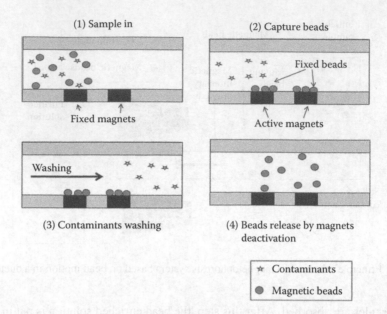

(1) Sample in

Fixed magnets

(2) Capture beads

Fixed beads

Active magnets

Washing

(3) Contaminants washing

(4) Beads release by magnets deactivation

★ Contaminants

● Magnetic beads

FIGURE 7.69 Principle scheme of a magnetophoresis system based on bed capture by fixed magnets.

in a regime of viscous motion, after a very brief transitory moves at a constant velocity at which the viscous resistance balance the active force. Thus, indicating with $\boldsymbol{F}$ the magnetic force given by Equation 7.221 we can write the magnetic induced flux of the beads Φ^M as

$$\Phi^M = \frac{c(\boldsymbol{r},t)}{\eta} \boldsymbol{F} \tag{7.272}$$

where $c(\boldsymbol{r}, t)$ is the beads' density, so that the convection diffusion equation writes in this case

$$\frac{\partial c(\boldsymbol{r},t)}{\partial t} = D\nabla^2 c + v_w \cdot \nabla c + \frac{c(\boldsymbol{r},t)}{\eta} \boldsymbol{F} \tag{7.273}$$

This model loses its validity if the beads concentration becomes not very small, as in many practical cases. Here, the hydrodynamic drag due to the beads cannot be neglected and the beads presence influences the bulk fluid motion.

In the extreme case of very small (e.g., with a radius of about 1 μm) and very concentrated beads it is conceivable that the environmental liquid is completely dragged by the beads [108], so that the magnetic force manifest itself like a volume force acting on all the liquid body. In this case, a suitable approximation is to set up a model where both the fluid velocity field and the bead concentration are unknown and the available equations are Equation 7.273 and the Navier–Stokes Equation 7.36 where the magnetic force is inserted among the volume forces acting on the fluid bulk. This is, in general, a quite difficult problem to solve, but it is not beyond the capability of fluid dynamics numerical methods once suitable boundary and initial conditions are set.

As far as the boundary conditions are considered, it is to take into account that, imposing the no-slip condition in this case requires that the bead in contact with the walls are still too, that is not true in several cases. Thus, finding suitable boundary conditions can be not at all easy.

REFERENCES

1. Poznikidis C., *Introduction to Theoretical and Computational Fluid Dynamics*, Oxford University Press, USA; 2nd edition (September 28, 2011), ISBN-13: 978-0199752072.
2. Shivamoggi, B., K., *Theoretical Fluid Dynamics*, Wiley-Interscience; 2nd edition (January 15, 1998), ISBN-13: 978-0471056591.
3. Bruus H., *Theoretical Microfluidics*, Oxford University Press, USA (November 17, 2007), ISBN-13: 978-0199235094.
4. Aris R., *Vectors, Tensors and the Basic equations of Fluid Mechanics*, Dover Publications (January 1, 1990), ISBN-13: 978-0486661100.
5. Milne-Thomson L. M., *Theoretical Aerodynamics*, Dover Publications (February 17, 2011), ISBN-13: 978-0486619804.
6. De U. C., *Tensor Calculus*, Alpha Science Intl Ltd; 2nd edition (December 30, 2007), ISBN-13: 978-1842654484;
7. Daintith J., *Oxford Dictionary of Chemistry*, Oxford University Press, USA; 6 edition (April 15, 2008), ISBN-13: 978-0199204632;
8. Atkin, J., Fox N., *An Introduction to the Theory of Elasticity*, Dover Publications Inc. (August 25, 2005), ISBN-13: 978-0486442419.
9. Brush, S.G., Theories of liquid viscosity. *Chemical Review*, vol. 62, pp. 513–54, 1962.
10. Evans D. J., Morriss D. G., *Statistical Mechanics of Nonequilibrium Liquids*, Cambridge University Press; 2nd edition (May 8,2008), ISBN-13: 978-0521857918.
11. Eisenberg D., Kauzmann W., *The Structure and Properties of Water*, Oxford University Press, USA (December 8, 2005), ISBN-13: 978-0198570264.
12. Lauga E., Brenner M. P., Stone H. A., Microfluidics: The no-slip boundary condition, in Springer Handbook of Experimental Fluid Mechanics (Chapter 15), Tropea C, Yarin A. L., Foss J. F. editors, Springer; 2007, ISBN-13 978-3540251415.
13. Kleinstein G. G., On the derivation of boundary conditions from the global principles of continuum mechanics, *Quarterly of Applied Mathematics*, vol. 63, pp. 469–478, 2005.
14. Tretheway D. C., Meinhart C. D., Apparent fluid slip at hydrophobic microchannel walls, *Physics of Fluids*, vol. 14, pp. L10–L12, 2002.
15. Bocquet L., Barrat J.-L., Flow boundary conditions from nano- to micro-scales, *Soft Matter*, vol. 3, pp. 685–693, 2007.
16. Priczjev N. V., Troian S. M., Influence of periodic wall roughness on the slip behaviour at liquid/solid interfaces: Molecular-scale simulations versus continuum predictions, *Journal of Fluid Mechanics*, vol. 554, pp. 25–46, 2006.
17. Brenner H., Beyond the no-slip boundary condition, *Physical Review E*, vol. 84, pp. 046309-1–046309-8, 2011.
18. Bing D., Bakir, M. S., Sekar, D. C., King, C. R., Meindl, J. D., Integrated microfluidic cooling and inter-connects for 2D and 3D chips, *IEEE Transactions on Advanced Packaging*, vol. 33, pp. 79–87, 2010.
19. Paik P. Y., Pamula V. K., Chakrabarty, K., Adaptive cooling of integrated circuits using digital microfluid-ics, *IEEE Transactions on Very Large Scale Integration (VLSI) Systems*, vol. 16, pp. 432–443, 2008.
20. Waite L., Fine J., *Applied Biofluid Mechanics*, McGraw-Hill Professional; 1st edition (May 31, 2007), ISBN-13: 978-0071472173.
21. Bowman F., *Introduction to Bessel Functions*, Dover Publications (reprinted on October 18, 2010), ISBN-13: 978-0486604626.
22. Neit J.-C., Wender A., Lachet V., Malfreit P., Prediction of the temperature dependence of the surface tension of SO_2, N_2, O_2, and Ar by monte carlo molecular simulations, *Journal of Physical Chemistry B*, vol. 115, pp. 9421–9430, 2011.
23. Lu H. M., Jiang Q., Surface tension and its temperature coefficient for liquid metals, *Journal of Physical Chemistry B*, vol. 109, pp. 15463–15468, 2005.
24. Ayyad A., Aqra F., Theoretical consideration of the anomalous temperature dependence of the surface tension of pure liquid gallium, *Theoretical Chemistry Accounts: Theory, Computation, and Modeling (Theoretica Chimica Acta)*, vol. 127, 5–6, pp. 443–448, 2010.
25. Desjonqueres M.-C., Spanjaard D., *Concepts in Surface Physics*, Springer; 2nd edition (March 13, 2002), ISBN-13: 978-3540586227.
26. Speight J., *Lange's Handbook of Chemistry*, McGraw-Hill Professional; 16 edition (December 20, 2004), ISBN-13, 978-0071432207.

27. Jasper J. J., The surface tension of pure liquids compounds, *Journal of Physical Chemistry Reference Data*, vol. 1, pp. 841–1009, 1972.

28. O'Neill B., *Elementary Differential Geometry*, Academic Press; 2nd edition (April 10, 2006), ISBN-13: 978-0120887354.

29. Nishida T., Equations of fluid dynamics—free surface problems, *Pure and Applied Mathematics,* vol. 39, pp. S221–S238, 1986.

30. Preisig M. Zimmermann T., Free-surface fluid dynamics on moving domains, *Computer Methods in Applied Mechanics and Engineering*, vol. 200, pp. 372–382, 2011.

31. de Gennes, P. G., Wetting: Statics and dynamics, *Reviews of Modern Physics*, vol. 57, pp. 827–863, 1985.

32. McHale G., Shirtcliffe N. J., Newton M. I., Contact-angle hysteresis on super-hydrophobic surfaces, *Langmuir*, vol. 20, pp. 10146–10149, 2004.

33. Marmur A., Wetting of hydrophobic rough surfaces: To be heterogeneous or not to be. *Langmuir* vol. 19, pp. 8343–8348, 2003.

34. Lin F., Zhang Y, Xi J, Zhu Y, Wang N, Xia F, Jiang L, Petal effect: Two major examples of the cassie–baxter model are the "petal effect" and "lotus effect." A superhydrophobic state with high adhesive force, *Langmuir*, vol. 24, pp. 4114–4119, 2008.

35. Ebert D., Bhushan D, Wear-resistant rose petal-effect surfaces with superhydrophobicity and high droplet adhesion using hydrophobic and hydrophilic nanoparticles, *Journal of Colloid and Interface Science*, vol. 384, pp. 182–188, 2012.

36. Sumesh P. T., Govindarajan R., The possible equilibrium shapes of static pendant drops, *Journal of Chemical Physics*, vol, 133, pp. 144707–14715, 2010.

37. Vacèk V., Determination of the shape of pendant drops, *The Chemical Engineering Journal*, vol. 9, pp. 167–169, 1975.

38. Berthier J., Brakke K., *The Physics of Microdroplets*, Wiley-Scrivener; 1st edition (May 8, 2012), ISBN-13: 978-0470938805.

39. Gardas R. L., Ge R., Ab Manan N., Rooney D. W., Hardacre, Interfacial tensions of imidazolium-based ionic liquids with water and n-alkanes, *Fluid Phase Equilibria*, vol. 294, pp. 139–147, 2010.

40. Yang D., Xu Z., Liu C., Wang L., Experimental study on the surface characteristics of polymer melts, *Colloids and Surfaces A: Physicochemical and Engineering Aspects*, vol. 367, pp. 174–180, 2010.

41. Fujikawa S., Yano T., Watanabe M., *Vapor-Liquid Interfaces, Bubbles and Droplets: Fundamentals and Applications*, Springer; 1st edition (May 4, 2011), ISBN-13: 978-3642180378.

42. Baroud C. N., Gallaire F., Dangla R., Dynamics of microfluidic droplets, *Lab on a Chip*, vol.10, pp. 2032–2045, 2010.

43. Fua T., Wua Y., Ma Y., Li H. Z., Droplet formation and breakup dynamics in microfluidic flow-focusing devices: From dripping to jetting, *Chemical Engineering Science*, vol. 84, pp. 207–217, 2012.

44. Schneider T., Burnham D. R:, Van Orden J., Chiu D. T., Systematic investigation of froplet generation at T-junctions, *Lab on a Chip*, vol. 11, pp.2055–2059, 2011.

45. Eggers, J. Nonlinear dynamics and breakup of free-surface flows. *Reviews of Modern Physics*, vol. 69, pp. 865–927, 1997.

46. Aslanov, S., Theory of breakup of a liquid jet into droplets, *Technical Physics*, vol. 4, pp. 1386, 1999.

47. Mead-Hunter R., King A. J. C., Mullins B. J., Plateau rayleigh instability simulation, *Langmuir*, vol. 28, pp. 6731–6735, 2012.

48. Chhabra R. P., J. Richardson F., *Non-Newtonian Flow and Applied Rheology*, Butterworth-Heinemann; 2nd edition (September 25, 2008), ISBN-13: 978-0750685320.

49. Chhabra R. P., *Bubbles, Drops, and Particles in Non-Newtonian Fluids*, CRC Press; 2nd edition (July 25, 2006), ISBN-13: 978-0824723293.

50. Graessley W. W., *Polymeric Liquids & Networks: Structure and Properties*, Garland Science; 1st edition (November 20, 2003), ISBN-13: 978-0815341697.

51. Dealy J., Larson R., *Structure and Rheology of Molten Polymers*, Hanser Publications (March 1, 2006), ISBN-13: 978-1569903810.

52. Nguyen Q. D., Uhlherr P. H. T., *Thixotropic Behaviour of Concentrated Real Mud Suspensions.* Proceedings of the 3rd NationalConference on Rheology, Melbourne, pp. 63–67, 1983.

53. Cussler E. L., *Diffusion: Mass Transfer in Fluid Systems*, Cambridge University Press; 3rd edition (February 2, 2009), ISBN-13: 978-0521871211.

54. Vasko F. T., Raichev O. E., *Quantum Kinetic Theory and Applications: Electrons, Photons, Phonons*, Springer; Reprint of 2005 1st edition 2005 (October 15, 2010), ISBN-13: 978-1441920775.

55. Westrum Jr. E. F., *Phonon Dispersion Treatment of the Thermodynamic and Physical Properties of Vitreous and Disordered Solids*, CreateSpace Independent Publishing Platform, 1st edition (September 14, 2011), ISBN-13: 978-1463520236.

56. Yamashita T., Peng Y., Knight C., Voth G. A., Computationally efficient multiconfigurational reactive molecular dynamics, *Journal of Chemical Computational Theory*, vol. 8, pp. 4863–4875, 2012.

57. Singharoy A., Joshi H., Ortoleva P. J., Multiscale macromolecular simulation: Role of evolving ensembles, *Journal of Chemical Information Models.*, vol. 52, pp. 2638–2649, 2012.

58. T. J. O'Leary, Concentration dependence of protein diffusion, *Biophysical Journal*, vol. 52, pp. 137–139, 1987.

59. Ribeiro A. C. F. et al., Binary mutual diffusion coefficients of aqueous solutions of sucrose, lactose, glucose, and fructose in the temperature range from (298.15 to 328.15) K, *Journal of Chemical Engineering Data*, vol. 51, pp. 1836–1840, 2006.

60. Wang A., Li C., Pielak G. J., Effects of proteins on protein diffusion, *Journal of American Chemical Society*, vol. 132, pp. 9392–9397, 2010.

61. Baune D., Kim S., Predicting protein diffusion coefficients, *Proceedings of the USA National Acccademy of Science*, vol. 90, pp. 3835–3839, 1993.

62. Gaigalas A. K., Reipa V., Hubbard J. B., Edwards J., A non-perturbative relation between the mutual diffusion coefficient, suspension viscosity, and osmotic compressibility: Application to concentrated protein solutions, *Chemical Engineering Science*, vol. 50, pp. 1107–1114, 1995.

63. Pfeiffer W. F., Krieger I. M., Bubble solution method for diffusion coefficient measurements. experimental evaluation, *Journal of Physical Chemistry*, vol. 78, pp. 2516–2521, 1974.

64. Wen W., Zhao H., Zhang S., Pires V., Rapid photoelectrochemical method for in situ determination of effective diffusion coefficient of organic compounds, *Journal of Physical Chemistry* vol. 112, pp. 3875–3880, 2008.

65. Komiya A., Maruyama S., Precise and short-time measurement method of mass diffusion coefficients, *Experimental Thermal and Fluid Science*, vol. 30, pp. 535–543, 2006.

66. Torres J. F., Komiya A., Shoji E., Okajima J., Maruyama S., Development of phase-shifting interferometry for measurement of isothermal diffusion coefficients in binary solutions, *Optics and Lasers in Engineering*, vol. 50, pp. 1287–1296, 2012.

77. Davis H. E., Leach J., K., Designing bioactive delivery systems for tissue regeneration, *Annals of Biomedical Engineering*, vol. 39, pp. 1–13, 2011.

78. Liu M.-K., Li P., Giddings J. C., Rapid protein separation and diffusion coefficient measurement by frit inlet flow field-flow fractionation, *Protein Science* vol. 2, pp. 1520–1531, 1993.

79. Freitas Jr. R. A., *Nanomedicine, Volume I: Basic Capabilities*, Landes Bioscience, 1999, ISBN-13: 978-157059645-X

80. Johnson E. M., Berk D. A., Jain R. K., Deen W. M., Diffusion and partitioning of proteins in charged agarose gels, *Biophysical Journal*, vol. 68, pp. 1561–1568, 1995.

81. Stakgold I., Holst M. J., *Green's Functions and Boundary Value Problems*, Wiley; 3rd edition (February 8, 2011), ISBN-13: 978-0470609705.

82. Lawler G. F., Limic V., *Random Walk: A Modern Introduction*, Cambridge University Press (July 26, 2010), ISBN-13: 978-0521519182.

83. Abramowitz, M., Stegun I. A., *Handbook of Mathematical Functions with Formulas, Graphs, and Mathematical Tables*, Dover Publications (June, 1965), ISBN-13: 978-0486612720.

84. Smith G. D., *Numerical Solution of Partial Differential Equations: Finite Difference Methods*, Oxford University Press, USA; 3rd edition (January 16, 1986), ISBN-13: 978-0198596509.

85. Johnson C., *Numerical Solution of Partial Differential equations by the Finite Element Method*, Dover Publications (January 15, 2009), ISBN-13: 978-0486469003.

86. Brown J, Churchill R., *Fourier Series and Boundary Value Problems*, McGraw-Hill; 8 edition (February 8, 2011), ISBN-13: 978-0078035975.

87. Boyce W. E., DiPrima R. C., *Elementary Differential Equations and Boundary Value Problems*, Wiley; 9 edition (October 27, 2008), ISBN-13: 978-0470383346.

88. Smoller J., *Shock Waves and Reaction-Diffusion Equations*, Springer; 2nd edition (October 14, 1994), ISBN-13: 978-0387942599.

89. Jackson J. D., *Classical Electrodynamics*, Wiley; 3rd edition (August 10, 1998), ISBN-13: 978-0471309321.

90. Di Bartolo B., *Classical Theory of Electromagnetism*, World Scientific Publishing Corporation; 2nd edition (November 2004), ISBN-13: 978-9812382191.

91. Rindler W., *Introduction to Special Relativity*, Oxford University Press, USA; 2nd edition (July 11, 1991), ISBN-13: 978-0198539520.

92. Raab L. E., Lange O. L., *Multipole Theory in Electromagnetism: Classical, Quantum, and Symmetry Aspects, with Applications*, Oxford University Press, USA (January 6, 2005), ISBN-13: 978-0198567271.

93. Agmon N., Mechanism of hydroxide mobility, *Chemical Physics Letters*, vol. 319, pp. 247–252, 2000.

94. Codorniu-Hernández E., Kusalik P. G., Mobility mechanism of hydroxyl radicals in aqueous solution via hydrogen transfer, *Journal of American Chemical Society*, vol. 134, pp. 532–538, 2012.

95. Delgado A. V., González-Caballero F., Hunter R. J., Koopal L. K., Lyklema J., Measurement and interpretation of electrokinetic phenomena, *Pure and Applied Chemistry*, vol. 77, pp. 1753–1805, 2005.

96. Teschke O., de Souza E. F., Ceotto G., Double layer relaxation measurements using atomic force microscopy, *Langmuir*, vol. 15, pp. 4935–4939, 1999.

97. Zhang H., Hassanali A. A., Shin Y. K., Knight C., Singer S. J., The water-amorphous silica interface: Analysis of the stern layer and surface conduction, *Journal of Chemical Physics*, vol. 134, pp. 024705, 2011.

98. Tadmor R., Hernández-Zapata E., Chen N., Pincus P., Israelachvili J. N., Debye length and double-layer forces in polyelectrolyte solutions, *Macromolecules*, vol. 35, pp 2380–2388, 2002.

99. Kohonen M. M., Karaman M. E., Pashley R. M., Debye length in multivalent electrolyte solutions, *Langmuir*, vol. 16, pp. 5749–5753, 2000.

100. Zaucha M.,Adamczyk Z., Barbasz J., Zeta potential of particle bilayers on mica: A streaming potential study, *Journal of Colloid and Interface Science*, vol. 360, pp. 195–203, 2011.

101. Boas M. L., *Mathematical Methods in the Physical Sciences*, Wiley; 3rd edition (July 22, 2005), ISBN-13: 978-0471198260.

102. Mugele F., Baret J. C., Electrowetting: From basics to applications, *Journal of Physics: Condensed Matter*, vol. 17, pp. R705–R774, 2005.

103. Jakeway S. C., de Mello A. J., Russell E. L. Miniaturized total analysis systems for biological analysis, *Fresenius' Journal of Analytical Chemistry*, vol. 366, pp. 525–539, 2000.

104. Klarman D., Andelman D., Urbakh M., A model of electrowetting, reversed electrowetting and contact angle saturation, *Langmuir* vol. 27, pp. 6031–6041, 2011.

105. Shevkoplyas S. S., et al., The force acting on a superparamagnetic bead due to an applied magnetic field, *Lab on a Chip*, vol. 7, pp. 1294–1302, 2007.

106. Mikkelsen C., Hansen M. F., Bruus H., Theoretical comparison of magnetic and hydrodynamic interactions between magnetically tagged particles in microfluidic systems, *Journal of Magnetism and Magnetic Materials*, vol. 293, pp. 578–583, 2005

107. Weddemann A., Wittbracht F., Auge A., Hütten A., Positioning system for particles in microfluidic structures, *Microfluidics and Nanofluidics*, vol. 7, pp. 849–855, 2009.

108. Mikkelsen C., Bruus H., Microfluidic capturing-dynamics of paramagnetic bead suspensions, *Lab on a Chip*, vol. 5, pp. 1293–1297, 2005.

8 Microfluidic Building Blocks

8.1 INTRODUCTION

In this chapter, we will introduce the main elements of the microfluidic circuit of a lab on chip. A large number of different architectures have been proposed for key elements, such as valves and pumps, and it is almost impossible to name and analyze them all from the point of view of performance and technology [1–5]. We will carry out a more detailed analysis for a selected number of building blocks, both to provide an idea of the performances that can be attained by these kinds of microsystems and to present examples of application of general methods to this particular field. We will also present a number of other examples without a detailed analysis of their performances to give an idea of the great variety of possibilities that arc at the designer's disposal when selecting the building blocks for microfluidic circuits inside a lab on chip.

With the intent of providing an idea of the performances attained by each architecture we will present a summary of average performances attained by summarizing the huge literature reporting specific implementations. In general, this is only an order of magnitude indication and sensible deviations can be present in particular prototypes. In any case, we have preferred this approach with respect to referring few specific implementations that unavoidably present specific performances. A large bibliography with reference to specific articles on prototypes and proofs of concept of different techniques is reported in the general books and articles we cite from in References [1–5]. The reader interested in a wide analysis of particular implementation is encouraged to consult as a starting point such articles. We will not try to summarize here all the interesting implementations reported in the literature, but will use the references more as a support for the discussion that we will carry out.

The chapter is mainly devoted to building blocks for microfluidic circuits when continuous flow happens, but elements of droplet-based microfluidics are also considered.

8.2 FLUID FLOW CONTROL: MICROVALVES

Valves are a kcy element to control fluid-dynamic systems, from macroscopic fluids plants to microfluidic-based circuits. Microvalves can be essentially divided into two types: control valves and active valves. Control valves are passive systems: they do not need power feeding to work. Their role is generally to allow fluid flow in a particular direction so as to prevent, for example, spurious flows from entering into pumps or other elements to perturb them. Control valves can also have more complex functionalities, such as deviating the flux from a channel to the other when it overcomes a given flow rate. Active microvalves are configured by an external command signal so as to assume a configuration functional to the wanted behavior of the circuit they belong to.

8.2.1 CONTROL MICROVALVES

The main element of many control microvalves is a membrane, and generally the membrane elasticity is exploited to obtain the wanted working. An example of process flow for the construction of a membrane on a silicon circuit is considered in Chapter 4 and its scheme is presented in Figure 4.11. This is quite a complex process that, when the valve is inserted as a part of a microfluidic circuit, has to be integrated with all the processes that are needed to realize the other parts of the circuit.

Control valves can be divided in normally open and normally closed valves. Normally open valves are open in the complete absence of fluid flow and when the flow happens in the correct direction, while they close if the fluid flows in the incorrect direction. Contrarily, normally closed valves are closed in the absence of flow and they open when a flow in the correct direction presents itself.

Two main parameters are used as quality indices of a control valve: valve leakage and valve capacity. The valve leakage L_L is defined as the ratio between the flow rate Q_D that the valve can accommodate in the direct direction when open and the flow rate Q_I that the valve allows in the opposite direction when closed. Both flows have to be evaluated at the same pressure difference δp at the valve extremes. This means that

$$L_L(\delta p) = \frac{Q_D(\delta p)}{Q_I(\delta p)} \qquad (8.1)$$

This indicates that the leakage has to be high to have a good valve. In the literature, the inverse definition is also found; in that case, the leakage has to be small to have a good valve.

The valve capacity C_V is essentially intended to provide a measure of the maximum flow rate Q_{Max} that can be accommodated by the valve in correspondence with the maximum pressure δp_{Max} that can be applied to the valve without damaging it. The valve capacity is conventionally normalized as

$$C_V = \frac{Q_{Max}}{\sqrt{\delta p_{Max}/L \rho g}} \qquad (8.2)$$

where L is the characteristic length of the fluid path through the valve, ρ is the fluid density, and g is the acceleration due to gravity. The capacity defined as in Equation 8.2 has the dimensions of a flow rate and it is normalized with the ratio between the so-called input duct head and the input duct length. The valve head is the height that the fluid propagating into the valve would reach if pushed by valve maximum pressure upwards against gravity. This is a particular case of a more general definition of hydraulic head and we will again encounter this concept in Section 8.3 dealing with micropumps.

The simplest way of fabricating a control valve is to fabricate a membrane interposed across a vertical part of the microfluidic duct, as shown in Figure 8.1. The fluid goes up into the short vertical part of the duct due to both external pressure and capillarity, when it arrives at the membrane, the overall pressure has to be sufficient to open the membrane if the flux goes in the right direction, while a flux in the opposite direction cannot open the membrane due to its position. The valve can be completely realized in silicon that is passivized with a very thin silica layer of thermal oxide after the system fabrication.

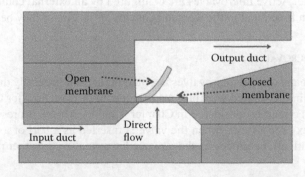

FIGURE 8.1 Vertical section of a control valve realized with an MEMs membrane on silicon.

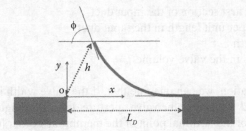

FIGURE 8.2 Geometrical parameters and reference system for the evaluation of the valve characteristics.

In order to carry out a performance analysis of such a valve, let us consider the reference system and the geometrical characteristics of the valve that are reported in Figure 8.2. The valve is generally closed due to the elastic force that is generated when the membrane is deformed. This is the force the fluid coming from the direct direction has to win to open the valve. Since we are dealing with a liquid, we can assume that pressure is distributed along all the directions in the same way so that the liquid operates at a uniform pressure on the membrane surface independently from the membrane shape.

Calculating the deformation of a membrane undergoing such a pressure is a well-known problem of elasticity theory [6]: the membrane uniformly deforms, assuming a shape described by the following formula on the x–y plane as represented in Figure 8.2:

$$y = \frac{\delta p\, d\, L^2}{24 \mathcal{E} J}\left[\left(\frac{x}{L}\right)^4 - 4\left(\frac{x}{L}\right) + 3\right] \tag{8.3}$$

where

δp is the applied pressure
d is the membrane width
L is the membrane length at rest along the x axis
$\mathcal{E}$ is the Young's modulus of the material
J is the membrane normalized inertia momentum $J = I/L^2$, where I is the inertia momentum of the structure

The pressure exerted by the fluid on the membrane is simply evaluated by starting from the initial duct section A_0, where we imagine that we have a Poiseuille flow, and the section of the membrane when it is closed, that is, $A_M = L_M d$; moreover, a pressure drop due to the ascending part of the duct has to be considered, that in a first approximation, neglecting hydraulic losses, can be written as $p_L = \rho L d H$, where H is the vertical displacement between the axis of the input duct and the membrane when at rest. When the valve is open, the pressure across the valve is the sum of two components: a component causing the fluid motion Δp and a component maintaining the valve open. This pressure is obtained from the incoming fluid so that we can write a pressure balance as

$$p_{valve} = \Delta p + \delta p = \left(p_{in} - \frac{\partial p}{\partial x} L_D\right)\frac{A_0}{L_M d} - \rho L_M d H - p_{loss} \tag{8.4}$$

where

p_{valve} is the overall pressure on the open valve area
δp is the pressure that makes the valve open
Δp is the pressure causing liquid motion through the valve

p_{in} is the pressure at the first section of the input duct
$\partial p/\partial x$ is the prevalence per unit length in the input duct
L_D is the input duct length
p_{loss} is the hydraulic loss in the valve volume

In a very first approximation, we can imagine that, if the valve width is d, the valve aperture is a rectangle with sides h and d, where h is the valve aperture defined in Figure 8.2. The valve aperture is obtained as the ordinate of the terminal point of the membrane border [6] so that, considering that the membrane is in elastic regime

$$h \approx \frac{\delta p L_M^4}{8 \mathcal{E} J} \tag{8.5}$$

As expected, the valve aperture is proportional to the applied pressure. Since we are considering a membrane of pure crystal silicon, it is quite elastic. Nevertheless, beyond a maximum value of the curvature angle ϕ defined in Figure 8.2, the membrane breaks.

We can evaluate the angle formed by the deformed membrane to be extreme with the horizontal plane using the elastic theory obtaining

$$\phi = \frac{4h}{3L_M} \tag{8.6}$$

so that a maximum valve aperture corresponds to the maximum curvature angle, which increases with increasing length of the membrane border.

To provide an estimate of the valve capacity, let us imagine that the liquid flow rate through the valve aperture is given by the Poiseuille-like equation. The pressure causing the motion that has to be inserted in the expression of the flow rate can be derived from Equation 8.4; thus, we can write for the valve capacity

$$Q_l(\Delta p) = \frac{\pi}{8\eta} \frac{\Delta p}{L} R = \frac{\pi}{8\eta} \frac{\Delta p}{L} \left(\frac{hd}{h+d} \right) \tag{8.7}$$

where we have indicated the hydraulic radius as R and the characteristic length of the fluid flow through the valve as L. We can introduce a maximum value of the applicable pressure as

$$\delta p_{Max} = \frac{6 \mathcal{E} J \phi_{Max}}{L_M^3} \tag{8.9}$$

so that the valve capacity changing the overall pressure on the valve can be written as

$$C_V = \frac{\pi}{8\eta} \frac{p_{valve} - \delta p_{Max}}{\sqrt{p_{valve}}} \left(\frac{\dfrac{h_{Max}}{d}}{\dfrac{h_{Max}}{d} + 1} \right) \sqrt{\frac{\rho g}{L}} \tag{8.10}$$

The result is shown in Figure 8.3 using the parameters of Table 8.1 that are evaluated for (1, 0, 0) silicon. Different curves are provided, corresponding to different values of the maximum angle

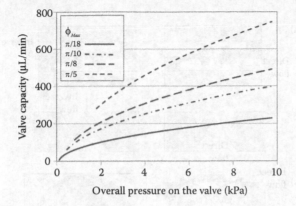

FIGURE 8.3 Control valve aperture for the valve shown in Figure 8.1 versus the aperture pressure δp. The system parameters are listed in Table 8.1.

ϕ_{Max}, due to the fact that ϕ_{Max} depends critically both on the passivation and on the technology process. Increasing the maximum angle, since the maximum pressure increases, a greater pressure is needed to open the valve at maximum opening. However, when the valve is completely open, the capacity grows more rapidly if the maximum angle is greater due to the greater openings of the valve.

Besides the valve that is shown in Figure 8.1, several other structures have been proposed for control valves [1]. A few of them are shown in section in Figure 8.4, but for the valve represented in Figure 8.4c where the top view of the valve is also needed to fully understand its architecture.

8.2.2 ACTIVE MICROVALVES

Differently from control microvalves, active microvalves are designed to assume a wanted configuration depending on a control signal. They can be divided into classes based on different properties.

An active valve is called normally closed if it is closed in the absence of a driving signal, and normally open if in that condition it is open or latching (sometimes also bistable) if, in the absence of driving signal, it remains in the last selected position, whatever it was. Latching microvalves are important in selected applications, where the system reliability requires that the current system configuration is maintained if the power goes off due to a failure of the power-feeding circuit.

An active valve is called switchable if it can be switched between two well-defined configurations that generally are closed and open. Differently, if the valve can assume a continuous set of

TABLE 8.1
Parameters for the Evaluation of the Performances of the Control Valve Sketched in Figure 8.1

Membrane length	L	40 μm
Membrane width	d	40 μm
Membrane thickness	w	2 μm
Valve flow characteristic length	L	
Young's modulus (bulk—100 plane)	$\mathcal{E}$	168 GPa
Inertia momentum (bulk)	J	26.6 μm⁴

Note: Material parameters are relative to silicon along (1, 0, 0) crystal orientation.

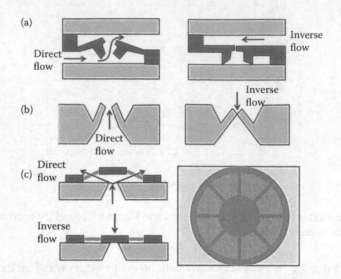

FIGURE 8.4 Different structures for control valves.

position so as to continuously regulate the duct section and the flow rate, it is said to be proportional. In this case, the valve driver has to produce an analog driving signal and has to be suitably biased to obtain the wanted effect.

In the case of active microvalves, the leakage and the capacity are defined as in the case of control microvalves, but in a slightly different manner. The leakage in particular is defined as the ratio between the flow rate traversing the valve when it is open and spurious flow rate that is present when the valve is closed. The capacity conversely is defined as the normalized maximum flow through the valve that corresponds to a given control signal.

Since active valves respond to a control signal, they have to be driven by an actuator, that is, a system converting the control signal in a suitable change of the valve configuration. All actuators have to be designed so as to assure a response time sufficient for the application, the capability to provide a reproducible behavior when used several times and a small required energy. Actuators used in proportional valves have more rigid requirements since they do not have to switch between two fixed positions, valve closed and open, but they have to be positioned on the ground of an analog driving signal in a position that corresponds to the wanted flow through the channel. Moreover, they have to be designed so as to maintain this position in time. Different actuators are characterized by different ranges of possible maximum pressure applied to the valve and response time to the command signal. Each actuator is also characterized by a minimum energy that is required to change the configuration. A qualitative actuator characterization under these points of view is provided in Table 8.2.

In general, it is possible to couple different types of actuators with several possible valve design, a few of them in common with control valves, thus obtaining a large number of active valves.

8.2.2.1 Electrostatic and Electromagnetic Microvalves

The basic scheme of a normally closed electrostatic actuated valve is reported in Figure 8.5a. The valve is essentially constituted by a duct that is interrupted by two vertical elements sustained by a membrane. The membrane deformation that opens the valve is obtained by creating a plane plate capacitor where one electrode is the membrane itself and the other is the ceiling of a chamber excavated above the duct. When an electrostatic tension is applied, the upper electrode and the membrane are charged with opposite signs and the membrane deforms so as to lift the vertical elements and to open the duct.

TABLE 8.2
Qualitative Characterization of Different Actuation Technologies for Active Microvalves

	Maximum Pressure (kPa)	Response Time (s)	Operational Energy (J/m³)
Electromagnetic	0.1–100	10^{-4}–10^{-3}	—
Disk piezoelectric	0.1–100	10^{-4}–10^{-3}	10^7
Electrostatic	0.1–100	10^{-5}	10^2–10^3
Electrochemical	0.1–100	1–10	10^2–10^4
Chemical	10–100	1–10	10^3
Pneumatic	10^2–10^3	1–10	10^6
Thermopneumatic	10^2–10^4	10^{-3}–1	10^6
Shape memory alloy	10^2–10^4	10^{-3}–0.1	10^7
Thermomechanic	10^2–10^4	10^{-3}–0.1	10^7
Stack piezoelectric	0.1–100	10^4–10^5	10^7

Source: Data from Meng E., *Biomedical Microsystems*, CRC Press; 1st edition (September 29, 2010), ISBN-13: 978-1420051223; Nguyen N.-T., Wereley S. T., *Fundamental and Applications of Microfluidics*, Artech House; 2nd edition (May 30, 2006), ISBN-13: 978-1580539722; Au A. K. et al., *Micromachines*, vol. 2, pp. 179–220, 2011; Oh K. W., Ahn C. H., *Journal of Micromechanics and Microengineering*, vol. 16, pp. R13–R39, 2006.

The first step to analyze such an actuator is to set up a model that allows us to evaluate the main actuators parameters. Since we are always in linear deformation regime, we can consider the model that is shown in Figure 8.5b [8]. The elastic characteristics and the shape of the deformable membrane are contained in the equivalent elastic constant, which has to be calculated starting from a structural analysis of the membrane itself. In particular, if we consider a circular membrane subject to a distributed uniform pressure due to the capacitor electrical field, the structure analysis of the system [6,7] results in an expression of the equivalent membrane elastic constant equal to

$$k = \frac{16\pi \mathcal{E} d_M^3}{3R^2(1-\nu^2)} \tag{8.11}$$

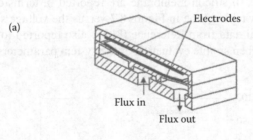

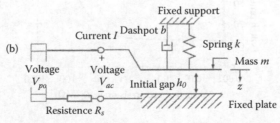

FIGURE 8.5 Example of an active valve with an electrostatic actuator (a) and discrete constant equivalent model for the actuator (b).

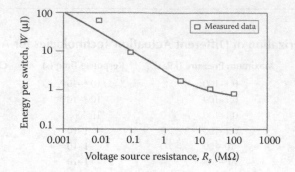

FIGURE 8.6 Switch energy in an electrostatic actuated valve based on a (1, 0, 0) silicon membrane versus the voltage source resistance. (With kind permission from Springer Science+Business Media: *Theory of Elasticity*, 2010, Maceri A.)

where R is the membrane radius, d_M the membrane thickness, and ν the Poisson ratio, which is the derivative of transverse strain versus the corresponding axial strain. If we substitute data for (1, 0, 0) silicon, we obtain $k = 3.01 \times 10^{12}(d_M^3/R^2)$, where d_M and R are measured in meters and k in N/m.

The equivalent circuit of Figure 8.5b allows us a complete analysis of the actuator once the values of the circuit parameters are correctly determined. In particular, since under an electrical point of view it is an RC-type circuit, the response time and the energy stored in the circuit when the membrane is open can be evaluated. As far as the energy is concerned, it can be readily evaluated by the capacitor formula obtaining

$$W = \frac{1}{2}\boldsymbol{D} \cdot \boldsymbol{E} \tag{8.12}$$

that in case of a plane plate capacitor with a homogeneous and isotropic dielectric medium and neglecting borders effects becomes simply $W = (\varepsilon/2)(V_{ac}^2/L_c^2)$, L_c being the distance between the capacitor plates and ε the dielectric constant of the capacitor medium. Results of the model from Figure 8.5b assuming a (1, 0, 0) silicon membrane are reported in terms of switching energy in Figure 8.6 and in terms of switching time in Figure 8.7 versus the voltage source resistance R_s. In both the figures, experimental data from Reference [8] are also reported to demonstrate the good behavior of the model even when simple evaluation of the system parameters is carried out.

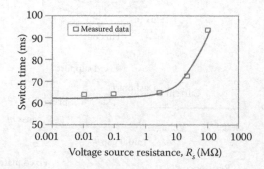

FIGURE 8.7 Switch time in an electrostatic actuated valve based on a (1, 0, 0) silicon membrane versus the voltage source resistance. (With kind permission from Springer Science+Business Media: *Theory of Elasticity*, 2010, Maceri A.)

(a)

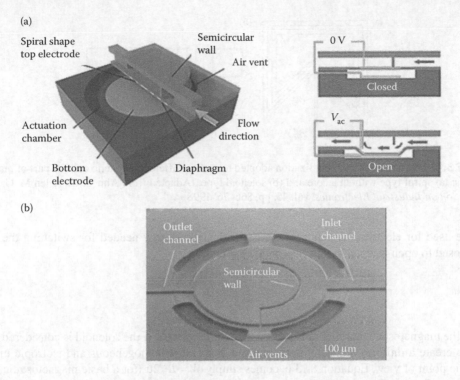

Spiral shape
top electrode

Semicircular
wall

Air vent

0 V

Closed

Actuation
chamber

Flow
direction

V_{ac}

Open

Bottom
electrode

Diaphragm

(b)

Outlet
channel

Inlet
channel

Semicircular
wall

Air vents   100 µm

FIGURE 8.8 Structure of a normally closed electrostatic valve based on the lift of a channel obstruction via a circular microcapacitor (a); scanning electronic microscope photos of the realized valve (b). (Reproduced from *Sensors and Actuators A: Physical*, vol. 83, Castañera L. et al., Pull-in time–energy product of electrostatic actuators: Comparison of experiments with simulation, pp. 263–269, Copyright 2000, with permission from Elsevier.)

Besides the simple structure of Figure 8.5, several different microvalve structures can be driven by electrostatic actuators. An example is given by the valve that was realized in Reference [9], whose scheme is reported in Figure 8.8a while a scanning electron microscope photo of the fabricated valve is reported in Figure 8.8b. Examples of fabricated microvalves based on the electrostatic actuation are reported in several research and engineering works. A large bibliography is reported in the reviews [3–5] while recent examples are References [10–12].

Besides electrostatic field, a magnetostatic field can also be used to activate microvalves [3,4,13]. This can be obtained for example, in the case of a normally closed valve, by building a magnetic core inside a solenoid over the membrane to be lift to open the channel. The principle scheme of such a valve is shown in Figure 8.9. The modeling of the actuator can be done using methods similar

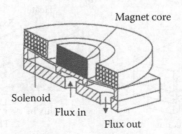

Magnet core

Solenoid

Flux in

Flux out

FIGURE 8.9 Principle scheme of a membrane valve with a magnetic actuator.

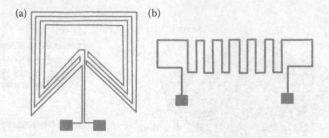

FIGURE 8.10 Structure of the metallization adopted to realize different magnetic coils as part of magnetic actuators: (a) spiral type without a core and (b) solenoid type. (Adapted from Ahn C. H., Allen M. G., IEEE *Transaction on Industrial Electronics*, vol. 45, pp. 866–76, 1998.)

to those used for electrostatic actuators. In particular, the energy needed for switching the valve from closed to open is given in this case by the expression

$$W = \frac{1}{2} \boldsymbol{B} \cdot \boldsymbol{H} \qquad (8.13)$$

that is, the magnetostatic parallel of Equation 8.12. In particular, if the solenoid is considered ideal, so as to create a uniform magnetic field, and the material is homogeneous and isotropic under a magnetic point of view, Equation 8.13 becomes simply $W = B^2/2\mu$ (for a basic magnetostatic introduction, see Section 7.6.1).

A critical point in building a magnetostatic actuator is the fabrication of the magnetic coil. Several techniques have been developed for planar integration of such components, whose detailed analysis is beyond the scope of this chapter [13,14]. An idea of a few structures that have been considered and fabricated is given in Figure 8.10, where the SEM photographs of different structures of planar integrated solenoids are reported from Reference [14]. Many examples of fabricated electromagnetic microvalves are reported in the reviews [3–5].

8.2.2.2 Pneumatic and Thermopneumatic Microvalves

Beside an electromagnetic force, the mechanical pressure caused by an expanding material can also close a normally open membrane valve, as shown in Figure 8.11a. In this case, a working fluid, either a gas or a liquid, is present in a chamber on top of the membrane to be deformed to close the valve. When the working fluid pressure is normal, the membrane is at rest, lifting the duct stopper so that the valve is open. When an external pressure operates on the fluid, it compresses the membrane that deforms and closes the valves. Considering the pressures constant all around the different surfaces, if we call A_{ac} the surface of the duct conducting the external pressure inside the actuator chamber

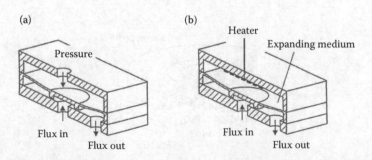

FIGURE 8.11 Pneumatic (a) and thermopneumatic (b) actuated membrane-based valve schemes.

and R the circular membrane radius, the pressure needed to activate the valve p_{ac} can be obtained by the force balance for the displacement d of the membrane center that is needed to close the valve. Indicating the inner pressure at rest with p_{in} and the chamber lower area with A_{in}, it is obtained

$$p_{ac} = p_{in} \frac{A_{in}}{A_{ac}} + k \frac{d}{\pi R^2} \qquad (8.14)$$

As an example, let us consider a membrane 1 μm thick with a radius of 300 μm fabricated using (1, 0, 0) silicon and accommodated in a square chamber with a side of 800 μm. The regulated duct height is 30 μm while the input opening of the membrane chamber used to convey the external pressure is circular with a radius of 300 μm. The equivalent elastic constant of the membrane is 2.11×10^6 N/m, while $p_{in} = 1$ atm $= 101.3$ kPa. The pressure that is needed to operate the valve is thus $p_{in} = 258$ kPa $= 2.5$ atm.

It is not difficult to understand that the pressure needed to operate the pneumatic valve increases if the valve gets smaller. This makes unsuitable the greater part of pumps compatible with microfluidic circuits to feed such valves so that the pressure source has to be frequently external. Having an external pressure source can be a problem in disposable systems due to the need of creating a good pressure interface between an external pump and the chip package that is plugged into the external device. For these reasons, thermopneumatic actuators are more frequently adopted for microvalves used in labs on chip.

The principle scheme of a membrane-based thermoactuated valve is presented in Figure 8.11b. The general principle is the same with respect to a simple pneumatic valve, but the pressure is operated on the membrane, not directly from an outside pump, but through the heating of a suitable material that is present inside the membrane chamber. In order to obtain this effect, a heater has to be constructed on top of the membrane change and driven by the valve driver.

Gas, liquid, and solid can all be used as working materials in a thermopneumatic valve. For example, if a gas is used, the pressure caused by an increase in temperature can be evaluated by using the gas constitutive law. Let us consider the valve sketched in Figure 8.11b. If the maximum membrane deformation is equal to d, the volume of the membrane chamber passes from $V_0 = A_{in}$ when the valve is at rest to $V = V_0 + \pi (R - R_d)^2 d$ when the valve is closed, where the so-called death radius R_d can be estimated by the structural analysis of the membrane deformation [6,7] and d_{ro} is the height of the membrane room. The pressure p_{in} operated on the membrane when the gas is heated at temperature T is then given by

$$T = \frac{(p_{ac} - p_{in})V_0 + \pi d(R - R_d)^2 p_{in}}{N_{Av} \kappa_B} \frac{V_M}{V_0} - T_0 \qquad (8.15)$$

where T_0 is the room temperature, N_{Av} is the Avogadro number, and V_M is the molar volume at standard conditions of the considered gas. If we consider a valve with the parameters of the previous example, we have to reach an operating pressure of 258 kPa. Imagining to use air as operating gas, setting $d_{ro} = 30$ μm and estimating $R_d \approx 10$ μm, since the molecular volume of an ideal gas at standard conditions is 24.5 m³/mole, we have $T \approx 336°C$, which is not a practical temperature to operate a similar valve.

It is possible to use materials that exert a greater pressure with respect to a perfect gas, but the best way to optimize the working of a thermopneumatic valve is to exploit the great change of volume happening when a system undergoes a state change. In this way, a smaller temperature increase causes much larger pressures on the membrane, rendering this kind of valve very useful for several applications.

The actuation material of the thermopneumatic valve can be gas, liquid, or solid. Owing to the large change in specific volume of the phase transition, thermopneumatic actuators can utilize the solid/liquid and liquid/gas phase change to obtain the maximum performance [15]. Figure 8.12

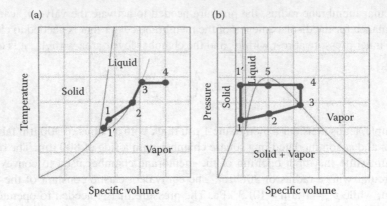

FIGURE 8.12 Example of thermodynamic cycle of a thermopneumatic valve using a liquid as working fluid both in the volume/temperature (V, T) (a) and in the volume/pressure (V, p) (b) thermodynamic planes.

represents the typical thermodynamic states of a thermopneumatic valve with a liquid as the initial actuating material [2,3]. The volume V and mass m determine the specific volume v and the density ρ of the working material in the actuation chamber. Considering that since the membrane chamber is sealed, the mass of the working material is constant. The state of the valve working process can be represented on the phase diagram of the working material as follows (see Figure 8.12):

Expansion in the liquid region (process 1′–1): In the initial state, the fluid in the actuator chamber is in the liquid phase. With the increasing temperature caused by the heater, the volume expands with an amount ΔV that is given by [15]

$$\Delta V = V_0 \gamma_f (T_2 - T_1) \tag{8.16}$$

where V_0 is the initial fill volume at temperature T_1, γ_f is the thermal expansion coefficient of the liquid, and T_2 is the operating temperature of the actuator. If in this state the valve membrane already closes the valve inlet and the specific volume remains constant, the pressure and temperature increase as a result. Based on the specific volume obtained by the valve geometry and the known operating temperature, the pressure inside the actuator chamber can be determined from the properties of compressed liquids.

Expansion in the liquid–vapor mixture region (process 1–2–3): If there is enough space inside the chamber, the fluid transforms into the liquid–vapor phase. If the valve is closed in this state, temperature and pressure increase as a result of the heat transfer. Because the pressure increases with temperature in state 3, keeping the temperature constant can close the valve with a constant pressure. In this state, the dryness fraction χ or the mass percentage of the vapor phase can be determined from the overall specific volume v and the specific volumes of saturated liquid v_f and saturated vapor v_g so that [15]

$$\chi = \frac{v - v_f}{v_g - v_f} \tag{8.17}$$

Expansion in the superheated vapor region (process 3–4): If the heat transfer continues, the fluid can jump from the liquid–vapor mixture region into the superheated vapor region. In this state, the generated pressure p in the actuator chamber can be evaluated by assuming the superheated vapor as a perfect gas and writing

$$p = p_0 \, e^{-\frac{\Theta_{ev}}{N_{av} \kappa_B T}} \tag{8.18}$$

where Θ_{ev} is the evaporation latent heat and p_0 the pressure at the entrance point of the cycle in the superheated vapor region.

To understand the potentiality of thermopneumatic valves, let us consider the valve we have analyzed at the beginning of this section. In order not to need an external pressure source, let us imagine that a thermopneumatic actuator is fabricated on top of the valve membrane and that liquid water is used inside the membrane chamber as working fluid. The valve is operated with the thermodynamic cycle of Figure 8.12.

In the first phase, water is heated from room temperature at 25°C to 100°C so as to enter into the liquid vapor equilibrium state at atmospheric pressure. The volume dilation is negligible, but when transition into the superheated gas region happens, the specific volume passes from $v_f = 0.001$ m^3/kg that is typical of liquid water up to about $v_g = 1.3$ m^3/kg, which is typical of superheated water vapor following the thermodynamic transformation.

Since the number of moles that are present in the membrane room does not change the pressure operated by the vapor when the transformation exits from the mixed zone at a temperature of 120°C is 200 kPa (as shown by looking at the phase diagram of water reported in Figure 8.13). At this point, the further temperature increase that is needed to reach the required activation pressure of 257 kPa can be evaluated using the perfect gas equation and taking into account that the transformation in the vapor zone is performed at constant volume. It is obtained that the final temperature of the state 4 is equal to 180°C, compared with the temperature of 336°C that would be needed if the working material would be a gas.

The scanning electronic microscope's photographs of two levels of a fabricated thermopneumatic valve [16] are presented in Figure 8.14. The valve has almost exactly the structure of Figure 8.11b and due to the use of tin-doped indium oxide (ITO) heaters, the valve can function reliably like a proportional valve with a characteristic time from open to close states or vice versa of the order of 20 s. The reaction time in the order of a few tens of second is characteristic of thermopneumatic valves due to both the slow pace of thermal processes and the dimensions that these valves generally have. Thus, they are not suited for fast response systems, while they are quite usable in case of systems where the overall wanted response time is of the order of 1 min. Numerous examples of fabricated thermopneumatic valves are reported in References [3–5].

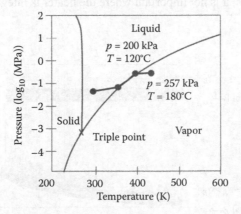

FIGURE 8.13 State diagram of water with the transformation relative to the thermopneumatic valve considered in the example of Section 8.2.2.2.

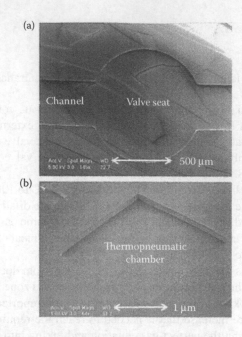

FIGURE 8.14 Scanning electronic microscope photos of a thermopneumatic valve: (a) duct and valve seat layer and (b) membrane chamber (called thermopneumatic chamber) before covering via bonding. (Reproduced from *Microelectronic Engineering*, vol. 73–74, Kim J. O. et al., A disposable thermopneumatic-actuated microvalve stacked with PDMS layers and ITO-coated glass, pp. 864–869, Copyright 2004, with permission from Elsevier.)

8.2.2.3 Thermomechanical Microvalves

The first types of thermomechanical actuated microvalves are those based on bimetallic actuators. Bimetallic actuation uses the difference in thermal coefficient of expansion of two bonded solids. This principle is often called thermal bimorph actuation [17,18]. As a matter of fact, when a structure composed of the superposition of two different metal thin layers is heated, it bends in the direction of the metal with the higher expansion coefficient as shown in Figure 8.15. The heater is usually integrated between the two solid materials or on one side of the bimorph. Because most bimorph structures are thin membranes, the temperature gradient along their thickness can be assumed to be zero. Thus, it is not important where the heater is integrated. Bimetallic actuators

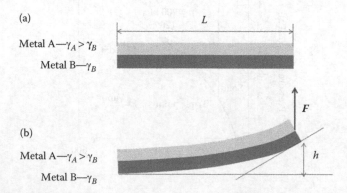

FIGURE 8.15 Scheme and definition of the main parameters of a thermal bimorph actuator: (a) rest configuration and (b) deformed configuration.

offer an almost linear deflection dependence on heating power. Their disadvantages are high power consumption and slow response typical of all thermal processes. Since a bimetallic actuator is able to bend a membrane as it was a large beam, it can be used to activate a flexible membrane valve like that shown in Figure 8.1.

The bimetallic actuator acts as if under the action of a bending force F whose value, for small deformations, depends linearly on the temperature difference from the steady state ΔT and on the difference between the two thermal expansion coefficients γ_A and γ_B as

$$F = F_0 \ (\gamma_A - \gamma_B)\Delta T \, \vartheta \tag{8.19}$$

where F_0 is constant with respect to temperature and the expansion coefficients and ϑ is the unit vector orthogonal to the plane of the actuator, which is parallel to the direction in which the actuator dimension is smaller.

Figure 8.15 shows that, for small deformations, the ordinate of the extreme point of the actuator h can be expressed as a function of the curvature radius R_c of the beam as

$$h \approx \frac{L^2}{2R_c} = \frac{L^2}{2}\kappa \tag{8.20}$$

where κ is the beam curvature.

The elastic analysis of the system beyond this simple conclusion is complicated by the fact that the two metals have different elastic and geometric parameters. The final result is that, assuming layers with the same width, that is reasonable since they form the closure plate of a valve, the beam curvature κ can be expressed as [19]

$$\kappa = \frac{6}{\delta_A + \delta_B} \frac{(\delta_B \mathcal{E}_B + \delta_A \mathcal{E}_A)}{3 \frac{\mathcal{E}_B}{\delta_B}(\delta_A + \delta_B)^2 + (\delta_B \mathcal{E}_B + \delta_A \mathcal{E}_A)\left[\left(\frac{\delta_A}{\delta_B}\right)^2 + \frac{\delta_A \mathcal{E}_A}{\delta_B \mathcal{E}_B}\right]}(\gamma_A - \gamma_B)\Delta T \tag{8.21}$$

where
δ_A, δ_B are the thicknesses of layers A and B, respectively
$\mathcal{E}_A, \mathcal{E}_B$ are the Young's modulus of layers A and B, respectively

In the regime of small deformation, the curvature is expected to be proportional to the bending force, as confirmed by the factor $(\gamma_A - \gamma_B)\Delta T$ appearing in Equation 8.21. As a matter of fact, the force intensity can be expressed as

$$F = \frac{3b}{4L} \frac{\delta_A + \delta_B}{\left(\dfrac{1}{\delta_A \mathcal{E}_A}\right) + \left(\dfrac{1}{\delta_B \mathcal{E}_B}\right)}(\gamma_A - \gamma_B)\Delta T \tag{8.22}$$

where b is the common width of the two layers.

An example of valve with a thermomechanical actuator is provided by a normally closed valve with the structure of Figure 8.16. Each of the radii sustaining the central membrane is constituted by a thermal bimorph actuator so that, when current flows through the actuators and they heat due to the Joule effect, the actuator deformation causes the valve opening.

Other types of thermomechanical actuators are simply based on the thermal expansion of a single metal [2] when current passes through a beam. In this case, the equivalent bending force is

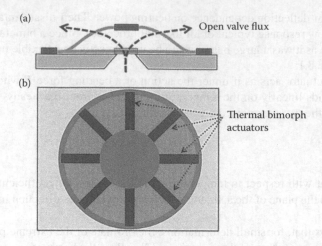

FIGURE 8.16 Example of the structure of a normally closed microvalve using thermal bimorph actuators; side view with open and closed configurations (a) and top view evidencing the actuators (b).

proportional to the product of a simple expansion coefficient and the temperature difference caused by the current flow, that is

$$F = F_0 \gamma \Delta T \vartheta \tag{8.23}$$

where F_0 is constant with respect to the temperature and the expansion coefficients and ϑ is the unit vector orthogonal to the plane of the actuator. Even if apparently the equivalent force can be higher in the case of a single metal, this type of actuators is not frequently used due to the great difficulty in designing effective electrodes and in controlling the dilation phenomenon. In Table 8.3, the thermal parameters used to design thermomechanical valves are listed for different materials.

TABLE 8.3
Thermal Parameters for Different Materials Used for Thermomechanical Microvalves

Material	Density (kg/m³)	Heat Capacity J/(kg K)	Conductivity W/(m K)	Thermal Expansion Coefficient 1/K × 10⁻⁶
Silicon	2330	710	156	2.3
Silicon oxide	2660	750	1.2	0.3
Silicon nitride	3100	750	19	2.8
Aluminum	2700	920	230	23
Copper	8900	390	390	17
Gold	19,300	125	314	15
Nickel	8900	450	70	14
Chrome	6900	440	95	6.6
Platinum	21,500	133	70	9
Parylene N	1110	837.4	0.12	69
Parylene C	1290	711.8	0.082	35
Parylene D	1418	—	—	30–80

Source: Data from Nguyen N.-T., Wereley S. T., *Fundamental and Applications of Microfluidics*, Artech House; 2nd edition (May 30, 2006), ISBN-13: 978-1580539722.

8.2.2.4 Shape Memory Alloy Microvalves

Shape memory alloy (SMA) microvalves are based on the specific properties of SMA materials [20,21] that render them suitable to be used as working materials in several types of both micro- and macroactuators. SMAs are metal alloys that exhibit two very unique properties, pseudoelasticity and the shape memory effect.

Shape memory is the effect of restoring the original shape of a plastically deformed sample by heating it. This phenomenon results from a crystalline phase change known as *thermoelastic–martensitic transformation*. At temperatures below the transformation temperature, SMAs are martensitic. In this condition, their microstructure is characterized by *self-accommodating twins*. The martensite is soft and can be deformed quite easily by detwinning. Heating above the transformation temperature recovers the original shape and converts the material to its high-strength austenitic state. An example of austenic and martensic crystal structure for a particular SMA is shown in Figure 8.17 while a graphical illustration of the martensic–austenic effect is reported in Figure 8.18 where the microscopic structure of a deformed martensite is compared with that of the nondeformed martensite and austenite. The similarity between stressed martensite and stressed austenite for a specific induced stress somehow justifies the fact that the martensic–austenic transition can also be induced by stress under specific conditions.

The transformation from austenite to martensite and the reverse transformation from martensite to austenite do not take place at the same temperature. A plot of the volume fraction of martensite as a function of temperature provides a curve of the type shown schematically in Figure 8.19. The complete transformation cycle is characterized by the following temperatures: austenite start temperature (T_{As}), austenite finish temperature (T_{Af}), martensite temperature (T_{Ms}), and martensite finish temperature (T_{Mf}).

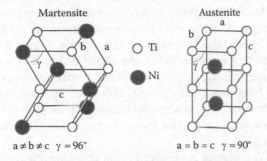

Martensite
b a
γ
c
a ≠ b ≠ c γ ≈ 96°

Austenite
a
b
γ
c
a = b = c γ ≈ 90°

○ Ti
● Ni

FIGURE 8.17 Martensic and austenic crystal structure of NiTi evidencing the different order degree of the two crystal arrangements.

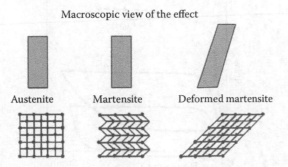

Macroscopic view of the effect

Austenite   Martensite   Deformed martensite

FIGURE 8.18 Qualitative explanation of shape memory effect based on the phase transition between martensic and austenic crystal structures.

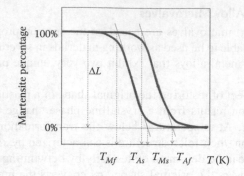

FIGURE 8.19 Percentage of martensic phase in a multiphase SMA versus temperature evidencing the relative hysteresis cycle. The extreme hysteresis temperatures are evidenced on the plot.

If a stress is applied to an SMA in the temperature range between T_{Af} and a maximum temperature T_{Md}, martensite can be stress-induced, as anticipated while discussing Figure 8.18. Less energy is needed to stress-induce and deform martensite than to deform the austenite by conventional mechanisms. Up to 10% strain can be accommodated by this process (single crystals of specific alloys can show as much as 25% pseudoplastic strain in certain directions). As austenite is the thermodynamically stable phase at this temperature, under no-load conditions, the material springs back into its original shape when the stress is no longer applied. This extraordinary elasticity is also called pseudoelasticity or transformational superelasticity. It becomes increasingly difficult to stress-induce martensite at increasing temperatures above T_{Af}. Eventually, it is easier to deform the material by conventional mechanisms than by inducing and deforming martensite. Above T_{Md}, the alloys undergo deformation like ordinary materials. Thus, superelasticity is only observed over a narrow temperature range.

The design of shape memory actuators is based on the distinctly different stress/strain curves of martensite and austenite, and their temperature dependence. Figure 8.20 shows tensile curves of a Ni–Ti alloy at various temperatures. While the austenitic curve ($T > T_{Md}$) looks like that of a normal material, the martensitic one ($T < T_{Mf}$) is quite unusual. On exceeding a first yield point, several percent strain can be accumulated with only little stress increase. After that, stress increases rapidly with further deformation. The deformation in the plateau region can be recovered thermally. Deformation exceeding a second yield point cannot be recovered. The material is then plastically deformed in a conventional way.

At temperatures $T > T_{Af}$, a plateau is observed again upon loading: in this case, it is caused by stress-induced martensite. Upon unloading, the material transforms back into austenite at a lower

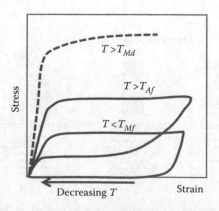

FIGURE 8.20 Typical temperature-dependent strain–stress plot of an SMA.

TABLE 8.4
Characteristics of Selected Shape Memory Alloys

Alloy	Composition	Transformation Temperature Range $(T_{Mf}; T_{Af})$ (°C)	Transformation Hysteresis $(T_{MF} - T_{As})$ (°C)
Ag–Cd	44/49 at.%Cd	(−190; −50)	15
Au–Cd	46.5/50 at.%Cd	(30; 100)	15
Cu–Al–Ni	14/14.5 wt.%Al, 3/4.5 wt.%Ni	(−140; 100)	35
Cu–Sn	≈ 15 at. %Sn	(−120; 30)	–
Cu–Zn	38.5/41.5 wt.%Zn	(−180; −10)	10
In–Ti	18/23 at.%Ti	(60; 100)	4
Ni–Al	36/38 at.%Al	(−180; 100)	10
Ni–Ti	49/51 at.%Ni	(−50; 110)	30
Mn–Cu	5/35 at.%Cu	(−250; −180)	25
Fe–Mn–Si	32 wt.% Mn 6 wt.%Si	(−200; 150)	100

Source: Data from Hodgson D. E., Wu M. H., Biermann R. J., *ASM Handbook, Volume 2: Properties and Selection: Nonferrous Alloys and Special-Purpose Materials*, ASM International; 10th edition (November 1, 1990), ISBN-13: 978-0871703781.

stress (unloading plateau). With increasing temperature, both loading and unloading plateau stress increase linearly. Characteristics of selected SMA that can be used in the design of SMA-based actuators for microvalves are reported in Table 8.4 [22]. In particular, an SMA actuator can be used to compress and release a membrane in a membrane based microvalve by changing its temperature. This is commonly done by using Joule effect generated by the current passage into the metal allot actuator.

A different type of microvalve that can be used to open or close flexible polymers microducts, such as those realized in PDMS, is shown in Figure 8.21 from Reference [23]. The microvalve actuator (Figure 8.21a) is an SMA piston realized by an SMA coil. When no current passes through the coil the SMA is in martensite state, while when current flows it transits in austenite state. The state change induces a rapid compression so as to retract the piston. The piston ends with a curved terminal protected by an SU8 termination.

The valve can be designed normally open if the terminal is positioned below the PDMS duct so as to compress and close it when it retracts; it is designed normally closed if at rest the terminal

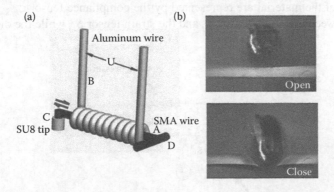

FIGURE 8.21 Principle of operation of a string-based SMA microvalve (a) and image before SU8 deposition of a close and opened valve configuration (b). (Reproduced from *Sensors and Actuators A: Physical*, vol. 168, Gui L., Ren C. L., Exploration and evaluation of embedded shape memory alloy (SMA) microvalves for high aspect ratio microchannels, pp. 155–161, Copyright 2011, with permission from Elsevier.)

compresses the duct and releases it when retracted. In order to avoid excessive stress accumulation in normally closed valves, the actuator can also be designed to push the wall of the duct against an internal obstacle when closed (see Reference [23]) and to release the wall when retracting so as to open the duct. A SEM photograph of the open and closed configuration of a normally open valve without the SU8 piston termination is shown in Figure 8.21b, where the underlying PDMS duct is 60 μm wide.

SMA actuators and related microvalves have attracted great research effort in the last few years; besides the many references reported in the reviews [3–5], recent achievements are reported in References [24–27].

8.2.2.5 Piezoelectric Microvalves

A piezoelectric substance is one that produces an electrostatic potential when a mechanical stress is applied, that is, the substance is squeezed or stretched. Conversely, a mechanical deformation is produced when an electric field is applied [28]. This effect is formed in crystals that have no electrical symmetry center for the charges distribution in the elementary cell. These crystals are said to have polar axes, which are crystal axes that cross the crystal cell so that the charge distribution along them creates a linear dipole.

Owing to the absence of a symmetry center, when stress produces a deformation of the periodic structure of the crystal along a polar axis, the charge equilibrium changes and a macroscopic dipole distribution is generated with the consequent generation of an electrical field. This effect is shown qualitatively in Figure 8.22 for an SiO_2 crystal (quartz) evidencing the polar axis in its tetrahedron structure that is generally used to compress the crystal and create the piezoelectric effect.

Conversely, an external electrical field acts on internal dipoles that are generally neutralized by their disposition in the unstrained structure by causing their alignment, with the consequent creation of a structural stress that expands or compresses the material bending if mechanical constrains are present.

The effect is reproducible and reversible, since the internal stress causes the microcrystals to return in a state of minimum energy corresponding to the initial state if the electrical field or the external stress is removed. Moreover, application of electrical fields with opposite directions causes opposite bending and application of opposite stresses causes opposite polarities.

Crystals that do not have a polar axis, such as NaCl, do not exhibit a piezoelectric effect. Conductors are never piezoelectric materials due to the fact that each dipole that is formed through a crystal lattice deformation is readily compensated by a change in the conduction electron population distribution, so that a macroscopic effect never arises.

Under a mathematical point of view, the piezoelectric effect creates a relationship between the mechanical and the electrostatic material constitutive equations. In a nonpiezoelectric material, the elastic properties of the material are represented by the compliance tensor $\sigma_{i,j,k,v}$ that establishes a linear relation between the stress tensor $\varsigma_{i,j}$ and the strain tensor $S_{i,j}$ while the dielectric properties

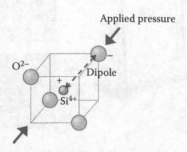

FIGURE 8.22 Elementary cell of the crystalline SiO_2 (quartz) and polar axis used to create the piezoelectric effect.

are represented by the dielectric constant tensor, relating the electrical displacement vector to the electrical field vector [28]. In the presence of a piezoelectric effect, a double cross dependence appears: strain-electrical field on one side and electrical displacement-stress on the other side. Thus the constitutive equations of the material appears as

$$S_{i,j} = \sigma_{i,j,k,v}\, \varsigma_{k,v} + d_{i,j,k}\, E_k \tag{8.24a}$$

$$D_i = \varepsilon_{i,j}\, E_j + d'_{i,j,k}\, \tau_{j,k} \tag{8.24b}$$

the tensors $d_{i,j,k}$ and $d'_{i,j,k}$ represents the piezoelectric effect in the case of application of an electrical field to generate a strain and of the application of a stress to generate an electrostatic displacement: they are called direct and inverse piezoelectric tensors. While expressions (8.24) are the most correct mathematical ways of expressing the constitutive equations of a piezoelectric material for small strains, generally, a different formalism is used exploiting the fact that only six elements of the stress and the strain tensor are different from zero since they are symmetric tensors [6,7]. Thus, equivalent six component stress and strain vectors are introduced by renumbering the tensor components as $11 \to 1; 22 \to 2; 33 \to 3; 23 \to 4; 13 \to 5; 12 \to 6$. As a consequence, the six elements of the compliance tensors that are different from zero can be renumbered accordingly to the new numeration of the stress and strain components. Finally, the piezoelectric tensors are rearranged as 6×3 and 3×6 matrixes. Equations 8.24 thus becomes

$$\hat{S}_\alpha = \hat{\sigma}_{\alpha,\beta}\, \hat{\varsigma}_\beta + \hat{d}_{\alpha,k}\, E_k \tag{8.25a}$$

$$D_i = \varepsilon_{i,j} E_j + \hat{d}'_{i,\beta}\, \hat{\tau}_\beta \tag{8.25b}$$

where the cap indicates reduced tensors and Greek indices run from 1 to 6. Such a relabeled notation is often called Voigt notation. For application in actuators for microvalves and other MEMs elements, the direct piezoelectric tensor is important since an electrical field is used to generate a material expansion or compression. If we set the z axis parallel to the direction of the electrical field and with opposite orientation (as shown in Figure 8.23), calculating from Equations 8.25 the strain components along the three axes directions, we get

$$\hat{S}_1 = \hat{S}_x = \hat{S}_y = \hat{d}_{3,1} E_3 \tag{8.26a}$$

$$\hat{S}_3 = \hat{S}_z = \hat{d}_{3,3} E_3 \tag{8.26b}$$

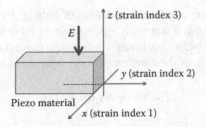

FIGURE 8.23 Reference system arrangement for the analysis of piezoelectric actuators.

TABLE 8.5
Characteristics of Selected Piezoelectric Materials Used in Valve Actuators

Material	$d_{3,1}$ (C/N $\times 10^{-12}$)	$d_{3,3}$ (C/N $\times 10^{-12}$)	Relative Dielectric Constant (ε_r)
Lead zirconate titanate (PZT)[a]	$-60 \div -270$	$380 \div 590$	1700
ZnO	-5	12.4	1400
Polyvinylidene difluoride (PVDF)[b]	$6 \div 10$	$13 \div 22$	12
BaTiO$_3$	78	190	1700
LiNbO$_3$[c]	-0.85	6	48.5 (average)

Source: Data form Nguyen N.-T., Wereley S. T., *Fundamental and Applications of Microfluidics*, Artech House; 2nd edition (May 30, 2006), ISBN-13: 978-1580539722.

[a] The PZT is an alloy with molecular formula Pb[Zr$_x$Ti$_{1-x}$]O$_3$ whose properties depend on the value of x.

[b] The exact properties depend on the polymeric form.

[c] The lithium–niobate dielectric constant varies sensibly (about 23%) with direction. The average value is reported to give an order of magnitude of dielectric characteristics.

where the strain in the x and y directions are assumed equal due to the homogeneity and macroscopic isotropy of the material. Thus, for our scope, only two elements of the direct piezoelectric tensor are needed to characterize the valve working material.

From now on, we will drop the cap from $\hat{d}_{3,1}$ and $\hat{d}_{3,3}$, calling them simply $d_{3,1}$ and $d_{3,3}$ as usual in the literature, but the nature of Equations 8.25 and 8.26 has always to be taken into account if they have to be combined with other electrostatic or mechanic elements. Piezoelectric characteristics of selected materials used for MEMs actuators are listed in Table 8.5.

Piezoelectric actuators generally generate small strain (usually less than 0.1%) and high stresses (several MPa). Therefore, they are suitable for applications that require large forces but small displacements.

Because of the large force and commercial availability, piezoelectric actuators were among the first to be used in microvalves. Since thin-film piezoelectric actuators do not deliver enough force for valve applications, all reported piezoelectric microvalves use external actuators, such as piezostacks, bimorph piezocantilevers, or bimorph piezodisks. Compared to a piezostack, bimorph piezocantilevers have the advantage of large displacements. The relatively small forces are not critical due to the small opening in microvalves. Figure 8.24 illustrates the use of a bimorph piezocantilever [2]. Several examples of fabricated piezoelectric microvalves from the literature are reported in References [3–5].

8.2.2.6 Electrochemical and Chemical Microvalves

Electrochemical microvalves are based on the creation of bubbles by water electrolysis. A possible scheme of a simple electrochemical normally open valve is reported in Figure 8.25. Voltage is applied to the two electrodes in order to generate an electrical current due to the ions that are present in the solution. The general form of the reaction of water hydrolysis is

$$2H_2O(l) \rightarrow 2H_2(g) + O_2(g) \tag{8.27}$$

However, this is the combined result of two reactions happening near the two electrodes: a reduction reaction takes place with electrons (e^-) from the cathode while an oxidation reaction occurs generating oxygen gas and giving electrons to the anode to complete the circuit.

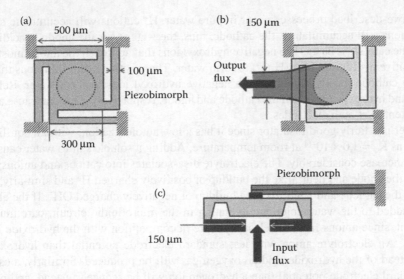

FIGURE 8.24 Example of a piezoelectric actuated valve: (a) top view of the membrane and valve sit layer; (b) top view of the output duct (the valve sit is above and represented in transparence); (c) side view.

The reactions can happen in the form balanced with acid as

$$2H^+(aq) + 2e^- \rightarrow H_2(g) \quad \text{(Cathode)} \tag{8.28a}$$

$$2H_2O(l) \rightarrow O_2(g) + 4H^+(aq) + 4e^- \quad \text{(Anode)} \tag{8.28b}$$

The same half reactions can also be balanced with base becoming

$$2H_2O(l) + 2e^- \rightarrow H_2(g) + 2OH^-(aq) \quad \text{(Cathode)} \tag{8.28c}$$

$$4OH^-(aq) \rightarrow O_2(g) + 2H_2O(l) + 4e^- \quad \text{(Anode)} \tag{8.28d}$$

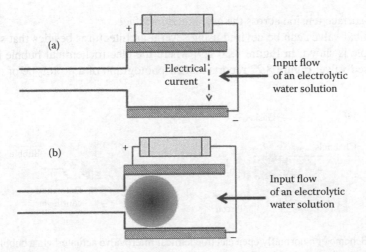

FIGURE 8.25 Working of an electrochemical microvalve: (a) valve open at rest and (b) valve closed by the electrolysis-generated gas bubble.

If the above-described processes occur in pure water, H⁺ cations will accumulate at the anode and OH⁻ anions will accumulate at the cathode; thus, the water near the anode is acidic while the water near the cathode is basic. The negative hydroxyl ions that approach the anode mostly combine with the positive hydronium ions (H_3O^+) to form water. The positive hydronium ions that approach the negative cathode mostly combine with negative hydroxyl ions to form water. Relatively few hydronium and hydroxyl ions reach the cathode and anode, respectively. This can cause a concentration over potential at both electrodes.

Pure water is a fairly good insulator since it has a low autoionization, with an equilibrium constant as low as $K_w = 1.0 \times 10^{-14}$ at room temperature. Adding a soluble salt to water causes the conductivity to increase considerably. The electrolyte disassociates into cations and anions; the anions rush toward the anode and neutralize the buildup of positively charged H⁺ and similarly, the cations rush toward the cathode and neutralize the buildup of negatively charged OH⁻. If the electrolyte is artificially added to the water solution circulating in the microfluidic circuit, care must be taken in choosing it, since anions from the electrolyte are in competition with the hydroxide ions to give up electrons. An electrolyte anion with less standard electrode potential than hydroxide will be oxidized instead of the hydroxide, and no oxygen gas will be produced. Similarly, a cation with a greater standard electrode potential than a hydrogen ion will be reduced instead, and no hydrogen gas will be produced. The following cations have lower electrode potential than H⁺ and are, therefore, suitable for use as electrolyte cations: Li^+, Rb^+, K^+, Cs^+, Ba^{2+}, Sr^{2+}, Ca^{2+}, Na^+, and Mg^{2+}. If ions are naturally present in the solution flowing in the circuit, they are generally ions suitable for electrolysis; for example, blood serum is rich in Na⁺ ions while containing also Ca^{2+}, and smaller quantities of other ions as Mg^{2+} and K⁺. Thus, water electrolysis happens in blood serum.

Once the gas bubble is formed and it is pushed toward the point where the duct section decreases, that in this case is the valve seat (see Figure 8.25), the valve pressure can be considered coincident with the surface pressure encountered traversing the bubble surface (see Section 7.3.5), since the fluid through the duct has to break the bubble surface to start to flow again. The pressure across the gas–liquid interface is given by Equation 7.122 that, assuming the bubble circular and with a radius equal to the radius of R_c the circle enclosed to the first duct section, can be approximately written as

$$p_{ac} = \frac{2\gamma_{lg}}{R_c} \tag{8.29}$$

where γ_{lg} is the surface tension across the gas–liquid interface.

Electrochemical valves can be devised using several architectures besides that shown in Figure 8.25. An example is shown in Figure 8.26 [29] where the electrochemical bubble is used to close a cantilever-based valve. Figure 8.27 reports a SEM photograph of a prototype of the valve whose

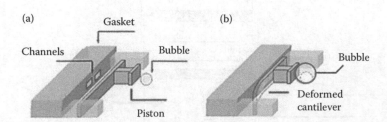

FIGURE 8.26 Scheme of a normally open electrochemical microvalve actuated via a bubble pushed cantilever: open valve (a) and closed valve (b). (Reproduced from *Sensors and Actuators B: Chemical*, vol. 155, Ezkerra A. et al., A microvalve for lab-on-a-chip applications based on electrochemically actuated SU8 cantilevers, pp. 505–511, Copyright 2011, with permission from Elsevier.)

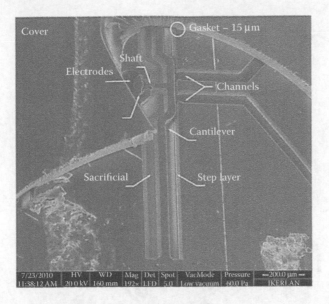

FIGURE 8.27 Scanning electron microscope photograph of a prototype of the valve described in Figure 8.26. (Reproduced from *Sensors and Actuators B: Chemical*, vol. 155, Ezkerra A. et al., A microvalve for lab-on-a-chip applications based on electrochemically actuated SU8 cantilevers, pp. 505–511, Copyright 2011, with permission from Elsevier.)

scheme is reported in Figure 8.26. Other types of architectures for electrochemical valves are reported in References [3–5].

We have, thus far, considered several ways to device active valves where the electrical current feeding the valve is transformed by an actuator in mechanical energy that either opens or closes the valve. In contrast, chemical actuators convert chemical energy into mechanical energy. Furthermore, the increasing use of polymers in the fabrication of microfluidic systems (see Chapter 3) is compatible with the integration of polymer-based chemical actuators. One of the major drawbacks of polymeric material in microfluidic systems is their swelling behavior. However, this behavior is attractive for actuator applications.

Hydrogels are polymers with high water content. Hydrogels can change their volume if changes in temperature, solvent concentration, and ionic strength are induced. The swelling behavior is controlled by water diffusion inside the polymeric matrix and thus is very slow in macroscopic equipment. In labs on chip, the response time to stimuli is drastically reduced due to the shorter diffusion path. Another advantage of this actuation scheme is that these polymers can be designed to suit conventional microfabrication technologies such as photolithography.

The mechanism causing hydrogel swelling due to water diffusion in the polymeric matrix can be explained by considering the simplest class of hydrogel polymers: those based on carboxyl acids. When a polymeric chain in water solution presents a carboxyl element, under suitable conditions, it can free a hydrogen ion so as to acquire a negative charge. The process arrives at equilibrium as shown in Figure 8.28a so that the polymer chain acquires an uneven charge distribution. The uneven positive charge in the polymeric chain creates a great number of polar bonds with the surrounding water molecules, as shown in Figure 8.28b, so as to produce a huge hydration of the polymer chain and the consequent swelling of the polymer. Penetration of water into the polymeric matrix can be attained by several methods:

- Simple water diffusion that is generally a slow phenomenon at standard temperature due to the difficulty of water molecules to penetrate into the polymeric matrix

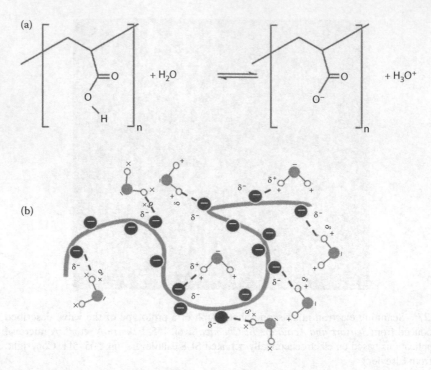

FIGURE 8.28 Hydrogel swelling effect: creation of negative charges along the chain for dissociation of carboxyl radicals (a) and water bond by polar bonding of water to the hydrogel chain (b).

- Change in solution pH that facilitates or thwarts the opening of the polymeric chains due to the electrostatic repulsion of charges along them
- Change of temperature that influences the value of the diffusion coefficient and the structure of the polymeric matrix
- Change in the concentration of the polymer molecules into the solution that renders more or less easy for water to penetrate into the gel

An example of hydrogel well adapted to the monolithic technologies used to fabricate labs on chip is PNIPAAm (poly-(*N*-isopropylacrylamide)) [30]. This polymer can be designed to have a compromise between film coating, UV polymerization, and working conditions at room temperatures. A hydrogel with a phase transition temperature T_{tr} of approximately 33°C that can be coated with a thickness of several tens of micrometers and cross-linked with conventional UV exposure is reported in Reference [31]. At room temperature below T_{tr}, the polymer is swollen. The polymer shrinks if the temperature increases above the transition temperature. Thus, together with a microheater, the hydrogel can be used as a thermomechanical actuator [31].

When a hydrogel sweep, due to the pH of the solution, it generally swells in alkali solution and shrinks in acidic solution. Examples of hydrogels that respond to changes in pH are polymethacrylic acid (PMAacid) tri-ethyleneglycol (pMAA-g-EG) [32], polyacrylic acid-2-hydroxymethylmethacrylate (pAA-2-HEMA) [33], and polyacrylamide-3-methaacrylamidophenylboronic acid (pAAm-3-MPBA) [34]. The transition region of pAA-2-HEMA and pMAA-g-EG is approximately 4 < pH < 7, while AAm-3-MPBA switches its volume at approximately 7 < pH < 9.

Hydrogel materials can be fabricated by either *in situ* photopolymerization [35] or *ex situ* polymerization techniques. Hydrogels fabricated *ex situ* require manual manipulation to incorporate them into devices, so that they can be used for research and small volume production, but cannot be adopted in high-volume production. *In situ* photopolymerization, which directly polymerizes the

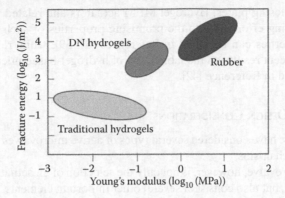

FIGURE 8.29 Relation between the energy needed to fracture a hydrogel using uniform pressure of one of its surfaces and the hydrogel Young's modulus for conventional and DN hydrogels compared with the same property of vulcanized rubber.

hydrogels inside microfluidic channels by liquid-phase photopolymerization, is much more suitable for the scope. Typically, a prepolymer solution consisting of monomer, cross-linker, and photoinitiator is flowed into the channel, and patterned by initiating polymerization via UV radiation through the mask.

A possible problem that can be encountered using hydrogels in very small structures such as microvalves is due to the brittle nature of these materials. If the material response time decreases greatly in a microstructure, the material tends to be fragile in these conditions. This problem can be solved by designing higher break energy materials specifically designed for this use. An example is provided by the so-called dense matrix (DM) polymers [36] that provide a resistance to fracture quite higher with respect to more traditional hydrogels, as shown in Figure 8.29 and only a bit smaller than that of traditional vulcanized rubber.

The simpler architecture for a normally closed hydrogel valve is reported in Figure 8.30a [35]; it is based on the use of a temperature responsive material. Two layers of a hydrogel material are used to internally coat a microduct. In the absence of heating, the gel is expanded and the valve is closed; when a heater rises, the temperature inside the gel shrinks and the valve opens. Typical response times for these structures are of the order of 15–40 s.

An hydrogel mass can also be used to deform a membrane in a membrane-based valve by inserting it into the membrane chamber as shown in Figure 8.30b or to move other types of actuators

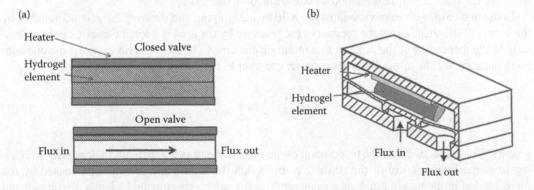

FIGURE 8.30 Coated duct (a) and membrane-based (b) hydrogel actuator valve scheme. Both valves are based on thermal actuated hydrogels.

such as cantilever or closing plates. Hydrogel MEM actuators and related valves are the focus of research and engineering efforts due to the promising properties of such materials; recent findings on hydrogel properties can be found in References [37–39], while reviews are presented in References [40,41]. Recent results on the fabrication of hydrogel-based microactuators and microvalves are also reported in Reference [42].

8.2.3 Microvalve Design Considerations

In the above section, we have considered several types of active microvalves focusing mainly on the different actuation mechanisms.

The design of a microvalve, however, is not only the selection of an actuation mechanism and the careful actuator design, but also consist of several other important elements. In this section, we will consider a few design elements to evidence different aspects of microvalve technology.

8.2.3.1 Valve Equivalent Spring and Bistable Valves (Latching Valves)

In most microvalve designs, the elastic deformation of the valve active element can be reproduced by substituting the effective distributed pressure by an equivalent elastic force applied at a suitable point of the active element. The elastic constant of this imaginary spring is generally called microvalve spring constant. The spring force closes the valve in normally closed valves while in normally open valves, the spring works against the actuator and decreases the closing force.

The spring constant of a microvalve can be obtained by starting from the effective distributed action of the actuator and performing a structural analysis of the system to find its deformation. Applying a constant pressure to the active element it will undergo a deformation so that a displacement can be defined for each active element point. Since the displacement is in any case finite and small with respect to the active element dimensions, a set of points corresponding with a maximum displacement can be individuate. Owing to the linearity of elastic equations, the maximum displacement z_{max} will depend linearly on the constant applied pressure p so that it is possible to write

$$z_{max} = fp \tag{8.30}$$

where f is a proportionality parameter depending on the valve characteristics, but not on the pressure. At this point, let us consider two cases that are the most relevant in microvalve study: the first is the case in which the maximum displacement is present in a single point of the active element, for example, at the center of a circular membrane that is constrained along its circumference and pushed by a uniform pressure, and the case in which the maximum displacement happens along a line, like the case of a square membrane constrained on one side.

In the first case, we can rewrite Equation 8.30 by multiplying and dividing the second member by the area A of the membrane: the product of the pressure by the area is a force F exerted perpendicularly to the membrane at the point of maximum displacement, while the ratio between the constant f and the area has the dimensions of an elastic constant k. Insulating the force we get

$$F = \frac{A}{f} z_{max} = k z_{max} \tag{8.31}$$

where k is called equivalent elastic constant of the membrane. It is not difficult to demonstrate starting from the linear nature of the elastic equations that the membrane deformation caused by the force applied in the maximum displacement point is the same experimented when a distributed and constant pressure is applied.

In the case in which maximum displacement is experimented along a segment on the active element surface, generally the surface can be reduced to a beam by considering that the displacement is the same along all the segments that are parallel to the maximum displacement segment. In this case, the reasoning bringing to the definition of the equivalent spring can be repeated for the beam.

We have already seen this principle in two particular cases. The square membrane of an electrostatic valve, where we introduced an equivalent elastic constant whose expression is provided in Equation 8.11 so that applying a force equal to the maximum displacement multiplied by the elastic constant to the center of the membrane, that is, the maximum displacement point, the deformation of the membrane is reproduced. In the case of a bimorph linear actuator, we said that the actuator deformation, which is clearly provoked by a distributed pressure caused by the different thermal expansion of the two materials, can be obtained by applying an equivalent force to the actuator extreme, that is, the maximum displacement point, so as to be able to introduce the expression (8.22) of the equivalent force.

The evaluation of the equivalent force for different types of active elements can be done using elastic theory of membranes and beams [6,7] and a few useful results are collected in Table 8.6.

In normally closed valves, the spring constant should be large to resist the inlet pressure. In normally open valves, the spring constant is to be optimized for a minimum value, which allows a larger closing force of the actuator. A small spring constant can be realized with a soft material such as rubber. The solution with soft materials offers a further advantage of excellent fitting characteristics. The leakage ratio can be improved from three to four orders of magnitude compared to those made of hard material such as silicon, glass, or silicon nitride.

TABLE 8.6

Equivalent Spring Constant for Different Shapes of the Microvalve Seat

Active Element Shape		Pressure	Point of Maximum Displacement
Rectangle fixed at two opposite sides	$F = k\delta z$	Distributed uniform	Rectangle center
Square suspended over four legs parallel to the square sides, legs fixed at the far end	$F = k\delta z$	Distributed uniform	Rectangle center
Square fixed on all the sides	$F = k\delta z$	Distributed uniform	Square center
Circle fixed on all the circumference	$F = k\delta z$	Concentrated in the circle center	Circle center
Circle fixed on all the circumference	$F = k\delta z$	Distributed uniform	Circle center

A bistable valve, different from a normally closed or normally open one, is stable without the intervention of an external force both in the close and open state, so maintaining its position if the power feed is interrupted. If the valve is designed for bistable operation, there is no need for a valve spring because the two valve states are structurally stable. Since the nonpowered state is undefined, a valve spring can still be considered for the initial, nonpowered state to assure safe operation. A bistable valve spring allows the valve active element to snap into its working position. In this case, the actuator just needs to be powered in a short period to have enough force to trigger the position change. The force generated by the spring is then high enough to seal the valve inlet.

A typical bistable valve can be constructed by prestressed membranes or beams [43,44]. For example, if a beam is blocked at the extreme between two constrains that are nearer than the beam length at rest, it accumulates an internal stress, implying the presence of an equilibrium curvature of the beam. If the beam is also constrained to belong to a plane containing its two extremes, two stable positions generate on opposite parts of the beam plane with respect to the straight line containing the extreme constrains (compare Figure 8.30).

If the beam is forced to compress so as to assume a straight position in between the two extreme constrains, it is in an instable equilibrium position that, theoretically, could last infinitely. In practice, however, the minimum perturbation of mechanical, thermal, or other types generate the relaxation toward one of the two stable equilibrium situations [45]. Since a microscopic perturbation is sufficient and its type and direction are random, it is not possible to forecast *a priori* what will be the stable position that the beam will assume and this is the reason why the nonpowered state is called undefined. A similar phenomenon happens for a prestressed membrane that is constrained in circular constrains with a radius a bit smaller than the membrane radius.

Considering the membrane case, assuming to remain in elastic regime of deformation, the point of maximum displacement of the membrane, due to circular symmetry, is its center. The center of the membrane can assume two possible positions, corresponding to the two stable equilibrium states of the membrane. Assuming a reference system with the membrane at rest on the (x, y) plane and the origin at the center of the membrane at rest, the two stable positions of the membrane center are given by [2]

$$z_{max} = \pm \frac{1}{24} \sqrt{105 \left(3R^2 |\varsigma_0| \frac{1 - v^2}{\varepsilon} \right) + 4\tau^2} \qquad (8.32)$$

where R is the membrane radius, τ the membrane thickness, and ς_0 the compressive (negative) stress of the membrane if compressed by the constrain while having a plane shape on the (x, y) plane.

Owing to the constrains, the membrane has to maintain a tangent plane coinciding with the (x, y) plane in every point common with the constrain; moreover, if we pass in cylindrical coordinates with coordinates (r, θ) on the (x, y) plane, the membrane equilibrium shapes do not have to depend on θ. A structural study of the problem generates the following expression of the membrane shape in the equilibrium configurations:

$$z(r) = z_{max} \left(1 - \frac{r^2}{R^2} \right)^2 \qquad (8.33)$$

If the membrane closes a valve, it will reach the valve seat before reaching the maximum deformation corresponding to the stable equilibrium point so as to exert a closure pressure on the valve seat. Considering a generic membrane center displacement z_0, the pressure p exerted by the membrane and the equivalent elastic force F are given by

$$p = p_0(z_0)z_0 = \frac{4\tau}{3R^4}\left(\tau^2\frac{\mathcal{E}}{1-\nu^2} + \frac{3}{2}R^2\varsigma_0 - \frac{32}{35}z_0^2\frac{\mathcal{E}}{1-\nu^2}\right)z_0 \tag{8.34}$$

$$F = -\frac{2\pi}{3R^2}\left(\frac{8}{3}\tau^3\frac{\mathcal{E}}{1-\nu^2} + 2\tau R^2\varsigma_0 + \frac{128}{105}\tau z_0^2\frac{\mathcal{E}}{1-\nu^2} - \frac{1}{2}p_0(z_0)R^4\right)z_0 \tag{8.35}$$

These equations allow the main characteristics of a bistable membrane to be evaluated. In a microvalve, generally the inlet has a smaller area with respect to the membrane, so the maximum pressure the closed valve can withstand can be evaluated by Equation 8.34 by multiplying by the membrane area πR^2 and dividing by the inlet area πR_{inlet}^2 so as to obtain

$$p = p_0(z_0)z_0 = \frac{4\tau}{3R^2 R_{inlet}^2}\left(\tau^2\frac{\mathcal{E}}{1-\nu^2} + \frac{3}{2}R^2\varsigma_0 - \frac{32}{35}z_0^2\frac{\mathcal{E}}{1-\nu^2}\right)z_0 \tag{8.36}$$

8.2.3.2 Valve Seat

The valve seat has to satisfy two main requirements: zero leakage and resistance against particles trapped in the sealing area. For a minimum leakage rate, the valve should be designed with a large sealing area, which has to be extremely flat. Softer materials such as rubber or other elastomers are generally more suited to satisfy these requirements.

Resistance against particles can be realized using different techniques:

- A hard valve seat can simply crush the particles if the valve closing force is sufficiently high. For this purpose, actuators like piezostacks exerting a large force are generally used in conjunction with a hard coating layer on the closing part of the valve seat such as silicon nitride, silicon carbide, or diamond-like carbon.
- The particles can be surrounded and sealed by a soft coating on the valve seat.
- Small particle traps such as holes or trenches can be fabricated on the valve seat or on the opposite valve base.

Potentially, a mix of the three methods can be used, and it is effectively used if the valve has to be opened and closed many times like it happens in microfluidic circuits that must have a long operating life. In disposable labs on chip, the valve design has to carefully balance the complexity, causing a higher fabrication cost, with the adoption of methodologies improving the chip reliability.

8.2.3.3 Fluid Flux through the Valve

In order to provide examples of microvalves, we have considered mainly vertical, membrane-based valves, where the liquid flux arrives vertically from the bottom part of the circuit just in front of the valve seat and it is made horizontal again inside the valve before the insertion in the exit duct (see, e.g., Figures 8.5, 8.11, and 8.16). This is not the only possible valve architecture and we have also introduced in Section 8.2.2 other possible architectures like those in Figure 8.25 or 8.29a.

Under an hydraulic point of view, an open valve constitutes a point of pressure drop due to the interruption of the duct continuity. This pressure drop should be minimized when designing the valve so as to allow the minimum fluid perturbation. Even if the Reynolds number is generally very small in the flow through the microvalves due to their small dimensions so that vortexes are generally avoided, death spaces where the fluid practically is still can be created, as shown in the example of Figure 7.14a near the point of duct section change. Besides creating a less efficient flow, death areas are dangerous if biological molecules are in solution in the flowing fluid. As a matter of fact, biological molecules tends to deposit more easily in still solution and a fat or protein deposit can be the seed for a more extended phenomenon that has to be avoided.

A first technique to avoid abrupt flow structure changes is to maintain the duct straight through the valve, avoiding angles, especially in the upward and downward direction. The first type of valves having straight ducts is the so-called direct action valve. These valves act on the duct itself without requiring its change of shape or direction when the valve is open. Generally, the action mechanism on the direct action valve is to operate a pressure on the external surface of the duct so as to flatten it and interrupt the flux. Examples of such valves are provided in Figures 8.21 and 8.26.

Under a fluid dynamic point of view, this kind of valve has the best performance since the liquid flow is almost unaffected when the valve is open; moreover, almost all actuators can be used for such a valve so that a very wide range of closing pressures can be realized. However, a soft duct wall is required so that these valves can be used practically only when the ducts are realized using soft polymers.

An example of the design of a horizontal flow membrane-based valve is presented in Figure 8.31a. The membrane is located below the main valve chamber and the inlet and outlet are at the same level. Here, the flux is somehow perturbed by the enlargement of the duct in correspondence of the valve seat, but a correct design of the transitions can minimize this effect. The drawback of this design is the intrinsic leakage due to the imperfect duct closure caused by the membrane curve deformation (compare Figure 8.32b).

A different architecture for a valve not requiring control duct curves is shown in Figure 8.32c. The valve closure is obtained by activating a piston interposing between the flux and closing the duct. This is quite a flexible design, suitable for actuation methods based either on elastic deformation or on expansion of the working material. However, the working material need not stick to the piston, so as not to provoke a valve failure due to the piston block. Drawbacks of this architecture can be due to the imperfect contact between the piston and the far duct wall causing leakage and to the penetration of the flowing liquid in the working material chamber if the piston is not perfectly adherent to the piston chamber walls.

A different class of valve design is conceived to solve the problem of the pressure loss due to the uprising flow by putting the incoming duct above the outcoming one, so that the flow during the change of duct level is supported by gravity. An example of a valve of this kind is reported in Figure 8.32d. This design decreases the pressure drop due to the passage of the liquid in the open valve while maintaining the horizontal membrane-based design, which is well consolidated in the MEMs industry, but dead spaces can still exist due to the valve structure.

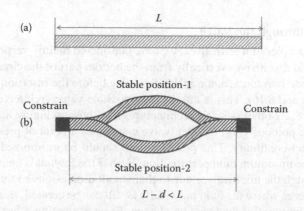

FIGURE 8.31 Bistable beam: beam at rest (a) and constrained beam with the two stable positions (b).

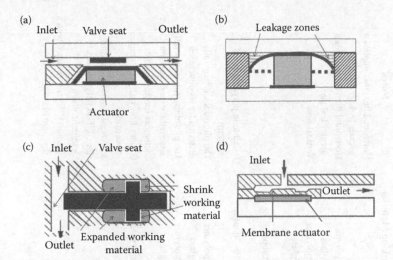

FIGURE 8.32 Schemes of the fluid flow through different types of valves: horizontal flow membrane valve: side (a) and front (b) sections; piston-based valve (c), and vertical flow valve with the inlet duct above the outlet (d).

8.2.4 MICROVALVE PERFORMANCE COMPARISON

In this section, we will carry out a comparison between different types of microvalves under a performance point of view. This comparison is intended only to provide a first evaluation of strength and limits of present microvalve technology. In general, before looking at the required valve performance, selection of a restricted list of possible technologies is performed on the ground of the target application. For example, if a valve is too big for a certain application, the fact that it provides a very good leakage is not relevant.

In compiling Tables 8.7 and 8.8, we have tried to give an indication of the characteristics that a certain design can provide without detailing too much the valve structure and the technological processes that have been performed to fabricate the valve. The reported figures thus have to be intended as orders of magnitude and specific realizations can deviate sensibly from them, especially if particular care or original design tricks have been used.

Valves are classified on the base of the type of actuator and the fluid flow structure. Data on these broad valve classes have been obtained by collecting several different references where similar valves have been fabricated and extracting from the reported data a sort of typical value. This is naturally a difficult and a bit arbitrary process, another reason why figures have to be intended as an indication of order of magnitude. However, we have preferred not to refer to specific realizations whose performances are frequently quite influenced by fabrication-specific techniques and details about the valve design.

Considering valve dimension, we have tried to report data regarding small valves, the reported dimensions thus have to be intended to be near the smallest possible dimension of the considered valve. However, it is frequently possible to obtain smaller valves of the indicated type, but probably not much smaller. The dimension indication should allow the reader to individuate in what microfluidic circuits a certain valve can be inserted and for what kind of application it is too big and a smaller valve is required.

Naturally, valves much greater than the dimensions we indicate in the tables can be realized, and if a greater valve is considered, the parameters depending on the valve size have to be scaled consistently. Scaling is not trivial however, since while dimension-related parameters, such as the pressure distributed on the valve area, scales with dimensions, the elastic parameters of the material do not scale. In order to perform a correct scaling, the equations provided in this section can be used.

As far as the working material is considered, the most common working material is reported and the data are obtained by referring to fabrication processes for that material. Finally, in the notes, we

TABLE 8.7

Comparison among Possible Performances of Different Types of Microvalves

Type	Size (mm × mm)	Fluid	Q_{max} (mL/min)	P_{clo} (kPa)	Leakage	V (V)	Power (mW)	Working Material	Notes
Electrostatic membrane	4 × 4	Air	100	12	24	30	—	Silicon	Horizontal flux, this implies a greater leakage
Electrostatic membrane	4 × 4	Water	1	20	12	40	—	Silicon/polymer Silicon/glass	Horizontal flux, this implies a greater leakage
Electrostatic membrane	4 × 4	Water	—	80	150	50	—	Silicon/polymer Silicon/glass	Vertical flux
Electromagnetic membrane	4 × 4	Air	500	—	—	—	1000	Silicon	
Electromagnetic polymer membrane	4 × 4	Air	—	10	100	—	1000	Silicon/rubber	
Electromagnetic needle based	5 × 5	Water	1	980	90	—	0.5	Silicon/Fe–Ni alloy	Possible in polymer-based systems
Piezostack membrane	15 × 15	Water	0.05	25	100	100	—	Silicon/polymer Silicon/glass	The piezostack is generally external for its dimension
Piezobimorph membrane with cantilever actuator	5 × 5	Water	1.5	10	200	150	—	Silicon/polymer Silicon/glass	The piezobimorph is generally external for its dimension. Other actuators forms possible
Thermomechanical membrane	8 × 8	Water	5	100	100	—	1000	Aluminum/silicon	Greater flow rate due to bigger dimension
Thermopneumatic piston	0.1 × 0.8	Water	0.3	1.4	100	—	100	Water	Also needle or duct flattening based if on polymers ducts
Thermopneumatic membrane	5 × 5	Water	1	6	30	—	200	Water	Membrane down to 2.5 mm × 2.5 mm realized with a flow rate of 0.3
Thermopneumatic membrane	5 × 5	Air	1500	700	20	—	200	Water	

Note: Considering the aspect ratio, small valves are considered. Thus, the reported aspect ratio is near to the minimum attainable with present technology. The maximum flow rate through the considered valve is indicated as Q_{max}, the maximum pressure the valve can withstand while closed with P_{max}, the leakage is intended at the maximum operating pressure, the operating electrical tension or power (depending on the valve type) are indicated with V and Power, respectively.

TABLE 8.8
Comparison among Possible Performances of Different Types of Microvalves

Type	Size (mm×mm)	Fluid	Q_{max} (mL/min)	P_{cfo} (kPa)	Leakage	V (V)	Power (mW)	Working Material	Notes
Pneumatic membrane	15×15	Air	120	241	300	—	—	Silicon	
Pneumatic piston	0.2×0.2	Water	0.26	100	10,000	—	—	Silicon/glass	The needle actuation technology can also be used with similar performances
Pneumatic membrane	1×1	Water	0.01	70	80	—	—	Silicon/rubber	
Thermal SMA membrane	1×1	Air	400	350	>100		110	Polymers	TiNiCd have greater power around 0.25 W; the membrane is an SMA thin film Membrane heater up to about 130°C
Thermal SMA radial beams	4×4	Air	1600	140	>100		110	TiNi or TiNiCu	The membrane is an SMA thin film Membrane heater up to about 50°C
Hydrogel duct coating	2×0.1	Water	—	450	>10,000			TiNi or TiNiCu	The coated duct is fabricated in polymer and 100 μm diameter. The flow rate depends on the duct flow. It can be either thermally and pH operated. Maximum temperature is 50°C
Hydrogel actuated membrane	0.4×0.4	Water	0.1	19	>100			PNIPAAm	Thermal and pH-based attuation possible. Maximum temperature is 50°C. PNIPAAm and other hydrogels are also frequently used, but performances vary greatly

Note: The parameters are the same of Table 8.7. AA/HEMA stands for PVA-AA cross-linked HEMA-based hydrogels.

report general observations that can be useful to evaluate the reported data or additional data that are relevant for the considered valve type.

The quantitative data reported in the tables are defined as follows:

- The maximum flow rate that the valve can withstand when open is called Q_{max}.
- The closure pressure, which is the maximum fluid pressure the valve can withstand when closed, is indicated as P_{clo}.
- The leakage factor as defined in this chapter is called *leakage*: it is increasingly better while getting exceedingly higher; in order to obtain the leakage defined as the ratio between the spurious flow rate and the maximum flow rate, the inverse has to be performed.
- The voltage needed to operate the valve, when the valve is voltage operated, is called V.
- The power needed to operate the valve, when a continuous power feed is needed, is indicated as *power*.

A first comment can be made about valve dimensions. The membrane-based valves have to be designed balancing the pressure provided by the actuator with the membrane dimension. The greater the membrane dimension, the greater the pressure the membrane can exert on the controlled duct when deformed, but also the greater the microfluidic chip hosting it. Moreover, the smaller the membrane, the greater the pressure that is needed to close it, while considering the overall exerted force, since it is proportional to the pressure and the area it increases with the membrane area.

The last element determining the membrane dimension is the actuator dimension itself, since a good contact has to be realized between the membrane and the actuator to effectively exploit the actuator force. Many actuators can manage squared or circular membranes made of silicon or rubber with an area of the order of 10–20 mm^2. Piezostack and other piezoelectric actuators are frequently capable of providing great closure pressures, but for their dimensions imply greater valves and even greater space to accommodate the actuator. Smaller membranes, up to 0.16 mm^2, can be realized with actuators based on expanding materials such as hydrogels or thermopneumatic chambers and SMAs.

Under a dimension point of view, valves based on different architectures can be quite smaller with respect to membrane-based valves. In-duct valves, like those realized by coating of hydrogels or levers that flatten a flexible duct, occupy space out of the duct, but do not perturb the flux once open. They can be as small as 0.04 mm^2 or even smaller if the great part of the valve is inside the duct as when the duct is coated with a hydrogel.

Hydrogel valves also have the property to be activated by a change of pH, besides the more traditional thermal actuation. If the valve has to be actuated on the ground of an external command, thermal actuation is more suitable while pH-based actuation allows the valve to close or open on the ground of chemical characteristics of the fluid flowing through it. This is an important property for biomimetic systems [46,47], where control is performed chemically instead of electrically. This is a wide and very promising field and, even if a complete discussion is beyond the scope of this book, mentioning it is for sure important.

As far as the maximum allowed flow rate is concerned, it depends mainly on the managed fluid. If it is a gas such as air, flows of the order of 100–500 mL/min can be easily obtained by membrane-based valves and even fluxes greater than 1500 mL/min can be attained if the membrane is sufficiently large. If water is concerned, the typical maximum flux of a membrane-based valve with an area around 16 mm^2 is of the order of 1 mL/min, even if variations are present due to the valve architecture.

Piston-based valves for water solutions flow control are constrained by the greater possible dimension of the piston and by the pressure the piston can withstand while avoiding a too large leakage. For this reason, these valves generally have a smaller allowed flow, of the order of 0.3 mL/min. In case of in duct valves, the flux naturally depends on the duct width, even if the maximum duct width is constrained by the ability of the working material to deform sufficiently to provide a good valve closure. Ducts of 100–150 µm can be closed by such valves, especially if they are realized with a polymeric material.

As far as the leakage is concerned, good leakage factor can be attained by membrane valves with vertical flux, generally in the order of 100–200, while membrane valves with horizontal flux provides leakage factors of the order of 25. The greater leakage factors are obtained by in-duct membrane realized using soft materials such as polymers, in this case, the leakage factor can be as high as 10,000.

Regarding the closure pressure, this spans a large range depending mainly on the managed fluid, on the actuator principle, and on the material constituting the valve seat. Values as high as 300–400 kPa can be obtained using soft material and expanding actuators or membrane actuators, while values of the order of 100 kPa or less are obtained when the material constituting the valve seat is quite hard. An exception is needle-based valves, providing a closure pressure as high as 1 MPa due to the actuator architecture itself.

Finally, electrostatic and piezoelectric valves do not theoretically require a continuous power to be operated, even if some power is needed in practice to balance current losses in the system. The driving voltage for electrostatic valves is in the order of 50 V, while it is greater than 100 V in the case of piezoelectric valves. Other valves need a continuous power feeding to be operated, which is either needed to activate a magnet or to work a heater. Electromagnetic valve needs a power of the order of 1 W, while thermally activated actuators generally are fed with a few hundred mWs.

8.3 FLUID FLOW GENERATION: MICROPUMPS

Pumping is an important functionality that has to be implemented in labs on chip microfluidic circuits. Unless an external hydraulic prevalence is provided, or gravity pushes the fluid downwards into the circuit, the fluid motion has to be generated by a system internal to the chip. Several principles are available to create micropumps that can be integrated in labs on chip so that a large range of pressures and flow rates can be obtained depending on the application. Several extensive reviews exist on micropump technologies containing a discussion of principles and an extensive bibliography [48–50].

A first category of micropumps is constituted by mechanical pumps, where the fluid motion is generated by the mechanical action of an MEMs system. Several types of mechanical pumps exist, using different types of actuators and different architectures to generate fluid motion. In this section, we will analyze check valve-based pumps, that generally use a membrane as actuator and peristaltic pumps. Other types of mechanical micropumps exist, such as rotating micropumps and centrifugal micropumps, but we will not detail their characteristics since they are less suitable for labs on chip due to both their dimension and the typical pressure and flow rate ranges.

A second category of micropumps is that of passive pumps, that is, pumps that do not require a continuous power feeding to work. These are quite useful pumps when the required prevalence and flow rate is in the range typical of these pumps. Almost all passive pumps are somehow based on the surface tension effect and we will analyze simple capillary pumps and transpiration pumps.

A third category is constituted by electromagnetic pumping, both electrostatic and electrodynamics. Electrostatic pumping can be based either on electroosmosis (see Section 7.5.4) or on electrophoresis (see Section 7.5.1), while electrodynamics pumps can exploit induction effect or magnetophoresis if the liquid is magnetically active or if a sufficient density of magnetic beads is present (see Section 7.6.1).

All the above pump categories are supposed to produce a continuous fluid flux. Specific pumps can be devised if the considered fluid is divided into droplets into an environmental fluid: in this category, we will consider thermocapillary and electrowetting-based pumps.

The most important quality parameters for micropumps are [2]

- The maximum flow rate Q_{max}, also called pump capacity, that is defined as the maximum volume per unit time of fluid the pump can inject in the inlet in the absence of back-pressure.
- The maximum back-pressure Π_{max}, that is, the maximum pressure the pump can work against: at this pressure, the flow rate of the pump becomes zero.

The term *pump head* is also often used as a parameter for pump performance. The hydraulic *head* relates the energy of an incompressible fluid to the height of an equivalent static column of that fluid. In particular, a pump head is the height that the fluid pushed by the pump can reach against the force of gravity. Head is thus expressed in units of height, that is, meters in the SI system [50,51].

The total energy at a given point in an incompressible fluid, in the absence of electromagnetic forces, is composed of three terms:

- The kinetic energy associated with the movement of the fluid
- The energy from the pressure in the fluid
- The energy from the height of the fluid relative to the arbitrary height reference

Corresponding to these three terms, we have three terms comprising the pumps head: the kinetic head, the pressure head, and the height head.

The kinetic head is given by the height corresponding to the fluid kinetic energy. If we define the square average velocity $\bar{v}$ across the section S of the duct where the fluid flows as

$$\bar{v}^2 = \int_S \left| v_j(x,y) n_j \right|^2 dx\, dy \tag{8.37}$$

where n_j is the unit vector perpendicular to the section, we can write the kinetic head H_k as

$$H_k = \frac{\bar{v}^2}{2g} \tag{8.38}$$

The pressure head H_p can be evaluated as the ratio of the energy related to the presence of a pressure prevalence different from zero and gravitational energy. The pressure-related energy is equal to the pressure multiplied by the area of the duct and by the average displacement per unit time, given by the average fluid velocity. The corresponding gravitational energy is given by the mass of the fluid, that is, volume by density, multiplied by the gravitational acceleration. In this case, the volume is equal to the product of the duct area by the average velocity since it is referred to the unit time. Simplifying the volume (area per velocity), we get

$$H_p = \frac{p}{\rho g} \tag{8.39}$$

Finally, if the center of mass of the duct section is at a level different from zero with respect to the reference, we have a height head equal to the center of mass height z of the fluid in the duct section. Thus, the total head H of an incompressible fluid flowing through a duct is

$$H = H_k + H_p + z \tag{8.40}$$

The pump head of a pump can be evaluated as the head difference between the pump output and the pump input; putting together the above head terms, we get

$$H = \left(\frac{p}{\rho g} + \frac{\bar{v}^2}{2g} + \bar{z} \right)_{out} - \left(\frac{p}{\rho g} + \frac{\bar{v}^2}{2g} + z \right)_{in} \tag{8.41}$$

where the first term is calculated at the pump output section and the second at the pump input section.

The maximum mechanical power P_{max} exercised by the pump on the fluid can be evaluated as a function of the maximum pressure exerted by the pump that coincides with the maximum backpressure Π_{max}, or as a function of the maximum flow rate and of the pump head as

$$P_{max} = \frac{\Pi_{max} Q_{max}}{2} = \frac{\rho g Q_{max} H}{2} \tag{8.42}$$

Another important performance parameter of a pump is the pump efficiency, which is the ratio of the power feeding the actuator and the power exerted on the fluid, that is,

$$\eta = \frac{\Pi_{max} Q_{max}}{2 P_{ac}} = \frac{\rho g Q_{max} H}{2 P_{ac}} \tag{8.43}$$

8.3.1 MECHANICAL MICROPUMPS

The first type of mechanical micropumps we will analyze are control valve-based micropumps. The general scheme of a control valve-based micropump is reported in Figure 8.33. The micropump accommodates two control valves. One control valve is placed at the pump inlet and allows the fluid to enter, but not to exit from the pump chamber. The second control valve is placed at the pump outlet and allows the fluid to exit, but not to enter into the pump chamber. A membrane is placed on top of the pump chamber and an actuator can flex or relax the membrane so as to decrease or increase the volume of the pump chamber.

The membrane is flexed and relaxed periodically; when the membrane is relaxed, the pressure difference between the in and out ducts and the pump chamber becomes negative. Owing to this pressure difference, the fluid tends to enter into the pump chamber, but due to the position of the valves, fluid can enter only from the inlet duct. When the membrane is flexed, the fluid exits from the pump chamber, and it can happen only from the output duct. Thus, the fluid is transferred from the inlet to

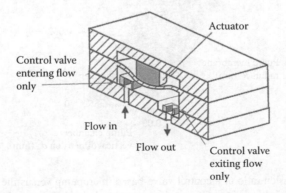

FIGURE 8.33 Control valve-based micropump.

the outlet periodically so that the flow can appear somehow discontinuous when similar valves are used. The volume pumped in a single period by such a valve is called stroke volume (V_S). The stroke volume can be estimated starting from Equation 8.33 that provide the shape of a deformed membrane as a function of the maximum displacement. The relation between the pressure applied by the actuator and the maximum displacement of the membrane center can be evaluated from Equation 8.34, substituting the maximum displacement to z_0 and considering that the last equation also holds in the zero prestress limit, that is, $\varsigma_0 = 0$. The critical parameter of a control valve pump is the compression ratio Ψ, which is the ratio between the stroke volume V_S, and the so-called death volume V_D, which is the volume of the pump chamber when the membrane is completely flexed downwards.

A reasonable compression ratio of a pump based on a circular valve is obtained imagining the pump chamber circular of the same radius of the membrane and the membrane deformation downwards at the limit of the elastic range of the membrane, which is equal to half the membrane thickness. Moreover, just to have orders of magnitude, we can imagine the depth of the pump chamber from 10 to 20 times the membrane thickness of the order of a few micrometers.

Staring from Equation 8.33, we can evaluate both the stroke and the death volumes obtaining the surfaces represented in Figure 8.34, where the compression ratio is represented versus the membrane radius and the chamber vertical dimension with membrane at rest for different ratios between the membrane thickness τ and the vertical chamber dimension. It is evident that a control valve-based micropump works with low compression ratios. Values of the order of 0.001 are normal for well-designed valves unless an actuator allowing the use of a particularly small membrane is adopted.

Moreover, for the working of a good pump both the input and the output control valves have to be easily opened by the fluid flow, so that we have

$$p_p - p_{in} > p_{cv} \tag{8.44a}$$

$$p_p - p_{out} > p_{cv} \tag{8.44b}$$

where

p_{in} is the pressure on the terminal surface of the inlet duct

p_{out} is the pressure on the section at the inlet of the output duct

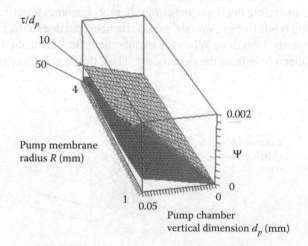

FIGURE 8.34 Compression ratio of a control valve-based micropump versus the circular membrane ratio R and the chamber vertical dimension with membrane at rest d_p for different ratios between the membrane thickness τ and the vertical chamber dimension d_p.

p_p is the overall pump created pressure
p_{cv} is the critical pressure needed to operate correctly the control valves

If the pump has to pump a liquid, the minimum compression ratio that allows the pump to work is the ratio providing a pump-generated pressure equal to the critical pressure p_{cv}, which is easily evaluated as

$$\Psi_{min} = \Theta p_{cv} \qquad (8.45)$$

where Θ is the liquid compressibility. It correctly results that for an ideal incompressible liquid, whatever compression ratio provokes the aperture of the control valves, creating on them an infinite pressure. Since in general, Θ is not zero, but it is very small for real liquids (it is about 0.5×10^{-8} m²/N for water) Equation 8.45 provides a very easy-to-fulfill condition if the pump is only full of liquid. In real systems however, it is quite frequent to have gas bubbles mixed with liquid, both caused by the process of liquid insertion and by the processing happening inside the lab on chip. In this case, the bubbles are much more compressible with respect to water and also a small percentage of air causes condition (8.45) not to be completely valid.

In Reference [52], the minimum compression ratio for a pump designed for gases is derived, and combining this result with Equation 8.45, calling ξ the gas percentage in water, we get

$$\Psi_{min} = (1 - \xi)\Theta p_{cv} + \xi \left[\left(\frac{p_0}{p_0 - p_{cv}} \right)^{1/k} - 1 \right] \qquad (8.46)$$

where p_0 is the atmospheric pressure and k is the ratio between the specific heats at constant pressure and at constant volume of the gas, being equal to 1.66 for a monoatomic perfect gas. Air behaves almost ideally as a two-atom perfect gas due to its composition at 99% of nitrogen and oxygen, so that $k = 1.4$ can be used with a very small error.

Setting, for example, Θ and k to values typical of water and air, respectively, and p_{cv} to 20 kPa, the ratio between the air and water contributions to Equation 8.46 is shown in Figure 8.35. It is clear that the air contribution is greater for an air percentage as low as 0.06% so that, in designing control valve-based pumps, the first contribution is neglected in Equation 8.46 and since a reliable value of ξ is generally unknown, ξ is set to one to obtain a robust design.

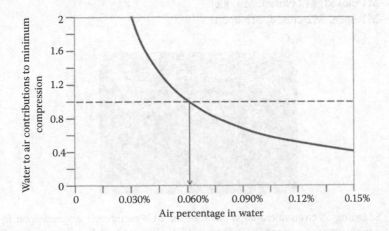

FIGURE 8.35 Ratio between the contribution of water and air in establishing a minimum needed compression ratio for a pump working with water/air mix.

The above conditions lead to the following design rules for control valve micropumps.

- Minimize the critical pressure p_{cv} by using more flexural valve design or valve material with a small Young's modulus.
- Maximize the stroke volume V_S by using actuators with a large stroke or more flexible pump membrane.
- Minimize the dead volume V_D.
- Maximize the pump pressure p_p by using actuators with large forces.

An example of fabricated polymeric micropump based on control valves is reported in Reference [53]. The micropump is made of SU-8 photoresist and PMMA. The key elements of the micropump are the microcontrol valves, which are fabricated in a 100-µm-thick SU-8 film. The SU-8 part is designed as a disk with 10 µm diameter. The check valves are 1 mm disks suspended on a spring with four arms as shown in Figure 8.36. The cross section of the spring beam has a dimension of 100 µm × 100 µm. The pump is designed as a stack of different layers, which are made of PMMA and SU-8. The low spring constant of the SU-8 check valves allows the use of relatively low drive voltages on the order of several 30 V for the piezodisk, which works as the pump's actuator. Pump rates up to 1 mL/min and back pressures up to 1.9 kPa have been achieved.

Peristaltic pumps are mechanical pumps based on a different principle with respect to check valve-based pumps. The pumping concept is based on the peristaltic motion of the pump chambers, which squeezes the fluid in the desired direction as shown in Figure 8.37a.

Theoretically, peristaltic pumps need three or more pump chambers each with its own actuator: most of the realized pumps have three chambers. Peristaltic pumps are easily implemented because of the lack of the complicated architecture requiring check valves. From an operational point of view, peristaltic pumps are active valves connected in series, so that all the technologies analyzed in Section 8.2 for active valves can be used in peristaltic pumps. The working of peristaltic pumps passes for a cycle of pumping constituted by six consecutive states of the three pump actuators. The transition from a pump state to the following in the pump cycle is obtained by activating a single actuator and it is never required simultaneous working of two or more actuators. The pump states are

- State 1—M1 open, M2 closed, M3 closed
- State 2—M1 open, M2 open, M3 closed
- State 3—M1 closed, M2 open, M3 closed
- State 4—M1 closed, M2 open, M3 open
- State 5—M1 closed, M2 closed, M3 open
- State 6—M1 open, M2 closed, M3 open

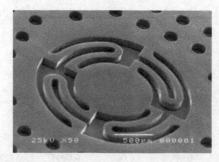

FIGURE 8.36 Scanning electron microscope photo of the SU8 membrane suspended on four spring legs realized for the micropumps described in Reference [53]. (Reproduced from *Sensors and Actuators B: Chemical*, vol. 97, Nguyen N. T., Troung T. Q., A fully polymeric Micropump with piezoelectric actuator, pp. 137–143, Copyright 2004, with permission from Elsevier.)

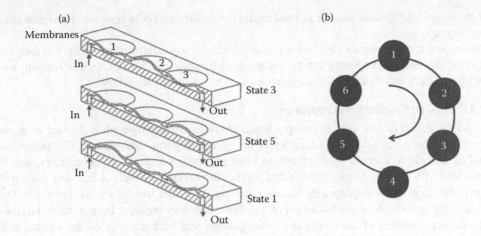

FIGURE 8.37 Scheme of a peristaltic pump based on membrane stages (a) and cyclic working of the pump constituted by the repletion of a specific sequence of its six states (b).

The pumping period as a sequence of states is represented in Figure 8.37b, while in Figure 8.37a, only the states 1, 3, and 5 are represented to give a view of the pumping action.

An advantage of the peristaltic pump is that, in contrast to the control valve-based pump, it can work in both directions, as a matter of fact, actuating the single chambers in the inverse order the system pumps in the opposite direction, if no control valve is present on the same duct where the pump is located.

The most serious problem of peristaltic micropumps is leakage. A small pressure difference between the outlet and the inlet will cause a backflow in the nonactuated state. A one-way check valve should be connected in series with a peristaltic pump for applications such as drug delivery systems and chemical analysis, which do not allow a backflow. The general optimization strategies for peristaltic pumps are maximizing the compression ratio and increasing the number of pump chambers. Since a peristaltic pump does not require a high chamber pressure, the most important optimization factors are the large stroke volume and the large compression ratio. This means that the single stage has to be designed looking to this elements first. Besides references reported in the cited reviews, recent results on peristaltic micropumps are reported in References [54–57].

8.3.2 Capillary Micropumps

The phenomenon exploited in capillary micropumps is simply surface tension of a liquid in a capillary duct. We have seen in Section 7.3.5 that a liquid in an ascending capillary arrives at a level determined by the equilibrium between the pressure difference across the contact surface between liquids and gravity. If the capillary is horizontal, the gravity effect is not present and the pressure difference across the interface provokes the advancement of the liquid through the capillary as far as the interface exists.

Passive capillary micropumps are pumping mechanism that does not require power feeding. This kind of pumps cannot reach the great pressure and flow rate typical of mechanical micropumps, but have several advantages, especially when small labs on chip are considered. Besides the absence of power feeding, capillary pumps can be very small with respect to mechanical pumps, as small as an array of ducts with a diameter of a few micrometers, and they can be effectively integrated with other systems both in polymer and in silicon technology. This is such an attractive set of properties that an entire labs on chip category, the so-called autonomous capillary systems [58,59], uses only or at least mainly capillary effect to move and process solution inside the chip.

The surface tension can also be actively controlled, so as to control the capillary effect. In this way, active capillary micropumps can be designed, as transpiration pumps. In this section, we will deal with capillary micropumps for the generation of a continuous fluid flow.

8.3.2.1 Passive Capillary Micropumps

The capillary effect can be used to pump a liquid from a reservoir through a channel as shown in Figure 8.38, where the geometric variables of the system are also introduced. The pump is constituted by an origin reservoir where the fluid to be pumped is inserted, by a capillary, and by an air reservoir. If we assume that at the initial instant the origin reservoir is full and the capillary is empty, the fluid starts to propagate through the capillary duct toward the air reservoir. During meniscus propagation, different forces act on the fluid: capillary pressure both in the capillary duct and on the fluid surface of the origin reservoir, gravity, and backpressure of the air that is compressed by the advancing liquid.

Thus, during meniscus propagation, the pressure p_{cap} acting on the liquid in the capillary can be written as (compare Equation 7.132)

$$p_{cap} = p_{duct} - p_{res} + p_{grav} - p_{air} \tag{8.47}$$

where

p_{duct} is the capillary pressure generated at the end interface of the duct connecting the reservoirs
p_{res} is the capillary pressure generated at the air–liquid interface of the reservoir
p_{grav} is the pressure due to gravity
p_{air} is the backpressure due to air compression

Capillary pressures can be evaluated using Equation 7.132 so that

$$p_{duct} - p_{res} = 4\pi\gamma\cos(\theta)\left(\frac{1}{\mathcal{P}_D} - \frac{1}{\mathcal{P}_R}\right) \tag{8.48}$$

where $\mathcal{P}_D$ and $\mathcal{P}_R$ are the duct and reservoir wetted perimeters and θ is the contact angle of the liquid with the duct and reservoir walls. The gravity pressure acting on the free liquid surface in the origin reservoir is written as

$$p_{grav} = \rho g h \tag{8.49}$$

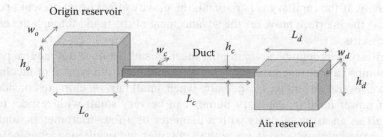

FIGURE 8.38   Scheme and definition of the main geometric variables of the elementary capillary micropump.

where h is the height of the liquid in the reservoir. The backpressure caused by air compression can be evaluated by considering air as a perfect gas obtaining

$$p_{air} = -n_a R_g T \int_{V_0}^{V_0 - \Delta V} \frac{dV}{V^2} = \frac{n_a R T}{2} \left[\frac{\Delta V}{V_0 (V_0 - \Delta V)} \right] = \frac{RT}{2 v_{air}} \frac{\Delta V}{V_0 - \Delta V} \qquad (8.50)$$

where

n_a is the number of air moles

T is the temperature, which is assumed constant

R_g is the gas constant

V_0 is the initial volume, which is the sum of volumes of the capillary and of the air reservoir

ΔV is the volume variation at a certain instant

v_{air} is the air molar volume at the considered temperature

If p_{cap} is positive, the liquid starts to move along the duct. In practical capillary pumps, the system is designed so that $\mathcal{P}_D \ll \mathcal{P}_R$; moreover, the liquid quantity is so small that the gravity term can be neglected, so that Equation 8.47 reduces to

$$p_{cap} = \frac{4\pi\gamma}{\mathcal{P}_D} \cos(\theta) - \frac{RT}{2 v_{air}} \frac{\Delta V}{V_0 - \Delta V} \qquad (8.51)$$

The air backpressure can be either exploited in the system working or made negligible by a suitable system design. For example, if the system has to be designed so that the liquid advancement through the capillary spontaneously stops inside the capillary itself, this can be obtained by exploiting the air backpressure without the need of an active valve.

Let us consider a PMMA system processing water in contact with air at atmospheric pressure and a 100-μm-long capillary duct with the dimension of 20 μm × 20 μm. Using data from Table 8.9, the capillary pressure results to be equal to 3.5 kPa. If the capillary is closed at the end without any reservoir, balancing the pressures in Equation 8.51, it is found that the meniscus advances through the capillary only 6.42 μm before being stopped by the air backpressure. The point where the meniscus stops can be controlled by suitably designing the air reservoir.

It is also possible to design the volume of the air reservoir sufficiently so that the air backpressure term can be neglected. In the example, if we design the air reservoir as a 400 μm × 400 μm × 400 μm

---

TABLE 8.9

Data for the Numerical Example on the Dynamics of an Elementary Capillary Pump

Destination reservoir width	w_d	500 μm
Destination reservoir length	L_d	500 μm
Feeding duct width	w_c	20 μm
Feeding duct length	L_c	100 μm
Feeding duct height	h_c	20 μm
Water–air surface tension	γ	0.072 N/m
Water–PMMA contact angle	θ	72°
Water dynamic viscosity	η	0.00089 Pa s
Air molar volume	v_{air}	0.02446 m³/mole
Temperature	T	300 K

chamber, the air backpressure is as small as 3% of the capillary pressure when the meniscus arrives at the end of the capillary, thus making the air backpressure be negligible.

If the air backpressure is to be made negligible, a suitable air vent can also be designed, so that the air is expelled from the microfluidic circuits while it is pumped by the advancing liquid. This solution, however, cannot be suitable for many applications, where protecting the inner part of the chip from contamination while providing an open access to the ducts for air requires a hermetic package that frequently results to be too expensive for a low cost, frequently disposable, device.

Assuming the air backpressure to be negligible, after a transient length of the order of magnitude of the capillary section dimensions, the capillary flux relaxes to a fully developed Poiseuille flux, so that the flow rate while the meniscus advances into the capillary can be evaluated in case of square ducts using Equation 7.90. In the case of Table 8.9, we obtain $Q = 11.64$ μL/min.

The process happening when the liquid arrives at the end of the capillary facing the air reservoir is driven by surface tension, that is, the dominant force at the dimensional scale of labs on chip. Here, the fluid experiments a sudden end of the contact with the solid wall. The fluid inertia would tend to push the fluid further, but it is counterbalanced by the fact that surface tension creates a force opposing to a change of the contact angle that would increase the overall system energy. In particular, there are two possible stable configurations: both corresponding to the same contact angle between the fluid and the duct walls: the sudden stop of the meniscus and the formation of a droplet out of the capillary duct. In particular, if the effect of the surface tension overcomes inertia and thwarts the contact angle change due to further fluid advancement, the meniscus comes to a sudden stop. If the inertia is sufficient to bring the meniscus from concave to convex, the surface tension induced force changes direction and a droplet starts to form from the capillary.

The inertial energy ΔG_{kin} of the liquid in the capillary can be evaluated as the kinetic energy of the fluid when the meniscus reaches the end of the duct; thus

$$\Delta G_{kin} = \frac{1}{2} \rho w_d h_d L_d v^2 \tag{8.52}$$

where v^2 is the average of the square velocity in the capillary duct section. This expression can be evaluated exactly using Equation 7.86 for the velocity field; however, in order to get simple results helping us to understand the meniscus dynamics we will approximately assume that the duct can be represented by a circular duct whose radius is the hydrodynamic radius $\mathcal{R}$ defined by Equation 7.72. Using the expression of the velocity field in a circular duct and the expression of the capillary pressure, we get

$$\Delta G_{kin} = \frac{1}{15} \rho \pi \frac{\mathcal{R}^4}{L_d} \frac{\gamma^2}{\eta^2} \cos^2(\theta) \tag{8.53}$$

The free energy increase that is needed to transform the curve meniscus to a plane can be evaluated in the case of a circular duct by using a similar procedure adopted in Section 7.3.5.2. The displacement of the meniscus center that is needed to transform the meniscus in a plane surface is considered small with respect to the geometrical dimensions of the problem and the free energy increase is evaluated by multiplying the free energy derivative with respect to the displacement by the displacement itself. The geometry allowing the evaluation of the displacement from the contact angle is reported in Figure 8.39. In particular, starting from the geometric relations reported in the figure and from the formula of the area of the spherical segment, we can evaluate the change of the surface for an infinitesimal change of the contact angle and then integrate it from the stable value to

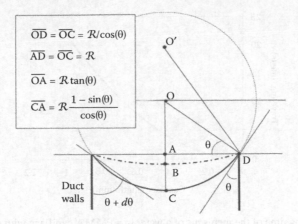

$$\overline{OD} = \overline{OC} = \mathcal{R}/\cos(\theta)$$

$$\overline{AD} = \overline{OC} = \mathcal{R}$$

$$\overline{OA} = \mathcal{R}\tan(\theta)$$

$$\overline{CA} = \mathcal{R}\frac{1 - \sin(\theta)}{\cos(\theta)}$$

FIGURE 8.39 Geometry of the meniscus change due to a small change in the contact angle.

zero. By observing that in this case the wetted surface of the duct walls does not change in area due to the change of the contact angle, we get

$$\Delta G_{cap} = 2\pi \mathcal{R}^2 \gamma \left[1 - \text{cotg}\left(\frac{\theta}{2} + \frac{\pi}{4} \right) \right] \qquad (8.54)$$

Thus, we can write the condition for droplet formation as

$$\Delta G_{kin} - \Delta G_{cap} = \frac{1}{15}\rho\pi \frac{\mathcal{R}^4}{L_d} \frac{\gamma^2}{\eta^2} \cos^2(\theta) - 2\pi \mathcal{R}^2 \gamma \left[1 - \text{cotg}\left(\frac{\theta}{2} + \frac{\pi}{4} \right) \right] > 0 \qquad (8.55)$$

By substituting the values in Table 7.8, we get $\Delta G_{kin} = 3.35 \times 10^{-15}$ J and $\Delta G_{cap} = 6.09 \times 10^{-10}$ J. This means that using PMMA for the duct, the inertial energy is by far smaller than the energy needed to revert the meniscus when the capillary flow arrives at the air reservoir. Thus, no droplet forms and the flow simply stops in front of the reservoir. If glass is used, the contact angle is almost zero, the computation can be carried out again with a contact angle that is very near to zero, depending on the glass surface state and, in case, on glass doping. As soon as the contact angle is a bit greater than zero, for example, for $\theta = 0.0001$, the meniscus stops in front of the reservoir. Since in real cases, the contact angle is at least one order of magnitude greater and the used approximations leads to an overestimation of the kinetic energy, we can conclude that a droplet out of the capillary does not form also in the case of a glass duct in the considered example. The relative energy difference is in any case smaller than that evaluated in the PMMA case.

Another important element of the dynamics of a capillary pump is the speed of advancement of the meniscus in the capillary duct. In the case of a rectangular capillary, the meniscus advancement rate can be derived by starting from Equation 7.90 for the flow rate and observing that dividing the flow rate by the duct section gives exactly the meniscus advancement velocity. Thus, indicating with x the meniscus position, we get

$$\frac{dx}{dt} = \frac{\pi\gamma}{6\eta} \frac{h_c^2}{(w_c + h_c)} \frac{1}{x} \cos(\theta) \left(1 - \xi_0 \frac{h_c}{w_c} \right) \qquad (8.56)$$

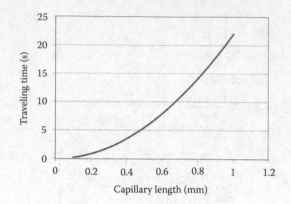

FIGURE 8.40 Traveling time of the meniscus of a water in a PMMA capillary with characteristics reported in Table 8.9.

This equation can be solved by variable separation obtaining

$$x(t) = \sqrt{\frac{\pi \gamma}{12\eta} \frac{h_c^2}{(w_c + h_c)} \cos(\theta) \left(1 - \xi_0 \frac{h_c}{w_c}\right) t} = L_c \sqrt{\frac{t}{\tau_L}} \quad (8.57)$$

where τ_L is the time needed to the meniscus to reach the end of the duct and it is expressed by

$$\frac{1}{\tau_L} = \frac{\pi \gamma}{12\eta} \frac{h_c^2}{(w_c + h_c)} \frac{1}{L_c^2} \cos(\theta) \left(1 - \xi_0 \frac{h_c}{w_c}\right) \quad (8.58)$$

The transient time depends on the square of the duct length and in the case of the parameters of Table 8.9 it is equal to 0.22 s, while if the duct would be 1 mm long the time to reach the end would be as long as 22 s as shown in Figure 8.40. This is an effect of the fact that, the capillary pressure is constant while the meniscus advances, the viscous force and the effect of the attrition on the duct walls increases greatly with the duct length.

Sometimes, elementary capillary pumps are not sufficient to assure the needed flow rate. As a matter of fact, the capillary pressure decreases with the duct dimension so that it cannot be increased too much. In order to obtain a higher flow rate from capillary pumps while maintaining a sufficient pressure, several capillary pumps can be put in parallel. They have to converge either in a reservoir or in a larger duct that is suitable to sustain such a flow rate. Naturally, such a convergence has to

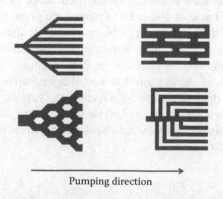

Pumping direction

FIGURE 8.41 Example of possible shapes of parallel capillary pumps. (Adapted from Zimmermann M. et al., *Lab on a Chip*, vol. 7, pp. 119–125, 2007.)

be performed in such a way as not to produce hydrodynamic death angles and excessive pressure losses. Examples of possible shapes of parallel capillary pumps are shown in Figure 8.41 [59].

8.3.2.2 Transpiration Micropumps

Transpiration micropumps are an example of biomimetic microsystems. Passive capillary effect, as described in the previous section, needs a liquid/gas surface to work. If the duct is filled, the liquid stops flowing. In nature, water supply to tree leaves still continues even when microchannels are completely filled, due to the phenomenon called transpiration: water lost by vaporizing through pores on the leaf surface is compensated by a fresh supply. Figure 8.42 shows the concept of pumping based on transpiration [60,61]. Liquid from a reservoir fills a horizontal duct due to passive capillary effect. The liquid meniscus is stopped by a hydrophobic patch at one end of the channel causing the vanishing of capillary pressure due to the contact angle equal to $\pi/2$ (see Equation 8.48). If the liquid is heated at the meniscus, the vapor pressure at the interface increases. Air supplied from an external source carries away the liquid vapor, and generates a gradient in vapor concentration as well as vapor pressure from the meniscus to the air flow channel. The gradient allows vapor to diffuse out and fresh liquid supply to flow into the channel. The velocity of the liquid can be controlled by the evaporation rate, which in turn is controlled by the vapor pressure or temperature at the meniscus controlled by an integrated heater. When the vapor is pushed by the air flow out of the heated area, it condenses again, forming a continuous flux of fluid out of the pump.

Let us indicate with A_c the area of the section S_c of the capillary and A_{ev} the area of the section S_{ev} of the evaporation duct, the balance between the supplied liquid and the evaporation can be written as

$$A_c \rho v = M A_{ev} \Phi_v \tag{8.59}$$

where an ideal incompressible liquid is assumed and

ρ is the liquid density
M is the liquid molar mass
Φ_v is the vapor flux from the meniscus for unit area due to evaporation

Moreover, the average velocity v in the capillary pump is defined as

$$v = \int_{S_c} v(x,y)\, dx\, dy \tag{8.60}$$

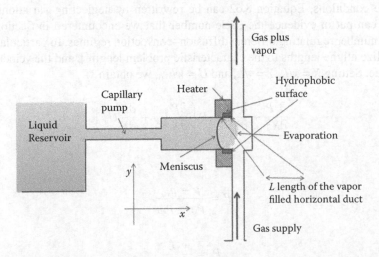

FIGURE 8.42 Principle scheme of a transpiration micropump.

Owing to Fick's law (7.160) and applying to the vapor the perfect gas state equation in the form $p_v = c_v N_a \kappa_B T$, where p_v is the vapor pressure, we can write

$$\Phi_v = D \frac{\partial c_v}{\partial x} = \frac{D}{N_a \kappa_B T} \frac{\partial p_v}{\partial x} \tag{8.61}$$

where D is the vapor diffusion coefficient, T indicates the temperature, V_v is the vapor volume, κ_B is the Boltzmann constant, and N_a is the Avogadro number. Moreover, the x and y axes are set as in Figure 8.42.

Equation 8.61 creates a relation between the pressure of the vapor and its concentration. The governing equation for the evolution of gas concentration in the vapor-filled horizontal duct and the point when the gas merges with the air flow is the diffusion–convection Equation 7.166. Substituting the relation (8.49) between the derivatives of the concentration and the pressure, we obtain the governing equation for the partial pressure of the vapor in the air flowing duct:

$$D \nabla^2 p_v - w \cdot \nabla p_v = \frac{\partial p_v}{\partial t} \tag{8.62}$$

where w is the air velocity, which has a maximum equal to $w_0 = w_0\, \mathbf{y}$ at the center of the air channel.

Under steady-state conditions, $\partial p_v/\partial t = 0$. Equation 8.62 has to be solved with the conditions

$$p_v(x, y) = p_{vl} \quad x = 0 \quad 0 \leq y \leq d \tag{8.63a}$$

$$p_v(x, y) = p_{v0} \quad x = L \quad 0 \leq y \leq d \tag{8.63b}$$

Equation 8.63a represents the condition on the meniscus, which we can approximate as almost a plane surface due to the presence of the hydrophobic walls for $0 \leq x \leq L$, where it is required that the vapor pressure is equal to the pressure of vapor of the liquid at the given temperature. Equation 8.63b represents the condition at the end of the horizontal duct, requiring that the pressure of the vapor is equal to the partial pressure of the vapor in the air flow. If we imagine the micropump represented in Figure 8.42 to be realized by rectangular ducts fabricated with planar technologies, generally, the dimension along the z direction is much smaller than that along the x and y directions. Moreover, no pressure gradient is present along z.

Under these conditions, Equation 8.62 can be rewritten by neglecting variations along the z. Moreover, we can put in evidence the Pécle number that we encountered in Section 7.4.5 as the dimensionless number regulating different diffusion–convection regimes. In particular, in this case, we can normalize all the lengths to the characteristic problem length L and the velocity of air to its maximum value. Setting $X = x/L$, $Y = y/L$, and $U = w/w_0$, we obtain

$$\frac{\partial^2 P}{\partial X^2} + \frac{\partial^2 P}{\partial Y^2} = P_e \left(\frac{\partial P}{\partial X} U_x + \frac{\partial P}{\partial Y} U_y \right) \tag{8.64}$$

where

$$P = \frac{p - p_{v0}}{p_{vl} - p_{v0}} \tag{8.65a}$$

$$P_e = \frac{w_0 L}{D} \tag{8.65b}$$

In cases like this, the Pécle number is always quite smaller than one, due to the system dimensions. The water vapor diffusion coefficient in air is about $D = 2 \times 10^{-5}$ m²/s. The characteristic length of the system is the width of the capillary duct so that $L = 50$ μm $= 5 \times 10^{-5}$ m and setting $w_0 = 1$ mm/s $= 10^{-3}$ m/s, we have $P_e = 2.5 \times 10^{-4}$. In this condition, Equation 8.64 has been studied extensively and its solutions have been reported, for example, in Reference [62].

Applying the correct boundary conditions to the solution of Equation 8.64, it is possible to evaluate the gas pressure in the gas-occupied horizontal duct and the gas flux from the meniscus, which results in

$$\Phi_v = \frac{D}{N_a \kappa_B T} \frac{\partial p_v}{\partial x} = \frac{D}{N_a \kappa_B T} \left(\frac{p_{v0} - p_{v1}}{L} \right) \left(1 + \sqrt{\frac{w_0 d_y}{D}} \right) \tag{8.66}$$

where d_y is the width of the part of the horizontal duct occupied by the meniscus. Calling R_{ev} the hydrodynamic radius, we can write, for a rectangular duct as we have assumed up to now

$$R_{ev} = \frac{d_y d_z}{d_y + d_z} \approx d_z \tag{8.67a}$$

$$d_y \approx \frac{d_y d_z}{d_z} = \frac{A_{ev}}{R_{ev}} \tag{8.67b}$$

Substituting expression (8.67b) in Equation 8.66 and the resulting expression of the flux in Equation 8.59, we can derive an expression of the velocity in the part of the duct filled with liquid, which gives a measure of the replenish rate of the liquid meniscus:

$$v = \frac{M A_{ev}}{A_c \rho} \frac{D}{N_a \kappa_B T} \left(\frac{p_{v0} - p_{v1}}{L} \right) \left(1 + \sqrt{\frac{w_0}{D} \frac{A_{ev}}{R_{ev}}} \right) \tag{8.68}$$

Equation 8.68 has been experimentally verified and, even if it has been obtained using several approximations, it reproduces quite well experimental results, so that it can be used to design transpiration pumps in practice.

8.3.3 Electromagnetic Micropumps

Electromagnetic micropumps are structures relying on electromagnetic forces, generally either electrostatic or magnetostatic, to transform the feeding power in mechanical fluid motion. A first category of electromagnetic pumps are pumps based on electromagnetic actuators such as electrostatic actuated control valve-based pumps or electrodynamics actuated peristaltic pumps. These pumps have been reviewed in Section 8.31. A second category, which we will consider here, are electromagnetic micropumps directly based on the interaction of the electromagnetic field with the fluid to be pumped, also called electrohydrodynamic (EHD) pumps. In Section 7.5, we have seen that the presence of an electromagnetic field influences even dielectric fluids via phenomena such as dielectrophoresis; thus, a large variety of possible electromagnetic pumps can be designed.

EHD pumps can be divided into electrostatic and electrodynamics pumps, depending on the possibility to use the electrostatic approximation to describe the interaction between the fluid and the electromagnetic field or the necessity to consider a relevant magnetic effect. In this case also, as it was underlined in Section 7.6, irradiative effects are negligible, thus strictly electrodynamic terms of the Maxwell equations are in any case neglected.

A great number of different electromagnetic micropumps have been proposed for different uses, from microfluidic circuits for microsystems cooling, to drugs dispensing to implantable circuits microsystems. In this section, we will review the main architectures having a direct application to labs on chip design. Owing to the difficulty to design electromagnets in planar technology and to the general small dimensions of labs on chip, they are mainly electrostatic pumps, even if magnetostatic pumps have also been proposed [2,3,62,63].

8.3.3.1   Electrostatic Micropumps

The expression of the volume force acting on a homogeneous fluid in the presence of an electrostatic field is provided by Equation 7.221 and it is constituted mainly by a Coulomb charge term and a dielectric term due to the polarization induced by the electrical field on the dielectric fluid particles.

However, this expression assumes that the fluid is homogeneous, while in several relevant cases, the coexistence of different fluid phases can generate situations in which a spatial dielectric constant gradient exists. In this case, further elements arise in the expression of the force exerted by the field at the interface between different fluid phases [2,62,63].

Several EHD micropumps based on simple Coulomb force acting on free charges in the fluid have been fabricated, exploiting different mechanisms to generate such free charge space distribution. Space charge can be produced essentially by exploiting three phenomena:

- Inhomogeneity of the fluid: in this case, the pump is called induction pump
- Dissociation of neutral particles: in this case, the pump is called conduction pump
- Direct charge injection: in this case, the pump is called injection pump

Similar to injection pumps are pumps simply working on fluids that possess a net charge due to their own composition. It is frequent in labs on chip that nonneutral solutions are used, for example, to enhance proteins or nucleic acids solubility or to favor electrophoresis with a suitable pH of the solution. In these, the pump can rely on a self-existing charge to work.

A spatial charge distribution can be induced in a multiphase fluid through the application of an electrical field transverse to the fluid motion, as it is represented in Figure 8.43. This is an effective means due to the fact that laminar motion into microfluidic ducts prevents rapid mixing of different phases. Moreover, in case of liquids, immiscible liquids can be used to maintain a stable phase separation. When the charges have been created at the interface between different fluids, the electrodes can be activated in a traveling wave configuration and axial components of the electric field result in net fluid flow due to viscous drag.

At present, conduction micropumps are not widely considered in the field of labs on chip. The fluid to be pumped in a lab on chip is generally a macromolecule solution; in order to create charges, strong chemical or electrical processes have to be generated in the solution, which risk damaging the macromolecules that have to be processed. Micropumps based on the injection of ions into the working fluid have also been reported. For specific electrode/liquid interfaces, typically, a metal electrode with sharp features in contact with a dielectric liquid, application of a very high electric field (generally >100 kV/cm) causes ions to be injected into the bulk fluid. The Coulomb force acts on the injected charges and viscous drag generates bulk flow. Also in these cases, the application of such a high electrical field can be detrimental in labs on chip.

The type of electrostatic pump that is more suitable for application in labs on chip is probably the electroosmosis-based pump, as anticipated in Section 7.5.4. Here we have seen that a typical electroosmosis fluid velocity of a diluted water solution is of the order of 1 mm/s, almost uniform in the duct section. If we imagine that the duct has a hydrodynamic radius of 50 μm and that, after the electroosmosis section, a fully developed Poiseuille flow is established with a negligible pressure loss, we can identify the electroosmosis velocity with the average Poiseuille flow velocity. The resulting hydraulic prevalence due to the pump is

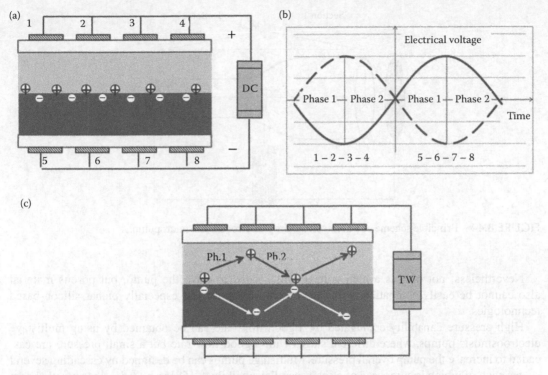

FIGURE 8.43 Working principle of an induction electrokinetic pump: creation of charges at the interface of two fluid phases (a); periodical variation of the voltage on electrodes during the creation of the pump effect (b); charge movement due to the periodical voltage variation (c). The bulk fluid movement is obtained by viscous drag due to charge movement.

$$\Delta p = \frac{\partial p}{\partial x} L_P = \frac{\varepsilon \psi_\zeta E_d}{R^2} L_P \tag{8.69}$$

where L_P is the length of the passive duct where the fluid is pushed by the pump and R is its hydrodynamic radius. Since the pressure difference depends on the inverse of the hydrodynamic radius, a high flow rate and a high prevalence cannot be simultaneously obtained. As a matter of fact, if R is high to accommodate a large flow rate, the pressure decreases too much and vice versa. Inserting in Equation 8.69 values relative to a diluted water solution, $\psi_\zeta = 100$ mV, $E_d = 10^5$ V/m, $R = 100$ μm, and $L_P = 400$ μm, we obtain $\Delta p = 2$ Pa, a too low prevalence for almost any kind of application.

The prevalence can be increased by increasing the electrical field. If the electrical field is increased to 10^6 V/m, at the expense of a much more complex structure of the electroosmosis pump [64], the prevalence becomes 20 Pa, always quite small. A more effective way of increasing the pump pressure is to put several electroosmosis pumps in parallel [65]. Even if it is quite difficult to fabricate a great number of parallel microchannels using planar technologies, porous materials [66,67] can be used, where more complex fluid patterns are created, somehow simulating a very large number of parallel electroosmosis pumps if subjected to an electrical field.

In this case, the prevalence is increased by the very small value of R, while a sufficient flow rate is also obtained since it is simply proportional to the number of parallel channels. Using Equation 8.69, the prevalence becomes equal to 1 kPa if ducts with a hydraulic radius of 200 nm are considered, while if their surface density is 75% (duct occupied area with respect to the area occupied on the surface of the porous material by the material itself), up to 250,000 ducts are present in the area providing a flow rate of the order of magnitude of 2 mL/min.

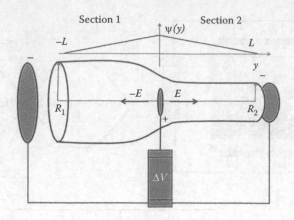

FIGURE 8.44 Principle scheme of a zero voltage drop electroosmosis micropump.

Nevertheless, not only is a high voltage still needed to drive the pump, but porous material also cannot be easily compatible with labs on chip technologies, especially planar silicon-based technologies.

High-pressure capability conjugated by a good flow rate can be obtained by using multistage electroosmosis pumps, where different stages with a good flow rate but a small pressure are cascaded to increase the pump overall pressure. Multistage pumps can be designed by cascading several stages each of which is composed of a set of parallel small ducts [68] or by using the so-called zero voltage electroosmotic pump [69], whose principle scheme is presented in Figure 8.44.

Let us introduce the ratio between the hydraulic radii of the two sections of the pump α: the second section hydraulic resistance r_2 (compare the definition in Section 7.3.4.2) and the electroosmosis flux in each of the pump sections Q_j ($j = 1, 2$). These parameters are defined as

$$\alpha = \frac{R_1}{R_2} \tag{8.70a}$$

$$r_2 = \frac{8\eta L}{\pi R_2^2} \tag{8.70b}$$

$$Q_j = -\frac{\pi \varepsilon R_j^2 \psi_\varsigma}{\eta} E \tag{8.70c}$$

where E is the electrical field intensity and the electroosmotic flow in a specific section of the pump is by definition the flow that would be realized if that section were alone and without any counterpressure.

The flow rate in the two pump sections have to be identical due to mass conservation. We have seen that in the presence of a counterpressure, the overall flow can be written as the electroosmosis flow minus the flow that would be created by the counterpressure (see Section 7.5.4), so that we can calculate the overall flow Q in both the pump sections as a function of the pressure $p(y)$ obtaining

$$Q = Q_1 - \frac{p(0)}{r_1} = -\alpha^2 Q_2 - \alpha^4 \frac{p(0)}{r_2} \tag{8.71a}$$

$$Q = Q_2 - \frac{p(L) - p(0)}{r_2} \tag{8.71b}$$

where the pressure reference is assumed at the inlet of the pump setting $p(-L) = 0$. Setting the pump flow rate equal to zero, we can evaluate the maximum pumping pressure P_{max}, that is, the pressure that the pump is able to exert in the absence of net flow, and the pump capacity Q_{max}, that is, the flow rate that the pump sustains in the absence of net hydraulic prevalence. We get

$$P_{max} = \left(\frac{1}{\alpha^2} - 1 \right) r_2 Q_2 \tag{8.72a}$$

$$Q_{max} = \frac{\alpha^2 - \alpha^4}{1 + \alpha^4} Q_2 \tag{8.72b}$$

Since we have obtained finite results, this means that the system, even in the absence of a net voltage drop at the extremes, is able to work as a pump. This is due to the different hydraulic resistance of the two pump sections that creates a different electroosmosis effect so that, when the two effects are subtracted, the net result is not zero. This is confirmed by the fact that if $\alpha = 1$, both maximum pressure and maximum flow rate become zero and that, greater α, greater the pumping effect, as shown in Figure 8.45.

From Figure 8.45, the main design parameters of a single stage of zero voltage drop pump are evident. While the maximum pressure monotonically decreases while the radii ratio passes from zero to one, the maximum flow rate has a maximum for $\alpha = \sqrt{(\sqrt{2} - 1)} \approx 0.6436$. The fact that the flow rate decreases if the radii ratio is decreased too much is quite intuitive, due to the increase of the effect of viscosity while the pump exit radius becomes smaller and smaller. The product $W = P_{max}Q_{max}/(r_2 Q_2^2)$, which can be somehow considered an overall performance indicator for this kind of pumps, is also shown in Figure 8.45.

The important characteristic of the zero-voltage drop electroosmosis pump is that different identical pump stages can be cascaded so as to maintain overall the cascade, the same flow rate by multiplying the pressure by the number of stages. Thus, the single stage can be designed at the maximum flow rate point even if the corresponding pressure is not sufficiently high. The principle scheme of such an electroosmosis multistage pump is shown in Figure 8.46. Considering data in Figure 8.45, we see that using $\alpha = \sqrt{(\sqrt{2} - 1)}$, the maximum flow through the multistage pump can be as high as $Q_2/5$ while using five stages the maximum pressure can theoretically arrive at $P_{max} \approx 25 r_2 Q_2$.

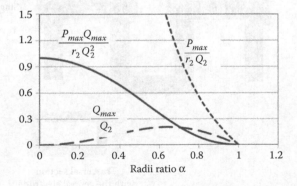

FIGURE 8.45 Universal characterization curve for a zero voltage drop electroosmosis single-stage pump. Symbols are defined in the text.

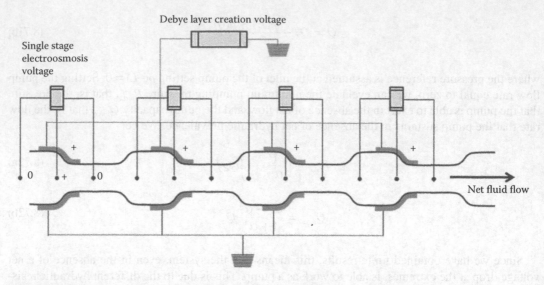

FIGURE 8.46   Principle scheme of a multistage zero voltage electroosmosis pump.

The critical element of the design of a multistage electroosmosis pump is the location of the stage electrodes, which in practice cannot be put just in the middle of the channel, and the pressure drop corresponding to the radius transitions of zero voltage drop stages and of channel curves.

A simple way to place electrodes in a planar implementation of a multistage pump is to use a serpentine channel, as shown in Figure 8.47. This also allows a simple electrical insulation of different electrodes, but has the disadvantage to increase the unwanted pressure drop since curves are added to the pump channel change of section. The effect of pressure drop can be seen clearly in experimental measures on multistage electroosmotic pumps. In Figure 8.48, the maximum pump pressure for a multistage serpentine electroosmosis pump is shown. The single stage is constituted by 10 parallel channels 800 μm long and with a dimension of 5 μm × 20 μm while the passive part of the serpentine is realized by a single channel having a section of 50 μm × 20 μm. Experimental data (from Reference [70]) are fitted with best-fit straight lines.

A detailed analysis of the multistage pump can be carried out with our electroosmosis model, adopting data for a diluted water solution, which is the fluid that was used in the experiment.

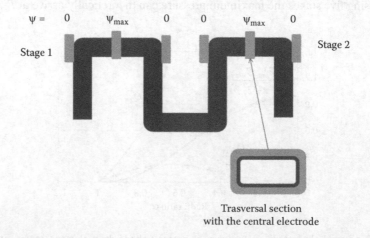

FIGURE 8.47   Possible planar implementation of a multistage electroosmotic pump.

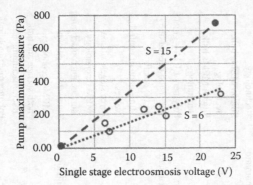

FIGURE 8.48 Maximum pump pressure for a multistage serpentine electroosmosis pump where S represents the number of stages. Dots represent experimental data and lines are obtained by data best fitting. (With kind permission from Springer Science+Business Media: *Theoretical Microfluidics*, 2007, Bruss H.)

Considering, for example, the case of an electroosmotic voltage of 10 V, we find a maximum pump pressure equal to 348 Pa in the six stages case and 870 Pa in the 15 stages case, while measured values are 150 and 350 Pa, respectively. A more detailed analysis of the pump structure reveals that this difference of about a factor 2.5 is due to different reasons such as spurious voltage drop not influencing electroosmosis. Among them, spurious pressure drop gives an important contribution.

8.3.4 COMPARISON AMONG DIFFERENT MICROPUMP ARCHITECTURES

A comparison between different types of micropumps that are suitable for application in labs on chip is provided in Tables 8.10 and 8.11. The tables are constructed by making a synthesis between a a number of bibliographies reporting fabricated micropumps so that the reported data are to be intended as indication of possible performances.

As we have already done for microvalves, we have pointed out performances of small pumps; even if not the smallest that has been realized. Bigger pumps have been realized, even if big micropumps whose dimensions are in the order of squared centimeters are frequently not suitable for lab on chip application.

The first observation is that if high pressures and high fluxes have to be obtained, mechanical pumps have to be selected, at the expenses of a greater real estate. The average maximum flux and pressure of mechanical pumps is 1.6 mL/min and 18.5 kPa while the same averages for electroosmotic and capillary pumps are 0.43 mL/min and 0.4 kPa. Moreover, capillary pumps are characterized by a particular way of working. While other pumps are devices that are able to create a pressure that is able to push the fluid through a duct external to the pump, capillary pumps coincide with the duct where the fluid has to propagate. Since the pressure due to the capillary effect is located at the fluid–environment interface, the longer the pump, the lower the exerted pressure per unit length.

These considerations on the possible flow rate and maximum pressure are to be traded off with the real space occupied by the pump. Rigorously, capillary pumps occupy no space, since the pump coincides with the propagation duct; however, in order to use capillary as propulsion pressure, the incoming fluid has to fill a previously gas-filled duct, so that a gas escape has to be foreseen in the chip design, either in one of the liquid reservoirs or somehow toward the external environment.

The average volume of electrokinetic pumps is about 0.4 mm³ with an average planar occupation of 20 mm², while the average planar occupation of mechanical pumps is about 40 mm². However, the planar occupation of control valve-based micropumps critically depends on the actuation mechanism, being smaller for electrostatic pumps and greater for piezoelectric and thermopneumatic pumps.

TABLE 8.10

Comparison among Possible Performances of Different Types of Micropumps

Type	Pump Chamber Length (mm)	Pump Chamber Height (μm)	Pump Chamber Width (mm)	Q_{max} (μL/min)	P_{max} (kPa)	f (Hz)	Power (mW)	Voltage (V)	Actuator	Notes
Control valve based	5	100–400	5	400	2.5	10–40	1000	—	Piezoelectric Thermopneumatic	Silicon MEMs technology
	4	100–400	4	800	30	1000	—	40	Electrostatic	Silicon MEMs bulk technology
	4	100–400	4	50	30	1	1000		SMA	Silicon MEMs bulk technology
	10	200–500	10	2100	11	100	1000	100	Piezoelectric Thermopneumatic	Polymers LIGA—great precision needed due to the small dimension of control valves
Peristaltic	0.5	4	0.5	10	0.6	1000	—	100	Electrostatic	Three stages, silicon MEMs technology, surface micromachining
	0.5	60	0.5		3.5	2	1000		Thermopneumatic	Three stages, silicon MEMs technology, both surface and bulk micromachining
	0.8	500	0.8	8000		100	—	100	Electrostatic	Polymer micromolding/hot embossing
Electrohydrodynamic	0.5	50		0.45	0.2	0.2	—	50	Induction	Silicon MEMs bulk technology
	3	200		15,000	0.5	0.5	—	100	Injection	Silicon MEMs bulk technology

Note: As far as the micropump aspect ratio "small" pumps are considered.

TABLE 8.11
Comparison among Possible Performances of Different Types of Micropumps

Type	Pump Length (mm)	Pump Height (μm)	Pump Width (mm)	Q_{max} (μL/min)	P_{max} (kPa)	Power (mW)	Voltage (V)	Principle	Notes
Electroosmotic	40	1	1	2.5	0.15	—	3000	Electroosmosis	Single capillary pump, glass or polymer technology
	0.3	50	83	1.8	5×10^{-4}	—	1500	Electroosmosis	Six parallel capillaries, glass or polymer technology
	0.8	20	0.05	0.012	750	—	20	Electroosmosis plus capillarity	15 serial stages each of which a parallel of 10 electroosmotic capillaries 20 μm × 50 μm. Polymer or glass technology can be used
	0.5	60	0.5	4	3.5	1000	—	Thermopneumatic	Three stages, silicon MEMs technology, both surface and bulk micromachining
Capillary	1	50	0.2	1000	18	—	—	Capillarity	The capillary is a duct 1 mm long that transports the fluid from one extreme to the other. It is not able to move the fluid out. Silicon planar technology
	1	10	0.01	300	400	—	—	Capillarity	The same as above. Parallel system of six parallel capillaries. Silicon planar technology
	25	5000	15	3.02	23.5	—	—	Transpiration	Polymer with micromolding or hot embossing (PMMA, PDMA mainly)

A small planar occupation is also attained by peristaltic pumps, due to the absence of control valves that are quite space consuming. We attain for this type of pumps the small average planar occupation of 0.4 mm², which is traded off with the small maximum pressure and flow rate attained by these pumps. An exception is represented by peristaltic micropumps designed using very deep pump chambers in polymer technology that allows high aspect ratios for large structures. In this case, the maximum pressure and flow rate are high due to the high volume of the pump chamber.

Transpiration pumps cannot be compared with the other types of micropumps since their scope is different. The target to reach if a transpiration pump is designed is not to provide high pressure or great flow rate, but providing a very small and very well-controlled flow rate at a small pressure. Thus, the more realistic quality parameter for transpiration pumps is the degree of control that can be realized when the pump works for a long time.

As far as the used technology is concerned, very complex mechanical micropumps are generally constructed either using silicon MEMs technology for all the structure or realizing part of the structure with silicon technology and part of the structure using polymers. Frequently, when complex structures as a large number of active valves or superimposed control vales have to be fabricated, surface MEMs technology is needed. Micropumps requiring a simpler structure, such as transpiration or electrokinetic micropumps, can be also fabricated using polymer technologies. In these cases, micromolding or hot embossing are convenient technologies for their low cost.

8.4   SAMPLE PREPARATION: MICROMIXERS

In macroscopic fluid systems, mixing different fluids is not a difficult task: microturbulence is almost always present and, if needed, macroscopic vortices can be easily caused. Turbulence causes a fast and effective mixing without any particular design attention. The situation is completely different in microfluidic systems, where the Reynolds number is very low and pure laminar flow is present. If we consider a mixing strategy simply based on injecting two different fluids to be mixed in the same channel from nearby ducts, at the start of the common channel, no mixing happens. Depending on the injection conditions, the fluids form either two parallel and disjoined laminar fluxes or droplets forms, while the higher pressure flow breaks the continuity of the lower pressure one. In the first case, while the nearby laminar flows propagate along the common channel, mixing happens due to diffusion; in the second case, diffusion slowly mix droplet with the environmental fluid.

In order to have an idea of the involved dynamics, let us imagine that mixing between parallel and continuous flows happens in a rectangular duct whose width d_y is much larger than the height d_z so that we can assume the duct as having two dimensions. Let us assume that the initial laminar flows come from similar ducts and are constituted by diluted water solutions of different macromolecules. For the system symmetry, the width of the individual fluxes aligned at the start of the mixing duct will be the same, as their average velocity v. Since the overall flow rate has to be constant in different sections of the common duct, the average velocity is not affected by the mixing phenomenon.

The typical diffusion length τ of one of the macromolecules up to the far wall of the duct can be written as

$$\tau \sim \frac{d_y^2}{D} \tag{8.73}$$

where D is the diffusion coefficient. Since the diffusion is asymptotically an exponential process, we can assume that diffusion is almost at equilibrium in a time that is of the order of five times τ. The distance L that is covered by the fluid due to convection in such a time is given by

$$L = 5v\frac{d_y^2}{D} \tag{8.74}$$

while the overall flow rate Q through the duct can be written approximately as in Equation 7.75

$$Q = \frac{1}{2} \frac{\Delta p}{L\eta} \frac{B^3}{\mathcal{P}^2} = \frac{1}{8} \frac{\Delta p}{L\eta} d_z^3 d_y \qquad (8.75)$$

and the Taylor diffusion coefficient D_T has to be considered instead of the particle diffusion coefficient where transversal diffusion during Poiseuille flow generates mixing.

The difficulty that is intrinsic in the design of mixers results from the simple Equations 8.73, 8.74, and 8.75. In order to obtain a short mixing length, the channels should be as small as possible, but a small channel section is not compatible with a high flow rate: in particular, asymptotically the mixer length tends to infinity as the square of the duct width while the flow rate tends to zero as the duct width itself. This means that either a clever design of the mixer has to be carried out in order to attain a good trade-off between these opposite trends or a different mixing mechanism has to be found. Mixers exploiting simple diffusion of one element into the other and adopting an elaborated design to obtain good performances are called lamination mixers [71–73].

8.4.1 Lamination Mixers

8.4.1.1 Basic Lamination Mixer Structures

The base structure of a lamination mixer, the so-called Y mixer, is reported in Figure 8.49a. The fluid dynamic governing equation is in this case a system of two convection–diffusion Equations 7.166, one for each of the incoming fluids. From now on, we will call fluid A and fluid B the fluids coming from the two inlets (ducts A and B) of the Y mixer and, if these fluids are solutions, we will call solute A and solute B the respective solutes.

This system is quite difficult to solve, in general. If we consider the convergence of two arbitrary fluxes into a common duct, it is quite intuitive that a large variety of possible regimes can be

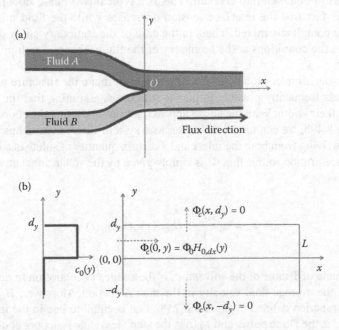

FIGURE 8.49 Principle scheme of a Y mixer (a) and rectangular shape of the region where the diffusion–convection equation governing the mixer working has to be solved (b). The coordinate system assumed for the system modeling is also shown.

generated, depending on the relative flow rates, on the hydrodynamic parameters of the converging fluids and on the geometry of the zones where the ducts join. In particular, if the flow rate of one of the liquids is much higher than the other or if the liquids have very different viscosities, the continuity of one of the fluxes can be broken, causing the generation of different types of droplets, as it is briefly discussed in Section 8.7.

A great simplification is attained in the case in which the two streams come from identical ducts and have the same hydrodynamic properties: the same viscosity, the same average velocity, and the same diffusion coefficient one into the other. These assumptions are not only useful to attain a mathematical model, but they also represent a quite important practical case: that of two diluted water solutions of similar molecules.

In this case, it is evident that no droplet forms due to the problem symmetry and that the diffusion of solute A in fluid B is exactly specular to the diffusion of solute B in fluid A, so that it is expected that the problem can be reduced to a single diffusion–convection equation. This is possible by modeling the system as a continuous and unperturbed solvent flow with continuous addition of one of the solutes from one of the input ducts: for example, of solute A from input duct A. The fact that solute B is also present is not relevant if the solutions are sufficiently diluted, since the diffusion coefficients do not depend on the macromolecule concentrations. At the end of the calculation, the evolution of solute B is simply obtained by symmetrizing the evolution of solute A.

It is to be noticed that the simple approach we adopt here is possible only when mixing of diluted solutions based on the same solvent is considered. In this case, but for the perturbation corresponding to the converging inlets that affects the flow for a distance of the order of the inlets hydraulic radius (compare Section 7.3.4.4), the flow can be considered almost coincident with a Poiseuille flow of the solvent itself. In several applications, different fluids are also mixed by using a Y mixer. In this case, the situation is much more complex due to the fact that when the fluids are inserted inside the main mixer duct, the flow of a single fluid cannot be determined using a no-slip boundary condition. The presence of the interface with the other fluid, where the slipping ratio is determined by the condition of continuity of the stress at the interface, that is, by the value of the surface tension, has to be taken into account. This is a typical two-phase flow problem, which is complicated by the fact that the interface tension decreases while the fluid mixes, to disappear when the fluids are completely mixed. Thus, in the case of the stationary study of a Y mixer mixing different fluids, the conditions at the boundary of the fluids changes with position, depending on the mixing rate.

Coming back to our simpler problem, we will also approximate the structure with a two-dimensional model, as it is frequently possible in planar structures, assuming that the depth of ducts is much smaller than their width. With the above approximations and using the coordinate system that is shown in Figure 8.49b, we can model the mixer as a system where continuous solvent flow happens with solvent arriving from both the inlets and a certain quantity of solute is added continuously at inlet A. This concentration source flux Φ_c is simply given by the solute concentration rate arriving from inlet A, that is

$$\Phi_c = c_0 \frac{v d_y d_z}{V_s} H_{0,d_x}(y)\delta(x)\eta_H(t) \tag{8.76}$$

where V_s is the volume of 1 mole of the solvent, c_0 is the solute concentration in duct A measured in moles/m³, and v is the average fluid velocity in the duct A section. Moreover, $H_{0,d_x}(y)$ is the rectangular Heaviside function defined in Equation 7.182 that is equal to one in the interval $[0, d_x]$ and zero otherwise, $\delta(x)$ is the Dirac pulse, and $\eta_H(t)$ is the step Heaviside function, equal to one for $t > 0$.

Equation 8.76 is simply obtained considering that $c_0 v$ is the number of moles entering per unit time and unit area into the main duct and that they are diluted in a solvent volume V_s, that is, the volume of 1 mole of the solvent. Moreover, the assumption of a constant concentration along the section of duct A is performed, which is justified under the condition of dominant Taylor dispersion in duct A (compare Section 7.4.5).

Neglecting the small variation of the average solute flow speed with the transversal coordinate, the transient solution of the problem is obtained by solving the diffusion–convection equation, which in this case is written as

$$\Phi_c - v\frac{\partial c}{\partial x} + D\left(\frac{\partial^2 c}{\partial x^2} + \frac{\partial^2 c}{\partial y^2}\right) = \frac{\partial c}{\partial t} \tag{8.77}$$

where the minus sign depends on the sign of the average speed. Equation 8.77 has to be solved with boundary conditions assuring a null flux through the main duct walls and zero concentration at the end of the infinitely long mixer, which is written as

$$\left.\frac{\partial c(x,y)}{\partial y}\right|_{y=-d_x} = \left.\frac{\partial c(x,y)}{\partial y}\right|_{y=d_x} = 0 \tag{8.78a}$$

$$c(\infty, y) = 0 \tag{8.78b}$$

Solving Equation 8.77 in a transient situation is quite difficult, practically requiring numerical algorithms; the stationary evolution of the mixed can be however determined analytically. In this, a stationary boundary condition can be added requiring that the concentration on the inlet A is constant and equal to c_0, thus representing the continuous replenishing of solutes from duct A.

Thus, the governing equation becomes

$$v\frac{\partial c}{\partial x} = D\left(\frac{\partial^2 c}{\partial x^2} + \frac{\partial^2 c}{\partial y^2}\right) \tag{8.79}$$

with the following boundary conditions:

$$c(0, y) = H_{0,d_x}(y)c_0 \tag{8.80a}$$

$$c(\infty, y) = c_0/2 \tag{8.80b}$$

$$\left.\frac{\partial c(x,y)}{\partial y}\right|_{y=-d_x} = \left.\frac{\partial c(x,y)}{\partial y}\right|_{y=d_x} = 0 \tag{8.80c}$$

Equation 8.79 can be solved by variable separation due to the rectangular geometry of the solution domain as it is shown in Figure 8.49b.

The solution obtained by eigenfunction superposition and imposition of the boundary conditions is written as

$$c(x,y) = \frac{c_0}{2} + \frac{2c_0}{\pi}\sum_{n=1}^{\infty}\frac{\sin(n\pi\alpha)}{n}\cos\left(n\pi\frac{y}{2d_y}\right)\exp\left(-\frac{2n^2\pi^2}{P_e + \sqrt{P_e^2 + 4n^2\pi^2}}\frac{x}{2d_y}\right) \tag{8.81}$$

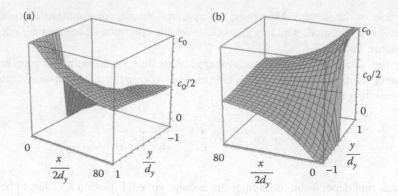

FIGURE 8.50 Stationary distribution of the concentration of one of the two solutions diffusing in an Y-shaped mixer seen from two different points of view evidencing the decrease of the concentration on the one side (a) and the increase on the other side (b).

where α is the ratio of the solution flow rates in the inlet A and in the mixing duct, which in our case is equal to 0.5 since the same flow rate arrives from both the ducts A and B, and P_e is the Pécle number, which is expressed in this case as $P_e = 2vd_y/D$.

The decay rate of the leading asymptotical term of Equation 8.81 is controlled by the Pécle number. This means that, since the diffusion coefficient is determined by the species to process, the mixing can be speeded by both decreasing the fluid average velocity and reducing the channel dimension. Both these measures however have to be traded off with the consequent reduction of the mixer flow rate. The typical distribution of the concentration in steady state in a Y mixer is shown in Figure 8.50 assuming $P_e = 300$, which can be obtained, for example, with a diffusion coefficient of 10^{-10} m²/s, an average velocity of 30 mm/min and a total width of the mixer channel of 60 μm.

8.4.1.2 Parallel, Sequential and Other Lamination Mixer Structures

From Figure 8.50, it is clear that even using quite small mixing ducts and small velocities, the mixing duct has to be quite long (about 5 mm in the case of the figure) to obtain a complete mixing. Two different strategies can be used to compact the mixing design: using a serpentine duct [74,75] as shown in Figure 8.51 or performing the mixing in a large number of parallel, small mixing ducts, as shown in Figure 8.52 [71]. The second system can be attained either fabricating a set of parallel channels as in the figure or, as in the case of electroosmotic pumps, by resorting to the use of porous materials, where percolation generates an effect very similar to that of a parallel of several ducts.

The profile of the concentration of one of the solutes in a parallel mixer is shown in Figure 8.53 using the same input flow parameters of Figure 8.50. The multiple flow mixing can be optimized by realizing strictly adjacent flows. This is a practical configuration when different flows are not created by different mixing ducts but by a structure that divides the flow coming from each inlet

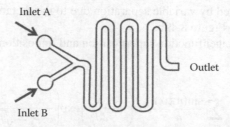

FIGURE 8.51 Schematic structure of a serpentine lamination mixer.

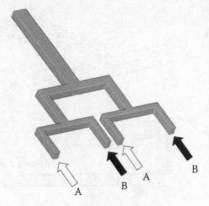

FIGURE 8.52   Schematic structure of a parallel lamination mixer.

duct and alternates them in the mixing duct to obtain a more efficient mixing. A possible scheme of an implementation arrangement of such a parallel lamination mixer is shown in Figure 8.54a. The two effects can also be combined by using a serpentine structure where every structure branch is a parallel of several small ducts.

Another possible arrangement to realize an efficient lamination micromixer is the so-called sequential micromixer. In this case, either active valves are used to start and stop the liquid flow in the two inlets of the mixer or the property of several micropumps to create a periodical fluid flow is exploited. The two flows are periodically started and stopped in such a way that when one is active, the other is nonactive. Such a micromixer feeding creates a sequence of fluids packets having a large interface area so as to cause fast diffusion. The scheme of a sequential lamination mixer is presented in Figure 8.54b.

In order to model the working of a sequential lamination mixer, let us observe that to improve the mixing efficiency, intuition tells us that the mixing channel has to be constructed quite wide, so that the contact between subsequent fluid packets is maximized, while the channel height is frequently dictated by the available technology. The velocity profile of the Poiseuille flow in a square channel with very different sides can be evaluated with Equation 7.88 and an example of such an evaluation is reported in Figure 8.55. With a ratio between the duct section dimensions of 7.5 the horizontal

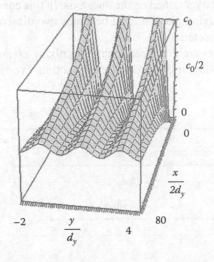

FIGURE 8.53   Stationary profile of the concentration in a parallel lamination mixer.

(a)

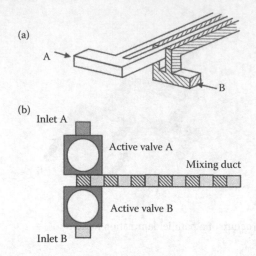

(b)

FIGURE 8.54 Alternative schemes for lamination micromixers: possible implementation scheme of a parallel micromixer (a) and principle scheme of a sequential micromixer (b).

velocity profile is almost constant but in the vicinity of the walls, while the vertical profile is a typical Poiseuille parabola. This trend is increasingly evident while horizontal to vertical dimension ratio increases, so it can be supposed that in case of very flat ducts, considering a constant horizontal velocity can be an accurate approximation.

This idea can be verified analytically by evaluating the Poiseuille flow among two infinite plates, that is a square duct infinitely wide, and using it to approximate the real profile in the flat duct. It is found (8.70) that the error in the flow rate is 7% for a dimension ratio of 10 and decreases up to about 2% for a dimension ratio of 30. Approximating the mixing channel as two infinite parallel plates allows us to write the velocity profile along the y axis as

$$v(y) = v_0 \left(1 - 4 \frac{y^2}{d_y^2} \right)$$
(8.82)

where v_0 is the maximum velocity attained on the duct axis. In this condition, the diffusion–convection equation governing the mixing phenomenon becomes two dimensional, since the time evolution in this case cannot be neglected.

While different fluid packets are displaced along the mixing channel, the solutes that are contained in each packet undergo Taylor dispersion during motion. We have seen in Section 7.4.5 that

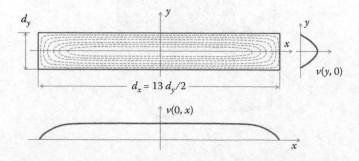

FIGURE 8.55 Velocity profile of the Poiseuille motion in a "flat" square duct.

the phenomenon of Taylor dispersion is regulated by an equivalent dispersion coefficient D_T that in the case of a flux between two parallel plates can be derived with a procedure completely parallel to those reported in Section 7.4.5 for a circular duct resulting in

$$D_T = D + \frac{d_y^2}{210D} v_0^2 \tag{8.83}$$

where the correction to the diffusion coefficient has the same dependence on the fluid dynamic parameter already found in the case of the circular duct, being 4.3 times smaller due to the smaller numerical multiplication factor.

Under the above hypothesis and taking into account Taylor dispersion, the convection diffusion equation is written as

$$\frac{\partial c}{\partial t} + v(y)\frac{\partial c}{\partial x} = D_T \frac{\partial^2 c}{\partial x^2} \tag{8.84}$$

In order to state the initial and boundary conditions for the solution of Equation 8.84, we have to determine the behavior of the valves. We will assume that the opening and closing of valves is instantaneous and that the valves are never both open. With these assumptions, the concentration of the solute entering from the inlet A is given by the square wave function represented in Figure 8.56. Assuming that the concentrations of the two solutes in the inlets are equal, the final concentration ratio is equal to the parameter α that characterizes the wave pulse length.

On the basis of the parameters defined in Figure 8.56, Equation 8.84 initial and boundary conditions can be written as

$$c(0,t) = c_0 \sum_{k=0}^{\infty} [H_{0,\alpha T/2}(t - kT) + H_{(1-,\alpha/2)T,T}(t - kT)] \tag{8.85a}$$

$$c(x,\infty) = \alpha c_0 \tag{8.85b}$$

$$c(x,0) = 0 \tag{8.85c}$$

Equation 8.84 with the conditions of (8.85) can be solved using the variable separation method, and imposing the conditions of (8.85) on the general solution obtained by the eigenfunctions superposition.

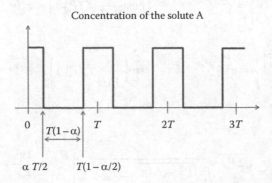

FIGURE 8.56 Concentration of the solute entering from the inlet A in a sequential lamination mixer.

The qualitative evolution of the phenomenon can be understood considering the system Pécle number that is written as

$$P_{eT} = \frac{2vd_y}{D_T} = \frac{1}{\dfrac{1}{P_e} + \dfrac{1}{P_{Tay}}} = \frac{810 P_e}{810 + P_e} \tag{8.86}$$

where $P_{Tay} = 410 \, D/v_0 d_y = 810/P_e$. The Pécle number in this case appears to be the parallel of two different nondimensional numbers: the standard Pécle number due to molecular diffusion and a Taylor number P_{Tay} accounting for the further dispersion effect due to the fluid motion. In a standard situation where $D \sim 10^{-10}$ m^2/s, $d_y \sim 10^{-4}$ m, and $v_0 \sim 1$ mm/s, we have $P_e = 1000$ and $P_{eT} = 447$. The result is that the Pécle number, which is the ratio between the effectiveness of the convection and that of the diffusion, is sensibly decreased by the mixer architecture so that we can expect that a shorter mixing duct will be needed if the sequential architecture is used with respect to the case of a pure Y lamination mixer.

The correctness of this analysis is confirmed by a quantitative evaluation of the solution of Equation 8.84. The solution is written as

$$c(x,t) = c_0 \alpha + \frac{2c_0}{\pi} \sum_{n=1}^{\infty} \frac{\sin(\alpha\pi n)}{n} \mathcal{Re}\left\{ e^{\frac{1}{2}\frac{x}{v_0 T}\left(P_{eT} - \sqrt{P_{eT}^2 + 8i\pi n P_{eT}}\right)} e^{2\pi i \frac{t}{T}} \right\} \tag{8.87}$$

where T is the sequential mixer period, i is the imaginary unit, and $\mathcal{Re}\{z\}$ indicates the real part of the imaginary number z. Just looking at the solution we see that the time behavior results to be periodic with period equal to T, since

$$\mathcal{Re}\left\{ z e^{2\pi i \frac{t}{T}} \right\} = \cos\left(2\pi \frac{t}{T} \right) \mathcal{Re}\{z\} - \sin\left(2\pi \frac{t}{T} \right) \mathcal{Im}\{z\} \tag{8.88}$$

where z is any complex number and $\mathcal{Im}\{z\}$ is the function extracting the imaginary part of a complex number. This is not surprising if we consider the periodicity of the boundary conditions at $x = 0$.

As far as the spatial evolution is concerned, it is a dumped oscillation with a leading dumping term corresponding to n = 1. To qualitatively analyze the spatial behavior of the solution, let us evaluate real and imaginary parts of the spatial transitory term. We have

$$\mathcal{Re}\left\{ e^{\frac{1}{2}\frac{x}{v_0 T}\left(P_{eT} - \sqrt{P_{eT}^2 + 8i\pi n P_{eT}}\right)} \right\} = e^{\frac{1}{2}\frac{x}{v_0 T}P_{eT} - \frac{x}{v_0 T}f_+(P_{eT})} \cos\left(\frac{x}{v_0 T}f_-(P_{eT}) \right) \approx e^{-\frac{4\pi^2}{P_{eT}}\frac{x}{v_0 T}} \cos\left(\frac{2\pi x}{v_0 T} \right) \tag{8.89a}$$

$$\mathcal{Im}\left\{ e^{\frac{1}{2}\frac{x}{v_0 T}\left(P_{eT} - \sqrt{P_{eT}^2 + 8i\pi n P_{eT}}\right)} \right\} = e^{\frac{1}{2}\frac{x}{v_0 T}P_{eT} - \frac{x}{v_0 T}f_+(P_{eT})} \sin\left(\frac{x}{v_0 T}f_-(P_{eT}) \right) \approx e^{-\frac{4\pi^2}{P_{eT}}\frac{x}{v_0 T}} \sin\left(\frac{2\pi x}{v_0 T} \right) \tag{8.89b}$$

where

$$f_\pm(P_{eT}) = \frac{\sqrt{2P_{eT}}}{4} \sqrt{\left(\sqrt{P_{eT}^2 + 64\pi^2} \pm P_{eT} \right)} \approx \begin{cases} \dfrac{P_{eT}}{2} + \dfrac{4\pi^2}{P_{eT}} & \text{for } f_+ \\ 2\pi & \text{for } f_- \end{cases} \tag{8.90}$$

and the approximation has an error smaller than 1% for $P_{eT} \geq 100$, which is in almost all the interesting cases. From Equation 8.89, the space behavior of the series leading term is clear; it oscillates with a period equal to $v_0 T$, which results to be the typical space scale of the phenomenon and is dumped exponentially with a characteristic length of $(v_0 T P_{eT})/4 \pi^2$. From the characteristic dumping length, we see that there are several ways to obtain a short mixing duct: it can be obtained by reducing the Pécle number, that is why the sequential architecture has been introduced, but it can also be obtained by increasing the switching frequency of the mixer valves, so that it is important in this kind of mixers to use valves with a fast response time, which do not have a great mass to move when operating. The faster among the mechanical valves are electrostatic valves, which can give good results in this case. Otherwise, some types of nonmechanical valves can be used to reduce the response time.

The spatial behavior of the solute concentration in the mixer duct is shown in Figure 8.57 for different Pécle numbers maintaining the same fluid average velocity in the duct, as is resulted by the fact that all the functions have the same pseudoperiod. The curves refer to the instant at the middle of the period in which the considered solute is injected in the duct. The approximate length L_{mix} of the needed mixing duct can be derived from the exponential dependence of the leading sum term by considering that the transient term is ended after π times the characteristic length of the phenomenon, where the exponential term is approximately equal to 0.043. Substituting the expression of the modified Pécle number, we get

$$L_{mix} = \frac{801}{2} \frac{\langle v \rangle^2 d_y T}{801 D + 2 \langle v \rangle^2 T} \tag{8.91}$$

Numeric values resulting from Equation 8.91 are reported in Figure 8.58 where the mixing length is shown versus the switching time and the fluid average velocity assuming $D = 10^{-10}$ m²/s and $d_y = 100$ μm. Quite fast switching rates are considered, to show how this is important to obtain short mixers.

Besides parallel and sequential lamination mixers, several other types of lamination mixers have been suggested, with complex designs intended to optimize the mixing performances. An example is the H lamination mixer [76] whose architecture is shown in Figure 8.59a besides the photograph of a prototype built using MEMs technologies (Figure 8.59b). This is an example of split and recombination mixer, which means that the fluxes of the two fluids are periodically split and recombined to achieve a better mixing efficiency.

The effect of the shape of curves that unavoidably are present in lamination mixers has also been optimized in order to improve mixing efficiency [77]. As a matter of fact, the perturbations

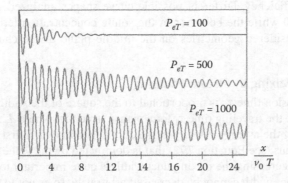

FIGURE 8.57 Concentration spatial dependence in a sequential lamination mixer for different values of the Pércle number modified to take into account Taylor dispersion.

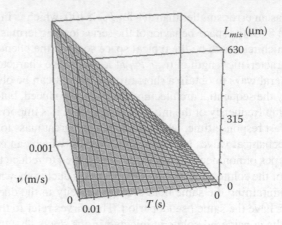

FIGURE 8.58 Sequential lamination mixer length versus fluid average velocity and switching rate.

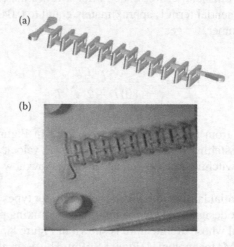

FIGURE 8.59 H-shaped lamination mixer structure (a) and scanning electron microscope image of a fabricated prototype (b). (Reproduced from *Journal of the American Institute of Chemical Engineers*, vol. 50, Jiang F. et al., Helical flows and chaotic mixing in curved micro channels, pp. 2297–2305, Copyright 2004, with permission from Elsevier.)

of the velocity field near curves are particularly important, especially in serpentine mixers to improve the mixing efficiency. Different possible curve shapes analyzed in Reference [77] are reported in Figure 8.60 while the behavior of the solute concentration (ethanol (C_2H_6O) in this case) for the three considered geometries on the middle plane of the channel cross section is reported in Figure 8.61.

8.4.1.3 Lamination Mixing by Stream Focusing

The characteristic diffusion time τ_D is proportional to the square of the width d of the mixing duct being $\tau_D \sim d_y^2/D$, while the traveling time τ_T for a planar structure, where $d_y \gg d_z$, weakly depends on the duct width, being the average velocity in the duct depending on a first approximation by the hydrodynamic duct radius (see Equation 7.72) that is dominated by the value of d_z. These considerations evidence while decreasing the mixing duct width is quite important to increase mixing efficiency. However, the duct width cannot be decreased arbitrarily, so as not to decrease the flow rate too much and due to technological limitations. As a matter of fact, even if ducts of a width of few hundreds of nanometers can be in principle fabricated on a silicon platform, the needed technology

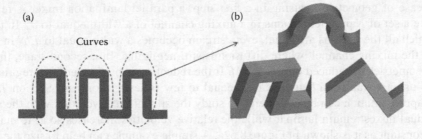

FIGURE 8.60   Different possible curve shapes for the design of a lamination serpentine mixer: mixer scheme (a) and curve shapes (b).

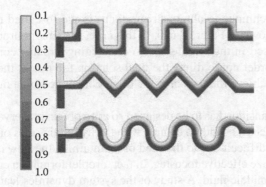

FIGURE 8.61   Solute concentration for the three geometries considered in Figure 8.60 on the middle plane of the channel cross section. (Reproduced from *Chemical Engineering Journal*, vol. 150, Hossain S., Ansari M. A., Kim K.-Y., Evaluation of the mixing performance of three passive micromixers, pp. 492–501, Copyright 2009, with permission from Elsevier.)

is much more complex requiring stepper lithography and phase masks instead of simple optical lithography as shown in Section 4.5.

An alternative way to realize a very small mixing flow width without the need of constructing submicrometer channels relies on the laminar nature of flux in microfluidic channels and it is called stream focus. Two different types of stream focus techniques can be used, as shown in Figure 8.62.

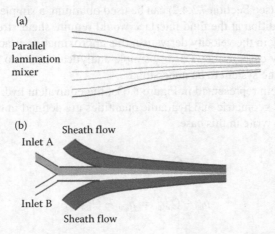

FIGURE 8.62   Principle of the working of a geometrical focus mixer (a) and of a hydrodynamic focus mixer (b).

In the case of geometric focusing in a first step, a parallel lamination mixer is realized, so as to create a set of N parallel streams in a mixing channel of a width equal to d_y. In the simple case in which all the streams are equal, every stream occupies a width equal to d_y/N in the initial section of the mixing channel, where diffusion is still negligible. In a second stage, the channel width is geometrically reduced of a factor M. If the reduction is performed by a regular channel shape and using a transition length at least equal to few times d_y (compare Section 7.3.4.4), an adiabatic approximation can be considered to study the spatial flux evolution with the result that the individual fluxes remain laminar while the relative velocities increases so as to maintain the flow rate constant as it is shown in Figure 8.62a. A simple example can help to size the potentiality of this technique. If we consider a parallel, 10 double streams mixer with a mixing channel 80 μm long and we restrict the channel to a width of 5 μm with a gradual evolution in a space of 240 μm, we have that the single solute stream becomes 250 nm wide, with a great improvement of the mixing efficiency.

The other available technique to obtain stream focus is the so-called hydraulic focus [78–80] and it is schematically shown in Figure 8.62b. In this case, the stream produced by a simple lamination mixer is compressed in the middle of two converging streams coming from lateral ducts at a higher pressure. In order not to dilute the final solution too much, the sheath streams, which are the streams used to achieve the focusing, are often constituted by a fluid immiscible with the solutions to mix.

Also in this case the transition has to be designed so as to obtain preservation of the laminar flow so that the inner flux reduces its width to comply with the hydraulic rules of the common flux in the central duct. This can be difficult due to the need of maintaining the flow rate of the shear streams as high as possible to realize effective focusing. In fact, droplet formation can arise due to the break of flow continuity of the middle fluid. A study of the system dynamics leads to the conclusion that the nondimensional number driving the process of droplet formation is the capillary number of the ducts, as detailed in Section 8.7, and that an accurate design of the system can either maintain steady-state laminar flow or drive the formation of well-controlled droplets. Delaying more details on the conditions for droplet formation to Section 8.7, here we assume that the system is designed so as to maintain continuous laminar flow of all the considered fluids.

Even if the conservation of laminar flow is assumed as an initial condition, a detailed study of mixing by hydrodynamic focus is very complex, requiring the study of Taylor diffusion while multiphase flow happens, especially when boundary conditions at the interface between fluids causes a sensible slip of one fluid with respect to the other [81]. An approximation of the final width of the focused beam can be attained if no slip at the fluids interface is assumed so as to assume continuity of the fluid velocity and of its derivative at the fluid interfaces. In this case, the electrical–hydrodynamic equivalence [79] (see Section 7.3.4.2) can be used obtaining a simple problem to solve. Since a correct boundary condition at the fluid interface would require shear stress continuity, generally implying a discontinuity in the velocity derivative, this approximation is accurate only in very particular situations. In any case, it allows a very simple analytical model to be derived allowing the qualitative behavior of the system to be understood.

Considering the system represented in Figure 8.63a, the equivalent hydraulic circuit is provided by Figure 8.63b. All the geometric and hydraulic quantities are defined in the figure.

Kirchhoff's relations write in this case

$$Q_{Tot} = Q_{in} + 2Q_s \tag{8.92a}$$

$$p_{in} - Q_{in}r_{in} = p_{out} - Q_{Tot}r_{out} \tag{8.92b}$$

$$p_s - Q_s r_s = p_{out} - Q_{Tot}r_{out} \tag{8.92c}$$

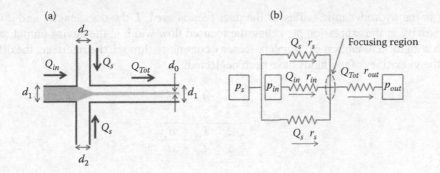

FIGURE 8.63 Structure of T-shaped stream hydrodynamic focus device (a) and equivalent hydrodynamic circuit (b). Hydraulic resistances of the different branches are represented with r, and flow rate and pressures with p and Q as usual.

where the hydraulic resistances of the different branches are indicated with r. The design parameters are generally the input pressure and the sheath fluid input pressure, p_{in} and p_s, respectively, besides the ducts geometry, the outside pressure, and the characteristics of the considered fluids. All the other parameters can be evaluated consequently.

In particular, we can calculate the input flow rates as

$$Q_{in} = \frac{p_{in} - p_{out}}{r_{in} + r_{out}} \tag{8.93a}$$

$$Q_s = \frac{p_s - p_{out}}{r_s + r_{out}} \tag{8.93b}$$

$$Q_{Tot} = \frac{p_{in} - p_{out}}{r_{in} + r_{out}} + 2\frac{p_s - p_{out}}{r_s + r_{out}} \tag{8.93c}$$

A Poiseuille flow will establish far from the T-shaped transition due to the assumed velocity continuity at the fluid interfaces.

Assuming that the width of the focused stream is much smaller than the width of the focusing duct (i.e., $d_0 \ll d_1$), we can suppose that the focused stream flow rate and the overall flow rate in the focusing ducts can also be written as

$$2Q_s \approx (d_1 - d_0)d_z v \tag{8.94a}$$

$$Q_{in} \approx 2d_0 d_z v \tag{8.94b}$$

Using Equations 8.93 and 8.94, we obtain

$$\frac{Q_{in}}{Q_s} = \frac{2d_0}{(d_1 - d_0)} = \frac{p_{in} - p_{out}}{p_s - p_{out}} \frac{r_s + r_{out}}{r_{in} + r_{out}} \tag{8.95}$$

evaluating the hydraulic resistance of rectangular channels from Equation 7.74 as

$$r = \frac{1}{8} \frac{\mathcal{R}^2 B}{L\eta} = \frac{d}{L\eta} \tag{8.96}$$

where $\mathcal{R}$ is the hydrodynamic radius, B the duct section area, L the duct length, and d the duct depth, we arrive at the expression providing the focused flow width at the device output, where in coherence with the assumption of complete velocity continuity through the interface, the difference between the viscosities of the fluids have been neglected:

$$d_0 = d_1 \frac{\dfrac{d_2}{d_1}}{2 \dfrac{\Delta p_s}{\Delta p_{in}} \dfrac{L_{in}}{L_s} + \dfrac{d_2}{d_1}} \tag{8.97}$$

Although quite approximated and usable only when using a sheath liquid at least approximately with the same viscosity of the processed liquid, Equation 8.97 is useful to simply evaluate the order of magnitude of the focusing that can be obtained through hydraulic focus.

The focused flow width mainly depends on three nondimensional ratios: $\bar{p} = \Delta p_s / \Delta p_{in}, \delta = d_2/d_1$, and $\lambda = L_s/L_{in}$. Generally, $\bar{p}$ is difficult to manage as a design parameter, since it is widely determined by other elements in the hydraulic circuit. The main system design parameters are δ and λ. To evidence their role, the focus ratio $\varphi = d_1/d_0$ can be expressed as

$$\varphi = \frac{2\bar{p}\lambda + \delta}{\delta} \tag{8.98}$$

and it is shown versus δ and λ in Figure 8.64 for two values of $\bar{p}$. Very high focusing ratios, up to 40 in the figure, can be obtained by having an input duct much longer than the ducts adducting the sheath liquid.

In case of the presence of a sheath liquid with a viscosity much larger than that of the focusing liquid, the simplified approach we have used here cannot be adopted and a fluid dynamic two-phase flow problem has to be solved to study stream focus mixers. Since the mixer is generally much longer than the transition region where the input channels converge, we can assume that the transition region can be neglected as far as the mixing effect is considered and the system works like a lamination mixer with a very small channel width.

A different approach can be used for a more accurate analysis of the stream focusing mixer in the case in which continuity of the fluid flows is assumed and focusing happens in a sufficiently short region where the effect of mixing can be neglected. In this case, the system can be modeled as the sequence of a stream focusing device and an equivalent lamination mixer.

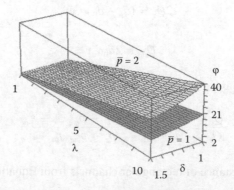

FIGURE 8.64 Focusing ratio with respect to the ratio between the width and the length of the input and lateral channels called δ and λ, respectively. Two values of the pressure ratio $\bar{p}$ are considered.

Whatever be the stream focus dynamics, far from the focusing region, the system has to establish a steady-state regime that is determined by the input parameters of the mixer, such as the input fluxes, the liquids viscosities and the input duct dimensions. In particular, let us assume that mixing between diluted water solutions has to be obtained and that an immiscible liquid of higher viscosity is used as a focusing liquid.

The stationary steady-state flux out of the focusing region can be viewed as the movement of three different fluid layers under the effect of a pressure difference Δp. To derive a mathematical model providing closed forms solutions for this flow, we also assume that the mixing region is constituted by a thin slab duct of length equal to L.

Since the contact surface between different liquids is flat, no Young–Laplace pressure drop creates on the surface; moreover, due to the translational symmetry of the system, the velocity field, since no flow continuity beak happens, has to be of the form $v = v(y)x$ and the pressure drop along the duct has to be linear, as it happens in the single-phase Poiseuille flow. Moreover, owing to the y inversion symmetry of the system, the velocity fields in the two high-viscosity fluids also must have a y inversion symmetry, while the velocity field in the low-viscosity fluid has to be an even function. The situation is shown in Figure 8.65.

The boundary conditions to be imposed on the Stokes equation, which has to be separately solved in each fluid layer, are no slip condition at the duct walls and the velocity and shear stress continuity at the fluid interface. The shear stress continuity is imposed by the fact that the local force density on the interface is equal to the shear stress derivative and it would be infinite if the derivative would be infinite due to a discontinuity of the shear stress. Owing to the expression (7.34) of the shear stress and to the particular system geometry, the shear stress continuity condition is written as

$$\eta_1 \left. \frac{\partial v_1(y)}{\partial y} \right|_{y=h} = \eta_2 \left. \frac{\partial v_2(y)}{\partial y} \right|_{y=h} \tag{8.99}$$

where condition (8.160) synthesize both the boundary condition at the fluid interfaces due to the symmetries of the functions $v_1(y)$ and $v_2(y)$.

Solving the Stokes equation and imposing the boundary conditions, we get

$$v_1(y) = \frac{1}{2\eta_1} \frac{\partial p}{\partial x}(H^2 - y^2) \quad (h < y < H) \tag{8.100a}$$

$$v_2(y) = \frac{1}{2\eta_2} \frac{\partial p}{\partial x}\left[\frac{\eta_2}{\eta_1}(H^2 - h^2) + h^2 - y^2 \right] \quad (0 < y < h) \tag{8.100b}$$

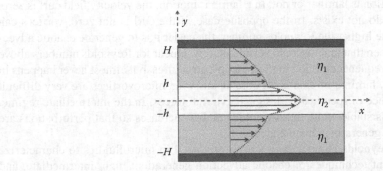

FIGURE 8.65 Multiphase Poiseuille flow in a straight duct: a fluid with small viscosity η_2 is enclosed in between two layers of a high-viscosity fluid with viscosity η_1; the speed field is also shown in the case of flow in a thin slab.

A plot of the velocity field in the case $\eta_2 = 0.00089$ Pa s, $\eta_1 = 0.01$ Pa s, $H = 200$ μm, and $h = 80$ μm is shown in Figure 8.65. In a realistic case, the fluxes are given besides the geometric characteristics of the system and the value of h is determined, besides the pressure field in the duct, by the hydrodynamic equations.

Evaluating the fluxes by the velocity field and imposing that the pressure drop per unit length in the multiphase flow and the thickness of the different phases are selected so as to sustain the input flow rates, the following expression is found for the layer separation coordinate h:

$$h = 2w \sqrt{\frac{\eta_2(Q_s + Q_{in})}{\eta_2 Q_{in} - Q_s(2\eta_1 - 3\eta_2)}} \sin\left\{ \frac{1}{3} arcsin\left[\frac{Q_{in}[Q_s(2\eta_1 - 3\eta_2) - \eta_2 Q_{in}]\sqrt{\dfrac{\eta_2(Q_s + Q_{in})}{\eta_2 Q_{in} - Q_s(2\eta_1 - 3\eta_2)}}}{\eta_2(Q_s + Q_{in})^2} \right] \right\}$$

$$(8.101)$$

where w is the mixing channel width, $Q_s = Q_1$ represents the flow of the focusing fluid and $Q_{in} = Q_2$ the flux of the fluids to be mixed. Once the width of the equivalent lamination mixer is found, the base lamination mixer theory can be used to analyze the stream focus mixer.

8.4.2 Chaotic Advection Micromixers

The transport of a solute substance within a moving fluid is called advection and it is another important cause of mixing among different solutions in macroscopic systems. As a matter of fact, in the presence of high Reynolds number, microvortices are always present and frequently macroscopic vortices appears. In the lamination micromixers, advection generally occurs in the direction of the laminar flow; hence it has no effect on the transversal transport of the substance. However, advection in other directions, the so-called chaotic advection [82–84], can generate components of the fluid velocity that are orthogonal to the average direction of motion, greatly improving the mixing efficiency in two contacting fluids. These "stirring" transverse flows can be generated by channel shapes that stretch, fold, break, and split the laminar flow over the cross section of the channel. This effect can be achieved using 2D curved [85–87], or 3D convoluted channels and by inserting obstacles and bas-reliefs on the channel walls. It must be noted that such type of chaotic flow could also be achieved by an active mixing strategy by a suitable external force acting on the fluid.

A key factor determining the most suitable design for a chaotic mixer is Reynolds number $\mathcal{R}_e$ (see Section 7.3.1.5). The Reynolds number represents the ratio between inertia and viscous forces and it determines if the motion is laminar or not. In a laminar motion, the velocity field curl is zero, so that closed streamlines do not exists. In the opposite case, if the curl is not zero, vortices can appear. It is intuitive that the higher the Reynolds number, the easier it is to generate chaotic advection. Experimentally, it is seen that macroscopic vortices surely appear for Reynolds numbers above about 2000, that is, a very frequent condition in macroscopic structures, but almost never happens in labs on chip. Below $\mathcal{R}_e = 1$, laminar motion is very stable and even microvortices are very difficult to be generated in the absence of specifically designed external forces. In the intermediate regime, laminar flow is less and less stable while the Reynolds number increases so that perturbations are more and more effective in generating chaotic advection.

Conventionally, three Reynolds number ranges are introduced in microfluidics to characterize the effectiveness of different techniques of chaotic advection generation: high, intermediate, and low Reynolds number regimes. If $\mathcal{R}_e \geq 100$, the motion happens in high Reynolds number regime. In case of water solutions $\mathcal{R}_e \approx 10^6 v_0 \ell_0$, so that $\mathcal{R}_e \geq 100$ is attained, for example, for ducts of the order of 10 mm width and average velocities of 10 mm/s. These parameters are at the limit of lab on chip applications, being, for example, possible in the case of labs on chip for cells processing.

The intermediate Reynolds number regime is characterized by $1 \leq \mathcal{R}_e \leq 100$; labs on chip realized in polymer technology are frequently within this regime, for example, if ducts with a width of 400 μm are realized and the average velocity of the fluid is of 5 mm/s. Pure laminar flow is generally established in this case, but it is not completely stable, so that sufficiently intense perturbations can cause chaotic advection generated by the effect of the nonlinear term in the motion equation.

The low Reynolds number regime is characterized by $\mathcal{R}_e \leq 1$; this is the most frequent regime labs on chip, when no reason exists to design the system for high fluid speed or with large channels. In this regime, the laminar motion is quite stable and very strong perturbations have to be introduced to see even a small effect of the motion equation nonlinear term. For this reason, chaotic advection in this regime is difficult unless a clever design of the system is performed.

While in the great majority of situations the Reynolds number is the main indicator to decide the formation and the stability of laminar regime, exceptions happen when the curvature of the duct where the fluid propagates is not negligible. It is quite intuitive that a sort of induce vortex can be created in a torus-shaped duct even at low Reynolds numbers and that curved ducts can be an effective way to create chaotic advection even when the Reynolds number is quite low [88,89].

The creation of vortices by using a curve shape of the duct where the fluid flows is a widely studied problem in fluid dynamics, since it recurs in many different problems. The main point of the problem is that, due to the contribution of the duct curvature to the instability of laminar flow, the Reynolds number is no more completely adequate to describe the motion due to the fact that it does not contain any information on the duct curvature. The problem of fluid propagation in curved ducts can be solved at the first order in the duct curvature obtaining the so-called Dean equations [90,91]. In their nondimensional forms, the Dean equation depends on a single nondimensional parameter, called the Dean number D_e, which is given by

$$D_e = \mathcal{R}_e \sqrt{R\kappa} \qquad (8.102)$$

where R is the hydrodynamic radius and κ is the duct axis curvature, which is the inverse of the curvature radius. It is evident that the Dean number is a correction of the Reynolds number that takes into account the duct curvature, in particular, relating it with the linear dimension characteristics of the duct section.

For weak curvature effects (small D_e), the Dean equations can be solved as a series expansion in D_e. The first correction to the leading-order axial Poiseuille flow is a pair of vortices in the cross section carrying flow from the inside to the outside of the bend across the center and back around the edges. This solution is stable up to a critical Dean number of about 965 [92]. For larger D_e, there are multiple solutions, many of which are unstable. Examples of Dean vortices in the flow of water in a coiled duct are shown in Figure 8.66. In the figure cases, the Reynolds number is as low as 15 and the vortices are created mainly due to the curvature effect.

8.4.2.1 Chaotic Advection Micromixers in a High Reynolds Number Regime

The simpler type of chaotic advection micromixers that works very well in the high Reynolds number regime are those designed by interposing obstacles on the fluid path into the duct. Obstacles can be etched in the duct floor, created on the walls, or generated by abrupt changes of the duct shape. Examples of these architectures are reported in Figure 8.67. In the figure, micromixers based on the creation of a sort of artificial vortex by a spiral shape of the mixing duct is also shown, which also provides good performances in the high Reynolds number regime. These kinds of structures exploit the formation of Dean vortices to obtain mixing by advection.

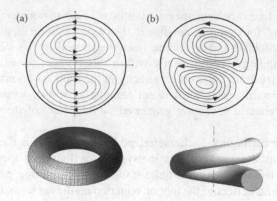

FIGURE 8.66 Example of Dean vortices in a curved channel: toroid channels and fully developed Dean vortices in the coil section (a) spiral channels and fully developed Dean vortices in the coil section (b), (Streamliner from (b) reproduced from *Chemical Engineering Science*, vol. 63, Mridha M., Nigam K. D. P., Coiled flow inverter as an inline mixer, pp. 1724–1732, Copyright 2008, with permission from Elsevier.)

8.4.2.2 Chaotic Advection Micromixers in an Intermediate Reynolds Number Regime

In the intermediate Reynolds number regime, to obtain chaotic advection simply by perturbation of the duct structure is more difficult. It can be done either with three-dimensional perturbations, as in C-shaped or L-shaped micromixers, whose architecture is shown in Figure 8.68a and b or by using the so-called split-and-recombine strategy such as in complex L-shaped structures. An example of complex L-shaped structure is reported in Figure 8.68c.

Two types of split-and-recombine strategy exist: in the first type, such as in Figure 8.68c, the whole flux, containing both the fluids to be mixed, is split and then recombined at the end of two different paths. The abrupt convergence of the two flows creates chaotic advection and enhances the mixing efficiency. In the second type of split and recombination mixers, the two fluids flows are split so that one fluid is sent to a path and the second to a different path. The two paths are then joined abruptly thus causing chaotic advection.

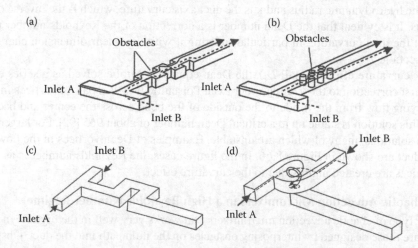

FIGURE 8.67 Example architectures for micromixers based on chaotic advection and designed to work in high Reynolds number regime: obstacles in the walls (a), obstacles etched on the duct floor (b), abrupt duct change of direction (c), and duct shape forming artificial vortices (d). (Reproduced from *Micromixers*, William Andrew; 2nd edition (November 3, 2011), ISBN-13: 978-1437735208; Nguyen N.-T., Chapter 6, Copyright 2011, with permission from Elsevier.)

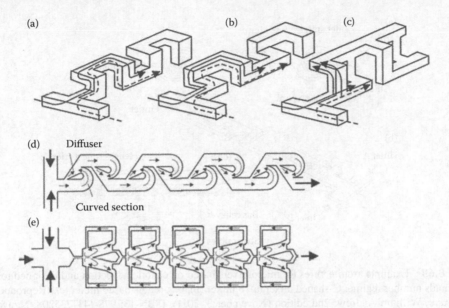

FIGURE 8.68 Example architectures for micromixers based on chaotic advection and designed to work in intermediate Reynolds number regime: C-shaped mixer (a), L-shaped mixer (b), double L-shaped mixer (or complex L-shaped mixer) (c), Tesla mixer with four mixing units (d), and recycle mixer with five mixing units (e). (Reproduced from *Micromixers*, William Andrew; 2nd edition (November 3, 2011), ISBN-13: 978-1437735208; Nguyen N.-T., Chapter 6, Copyright 2011, with permission from Elsevier.)

Split and recombination are also part of the working mechanism of micromixers shown in Figure 8.68d and e. In these cases, however, the effect of diffusion by rapid increase of duct section is also used in case (d) while Deans vortices are exploited in case (e) through the creation of closed loops in the mixer structure.

8.4.2.3 Chaotic Advection Micromixers in a Low Reynolds Number Regime

As the Reynolds number decreases, generating chaotic advection is more and more difficult, requiring more and more dense structures or very dense and abrupt changes of direction of the mixing duct. A few of the structures that are designed for intermediate Reynolds number also work for low Reynolds numbers; for example, the double L-shaped mixer that is shown in Figure 8.68c was fabricated in PDMS using a 100 μm × 70 μm channel achieving good mixing performances for Reynolds numbers as low as 0.1 [93].

A popular architecture to cause chaotic advection at low Reynolds number is to twist the flow by using suitable rips or grooves so as to force the fluid on helical trajectories that give rise to chaotic advection. Another possible strategy is to use very complex duct shapes that split and recombine the flux along twisted paths also creating artificial loops to exploit the creation of Dean vortices.

Examples of such structures are reported in Figure 8.69 [94]. In particular, Figure 8.69a shows a spiral micromixer exploiting successive spiral sections to generate Dean vortices and speed up the mixing. In Figure 8.69b, an example is provided of a mixer relying on a complex three-dimensional channel structure with frequent and abrupt changes of shape, in particular, the example architecture is called F channels mixer for the particular form of the mixing channel. Finally, in Figure 8.69c, a mixing based on bas-relieves on the mixing wall is shown. Bas-relieves forces the fluids to move along helical streamlines creating vortices inside the mixer and improving the mixing efficiency.

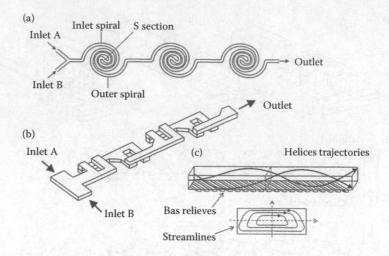

FIGURE 8.69 Example architectures for micromixers based on chaotic advection and designed to work in low Reynolds number regime: C-shaped mixer (a), F mixer (b), bas-reliefs based mixer (c). (Reproduced from *Micromixers*, William Andrew; 2nd edition (November 3, 2011), ISBN-13: 978-1437735208; Nguyen N.-T., Chapter 6, Copyright 2011, with permission from Elsevier.)

8.4.3 ACTIVE MICROMIXERS

Active micromixers are based on the application of an external force to cause effective mixing between the considered fluids. Different mechanisms can be used in a great number of possible mixer structures.

A first example is provided in Figure 8.70a, where the fluids containing an electrolyte are deviated toward electrodes that are allocated in spaces excavated into the mixing duct walls. This

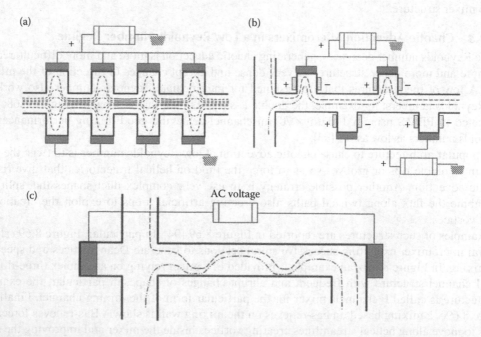

FIGURE 8.70 Examples of active mixers: electrostatic mixer (a), dielectrophoresis mixer (b), and electrokinetic mixer (c).

strong perturbation of the laminar flow provokes curved streamlines, thus increasing the mixing efficiency.

A second example of active mixer is provided in Figure 8.70b, where a principle scheme of the use of dielectrophoresis (see Section 7.5.5) is used to perturb the laminar flow in the mixing channel. As a last example, the principle scheme of an electroosmosis mixer (see Section 7.5.4) is reported in Figure 8.70c. It is worth observing that in the last two cases, in order to obtain an effective perturbation of laminar flow, an alternate voltage is used to obtain time-variable dielectrophoresis or electroosmosis.

When an alternate potential is used in EHD phenomena, the effect of the electromagnetic propagation delay can be neglected due to the electrostatic hypothesis. Electroosmosis and dielectrophoresis can then be analyzed using the same procedure we used in Chapter 7, but for the fact that the external potential has the form $\psi(r,t) = \psi_0(r)e^{i\omega t}$.

If we use this assumption in the study of dielectrophoresis, we obtain the following expression for the velocity of the dielectric particles, which is also the fluid velocity if it is due to the drag caused by the dielectric particles motion:

$$v_j = \frac{3}{2}\frac{\varepsilon_s}{\rho_0} K(\epsilon_s(\omega),\epsilon_L(\omega)) M E_k \frac{\partial E_j}{\partial x_k} \tag{8.103}$$

where the expression of the Clausius–Mossotti factor is the same as that found in the continuous case and, while ε_s is the dielectric constant of the sphere as in the continuous-wave case, $\epsilon_s(\omega)$ and $\epsilon_L(\omega)$ are the complex dielectric constants of the spheres and the liquid, respectively. In particular

$$\epsilon(\omega) = \varepsilon - i\frac{\sigma_c}{\omega} \tag{8.104}$$

where σ_c is the surface conductivity of the dielectric sphere and of the liquid in contact with the sphere itself. The conductivities are different from zero even if both the particle and the liquid are dielectric due to the accumulated surface charges that cause the dielectrophoresis phenomenon.

From Equation 8.104, it is clear that, in the case in which dielectrophoresis is superimposed to a laminar flow, a time-changing liquid deviation can be obtained, thus favoring the creation of chaotic advection. The study of AC electroosmosis is more complex than a simple extension of the continuous-wave case [95,96]. As a matter of fact, a pulsating double layer is created due to the external field, the double layer creates an internal pulsating field that follows the external field with the time scale typical of the formation of the Debye layer. In any case, a conclusion similar to that reached for dielectrophoresis can be attained.

8.4.4 Comparison among Different Micromixer Architectures

The base of the qualitative comparison we carry out among different micromixer technologies is the same already used for microvalves and micropumps: we try to make a synthesis of the great number of prototypes that are presented in the literature extrapolating, at least as an order of magnitude, what seems to be a common design trend.

However, if it is difficult to perform a comparison among different technologies to fabricate microvalves and micropumps, comparing different micromixers is even more difficult due to the great difference in working conditions, applications, materials, and, last but not least, requirements. For this reason, we have to limit the variety of the elements to consider in the comparison.

The first choice we do is to consider practically only micromixers for low Reynolds numbers. Since we are dealing with lab on chip applications, we do not expect high velocities and great lengths so that working with a Reynolds number greater than one is a rare occurrence. Even when

TABLE 8.12

Comparison among Possible Performances of Different Types of Micromixers Working in the Low Reynolds Number Regime

Type	Duct Width (μm)	Duct Height (μm)	Average Velocity (mm/s)	$\mathcal{R}_e$	P_e	Material	Notes
T-mixer	550	25	6	0.5	800	Silicon/glass	
Y-mixer	100	100	8	0.5	240	PDMS with glass cover	
Y-mixer	1000	50	0.27	0.02	150	PMMA	
Parallel lamination	80	5	0.7	0.0035	60	Silicon/glass	Three parallel double fluxes
Focusing mixer	10	10	50	0.5	500	PDMS or silicon/glass	Hydrodynamic focusing
Focusing mixer	1000	150	1	0.15	200	PDMS	Geometrical focusing
Serial lamination	300	30	10	0.3	150	Silicon/glass or polymer	Three liquid packets in the mixing duct
Serial lamination	50	50	2	0.1	14	Silicon/glass or polymer	16 liquid packets in the mixing duct
Chaotic advection	10	100	20	0.2	200	Silicon/glass or polymer	Based on cylindrical obstacles
Chaotic advection	72	31	0.6	0.024	15	Polymer	Based on bas-relieves patterned on the duct walls
Chaotic advection	100	70	1	0.1	10	PDMS	Based on a serpentine shape of the mixing duct
Active	50	25	0.5	0.02	25	Silicon/glass or polymer	AC frequency 1 Hz, based on AC dielectrophoresis
Active	200	25	0.5	0.01	100	Silicon/glass or polymer	Electroosmosis, AC = 1 Hz

relatively large ducts are used due to the need of analyzing cells, great speeds are to be avoided not to damage the biological sample.

In addition, we consider only a few active mixers architectures. Dealing with labs on chip limiting active elements is generally needed both to limit energy consumption and to simplify as much as possible the design. The results of a comparison carried out on the ground of these considerations are summarized in Table 8.12.

8.5   SAMPLE PURIFICATION: FILTERS

Sample purification is a key operation in labs on chip. Frequently, the inserted sample is a complex biological solution, containing the target species besides several other species such as macromolecules, small molecules such as peptides or simple sugars, ions, and greater particles such as cells or even bigger impurities such as small sand grains. No assay can be performed if the solution is somehow not purified and concentrated.

Purification and concentration can be performed using macroscopic systems, such as ultrafast centrifugation for cells and great particle elimination, chromatography, or electrophoresis. This procedure, however, is suitable for a research environment, but not if the lab on chip has to be used in the field. As a matter of fact, the main advantages of labs on chip field use are related to their small dimension and small quantity of required reagents. If a processing through a macroscopic equipment is needed before insertion of the sample in the lab on chip, several of such advances are lost. On-chip sample purification is thus a key enabler for labs on chip field use.

Several methods can be used for on-chip purification and concentration, exploiting different phenomena. Some of them are on-chip versions of macroscopic methods, such as electrophoresis; others exploit the specificity of working in a microenvironment.

A first group of purification systems exploits the fluid dynamics properties of labs on chip microfluidic systems to divide several different species and concentrate the resulting sample. Labs on chip sections implementing such methods are called hydrodynamic filters.

A second group of purification methods exploits the joint action of fluid motion in suitably designed structures and of the presence of electrical or magnetic field. Electrophoresis performed in specific electrophoresis chambers inside the chip is an example of a method belonging to this category, but several other methods have been introduced based on the exploitation of electrohydrodynamics or magnetohydrodynamics.

A third class of filter is based on the traditional concept of percolation, which is filtering by passage through a suitable porous material or artificially fabricated membrane. The simpler example of this procedure, used both in macroscopic arrangement and on chip, is dialysis filtration.

The selection of a method for sample purification depends on the type of impurities that have to be eliminated: frequently, several different filtration methods are adopted one after the other to progressively purify the sample from different kinds of impurities.

A general classification of the purification ability of different filtering methods is reported in Figure 8.71. Here, the particles to be eliminated from the sample are classified on the basis of their dimension and the type of filter more suitable to eliminate such particles is indicated. This classification is useful to provide a potential range of applications for the different filtering techniques; however, exceptions exist, frequently due to the fact that the filtering efficiency depends not just on the dimensions of the particles to be eliminated. This is the case of cells, whose elimination from anticoagulated blood is one of the most studied microfiltering problem. Cells membrane elasticity, allowing the cell to change shape answering to external stimuli, and cell activation typical, for example, of immune system cells, are important factors. As an example, if white cells are activated

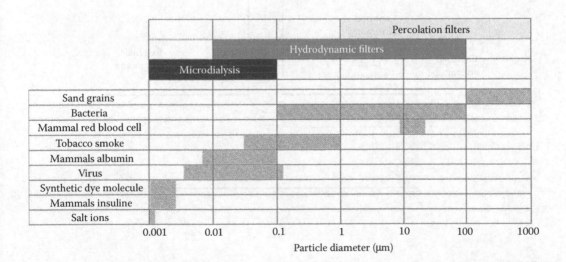

FIGURE 8.71 Application field of different classes of on-chip purification filters. (Data from Meng E., *Biomedical Microsystems*, CRC Press; 1st edition (September 29, 2010), ISBN-13: 978-1420051223.)

in blood during filtration, they generate great quantities of highly reactive enzymes greatly impairing the functionality of other biological macromolecules such as proteins.

8.5.1 HYDRODYNAMIC FILTERS

Hydrodynamic filters are based on the very properties of the fluid flow in carefully designed structures either shaping the streamline suitably to obtain filtering effect or exploiting the different diffusion coefficient of different solutes to divide them.

Several hydrodynamic filters exploit the fluid motion at the intersection between a main duct and a secondary duct much smaller than the main duct, as it is shown in Figure 8.72. Let us imagine a microfluidic circuit with a vertical dimension much smaller than the horizontal dimensions, so that it can be considered in a first approximation as two dimensional. The circuit is constituted by a main duct of width w_m where a secondary duct of width $w_l \ll w_m$ is orthogonally inserted in such a way that the axis of the secondary duct is the axis $y = 0$ of the reference system. The main duct, far from the intersection, sustains a Poiseuille flow with given velocity field (represented in the figure before and after the intersection) and flow rate. Owing to the intersection part of the fluid flowing through the main duct enters the secondary duct and, if the secondary duct is sufficiently long, establishes far from the intersection a Poiseuille flow whose velocity distribution is represented in the figure.

The fluid dynamics analysis of this system is not simple, owing to the fact that the abrupt intersection between the two ducts could create microvortices. This phenomenon, as described in Section 8.4.2, can be qualitatively understood through the Dean number. In principle, since the change in curvature ratio at the intersection is discontinuous, we should expect an infinite Dean number; in reality, infinitely sharp angles do not exist. Thus, we have to introduce an equivalent curvature at the angle, depending on the angle physical fabrication. Using this figure, we can qualitatively state that stable laminar flow in the system is attained only if the Dean number is quite smaller than one. Let us imagine that the Reynolds number is 0.01 and that the hydrodynamic radius is 20 μm. In order to obtain a Dean number equal to one from Equation 8.100, we get $\kappa = 5 \times 10^8$ that coincides with

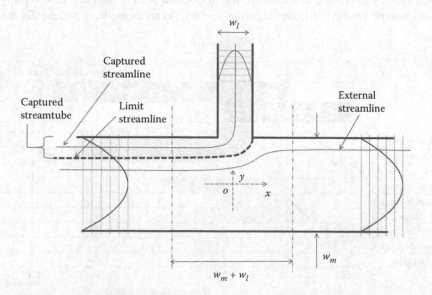

FIGURE 8.72 Flow of an incompressible liquid at the intersection between a main duct and a secondary duct of smaller dimension. Stationary laminar flow is assumed; the captured streamtube and the different types of streamlines are evidenced besides Poiseuille velocity distribution far from the intersection.

a curvature radius at the angle of 2 nm. In microfluidic circuits, this is a sharp curvature, so that it can still be called an angle.

Assuming to have a small Dean number, the flow in the system is laminar, implying that the velocity curl is everywhere equal to zero. Thus, the streamlines are never oriented against the average fluid motion. In this condition, the fluid in the main duct will be divided into two streamtubes: a captured streamtube that is adjacent to the main duct wall where the intersection is present and that ends with a limit streamline and a free streamtube, constituted by all the streamlines that are external to the limit streamline.

In Section 7.3.4.4, we have seen that the establishment of a fully developed Poiseuille flow after a perturbation happens in a characteristic length approximately equal to half the duct width so that the transition region length around the intersection can be evaluated as about $w_l + w_m$, while well outside this region the flux can be assumed a Poiseuille flux. The width of the captured streamtube can be evaluated by adopting the electrical equivalence introduced in Section 7.3.4.2. This is possible even if the flow is not Poiseuille like near the intersection, since the Poiseuille relations have to hold far from the intersections and the flow rate has to be conserved in each linear duct.

The electrical equivalent of the considered fluid dynamic circuit is shown in Figure 8.73 with the hydraulic resistances given by

$$r_1 = \frac{1}{4}\frac{1}{L_1}\frac{1}{\eta}B_m^2 \frac{\zeta_m}{\zeta_m^2 + 2\zeta_m + 1} \tag{8.105a}$$

$$r_2 = \frac{1}{4}\frac{1}{L_2}\frac{1}{\eta}B_m^2 \frac{\zeta_m}{\zeta_m^2 + 2\zeta_m + 1} \tag{8.105b}$$

$$r_d = \frac{1}{4}\frac{1}{L_d}\frac{1}{\eta}B_d^2 \frac{\zeta_d}{\zeta_d^2 + 2\zeta_d + 1} \tag{8.105c}$$

where

$$B_j = w_j z_j \quad (j = m, d) \tag{8.106a}$$

$$\zeta_j = \frac{w_j}{z_j} \quad (j = m, d) \tag{8.106b}$$

It is worth noting that the above equations do not contain the two-dimensional hypothesis; thus they also hold if the ducts are not slabs.

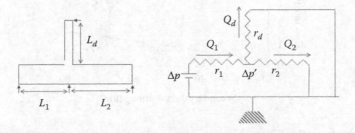

FIGURE 8.73 Electrical equivalent of the microfluidic circuit of Figure 8.71.

TABLE 8.13
Parameters of the Microfluidic Circuit Represented in Figure 8.71

L_1	400 µm	B_m	2.25×10^{-9} m²
L_2	400 µm	B_d	7.5×10^{-10} m²
L_d	140 µm	ζ_m	10
z_m	15 µm	ζ_d	3.33
z_d	15 µm	r_1	2.96×10^{-13} m³/(s Pa)
w_m	150 µm	r_2	2.96×10^{-13} m³/(s Pa)
w_d	50 µm	r_d	7.41×10^{-14} m³/(s Pa)
η	0.00089 Pa s		
Δp	50 kPa		

The corresponding circuit equations are readily solved obtaining the flow rates and the pressure in the intermediate point:

$$Q_1 = r_1 \Delta p \frac{r_2 + r_d}{r_1 + r_2 + r_d} \tag{8.107a}$$

$$Q_2 = r_2 \Delta p \frac{r_1}{r_1 + r_2 + r_d} \tag{8.107b}$$

$$Q_d = Q_1 - Q_2 \tag{8.107c}$$

$$\Delta p^{'} = \Delta p - \frac{Q_1}{r_1} \tag{8.107d}$$

In order to consider a numerical example, let us assume the parameters of Table 8.13 for the microfluidic circuit. The obtained flow rates are represented versus the width of the secondary duct in Figure 8.74; besides the expected increase of the flow rate in the side duct, the flow rate in the first part of the main duct also increases w_d increases due to the overall change of the circuit hydraulic resistance.

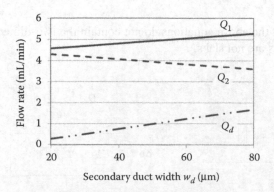

FIGURE 8.74 Flow rates at the different branches output of the microfluidic circuit represented in Figure 8.71 versus the width of the secondary duct; data in Table 8.13 have been used for the plot.

Once the flow rate Q_d is known, the distance L_{lim} of the limit streamline from the wall of the main duct, where the intersection is realized, can be evaluated with the equation

$$Q_d = \int_0^{z_w} \int_{L_{lim}}^{w_m/2} v(y,z)\, dydz \qquad (8.108)$$

where $v(y,z)$ is the module of the velocity distribution in the Poiseuille region of the main duct before the intersection that can be evaluated through Equation 7.86. With the values of Table 8.13, we obtain $L_{lim} = 37.57\ \mu m$.

8.5.1.1 Pure Hydrodynamic Filters

The initial sample to be purified is generally a diluted solution of several solutes composed of particles of very different size. The best example of this situation is anticoagulated blood.

In order to avoid blood coagulation, the first operation before any kind of processing is to dilute blood with a water solution composed of a substance inhibiting coagulation. A common way of doing this is to use Ca^{2+} chelation via ethylenediaminetetraacetic acid (EDTA) [97]. Typical blood dilutions are from 1:5 to 1:10, which is sufficient to practically eliminate the non-Newtonian characteristic of pure blood [98]. The obtained solution contains three types of solvents of very different nature: cells, macromolecules such as proteins, small molecules such as single peptides, and ions. Cells range from almost spherical bodies with a radius of 12–15 μm such as the neutrophils to red cells that are disks with a maximum diameter around 8 μm and a minimum dimension around 2 μm to platelet that are almost spherical with a diameter of about 2 μm. Blood proteins span to a weight of 16 kDa to more than 200 kDa and ions with a weight from 20 to 50 Da have a classical radius from 1 to 5 Å.

Let us thus assume that we feed the circuit of Figure 8.72 with a solution containing two kinds of particles that can be approximated as spheres with different radii ($d_1 = 12\ \mu m$ and $d_2 = 50\ nm$). A first possible approximation, allowing us to understand the qualitative working of the system is to assume that all particles travel with a speed coinciding with the local value of the velocity field in their center of mass. Assuming the main duct to be 80 μm wide and the secondary duct 8 μm wide, it is possible to find a practical condition in terms of applied pressure and duct lengths producing a captured streamtube width equal to 6.5 μm, as it is shown in Figure 8.75. In the figure, both small and large spheres are represented, with the relative velocity applied to the center of mass.

Owing to their dimension, the bigger particles are always linked to a streamline that is out of the captured streamtube, so that they cannot enter into the lateral duct, while smaller particles fit

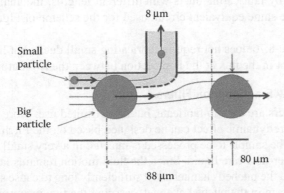

FIGURE 8.75 Particles of different dimensions in a pure hydrodynamic filter.

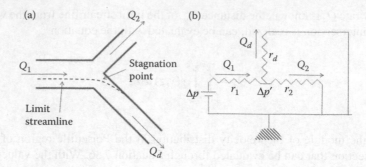

FIGURE 8.76 Pure hydrodynamic filter based on ducts with the same section and different flow rates; (a) scheme of a filter where the different flow rate is obtained by using ducts of different length, and (b) electrical equivalent of the microfluidic circuit.

into the captured streamtube thus being subdivided between the main and the lateral ducts. In this simple model, we can assume, due to Taylor dispersion (see Section 7.4.5), that the solute concentration is constant through the main duct; thus, the percentage of the number of particles captured by the secondary duct is equal to the ratio between the flow rate at the input of the system and the flow rate at the output of the secondary duct. This means that the fluid at the output of the secondary duct presents the same concentration of small particles with respect to the initial sample, but no big particles. The result is that the sample is purified eliminating one solute at the cost of greatly reducing the overall sample volume by maintaining the concentration of the target constant. Such a filter is called pure hydrodynamic filter.

The main characteristic of a pure hydrodynamic filter is the ability of eliminating from the sample particles whose dimensions are of the same order of magnitude of the dimension of the lateral duct; thus, it can be used essentially to eliminate contaminants such as small sand grains and cells from a biological sample, but it cannot select a specific type of macromolecule or even ions from macromolecules. Frequently, such filters represent the first stage of a purification system, for example, a stage in which diluted blood is transformed in plasma [99,100].

A different type of pure hydrodynamic filter can be built by leveraging on the difference between the flow rate in the output branches of the circuit instead of their dimensions [101]. A scheme of such a filter is reported in Figure 8.76a while the equivalent electrical circuit is reported in Figure 8.76b. The working mechanism is the same as that of the filter in Figure 8.72: since the sum of the exiting fluxes has to be equal to the input flux, a limit streamline creates, nearer to the wall from which the lower flow rate ducts departs. Bigger particles do not enter inside the captured streamtube and hence they cannot enter in the low flow rate duct. If different flow rates in the output ducts are obtained by fabricating ducts with different lengths, the analysis of the system can be carried out using the same equivalent circuit used for the scheme of Figure 8.72, as it is shown in Figure 8.76b.

The design of Figure 8.76 does not require fabricating small ducts, but has the disadvantage of creating a stagnant point in the flux at the intersection between the two output ducts.

8.5.1.2 Pinched Flow Fractionation Filters

Pure hydrodynamic filters are easy to fabricate, but has a limited use. More complex and performing filters based on hydrodynamic effect can be designed based on the Pitch effect [102,103] that is shown in Figure 8.77. The sample to be processed is injected in a very small microduct, the pitched channel, besides a higher-flow-rate liquid. Since the fluid motion remains laminar for the accurate design of the system and the pitched channel is not sufficiently long to cause sensible dispersion, two different streamtubes form in the pitched channel, carrying the two incoming fluxes. Particles that fit in the streamtube coming from the sample duct remain there; on the contrary, bigger particles are

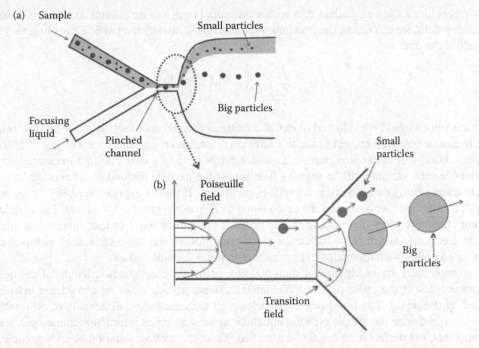

FIGURE 8.77 Hydrodynamic filter based on pitched duct separation: system scheme (a), and particular of the pitched duct with qualitative behavior of the velocity field inside the duct and at the transition with the larger filter area (b).

pushed by the pitched channel walls toward the center of the channel, inside the streamtube coming from the second duct; compare Figure 8.77b where the detain of the pitched channel is shown with a qualitative representation of the velocity fields within it and at its output.

When the pitched channel opens in a much larger channel, the velocity field opens so that the fluid fills all the larger area without destroying the separation between the two streamtubes. Depending on the position of the particles' center of mass, big and small particles are deflected from the pitched tube axis of a different angle, so that by suitably placing the output duct, only one type of particles can be selected.

From the description of this method, it appears that it has the potentiality not only to provide a way for sample purification, but also to divide sample components on the ground of their dimensions, that can be correlated to their mass once the stereography of the single molecule is known. This can be done, for example, by opening at the end of the separation part of the circuit several output channels, in correspondence of the arrival point of each considered composite.

However, if a very rough description of the particle motion is sufficient for a pure hydrodynamic filter to be described, this is not true for pitched effect-based filters. As a matter of fact, the trajectory of a specific type of particle depends on the exact particle motion so that if quantitative measures are needed, it has to be analyzed. The critical factor determining the complexity of the particle motion is the presence of an appreciable velocity gradient over the typical dimensions of the particle. As a matter of fact, if the particle is so small that the velocity field is essentially constant within the particle dimension, the particle can be considered as a point body and its motion can be simply assumed to be determined by its belonging to a certain streamline. On the contrary, if a velocity gradient exists, besides the translational force applied to the particle center of mass, a momentum also appears causing particle rotation. A relevant rotation causes the particle trajectory to be different from the trajectory caused by simple drag from the fluid so that the particle arrives at the end of the filter in a different position.

If we consider a squared pitched duct with a side equal to d_s and we assume expression (7.86) for the velocity field, we can define the maximum dimension d_{par} at which a particle traveling very near to a wall of the duct as

$$v\left(d_{par}, \frac{d_s}{2}\right) = (1 + \varepsilon)v\left(\frac{d_{par}}{2}, \frac{d_s}{2}\right) \tag{8.109}$$

where the velocity field is evaluated in radial coordinates in the duct section plane and the relative result is maximized with respect to the angular coordinate and ε is a small number (e.g., 0.001) setting the accuracy of the approximation. Equation 8.109 is simply derived from imposing that the ratio between the variation of the velocity field across the particle divided by its average has to be equal to ε and setting the velocity at the wall equal to zero. If we use expression (7.86) for the velocity field, $\varepsilon = 10^{-3}$ and we assume a duct side equal to 20 μm we get $d_{par} \approx 800$ nm. The conclusion does not change sensibly if we change ε one order of magnitude more or less: macromolecule and even smaller particles can be considered for sure point bodies, but large cells, such as blood cells, and other particles, such as small sand grains, are in no case point bodies.

Macromolecules are much smaller than 800 nm, being the characteristic length of the heavier macromolecules of the order of a few nanometers, these particles can be considered effectively dragged by the liquid. The trajectory of particles with a characteristic dimension of 500–600 nm can be analyzed with the simple Newton equation, at least as far as interaction among particles is not important, but perfect drag cannot be assumed. Thus, the motion equation of each particle is

$$F_{Drag} = \frac{1}{m}\frac{dP}{dt} \tag{8.110}$$

where P is the particle momentum and m its mass. The force exerted by the flowing fluid on the particles is indicated by F_{Drag}.

The case of bigger particles, for example, particles of a dimension of the order of 10 μm, is much more complex; they not only have to be considered extended bodies, but they are not even rigid, since deformability of cells is not small. If we assume, however, in a first approximation that big bodies can be considered rigid so as to study their motion with Euler equations

$$F_{Fj} = \frac{1}{m}\frac{dP_{cj}}{dt} \tag{8.111a}$$

$$\mathcal{U}_{i,j}M_{Fj} = I_{i,j}\frac{d\omega_j}{dt} + \epsilon_{i,j,k}I_{k,h}\omega_j\omega_h \tag{8.111b}$$

where

$I_{i,j}$ is the inertia momentum tensor expressed in the reference of its eigenvectors; this means that is a diagonal tensor
ω_j is the instantaneous angular velocity
P_{cj} is the center of mass momentum
F_{Fj} and M_{Fj} are the resultant of forces and force momenta exerted by the fluids on the body
$\mathcal{U}_{i,j}$ is the rotation tensor, an orthogonal tensor defined by the equation

$$\epsilon_{i,j,k}q_j\omega_k = \frac{d\mathcal{U}_{i,j}^{-1}}{dt}\mathcal{U}_{j,k}q_k \tag{8.112}$$

that has to hold whatever is the vector **q**.

If the particle can be assumed to be spherical, the tensor of the principal inertia momenta becomes a scalar and Equation 8.111b simplifies further. However, practical cases exist where this approximation cannot be performed, like in the case of red cells in diluted blood. Experimental evidence exists [102] that rotation of the red cell plane is important for the exact determination of red cell trajectories in this category of filters. As a matter of fact, while in a wide channel, red cell orientation is random, in a rectangular pinched channel, they tend to orient so as to be parallel to the channel wider dimension, in such a way that prevision based on a spherical red cell shape provides wrong results.

Once Euler equations have been adapted at the considered case, an expression has to be found for F_{Dj} and M_{Dj}, which are the terms characterizing the interaction between the particle and the environmental fluid. The total force acting on a single point of the particle can be divided into two terms [103,104], the first taking into account the variation of the macroscopic velocity field of the flowing fluid and the other related to much faster fluctuations of the local fluid stress tensor.

The velocity field-related force is dominated by the fluid drag force F_D that can be considered applied to the particle center of mass and is written as

$$F_{D,j} = \beta(u_j - v_j) \tag{8.113}$$

where u and v are the instantaneous particle velocity and the average of the velocity field in the particle occupied space. The fluid drag force is generally corrected by inserting phenomenological terms taking into account the so-called added mass force and the history force. The first term is due to the difference between the fluid and the particle density causing a force to arise to avoid a fluid mass substitution by the particle, the second somehow models the fact that the real force depends not only on the instantaneous values of the system parameters, but also on passed values.

The force F_s depending on the local stress can be written as the stress gradient multiplied by a constant as

$$F_{Sj} = \varphi \frac{d}{dx_k}(p\delta_{j,k} + \gamma'_{j,k}) \tag{8.114}$$

where φ is the local particle volume fraction, that is, the local ratio between the volume occupied by particles and the total fluid volume [105,106]. As evident from the expression of $\gamma'_{j,k}$ (7.33) of the viscosity tensor, the term F_{Sj} takes into account the velocity field variation inside the space occupied by the body.

The procedure of solving the Navier–Stokes equation in the system to determine the whole fluid motion and thereafter the Euler equations to find the particle trajectories is quite complex and generally require numerical simulation; nevertheless, obtained results are quite in agreement with experience and allows effective systems using pitched channel-based separation to be designed.

In order to introduce an example of dependence of the trajectories of different particles on particle dimension, let us consider the system represented in Figure 8.78. The dynamics of the two kinds of considered particles in diluted water solution are simulated in such a system in different conditions [107], obtaining results such as those represented in Figure 8.79. Here, the trajectories of small and large particles are shown from a point well inside the incoming duct, where their centers of mass occupy the same point, through the pitched duct to the core of the separator, where the particles trajectories are well divided. While the small particle, which is smaller than the pitched duct radius, practically follows the streamline both in the pitched duct and in the separation zone, the dynamics of the large particle is different. While the particle reaches near the insertion of the pitched duct, its trajectory abruptly leaves the streamline due to the fact that it has to fit the pitched duct section; thus, it relaxes on a different streamline in the duct. Moreover, once the particle

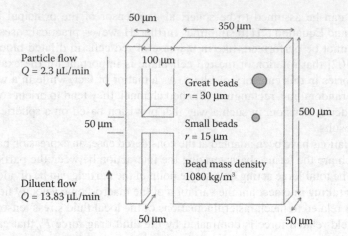

FIGURE 8.78 Scheme and parameters of the pitched channel effect fractional device considered in the numerical example of the text. The base fluid in the system is pure water.

leaves the pitched duct, its trajectory does not follow the streamline at the duct output, but it deviates toward positive y, relaxing after the end of the separation region on a different streamline. This effect is due to a combined action of inertia and particle rotation induced by interaction with the liquid.

Owing to the simplicity and effectiveness of the pitched channel effect, many variations have been proposed to further enhance the effectiveness of this purification method or to adapt it to particular situations. The design of the channels at the output of the separation zone has been optimized in order to improve the separation range [108] and both magnetic [109] and optical [110] interactions have been exploited in conjunction with pitched effect fractionation to obtain more complex functionalities like further separation among particles with similar dimensions.

8.5.1.3 Diffusion-Based Filters

Hydrodynamic filtering can be based not only on a suitable shape of the streamlines due to the design of microchannels, but also on the different diffusion properties of particles with different dimensions.

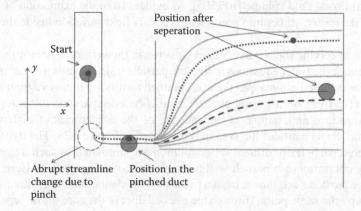

FIGURE 8.79 Trajectories of small and big particles in the fractional system of Figure 8.77. The middle section of the device along the z axis is shown in the figure and the water streamlines are represented in light gray. Particle trajectories are compared with the streamlines to whom the particle belongs at the output of the pitched duct that are represented with dashed black lines. (Data from Shardt O., Mitra S. K., Derksen J. J., *Chemical Engineering Science*, vol. 75, pp. 106–119, 2012.)

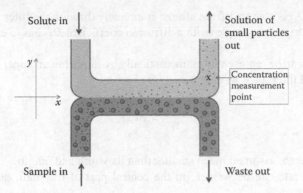

FIGURE 8.80 Principle scheme of the H filter and graphical illustration of its working based on different diffusion coefficients of particles with different dimensions.

The simpler type of diffusion-based filter is the so-called H filter, whose name derives from its form [1,2]. The shape of this filter is reported in Figure 8.80 besides a graphical illustration of its working. The H filter is essentially a laminar mixer, where a solution containing different particles is injected from one input and the simple solvent is injected from the other side. The analysis carried out for the laminar mixed in Section 8.4.1.1 can be used to analyze the behavior of the basic H filter structure. Its filter characteristics depend on the fact that particles with smaller dimensions have higher diffusion coefficient; thus, if the filter length is carefully designed, small particles can be equally shared between the two exit ducts while big particles remain essentially in one of the ducts.

The concentration of the solute present in the input sample versus the H filter length and the solute diffusion coefficient is reported in Figure 8.81 as measured at the center of the exit H filter channel. Dispersion coefficients range from values typical of big proteins and nucleic acids to typical values of cells and small beads. From the figure, it is clear that about 40% of the initial proteins and nucleic acids concentration is captured by a filter few millimeters long, while cells or beads are almost absent in the flux at the selected output. If the filtering efficiency of a single filter is not sufficient, multiple H stages can be put in cascade to achieve better purification of the sample.

Three key points regulate the working of an H filter, the condition of laminar flow, the possibility of sustaining a minimum required flow rate and the fact that the particle to be purified (with a

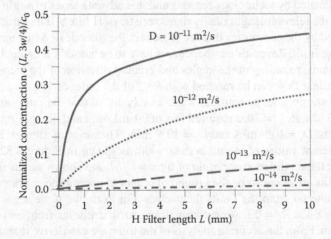

FIGURE 8.81 Concentration of a solute captured at the output of an H filter normalized to the initial sample concentration c_0; the measurement point is half of the existing filter duct (this point is marked in Figure 8.79); L indicates the main duct length and w its width.

diffusion coefficient D_1) is able to diffuse almost completely through the filter width, while the particle to be eliminated from the sample (with a diffusion coefficient D_2) has to experiment negligible diffusion [111].

The first condition can be represented mathematically by imposing an upper limit to the Reynolds number in the main H filter duct, writing

$$\frac{\rho v h}{\eta} \le Re_{lim} \tag{8.115}$$

where h is the filter depth, assumed much smaller than its width and length.

The required flow rate can be written, in the central part of the main duct where we have a Poiseuille flow

$$Q_{req} = vhw = w\,Re_{min}\frac{\eta}{\rho} \tag{8.116}$$

where w is the main filter duct width and Re_{min} is the minimum Reynolds number assuring the wanted flow rate. On the diffusion side, the requirements on diffusion are written as

$$\sqrt{D_2\frac{L}{v}} \ll w \ll \sqrt{D_1\frac{L}{v}} \tag{8.117}$$

where L/v is the time taken by a fluid element to traverse the filter. Considering equations in Equations 8.113 and 8.14, substituting the obtained value of v in Equation 8.117, we can get the design equations for the H filter

$$\sqrt{\frac{D_2}{Re}\frac{\rho}{\eta h^2}} \ll \frac{w}{\sqrt{hL}} \ll \sqrt{\frac{D_1}{Re}\frac{\rho}{\eta h^2}} \tag{8.118a}$$

$$Re_{min} \ll Re \ll Re_{lim} \tag{8.118b}$$

Generally, h is dictated by technology reasons and it is advantageous to attain a low value of the aspect ratio, due to the relevant length that is characteristic of H filters. The limit Reynolds number is largely determined by the curvatures that are present in the filter design (see Section 8.4.2) so that in order to have large limit, Reynolds number curves have to be smoothed as much as possible in the filter design. By suitable rounding of the angles and gradual insertion of the incoming and outcoming ducts, stable laminar flow can be reached with Re_{lim} of the order of 100.

For a numerical example, let us consider water as solvent, so that the ratio ρ/η is about 1.124 at 25°C. Assume $h = 5$ μm, $Re_{lim} = 20$, a required flux of 0.1 mL/min and, imagining that proteins have to be divided by cells, $D_1 = 10^{-11}$ m²/s and $D_2 = 10^{-13}$ m²/s. The range of allowed Reynolds numbers with respect to different values of the main duct width is shown in Figure 8.82a while in Figure 8.82b, the limits for the modified aspect ratio of filter $w/\sqrt{hL}$ are shown versus the Reynolds number. Since these limits are deduced on the ground of orders of magnitude considerations, the design has to be located quite far from the limits themselves. For example, if we set $w = 100$ μm and we choose from Figure 8.82a $Re = 0.1$, we get, remaining sufficiently far from extremes, $w/\sqrt{hL} = 1$ that means $L = 2$ mm. From the accurate analysis of the filter, we can derive that this design collects in the output duct about 33% of the sample protein concentration by maintaining only 1% of the cell concentration. If we cascade two such stages, we reduce the cell concentration below 0.01% at the expense of reducing the protein concentration to about 11% of the initial value.

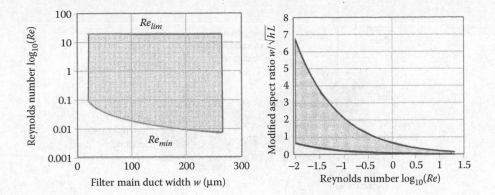

FIGURE 8.82 Design plots of an H filter with the parameters provided in the text numerical example: range of possible Reynolds number versus the main duct width (a) and modified aspect ratio versus the Reynolds number (b).

8.5.1.4 On-Chip Chromatography

The most used macroscopic method of mechanical separation between chemical species of different mass is chromatography, as discussed in Section 3.5. Chromatography has been the first filtering technique that was transported in labs on chip: the first lab on chip prototype was a gas chromatograph integrated into a whole silicon wafer [112]. Since this pioneering work, several different types of chromatography have been integrated in labs on chip attaining very good performances [113–115] and even commercial labs on chip exist implementing chromatographic separation [116].

However, on-chip chromatography has an essential drawback with respect to other separation techniques: the high pressure that is needed to obtain effective separation. Such a high pressure is practically not attainable with integrated pumps and the chip has to be connected with an external pump to work at best. Several solutions have been proposed to this problem [117] both designing chromatography so as to minimize the required pressure and suggesting integrated systems capable of providing the required pressure gradient [117].

As far as the insertion of fixed phase in microfluidic ducts is concerned, it has no principle problem, but it could be a limiting factor if the chip has to be produced in very large volumes. For this reason, it has been proposed to create the required solid phase by a suitable monolithic fabrication of the chromatograph channel. Typically, the channel is fitted with small obstacles, such as columns or other elements, so as to simulate the structure of the chromatographic liquid phase [118].

8.5.2 Electrophoresis Filters

Electrophoresis separation systems are based either on the effect of an electrical field or on the combined effect of the electrical field and of the hydrodynamic velocity distribution to divide different species in a sample, so as to purify the target species for an assay.

The simpler way of performing such an operation is to transport gel electrophoresis from its base macroscopic arrangement (see Section 3.6) to a microscopic on-chip design [119,120]. This is in principle not difficult if a suitable electrophoresis chamber is prepared in the chip and gel is injected into it during the back-end chip fabrication stage. An example of such an arrangement is shown in Figure 8.83. Here, a sample is injected into a gel-filled electrophoresis chamber from a feeding duct.

In a first phase, the valve regulating the access to the electrophoretic chamber is closed while the duct is filled with the sample under analysis. In a second phase, the valve is opened and the voltage is applied to the electrodes: the sample is thus first injected in the electrophoresis chamber by the field and then migrates in the gel to obtain electrophoretic separation. In a third phase, the orthogonal electrodes are activated so as to extract from the electrophoretic chamber the separated species.

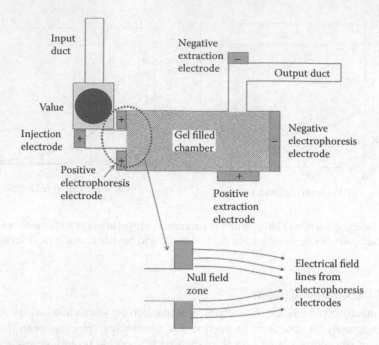

FIGURE 8.83 Possible scheme of an integrated gel electrophoresis chamber where the electrodes and the electrical field lines near the electrophoresis chamber are evidenced.

An important advantage of on-chip electrophoresis is its high speed with respect to its macroscopic counterpart. Assuming to perform on-chip electrophoresis with the same gel and the same field intensity that is used in an equivalent macroscopic setup, the macromolecule migration time scales down linearly with the electrophoresis chamber length reduction while the line resolution is decreased from the order of millimeters to the order of micrometers, that is three orders of magnitude, due to the use of microducts for the macromolecule extraction from the separation chamber.

Moreover, in order to obtain the same electrical field in the gel the required voltage also scales down linearly with the separation chamber length. For example, a macroscopic electrophoresis performed in half an hour in a macroscopic cell 20 cm long with an applied voltage of 200 V can be performed in a microscopic cell of a length of 1 mm using an applied voltage of 1 V in about 10 s. The line separation also scales down to a factor of 200, which is counterbalanced by the ability of extracting the selected macromolecules through microducts.

A particular aspect of the electrode configuration reported in Figure 8.83 is insertion and extraction from the electrophoretic chamber via ducts lying in the same plane of the chamber itself. On the contrary, in the macroscopic case, these operations are preformed accessing to suitable spots orthogonally to the electrophoresis plane. This circumstance causes the fact that electrodes cannot cover continuously the side of the electrophoresis chamber, causing a zone of very low electrical field, as shown in Figure 8.83. Thus, in order to both inject and extract the molecules and to overcome the low field zone, electrodes also have to be placed on the side of the insertion/extraction ducts.

For these reasons, even if two orthogonal fields are present in the design of Figure 8.83, the system realizes standard, not two-dimensional, electrophoresis. The field that is activated in the second separation phase is only used for the extraction of the molecules from the electrophoretic chamber, injecting them in a suitable solution, generally for the final detection or for a subsequent stage of the assay. Two-dimensional electrophoresis can be in any case performed on chip with similar arrangements slightly modifying the electrophoresis chamber design.

A last important element relates to the gel insertion during the chip fabrication. This is not a problem if the chip is used for research purposes, so as to be stored for a relatively short time and in a suitable environment, for example, at low temperature such as 4°C. Differently, if the chip has to be stored for long periods, like years, in uncontrolled conditions, it is important to use a gel with a very high water retention ability, so as to avoid gel drying, especially if the external microfluidic circuit is not filled with a liquid before the use. In order to completely avoid this problem, direct on-chip gel synthesis has been proposed [121] where the gel is synthesized immediately before the assay.

Since electrophoresis on chip is generally used to fractionate the different components of a mix, it is important to define and evaluate the electrophoresis resolution. Let us imagine to have two different species A and B that are characterized by different electrophoresis mobility and diffusion coefficients in the gel. At the end of electrophoresis, each species will generate a line on the electrophoresis diagram that will be characterized by a center of mass position (x_A and x_B, respectively) and a standard deviation (σ_A and σ_B, respectively). The two species can be resolved via electrophoresis if the centers of mass of the two lines are sufficiently far to allow a quantitative line identification and, in case, the possibility to extract from the electrophoresis chamber one species besides a very small quantity of the other.

Following this idea, the electrophoresis resolution δ of the two species A and B can be defined as

$$\delta = \frac{\sigma_A + \sigma_B}{x_A - x_B} \tag{8.119}$$

On the ground of this definition, approximating the electrophoresis line with a Gaussian curve, the presence of the two substances with similar concentrations is clearly recognized and quantified if $\delta \approx 1.5$, as shown in Figure 8.84. If the concentrations are quite different, the value of δ allowing to have a given contrast of the electrophoresis diagram, that is, a given ratio between the peak of the line to be detected to the minimum of the electrophoresis diagram is reported in Figure 8.85, where σ_A and $x_A - x_B$ are fixed and σ_B is changed to obtain different values of δ.

If we want to evaluate the resolution allowing us to extract one substance, for example, A, and reduce the other of a known factor ε, such as, for example, 0.1%, the form of the electrophoresis line and the width of the extraction channel have to be known. If we approximate electrophoresis lines like Gaussian lines and we call w the extraction channel width, we found that the fractions f_A and f_B of the two substances after extraction are provided by

$$f_A = \mathrm{erf}\left(\frac{w}{2\sigma_a}\right) \tag{8.120a}$$

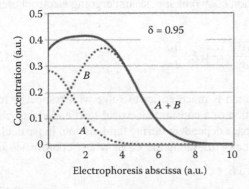
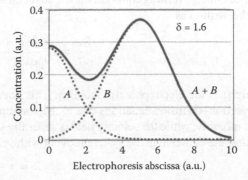

FIGURE 8.84 Two electrophoresis interfering lines corresponding to species having similar concentrations in the sample and to different values of the electrophoresis resolution.

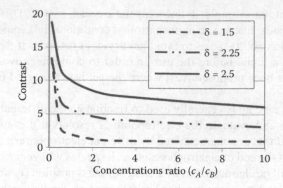

FIGURE 8.85 Contract in the detection of two nearby electrophoresis lines versus the ratio of the species concentrations for different electrophoresis resolutions. In the figure, σ_A and $x_A - x_B$ are fixed and σ_B is changed to obtain different values of δ.

$$f_B = \frac{1}{2}\,\mathrm{erf}\left(\frac{x_B - x_A - w}{2\sigma_B}\right) \qquad (8.120b)$$

From Equation 8.120, it is quite evident that, once the electrophoresis parameters are given, a trade-off has to be performed between the quantity of A and B that are extracted from the electrophoresis chamber.

An evaluation of the electrophoresis resolution parameters can be carried out once the electrophoresis mobility of the considered substances is known such as their diffusion constant in the considered gel (see Section 7.4.2).

Let us assume that the sample is injected into the electrophoresis chamber by a fast electrical field action that does not provoke sensible separation, so that after insertion the sample occupies a squared area $\mathbb{A}$ in the electrophoresis chamber with

$$\mathbb{A} \equiv \left\{ \left[-\frac{x_M}{2}, \frac{x_M}{2} \right], \left[-\frac{y_M}{2}, \frac{y_M}{2} \right] \right\}$$

Each charged particle experiments an electrical-induced drag causing a constant speed average motion and a diffusive effect. Deducing the equation for the particle concentration with the usual method of the fluxes, we derive an equation completely analogous to the diffusion–convection Equation 7.166 since the derivation procedure of Section 7.4.1 does not change if the drag velocity is exerted by a moving fluid or by other sources.

Thus, the governing equation for the concentration $c(x,y,t)$ of species undergoing electrophoresis can be written as

$$\frac{\partial c}{\partial t} = D\left(\frac{\partial^2 c}{\partial x^2} + \frac{\partial^2 c}{\partial y^2} \right) + \mu E_x \frac{\partial c}{\partial x} \qquad (8.121)$$

where μ is the electrophoretic mobility. This equation is much easier to solve with respect to real convection–diffusion equations due to the assumption of a constant electrical field and electrophoretic mobility, while the velocity field is generally space dependent during fluid motion. In particular, writing the equation in the system moving with velocity μE_x along the x axis whose coordinates are

$$\bar{x} = x - \mu E_x t$$
$$\bar{y} = y \qquad (8.122)$$
$$\bar{t} = t$$

Equation 8.121 becomes

$$\frac{\partial c}{\partial t} = D\left(\frac{\partial^2 c}{\partial \bar{x}^2} + \frac{\partial^2 c}{\partial \bar{y}^2}\right) \tag{8.123}$$

which is a simple diffusion equation. In this case, diffusion happens with a good approximation in an infinite two-dimensional environment, at least if the electrophoresis has a good resolution, so that Equation 8.122 can be solved using the Green formula and the initial conditions

$$c(\bar{x},\bar{y},0) = c_0 H_{-y_M,y_M}(\bar{y}) H_{-x_M,x_M}(\bar{y}) \tag{8.124}$$

where the rectangular function $H_{a,b}(y)$ is defined in Equation 7.182. The resulting integral can be solved in closed form and returning to the laboratory system we get (see Equation 7.173):

$$c(r,t) = c_0\left[\text{erf}\left(\frac{x - \mu E_x t - x_M}{\sqrt{4Dt}}\right) - \text{erf}\left(\frac{x - \mu E_x t + x_M}{\sqrt{4Dt}}\right)\right]\left[\text{erf}\left(\frac{y - y_M}{\sqrt{4Dt}}\right) - \text{erf}\left(\frac{y + y_M}{\sqrt{4Dt}}\right)\right] \tag{8.125}$$

The meaning of Equation 8.125 is quite clear: owing to the constant drag velocity, the diffusion effect is not altered by the migration of molecule population so that the molecule distribution gradually widens due to diffusion while they migrate in the electrophoresis chamber.

If a square injection side is assumed, that is, $x_M = y_M$, the electrophoresis line has the same variance along the x and y axes, which is given by

$$\sigma_c^2 = \frac{x_M^2}{3} + \frac{D x_f}{\mu E_x} \tag{8.126}$$

where x_f is the final position of the electrophoresis distribution center of mass. The first term in Equation 8.126 is called injection dispersion and the second is called diffusion dispersion.

From Equation 8.125, it is also possible to individuate a condition, allowing the electrophoresis line to be considered Gaussian: it happens when the linewidth is dominated by diffusion instead of the width of the original distribution. Considering that separation among different substances is obtained along the field axis, that is, along x, this happens when

$$\sqrt{4D t_M} \gg x_M \tag{8.127}$$

where t_M is the electrophoresis duration. This is a desired condition in general, since once the gel and the sample are given, it allows the resolution to be optimized simply by suitably charging the sample into the electrophoresis chamber. In this condition, the injection resolution is negligible and diffusion is practically the only element limiting on-chip electrophoresis resolution. This is also an evidence of the advantage of on-chip electrophoresis with respect to the analogous macroscopic procedure. As a matter of fact, the small values of the electrical field needed to obtain electrophoresis in microchambers render negligible all effects related to Joule heating of the electrophoretic gel, which are another important element in evaluating the resolution of macroscopic electrophoresis [121].

An example of on-chip gel electrophoresis measurement of fragments of human IgG4 (a subtype of IgG immunoglobulin) [122] is reported in Figure 8.86 evidencing the format of results completely analogous to that provided by macroscopic electrophoresis and the very good resolution of the applied method.

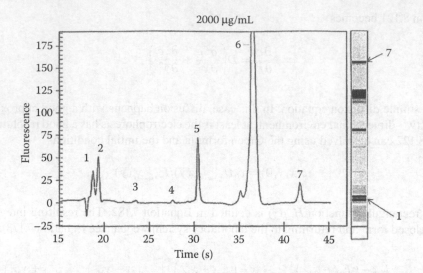

FIGURE 8.86 On-chip electrophoresis diagram measured using a fluorescence technique, of the IgG4 reference drug substance solution with a concentration of approximately 2 mg/mL. 1, Lower marker; 2, system peak; 3, light chain; 4, heavy chain; 5, half-antibody; 6, IgG4 antibody; and 7, molecular weight marker, 210 kDa (upper marker). The band positioned at the right side of the diagram shows the corresponding on chip gel presentation. (Andrews A. T., *Electrophoresis: Theory, Techniques, and Biochemical and Clinical Applications*, (April 24, 1986), 2nd edition, ISBN-13: 978-0198546320, by permission of Oxford University Press.)

Even if standard gel electrophoresis produces good results even when applied to labs on chip, it does not exploit either the microfluidic environment or the possibility of building very small structures that are typical of labs on chip. In order to exploit these characteristics, different types of electrophoresis processes can be used in labs on chip: free-flow electrophoresis and capillary electrophoresis.

8.5.2.1 Free-Flow Electrophoresis

Free-flow electrophoresis is a separation technique where electrophoresis happens while the sample is traveling through a microfluidic duct where Poiseuille flow of a neutral liquid phase happens. The electrical field generating electrophoresis is orthogonal to the fluid flow, and the sample is inserted at the side of the duct section. While different species are displaced by electrophoresis to the duct center, they also accelerate due to the gradient of the velocity field. This hydrodynamic effect enhances the separation among different species, allowing effective electrophoresis without a very high viscosity buffer like a gel [123–125]. The scheme of this separation technique is shown in Figure 8.87.

This is a more complex scheme with respect to simple gel electrophoresis that adapts well to use in labs on chip due to the possibility to be implemented also without the use of an electrophoretic gel. Since we are considering molecule separation, we can assume that all the solutes are dragged by the fluid so that their velocity in the absence of electrical field corresponds to the local fluid velocity (see Section 8.5.1.2). Assuming that the sample is injected in a channel with axis in $x = x_0$ and using for the fluid buffer velocity field Equation 7.88 for an infinite slab, the average motion equation of a solute molecule is given by

$$\frac{d\mathbf{r}}{dt} = v_0 \left(1 - \frac{x}{w}\right)\frac{x}{w}\mathbf{y} + \mu E_x \mathbf{x} \tag{8.128}$$

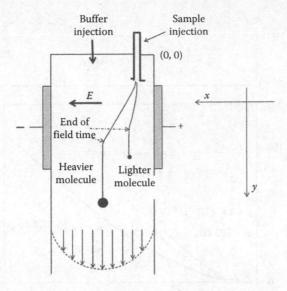

FIGURE 8.87 Principle scheme of free-flow electrophoresis.

where v_0 is the maximum buffer speed, $E_x = \psi/w$ the electrophoresis field, w the electrophoresis channel width, and x, y the axes unit vectors. The resulting average trajectories in the electrophoretic duct are given by

$$y(x) = \frac{v_0(x - x_0)^2(3w - 2(x - x_0))}{6\psi\mu w}$$ (8.129)

and the instant t at which the position corresponding to a certain coordinate is given by

$$t = \frac{w}{\mu\psi}(x - x_0)$$ (8.130)

The average trajectories are shown in Figure 8.89 assuming $x_0 = 10$ μm, $w = 300$ μm, $\psi = 5$ V, and $v_0 = 500$ μm/s for different values of mobility for proteins in ionized water associated with proteins of different masses. The separation advantage due to the hydrodynamic drag during electrophoresis is clearly evident from the figure. For example, in a standard electrophoresis with the same parameters, the separation between the molecules weighing 20 and 100 kDa will be 30 μm after 2.2 s electrophoresis, while in the free flow case, it results to about 150 μm.

As in the case of standard electrophoresis, fluctuations happen around the average particle trajectories so that the electrophoresis mark is not a single point but a shaded area where the molecule concentration gradually passes from a maximum to zero. Besides the causes of electrophoresis mark spread we have already considered in the above section, hydrodynamic spread also happens in free-flow electrophoresis due to the fact that any spread of the molecule population along the y direction also causes them to move with different drag velocities, thus causing a spread along the x direction [126].

Both diffusive and hydrodynamic spreads can be included into the dynamic equation of the molecule concentration, which can be derived similarly to Equation 8.121 and is written as

$$\frac{\partial c}{\partial t} = D\left(\frac{\partial^2 c}{\partial x^2} + \frac{\partial^2 c}{\partial y^2}\right) + \mu E_x \frac{\partial c}{\partial x} + v_y(x)\frac{\partial c}{\partial y}$$ (8.131)

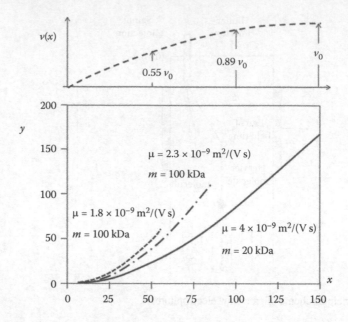

FIGURE 8.88 Average trajectories of molecules with different masses and electrophoretic mobility in the free-flow electrophoresis system that is detailed in the text. The trajectories stop when they reach the point corresponding to 2.2 s of electrophoresis. The fluid buffer velocity distribution is also evidenced.

This is a complex equation and generally numerical solution is needed to obtain an accurate determination of the concentration dynamics during electrophoresis. It is, however, more intuitive than an approximate solution of Equation 8.131 can be attempted under the validity conditions of the Taylor dispersion approximation listed in Section 7.5.4, which are frequently valid for free-flow electrophoresis [127]. Solving Equation 8.131 in the system moving with the concentration center of mass in the x direction, it is derived that the maximum spread of the concentration distribution happens in the x direction and the corresponding concentration variance is given by

$$\sigma_{c,x}^2 = \frac{y_M^2}{3} + \frac{2Dy_f}{v_0} + \frac{w^2 v_0}{105D}\overline{x} \qquad (8.132)$$

where y_f is the ordinate of the final electrophoresis distribution and $\overline{x}$ is an electrophoresis condition-dependent length. The expression of $\overline{x}$ depends on the abscissa of the middle of the input duct x_0 and on the center of mass of the final electrophoresis distribution x_f as

$$\overline{x} = \frac{(x_f - x_0)}{3w(x_f + x_0) - 2(x_f^2 + x_0^2 + x_f x_0)} \approx \frac{1}{3w - 2x_f} \qquad (8.133)$$

where the approximation holds when $x_f \gg x_0$. The structure typical of the Taylor dispersion is clear in Equation 8.134 and the three terms are the injection dispersion, the diffusion dispersion, and the hydrodynamic dispersion.

8.5.2.2 Capillary Electrophoresis

Capillary electrophoresis is a process for the separation of charged species in a sample during their migration by electroosmosis in a capillary. The principle scheme of an on-chip arrangement for capillary electrophoresis is shown in Figure 8.89a [128–130]. The sample containing charged species, for example, proteins or nucleic acids, is injected into a buffer-filled electrophoretic

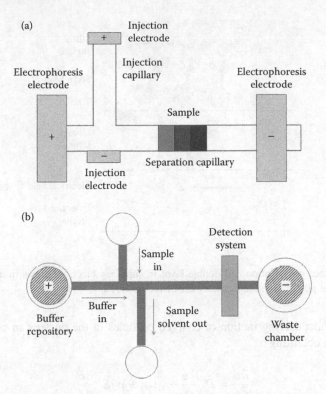

FIGURE 8.89 Principle scheme of on-chip capillary electrophoresis with electrokinetic injection of the sample in the electrophoresis duct (a) and practical arrangement of a capillary electrophoresis chip (b).

capillary near one of the two electrophoretic electrodes. In Figure 8.89a, injection is realized by moving the charged species with a suitable electrostatic field in a sufficiently short time so as not to cause electrophoretic spurious effects, but any other injection methods can be devised. The separation capillary starts and terminates with two electrodes generating a high voltage electrical field and is filled with a suitable buffer containing electrolytes so as to obtain the desired pH for electrophoresis. The field that generates inside the buffer orients the surface molecules of the capillary surface so as to create a dipole and consequently a secondary field orthogonal to the capillary walls. This secondary field attracts the ions of the buffer so as to form an electrical double layer, as described in Section 7.5.2: this effect is schematically shown in Figure 8.90 in the case of an SiO_2 capillary.

The creation of a double layer induces electroosmotic flow in the capillary (see Section 7.5.4) with the typical almost flat velocity profile. When the sample is injected in the electrophoresis capillary and the field is switched on, the electroosmosis flow is sufficiently strong to drag all the charged particles toward the same electrode, independently of their charge. Nevertheless, each particle is subject to an individual electrostatic force that superimposes to the fluid induced drag and that depends on the particle charge. This force influences the particle velocity thus causing separation between particles having different charge and mobility in the buffer. Besides electrical forces, diffusion also operates, creating a wide distribution of the different particle populations even if injection ideally happens in a single point.

In practical on-chip capillary electrophoresis, the electroosmotic flow of the buffer through the capillary is frequently exploited to inject not only the sample, but also the buffer into the capillary at the start of the separation process, thus avoiding long storage of the buffer into a small capillary with possible problems related to its stability. In this case, the electrophoresis chip arrangement is similar to that shown in Figure 8.89b.

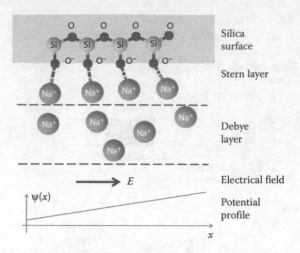

FIGURE 8.90 Surface polarization and double layer in capillary electrophoresis in a glass capillary. The electrical field and the potential in the capillary are also evidenced.

The different effect driving motion of charged particles in the buffer can be summarized in a governing equation obtaining

$$\frac{\partial c}{\partial t} = D\frac{\partial^2 c}{\partial x^2} + (\mu_{EO} + \mu)E_x\frac{\partial c}{\partial x} \tag{8.134}$$

where diffusion in the capillary section has been neglected due to the fact that separation happens along the capillary axis x, μ_{EO} represents the buffer electroosmosis mobility (see Equation 7.240), and μ the electrophoretic mobility of the considered species in the buffer. The solution of Equation 8.134 is simply obtained by setting $\bar{x} = x - (\mu_{EO} + \mu)E_x t$. The solution in case of uniform initial concentration in the interval $[0, x_M]$ is written as

$$c(x,t) = c_0\left[\operatorname{erf}\left(\frac{x - \mu E_x t - \mu_{EO}E_x t - x_M}{\sqrt{4Dt}}\right) - \operatorname{erf}\left(\frac{x - \mu E_x t - \mu_{EO}E_x t}{\sqrt{4Dt}}\right)\right] \tag{8.135}$$

so that the variance of the electrophoretic distribution at a certain instant can also be written in this case as a sum of an initial dispersion and of a diffusion dispersion as

$$\sigma_c^2 = \frac{x_M^2}{3} + \frac{Dx_f}{(\mu_{EO} + \mu)E_x} \tag{8.136}$$

In the case of capillary electrophoresis, the electrophoresis definition is frequently expressed in terms of theoretical plates, as it is done in the case of chromatography (see Section 3.5.1). Since the number of theoretical plates N_x is related to the correlation between nearby points of the electrophoresis diagram (or the chromatograph diagram in the case of chromatography), it can be expressed as the square distance traveled in the capillary by the considered species divided by the concentration variance. In the case of diffusion-limited resolution, we get

$$N_x = \frac{(\mu_{EO} + \mu)E_x x_f^2}{Dx_f} = \frac{(\mu_{EO} + \mu)\psi_x}{D} \tag{8.137}$$

where ψ_x is the potential experienced by the species during electrophoresis, which coincides with the electrophoresis potential if detection is performed at the end of the capillary. The efficiency of capillary electrophoresis separations is typically much higher than the efficiency of HPLC, which explains its wide use in labs on chip, besides the fact that its architecture is much more suitable for on-chip integration. Unlike HPLC, in capillary electrophoresis, there is no mass transfer between phases (see Section 3.5.2). Moreover, the buffer velocity profile in EOF-driven systems is almost constant, while in HPLC it is in a very first approximation parabolic. A velocity profile changing along the separation duct section introduces a Taylor-like effect, that is, an hydrodynamic spread of the concentration distribution that does not exist on capillary electrophoresis. As a consequence, on-chip capillary electrophoresis can have more than ten thousand theoretical plates, one or two order of magnitudes more than HPLC implemented in a similar geometry [131].

8.5.3 MEMBRANE FILTERS

Perhaps, the most traditional filters in biochemical and fluid-based systems are based on membranes allowing the passage of selected substances while blocking other. Membrane-based filters have a wide range of performances, depending on the type of substances to be filtered and on the type of used membrane.

In this section, we will deal with two types of membrane filters that can be used in labs on chip: artificial membrane filters and microdialysis filters. Artificial membrane filters rely on the capabilities of microtechnologies to fabricate artificial porous membranes with well-controlled properties. These membranes are used to filter large particles from the sample before further processing it into the lab on chip. Conversely, microdialysis filters adopt semipermeable membranes to filter small molecules from the sample by the use of reverse osmosis, being able even to partially purify the sample from ions and small inorganic molecules such as carbonates.

8.5.3.1 Size-Exclusion Membrane Filters

The working principle of this type of filter is quite simple: the sample is passed through a membrane, in case under a sufficient pressure to obtain a good filtering action, so that particles larger than the membrane holes are blocked by the membrane while the rest of the sample is passed through [132,133].

The main membrane fabrication parameters, besides the properties of the material constituting the membrane itself, are the hole area A_H, the hole compactness χ_H, and the membrane opening factor M_o. The form factor of the holes is defined as

$$\chi_H = \frac{\mathcal{P}_H^2}{4\pi A_H} \tag{8.138}$$

where $\mathcal{P}_H$ is the hole perimeter. The hole compactness is important when the membrane has to filter particles whose shape is significantly different from a sphere, such as red cells. In this case, the fraction of the filtered particles depends critically on their orientation in the sample and on the hole compactness. The membrane opening factor is defined as

$$M_o = \frac{N_H A_H}{A_M} \tag{8.139}$$

where N_H is the hole number and A_M the overall membrane area. The opening factor is the main factor determining both the pressure drop on the membrane, which is an important factor when it is inserted in a more complex microfluidics circuit, and the membrane break pressure. This is the maximum pressure the membrane can withhold before breaking.

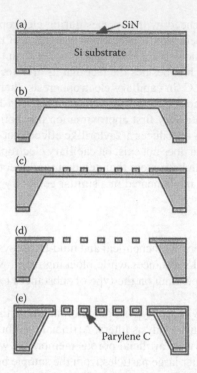

FIGURE 8.91 High-level process flow for the fabrication of a filtering membrane using SiN as fabrication material and Parylene C as protecting polymer. (a) SiN deposition, (b) KOH etching, (c) SiN patterning, (d) Si etching, and (e) Parylene C deposition. (Reproduced from *Sensors and Actuators A: Physical*, vol. 73, Yang X. et al., Micromachined membrane particle filters, pp. 184–191, Copyright 1999, with permission from Elsevier.)

The fabrication of suspended membrane in silicon technology is a standard MEM process (see Section 4.2.19, widely used for fabrication of microvalves and micropumps). Using anisotropic etching holes can be created in the suspended membrane so as to create a membrane filter. The sample can be then forced to pass through the membrane using a vertical channel, such as in a valve (see Figure 8.1).

In order to optimize the membrane elasticity and its capacity to withstand the needed pressures, different methods can be used. A possibility is to build the membrane in a suitable material that can be deposited like a film on silicon and to protect the membrane with a protective polymer after fabrication. A high-level process flow for the fabrication of a filtering membrane using SiN as fabrication material and Parylene C as protecting polymer is reported in Figure 8.91 [134] and photographs of different types of membrane realized using such a process are shown in Figure 8.92 [134]. Such membranes have been fabricated by varying hole dimensions from 6 to 12 μm to obtain different opening factors and experimental curves for the pressure drop of such membranes [134] are reported in Figure 8.93. In the example, rectangular holes have a compactness of 2.29 while the compactness of a regular hexagon is 11,026.

Membrane filters can also be realized using polymers [135]. These membranes are generally deployed horizontally over a solid polymer or glass layer where the microfluidic circuit is realized and performs filtration between a repository fabricated over them and the circuit themselves. This is frequently realized during the fabrication process itself, as shown in the example reported in Figure 8.94 and that has been used to fabricate the membrane whose electron microscope photo is reported in Figure 8.95.

Porous polymeric materials can also be directly deposited on silica or other silicon compatible materials, so as to provide direct filtration effect [136]. This technique allows smaller particles to be filtered, like big macromolecules.

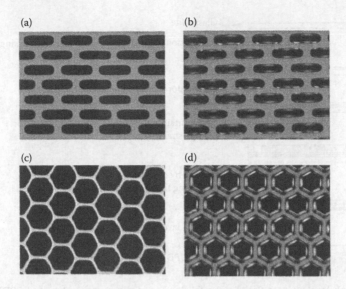

FIGURE 8.92 Scanning electron microscope photographs of different types of membrane realized using the process presented in Figure 8.90. (a) A SiN membrane filter with rectangular holes. (b) The filter after Parylene coating. (c) A SiN membrane filter with hexagonal holes. (d) The filter after Parylene coating. (Reproduced from *Sensors and Actuators A: Physical*, vol. 73, Yang X. et al., Micromachined membrane particle filters, pp. 184–191, Copyright 1999, with permission from Elsevier.)

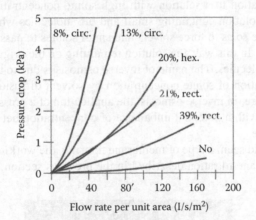

FIGURE 8.93 Pressure drop through membranes like those shown in Figure 8.91 for different values of the membrane opening factor and for different shapes of the holes; circ, circular holes; hex., hexagonal holes; rect., rectangular holes. The opening factor is indicated in percent of the membrane area. (Data from Yang X. et al., *Sensors and Actuators A: Physical*, vol. 73, pp. 184–191, 1999.)

8.5.3.2 Microdialysis Filters

Dialysis is a process of elimination of small molecules from a solution that in biochemistry is frequently used, for example, to eliminate ions and other small organic molecules from a protein solution. The main characteristic of dialysis is its unique ability to eliminate very small contaminants that cannot be filtered out with other techniques [137–139].

The base mechanism of dialysis is the so-called inverse osmosis [140]: while during a normal osmosis process, we have passage of a solvent through a semipermeable membrane from a solution

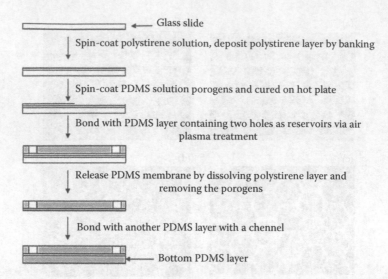

Glass slide

Spin-coat polystirene solution, deposit polystirene layer by banking

Spin-coat PDMS solution porogens and cured on hot plate

Bond with PDMS layer containing two holes as reservoirs via air plasma treatment

Release PDMS membrane by dissolving polystirene layer and removing the porogens

Bond with another PDMS layer with a chennel

Bottom PDMS layer

FIGURE 8.94 High-level process flow for the fabrication of filtering membranes in PDMS via deposition of PDMS over a polystyrene support presenting particle generating holes in the deposited layer. (Reproduced from *Analytica Chimica Acta*, vol. 662, Oua J., Rena C. L., Pawliszyn J., A simple method for preparation of macroporous polydimethylsiloxane membrane for microfluidic chip-based isoelectric focusing applications, pp. 200–205, Copyright 2010, with permission from Elsevier.)

with low solute concentration to a solution with high solute concentration, in reverse osmosis, a pressure is applied to a solution containing small and big molecules while it is in contact with a semipermeable membrane so as to force solvent and small solutes to pass the membrane, while big molecules cannot do that. In this way, the solution remaining on the original side of the membrane is purified from small molecules. The name of inverse osmosis is due to the fact that, while in normal osmosis the equalization of solute concentration by solvent diffusion through the membrane creates an osmosis pressure, in inverse osmosis, the application of a pressure causes the passage of solvent and small solute with a potential unbalance of concentration between the two sides of the semipermeable membrane.

While the dialysis could seem a type of membrane filtering, the working mechanism is in reality quite different. In membrane filtration described in the previous section, the selection mechanism

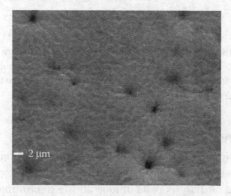

2 μm

FIGURE 8.95 Electron microscope photograph of a membrane fabricated with the process presented in Figure 8.93. (Reproduced from *Analytica Chimica Acta*, vol. 662, Oua J., Rena C. L., Pawliszyn J., A simple method for preparation of macroporous polydimethylsiloxane membrane for microfluidic chip-based isoelectric focusing applications, pp. 200–205, Copyright 2010, with permission from Elsevier.)

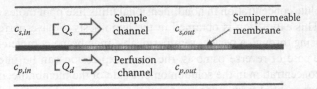

FIGURE 8.96 Principle scheme of on-chip dialysis.

is essentially based on size exclusion: large molecules cannot pass through the membrane holes due to their size. For this reason, complete exclusion of selected species from one side of the filter is possible, while on the other hand, the dimension of the membrane pores directly determines what substances are blocked and what substances are passed through. Dialysis is based on a diffusion mechanism enabled by the presence of the membrane; this causes both a statistical nature of the filtration, which cannot reach perfect exclusion or perfect retention of selected species, and the fact that the dimension of the membrane pores is only indirectly related to the species that are filtered during the process.

The typical structure of an on-chip dialysis system is presented in Figure 8.96: two parallel microchannels host the flow of the sample and that of the so-called perfusion liquid, that is, the liquid that will remove the waste from the sample. The separation surface between the two channels is constituted for the length of the dialysis filter by a semipermeable membrane with characteristics designed for the wanted filtering action. If the channels have similar sections, as it is almost always the case, the flow rate of the sample is maintained much higher than the flow rate of the perfusion liquid, so as to create the wanted difference of pressure through the membrane and create inverse osmosis. Besides the basic arrangement that is shown in Figure 8.96, several other arrangements are possible, for example, the sample and the perfusion liquid can flow in opposite directions in the parallel channels [141] or the channels can be constructed one on top of the other, for example, in two different wafers of polymer slabs before bonding. The last arrangement can be useful when the membrane is deposited on top of one of the channels so as to constitute its roof [142].

A complete modeling of a dialysis filter is quite complex due to the need of not only modeling the membrane working, but also the hydrodynamic boundary conditions at the membrane interface. Such modeling is possible via the solution of the Navier–Stokes equation with suitable boundary conditions in a first step to determine the fluid velocity field in the system and then the diffusion–convection equation to obtain the evolution of the solutes concentrations [143,144]. Explicit results from such models can be obtained by numerical simulation; here we prefer to introduce a quite simplified model, which nevertheless allows an insight into the phenomenon dynamics.

The first step is to assume that the fluid flow in the two parallel ducts is a Poiseuille flow and that at the end of both ducts, the pressure is equal to the zero reference pressure. Different pressures can be applied at the duct inputs and the ducts can have different dimensions so that the flow rates in the two ducts are, in general, different. Since we are not interested in the distribution of the solute in the ducts, but in the passage of solutes from a duct to the other, we will model the system as a one-dimensional system. The space variable along the duct axes will be called x. Since in order to obtain effective dialysis, the speed of the fluids in the ducts does not have to be very high, this is a good approximation since Taylor dispersion tends to maintain the solute concentration almost constant in the duct sections.

Under a thermodynamic point of view, osmosis and reverse osmosis can be analyzed by starting from the equilibrium of the chemical potential on the two sides of the semipermeable membrane [145]. From this analysis, the classical expression of the osmosis pressure P can be obtained:

$$P = \left(\frac{RT}{V}\right) \ln(c) \qquad (8.140)$$

where $c(x,t)$ is the solute concentration in nondimensional units like ppm moles and V is in this case the molar volume. This expression is obtained in the hypothesis to have perfect solvent osmosis, that is, a solvent passing through a perfect semipermeable membrane completely preventing solute to traverse it. In the case of reverse osmosis, the same expression can be interpreted as the link between the solute concentration in the solution on one side of the membrane and the applied pressure. Passing to an exponential form evidencing that the pressure is the external driver, we get

$$c = \exp\left(\frac{PV}{RT}\right) \tag{8.141}$$

If we change the applied pressure a bit, the solute concentration also changes so as to restore the balance between the chemical potential on the two membrane sides causing a solvent flux through the membrane, whose expression can be evaluated by differentiation (8.141) with respect to P so that

$$\frac{dc}{dP} = \frac{V}{RT}\exp\left(\frac{PV}{RT}\right) = \frac{V}{RT}c \tag{8.142}$$

Using Equation 8.142, a set of governing equation for the concentrations in the two ducts of the dialysis filter can be obtained directly balancing the fluxes in the system as usual. In doing that we have to add to thermodynamic and fluid-dynamic equations the characteristic equation of the membrane, relating the external pressure to the material flow through the membrane in time. If the applied pressure is not too high and if no anisotropy exists between the fluxes through the membrane in the two possible directions, a linear characteristic equation is generally well suited to represent the membrane behavior, so that we can characterize the membrane by the equation

$$\frac{\partial c}{\partial t} = \alpha S_M \frac{\partial c}{\partial P} = \alpha S_M \frac{V}{RT}c \tag{8.143}$$

where S_M is the membrane area and α is the membrane permeability per unit area, and it is measured in Pa/s/m^2. The permeability of the membrane depends on the solute molecules critical dimension and shape so as to determine the dialysis filtering action. Using Equation 8.143, the governing equations derived by the fluxes balance is written as

$$\frac{\partial c_s}{\partial t} + \bar{v}_s \frac{\partial c_s}{\partial x} = -\frac{\alpha S_M V}{RT}c_s + \frac{\alpha S_M V}{RT}c_p \tag{8.144a}$$

$$\frac{\partial c_p}{\partial t} + \bar{v}_p \frac{\partial c_p}{\partial x} = \frac{\alpha S_M V}{RT}c_s - \frac{\alpha S_M V}{RT}c_p \tag{8.144b}$$

where the indexes s and p indicate the sample and the perfusion fluid and $\bar{v}_s$, $\bar{v}_p$, are the average fluid velocities in the sample and perfusion channels, respectively. Since the fluid fluxes are generally considered instead of the average velocities, it is useful to express Equations 8.144 using the flow rates Q_s and Q_p and the duct sections S_s and S_p. To find a stationary state solution of Equations 8.144, we have to set to zero the time derivatives, obtaining the intuitive relation

$$\frac{Q_s}{S_s}\frac{\partial c_s}{\partial x} = -\frac{Q_p}{S_p}\frac{\partial c_p}{\partial x} \tag{8.145}$$

Setting the initial conditions to $c_s(0) = c_0$ and $c_p(0) = 0$ we get

$$c_s(x) = c_0 - \frac{S_s}{S_p} \frac{Q_p}{Q_s} c_p(x) \tag{8.146}$$

Substituting in Equation 8.141a, we find the following solution for the concentrations:

$$c_s(x) = \frac{c_0}{Q_s S_p + Q_p S_s} \left[Q_s S_p + Q_p S_s e^{-\frac{x}{x_D}} \right] \tag{8.147a}$$

$$c_p(x) = c_0 \frac{Q_s S_p}{Q_s S_p + Q_p S_s} \left[1 - e^{-\frac{x}{x_D}} \right] \tag{8.147b}$$

where the dialysis characteristic length x_D is given by

$$x_D = \frac{RTQ_sQ_p}{\alpha S_M V(S_s Q_p + S_p Q_s)} \tag{8.148}$$

Equation 8.148 is in reality only an implicit definition of the dialysis filter characteristic length, since the membrane surface is present at the denominator, which in our case also depends on the filter length. If we ideally imagine to occupy all the channel side with the membrane, we can set $S_M = Lh = \xi h x_D$, where L is the filter length, h is the channel depth, and ξ is the parameter determining the ratio between the filtration capability of the real filter and the ideal filtration capability of an infinitely long filter. Substituting in Equation 8.148 and solving for the filter length L, we get

$$L = \sqrt{\frac{\xi RTQ_sQ_p}{\alpha hV(S_s Q_p + S_p Q_s)}} \tag{8.149}$$

The filter characteristic length is inversely proportional to the membrane permeability, moreover it increases with temperature since the thermal motion renders the diffusion through the membrane less effective.

The equilibrium distribution of the solute does not depend on the permeability, since it is theoretically reached only for an infinitely long filter. The effectiveness of the dialysis filter is generally evaluated by the so-called capture ratio Γ, which is defined as the fraction of the input solute captured by the perfusion fluid. From our model, it results that

$$\Gamma = \frac{Q_s S_p}{Q_s S_p + Q_p S_s} \tag{8.150}$$

which further simplifies in the common case of channels with the same section and the same length as

$$\Gamma = \frac{Q_s}{Q_s + Q_p} = \frac{P_s}{P_s + P_p} \tag{8.151}$$

where P_s and P_p are the applied pressures at the input of the filter channels. The capture ratio is determined only by design variables of the filter, that is, the geometry of the channels and the flow rates. In particular, as anticipated, the flow rate in the sample channel has to be much higher than the flow rate in the perfusion channel.

If we consider a dialysis filter with channels with the same section and the same length where the flow rate is 100 μL/min in the sample channel and 1 μL/min in the perfusion channel, a capture rate as high as 90.9% can be obtained. As far as the filter length is concerned, assuming $h = 8$ μm, $V = 18$ mL, $T = 300$ K, $S_s = S_p = 1600$ μm^2, $\xi = 3$, and $\alpha = 50$ kPa/s/μm^2, we get $L \approx 3$ mm, which is a dimension compatible with labs on chip applications.

A microdialysis membrane is very similar in structure and function to a conventional filtering membrane: it has a rigid, highly voided structure with randomly distributed, interconnected pores. However, the pores differ from those in a conventional filter by being extremely small, as average pore sizes are on the order of 10–100 nm in diameter.

A requirement of any dialysis membrane is that the pores must be filled with the solvent liquid during use; therefore, wettability of the membrane material is a needed characteristic. Hydrophilic polymers combine a good compatibility with labs on chip production technologies and very good wettability by water, so being by far the most used materials for microdialysis membrane fabrication.

The first method that has been used to integrate dialysis membranes in labs on chip systems is to include them between ducts fabricated on different wafers during wafer bonding. This method has the advantage of exploiting well-experimented membranes, but requires a careful wafer bonding process not to damage the membrane [146–148]. Cellulose acetate has been one of the early membrane materials used for reverse osmosis; these membranes are relatively easy to manufacture, are cost effective, and result in membranes with a high flux. Cellulose acetate is prepared from cellulose by acetylation, that is, in a reaction with acetic anhydride, acetic acid, and sulfuric acid. Cellulose acetate drawbacks include a fairly narrow temperature range of usage (maximum 30°C), a narrow pH range restricted to pH 2–8, and high biodegradability. At low pH, the beta-glucosidic linkages in the backbone of the cellulose polymer can be degraded, reducing the effective molecular weight and causing loss of structural integrity, while at high pH, cellulose acetate membranes can deacetylate [149]. This has made other polymer materials such as polysulfone (PS) [150,151], polyethersulfone (PES) [151], and regenerated cellulose [152].

PS is a name describing a family of thermoplastic polymers that are suitable for manufacturing of membranes with pores up to 40 nm average diameter. They contain the subunit aryl-SO_2-aryl, the defining feature of which is the sulfone group, the molecular formula of the base PS polymer is reported in Figure 8.97. These polymers are rigid, high-strength, and transparent, retaining these properties between −100°C and 150°C. They have very high dimensional stability; the size change when exposed to boiling water or 150°C air or steam generally falls below 0.1%. Its glass transition temperature is 185°C.

PES is another polymer of the PS family that is frequently used for microdialysis membranes; the structure formula and an electron microscope photo of a dialysis membrane realized using this polymer are reported in Figure 8.98. PES membranes, due to the insufficient water wetting property of PES, usually contain a small amount of polyvinylpyrrolidone (PVP) as an alloying agent. The PVP provides the requisite wetting, although there may still be very small diameter pores that are inactive during dialysis because of the exclusion of water. PES membrane filters have excellent flow speeds and, connected to it, a high filterable volume. They work properly in the wide pH range 2–12 and manifest a much smaller tendency to absorb proteins with respect to basic PS membranes.

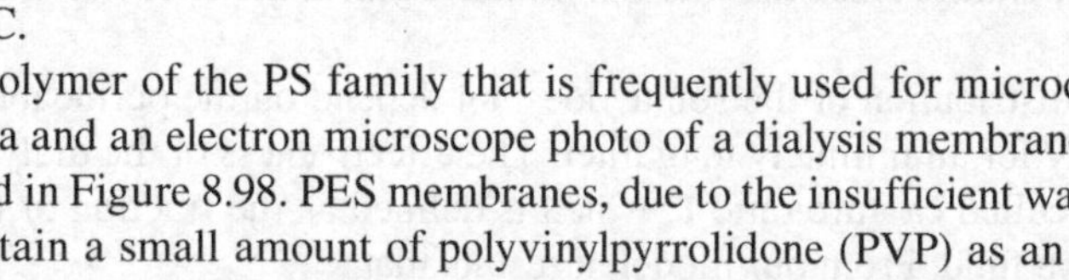

FIGURE 8.97 Structure formula of the base polysulfone polymer.

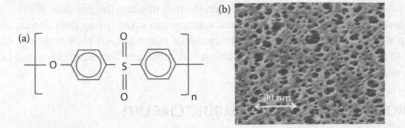

FIGURE 8.98 Polyethersulfone structure formula (a) and electron microscope photo of a dialysis membrane realized using this polymer (b).

The membrane in widest use for microdialysis is regenerated cellulose; this can be fabricated from cellulose acetate by performing an additional hydrolysis step, using an alkaline solution that deacetylates the membrane and reverts it to cellulose. Deacetylation affects selectivity and integrity, and is known to increase the porosity of bulk dialysis membranes [153]. The regenerated cellulose membranes are atypical in that they contain a high percentage of water, yet do not lose their mechanical integrity unless they dry out.

Several techniques have also been devised for *in situ* fabrication of the microdialysis membrane during the lab on chip fabrication process. Cellulose acetate membranes can be directly built on chip using a phase separation technique [142], the high-level process flow is represented in Figure 8.99. After the creation of the dialysis channels via wet etching, the cellulose acetate polymer solution is spun on the wafer. After spinning, the sample is transferred to room temperature for a deionized water bath. The polymer undergoes precipitation in the nonsolvent water, as the solvent is displaced from the film. The sample is then left in the bath overnight to remove any remaining solvent and dried by air flow exposure. At the end of the processing a semiclear, conformal polymer coating is formed on the silicon substrate.

Pores are formed in the polymer film by the phase separation process. During the immersion precipitation, the composition of the polymer enters the two-phase region in the phase diagram and phase separation occurs, producing a polymer-rich phase, containing mainly polymer and less solvent, and a polymer-lean phase, containing mainly solvent and less polymer. The polymer-rich phase represents the structural walls of the coating while the polymer-lean phase represents the porous regions in the coating. By varying the polymer concentration, the precipitation medium, and the temperature, a large variety of pore sizes can be attained.

The polymer's wetting characteristics are largely responsible for its ability not to fill the underlying dialysis channels. The main force driving the polymer into a cavity is capillary action while the main

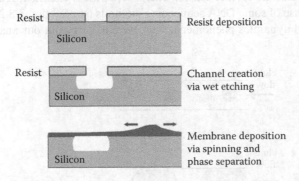

FIGURE 8.99 *In situ* fabrication of a cellulose acetate microdialysis membrane by spinning and phase separation.

opposing forces include the cohesive forces within the polymer and the pressure of the gas trapped in the cavity. Thus, a correct design of the spinned solution can avoid filling the microchannels.

Another possible technique for *in situ* fabrication of microdialysis membranes is direct polymerization of the polymer precursor once spun on the substrate, for example, using laser-induced polymerization [154].

8.6 MICRODROPLETS IN MICROFLUIDIC CIRCUITS

Control of volumes in labs on chip is a critical element. Several detection systems can be roughly depicted as molecule counts systems and if concentrations have to be measured, the fluid volume has to be strictly controlled. In continuous-flow systems, this can be achieved by a strict control of the exerted pressures and by in-line flow rate control; in addition, experimental calibration curves are often used in practice for a specific device.

An alternative way to achieve a very good volume control is to process the sample in the form of droplets immersed in an environmental fluid that has the only role of providing flow continuity with the suitable fluid dynamic properties [155,156]. In Chapter 7, it has been underlined as the volume and the form of droplets is determined by the generation mechanism and by the physical and chemical conditions occurring during droplet generation. These elements can be controlled with a very good accuracy so that the form and volume of droplets can be accurately defined at the moment of the lab on chip design.

Operating with droplets in the vast majority of cases also has the advantage of further reducing the needed sample volume, thus allowing the process of very small samples that are typical of selected applications. Last but not least, the use of droplets frequently allows the quantities of reagents to be reduced, with a further economic advantage with respect to continuous-flow systems.

The fact that droplets-based system have emerged as a possible alternative to continuous-flow-based system depends on the fact that in the microscale, droplets are stable and highly reproducible, allowing both a very good sample volume control and the design of suitable processing elements. Two different kinds of droplets could be generated in microfluidic circuits: the so-called free droplets that are completely dragged by the environmental fluid without interaction with the duct walls, and the constricted drops that are in contact both with the duct walls and with the environmental fluid, as shown in Figure 8.100. In lab on chip applications, constrained droplets are generally used, even if cases of the exploitation of free droplets are not absent.

8.6.1 DROPLET STABILITY AND BREAKING DOWN

The energy of a droplet at constant temperature $\mathcal{E}_{tot}$ is formed by three terms: the internal energy, the kinetic energy $\mathcal{E}_k$, and the surface tension energy $\mathcal{E}_s$. Unless chemical reactions happen inside the droplet, as in the case of some DNA sequencing methods (see Section 3.8.2), the internal energy is not changed by fluid dynamics phenomena; thus, we can carry out our analysis considering the

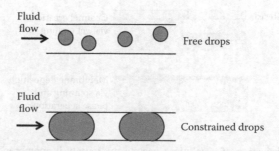

FIGURE 8.100 Different droplets types in a microfluidic duct.

sum of the kinetic energy and the surface tension energy. If the droplet temperature is changed, for example, by a heater, the added thermal energy has to be added to the total droplet energy.

Starting from a constant temperature situation, assuming that the droplet translates with velocity v_d with no rotation, which is a quite reasonable assumption in a microfluidic circuit and calling S and V the droplet surface and volume, respectively, we can write

$$\mathcal{E}_{tot} = \mathcal{E}_K + \mathcal{E}_s = \frac{1}{2}\rho V v_d^2 + S\gamma \tag{8.152}$$

This relation is the base of the stability analysis of a microfluidic droplet. In general, to better define various droplet states, the so-called Weber number We is defined, which is a nondimensional number related to the ratio between the droplet kinetic and surface energy. It is defined as

$$We = \frac{6\rho V v_d^2}{S\gamma} = \frac{\rho L_d v_d^2}{\gamma} \tag{8.153}$$

where L_d is the droplet characteristic dimension that coincides with three times the volume-to-surface ratio. In the frequent case of spherical droplets, we simply have $L_d = d_d$, where d_d is the droplet diameter. This simple relation also explains the presence of the factor six in the definition of the Weber number for droplets. In the case of microfluidic ducts, however, constrained droplets are frequently more important than free droplets, whose surface is generally spherical with a good approximation. An approximated value of the Weber number for a constrained droplet can be obtained considering a circular duct of radius equal to R and a droplet wetting the duct walls for a length equal to l, as shown in Figure 8.101.

In this case, the Weber number can be explicitly evaluated due to the fact that the extreme parts of the droplet are sphere segments due to the symmetry of the problem. The following expression results for the droplet characteristic length:

$$L_d = 2R\frac{6R\cos^3(\theta) - 8R\cos^2(\theta) - 2R\cos(\theta) + 3l + 4R}{2l + 4R - 4R\cos(\theta)} \tag{8.154}$$

From Equation 8.154, it results that a correction factor appears in the case of constrained droplets that depends on the contact angle between the liquid and the duct walls and in general cannot be neglected. The value of the droplet characteristic length versus the duct diameter for constrained droplets is plotted in Figure 8.102 versus the contact angle for different values of the ratio R/l. From the figure it is evident that if the droplet is longer than the channel radius, the characteristic length dependence on the contact angle can be neglected due to the fact that both the surface and the volume are very little influenced by the menisci at the ends of the droplet. On the contrary, if the

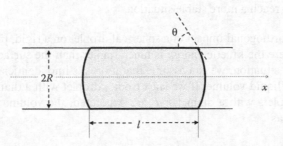

FIGURE 8.101 Geometry of a constrained drop in a microchannel.

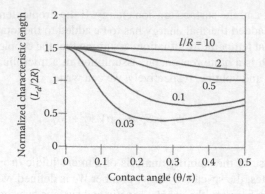

FIGURE 8.102 Characteristic length of a constrained droplet in a circular microchannel versus the contact angle for different ratios between the length of the wetted channel wall and the channel radius.

droplet is of the same order of magnitude or smaller, the dependence on the contact angle cannot be neglected.

The total droplet energy can be rewritten substituting the expression of the Weber number in Equation 8.149 as

$$\mathcal{E}_{tot} = S\gamma\left(\frac{1}{12}We + 1\right) \tag{8.155}$$

In order to break the droplet due to the droplet motion, it is necessary that the kinetic energy is greater than the surface tension energy, so that the motion inertial effect causes the surface breakage. On this ground, we can individuate three motion regimes for a droplet, depending on the characteristic Weber number:

- $We \ll 12$: This is the stable regime—the kinetic energy is never sufficient to overcome the surface tension or even to induce sensible deformation in the droplet surface, the droplet is stable and moves in an essentially rigid motion; even if the droplet is suddenly stopped by the impact with a rigid surface and all the kinetic energy is transformed in surface deformation, it does not break and, after the impact, it returns to equilibrium.
- $We \approx 12$: The kinetic energy is sufficient to induce relevant deformation of the droplet shape during motion and the droplet could break into two smaller droplets if it impacts a solid surface; the fluid behavior after the impact in this transition region is essentially determined by side factors such as surface roughness, the impact angle, and so on.
- $We \gg 12$: In this regime, the droplet is not stable, its shape depends on the motion conditions, and it breaks in several smaller droplets after the impact with a solid surface. If the Weber number is very high, the droplet itself becomes instable and it can break due to the simple motion to reach a more stable situation.

Let us imagine the orthogonal impact of a spherical droplet on a rigid, perfectly smooth surface in instable regime, where the kinetic energy is much higher than the surface tension energy [157]. In a perfectly isotropic situation, we can assume that it breaks into identical smaller droplets while conserving the overall liquid volume. If we start from a droplet with a diameter equal to d_0 and at the end N smaller droplets with a diameter d_1 are generated, the volume conservation condition allows us to deduce d_1 as

$$d_1 = \frac{d_0}{\sqrt[3]{N}} \tag{8.156}$$

The overall surface thus passes from $S_0 = 4\pi d_0^2$ to $S_1 = 4N\pi d_1^2$, thus causing an increase $\Delta\mathcal{E}_s$ in the surface energy that is equal to

$$\Delta\mathcal{E}_s = 4\pi\gamma \, (N d_1^2 - d_0^2) = 4\pi\gamma d_0^2 \, (\sqrt[3]{N} - 1) \tag{8.157}$$

The increase in the surface energy, due to the rigid nature of the surface, has to be created at the expense of the kinetic energy of the droplets, so that it has to be equal to the difference in kinetic energy before and after the fragmentation. Calling v_0 the droplet velocity before the fragmentation, v_1 the droplets velocity after the fragmentation, and assuming that no rotation is generated to absorb further energy, the kinetic energy gap $\Delta\mathcal{E}_k$ is given by

$$\Delta\mathcal{E}_K = \frac{2}{3}\rho\pi d_0^3 v_0^2 - \frac{2}{3}\rho N\pi d_1^3 v_1^2 = \frac{2}{3}\rho\pi \, (d_0^3 v_0^2 - N d_1^3 v_1^2) \tag{8.158}$$

Moreover, we can imagine that the after fragmentation, the new droplets are in the stable region, that is, the new Weber number is equal to 12. Thus, we have the equation

$$\frac{\rho d_1 v_1^2}{\gamma} = 12 \tag{8.159}$$

Equations 8.156, $\Delta\mathcal{E}_s = \Delta\mathcal{E}_K$, and Equation 8.159 constitute a system of three equations with three unknown variables: N, d_1, and v_1; thus, all the characteristics of the set of secondary droplets can be calculated.

In particular, we get

$$N = \left(\frac{1}{6}We - 1\right)^3 \tag{8.160a}$$

$$d_1 = \frac{6 d_0}{(We - 6)} \tag{8.160b}$$

$$v_1 = v_0 \sqrt{2\frac{We - 6}{We}} \tag{8.160c}$$

From Equation 8.160, the fact that the Weber number is the fundamental parameter determining the stability of a droplet results clearly. If the Weber number is smaller than 12, the number of secondary droplets loses the physical meaning, thus indicating that the droplet does not break.

Let us now substitute typical parameters of a microfluidic system into the expression of the Weber number to state the stability degree of the droplet in this environment. Considering constraint droplet, let us use Equation 8.154 with $\theta = 72°$ ($2\pi/5$). The resulting values of the Weber number are plotted in Figure 8.103 versus the ratio l/R between the length of the duct wall wetted by the droplet and the duct radius for different values of the velocity of the droplets in the typical microfluidic range. The obtained values are many orders of magnitude smaller than one, so that it can be concluded that the droplets, once created, are very stable in such a system, moving almost as a rigid body, without any noticeable change of shape.

This is also in agreement with the fact that both the Reynolds number and the capillary number are generally quite small in microfluidic circuits of labs on chip. As seen in Chapter 7, a small

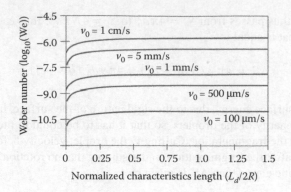

FIGURE 8.103 Logarithm of the Weber number for water constrained droplets in a circular PMMA microduct (contact angle 72°). The environmental liquid is assumed completely immiscible with water and different droplets velocities in the typical range of microfluidic circuits are considered.

Reynolds number means that fluid motion is driven by pressure and viscous forces and vortex does not form in the system. The capillary number conversely is defined as the ratio between viscous forces and capillary forces and it is defined as

$$Ca = \frac{\eta \bar{v}}{\gamma} \tag{8.161}$$

where $\bar{v}$ is the fluid characteristic velocity. In a typical lab on chip case, where $\eta = 0.00089$ Pa s, $\bar{v} = 100\,\mu\text{m/s}$, and $\gamma = 0.072$ Pa m, the capillary number is as low as 1.2×10^{-6}, so that viscous forces are much smaller than forces related to the surface tension and they are not sufficiently strong to influence, for example, the shape of menisci.

8.6.2 Microdroplet Break

The fact that droplets are extremely stable in microfluidic circuits also implies that droplet breaking is very difficult and if this is a beneficial effect, it has to be provoked in different ways that causes collisions with hard walls. A possible way of forcing a microdroplet breakup is to shape suitably the microfluidic circuit geometry. We will consider as examples two structures causing droplet breaking: the T junction and the stream focusing device that we have already encountered in Section 8.4.1 dealing with laminar mixing. A third structure, the so-called λ junction, will also be briefly presented.

8.6.2.1 T Junction

The simpler structure that can be used to force droplet breaking through the microfluidic circuit geometry is the so called T junction [158] that is shown schematically in Figure 8.104. If we imagine that a continuous flow of constrained droplets arrive at the intersection between the two ducts, two different regimes can be observed: droplet breakup and droplet propagation toward one of the side channels as it is shown in Figure 8.105.

Even if at a first glance it would seem that droplets breakup is forced by the complete symmetry of the situation, this is not correct. As a matter of fact, when droplets do not break they are alternatively directed toward one or the other of the T junction exit ducts, thus recreating the symmetry in the fluid flow that is required by the structure geometry.

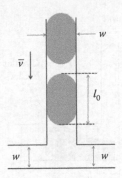

FIGURE 8.104 Scheme of a T Junction for liquid droplets breakup.

Several assumptions can be done on the structure of the droplet shape when impact with the T junction wall happens if the capillary number is sufficiently short as in microfluidic applications that are well respected in practice. As in many microfluidic applications, imagining that the system is a slab with a very small depth, the two-dimensional approximation can frequently be adopted. In this case, it is possible to assume that the pressure drop in the flow past a stationary droplet at the T junction near breakup is concentrated in a narrow gap, as shown in Figure 8.106. Outside this region, the shape of the droplet is determined by surface tension alone, so that the droplet interface is shaped as a circular arc with the curvature determined by the ambient pressure. Owing to the pressure drop across the gap, the droplet is convex at its outside tips and concave in the middle depression region [159]. It turns out to be impossible to attain a too high negative curvature at a fixed droplet volume. This leads to a critical condition determining droplet breakup.

This model of the droplet shape allows the hydrodynamic problem to be simplified by the use of the lubrication approximation [160] in the analysis of droplet evolution [159]. Lubrication theory describes the flow of fluids in a geometry in which one dimension is significantly smaller than the others. Mathematically, lubrication theory can be seen as exploiting the disparity between two length scales to simplify the fluid dynamics equations.

The obtained results are well verified by experiments [158,161] and constitute a design guide for T junctions either in the case in which droplet breakup is desired or in the case where it has to be

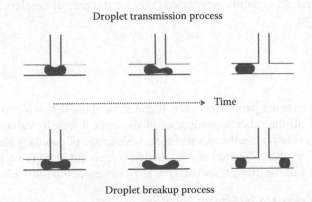

FIGURE 8.105 Schematics of the process of droplet transmission and droplet breakup in a T Junction. The so-called channeled droplet breakup is considered since the environmental fluid continues to be transmitted through the junction while the droplet splitting. If the droplet would completely obstruct the junction while splitting, obstructing droplet breakup would happen.

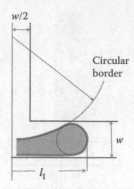

FIGURE 8.106 Shape of a droplet after the impact on the T junction wall.

avoided. The T junction behavior can be represented on a phase diagram reporting on the abscissa the length of the droplets in the input channel l_0 normalized to the channels width w, which is assumed the same for all the channels, and in the ordinate the capillary number of the system Ca. Three different regimes can be individuated on the phase plane:

- *Droplet transmission* (no breakup occurs)
- *Channeled droplet breakup*, characterized by the fact that during breakup the environmental fluid is also transmitted through the junction
- *Obstructing droplet breakup*, characterized by the fact that during breakup the environmental fluid is not transmitted through the junction that is obstructed by the splitting droplet

Two main parameters represent the dynamics of the T junction, the normalized characteristic droplets length $\overline{l}_0/w$ and the limit droplet length l_{lim}. The characteristic droplet length essentially depends on the capillary number and divides the droplet transmission by the droplet channeled breakup up to the limit droplet length. As far as the limit droplet length is concerned, available measurements present an almost constant value of the capillary number, as far as the system can be considered two-dimensional and the capillary number is small. This result is compatible with a theoretical evaluation [162] that reports the existence of a small dependence of l_{lim} on the capillary number.

A simple semiempirical equation is reported [158] for the critical droplets length as a function of the capillary number:

$$\frac{\overline{l}_0}{w} = \beta Ca^{-\varphi} \tag{8.162}$$

where φ is an almost constant parameter that is found to be about 0.21 while β is a parameter near one that summarizes all the other dependencies of the critical length. Values of β between 0.98 and 1.3 are found in many practical cases and for a wide range of capillary numbers in Reference [161]. An example of the phase diagram of a T junction is reported in Figure 8.107 in case of a ratio between the viscosities of the droplet fluid and the environmental fluid of 1.67.

8.6.2.2 Droplets Break-Up by Stream Focusing

Another way of generating droplet breakup is to operate hydrodynamic stream focusing by using a focusing liquid to shrink the main liquid stream, as already considered in Section 8.4.1 dealing with lamination mixers. While a mixer is designed so as to preserve flux continuity for all the involved fluids, if droplet break is desired, pressures and device dimensions have to be designed so as to obtain the periodic interruption of the main flux.

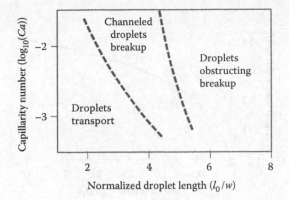

FIGURE 8.107 Phase diagram of droplets dynamics in a T junction in case of a ratio between the viscosities of the droplet fluid and the environmental fluid of 1.67. (Data from Jullien M.-C. et al., *Physics of Fluids*, vol. 21, pp. 072001-1–072001-6, 2009).

Let us imagine a device such as those schematically sketched in Figure 8.108: a periodical droplet flux composed of droplets of a low-viscosity fluid in an intermediate-viscosity environmental fluid enters into a stream focusing device (see Section 8.4.1.3) where focusing is operated by a high-viscosity fluid, such as a high-viscosity oil [163].

The phenomena happening when the droplet containing stream is focused can be better understood if we consider the velocity field that is created during the multiphase continuous flow of a low-viscosity fluid within two layers of high-viscosity fluid that we have analyzed in Section 8.4.1, as sketched in Figure 8.65. A droplet entering the viscosity-stratified field experiences a deformation of its front end-cap. The droplet nose first becomes elongated due to the additional viscous stresses caused by the side flow. If the deformation of the front end-cap is large enough, a neck appears along the droplet core and capillary forces induce breakup to reduce interfacial area. For long droplets ($d_0/h \gg 1$, see Figure 8.109), this mechanism can repeat itself on the remaining initial droplet volume and, eventually, a mother droplet can breakup into an array of n smaller daughter droplets.

In the absence of viscous stratifications ($\eta_2 = \eta_1$), three regimes of droplet behavior have been experimentally identified [164]:

- Relaxing deformation for small shear fluid flow rate Q_1
- Convective breakup for moderate Q_1
- Absolute breakup for large Q_1

The term convective breakup refers to a droplet splitting mechanism that occurs downstream from the junction and the term absolute breakup corresponds to a droplet fragmentation process localized at the junction, similar to the dripping regime.

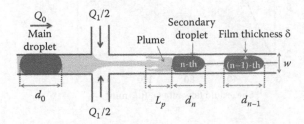

FIGURE 8.108 Droplet splitting by stream focus; the geometric variable that is relevant for the system analysis is evidenced.

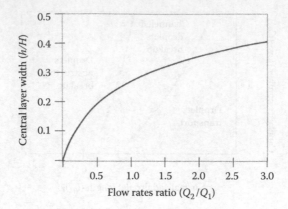

FIGURE 8.109 Layers width versus the ratio between the input flow rates of the low- and the high-viscosity fluids setting $\eta_2 = 0.00089$ Pa s, $\eta_1 = 0.01$ Pa s, $H = 200$ μm, $Q_1 = 100$ μL/s.

In the case in which viscosity stratification is present ($\eta_2 \ll \eta_1$) and for strictly identical flow rates $Q_1 = Q_2$, increasing η_1 produces a larger number of secondary droplets, as it is shown in Figure 8.110 that was interpolated from the experimental data reported in Reference [163]: overall, the number of secondary droplets appears to be roughly proportional to Q_1.

In order to conserve the mass of the initial droplet, the typical size of daughter droplets decreases with n. The presence of viscous stratifications effectively changes the environment of droplets. In particular, the sharp increase in the viscosity of the external phase modifies the ratio of capillary to viscous stresses exerted at the droplet interface and triggers a variety of dynamics. To model this effect, it is useful to define the capillary number Ca_1 associated with the side flow as

$$Ca_1 = \frac{\eta_1 Q_1}{\gamma h} \tag{8.163}$$

where γ is the surface tension at the interface between the droplet fluid and the shear fluid. For a fixed inlet flow, droplets deform for small Ca_1 and breakup for large Ca_1. The droplet dynamic response also depends on the relative change of Ca_1 compared to the inlet flow.

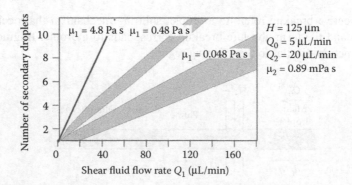

FIGURE 8.110 Variability of the number of secondary droplets formed after the junction versus the viscosity of the shear fluid. (Data from Garstecki P. et al. *Lab on a Chip*, vol. 6, pp. 437–446, 2006.)

For instance, if Ca_1 is fixed, a change in Q_2 will yield different transitions between droplet regimes. To quantify this relative change, it is useful to introduce a third flow rate value: the flow rate of the environmental fluid before the intersection, whose viscosity is intermediate between η_2 and η_1, which we call Q_0. A useful set of dimensionless quantities is the homogeneous flow fractions q_j $(j = 0, 1, 2)$ that can be defined as

$$q_j = \frac{Q_j}{Q_1 + Q_2 + Q_3} \quad (j = 0,1,2) \tag{8.164}$$

For a given viscosity ratio η_2/η_1, droplet regimes can be located on a phase diagram where d_0/h is plotted as a function of the so-called modified capillary number of the shear phase Ca_M that is defined as

$$Ca_M = \frac{\tilde{\eta}\bar{v}}{\gamma} = \sqrt{\frac{\eta_2}{\eta_1}}\, q_1\, Ca_1 \tag{8.165}$$

where $\tilde{\eta} = \sqrt{\eta_1 \eta_2}$ is the effective multiphase flow viscosity and $\bar{v} = q_1(Q_1/h^2)$ is the velocity of the shear phase at the phases interface weighted by its homogeneous flow fractions.

This is a similar technique adopted for the droplet breakup in a T junction; the modified capillary number is taken into account instead of the capillary number in this case. This because in this arrangement both the flow rates and the degree of viscous shear, represented by the ratio between η_1 and η_2 have to be taken into account.

By plotting in the considered phase diagram as it is shown in Figure 8.111, the results of several tests with the considered device [163], a clear separation between a droplet transmission and a droplet breakup zone is found in correspondence with the critical droplet length individuated by the relation

$$\frac{d_0}{h} = \alpha\, Ca_M^{-\beta} \tag{8.166}$$

with $\alpha \approx 0.58$ and $\beta \approx 0.3$.

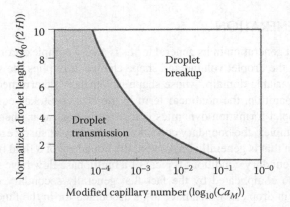

FIGURE 8.111 Droplet transmission and droplet breakup zones on the system phase diagram plotted using the modified capillary number Ca_M; the existence of a critical droplet length is clearly identified.

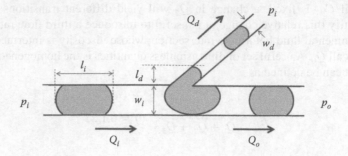

FIGURE 8.112 Scheme of a λ junction with an example of droplet transit through the junction.

8.6.2.3 λ Junction

The principle scheme of a λ junction is shown in Figure 8.112 [165]. A continuous flow of constrained ducts proceeds along a main channel under the action of an input pressure. At a certain point, a secondary channel departs from the continuous channel with an axis, forming an acute angle with the main channel axis (from which is derived the λ junction name). When a droplet arrives at the junction, part of it enters the lateral channel due to the shape of the streamlines (see Section 8.5.1). At this point, two situations are possible: a secondary drop detaches from the main drop and advances along the secondary channel as depicted in Figure 8.112 or the drop remains compact due to the effect of the surface tension and the liquid that during the transit in the junction enters into the secondary channel is dragged in the main channel again while the main drop advances. Breakup can happen through the Rayleigh–Plateau instability (see Section 7.3.5) if the thickness of the droplet between its back side and the sharp top right corner of the junction becomes small enough. This will happen if the volume of the droplet finger is allowed to advance sufficiently in the secondary channel without allowing the environmental fluid to penetrate in the secondary channel from the droplet side and to pass around it by generating sufficient flow to feed the secondary channel.

As in other cases, the complete hydrodynamic treatment of the phenomenon through the two-phase flow study and the determination of the droplet shape during transition is quite complex, but an approximate condition for the drop breakup can be determined by using the technique of the critical droplet length that has been used in the two cases considered in the above sections. We do not repeat here the whole analysis; data and comments are reported in Reference [165].

8.7 DROPLET GENERATION

The problem of droplet generation in its general terms is a very complex problem. Owing to the fact that during generation the droplet volume and shape change, it implies the solution of the Navier–Stokes equation in a variable domain, whose shape is somehow determined by the solution itself [157,166]. In such a condition, the nonlinear term in the Navier–Stokes equation is generally not negligible and the droplet formation dynamics is a strongly nonlinear phenomenon. To make the situation even more complex, the boundary conditions at the droplet surface are in no case as simple as the no-slip condition that is generally imposed at the boundary of a fluid mass flowing in contact with a solid surface. Boundary conditions typical of a multiphase flow have to be used [167,168].

The problem is also complicated by the fact that generally secondary droplets are generated besides the desired main droplets, which have to be accounted for in the fluid dynamics analysis of the system.

In this section, we will not face the whole complexity of the system, but we will adopt an analysis similar to that carried out in the last section for droplet breakup, providing design hints and a synthesis of available results.

8.7.1 T Junction Droplet Generator

Droplet generation is attained in a T junction generally designing the junction geometry so that the T channel is much wider than the feeding channel, as shown in Figure 8.113 [169,170]. The droplet fluid is then fed to the junction from the smaller channel while the environmental fluid from the T channel with flow rates Q_d and Q_c, respectively. In a first moment, we will consider a planar junction, where the depth h of all the channels is much smaller than their width and an environmental fluid wetting the device walls better than the droplet fluid. This means that the contact angle at the droplet meniscus is smaller than 90° as shown in Figure 8.100 and the meniscus is concave.

The experimental data collected on the working of such a system can be well represented by a phase graph, as it was done in the case of microfluidic circuits for droplets breakup [170,171]. The most intuitive way of plotting such a phase graph is to use the capillary number and the droplet fluid flow as coordinates, thus obtaining a graph similar to that in Figure 8.114.

In the phase graph, three different regimes of droplet formations can be identified, divided by threshold values of the capillary number that weakly depends on the flow rate of the droplet fluid.

Plug flow or squeezing regime: This is the regime characterized by low capillary numbers, smaller than the first threshold ($Ca_{th1} \approx 0.002$ in the example of Figure 8.114). In this regime,

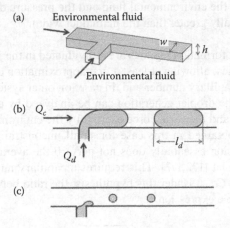

FIGURE 8.113 Droplet generation in a microfluidic T junction; scheme of the T junction for droplet generation (a), generation of constrained droplets in the transition regime (b), and generation of unconstrained droplets in the dripping regime (c).

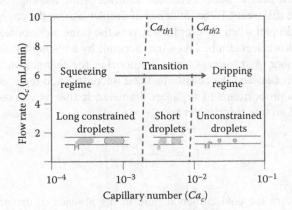

FIGURE 8.114 Phase diagram of a T junction for droplet generation.

very long droplets are generated, to arrive at an injection of the droplet fluid into the main channel in an almost continuous laminar flow. In this regime, the droplet length is always greater than twice the width of the main channel. In this regime, the surface tension at the interface between the two fluids dominates the shear force due to the environmental fluid push on the droplet fluid, and the dynamics of breakup is dominated by the pressure drop across the plug as it forms.

Drop flow or dripping regime: In this regime, the cross-flow shear force is large enough to play an important role in the process of breakup, and the dynamics of breakup is dominated by the balance of forces between shear force and surface tension. In this regime, the droplet dimension is smaller than the main channel width and unconstrained droplet appears either at the critical capillary number for sufficiently high capillary number ($Ca_{th1} \approx 0.01$ in the example of Figure 8.114) or for higher capillary numbers depending on the contact angle between the droplet fluid and the channel walls. The dripping regime is maintained up to the moment in which the hypothesis that are at the base of this analysis are no more true, that is, either the capillary number is too high and the surface tension starts to be less significant in the fluid dynamics inside the channel or the laminar flow is no more stable due to a too high Reynolds number.

Transition regime: In this intermediate regime, droplet formation is possible due to both the shear force exerted by the environmental fluid and the pressure drop across the plug. The droplet length is generally greater than the main duct width.

Once the different droplet formation regimes are individuated in the junction phase diagram, it is important to drive design rules, allowing at least a first approximation determination of the droplet length as it depends on the capillary number and, in case, on other system characteristics.

In the dripping regime, the droplet generation can be analyzed by considering the equilibrium between the surface tension and the shear force exerted by the environmental fluid. A very simple approximate result can be obtained in this case for small unconstrained droplets whose form is spherical and whose dimension essentially does not perturb the average velocity of the environmental fluid around the droplet [172,173]. This requires a capillary number sufficiently high, frequently sensibly higher than Ca_{th2}. Under this hypothesis, the ratio between the droplet radius can be approximated with a simple expression

$$R_d = \frac{\sqrt{h^2 + w^2}}{Ca} \tag{8.167}$$

This approximation results to be less and less accurate while the capillary number decreases. The main reason for the difference is the influence of droplet size on the environmental fluid velocity across the forming droplet when the droplet size is of the same order of magnitude of the microchannel dimensions. This effect can be taken into account by a phenomenological expression of a modified capillary number. A spherical droplet that touches the channel walls can be considered a sort of transition droplet between the constrained and unconstrained regimes. The cross-sectional area of such a droplet is proportional to its square diameter, so that we can set the average speed of the environmental fluid around this droplet as

$$\bar{v}_c = v_c \frac{wh}{wh - \pi R_d^2} \tag{8.168}$$

where v_c is the velocity of the environmental fluid in the absence of droplets. This introduces a modified capillary number Ca_{cM} of the environmental fluid [170]

$$Ca_{cM} = \eta_c \frac{v_c}{\gamma_c} \frac{wh}{wh - \frac{\pi}{4}l_d^2} = Ca\frac{wh}{wh - \pi R_d^2} \qquad (8.169)$$

Inserting this version of the modified capillary number in Equation 8.167 and solving for the droplet radius, we get

$$R_d = \frac{wh}{\pi\sqrt{w^2 + h^2}} Ca\sqrt{1 + \frac{4\pi(w^2 + h^2)}{whCa^2}} \qquad (8.170)$$

Equation 8.170 provides a good approximation for the droplet radius in almost all the dripping region, as it is shown in Figure 8.115, where the dispersion of measured drops dimensions in the transition region reported in the literature are plotted versus the theoretical value of Ca_{cM} provided by substituting Equation 8.170 in Equation 8.169.

When the two-phase flow is in the squeezing regime, the dynamics of breakup is dominated by the pressure drop across the plug as it forms. Dynamic observations of breakup process [174] allow to state that the final length of a droplet is built by a two-step process, whose mechanics is depicted in Figure 8.116. In the first phase, the tip of the droplet fluid enters the main channel and blocks it. When blocking happens, the length of the plug $L_1 = \varepsilon w$, where ε depends on the geometry of the channel, which is generally very near to one if not exactly one. Owing to the main channel obstruction, the pressure of the environmental fluid increases and squeezes the neck of the plug. The thickness of the neck decreases at a rate approximately equal to the mean speed of the environment fluid $v_c = Q_c/(hw)$. During this process, the plug elongates at a rate $v_d = Q_d/(hw)$ so that the squeeze length L_s of the plug can be written as

$$L_2 \approx d\frac{v_d}{v_c} = d\frac{Q_d}{Q_c} \qquad (8.171)$$

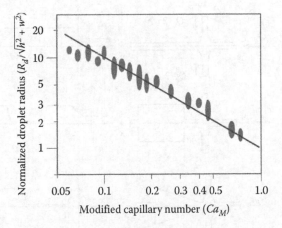

FIGURE 8.115 Dispersion of droplet radius measurement presented in the literature versus the inverse of the modified capillary number compared with a semiempirical theoretical prediction. (Experimental data from Szeri A. Z., *Fluid Film Lubrication: Theory and Design*, Cambridge University Press (February 17, 2005), ISBN-13: 978–052161945.)

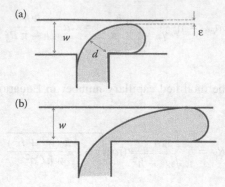

FIGURE 8.116 Phases of the droplet formation in the squeezing region: (a) plug formation and (b) plug extension.

where d is the length of the plug characteristic with that defined in Figure 8.117. The final length of the plug is therefore equal to $l_d = L_1 + L_2$. Substituting to L_1 and L_2 the relative expression and normalizing to the main channel width, we get

$$\frac{l_d}{w} - \varepsilon = \frac{d}{w}\frac{Q_d}{Q_c} \tag{8.172}$$

This equation can be intended as a semiempirical equation for the droplet length in the squeezing regime, where ε and d have to be intended as fitting parameters, depending on the structure, but not on the fluid motion characteristic, which is independent of the flow rates. The linear dependence of the droplet length on the flow rate ratio is well satisfied by experimental data [170] when a simple fitting of the two parameters ε and d. It is however observed that the spreading in the fitted values of ε is much larger than that expected by the physical meaning of this parameter, ranging at least from 0.9 to 1.9. This is the sign that the model represents only the main part of the complex dynamic of droplet formation, even if an overall linear dependence on the flow rate ratio is globally very well fulfilled.

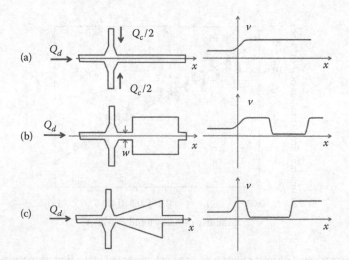

FIGURE 8.117 Different structures for stream focus droplet generation: simple injection in a T junction (a), injection in a T junction terminating with a very large channel (b), and injection in a T junction termination with a diverging nozzle (c). The qualitative plot of the fluid velocity along the x axis of each structure in single-phase regime is also shown.

In the transient regime, both the mechanisms contribute with similar impacts on the dynamics of droplet formation. We have found analyzing the two extreme regimes that the dynamic breakup of the interface is mainly driven by the flow rate ratio, while the equilibrium between shear stress and surface tension is mainly driven by the environmental fluid capillary number. This observation suggests the following empirical equation for the prevision of the droplet length in the transition regime:

$$\frac{l_d}{w} - \varepsilon = \delta \left(\frac{Q_d}{Q_c} \right)^\alpha \left(\frac{1}{Ca_c} \right)^\beta \qquad (8.173)$$

where α and β represent exponential weights for the two droplet formation concurring mechanisms. Equation 8.173 has been used to fit satisfactory exponential results [170], but the presence of four fitting parameters makes the fit less significant with respect to the previous case. Results also show that different geometries and wetting properties would cause the different values of parameters in Equation 8.173. This constitutes a limitation of the model, which should be modified for more generality in the forms and the exponents by considering the effects of geometries and the wetting properties.

8.7.2 Stream Focus Droplet Generator

The stream focus method that was already considered for droplet breakup can also be used for droplet generation. Let us consider, as in the previous section, a slab device and two fluids that are chosen so that the environmental fluid coming from the side ducts of the focusing device wets the ducts walls better with respect to the droplet fluid. We also will assume operation with an environmental fluid flow rate much higher than the droplet fluid and relatively high capillary numbers of the environmental fluid, similar to the dripping regime introduced in the analysis of the T junction. In this regime, unconstrained droplets are generated and the generation parameters have a small dependence on Q_d, becoming smaller and smaller by increasing Q_c.

Different geometries can be used to create droplets using a stream focus device; a few of them are represented in Figure 8.117. The profile of the fluid velocity along the x axis in case of single-phase flow in the structure is also shown in the figure.

Experimental observations detect droplet formations in all the structures that are shown in Figure 8.117 but the observed dynamics is different, mainly regarding the number of generated droplet per second and its fluctuations if the systems are operated in the same conditions [175,176].

The droplet generation dynamics in the structures of Figure 8.117 is dominated by the ratio between the shear stress on the droplet fluid due to the environmental fluid flow and the surface tension, so that in general we have to expect the formation of unconstrained droplets whose dimension is in a first approximation dependent on the inverse of some power of the capillary number, as it happens in analogous structures when small droplets are formed by breakup of larger droplets (see Section 8.6.2.2). Since the focusing effect due to the shear stress depends on the velocity of the environmental fluid, as far as the droplets are not so great to change substantially, the environmental fluid speed in the system looking at the velocity field in a single-phase regime is useful to understand the variability of the droplet formation point and number in the different systems. The value of the velocity field along the symmetry axis of the system (x axis) is reported in Figure 8.117.

We can imagine that droplet formation happens more probably in the region in which the environmental fluid velocity is greater so that we can expect that the more concentrated the velocity peak, the less variable the droplet formation point and the droplet number. This simple observation leads to conclude that the structures in Figure 8.117b and c are more suited for a precise droplet control than the structure of Figure 8.117a, due to the fact that particular care is taken in the structure design of the concentration of the environmental fluid velocity in a small length of the system. The best of these structures is not easy to be individuated due to the fact that dimensions and wetting properties can change from case to case and individuation of a general rule is quite difficult.

A simple empirical law [175] for the dependence of the unconstrained droplet radius R_d in the structure of Figure 8.117b can be written as

$$\frac{R_d}{w} = \frac{\delta}{2}\frac{1}{Ca_c} = \frac{\delta}{2}\frac{\gamma_c}{\eta_c \bar{v}} \tag{8.174}$$

where w is the width of the channel between the injection plane and the opening of the larger channel, $\bar{v}$ is the average velocity of the environmental fluid, δ is a fitting parameter taking into account structural factors and the wetting properties of the considered fluids, and the equation has to be considered valid down to a limit capillary number $Ca_{c,l}$ whose empirical expression can be written as

$$Ca_{c,l} \sim \frac{\alpha}{20} \tag{8.175}$$

where α is a fitting parameter frequently of the order of one. This condition is not surprising since a similar behavior has been already found in Section 8.7.1. The condition (8.175) can be rewritten as a condition on the environmental fluid flow rate, stating that once the fluid characteristics are given, there exists a minimal flow rate above which Equation 8.174 can be used that is written as

$$Q_{min} = \frac{\alpha}{20}wh\frac{\gamma_c}{\eta_c} \tag{8.176}$$

Equation 8.174 is very similar to Equation 8.167 if we can neglect the channel depth with respect to the channel width, approximation that is in general valid for planar microfluidic structures, and it can be justified in the same way. A fit of experimental data with Equation 8.174 is presented in Figure 8.118. Different values of δ correspond to different environmental fluids (Dynalene SF made by Synthetic Alkylated Aromatics [177] for the curve with $\delta = 1$ and Pentafluorophenol for the curve with $\delta = 2.17$), reflecting mainly their different abilities to wet the PDMS walls of the considered fluidic circuit.

Equation 8.174 is also quite useful to understand the impact of temperature on the dimension of the generated droplets [178]. As a matter of fact, if a great impact of temperature can be detrimental

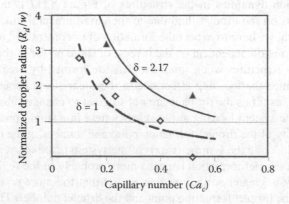

FIGURE 8.118 Fit of experimental data with the droplet dimension evaluated by the equation reported in the text. (Data from Tan Y.-C., CristiniV., Lee A. P., *Sensors and Actuators B: Chemical*, vol. 114, pp. 350–356, 2006.)

in selected cases, where temperature cannot be controlled, it can also be used as an active way to control the droplet dimension by integrating a microheater on the chip (see Section 6.6.3). From Equation 8.176, we see that both the viscosity and the surface tension of the environmental fluid generally decrease with temperature; thus, the behavior of the capillary number and consequently of the droplet radius depends on which of these parameters decreases faster. In any case, if the scope is to limit the droplet size temperature dependence, an environmental fluid with a small variation of the capillary number has to be used, while if the temperature has to be exploited as a control parameter of the system, the environmental fluid has to be selected so that either the viscosity or the surface tension depends quite rapidly on the temperature, while the other parameter dependence is slow.

The droplet generation circuit of Figure 8.117b sometimes is limited in its capability of concentrating the zone in which the environmental fluid velocity is maximum by the fact that selected technologies cannot build very short ducts. The circuit scheme of Figure 8.117c does not have this limitation since the output diverging nozzle has a progressive width increase that is easier to be fabricated.

Since the region in which the droplet fluid experiments the maximum shear stress is more concentrated, the diverging nozzle architecture operates an abrupt break of the droplet fluid flow. Moreover, smaller environmental fluid flow rates are frequently needed, below the validity limit of a simple inverse proportionality of the droplet radius from the capillary number. For these reasons, the droplet radius in measured devices results to be less dependent on the capillary number of the environmental fluid, so that an empirical relation has been used [176] that is written as

$$\frac{R_d}{w} = \frac{\alpha'}{Ca_c^\beta} = \frac{\alpha}{Q_c^\beta} \tag{8.177}$$

where α' and α are suitable fitting parameters and the exponent β is of the order of 0.3, with measured values fluctuating between 0.25 and 0.37.

We have seen that, in semiempirical expressions of the droplet dimensions, the wetting characteristics of the two fluids used in a droplet generation circuit are very important. Up to now we have assumed an environmental fluid wetting the device walls better than the droplet fluid. If we consider the opposite case, that is, a droplet fluid wetting the device walls better than the environmental fluid, the situation is much different. The adhesion of the droplet fluid to the device walls is so strong that practically droplets do not form and the droplet fluid is injected in a continuous stream into the main duct that flows in contact with one or both the system walls. As a matter of fact, complete substitution of the environmental fluid in contact with the walls allows the overall surface energy to be minimized. This means that if we consider a state diagram of a stream focus droplet generation system on the plane $\theta - Ca_c$, it is simply divided into two zones: $\theta < \pi/2$, where droplets are generated, and $\theta > \pi/2$, where no droplets are generated, independently from other conditions.

The situation completely changes if the T junction is fabricated with channels of different depths as represented in Figure 8.119 [179]. In this structure, unconstrained droplets can form even if the angle θ is greater than $\pi/2$. This is essentially due to the fact that during droplet formation out of the incoming duct, the droplet fluid does not touch the lateral walls of the main duct, thus not being stuck to them due to the high adhesion with respect to the environmental liquid.

To study droplet formation in this regime, the critical flow rate of the environmental fluid Q_c that separates drop formation from the regime in which a continuous flow of the droplet fluid is generated along the walls of the main duct without forming droplets has to be determined. A very evident Q_c hysteresis cycle can be observed by several experimental data [179], where the critical value of Q_c found starting from a situation in which droplets are not generated and increasing the flux can be up to 10 times greater than the critical value measured starting from a situation where droplet forms and decreasing Q_c. Moreover, as expected, the flow rate of the droplet fluid is not dependent on the critical value of Q_c as long as it is much smaller than Q_c, while as long as the flow rate of the droplet

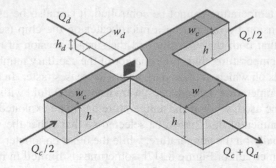

FIGURE 8.119 Structure of a T junction with microchannels of different depths.

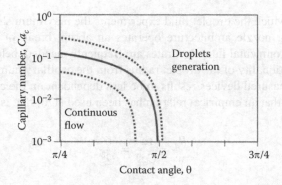

FIGURE 8.120 Phase diagram of a stream focus ducts generator with ducts of different depths at its first use; dotted lines individuate the area where experimental measures reported in Reference [179] are located and the continuous line reports the analytical approximation for the critical capillary number.

fluid becomes similar or even smaller than the flow rate of the environmental fluid, the critical value of Q_c is more and more dependent on Q_d.

Owing to the importance of disposable chips, it is interesting to characterize the behavior of never-used chips, where the main channel is occupied by the flow of the environmental fluid and the droplet fluid is inserted in the chip the first time. In this case, the phase diagram of the system appears as in Figure 8.120: droplets are formed for any value of the capillary number Ca_c in the regime $\theta < \pi/2$, while a critical value of the environmental fluid capillary number can be found in the zone $\theta > \pi/2$, dividing a regime of droplet formations and a regime of continuous flow of the droplet fluid in contact with the main duct walls. In a first approximation, the critical capillary number can be written as

$$Ca_c = K \cos(\theta) \tag{8.178}$$

where K is a fitting variable.

8.8 MICROPUMPS FOR DROPLET FLOW

Once a droplet flow is obtained, the flow that microfluidic processing presents needs to be similar to those of continuous-flow processing. In particular, both to compensate pressure drops due to various microfluidic elements and to reach the pressure needed to perform selected operations, pumps are needed.

In case of droplets, lab on chip pumps are also sometimes needed to decouple the pressure that is present in the droplet generation section to the pressure that is required in subsequent microfluidic elements, due to the fact that flow rate is often used in the generation element as a control variable to determine droplet dimension and generation rate.

Micropumps for continuous flow can be used for this scope: owing to the fact that breaking droplets in a microfluidic system is quite difficult, the greater part of micropumps simply propels the environmental fluid and the droplet at the same pressure. Dealing with droplets also opens up other possibilities, directly related to the particular behavior of microdroplets. In this section, we will describe two micropumps whose working principle is directly related to the fact that they deal with a droplet flow.

8.8.1 THERMOCAPILLARY MICROPUMPS

Thermocapillary micropumps are based on the so-called Marangoni force. Marangoni force rises when a gradient in the surface tension is generated through the interface between different fluids. In this case, analogously to the creation of a volume force due to a pressure gradient, a surface force is created due to the gradient of the surface tension. This is a force acting on each point of the interface and tending to reduce as much as possible the part of the interface where the surface tension is greater so as to minimize the surface free energy.

Let us indicate with $x_i = x_i(\xi,\zeta)$ the parametric equations of the interface between the fluids, which is assumed to be regular so as to have a finite normal vector and tangent plane in each point. The normal unit vector $\boldsymbol{n}$ to the surface can then be written as

$$n_i = \frac{\epsilon_{i,j,k} \dfrac{\partial x_j}{\partial \xi} \dfrac{\partial x_k}{\partial \zeta}}{\mathrm{I}_i \left| \epsilon_{i,j,k} \dfrac{\partial x_j}{\partial \xi} \dfrac{\partial x_k}{\partial \zeta} \right|^2} \tag{8.179}$$

where I_i is equal to one for each value of i. Once the normal unit vector in a surface point is determined, two unit orthogonal vectors ξ and ζ can be determined on the plane tangent to the surface in that point that constitute the intrinsic surface reference system in that point. The intrinsic reference system will change from point to point, but we will assume that it is set so as to change in a continuous way, which is possible due to the surface regularity.

Using the above definitions, the Marangoni force $\boldsymbol{F}_M$ can be written as

$$F_M = \nabla_s \gamma(\xi,\zeta) = \frac{\partial \gamma}{\partial x_i}\left(\frac{\partial x_i}{\partial \xi}\xi + \frac{\partial x_i}{\partial \zeta}\zeta \right) \tag{8.180}$$

where ∇_s indicates the gradient on the surface.

Considering a constrained droplet, essentially two different ways exists to create a gradient of surface tension in the interface between a droplet and the environmental liquid: creating a temperature gradient along the microchannel where the droplet propagates in such a way that the two opposite interfaces between the droplet and the environmental fluid are at different temperatures and introducing in the two separate volumes of environmental liquid in contact with the droplet different concentrations of surfactant (e.g., a suitable detergent) whose presence greatly influences the surface tension [180,181].

In general, increasing the temperature of a liquid will decrease its surface tension when it is in contact with an environmental fluid, eventually reaching some critical temperature at which the surface tension goes to zero. The surface tension dependence on temperature is very difficult to be

---

TABLE 8.14

Values of the Phenomenological Parameters to Insert in Equation 9.31 to Obtain an Accurate Fit of the Dependence of Water–Air Surface Tension on Temperature at Critical Pressure

Parameter	Dimensions	Value
γ_0	mN/m	235.8
ϑ	Nondimensional	1.256
T_c	K	647.15
β	Nondimensional	−0.625

---

evaluated in general form starting from prime principles, but a well-established empirical formula is written as [182]

$$\gamma(T) = \gamma_0\left(1 - \frac{T}{T_c}\right)^{\vartheta}\left[1 + \beta\left(1 - \frac{T}{T_c}\right)\right] \tag{8.181}$$

where T_c is the critical temperature, γ_0 is a constant, and ϑ is an exponent generally quite near to one, both dependent on the fluid characteristics. Accurate data for water in contact with air at the critical pressure are reported in Table 8.14 [182], while for a wide range of organic liquids, $\vartheta = 11/9$ and $\beta = 0$ allows experimental values to be satisfactory reproduced. An example of surface tension variation with temperature for two liquids (water and benzene) in equilibrium with its own vapor at the critical pressure is provided in Figure 8.121.

Since the temperature gradient are generally small in microfluidic circuits and due to the value of ϑ the order of one, a linear approximation of Equation 8.181 can be generally used in microfluidic cases, thus setting

$$\gamma(T) = \gamma_0(1 - \alpha T) \tag{8.182}$$

Values of the surface tension and of the temperature coefficient α are reported in Table 8.15 for different fluids used in lab on chip applications.

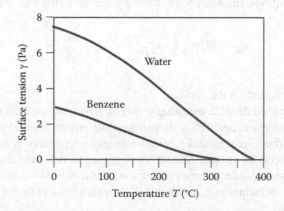

FIGURE 8.121 Example of surface tension variation with temperature for two liquids (water and benzene) in equilibrium with its own vapor at the critical pressure.

TABLE 8.15
Values of Surface Tension at the Interface with Air of Different Liquids Used in Lab on Chip Applications and of Its Temperature Coefficient α

Liquid	γ (mN/m)	α (mN/m/K)
Acetone	25.2	0.112
Benzene	28.9	0.129
Ethanol	22.1	0.0832
Glycerol	64.0	0.060
Mercury	425.4	0.205
Water	72.8	0.1514

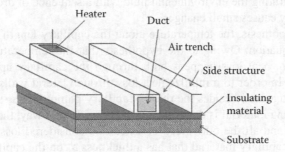

FIGURE 8.122 Three-dimensional representation of a possible architecture for a thermocapillary pump evidencing the heater, the microchannel, and the lateral trenches limiting lateral heat dispersion.

To show an example of thermocapillary pump for droplet flow, let us consider the system that is shown in Figure 8.122. The definition of the geometrical variables of the structure of Figure 8.122 is provided in Figure 8.123. A slab capillary of depth d and width w is heated on one side by a heater much shorter than the capillary itself. The heater establishes on the outside capillary surface a radially uniform temperature so that a temperature gradient establishes along the capillary. Owing to the capillary small dimension and to the fact that we want to study the stationary system regime, we can assume that the temperature field is uniform all along the capillary section, so as to be a function of the axial coordinate x and, in the transient, of time.

We will also assume that a train of identically constrained droplets are traveling with uniform velocity along the capillary, each droplet length l_d much longer than the length of the menisci

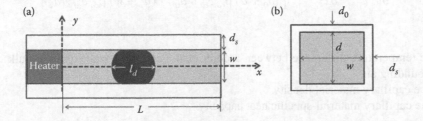

FIGURE 8.123 Geometrical variables used in the analysis of the structure of Figure 9.25: top view (a) and front view (b) of the microchannel. A droplet traversing the pump is represented in dark gray in the channel top view.

terminating the droplet, much longer than the heater length and much shorter than the capillary length L_c. Last, but not least, we will assume that the droplet flow does not sensibly alter the temperature field inside the capillary. This condition is satisfied if

$$\frac{l_d (C_d - C_c)}{(L_+ + l_d)C_c} \ll 1 \tag{8.183}$$

where

l_d is the single droplet length
L_d is the distance between two successive droplets
C_d is the thermal capacity of the droplet fluid
C_c is the thermal capacity of the environmental fluid

since in this case substituting the environmental fluid with a sequence of droplets, the temperature field inside the capillary causes small changes.

Under the above hypothesis, the temperature along the capillary length can be determined by the heat conduction equation. Owing to the hypothesis that the temperature is the same in the whole capillary section, heat loss happens both through the capillary upper wall and through lateral walls and floor. In order to minimize heat loss through lateral walls and floor, we assume that air trenches are excavated besides the thermocapillary pump duct as shown in Figure 8.123 and a perfectly insulating material is deposited on the floor. In this way, the heat loss through the floor can be neglected and all the other heat losses can be considered losses toward an air mass through a thin film of capillary material that has a thickness d_0 on the capillary cap and d_s on the capillary sides. The heat loss term in the temperature conduction equation can be modeled by a constant heat transfer coefficient due to the small difference of temperature along the capillary length with respect to the gradient of temperature between the capillary and the bulk of the air and chip volume. Under these conditions, assuming natural air convection, we can simply write the heat transfer coefficients H_A toward air as [183,184]

$$H_H = \frac{\kappa_a}{d_j} \quad (j = 0, s) \tag{8.184}$$

where k_a is the air heat conduction coefficient at normal conditions. Using Equation 8.184, the governing equation of the temperature field inside the capillary walls is written as

$$\frac{\partial T}{\partial t} = D_T \frac{\partial^2 T}{\partial x^2} - \kappa_a \left[\frac{1}{(d_0 + d)} \frac{(d_0 + d)}{\rho_{ca} c_{ca} w d_0} + \frac{2}{(d_s + w)} \frac{(d_s + w)}{\rho_{ca} c_{ca} w d_s} \right] T \tag{8.185}$$

where

T is the temperature difference between a point of the capillary walls and the bulk of the surrounding air
ρ_{ca} is the capillary material density
c_{ca} is the capillary material-specific heat capacity

At steady state, the time derivative has to be set to zero and the initial condition at $x = 0$ is simply written as $T(0) = T_0$, where T_0 is the temperature difference with the surrounding imposed by the integrated heater. Defining the characteristic length $\bar{x}$ of the thermocapillary pump as

TABLE 8.16

Typical Data for Glass and PMMA Capillaries in Air at Standard Conditions Used for Numerical Examples of Thermocapillary Pumps

			Glass	PMMA
Capillary floor thickness	d_0	15 μm		
Capillary walls thickness	d_s	15 μm		
Capillary depth	d	20 μm		
Capillary width	w	200 μm		
Air thermal conductivity	κ_a	0.024 W/m/K		
Density	ρ_c		2500 kg/m³	1180 kg/m³
Specific heat capacity	c_{ca}		840 J/kg/K	1466 J/kg/K
Thermal conductivity	κ_c		1 W/m/K	5 W/m/K

$$\bar{x} = \sqrt{\frac{D_T \rho_{ca} c_{ca} w (d_0 + 2 d_s)}{\kappa_a}} = \sqrt{w (d_0 + 2 d_s) \frac{\kappa_c}{\kappa_a}} \tag{8.186}$$

where κ_c is the thermal conductivity of the capillary material, the stationary solution of Equation 8.186 is written as

$$T(x) = T_0 e^{-x/\bar{x}} \tag{8.187}$$

The value of $\bar{x}$ represents an order of magnitude for the needed length of the capillary. Assuming typical data for glass and PMMA capillaries in air at standard conditions (see Table 8.16), we see that the characteristic length is about 612 μm for a glass capillary and 1118 μm for a PMMA capillary. The characteristic length increases by increasing the capillary radius and decreases by decreasing the capillary wall thickness, in fact it minimizes heat dispersion toward the surrounding air. For example, reducing the capillary wall thickness to 10 μm, we get in the above conditions 500 and 913 μm in the glass and PMMA cases, respectively. Equation 8.185 can also be solved analytically with quite a complex procedure in the transient case [185,186] to determine the characteristic time for the instauration of the stationary regime.

We can determine the motion of the droplets in the thermocapillary pump by assuming it to move almost as a rigid body so that determination of the center of mass motion is sufficient. The forces acting on the droplets are the inertia force F_i due to its mass, the force F_p due to the fluid viscosity and interaction with the duct walls, and the resultant F_s between the different forces acting on the droplet menisci. Since the inertia force is proportional to the mass of the droplet and its acceleration, we can write

$$F_i = -\rho_d l_d w d \frac{d^2 x}{dt^2} \tag{8.188}$$

where x is the position of the droplet center of mass. Using as a model to relate the viscosity and walls adhesion effect to the fluid velocity, the characteristic equation of the Poiseuille flow, the viscosity friction, can be written using Equation 7.90 as

$$F_p = d w l_d \frac{\partial p}{\partial x} = l_d Q \frac{12 \eta}{d^2 \left(1 - \xi_0 \frac{d}{w}\right)} = 12 \eta \frac{l_d w}{d \left(1 - \xi_0 \frac{d}{w}\right)} \frac{dx}{dt} \tag{8.189}$$

Finally, the force due to the effect of the temperature gradient on the droplet menisci can be written as

$$F_s = 2(d + w)\left[\gamma\left(x + \frac{l_d}{2}\right)\cos\theta\left(x + \frac{l_d}{2}\right) - \gamma\left(x - \frac{l_d}{2}\right)\cos\theta\left(x - \frac{l_d}{2}\right)\right] \qquad (8.190)$$

Equation 8.189 reflects the fact that, due to the temperature dependence on x, both the surface tension and the contact angle depend on x too.

The droplet motion equation is obtained by balancing the inertia force given by Equation 8.188 with dissipative and menisci forces provided by Equations 8.189 and 8.190. It is obtained

$$\frac{d^2x}{dt^2} + \frac{12\eta}{\rho_d\, d^2\left(1 - \xi_0\dfrac{d}{w}\right)}\frac{dx}{dt} + 2\frac{(d + w)}{\rho_d\, d\, l_d\, w}$$

$$\times\left[\gamma\left(x + \frac{l_d}{2}\right)\cos\theta\left(x + \frac{l_d}{2}\right) - \gamma\left(x - \frac{l_d}{2}\right)\cos\theta\left(x - \frac{l_d}{2}\right)\right] = 0 \qquad (8.191)$$

This equation has to be integrated by substituting

$$\gamma(x) = \gamma_0\left(1 - \alpha\, T_0 e^{-x/\bar{x}}\right) \qquad (8.192a)$$

$$\cos\theta(x) = \frac{\gamma_{ec} - \gamma_{dc}}{\gamma_{de}} = \frac{\gamma_{ec0}(1 - \alpha_{ec}T_0 e^{-x/\bar{x}}) - \gamma_{dc0}(1 - \alpha_{dc}T_0 e^{-x/\bar{x}})}{\gamma_{ed0}\,(1 - \alpha_{ed}T_0 e^{-x/\bar{x}})} \qquad (8.192b)$$

and with the initial conditions

$$x(0) = 0 \qquad (8.193a)$$

$$\left.\frac{dx}{dt}\right)_{t=0} = v_0 \qquad (8.193b)$$

In Equation 8.192b, the surface tensions relative to different interfaces are indicated as

- γ_{ec}: surface tension at the environmental fluid–capillary wall interface
- γ_{dc}: surface tension at the droplet fluid–capillary wall interface
- γ_{dc}: surface tension at the interface between the two fluids

and similar indexes are used for the temperature coefficients and the surface tension constants.

Equation 8.191 can be integrated analytically by adding the general solution of the homogeneous equation to a particular solution of the nonhomogeneous equation; it can be found starting from a test solution composed of a linear term plus a rational function of the decay exponentials that are present in the expression of the surface tension-induced force. The solution obtained in this way is a very long expression and often numerical integration is a more direct way to solve specific cases. In order to provide a numerical example, we consider the parameters reported in Table 8.17 that are relative to a capillary containing 300-μm-long water droplets in an artificial oil and we assume that the heater is at a temperature of 75°C while the room temperature is 25°C. The initial flow rate is

TABLE 8.17

Surface Pressure-Related Data for the Numerical Example of Performances of a Thermocapillary Pump

	Surface Tension (mN/m)	Temperature Coefficient (mN/m/K)	Surface Tension Constant (mN/m)
Oil–water	44.3	0.10	45.67
Water–glass	41.0	0.15	42.93
Oil–glass	12.52	0.06	12.74

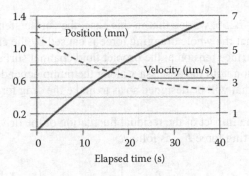

FIGURE 8.124 Position and velocity of a droplet during stationary state working of the thermocapillary pump considered in the numerical example of the text.

assumed to be $Q_0 = 0.1$ μm/min. Plots of the position of the droplet center of mass of the droplet velocity are given in Figure 8.124 for a case of an initial droplet velocity equal to zero. The droplet undergoes an abrupt acceleration as it traverses the electrode since the maximum temperature gradient is present at the beginning of the pump, advancing the velocity drops through the capillary.

8.8.2 ELECTROWETTING MICROPUMPS

A different way to control the surface tension at the interface between immiscible liquids and a solid channel is to use an electrostatic field through electrowetting, and in particular electrowetting on dielectric (EWOD). In Section 7.5.6, we have seen that electrowetting is an electrostatic effect due to the contribution of electrostatic energy accumulated in the electrical double layer between a charged liquid droplet and a conducting solid surface to the interface tension of a liquid. In particular, in case of EWOD, a better control of the effect is achieved by interposing between the droplet and the conducting interface a thin dielectric layer.

Let us now consider the system that is represented in Figure 8.125 [187,188]: a flow of constrained droplets of length l_d traverses a rectangular channel. The droplets are constituted by an electrolyte solution. A set of electrodes whose length is much smaller than the droplet length are deposited under the channel floor and activated one after the other while the front meniscus of the droplet passes over them. The activation of an electrode causes electrowetting, changing selectively the surface tension of the front meniscus of the droplet and causing the generation of a net force moving toward the droplet.

The effect is similar to those existing in a thermocapillary pump, with the advantage that here there is no attenuation of the drag force while the droplet advances through the pump so that the pump length is a design parameter of the system besides the electrode length, the electrode voltage, and the dielectric film thickness.

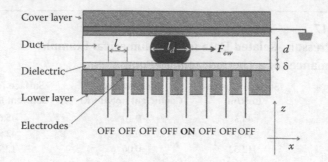

FIGURE 8.125 Principle scheme of an electrowetting droplet pump.

Starting from Equation 7.256, we see that in this case, the surface tension between the two liquids does not change, so that the whole dragging force is caused by the change in the contact angle due to the change in the surface tension at the droplet fluid channel surface. The exact dependence of the contact angle variation with the abscissa x along the pump depends on the shape of the electrodes driving command, that will be designed so as to make the drag force as much constant along the pump as possible.

To provide an idea of the impact of the residual fluctuation of the driving force along the pump, let us model the electrowetting force F_{ew} as follows:

$$F_{ew} = 2(d + w)\varepsilon_0 \frac{\varepsilon_l}{\delta} \Delta\psi^2 \left[(1 - \xi) + \xi\cos\left(2\pi\frac{x}{l_e}\right)\right] \qquad (8.194)$$

where
  $\Delta\psi$ is the potential applied to the electrode that is on in a certain instant
  ε_0 is the dielectric constant of vacuum
  ε_l is the dielectric constant of the dielectric thin film
  d is the thickness of the dielectric film
  ξ is a design constant representing the fact that we have not ideal electrodes
  δ is the distance between the middle section of adjacent electrodes

In this case, following a procedure similar to that used in the above section, the motion equation of the droplets is written as

$$\frac{d^2x}{dt^2} + \frac{12\eta}{\rho_d d^2\left(1 - \xi_0\frac{d}{w}\right)}\frac{dx}{dt} + 2\frac{(d + w)}{\rho_d d l_d w}\varepsilon_0\frac{\varepsilon_l}{\delta}\Delta\psi^2\left[(1 - \xi) + \xi\cos\left(2\pi\frac{x}{l_e}\right)\right] = 0 \quad (8.195)$$

If $\xi = 0$, that is, in the case of perfect design of the pump, this equation can be easily solved in closed form. Setting

$$\tau = \frac{\rho_d d^2\left(1 - \xi_0\frac{d}{w}\right)}{12\eta} \qquad (8.196a)$$

$$a_{ew} = \frac{F_{ew}}{M_d} = 2\frac{(d + w)}{\rho_d d l_d w}\varepsilon_0\frac{\varepsilon_l}{\delta}\Delta\psi^2 \qquad (8.196b)$$

we get

$$v(t) = \tau a_{ew} + (v_0 - \tau a_{ew})e^{-t/\tau} \tag{8.197}$$

This is indeed an expected result, since if the design parameter ξ is equal to zero, the force dragging the droplet along the pump is a constant force, depending only on the electrowetting parameters. This force is thwarted by the viscous attrition and it is well known that in such a condition after a transient a steady-state constant velocity is reached, only depending on the operating force and on the viscosity drag, which in our case is a resultant of both the droplet adhesion to the walls of the duct and of the internal fluid viscosity. In Equation 8.197, the physical meaning of the parameters is clear: τ is the transient characteristic time, while a_{ew} is the characteristic acceleration due to the electrowetting force alone, so that the steady-state velocity is given by the term τa_{ew}.

With further integration we get the expression of the droplet position in time

$$x(t) = \tau(a_{ew}(t - \tau) + v_0) + \tau(\tau a_{ew} - v_0)e^{-t/\tau} \approx \tau(a_{ew}(t - \tau) + v_0) \tag{8.198}$$

where the approximation is valid for $t \gg \tau$. With the parameters we used in the case of the thermocapillary pump, we obtain $\tau \approx 35$ µs, which as expected is an almost instantaneous time on the typical time scale of lab on chip phenomena.

The impact of the parameter ξ is to reduce the effectiveness of the electrowetting force. If this parameter is different from zero, Equation 8.195 can be solved in closed form again using the fact that the solution can be decomposed in the sum of the solution of the corresponding homogeneous equation and a particular solution of the nonhomogeneous equation, which can be found in the form

$$x(t) = K_1 t + K_2 \cos\left(2\pi \frac{x}{l_e}\right) + K_3 \cos\left(2\pi \frac{x}{l_e}\right) \tag{8.199}$$

where the constants K_j can be determined by direct substitution. Assuming that the length of an electrode is much shorter than the length of a droplet and that the parameter ξ is much smaller than one, it is possible to approximate the oscillating electrowetting force with its average and analyze the pump as if the electrowetting force would be constant. Since the average of the oscillating part is zero, the average electrowetting force is simply proportional to $(1 - \xi)$, so that ξ is simply the pump efficiency parameter, measuring how much the effective electrowetting force deviates from the ideal force that corresponds to the given structure parameters.

REFERENCES

1. Meng E., *Biomedical Microsystems*, CRC Press; 1st edition (September 29, 2010), ISBN-13: 978-1420051223.
2. Nguyen N.-T., Wereley S. T., *Fundamental and Applications of Microfluidics*, Artech House; 2nd edition (May 30, 2006), ISBN-13: 978-1580539722.
3. Au A. K., Lai H., Utela B. R., Folch A., Microvalves and Micropumps for BioMEMS, *Micromachines*, vol. 2, pp. 179–220, 2011.
4. Oh K. W., Ahn C. H., A review of microvalves, *Journal of Micromechanics and Microengineering*, vol. 16, pp. R13–R39, 2006.
5. Zhang C., Xing D., Li Y., Micropumps, microvalves, and micromixers within PCR microfluidic chips: Advances and trends, *Biotechnology Advances*, vol. 25, pp. 483–514, 2007.
6. Saada A. S., *Elasticity: Theory and Applications*, J. Ross Publishing, Inc.; 2nd edition (March 9, 2009), ISBN-13: 978-1604270198.

7. Maceri A., *Theory of Elasticity, Springer*; 1st edition (August 10, 2010), ISBN-13: 978-3642113918.

8. Castañera L., Rodri´gueza A., Ponsa J., Senturia S. D., Pull-in time–energy product of electrostatic actuators: Comparison of experiments with simulation, *Sensors and Actuators A: Physical*, vol. 83, pp. 263–269, 2000.

9. Yildirim E., Arikan M. A. S., Külah H., A normally closed electrostatic parylene microvalve for micro total analysis systems, *Sensors and Actuators A: Physical*, vol. 181, pp. 81–86, 2012.

10. Petrov D., Lang W., Benecke W., A nickel electrostatic curved beam actuator for valve applications, *Procedia Engineering*, vol. 5, pp. 1409–1412, 2010.

11. Yoshida K., Tanaka S., Hagihara Y., Tomonari T., Esashi M., Normally closed electrostatic microvalve with pressure balance mechanism for portable fuel cell application. Part I: Design and simulation, *Sensors and Actuators A: Physical*, vol. 157, pp. 299–306, 2010.

12. Patrascu M., Gonzalo-Ruiz J., Goedbloed M., Brongersma S. H., Crego-Calama M., Flexible, electrostatic microfluidic actuators based on thin film fabrication, *Sensors and Actuators A: Physical*, vol. 186, pp. 249–256, 2012.

13. Oh K. W., Ahn C. H., Magnetic actuation, *in Comprehensive Microsystems, Y. B. Gianchandani, Tabata O., Zapp H., editors, Elsevier Science; 1st edition (December 19, 2007)*, vol. 2 of a 3 volumes set, pp. 39–68, ISBN-13: 978-0444521941.

14. Ahn C. H., Allen M. G., Micromachined planar inductors on silicon wafers for MEMS applications, *IEEE Transaction on Industrial Electronics*, vol. 45, pp. 866–76, 1998.

15. Solé R. V., Phase Transitions, Princeton University Press (July 25, 2011), ISBN-13: 978-0691150758.

16. Kim J. O. et al., A Disposable thermopneumatic-actuated microvalve stacked with PDMS layers and ITO-coated glass, *Microelectronic Engineering*, vol. 73–74, pp. 864–869, 2004.

17. Cappelleri D. J., Frecker M. I., Simpson T. W., Design of a PZT bimorph actuator using a metamodel-based approach, *Journal of Mechanical Design*, vol. 124, pp. 354–357, 2002.

18. Oldfield M. J., Atherton M. A., Bates R. A., Perry M. A., Wynn H. P., Modal validation of a cantilever-plate bimorph actuator illustrating sensitivity to 3D characterisation, *Journal of Electroceramics*, vol. 25 pp. 45–55, 2010.

19. Chu, W. H., Mehregany, M., Mullen, R. L., Analysis of tip deflection and force of a bimetallic cantilever microactuator, *Journal of Micromechanics and Microengineering*, vol. 3, pp. 4–7, 1993.

20. Shape Memory Alloys: *Modeling and Engineering Applications*, Lagoudas D. C. editor, Springer; Reprint of 2008 edition (November 4, 2010), ISBN-13: 978-1441942975.

21. *Shape Memory Alloys: Manufacture, Properties and Applications*, Chen H. R. editor, Nova Science Pub Inc (April 30, 2010), ISBN-13: 978-1607417897.

22. Hodgson D. E., Wu M. H., Biermann R. J., Shape Memory Alloys, *in ASM Handbook*, volume 2: Properties and Selection: Nonferrous Alloys and Special-Purpose Materials, ASM International; 10th edition (November 1, 1990), ISBN-13: 978-0871703781.

23. Gui L., Ren C. L., Exploration and evaluation of embedded shape memory alloy (SMA) microvalves for high aspect ratio microchannels, *Sensors and Actuators A: Physical*, vol. 168, pp. 155–161, 2011.

24. Barth J., Megnin C., Kohl M., A bistable shape memory alloy microvalve with magnetostatic latches, *Journal of Microelectromechanical Systems*, vol. 21, pp. 76–84, 2012.

25. Merzouki T., Duval A., Ben Zineb T., Finite element analysis of a shape memory alloy actuator for a micropump, *Simulation Modelling Practice and Theory*, vol. 27, pp. 112–126, 2012.

26. Barth J., Kohl M., A bistable magnetically enhanced shape memory microactuator with high blocking forces, *Physics Procedia*, vol. 10, pp. 189–196, 2010.

27. Gradin H. et al., A low-power high-flow shape memory alloy wire gas microvalve, *Journal of Micromechanics and Microengineering* vol. 22, 2012.

28. Tichy' J., Erhart J., Kittinger E., Prívratská J., *Fundamentals of Piezoelectric Sensorics: Mechanical, Dielectric, and Thermodynamical Properties of Piezoelectric Materials*, Springer; 1st edition (August 18, 2010), ISBN-13: 978-3540439660.

29. Ezkerra A., Fernández L. J., Mayora K., Ruano-López J. M., A Microvalve for lab-on-a-chip applications based on electrochemically actuated SU8 cantilevers, *Sensors and Actuators B: Chemical*, vol. 155, pp. 505–511, 2011.

30. Hoffmann, J., et al., Photopatterning of thermally senstive hydrogels useful for microactuators, *Sensors and Actuators A*, vol. 77, pp. 139–144, 1999.

31. Richter, A., et al., Electronically controllable microvalves based on smart hydrogels: Magnitudes and potential applications, *Journal of Microelectromechanical Systems*, vol. 12, pp. 748–753, 2003.

32. Cao X., Lai S., Lee L. J., Design of a self-regulated drug delivery device, *Biomedical Microdevices*, vol. 3, pp. 109–118, 2001.

33. Liu R. H., Yu Q., Beebe D. J., Fabrication and characterization of hydrogel-based microvalves, *Journal of Microelectromechanical Systems*, vol. 11, 2002, pp. 45–53.

34. Baldi A., et al., A hydrogel-actuated environmentally sensitive microvalve for active flow control, *Journal of Microelectromechanical Systems*, vol. 12, pp. 613–621, 2003.

35. Beebe D. J., Moore J., Bauer J., Yu Q., Liu R. H., Devadoss C., Jo B. H., Functional hydrogel structures for autonomous flow control inside microfluidic channels, *Nature*, vol. 404, pp. 588–590, 2000.

36. Naficy S., Brown H. R., Razal J. M., Spinks, G. M.,Whitten P. G., Progress toward robust polymer hydrogels, *Australian Journal of Chemistry*, vol. 64, pp. 1007–1025, 2011.

37. Bassil M., Ibrahim M., El Tahchi M., Artificial muscular microfibers: Hydrogel with high speed tunable electroactivity, *Soft Matter*, vol. 7, pp. 4833–4838, 2011.

38. Naficy S., Razal J. M., Spinks G. M., Wallace G. G., Whitten P. G., Electrically conductive, tough hydrogels with pH sensitivity, *Chemical Materials*, vol. 24, pp. 3425–3433, 2012.

39. Chang C., He M., Zhou J., Zhang L., Swelling behaviors of pH- and salt-responsive cellulose-based hydrogels, *Macromolecules*, vol. 44, pp. 1642–1648,2011.

40. Pal K., Banthia A. K., Majumdar D. K., Polymeric hydrogels: Characterization and biomedical applications–a mini review, *Designed Monomers and Polymers*, vol. 12, pp. 197–220, 2009.

41. Jonker A. M., Löwik D. W. P. M., van Hest J. C. M., Peptide- and protein-based hydrogels, *Chemistry of Materials*, vol. 24, pp. 759–773, 2012.

42. Deligkaris K., Shiferaw T., Olthuis W., van den Berg A., Hydrogel-based devices for biomedical applications, *Sensors and Actuators B: Chemical*, vol. 147, pp. 765–774, 2010.

43. Qiu J., Lang J. H., Slocum A. H., A curved-beam bistable mechanism, *Journal of Microelectromechanical Systems*, vol. 13, pp. 137–146, 2004.

44. Malhaire C., Didiergeorges A., Bouchardy M., Barbier D., Mechanical characterization and reliability study of a bistable SiO2/Si membrane for microfluidics applications, *Sensors and Actuators A: Physics*, vol. 99, pp. 216–219, 2002.

45. Arecchi F. T., Politi A., Transient fluctuations in the decay of an unstable state, *Physics Review Letters*, vol. 45, pp. 1219–1222, 1980.

46. Nosonovsky M., Rohatgi P. K., *Biomimetics in Materials Science: Self-Healing, Self-Lubricating, and Self-Cleaning Materials*, Springer; 2012 edition (December 6, 2011), ISBN-13: 978-1461409250.

47. *Biomimetics: Biologically Inspired Technologies*, Bar-Cohen Y. editor, CRC Press; 1st edition (November 2, 2005), ISBN-13: 978-0849331633.

48. Iverson B. D., Garimella S. V., Recent advances in microscale pumping technologies: A review and evaluation, *Microfluidics and Nanofluidics*, vol. 5, pp. 145–174, 2008.

49. Au A. K., Lai H., Utela B. R., Folch A., Microvalves and micropumps for BioMEMS, *Micromachines*, vol. 2, pp. 179–220, 2011.

50. Mulley R., *Flow of Industrial Fluids: Theory and Equations*, CRC Press; 1st edition (April 30, 2004), ISBN-13: 978-0849327674.

51. Chanson H., *The Hydraulics of Open Channel Flow: An Introduction*, John Wiley & Sons; 1st edition (September 15, 1999), ISBN-13: 978-0470361030.

52. Richter M., Linnemann R., Woias P., Robust design of gas and liquid micropumps, *Sensors and Actuators A, Physics*, vol. 68, pp. 480–486, 1998.

53. Nguyen N. T., Troung T. Q., A fully polymeric micropump with piezoelectric actuator, *Sensors and Actuators B: Chemical*, vol. 97, pp. 137–143, 2004.

54. Fuchs O., et al., A novel volumetric silicon micropump with integrated sensors, *Microelectronic Engineering*, vol. 97, pp. 375–378, 2012.

55. Trenklea F., Haeberleb S., Zengerlea R., Normally-closed peristaltic micropump with re-usable actuator and disposable fluidic chip, *Sensors and Actuators B: Chemical*, vol. 154, pp. 137–141, 2011.

56. Leea K. S., Kimb B., Shannon M. A., An electrostatically driven valve-less peristaltic micropump with a stepwise chamber, *Sensors and Actuators A: Physical*, vol. 187, pp. 183–189, 2012.

57. Chia B. T., Liao H.-H., Yang Y.-J., A novel thermo-pneumatic peristaltic micropump with low temperature elevation on working fluid, *Sensors and Actuators A: Physical*, vol. 165, pp. 86–93, 2011.

58. Juncker D. et al., Autonomous microfluidic capillary system, *Analytical Chemistry*, vol. 74, pp. 6139–6144, 2002.

59. Zimmermann M., Schmid H., Hunziker P., Delamarche E., Capillary pumps for autonomous capillary systems, *Lab on a Chip*, vol. 7, pp. 119–125, 2007.

60. Namasivayam V., Larson R. G., Burke D. T., Burns M. A., Transpiration-based micropump for delivering continuous ultra-low flow rates, *Journal of Micromechanics and Microengineering*, vol. 13, pp. 261–271, 2003.

61. Li J.-M., et al., Bio-Inspired micropump based on stomatal transpiration in plants, *Lab on a Chip*, vol. 11, pp. 2785–2789, 2011.
62. Cussler E. L., *Diffusion: Mass Transfer in Fluid Systems*, Cambridge University Press, 3rd edition (February 2, 2009), ISBN-13: 978-0521871211.
63. Fuhr G., Schnelle T., Wagner B., Travelling wave-driven microfabricated electrohydrodynamic pumps for liquids, *Journal Micromechanics Microengineering*, vol. 4, pp. 217–226, 1994.
64. Zeng S., Chen C.-H., Mikkelsen Jr. J. C., Santiago J. G., Fabrication and characterization of electroosmotic micropumps, *Sensors and Actuators B: Chemical*, vol. 79, pp. 107–114, 2001.
65. Yairi M., Richter C., Massively parallel microfluidic pump, *Sensors and Actuators A: Physical*, vol. 137, pp. 350–356, 2007.
66. Kivanc F. C., Litster S., Pumping with electroosmosis of the second kind in mesoporous skeletons, *Sensors and Actuators B: Chemical*, vol. 151, pp. 394–401, 2011.
67. Seibel K., Schöler L., Schäfer H., Böhm M., A programmable planar electroosmotic micropump for lab-on-a-chip applications, *Journal of Micromechanics and Microengineering*, vol. 18, 2008.
68. Takamura Y., Onoda H., Inokuchi H., Adachi S., Oki A., Horiike Y., Low-voltage electroosmosis pump for stand-alone microfluidics devices, *Electrophoresis*, vol. 24, pp. 185–92, 2003.
69. Brask A., Goranovic´ G., Bruus H., Theoretical analysis of the low-voltage cascade electro-osmotic pump, *Sensors and Actuators B: Chemical*, vol. 92, pp. 127–132, 2003.
70. Bruus H., *Theoretical Microfluidics*, Oxford University Press, USA (November 17, 2007), ISBN-13: 978-0199235094.
71. Nguyen N.-T., Wu Z., Micromixers—a review, *Journal of Micromechanics and Microengineering*, vol. 15, pp. R1–R16, 2005.
72. Lee C.-Y., Chang C.-L., Wang Y.-N. Fu L.-M., Microfluidic mixing: A review, *International Journal of Molecular Science*, vol. 12, pp. 3263–3287, 2011.
73. Capretto L., Cheng W., Hill M., Zhang X., Micromixing within microfluidic devices, *Topics in Current Chemistry*, vol. 304, pp. 27–68, 2011.
74. Liu R. H. et al., Passive mixing in a three-dimensional serpentine microchannel, *Journal of Microelectromechanical Systems*, vol. 9, pp. 190–197, 2000.
75. Kim D. S., Lee S. H., Kwon T. H., Ahn C. H., A serpentine laminating micromixer combining splitting/recombination and advection, *Lab on a Chip*, vol. 5, pp. 739–747, 2005.
76. Nimafar M., Viktorov V., Martinelli M., Experimental comparative mixing performance of passive micromixers with h-shaped sub-channels, *Chemical Engineering Science*, vol. 76, pp. 37–44, 2012.
77. Hossain S., Ansari M. A., Kim K.-Y., Evaluation of the mixing performance of three passive micromixers, *Chemical Engineering Journal*, vol. 150, pp. 492–501, 2009.
78. Knight J. B., Vishwanath A., Brody J. P., Austin R. H., Hydrodynamic focusing on a silicon chip: Mixing nanoliters in microseconds, *Physical Review Letters*, vol. 80, pp. 3863–3866, 1998.
79. Stiles T., Fallon R., Vestad T., Oakey J., Marr D. W. M., Squier J., Jimenez R., Hydrodynamic focusing for vacuum-pumped microfluidics, *Microfluidics and Nanofluidics*, vol. 1, pp. 280–283, 2005.
80. Dziubinski M., *Hydrodynamic Focusing in Microfluidic Devices*, in Advances in Microfluidics, Kelly R. editor, In Tech Inc.; 1st edition (2012), ISBN-13: 978-953510106-2.
81. Lee G.-B., Chang C.-C., Huang S.-B., Yang R.-J., The hydrodynamic focusing effect inside rectangular microchannels, *Journal of Micromechanics and Microengineering*, vol. 16, pp. 1024–1031, 2006.
82. Ottino J. M., Mixing, chaotic advection, and turbulence, *Annual Reviews of Fluid Mechanics*, vol. 22, pp. 207–253, 1990.
83. Cartwright J. H. E., Feingold M., Piro O., Chaotic advection in three dimensional unsteady incompressible laminar fow, *Journal of Fluid Mechanics*, vol. 316, pp. 259–284, 1996.
84. Kuznetsov l., Zaslavsky G. M., Regular and chaotic advection in the flow field of a three-vortex system, *Physical Review E*, vol. 58, pp. 7330–7349,1998.
85. Mengeaud V., Josserand J., Girault H., Mixing processes in a zigzag microchannel: Finite element simulations and optical study, *Analytical Chemistry*, vol. 74, pp. 4279–4286, 2002.
86. Jiang F., Drese K., Hardt S., Kupper M., Scheonfeld F., Helical flows and chaotic mixing in curved micro channels, *Journal of the American Institute of Chemical Engineers*, vol. 50, pp. 2297–2305, 2004.
87. Scheonfeld F., Hardt S., Simulation of helical flows in microchannels, *Journal of the American Institute of Chemical Engineers* vol. 50, pp. 771–778, 2004.
88. Stremler M. A., Haselton F. R., Aref H., Designing for chaos: Applications of chaotic advection at the microscale, *Philosophical Transactions of the Royal Society A*, vol. 362, pp. 1019–1036, 2004.
89. Sui Y. Teo, C. J., Lee P. S., Chew Y. T., Shu C., Fluid flow and heat transfer in wavy microchannels, *International Journal of Heat and Mass Transfer*, vol. 53, pp. 2760–2772, 2010.

90. Berger S. A., Talbot L., Yao L. S., Flow in curved pipes, *Annual Review of Fluid Mechanics*, vol. 15, pp. 461–512, 1983.

91. Gammack D., Hydon P., Flow in pipes with non-uniform curvature and torsion, *Journal of Fluid Mechanics*, vol. 433, pp. 357–382, 2001.

92. Dennis C. R., Ng M., Dual solutions for steady laminar-flow through a curved tube, *Quarterly Journal of Mechanics and Applied Mathematics*, vol. 35, pp. 305, 1982.

93. Mridha M., Nigam K. D. P., Coiled flow inverter as an inline mixer, *Chemical Engineering Science*, vol. 63, pp. 1724–1732, 2008.

94. Nguyen N.-T., *Micromixers*, William Andrew; 2nd edition (November 3, 2011), ISBN-13: 978-1437735208; Chapter 6.

95. Erickson D., Li D., Analysis of alternating current electroosmotic flows in a rectangular microchannel, *Langmuir*, vol. 19, pp. 5421–5430, 2003.

96. Ramos A., Morgan H., Green N. G., Gonzalez A., Castellanos A., Pumping of liquids with traveling-wave electroosmosis, *Journal of Applied Physics*, vol. 97, pp. 1063–1071, 2005.

97. Hart J. R., *Ethylenediaminetetraacetic Acid and Related Chelating Agents* in Ullmann's Encyclopedia of Industrial Chemistry, Wiley-VCH, 7th edition (2005), ISBN-13 978-3527306732.

98. Říha P., The unified description of viscoelastic and thixotropic properties of human blood, *Rheologica Acta*, vol. 21, pp. 650–652, 1982.

99. Yamada M., Seki M., Hydrodynamic filtration for on-chip particle concentration and classification utilizing microfluidics, *Lab on a Chip*, vol. 5, pp. 1233–1239, 2005.

100. Rodríguez-Villarreal A. I., Arundell M., Carmonaab M., Samitier J., High flow rate microfluidic device for blood plasma separation using a range of temperatures, *Lab on a Chip*, vol. 10, pp. 211–219, 2010.

101. Yang S., Ündarb A., Zahnc J. D., A microfluidic device for continuous, real time blood plasma separation, *Lab on a Chip*, vol. 6, pp. 871–880, 2006.

102. Yamada M., Nakashima M., Seki M., Pinched flow fractionation: Continuous size separation of particles utilizing a laminar flow profile in a pinched microchannel, *Analytical Chemistry*, vol. 76, pp. 5465–5471, 2004.

103. Vig A. L., Kristensen A., Separation enhancement in pinched flow fractionation, *Applied Physics Letters*, vol. 93, pp. 203507–203510, 2008.

104. Derksen J. J., Sundaresan S., Direct numerical simulations of dense suspensions: Wave instabilities in liquid-fluidized beds, *Journal of Fluid Mechanics*, vol. 587, pp. 303–336, 2007.

105. Yang J., Renken A., A generalized correlation for equilibrium of forces in liquid–solid fluidized beds, *Chemical Engineering Journal*, vol. 92, pp. 7–14, 2003.

106. Lecuona A., Sosa P. A., Rodríguez P. A., Zequeira R. I., Volumetric characterization of dispersed two-phase flows by digital image analysis, *Measurement Science and Technology*, vol. 11, pp. 1152, 1156, 2000.

107. Shardt O., Mitra S. K., Derksen J. J., Lattice boltzmann simulations of pinched flow fractionation, *Chemical Engineering Science*, vol. 75, pp. 106–119, 2012.

108. Takagi J., Yamada M., Yasuda M., Seki M., Continuous particle separation in a microchannel having asymmetrically arranged multiple branches, *Lab on a Chip*, vol. 5, pp. 778–784, 2005.

109. Mitamura R., Toyama K., Mizuno M., Yamada M., Seki M., *Magnetophoresis-Assisted Hydrodynamic Filtration System for Continuous Two-Dimensional Cell Sorting*, Proceedings of 15th International Conference on Miniaturized Systems for Chemistry and Life Sciences, Seattle USA, 2011, pp. 2037–2039.

110. Lee K. H., Kim S. B., Lee K. S., Sung H. J., *Adjustable Particle Separation in Pinched Flow Fractionation with Optical Force*, Proceedings of ISFV14—14th International Symposium on Flow Visualization, Daegu, Korea, 2010, pp. 1–6.

111. Brody J., *Maximum Throughput in the H Filter*, Personal Communication, February 11, 2013.

112. Terry S. C., Jerman J. H., Angell J. B., A gas chromatographic air analyzer fabricated on a silicon wafer, *IEEE Transaction on Electronic Devices*, vol. 26, pp. 1880–1886, 1979.

113. Chen J., Abell J., Huang Y.-W., Zhao Y., On-chip ultra-thin layer chromatography and surface enhanced raman spectroscopy, *Lab on a Chip*, vol. 12, pp. 3096–3102, 2012.

114. Sainiemi L., Nissilä T., Kostiainen R., Franssila S., Ketola R. A., A microfabricated micropillar liquid chromatographic chip monolithically integrated with an electrospray ionization tip, *Lab on a Chip*, vol. 12, pp. 325–332, 2011.

115. Bynum M. A., Characterization of IgG N-glycans employing a microfluidic chip that integrates glycan cleavage, sample purification, LC separation, and MS detection, *Analitical Chemistry*, vol. 81, pp. 8818–8825, 2009.

116. Yin H., Killeen K., The fundamental aspects and applications of agilent HPLC-chip, *Journal of Separation Science*, vol. 30, pp. 1427–1434, 2007.

117. Brennen R. A., Yin H., Killeen K. P., Microfluidic gradient formation for nanoflow chip LC, *Analytical Chemistry*, vol. 79, 9302–9309, 2007.

118. Noguchi M., Tsunoda M., Mizuno J., Funatsu T., Shoji S., *MEMS Fabricated Liquid Chromatography Microchip for Practical uses*, Proceedings of IEEE 23rd International Conference on Micro Electro Mechanical Systems (MEMS) 2010, pp. 911–914.

119. Herr A. E., Throckmorton D. J., Davenport A. A., Singh A. K., On-chip native gel electrophoresis-based immunoassays for tetanus antibody and toxin, *Analytical Chemistry*, vol. 77, pp. 585–590, 2005.

120. Tran N. T., Ayed I., Pallandre A., Taverna M., Recent innovations in protein separation on microchips by electrophoretic methods: An update, *Electrophoresis*, vol. 31, pp. 147–173, 2010.

121. Andrews A. T., *Electrophoresis: Theory, Techniques, and Biochemical and Clinical Applications*, Oxford University Press; 2nd edition (April 24, 1986), ISBN-13: 978-0198546320.

122. Forrer K., Hammer S., Helk B., Chip-based gel electrophoresis method for the quantification of half-antibody species in IgG4 and their by- and degradation products, *Analytical Biochemistry*, vol. 334, pp. 81–88, 2004.

123. Zhang C.-X., Manz A., High-speed free-flow electrophoresis on chip, *Analytical Chemistry*, vol. 75, pp. 5759–5766, 2003.

124. Song Y.-A., et al., Free-flow zone electrophoresis of peptides and proteins in PDMS microchip for narrow pI range sample prefractionation coupled with mass spectrometry, *Analytical Chemistry*, vol. 82, pp. 2317–2325, 2010.

125. Turgeon R. T., Fonslow B. R., Jing M., Bowser M. T., Measuring aptamer equilibria using gradient micro free flow electrophoresis, *Analytical Chemistry*, vol. 82, pp. 3636–3641, 2010.

126. Turgeon R. T., Bowser M. T., Micro free-flow electrophoresis: Theory and applications, *Analytical and Bioanalytical Chemistry*, vol. 394, pp. 187–198, 2009.

127. Fonslow B. R., Bowser M. T., Optimizing band width and resolution in micro-free flow electrophoresis, *Analytical Chemistry*, vol. 78, pp. 8236–8244, 2006.

128. Chim W., Li P. C. H., Repeated capillary electrophoresis separations conducted on a commercial DNA chip, *Analytical Methods*, vol. 4, pp. 864–868, 2012.

129. Jha S. K., et al., An integrated PCR microfluidic chip incorporating aseptic electrochemical cell lysis and capillary electrophoresis amperometric DNA detection for rapid and quantitative genetic analysis, *Lab on a Chip*, vol. 12, pp. 4455–4464, 2012.

130. Pumera M., Analysis of nerve agents using capillary electrophoresis and laboratory-on-a-chip technology, *Journal of Chromatography A*, vol. 1113, pp. 5–13, 2006.

131. Andreev V. P., Lisin E. E., *On the Mathematical Model of Capillary Electrophoresis*, *Chromatographia*, vol. 37, pp. 202–210, 1993.

132. Wang S. Q., et al., Simple filter microchip for rapid separation of plasma and viruses from whole blood, *International Journal of Nanomedicine*, vol. 7, pp. 5019–5028, 2012.

133. Wei H., et al., Particle sorting using a porous membrane in a microfluidic device, *Lab on a Chip*, vol. 11, pp. 238–245, 2011.

134. Yang X., Yang J. M., Tai Y.-C., Ho C.-M., Micromachined membrane particle filters, *Sensors and Actuators A: Physical*, vol. 73, pp. 184–191, 1999.

135. Oua J., Rena C. L., Pawliszyn J., A simple method for preparation of macroporous polydimethylsiloxane membrane for microfluidic chip-based isoelectric focusing applications, *Analytica Chimica Acta*, vol. 662, pp. 200–205, 2010.

136. Mohamed h., et al., Development and characterization of on-chip biopolymer membranes, *Journal of Chromatography A*, vol. 1111, pp. 214–219, 2006.

137. Hsieh Y.-C., Zahn J. D., On-chip microdialysis system with flow-through sensing components, *Biosensors and Bioelectronics*, vol. 22, pp. 2422–2428, 2007.

138. Torto N., A review of microdialysis sampling systems, *Chromatographia*, vol. 70, pp. 1305–1309, 2009.

139. Kurita R., Yabumoto N., Niwa O., Miniaturized one-chip electrochemical sensing device integrated with a dialysis membrane and double thin-layer flow channels for measuring blood samples, *Biosensors and Bioelectronics*, vol. 21, 15 pp. 1649–1653, 2006.

140. Tosun I., *The Thermodynamics of Phase and Reaction Equilibria*, Elsevier; 1st edition (September 2012), ISBN-13: 978-0444594976.

141. An Y.-H., Song S., Fabrication of a CNT filter for microdialysis chip, *Molecular and Cellular Toxicology*, vol. 2, pp. 279–284, 2006.

142. Lopez G. C., Fedder G. K., *Suspended, Porous Cellulose Acetate Membranes for Microdialysis Use*, Proceedings of 8th International Conference on Miniaturized Systems for Chemistry and Life Science, Malmö, Sweden 2004, pp. 252–254.

143. Bungay P. M., Sumbria R. K., Bickel U., Unifying the mathematical modeling of in vivo and in vitro microdialysis, *Journal of Pharmaceutical and Biomedical Analysis*, vol. 55, pp. 54–63, 2011.

144. Annan K., Mathematical modeling for hollow fiber dialyzer: Blood and –dialysate flow characteristics, *International Journal of Pure and Applied Mathematics*, vol. 79, pp. 425–452, 2012.

145. Kucera J., *Reverse Osmosis: Design, Processes, and Applications for Engineers*, Wiley-Scrivener; 1st edition (April 5, 2010), ISBN-13: 978-0470618431.

146. Xu N., Lin Y., Hofstadler S. A., Matson D., Call C. J., Smith R. D., A Microfabricated dialysis device for sample cleanup in electrospray ionization mass spectrometry, *Analytical Chemistry* vol. 70, pp. 3553–3556, 1998.

147. Lamoree M. H., Van Der Hoeven R. A. M., Tjaden U. R., Van Der Greef J., Application of microdialysis for on-line coupling of capillary isoelectric focusing with electrospray mass spectrometry on a magnetic sector instrument, *Journal of Mass Spectrometry* vol. 33, pp. 453–460, 1998.

148. Jiang Y., Wang P.-C., Locascio L. E., Lee C. S., Integrated plastic microfluidic devices with ESI-MS for drug screening and residue analysis, *Analytical Chemistry* vol. 73, pp. 2048–2053, 2001.

149. McCray S. B., Glater J., Effects of hydrolysis on cellulose acetate reverse osmosis transport coefficients, *ACS Symposium Series*, vol. 281 (Reverse Osmosis Ultrafiltration), pp. 141–151, 1985.

150. Hickner M. A. et al. Alternative polymer systems for proton exchange membranes (PEMs), *Chemical Reviews*, vol. 104, pp. 4587–4611, 2004.

151. Parker D. et al., *Polymers, High-Temperature* in Ullmann's Encyclopedia of Industrial Chemistry, vol., Wiley-VCH; 7th Edition, 40 Volume Set edition (September 26, 2011), ISBN-13: 978-3527329434.

152. Fink H.-P., Weigel P., Purz H. J., Ganster J., Structure formation of regenerated cellulose materials from NMMO-solutions, *Progress in Polymer Science*, vol. 26, pp. 1473–1524, 2001.

153. Rubinson K. A., A dialysis electrode for microelectrochemistry, *Analytical Chemistry*, vol. 53, pp. 932–934, 1981.

154. Song S., Singh A. K., Timothy Shepodd J., Kirby B. J., Microchip dialysis of proteins using in situ photopatterned nanoporous polymer membranes, *Analytical Chemistry*, vol. 76, pp. 2367–2373, 2004.

155. Sterling J. D., Nadin A., *Droplet Based Lab on chip Devices*, in Encyclopedia of Microfluidics and Nanofluidics, Dongqing Li Editor, Springer; 2008 edition (August 6, 2008), ISBN-13: 978–0387324685.

156. The S. J., Lin R., Hung L. H., Lee A. P., Droplet microfluidics, *Lab on a Chip*, vol. 8, pp. 198 220, 2008.

157. Eggers J., Drop formation: An overview, *Applied Mathematics and Mechanics*, vol. 85, pp. 400–410, 2005.

158. Link D. R., S. L. Anna S. L., Weitz D. A., Stone H. A., Geometrically mediated breakup of drops in microfluidic devices, *Physical Review Letters*, vol. 92, pp. 054503–1-054503–4, 2004.

159. Leshanskya A. M., Pismen L. M., Breakup of drops in a microfluidic T junction, *Physics of Fluids*, vol. 21, pp. 023303-1—023303-6, 2009.

160. Szeri A. Z., *Fluid Film Lubrication: Theory and Design*, Cambridge University Press (February 17, 2005), ISBN-13: 978–052161945.

161. Jullien M.-C., Tsang Mui Ching M.-J., Cohen C., Menetrier L., Tabeling P., Droplet breakup in microfluidic T-junctions at small capillary numbers, *Physics of Fluids*, vol. 21, pp. 072001-1–072001-6, 2009.

162. Leshansky A. M., Afkhami S., Jullien M.-C., Tabeling P., Obstructed breakup of slender drops in a microfluidic T junction, *Physical Review Letters*, vol. 108, pp. 0264502–1–264502–4, 2012.

163. Cubaud T., Jose M. B., Darvishi S., Sun R., Droplet breakup and viscosity-stratified flows in microchannels, *International Journal of Multiphase Flow*, vol. 39, pp. 29–36, 2012.

164. Cubaud, T., Deformation and breakup of high-viscosity droplets with symmetric microfluidic cross flows, *Physical Review E, Statistical, Nonlinear and Soft Matter Physics*, vol. 80, pp. 026307, 2009.

165. Ménétrier-Deremble L., Tabeling P., Droplet breakup in microfluidic junctions of arbitrary angles, *Physics Review E, Statistical, Nonlinear and Soft Matter Physics*, vol. 74, part 2, pp. 035303, 2006.

166. Richards J. R., Beris A. N., Lenhoff A. M., Drop formation in liquid-liquid systems before and after jetting, *Physics of Fluids*, vol. 7, pp. 2617–2630, 1995.

167. Brennen C. E., *Fundamentals of Multiphase Flow*, Cambridge University Press; 1st edition (August 24, 2009), ISBN-13: 978-0521139984.

168. Faghri A., Zhang Y., *Transport Phenomena in Multiphase Systems*, Academic Press; 1st edition (June 8, 2006), ISBN-13: 978-0123706102.

169. Garstecki P., Fuerstman M. J., Stonec H. A., Whitesides G. M., Formation of droplets and bubbles in a microfluidic T-junction—scaling and mechanism of break-up, *Lab on a Chip*, vol. 6, pp. 437–446, 2006.
170. Xu J. H., Li S. W., Tan J., Luo G. S., Correlations of droplet formation in t-junction microfluidic devices: From squeezing to dripping, *Microfluidics and Nanofluidics*, vol. 5, pp. 711–717, 2008.
171. Xu Q., Nakajima M., The generation of highly monodisperse droplets through the breakup of hydrodynamically focused microthread in a microfluidic device, *Applied Physics Letters*, vol. 85: pp. 3726–3728, 2004.
172. Thorsen T., Roberts R., Arnold F., Quake S., Dynamic pattern formation in a vesicle-generating microfluidic device, *Physical Review Letters*, vol. 86, pp. 4163–4166, 2001.
173. Cristini V., Tan Y. C. Theory and numerical simulation of droplet dynamics in complex flows–a review, *Lab on a Chip*, vol. 4, pp. 257–264, 2004.
174. Garstecki P., Fuerstman M. J., Stonec H. A., Whitesides G. M. Formation of droplets and bubbles in a microfluidic t-junction—scaling and mechanism of break-up. *Lab on a Chip*, vol. 6, pp. 437–446, 2006.
175. Anna S. L., Mayer H. C., Formation of dispersions using "flow focusing" in microchannels, *Applied Physics Letters*, vol. 82, pp. 364–366, 2003.
176. Tan Y.-C., Cristini V., Lee A. P., Monodispersed microfluidic droplet generation by shear focusing microfluidic device, *Sensors and Actuators B: Chemical*, vol. 114, pp. 350–356, 2006.
177. Description and technical data sheet on http://www.dynalene.com/heattransferfluids/sf.html last accessed on March 3, 2013.
178. Stan C. A., Tang S. K. Y., Whitesides G. M., Independent control of drop size and velocity in microfluidic flow-focusing generators using variable temperature and flow rate, *Analytical Chemistry*, vol. 81, pp. 2399–2402, 2009.
179. Rotem A., Abate A. R., Utada A. S., Van Steijnd V., Weitz D. A., Drop formation in non-planar microfluidic devices, *Lab on a Chip*, vol. 12, pp. 4263–4268, 2012.
180. Ogino K., Onoe Y., Abe M., Ono H., Bessho K., Reduction of surface tension by novel polymer surfactants, *Langmuir*, vol. 6, pp. 1330–1330, 1990.
181. Darhuber A. A., Troian S. M., Principles of microfluidic actuation by modulation of surface stresses, *Annual Review of Fluid Mechanics*, vol. 37, pp. 425–455, 2005.
182. Vargaftik N. B., Volkov B. N., Voljak L. D., International tables of the surface tension of water, *Journal of Physical and Chemical reference Data*, vol. 12, pp. 817–820, 1983.
183. Lienhard V. J. H., Lienhard IV J. H., *A Heat Transfer Textbook*, Dover Publications; 4th edition (17 March 2011), ISBN-13: 978-0486479316.
184. Nellis G., Klein S., *Heat Transfer*, Cambridge University Press; 1st edition (December 22, 2008), ISBN-13: 978-0521881074.
185. Nguyen N. T., and Huang X. Y., Thermocapillary effect of a liquid plug in transient temperature fields, *Japanese Journal of Applied Physics*, vol. 44, pp. 1139–1142, 2005.
186. Nguyen N.-T., Chen J.-C., Effect of slippage on the thermocapillary migration of a small droplet, *Biomicrofluidics*, vol. 6, pp. 012809–012822, 2012.
187. Mugele F., Barret J. C., Electrowetting: From basics to applications, *Journal of Physics, Condensed Matter*, vol. 27, pp. R-705-R-711, 2005.
188. Song J. H., Evans R., Lin Y.-Y., Hsu B.-N., Fair R. B., A scaling model for electrowetting-on-dielectric microfluidic actuators, *Microfluidics and Nanofluidics*, vol. 7, pp. 75–89, 2009.

9 Surface Functionalization

9.1 INTRODUCTION

In order to detect, quantify, and study the target, it has to be purified and prepared in a suitable state for detection. This state has to assure specific detection of the target, minimizing the interference from other molecules, and noise from the environment or the detection system.

Several detection mechanisms operate on purified and concentrated solutions containing the target. Another widely diffused technique to obtain a specific response to the detection stimulus is to fix the target to a suitably prepared surface, either via an intermediate molecule, as in the ELISA assay (see Section 3.7.5) or directly, like in the technique of spin column-based nucleic acid extraction (see Section 3.2.2.2), where DNA strands are directly bonded to silica through a salt bridge after disruption of their hydration shell (see Figure 3.3). Such a technique is also widely used in labs on chip, with a significant difference with respect to the macroscopic case.

During a macroscopic assay, biomolecules are bonded to an activated surface to allow it to catch the target immediately before the assay. Stability of the bonding over long times and wide temperature ranges are not required due to the short assay duration and the stable laboratory environmental conditions. A lab on chip is a closed subsystem, which is frequently meant for use out of a laboratory. For this reason, the whole procedure of inserting the binding molecules, in case washing the assay chamber, and inserting the sample cannot be performed immediately before the assay. The binding molecules have to be inserted into the system and fixed to the activated surface during chip fabrication, potentially years before the chip use. Thus, the requirements of stability and tolerance to mechanical vibrations and temperature changes are much more severe for lab on chip systems. For these reasons, a large number of different techniques for surface activation and functionalization have been developed.

Functionalized micro and nanoparticles are also used in labs on chip. These are the particles whose surface has been functionalized so as to capture the assay target. Different from functionalized surfaces, functionalized particles can move through the microfluidic circuit of the lab on chip either dragged by the environmental fluid or due to the action of electromagnetic forces, so allowing, for example, target insulation from the original solution and detection in a more suitable environment.

In this chapter, we will briefly review the techniques for surface activation and functionalization. We will call activation as the procedure of modifying the physical and chemical surface properties so as to allow successive surface functionalization. Activation can be achieved either with simple physical meanings or by chemical surface modification. As we have seen in Chapter 4, ion bombing a surface with suitable ion flux and energy creates open chemical bonds on the surface that render it chemically active. A similar result can be obtained by a chemical bath in a solution of strong acid or base with subsequent washing of the surface. Sometimes, these physical procedures are sufficient to allow surface functionalization.

Many times, however, surface activation is performed by creating a mono or multiple molecular layer on the surface itself, so as to have chemically active elements.

Surface functionalization is obtained over an activated surface by fixing on the surface a monolayer of molecules that specifically bond the target. In this way, when the target enters in contact with the surface it is captured and immobilized for the subsequent assay. The most common molecules used for this scope are either antibodies or aptamers, for their ability to create very specific bonds.

In this chapter, we will briefly review activation and functionalization of lab on chip detection room surfaces. We will also devote a very brief discussion too on the nanoparticle surfaces activation.

9.2   SURFACE ACTIVATION FOR LABS ON CHIP

Self-assembled monolayers (SAMs) of organic molecules are molecular assemblies formed spontaneously on surfaces by adsorption and are organized into ordered domains as discussed in Section 5.2.1.1 [1,2]. In some cases, the molecules that form the monolayer do not interact strongly with the substrate. This is the case, for instance, of the so-called two-dimensional supramolecular networks [3]. In other cases, the molecules possess a functional group that has a strong affinity to the substrate and anchors the molecule to it [2]. Such an SAM consisting of a head group, tail, and functional group is shown in Figure 9.1, and it is mostly used for chemical activation of surfaces and microparticles in labs on chip.

Under a thermodynamic point of view, the generation of SAM happens because the surface energy is decreased due to the absorption of the heads of the monolayer molecules, while it is increased due to the proximity of the monolayer molecules functional group. In this balance, generally, the intermediate chain of the monolayer molecules has only the role of increasing the distance from the surface to the functional group, even if, in selected case, a small contribution to the surface energy can also be present.

Thus, indicating with A the surface element, we can express the thermodynamic condition for the formation of the monolayer as

$$\left.\frac{\partial G_{free}}{\partial A}\right)_{p,T,M} - \left.\frac{\partial G_{mono}}{\partial A}\right)_{p,T,M} > 0 \tag{9.1}$$

where G_{free} is the free energy of the free surface and G_{mono} is the free energy of the monolayer. Equation 9.1 also provides a thermodynamic explanation of the utility of procedures, like ion bombing to create a stable monolayer; ion bombing and similar procedures increase the free surface energy G_{free}, rendering the difference in Equation 9.1 to be greater and thus the monolayer more stable.

From Equation 7.112 we can recognize that Equation 9.1 can also be interpreted in terms of surface tension of the surface in contact with a reference liquid and air. Generally, the reference liquid is water, so that the monolayer is formed, and the surface tension of the free surface in contact with water is greater than the surface tension of the monolayer in contact with water. Moreover, if we

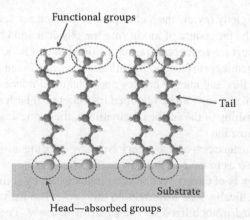

FIGURE 9.1 Self-assembled monolayer consisting of organic molecules with a head group, a tail, and a functional end group.

consider instead of a continuous interface between water and the considered material a water droplet on the material surface, we can substitute the surface tension with the contact angle, since the surface tension between air and water does not change due to the monolayer. Thus, we can say that the monolayer is stable if the contact angle decreases due to the monolayer formation with respect to the contact angle between water and the original surface. In this form condition (9.1) also writes

$$\theta_{free} > \theta_{mono} \tag{9.2}$$

Expressing the monolayer stability condition in terms of contact angles is particularly useful because the contact angle can be measured directly in almost all conditions. The reduction of the contact angle due to the SAM generation is a direct measure of the SAM stability, linked to the associated reduction of the surface energy. A qualitative description of common traits of SAM growth on a suitable surface is reported in Section 5.2.2.1 and sketched in Figure 5.3.

In Section 5.3.4, we have described the method of Langmuir–Blodget deposition for SAMs, which can be applied to almost all surfaces compatible with such functionalization. However, while widely used in macroscopic applications, Langmuir–Blodget deposition is not suitable for labs on chip applications due to the difficult integration of Langmuir–Blodget procedure with the lab on chip fabrication process, both in the case of use of polymer and of silicon substrates, and due to the insufficient stability of the obtained structures [4,5]. The creation of SAMs in labs on chip is generally performed by other techniques, depending on the substrate to be functionalized.

9.2.1 Noncovalent Chemical Surface Activation

Classical adsorption of biochemical compounds on surfaces, in case after a suitable surface physical pretreatment, involves noncovalent bonds between the surface material and the fixed molecules. Ionic bonds, hydrophobic interactions, and hydrogen bonds can all create monolayers on suitable surfaces. The method to create such monolayers is simple: in the most frequent case, absorption is obtained by a prolonged contact of the surface with a solution of the adsorbate. Due to the kind of link between the surface and the adsorbed molecules, any active site in the molecule structure results to be accessible from outside the surface and no sensible modification is induced in the adsorbed molecule.

On the other hand, the adsorbed monolayers are not particularly stable, being prone to desorption due to change in temperature or pH or due to mechanical vibrations. If proteins or artificial polymer chains are adsorbed on the surface, stabilization of the monolayer can be achieved by molecules cross-linking, induced after the monolayer formation. When a great cross-link density is obtained, they shield the major part of the chains internal groups, in case creating a change in the tertiary structure of the molecules.

As a rule, adsorption of proteins on a surface follows the Langmuir–Blodget isotherm behavior (see Section 5.3.4). If we indicate with $\bar{c}$ the surface concentration of the adsorbed proteins and with c their volume concentration in the solution where the surface is immersed during the monolayer formation, we can deduce the equilibrium condition of the adsorption process by starting from the general mass action law [1,2]. In particular, let S represent an active site on the surface, M a molecule that can be adsorbed, and SM the complex of the molecule and of the absorption site, then we can express the adsorption process with the following equation:

$$S + M \rightleftarrows SM \tag{9.3}$$

Applying the mass action law to the above equation, we get

$$k = \frac{\bar{c}}{c_S \, c} \tag{9.4}$$

where $\bar{c}$ and $\bar{c}_S$ are the surface concentrations of bonded molecules (SM sites) and of the free bonding sites (S sites), while c is the volume concentration of molecules in the solution from which the monolayer is generated. If we indicate with $\bar{c}_{max}$ the total concentration of active sites on the surface, we have

$$\bar{c}_S = c_{max} - \bar{c} \tag{9.5}$$

Substituting Equation 9.5 into Equation 9.4 and rearranging the resulting equation, we get

$$\bar{c} = \frac{\bar{c}_{max}(kc)}{1 + kc} \tag{9.6}$$

where $\bar{c}_{max}$ is the maximum attainable surface density, which essentially depends on the surface state, k is the equilibrium constant of the adsorption process. Generally, the so-called surface coverage Θ is defined as the ratio between the effective protein surface density and its maximum value, so that it results in

$$\Theta = \frac{kc}{1 + kc} \tag{9.7}$$

9.2.2 Covalent Chemical Surface Activation

Much more stable chemical surface activation can be obtained if the activating molecules are covalently bonded to the surface [4,5]. The first and simplest technique that can be used to grow covalent monolayers in selected areas of a lab on chip is pretreating the area through a process that increases its surface energy like inert ion bombing or a suitable chemical treatment and subsequent selective exposure to a solution in which the molecules that are intended to form the monolayer are dissolved. This wet treatment requires generally more time both for permanence of the substrate in the solution and for drying and reassembly of the molecules population, but the exposure area is easily controllable through masking, similar to the technique adopted in wet etching processes (see Section 4.7.1). An effective alternative technique that allows reduction of process time without decreasing the control is micro contact printing, which is mainly used if a polymer substrate is adopted. This methodology has been described in detail in Section 5.2.1, besides the corresponding monolayer growing process.

Commonly, the active groups involved in covalent activations are hydroxyl, carboxyl, primary amine, and sulfhydryl groups that are present in great number in almost all the proteins. Bonding can be performed directly if the surface material and the activation molecule react directly, or it can be performed by using a cross-linker, that is an intermediate molecule, if this does not happen.

9.2.2.1 Covalent Activation by Zero-Length Crosslinkers

A zero-length crosslinker is a single atom of a molecule that is covalently attached to an atom of another molecule via a condensation reaction. For example, a bond between a carboxyl group, belonging to a polymeric surface, with a molecule **B** through an amide link can be obtained by compounds of the carbodiimide class. An example of such a reaction happening on a polymeric surface is reported in Figure 9.2.

The typical reagents used in such reactions are 1-ethyl-3-(3-dimethylaminopropyl)carbodiimide) hydrochloride (EDC) and N,N'-dicyclohexylcarbodiimide (DDC), whose molecular formulas are shown in Figure 9.3. These reagents react first with a carboxyl group to provide an intermediate product that reacts next with a primary amine group providing an amine link. EDC coupling better occurs if sulfo-N-hydroxysuccinimide (sulfo-NHS) is present in the solution, since it improves the solubility of the intermediate product and eases the amine attack. The structure formula of sulfo-NHS is shown in Figure 9.4.

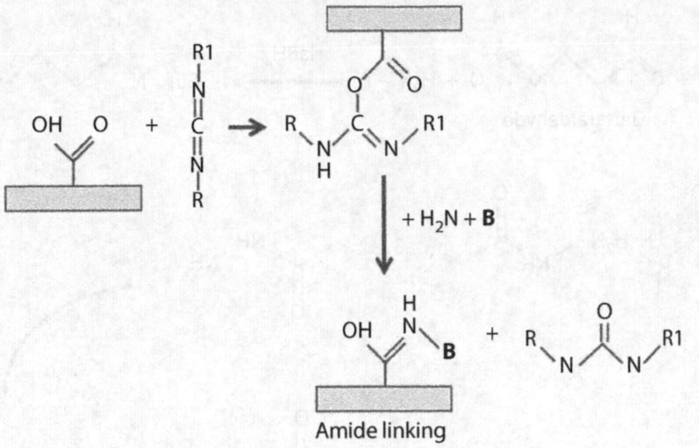

FIGURE 9.2 Covalent bond between a carboxyl group belonging to a polymeric surface and a molecule B via an amide link created using a carbodiimide crosslinker.

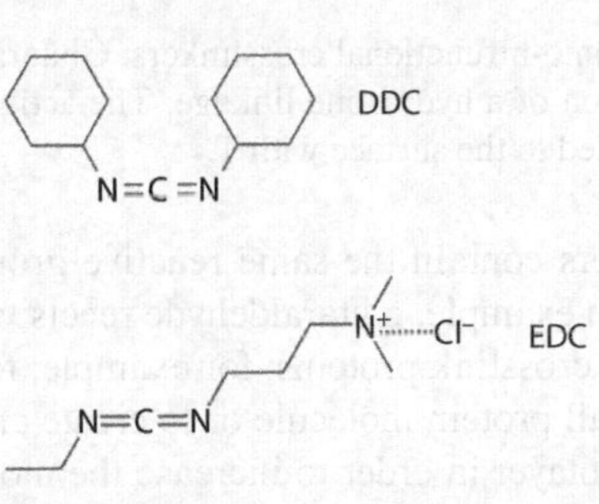

FIGURE 9.3 Structure formulas of DDC and EDC. In the DDC formula each carbon atom of the hexagon links three hydrogens, but the atom is linking the nitrogen, so that the typical benzene structure with six completely delocalized electrons in the ring is not present.

9.2.2.2 Bifunctional Crosslinker

Bifunctional crosslinkers are generally small molecules having two functional groups at the end of the molecular chain. These molecules are able to link a target to one functional group, while the other is covalently bonded to the surface; thus introducing a short spacer, that is, the molecular chain between the substrate and the activating molecule.

The presence of a spacer arm generally has particular advantages, since the activating molecule has a greater mobility with respect to the case of zero-length crosslinking. This allows both an enhanced reaction velocity and a greater activity due to a smaller steric hindrance. In addition, the spacer introduces a distance between the surface and the activating molecule, assuring a smaller interaction between this molecule and the surface microenvironment.

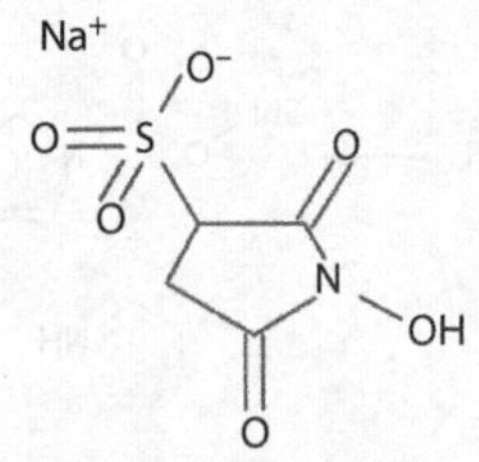

FIGURE 9.4 Structure formula of sulfo-NHS.

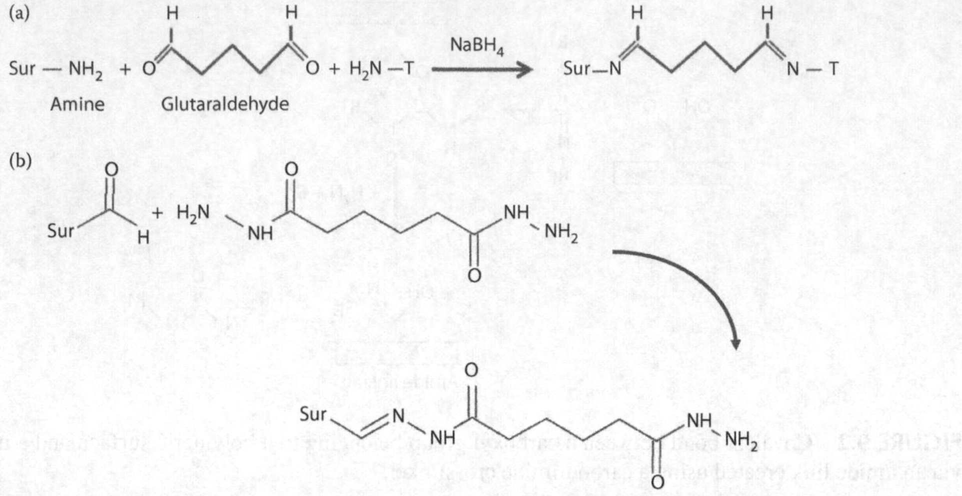

FIGURE 9.5 Crosslinking with homo-bifunctional crosslinkers: Glutaraldehyde linking (a) and adipic acid dihydrazide (AAD) mediated creation of a hydrazone linkage. The active group on the surface is indicated with Sur and the molecule to be linked to the surface with T.

Homo-bifunctional crosslinkers contain the same reactive group at both ends and are used to conjugate similar elements. As an example, glutaraldehyde reacts with the amino group of lysine in protein and is frequently used to crosslink proteins; for example, for the creation of a protein layer on a surface activated with a small protein molecule or to create crosslinking between nearby proteins belonging to the same monolayer in order to increase the monolayer stability. The scheme of this frequent linking reaction is provided in Figure 9.5a. Enzymes are also frequently immobilized on protein-activated surfaces by using glutaraldehyde crosslinking when surface catalysis is needed.

Homo-bifunctional hydrazides are widely used to conjugate molecules that contain carbonyl or carboxyl groups, which are frequent on the exposed surface of several polymers after treating with chemical attacks or ion bombing. Such reagents spontaneously react also with aldehydes to form hydrazone linkages, as shown in Figure 9.5b. This reaction is used to attach polysaccharides to amine groups that can be present on the surface or has been attached to the surface itself in a previous activation process. This is generally done after oxidation of the saccharide with periodate, which creates aldehyde groups.

Another frequently used crosslinker is 1,1'-carbonyldiimidazole (CDI), whose formula is reported in Figure 9.6a. It acts as crosslinkers of hydroxyl groups that can be generated on a surface after physical activation, with amine derivatives via a carbamate spacer, as shown in Figure 9.6b.

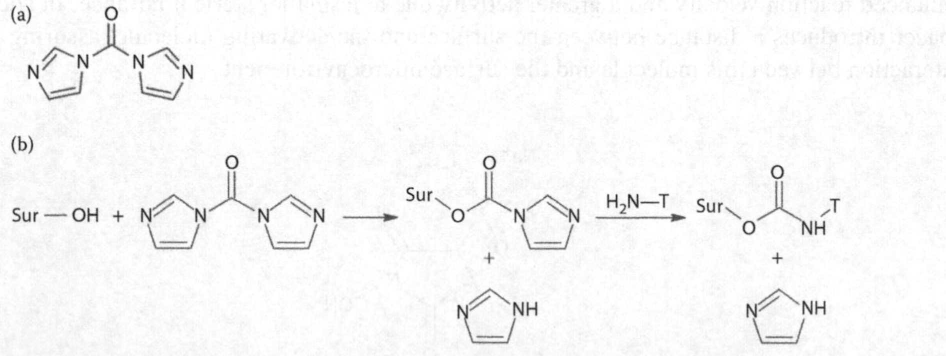

FIGURE 9.6 CDI structure formula (a) and example of crosslinking of a target T to an active hydroxyl group on a surface Sur via a carbamate link generated through CDI chemical mediation (b).

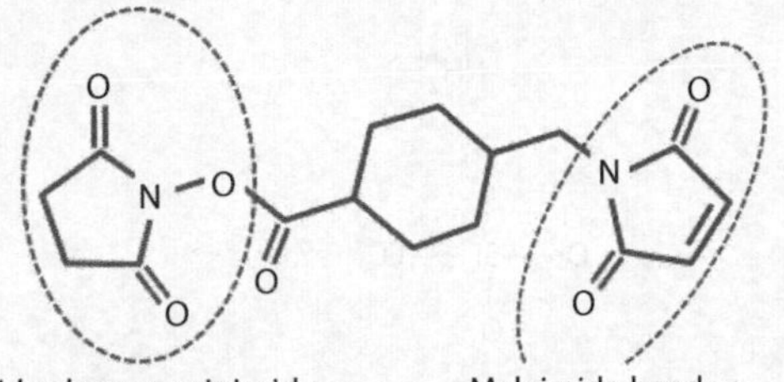

N-hydroxysuccinimide
(NHS) head

Maleimide head

FIGURE 9.7 SCCM structure formula evidencing the different active heads.

Coupling with amide and thiol derivatives can be achieved by means of hetero-bifunctional reagents, having different reactive groups at the extremes of the molecular chain. An example of such a material is *N*-succinimidyl-4-(maleimidomethyl)cyclohexane-1-carboxylate (SCCM), whose structure formula is shown in Figure 9.7. This molecule contains an amine reactive NHS ester on one end, and a maleimide functional group that can be utilized to react specifically with sulfhydryl (–SH) moieties at the other end. The maleimide functional group does not readily react with amino group (–NH$_2$) as found on lysine residues, thus maleimide-activated conjugates can be formed. For example, the maleimide group can react with the sulfur extreme of a thiol to create a long spacer in the generated monolayer. In this case, the NHS group reacts with a primary amine group to create a reactive intermediate that further reacts via the maleimide fragment with the thiol. As antibodies contain a large number of thiol groups, this method is also used frequently to create antibody–enzyme conjugates.

9.3 ACTIVATION OF DIFFERENT SUBSTRATES

In lab on chip application, three families of substrates have a relevant interest: (i) glass of different types, (ii) polymers like PMMA and S8, and (iii) metals, mainly gold layers deposited over silicon or glass, but also aluminum and other metals.

9.3.1 Glass Surface Activation

A glass surface, either directly from glass wafers or created by silica deposition on a silicon wafer, is an inert surface so that it has to be prepared for deposition of an activating SAM by creating a suitable density of active sites on the glass surface where the activating molecules can absorb to start the formation of the monolayer.

The process of activating a glass surface thus generally comprises two steps: In the first step, an extensive break of surface bonds between silica atoms, for example, by plasma bombardment obtained by a suitable plasma machine (see Section 4.7.2) is performed. This step is generally called physical activation. If the molecule that will be used for surface functionalization can be directly fixed to the physically activated surface, functionalization is directly performed. Otherwise, a second step of chemical activation is needed, creating amino layer suitable to fix the functionalizing molecule. During chemical activation the head of the activating molecule combines with the free bonding sites created by physical activation, and the functional group, mostly a nitrogen group, is left on the top of the monolayer, as shown in Figure 9.8. The monolayer is commonly obtained by exposing the physically activated surface to a solution in which silanes hydrolysis happens.

Silanes are molecules with an amine core, three radicals in substitution of three free hydrogens of the original amine and a silane group at one extreme. Due to hydrolysis the radicals are substituted by hydrogen, thus forming a trisilanol. In this form, the molecule becomes active and the silane head bonds to the silica surface. After crosslinking of silica molecules the surface functionalization is obtained. An example of such a reaction using trialkoxysilane is reported in Figure 9.9 [6,7].

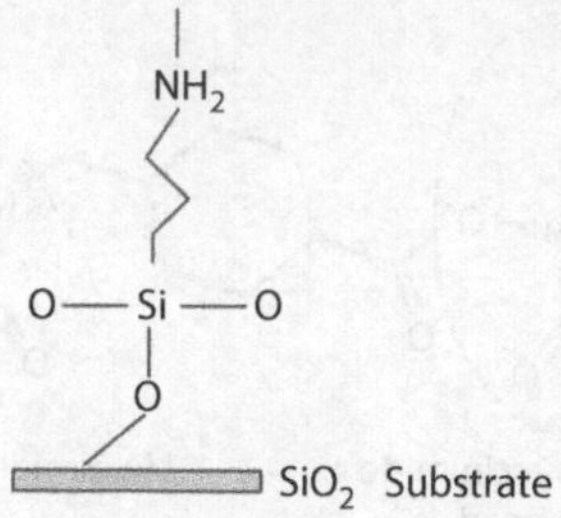

FIGURE 9.8 Chemical functionalization of an ion bombed glass surface with amine.

A glass surface that has been functionalized with amine molecules can be used to capture a variety of molecules. It has been used for functionalization with DNA strands [8,9], proteins [10], and even small molecules such as acid chloride, acetyl chloride, and methylene chloride [11]. Capture of the target molecule by the activated surface generally happens via a linker, either zero-length or bifunctional linkers are used when glass surfaces are activated. An example where a protein, biotin in this case, is fixed via a bifunctional polymer linker is shown in Figure 9.10, where the capture of a biotin molecule by a glass-activated surface mediated by a PEG_{12} polymer and NHS ester is shown. The NHS–PEG_{12}–biotin complex is present as a unique molecule in the solution. Due to the reaction of the NHS end with the amine end of the monolayer, the NHS detaches from the complex and the PEG_{12} remains as a bridge attached on one side to the functionalized surface and on the other side to the biotin molecule.

The choice of the mediation molecules is very important to obtain a reliable and useful adsorption of the target on the activated surface. If the bond is too weak, the target can detach partially from the surface, thereby introducing uncertainty in the following assay; if the bond is too strong, or the target is too near to the glass surface to undergo weak bonds with the surface itself, the target properties could be altered by bonding with the surface. In this case, the target could lose the specific affinity with the assay target. Moreover, the assay response intensity, from whom the assay accuracy and resolution depends, is a function of the bond type between the surface and the target. Thus, if different strategies to bond a certain target to a glass surface are known, the most effective strategy in terms of stability and assay quality has to be chosen [10]. A possible way to obtain

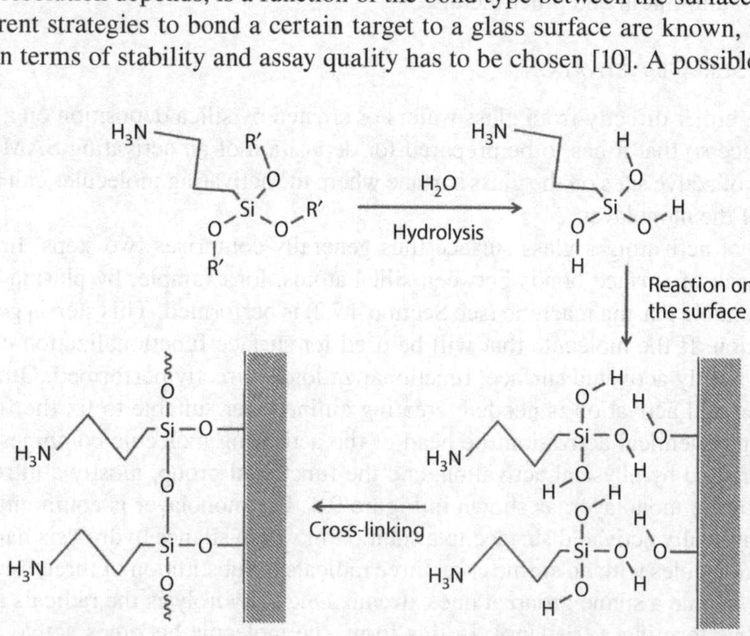

FIGURE 9.9 Functionalization of a glass surface activated with trialkoxysilane through ion bombing: The three steps of the reaction are evidenced: Hydrolysis, reaction on the surface, and cross-linking.

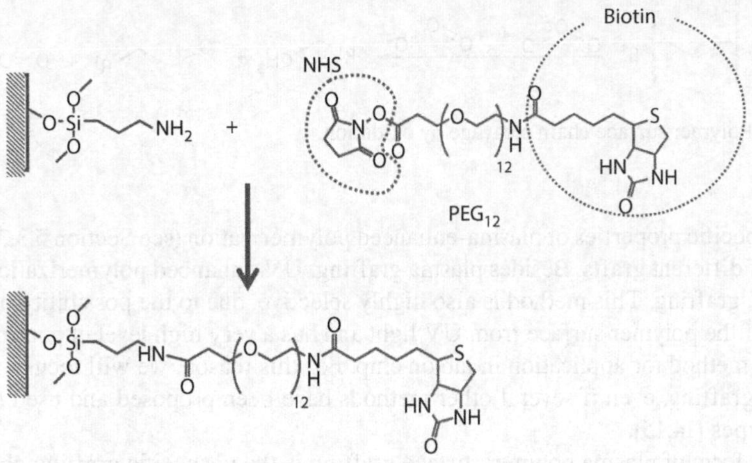

FIGURE 9.10 Biotin absorption on a glass functionalized surface from the NHS–PEG$_{12}$–biotin complex.

sufficiently strong bonds between the target and the surface, without bringing the target too near to the surface itself, is to use spacer molecules, as happens when bifunctional linkers are used, like the PEG$_{12}$ polymer in the example of Figure 9.10. If spacers are useful to maintain the target far from the surface and to mediate the target–surface bond, they have to be chosen not to alter the assay response providing nonspecific signals.

9.3.2 POLYMER SURFACE ACTIVATION

If a polymer like PMMA, SU8, or PDMS is the base material from which the lab on chip is fabricated, chemical techniques like those used for glass surfaces cannot be used to activate selected parts of the polymer surface. One of the most important advantages of polymers is their inert nature, assuring a very good chemical resistance. On the other hand, this property also renders surface chemical activation quite difficult. More specific processes have to be used, frequently causing a great increase of the surface energy of the polymer. The ensemble of such techniques is called grafting in the framework of polymer chemistry.

Grafting techniques are divided into two main classes: (i) *grafting onto* and (ii) *grafting from* [12,13]. In a *grafting onto* mechanism polymer chains adsorb onto a surface out of a solution; in a *grafting from* mechanism, a polymer chain is initiated and propagated at the surface. Since prepolymerized chains used in the *grafting onto* methods must have a thermodynamically favored conformation in solution in order to avoid their precipitation with no grafting result, their adsorption density is self-limiting. The *grafting from* technique circumvents this phenomenon and allows for greater grafting densities. Since in lab on chip technology the grafting density is a key issue due to the need of reaching a good efficiency in trapping target molecules and to the small available areas, almost only *grafting from* techniques are used in this application.

Grafting has to be assisted by a process of increasing the polymer surface energy by cleaving the surface polymeric chains and making available active sites for the grafts development. Different techniques can be used to perform this step, for example, plasma processing like in the glass case, high-energy UV illumination, corona treatment, and flame treatment. All these methods involve cleavage of polymer chains in the material and the incorporation of carbonyl and hydroxyl functional groups. The incorporation of oxygen into the surface creates a higher surface energy. A quite general chemical form of polymer chain cleavage by oxidation is represented in Figure 9.11.

While plasma oxidation is not diffused in general polymer industry due to the complexity and cost of the process besides nonuniformity on large surfaces, this is a suitable treatment for grafting of small polymeric surfaces in lab on chip, due to its ability of working on a very small surface and

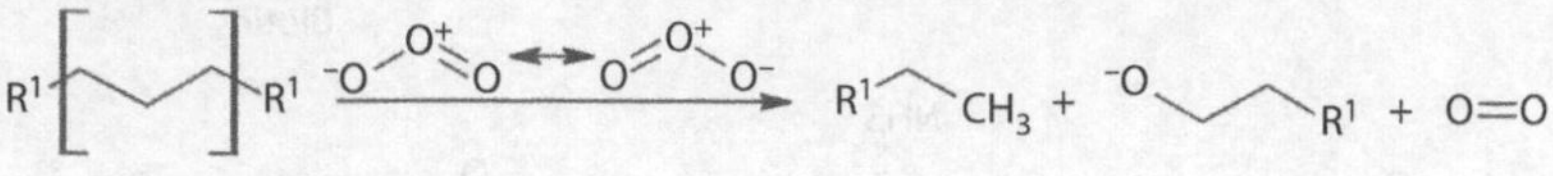

FIGURE 9.11 Polymer surface chain cleavage by oxidation.

to exploit the specific properties of plasma-enhanced polymerization (see Section 5.3.3) to produce a large variety of different grafts. Besides plasma grafting, UV-enhanced polymerization can be used to generate UV grafting. This method is also highly selective, due to the possibility of using masks to shield part of the polymer surface from UV light and has a very high level of control, resulting in a very suitable method for application in lab on chip. For this reason, we will focus on plasma- and UV-enhanced grafting, even if several other methods have been proposed and used to develop lab on chip prototypes [14,15].

The simpler form of plasma polymer surface grafting is the unspecific grafting obtained simply by bombing the polymer surface by an oxygen plasma of suitable energy. In this case, besides base oxidation of the surface several oxygen groups are created at the oxidation sites, in case also incorporating carbon atoms occasionally freed from polymer chains. A set of typical groups that can be obtained with unspecific grafting is reported in Figure 9.12. The grafting density typical of these processes is of 20–30%, that is, 20–30 grafts every 100 surface C atoms.

Besides the random nature of the process, the main cause of the great variety of grafting products is due to the fact that the energy that is needed to sustain the plasma is much higher than the typical activation energy needed to create a specific graft molecule, thus a great number of different products compete for generation, and the final process generates a random combination of them all [16]. An example of the relation between the energy of plasma particles and the activation energy of relevant chemical reactions is provided in Figure 9.13, where the electron energy distribution typical of a low-temperature plasma is compared with the activation energy of several chemical reactions that could lead to graft formation. Even if electrons are not used to bomb the polymer surface, the fact that relatively slow electrons have already an energy of the order of magnitude of C–H and C–C bonds energy is relevant.

Since plasma cannot be sustained at a lower energy, simple oxygen plasma grafting cannot give rise to a well-defined type of grafting molecules and a more complex process has to be used. The first category of such methods relies on the use of plasma to activate the surface followed by chemical grafting. Two procedures of this kind are briefly described here.

A possible way to obtain a specific activation of the polymer surface starting from the unspecific activation obtained through oxygen plasma treatment is to operate wet surface reduction, for example, by B_2H_6 or $LiAlH_4$. This operation generates a series of reduced composites by leaving a series of OH groups on the surface. Thus, selective OH activation is obtained in this way. The principle scheme of this process is reported in Figure 9.14a. Experimental observations indicate that, while after unselective surface activation the percentage of OH groups on the surface is as low as about 10%, the subsequent reduction process increases them to about 65% of all functional groups [17]. At the end, the final OH graft density is of the order of 15%.

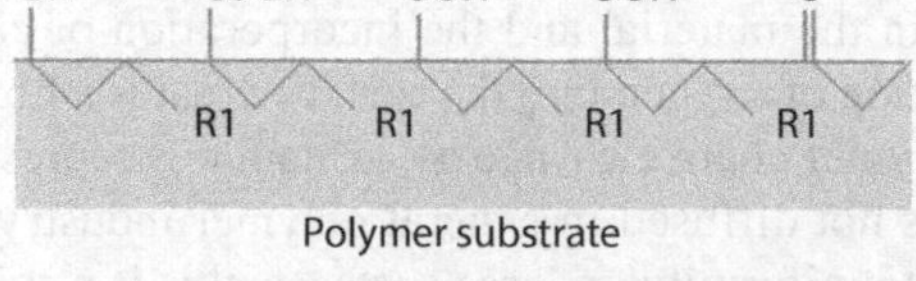

FIGURE 9.12 Typical groups forming the surface unspecific grafting on a polymer surface.

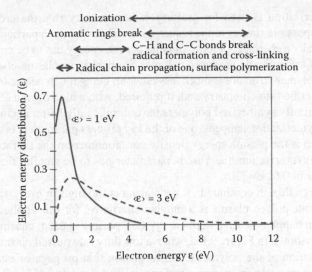

FIGURE 9.13 Comparison between typical electronic energy distribution in a low-temperature plasma and activation energy for selected chemical processes relevant for grafting.

More complex surface activation can be thus achieved by exposure of the surface with a solution of molecules reacting with the OH surface groups to provide more complex grafting.

If a neutral plasma, like Ar plasma, is adopted to bomb the polymer surface instead of the reactive O_2 plasma, the net effect is the break of a certain number of C–C and C–H bonds, activating the surface similar to what is done with a glass surface. These broken bonds can be exploited with a subsequent wet process to create a chemical grafting. Grafting with complex molecules can be created in this way, with an almost complete absence of spurious grafts. Spacers can also be used in this case analogously to what is done on silica surfaces by inserting suitable linkers in the reaction for chemical activation. The principle scheme of this method is shown in Figure 9.14b. The limitation of this technique is that the plasma energy cannot be increased beyond a threshold at which plasma treatment causes deep damage to the surface while the grafting density at compatible plasma energy is as low as 5% [16].

An alternative way to obtain plasma-enhanced grafting is by using plasma polymerization (see Section 5.3.2.3) to obtain creation and propagation of polymer chains on the original polymeric surface [18,19].

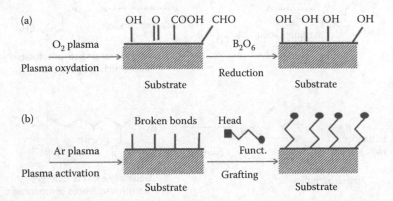

FIGURE 9.14 Principle schemes of plasma oxidation followed by wet chemical reduction (a) and of plasma bombing followed by chemical grafting (b).

If plasma polymerization is used for grafting, it is necessary that the created polymer has a structure as much as possible similar to the required one. This means, in particular, that polymerization has to be essentially a chemical process and that plasma energy has to be only the process initiator. The advantage of a chemically produced polymer compared to a plasma-chemically synthesized material is that the polymer structure is much less random, being much nearer to the desired defined structure, with a prescribed stoichiometry and, if required, with a high degree of internal crystallization. Moreover, chemically synthesized polymers have significantly better ageing stability.

When plasma polymerization happens, one of the key process parameters is the so-called Yasuda parameter [20], which is the plasma energy density per monomer on the surface. In order to obtain essential chemical polymerization, the Yasuda parameter has to be smaller than a threshold value, generally of the order of 0.01 eV [20].

The constant energy flux in continuous wave plasma is too high in every self-sustained plasma state, thus low duty rate pulsed plasma is a suitable alternative for this application. While chaotic plasma fragmentation happens when a high-energy CW plasma is used, causing a chaotic polymer chain propagation, as shown in Figure 9.15a, when a low duty rate pulsed plasma is used the plasma pulses generate activation of the polymer chain formation that propagates essentially due to gas-phase chemical polymerization in the gas envelope created near the surface by the plasma pulse, as shown in Figure 9.15b. Using chemically reactive monomers undergoing chemical radical chain propagation, only one energetic activation event is required to start a chain polymerization with a resulting molar polymerization degree greater than 1000. In the example of Figure 9.15b, the threshold energy for chain initiation is 1.5 eV [17].

In the previous section, we have seen that activation with NH_3 groups is particularly useful in lab on chip applications due to the ability of such groups to combine with several macromolecules. This is possible using pulsed plasma grafting in several ways. The density of the graft is determined mainly by the adopted monomers that also drive the type of grafting generating process, homo-polymerization, or copolymerization, and the density of cross-links among the different chains that are present in the graft. Examples of different processes for this type of plasma graft are reported in Figure 9.16 [17].

Alternatively to plasma-induced grafting, UV-induced grafting can be adopted for graft from generation on polymers small areas like those present in labs on chip. The base process relies on photo-induced polymerization of monomers that are patterned on the surface starting from surface-active sites, which in this case are generally constituted by C-links. In general, UV grafting is much slower with respect to plasma-induced grafting, but has the great advantage to be able to generate

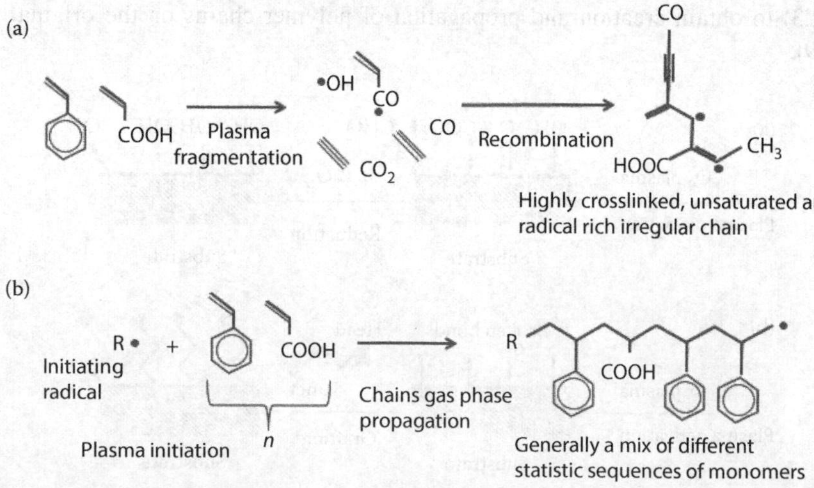

FIGURE 9.15 Different types of plasma copolymerization: CW plasma (a) and low duty rate pulsed plasma (b). Example monomers are styrene and acrylic acid.

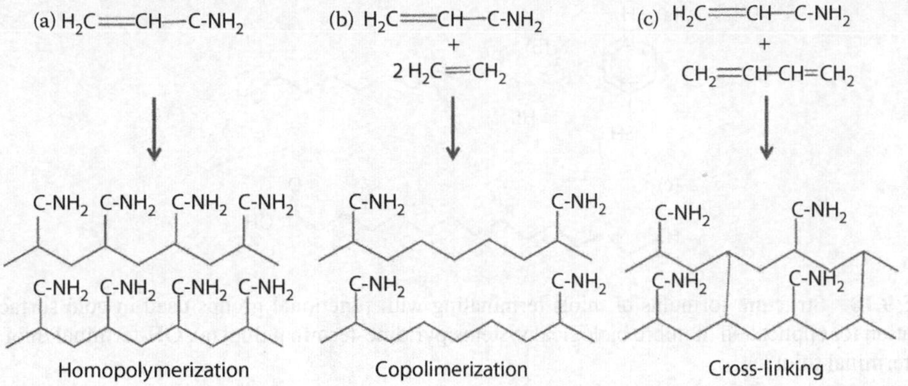

(a) $H_2C{=}CH{-}C{-}NH_2$ (b) $H_2C{=}CH{-}C{-}NH_2$ (c) $H_2C{=}CH{-}C{-}NH_2$
                                    $+$ $+$
                              $2\,H_2C{=}CH_2$ $CH_2{=}CH{-}CH{=}CH_2$

C-NH₂ ... Homopolymerization   Copolimerization   Cross-linking

FIGURE 9.16 Different reactions generating polymer grafting with NH_2 reactive groups through homopolymerization (a) and co-polymerization (b). Mechanism of cross-link formation through different grafting molecules (c).

dense and deep grafts without the risk of damaging the polymer surface [14]. Moreover, the use of UV-driven polymerization allows use of UV masks for the definition of the graft area, so rendering the process ease to integrate with traditional lithography.

The basic principle of the process is similar to that of plasma-initiated grafting: after deposition or patterning of the monomers on the surface, UV light is used to initiate graft from process while chains propagation is essentially chemical, so as to obtain an ordered and reproducible graft. Photografting has been used to coat the surface of polymers with active groups like $-NH_2$ or $-COOH$ allowing to fix both proteins like biotin and DNA strands [21,22].

9.3.3 METAL LAYER ACTIVATION

Thiols are very interesting molecules for surface activation. A thiol is an organic compound of sulfur that contains a carbon-bonded sulfhydryl $-C-SH$ group, as shown in Figure 9.17. The carbon is generally at the extreme of a more complex organic radical like an alkane or alkene. In some ways thiols are the sulfur analogue of alcohols in the sense that sulfur takes the place of oxygen in the hydroxyl group of an alcohol. The $-SH$ functional group itself is referred to as either a thiol group or a sulfhydryl group.

The thiols structure is characterized by a sulfur head that is quite reactive with metal surfaces, assuring for example very good covalent bond on gold single crystal surfaces, and a functional part that can be changed by selecting different organic compounds so as to fit the functional required characteristics. Examples of thiols terminating with pyridine, OH, and COOH groups are shown in Figure 9.18.

(a)   (b)

$R{-}S$
      $\backslash$
       H

SH

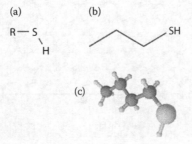

(c)

FIGURE 9.17 General structure formula of thiol molecules (a), structural (b), and stereographic (c) representation of the propanethiol molecule.

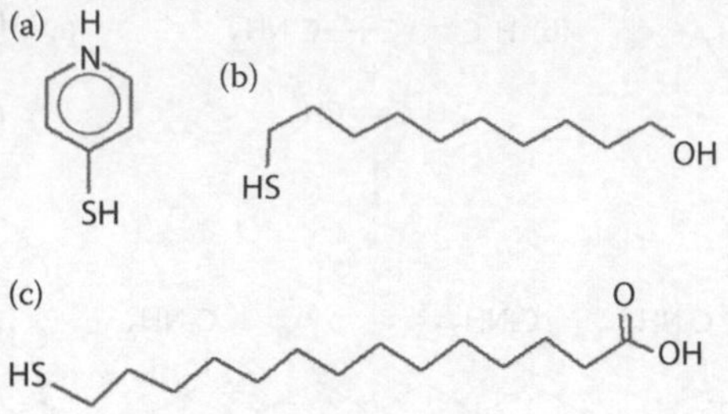

(a) H

SH

(b)

HS

OH

(c)

HS

O

OH

FIGURE 9.18 Structure formulas of thiols terminating with functional groups used in gold surface functionalization for application in micro biological systems:pyridine-terminal thiol (a), OH-terminal thiol (b), and COOH-terminal thiol (c).

Among the many metals that absorb thiols, gold is by far the most used. This is due to several reasons, besides the fact that absorption of thiols on gold is a well-known process [23]. Gold is a quite inert surface that adapts easily in order to be used in lab on chip without contaminating the ongoing chemical processes; moreover, the process of gold deposition is well known due to the wide use of gold in electronic and microwave applications for its characteristics of conduction and durability. The sulfur–gold interaction is semi-covalent and has a strength of approximately 45 kcal/mol, a good premise to obtain dense and stable SAM. Gold crystal cell is a face-centered-cubic with a side length of 4.07 Å, better thiols SAM can be grown on the (1, 1, 1) crystal plane, and this deposition direction is generally used for this application.

Surface activation obtained by gold deposition on silicon, glass, or polymer has been extensively studied [5,24,25] and used to build micro-sensors [26].

Owing to van der Waals interaction between the thiols heads, the monolayer assumes a very ordered structure that is typical of SAMs (see Section 5.3.4), with the thiols chains disposed at an angle of 30° from the surface plane, as schematically shown in Figure 9.19. Thiols monolayers can be grown on metals different from gold, such as silver and platinum, and other sulfur derivatives such as thiones or thiocarboxylic acid, whose structure formula is reported in Figure 9.20 that behave similarly [5]. Selenols, see Figure 9.20, also form SAM on gold surfaces [5].

Gold electrodes and gold surfaces have been widely used in the design of lab on chip to obtain functionalized surfaces by attaching active biomolecules to the thiol exposed head. A simpler way to obtain this result is by simple hydrophobic interaction between the exposed thiol head and the target molecule. If the end group of the thiol layer bears an electrical charge, as happens for COO^- or NH_3^+ terminating thiols, charged molecules can be attached by electrostatic action.

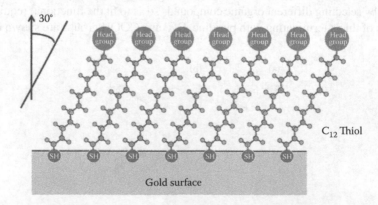

FIGURE 9.19 Schematic representation of SAM molecules of a sample thiols (the C_{12} thiol) on a gold (1, 1, 1) surface.

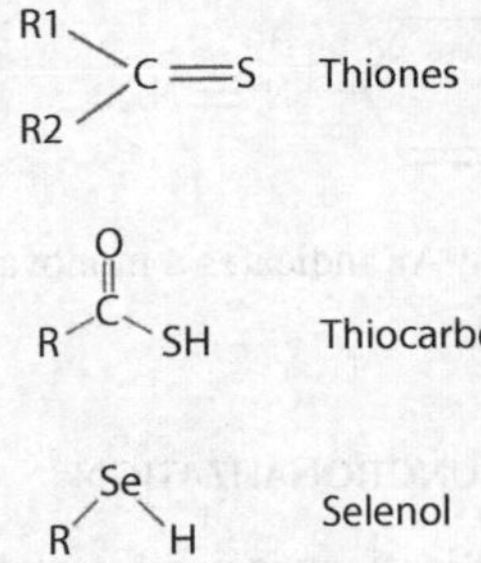

R1
R2
C═S   Thiones

O
‖
R—C—SH   Thiocarboxylic acid

Se
R   H   Selenol

FIGURE 9.20 Selected molecules that also give rise to SAM on a crystal gold surface.

A more stable functionalization of a thiol-activated gold surface can be attained by covalent bond of the thiol terminal group with the target molecule. This can be either directly obtained or mediated by a crosslinker that attaches on one side to the thiol terminal group, on the other side to the target molecule.

The so-called molecular wires [4,5] can also be attached to gold surfaces by thiol chemisorption. A molecular wire is a linear molecule containing a system of conjugated π molecular bonds (see Section 3.6.3 and Figure 3.36). Due to delocalization the π-electrons can flow along the molecule so as to create a contact between the metal and a RedOx species that has to be immobilized on the monolayer. An example of molecular wire is shown in Figure 9.21.

Sometimes, the thiol-functionalizing molecule compound is present in the solution before the generation of the thiol monolayer on the metal surface. In this case, chemical activation and functionalization happen together when the composite absorbs on the metal surface from the solution. Many proteins contain thiol groups in the cysteine residues so that they directly generate a SAM on gold. If such a group is not present, it is possible to artificially add a short thiol tail on the amino residues of almost all proteins by reaction with 2-iminothiolanel (also called Traut's reagent). Similar procedures can be repeated for many types of molecules. In case of large molecules, like many enzymes, more than one thiol group is attached to the molecule, in order to obtain a more stable gold surface functionalization.

The procedure of initially creating a thiol–target composite in the solution and then the functionalization layer has, however, a few disadvantages with respect to the immobilization of functionalizing molecules on a thiol-activated surface, especially if the functionalizing molecule is a large molecule like an enzyme. Very dense and well-oriented monolayers are only obtained if long thiol chains are directly fixed to the gold surface. If a large molecule with a thiol tail is used, the resulting monolayer is generally looser, leaving portion of the available surface nonoccupied. If nonspecific interactions of the nonoccupied surface areas need to be prevented, then they can be saturated after the functionalization with a newly created thiols layer.

An alternative method to generate SAM on a metal surface relies on the use of the aryl diazonium salt, whose structure formula is reported in Figure 9.22 [27]. When electrochemically reduced near a gold electrode (see Section 10.3) the salt deposits on the electrode, forming a thick layer that adheres quite well to the metal surface. The resulting diazonium salt layer can be functionalized by linking to the positive nitrogen negatively charged molecules, like polypeptides.

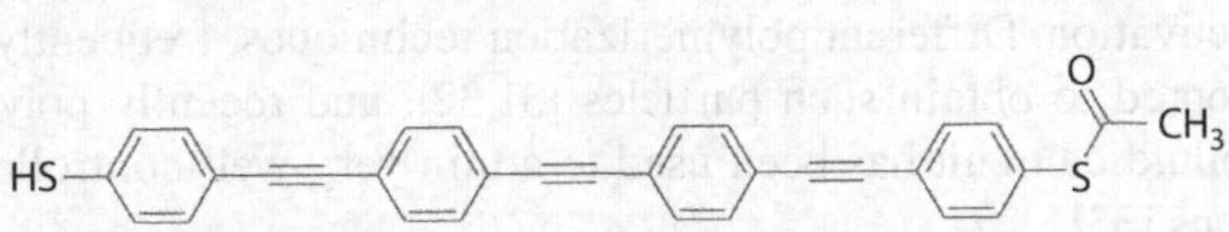

HS— ═ ═ ═
O
‖
S—CH₃

FIGURE 9.21 Structure formula of an example of molecular wire.

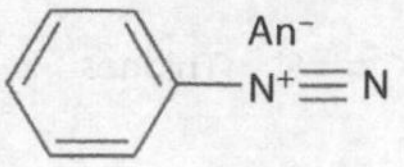

FIGURE 9.22 Example of aryl diazonium salt; An indicates a monovalent anion.

9.3.4 Nanoparticle Activation and Functionalization

Surface functionalization in lab on chip applications is used to attach the molecules under test to the surface of the reaction chamber of the lab on chip in order to purify them and render them available for the assay reaction. This is a widely diffused principle in macroscopic assays, for example in immunoassays like the various ELISA versions (see Section 3.7.5).

In a lab on chip, where generally a microfluidic circuit is present, attaching molecules to movable particles can be however quite useful. As a matter of fact, magnetic- or electrically charged particles can be moved with the help of suitable fields through the lab on chip where they are processed before detection. In other cases, particles are dragged by the moving fluid being guided by suitable streamlines (see, e.g., Section 8.5.1).

In principle, the techniques used for particles functionalization are not different from those adopted for surface functionalization, due to the fact that it is the particle surface to be functionalized in order to exhibit suitable active elements. However, the fact that we are dealing here with very small particles, frequently with a diameter under 1 μm, creates several practical-specific aspects of the process.

The first element is related to the surface activation, a preliminary step to chemical functionalization. No plasma bombing or aggressive chemical etching is possible on nanoparticles. Thus, the particle surface has to be active due to its own structure. However, the nanoparticle has no structural role in the lab on chip, different from the floor surface of a reaction room. Thus, a wider range of materials can be used in order to provide suitably active surfaces.

The first possible choice is to select gold crystal nanoparticles, whose surface can capture thiols and other molecules terminating with a sulfur. Generally, gold nanoparticles are produced by the so-called colloidal or liquid chemical synthesis, by the reduction of chloroauric acid $HAuCl_4$ solution in water. After dissolving $HAuCl_4$, the solution is rapidly stirred while a reducing agent is added. This causes Au^{3+} ions to be reduced to neutral gold atoms. As increasing number of these gold atoms form, the solution becomes supersaturated, and gold gradually starts to precipitate in the form of sub-nanometer particles. The remaining gold atoms that form stick to the existing particles, and, if the solution is stirred vigorously enough, the particles will be fairly uniform in size.

To prevent the particles from aggregating, some stabilizing agent that sticks to the nanoparticle surface is usually added. Alternatively, gold colloids can be synthesized without stabilizers by laser ablation in liquids [28]. Particles with a quite accurate spherical form with a diameter in the range of 3–10 nm can be obtained easily, that are suitable for use in labs on chip.

Once created, the colloidal gold nanoparticles can be functionalized with a large variety of moieties that attaches to their surface [29,30]. A list of selected moieties used for gold particles functionalization is reported in Tables 9.1 and 9.2.

A very diffused alternative to gold nanoparticles is the use of polymeric particles with a very porous surface. Pores create a high surface energy due to the small curvature radius and render the surface suitable for activation. Different polymerization techniques, frequently performed in liquid phase, have been adopted to obtain such particles [31,32], and recently polymerization in liquid phase within a microfluidic circuit has been used to attain very well-controlled surface properties and particle dimensions [33].

TABLE 9.1

List of Selected Biological Hydrophobic Moieties That Can be Used to Functionalized Gold Nanoparticles Obtained by Liquid Chemical Synthesis (Colloidal Gold)

Trioctylphosphine oxide	TOPO	
Triphenylphosphine	TPP	
Dodecanethiol	DDT	
Tetraoctylammonium bromide	TOAB	
Oleic acid	OA	

TABLE 9.2

List of Selected Biological Hydrophilic Moieties That Can be Used to Functionalized Gold Nanoparticles Obtained by Liquid Chemical Synthesis (Colloidal Gold)

Mercaptoacetic acid	MAA	
Mercaptopropionic acid	MPA	
Mercaptosuccinic acid	MSA	
Dihydrolipic acid	DHLA	

9.4   SURFACE ACTIVATION USING CARBON NANOTUBES

A recent and very interesting intermediate structure considered for the functionalization of lab on chip surfaces is the carbon nanotube. A large variety of structures can be designed using both stand-alone and surface-grafted carbon nanotubes having different biochemical functions.

9.4.1   CARBON NANOTUBE NATURE AND GROWTH

Carbon nanotubes are allotropes of carbon with a cylindrical nanostructure [34,35]; a pictorial representation of a sample carbon nanotube is reported in Figure 9.23a. Nanotubes have been constructed with length-to-diameter ratio of up to $1.32 \times 10^8{:}1$, significantly larger than for any other material. Many of the unusual properties of these structures are due to the particular kind of bonds existing between the nearby atoms: these are completely due to sp^2 hybridization, similar to those of graphite. While sp^3 hybridization produces tetrahedral bonds, like those found in methane and diamond, sp^2 hybridization produces three planar bonds at 120°, allowing planar carbon structures to be developed. This property is shown schematically in Figure 9.24. Moreover, sp^2 bonds are stronger than sp^3 bonds and are the base of many nanotubes properties, starting from their unique mechanical strength.

The first classification of nanotubes is the so-called single-walled nanotube, in which the structures are constituted by a single curved sheet of carbon atoms, whereas the structures constituted by multiple sheets accommodated one into the other are called multi-walled nanotubes. The nanotube represented in Figure 9.23a is a single-walled structure; a multi-walled structure is represented in Figure 9.23b. Most single-walled nanotubes have a diameter close to 1 nm, with a tube length that can be many millions of times longer.

Each sheet constituting a nanotube can be ideally obtained by rolling a plane graphene sheet. The way the graphene sheet is wrapped is represented by a pair of indices (n,m), once the standard reference system composed by the vectors $\boldsymbol{a}_1$ and $\boldsymbol{a}_2$ is set on the sheet plane (see Figure 9.25). In particular, we can define the roll-up vector $\boldsymbol{C}$ of the nanotube as the vector joining two points in the plane sheet that will be coincident with the rolled-up form of the nanotube. The roll-up vector cannot be arbitrary, due to the need of preserving the two-dimensional crystal structure to obtain a stable nanotube and it can be verified that the most general expression of the roll-up vector is

$$C = na_1 + ma_2 \tag{9.8}$$

where n and m are integer numbers. If $m = 0$, the nanotubes are called zigzag nanotubes, and if $n = m$, the nanotubes are called armchair nanotubes. Otherwise, they are called chiral. The diameter d of an ideal nanotube can be calculated from its (n,m) indices as follows:

$$d = \frac{\alpha}{\pi}\sqrt{n^2 + nm + m^2} \tag{9.9}$$

where $\alpha \approx 0.246$ nm.

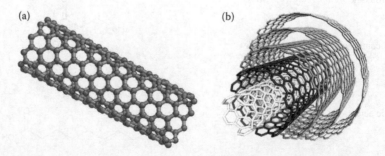

(a)   (b)

FIGURE 9.23   Pictorial representation of a carbon nanotube structure: single-walled nanotube (a) and multi-walled nanotube (b).

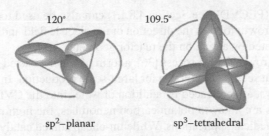

sp²–planar   sp³–tetrahedral

FIGURE 9.24 Pictorial representation of sp² and sp³ hybrid orbitals of the carbon atom generating the corresponding graphite and diamond bonds.

There are two models that can be used to describe the structures of multi-walled nanotubes. In the Russian doll model, sheets of graphite are arranged in concentric cylinders as shown in Figure 9.23b. For example, a (0,8) single-walled nanotube can be inserted within a larger (0,17) nanotube. In the parchment model, a single sheet of graphite is rolled in around itself, resembling a scroll of parchment or a rolled newspaper. The interlayer distance in multi-walled nanotubes is close to the distance between graphene layers in graphite, approximately 3.4 Å.

Several processes are able to produce standalone carbon nanotubes, but if they are to be grown out of a substrate surface, chemical vapor deposition (CVD) is almost the only industrial available technique (see Section 4.8.1). During CVD, a layer of metal catalyst particles is deposited on the surface, most commonly nickel, cobalt [36], iron, or a combination of them [37]. Besides simple deposition, the catalyst metal particles can be produced on the surface by the deposition of a continuous metal film followed by a controlled film etching, for example, by low-energy reactive ion etching (RIE). The use of low-energy RIE is advantageous for its ability to control well the dimensions of the residual metal particles and, as a consequence, of the diameter of the nanotubes that will be created.

After metal particle deposition, the substrate is heated to approximately 700°C. To initiate the growth of nanotubes, two gases are bled into the reactor: a process gas, such as ammonia, nitrogen, or hydrogen, and a carbon-containing gas, such as acetylene, ethylene, ethanol, or methane. Nanotubes grow at the sites of the metal catalyst; the carbon-containing gas is broken apart at the surface of the catalyst particle, and the carbon is transported to the edges of the particle, where it forms the nanotubes. The details of this growing mechanism are still under investigation [38]: the catalyst particles can stay at the tips of the growing nanotube during the growth process, or remain at the nanotube base, depending on the adhesion between the catalyst particle and the substrate [39].

If standard CVD is used to grow nanotube, they are generally randomly oriented with respect to the surface, even if more regular configurations can be observed in specific situations.

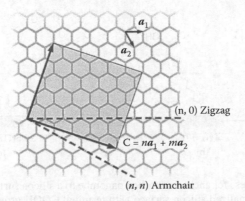

FIGURE 9.25 Standard reference system on the graphene sheet of a carbon nanotube and the roll-up vectors for zigzag and armchair nanotubes.

Plasma-enhanced CVD (PECVD) (see Section 4.8.1.1) can also be used to grow nanotubes [40]. In this case, the nanotube growth follows the direction of the electric field and the angle they form with the surface can be regulated by acting on the reactor geometry.

The so-called super-growth CVD process [36], a form of water-assisted CVD, is an efficient way of creating nanotubes that seem to be suitable for large-scale production. In this process, the activity and lifetime of the catalyst are enhanced by addition of water into the CVD reactor.

While metal catalysts are a key to obtain carbon nanotubes, the high metal reactivity can constitute a problem in biomedical applications. While un-encapsulated catalyst metals may be readily removable by acid washing, encapsulated ones require oxidative treatment for opening their carbon shell [36]. The effective removal of catalysts, especially of encapsulated ones, while preserving the nanotube structure is a challenge, and many possible solutions have been proposed [41–43].

9.4.2 Carbon Nanotube Functionalization

Two main methods have been introduced to functionalize surfaces by using carbon nanotubes as intermediate structures: either using standalone nanotubes that are on one side grafted with functional groups and on the other side bonded to the surface by a linker molecule or by directly functionalizing nanotubes growth on the target surface.

If carbon nanotubes cannot be grown starting from the considered surface, or if nanotubes activation has to be done on free nanotubes, nanotubes can be fixed to the surface by using a suitable intermediate molecule, as shown in Figure 9.26, where a (1, 1, 1) silicon surface is considered [44]. This approach is based on a surface amidation reaction between soluble amino sidewall functionalized multi-walled carbon nanotubes and the NHS head groups of an alkyl monolayer covalently bonded to p-type Si (111) surface. The monolayer can be prepared by surface activation obtained through wet etching in order to break surface crystal bonds and terminating them with hydrogen atoms. After etching, the silicon is immersed into a solution containing undecylenic acid, which under UV irradiation causes substitution of the H terminals with a COOH-terminated alkyl monolayer. Then, the terminal COOH groups were activated with NHS by immersing the modified silicon surface on a suitable NHS solution.

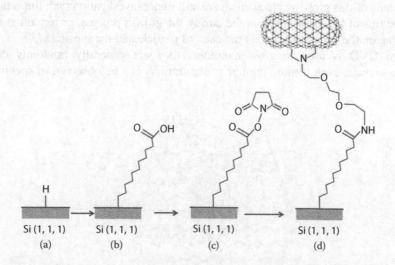

FIGURE 9.26 Sample process for anchoring carbon nanotube to a silicon surface; H grafted silicon surface after wet etching (a), functionalized silicon surface with terminal COOH groups (b), functionalized silicon surface with terminal NHS groups (c), and standalone nanotube anchored to the surface via the NHS group opening (d).

The process allowing to bond standalone nanotubes to a surface after nanotubes functionalization has two main advantages: it allows the use of closed nanotubes and the use of activation techniques that otherwise would detach the nanotubes from the surface where they are built. In particular, closed nanotubes are generated when the two ends of a single-walled nanotube are closed by two nanotube caps whose structure is different from the nanotube walls [45]. This structure is energetically favorable when the nanotube is created from separated catalytic particles or when it is detached from the original surface at the very initial phase of growth, since it avoids the high-energy contribution of the open carbon bonds at the nanotube extremes. The structures of the caps in both armchair and zigzag nanotubes are shown in Figure 9.27.

The presence of five-membered rings at the caps leads to a relatively higher reactivity at these points, comparable to the reactivity of the regular graphene framework of the walls [46]. By comparison, functionalization of the sidewall comprising the regular graphene framework is more difficult to accomplish. In general, addition reactions to the partial carbon–carbon double bonds cause the transformation of sp_2- into sp_3-hybridized carbon atoms, which is associated with a change from a trigonal–planar local bonding geometry to a tetrahedral geometry. This process is energetically more favorable at the caps due to their pronounced curvature in two dimensions.

The main disadvantage of this technique is that the long-chain anchoring the carbon nanotube to the surface is structurally less resistant than direct anchoring and functionalization of the surface results to be unavoidably less reliable when realized in this way.

More frequently, however, carbon nanotubes are directly grown and activated on the target surface. In this case, the activation method has to be suitable not to detach the nanotubes from the surface while creating the wanted graft on their surface.

Three methods exist to create a functional graft on a nanotube surface: thermal methods, generally based on the nanotube surface oxidation, electrochemical methods, and photochemical methods. Both single- and multi-walled nanotubes can be functionalized in these ways [47,48], obtaining a large variety of active structures, that are different not only for their chemical properties, but also for mechanical and electronic behavior.

An efficient oxidation process of single-walled free nanotubes involves extensive ultrasonic treatment in a mixture of concentrated nitric and sulfuric acid [49]. Such drastic conditions lead to the opening of the tube caps as well as the formation of holes in the sidewalls, followed by an

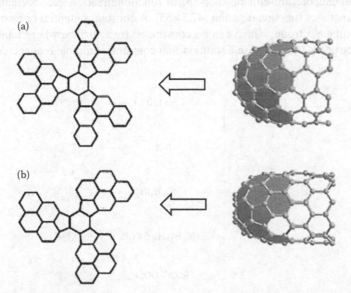

FIGURE 9.27   End cap of an armchair (a) and of a zigzag (b) single-walled nanotube. Each cap is represented in a three-dimensional plot and developed by putting all the faces on the same plane.

oxidative etching along the walls with the concomitant release of carbon dioxide. The final products are nanotube fragments with lengths in the range of 100–300 nm, whose ends and sidewalls are decorated with a high density of various oxygen containing groups, such as CO, COOH, and OH.

Under less energetic conditions, such as refluxing in nitric acid, the shortening of the tubes can be minimized. The chemical modification is limited in this case, mostly due to the opening of the tube caps and the formation of functional groups at defect sites along the sidewalls. Nanotubes functionalized in this manner basically retain their pristine electronic and mechanical properties. The carboxyl groups introduced by oxidation represent useful sites for further modifications, as they enable the covalent coupling of molecules through the creation of amide and ester bonds [47]. In both these cases naturally, free functionalized single-walled nanotubes are obtained, that have to be anchored to the surface to be functionalized.

Multi-walled nanotubes can be functionalized by oxidation too [50,51]. Less destructive oxidation conditions can also be used on multi-walled nanotubes while they are fixed on a surface by avoiding the nanotube detachment through a rigorous process control.

While the two-step functionalization of nanotubes through the oxidative introduction of carboxyl groups followed by the formation of amide or ester linkages does allow for a stable chemical modification, it has only a relatively weak influence on the electrical and mechanical properties of the nanotubes. By comparison, addition reactions enable the direct coupling of functional groups onto the π-conjugated carbon framework of the tubes. The required reactive species, like atoms, radicals, carbenes, or nitrenes, are in general made available through thermally activated reactions. Carbenes and nitrenes, in particular, are quite useful to obtain high reactivity grafts. A carbene is a molecule containing a neutral carbon atom linking one or two organic radicals and having two unshared valence electrons. The general formula is either $\mathbf{R}' - (\mathbf{C}{:}) - \mathbf{R}$ or $(\mathbf{C}{:}) = \mathbf{R}$. A nitrene is the nitrogen analogue of a carbene. Since nitrogen has six valence electrons, a nitrene has four unshared valence electrons; the two possible nitrene formulas are either $\mathbf{R} - (\mathbf{\ddot{N}}{:}) - \mathbf{R}$ or $(\mathbf{\ddot{N}}{:}) = \mathbf{R}$.

Addition reactions are compatible with nanotube sets that are directly grown on the surface to be functionalized, not requiring subsequent nanotube anchoring. A series of addition reactions have been well documented [47,52,53], the most important of which is listed in Figure 9.28. The most efficient functionalization procedures attain a good graft density, like one graft every 100 surface carbon atoms.

In alternative to temperature-enhanced chemical functionalization, electrochemical procedures can be used for nanotubes functionalization [47,54,55]. A constant potential or a constant current is applied to a nanotube electrode, which can be constituted by a surface where nanotubes are present, while the electrode is immersed in a solution that contains a suitable reagent. A highly reactive

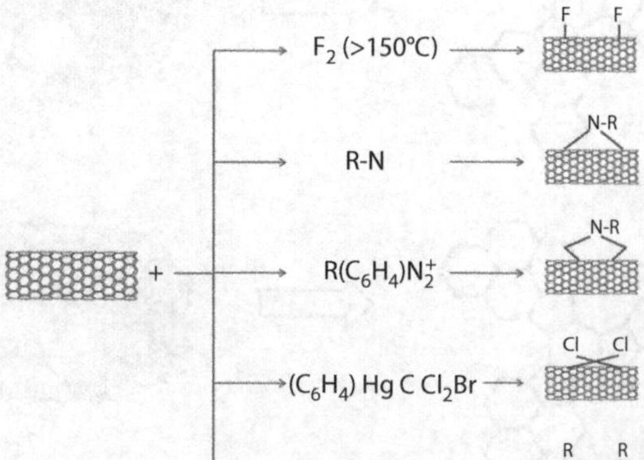

FIGURE 9.28 Principle scheme of possible substitution reactions generating grafting on the surface of a single-walled carbon nanotube.

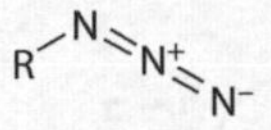

$$R^{N} \diagdown_{N} \diagup^{N^+} \diagdown_{N^-}$$

FIGURE 9.29 General structure formula of an azido compound.

radical is generated through electron transfer between the nanotubes and the reagent generating self-polymerization or cross-polymerization with the initial reagent. This results in a polymer coating on the nanotubes.

Depending on the used reagent, the polymeric layer may or may not be bonded in a covalent manner onto the nanotube sidewall. In addition to being simple, clean, and efficient, electrochemical modification schemes are quite versatile in that they allow for an accurate control over the extent of film deposition through the choice of suitable electrochemical conditions, that is, the duration and magnitude of the applied potential. Moreover, by utilizing reagents containing appropriate substituents, the surface properties of the coated tubes can be tailored, for example, from highly polar to predominantly hydrophobic.

This method is able to reach very high-density grafts on single-walled nanotubes [56], up to one graft every 20 surface carbon atoms.

In contrast to the chemical functionalization routes based on thermal activation or electrochemistry, photochemical approaches have been employed to a much lesser extent up to now. Photoirradiation has been used to generate reactive species such as nitrenes in the course of sidewall addition reactions [57] for single-walled nanotubes functionalization. In these cases, however, the photoactivation exclusively employs an azido compound as the nitrene precursor. The general formula of azido compounds is reported in Figure 9.29. Direct photo-induced functionalization of multi-walled nanotubes has been used to obtain different types of grafts [58] and is a quite promising technique, completely suitable to directly functionalize surface attached nanotubes.

9.5 ANTIBODY AND APTAMER SURFACE FUNCTIONALIZATION

Even if the simple surface activation is sufficient to create a selective binding site for the assay target, this is not the case, generally. As an example, the very common functionalization with NH_3 or COOH terminals in suitable conditions has the potential to bind all proteins that exhibit a steric access to the N or C terminal of the peptide chain. In order to obtain a very specific binding capacity, the activated surface has to be engineered for the wanted target.

Several methods have been devised [5] for this task, the most diffused and effective techniques are based on the deposition of monolayers of specific antibodies or aptamers.

9.5.1 ANTIBODY MONOLAYERS ON ACTIVATED SURFACES

Monoclonal antibodies are characterized by very specific binding sites on their branches that are devoted to the recognition of their target antigens (see Section 2.4). Moreover, antibodies have accessible binding sites on their tail that are used to block them on immunity system cells in several immunity system operations [59]. It is thus possible to device systems to fix the antibody tail to the monolayer that is grown on the activated surface so as to expose the specific binding sites on the branches.

Various methods can be used to immobilize antibodies on an activated surface, like covalent bonding to the NH_3 or COOH terminals of the graft on the surface, or affinity links. In particular, a common way of creating affinity immobilization is by grafting Protein A on the activated surface, frequently through covalent bonds. The protein A binds the Fc region of immunoglobulins through interaction with the heavy chain by leaving the antigen-binding sites exposed on top of the monolayer.

The avidin–biotin system is also a widely diffused method to fix antibodies in a monolayer. Streptavidin, the most common protein containing the avidin structure, is a homotetrameric eight-stranded β-barrel protein, as shown in Figure 9.30 with deepbinding pockets to accommodate

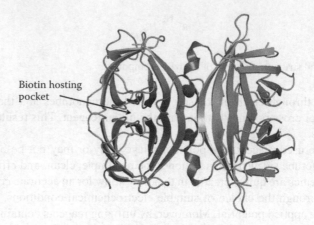

FIGURE 9.30   Streptavidin tertiary structure with one of the biotin hosting pockets evidenced.

biotin. In this technique, the avidin is generally bonded to the activated surface while the antibodies are separately coupled with biotin through its COOH group, as shown in Figure 9.31. This coupling exposes the biotin group fitting the streptavidin pocket so that, when the activated surface is exposed to the biotinylated antibodies they are bonded to the surface via the avidin–biotin system [5].

Depending on the surface functionalization and on the monolayer growing process, the antibodies can be either randomly oriented or oriented in a well-defined direction [60]; the oriented antibodies' monolayers generally assure better performances, but applications are possible where the easier process needed to generate randomly oriented monolayers is at premium with respect to the monolayer performances in terms of antibodies' density and activity. A schematic illustration of various types of antibody monolayers on an activated surface is shown in Figure 9.32.

Frequently, monolayers of antibodies fragments are created instead of using the whole immunoglobulin molecule [5]. In this case, a single antibody Fab + Fc region is attached to the functionalized surface, exploiting the active site that are present in the hinge region binding carbohydrates in the complete molecule. In this case, a reduction of the binding energy is obtained, due to the fact that the single Fab active site has a lower bonding energy with respect to the bivalent molecule (see Section 3.7.1) that can be partially compensated by the higher monolayer density.

9.5.2 APTAMER MONOLAYERS ON FUNCTIONALIZED SURFACES

Aptamers [61] are either short, single-stranded DNA or RNA molecules or peptide molecules that bind to a specific target molecule. Aptamers are generally synthesized artificially by researching the wanted target affinity within a pool of test molecules; however, natural aptamers also exist,

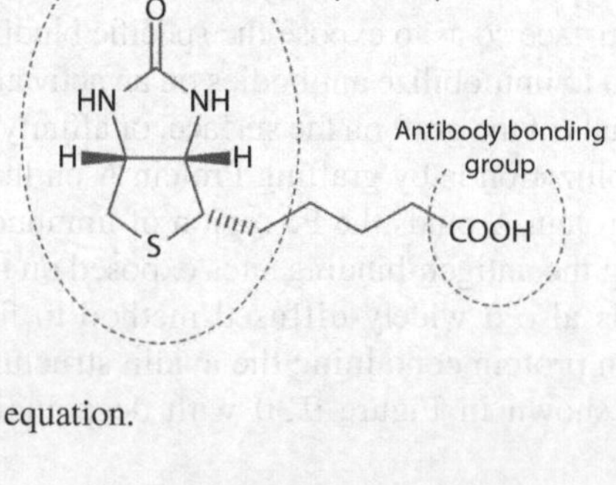

FIGURE 9.31   Biotin structure equation.

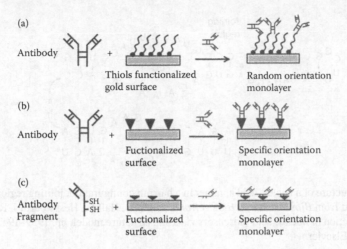

FIGURE 9.32 Schematic illustration of different types of antibody monolayers on an activated surface; randomly oriented monolayer (a), monolayer oriented in a specific direction obtained using complete IgG antibodies (b), monolayer oriented in a specific direction obtained using antibodies fragments (c).

for example, in ribo switches that are regulatory segments of a messenger RNA that binds a small molecule, resulting in a change in production of the proteins encoded by the mRNA.

An example of nucleic acid-based aptamer molecule, the biotin RNA aptamer, is presented in Figure 9.33. The aptamer is represented superimposing stick and volume representations, while the biotin molecule is represented in volume representation. From the figure the importance of the tertiary structure of the aptamer in creating a suitable binding site for the conjugate molecule results clearly. The fact that steric effects related to the molecule tertiary structure are quite important is a common property of almost all aptamers. Small molecules are generally hosted into aptamers' packets in order to be strongly bonded to the aptamer due to the final steric configuration.

Nucleic acid aptamers are frequently bonded to a functionalized surface in an hairpin configuration. An example of aptamer in hairpin configuration is reported in Figure 9.34 [62]. An hairpin is constituted by a sequence of joining regions, where the nucleobases of different segments of the single-stranded molecule are connected by hydrogen bonds so as to close the structure, and pockets, where the nucleobases are free. Small molecules are generally hosted in pockets in an hairpin

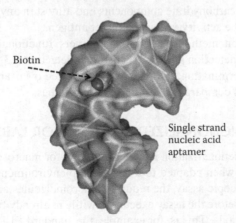

Biotin

Single strand
nucleic acid
aptamer

FIGURE 9.33 Example of nucleic acid-based aptamer molecule: Biotin RNA aptamer binding a biotin molecule. The aptamer is represented superimposing stick and volume representations while the biotin molecule is represented in volume representation.

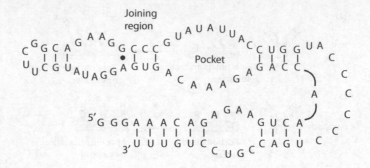

FIGURE 9.34 Structure of a nucleic acid aptamer in a hairpin configuration, joining regions and pockets are evidenced. (Adapted from *Biosensors and Bioelectronics*, vol. 22, Hall B., Hesselberth J. R., Ellington A. D., Computational selection of nucleic acid biosensors via a slip structure model, pp. 1939–1947, Copyright 2007, with permission of Elsevier.)

aptamer, to be strongly bonded to the molecule. Applications also exist where the target molecule has a high affinity with the hairpin aptamer and bonds with it while opening the strand, that generally happens when a single joining region exist. In this case, the hairpin structure of the free aptamer is changed by the bonding with the target, so greatly changing the functionalized surface properties.

Theoretically, aptamers can be developed for any kind of molecules, nucleic acids, proteins, and small molecules like single peptides. The fact that aptamers can be created with high affinity with small molecules is one of their advantages over antibodies, when these kinds of targets have to be bonded. This advantage is particularly evident when toxins have to be detected, since antibodies are not sensible to toxins due to their small dimension and poor structure.

The fact that aptamers can be artificially synthesized by an in vitro selection process while monoclonal antibodies require the use of living organisms for generation is another advantage of aptamers, besides the small aptamer dimension with respect to antibodies. For example, a human IgG has a molecular mass of about 150 kDa, while many aptamers ranges from 350 to 600 Da. Last, but not the least, aptamers are much less sensible to temperature variations with respect to antibodies.

Aptamers also have disadvantages, mainly related to the fact that the tertiary structure of this small molecule is very dependent on the solution where they are dissolved, so that in specific conditions they lose their affinity to the target molecule due to steric effects. This happens typically when aptamers are solved in blood. Antibodies on the contrary have a very stable tertiary structure due to the structural role of their carbohydrate components and almost in any circumstances expose the active sites so to maximize the activity versus the target antigen.

Several types of detection methods based on aptamers functionalized surfaces have been designed, both using optical detection and electrochemical detection [63]. Aptamers can be bonded to the OH, NH_3, or COOH termination of monolayers fabricated over target surfaces and results to have adhesion characteristics comparable with those of antibodies.

9.6 STABILITY OF FUNCTIONALIZED SURFACES FOR LABS ON CHIP

Surface and nanoparticle functionalization is widely adopted for macroscopic assays, but the assay process is sensibly different when adapted to a lab on chip environment. When surface functionalization is used in a macroscopic assay, the required macromolecules are absorbed on the macroscopic surface immediately before the assay execution, while in already functionalized surface they are rarely stored for long periods. This is, for example, the standard ELISA procedure, as reported in Section 3.7.5.

If a lab on chip is considered, surface functionalization immediately before the assay execution requires a suitable microfluidic access for the functionalizing solution and frequently a dedicated microfluidic circuit, besides the availability of a suitable functionalizing solution at the time of the assay. In addition, since the functionalizing solution has to be washed out from the assay chamber before the assay, a suitable wash has also to be executed. Such conditions, that can be realized only if the lab on chip is used in a laboratory environment, require in any case a more complex chip structure which impacts on both cost and yield.

For such reasons, surfaces are normally functionalized during the lab on chip fabrication, as a part of the front-end fabrication or in any case before closing of the microfluidic circuit. This renders the lab on chip use much easier and allows field assay execution, but has an important drawback. A lab on chip can experience a few years storage after fabrication before it is used. If standard storage conditions are considered, it undergoes temperature and humidity fluctuations besides mechanical vibrations during transport. Thus, for long-term stability of functionalized surfaces it has to be carefully assessed.

Quite different results can be obtained depending on the considered functionalized surface and the adopted conditions. For example, in selected cases, monolayers are stored in the lab on chip in a dry environment, but more often they are in the presence of a buffer solution that fill the whole microfluidic circuit. This depends both on the kind of assay that is realized in the chip and on the method that is chosen for fluid movement. In capillary-based systems, since an interface between advancing liquid and air has to be maintained while the fluid moves, it is probable that an activated surface that is present in the reaction room is in dry condition for all the storage duration. On the contrary, if fluid movement is attained by a micropump or the target and test species diffuses through a still buffer, the buffer will be present for all the storage time.

In general, the fabrication procedures and the length of the surface attached chain play a key role in assuring stability under thermal cycling [64,65]. If the monolayer is obtained by a patterning technique during front-end fabrication, the characteristics of the photoresist removal process following the patterning seem to have a key importance in avoiding a weakening of the SAM adhesion to the surface. In particular, aggressive chemical processes or plasma photoresist removal should be avoided, even if the monolayer is suitably masked during such processes [64]. Moreover, high-temperature processes, like thermal wafer bonding (see Section 4.9.3), are not suggested after the monolayer patterning. Under this point of view, SAMs should be created immediately before the microfluidic circuit closing with a cap layer, followed only by an adhesive closing of the chip.

If the SAM is stored while immersed in a biological buffer, the length of SAM chains influences the SAM stability. It seems from some studies that SAM stability under thermal cycles is favored by the presence of longer chains [64], but it is not completely clear if this result can be generalized beyond the specific cases reported in the literature.

Long-term thermal stability has been studied extensively for alkanethiol SAM on gold by comparing it both with the stability of polymeric monolayers used for different applications and analyzing the stability dependence on the attached molecule. Alkanethiol SAM results in much less resistance to thermal fluctuations with respect to monolayers of biologically inactive polymers on gold, if we consider aging accelerations through extreme thermal cycling, thermal excursions to 200°C, and exposure to hot base. For example, a 1:1 mixture of ethanol and 1.0 mole of KOH in water solution at 100°C completely strip n-alkanethiol SAMs from the gold substrates [66], while photo-polymerized SAMs are resistant to these extreme conditions.

Observations on SAMs created with different thiol molecules suggest that a correlation exists between film stability under thermal cycling and the degree of chelation in the covalent bond between the gold surface and the thiol head [67]. This suggests that chelating thiols should be preferred in order to obtain a better thermal stability of SAMs on gold.

The situation is different for alkanethiol SAMs in air, as it can happen in lab on chip based on capillary effect for fluid motion. The sulfur thiol heads start to oxidize only after hours of air exposure, and even if oxidized alkanethiol SAMs retain blocking characteristics toward electron transfer, they could weaken greatly the SAM stability versus other stressing factors [68]. Experiments suggest ozone as the primary oxidant in environmental air, which causes rapid oxidation of the thiolate moiety. Thus, if part of the microfluidic circuit has to be filled with a gas during storage, an inert gas as helium is strongly suggested.

Finally, the stability of the monolayer when immersed for a long time in different types of biological active buffers has been explored. Different types of buffers have been adopted for this study like phosphate-buffered saline serum and calf serum [69] or 10% fetal bovine serum solution [70]. In both cases, the stability of the order of 20–30 days is detected, depending on the buffer, in the absence of thermal cycling.

The major problem in this case is the oxidation of the thiol head, altering the surface properties, even if in selected case also interaction of the functional group of the SAM with the buffer solution could occur.

As far as SAMs on silicon oxide are concerned, the experimental results [71] indicate a poor stability versus high temperature and accelerated aging. SAMs that are stable for short time at room temperature are at risk of extensive damage by storage for few hours at 125°C–160°C; moreover, a longer time-scale evolution seems also present that induces a further degradation of the surface. The observed effect seems driven mainly from the hydrolysis of the organic molecules by water molecules existing at the monolayer–substrate interface. This means that the stability is improved by preliminary silica annealing and storage of the SAM in dry situation. This is not compatible with lab on chip where the SAM is immersed in a biological buffer, which is the most critical situation for this kind of monolayers. SAMs containing hydrogen bonds have also been observed [72] to form a network of lateral crosslinks within the SAM which could improve the stability. Thus, spacers having this characteristic may improve stability without affecting the nature of the functional group, which is generally dictated by the application, and of the reactive head, which is selected on the ground of its affinity with the silica substrate. Crosslinks between functional heads have instead to be avoided, due to the reduction of the surface functionality.

Polymer functionalized surfaces are used for a wide variety of applications, from textile industry to biocompatible materials; thus, a huge number of functional molecules can be attached to a polymer surface using different techniques [73]. Extremely stable and durable graft can be obtained by graft from techniques based on surface polymerization, but generally these SAMs are difficult to be adapted to assay applications in lab on chip. The requirements for this application are strong affinity to the molecules to be attached and low probability of unspecific bonds. Considering polymer grafts for this particular application, stability issues arise, similar to those present for thiols on gold SAMs.

PMDS surfaces grafts are widely studied owing to their importance in biological applications [74,75]. Several methods both for graft on and graft from are available and good stability results even for long time periods can be obtained when hydrophobic surfaces have to be obtained or when unspecific absorption of proteins and nucleic acids have to be avoided. On the contrary, long-term stability is not yet clear for structure designed for specific absorption of biomolecules.

All the above results suggest that SAM functionalized lab on chip surfaces are very effective in supporting on-chip biological assays if they can be used immediately after their creation though suitable care is needed during their fabrication. On the contrary, obtaining functionalized surfaces that are able to withstand the stress derived from a long-term storage under temperature and, in case, mechanical stress is still a challenge that has to be addressed. Nevertheless, a strong research effort is still present in the field, and the evolution toward the use of SAMs in a wider range of applications is well possible in the near future.

9.7 ON-CHIP CELLS IMMOBILIZATION

An important aspect of functionalized surfaces is their ability to immobilize living cells, allowing a wide array of on-chip cells assays [76,77]. Different mechanisms have been proposed for cell adhesion on a lab on chip surface, and in many cases a suitable surface functionalization has to be realized. Adsorption of adhesion cells on the surface, adhesion of the cell membrane, entrapment in artificial surface structures, and crosslinking of adhesion cells are all possible mechanisms.

9.7.1 IMMOBILIZATION THROUGH ADHESION MOLECULES

In any chemical-driven cell adhesion mechanism, a key role is played by the so-called adhesion molecules that are found on the cell surface and assure the mutual adhesion of different cells composing a tissue [78–80]. They can be adsorbed on the surface or cross-linked through suitable surface functionalization. The position of adhesion molecules on the cell membrane is shown schematically in Figure 9.35. Typical cells adhesion molecules are selectins, integrins, or cadherins.

9.7.1.1 Adhesion Molecule Families

There are three subsets of selectins [81–83]:

- E-selectin (in endothelial cells)
- L-selectin (in leukocytes)
- P-selectin (in platelets and endothelial cells)

L-selectin is the smallest of the vascular selectins, expressed on all granulocytes and monocytes and on most lymphocytes, and can be found in most leukocytes. P-selectin, the largest selectin, is stored in α-granules of platelets and in Weibel–Palade bodies of endothelial cells, and is translocated to the cell surface of activated endothelial cells and platelets. E-selectin is not expressed under baseline conditions, except in skin microvessels, but is rapidly induced by inflammatory cytokines.

These three types share a significant degree of sequence homology, except in the transmembrane and cytoplasmic domains, and among different mammal species. All three members of the selectin family share a similar cassette structure: an N-terminal, calcium-dependent lectin domain, an epidermal growth factor (EGF)-like domain [84,85], a variable number of intermediate units (2, 6, and 9 for L-, E-, and P-selectin, respectively), a transmembrane domain (TM) passing through the cell membrane and an intracellular cytoplasmic tail. The lectin domain, which binds sugars is quite similar in all the selectins, suggesting that they bind similar sugar structures. The transmembrane and cytoplasmic parts are instead different in different selectins. Though they share common elements, their tissue distribution and binding kinetics are quite different, reflecting their divergent roles in various processes.

The strip model of P-selectin while binding a sugar molecule, represented in stick model, is shown in Figure 9.36.

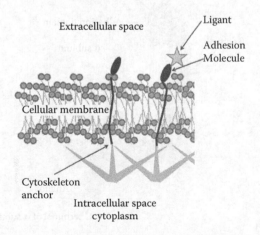

FIGURE 9.35 Schematic representation of the adhesion molecule position on the external surface of the cellular membrane.

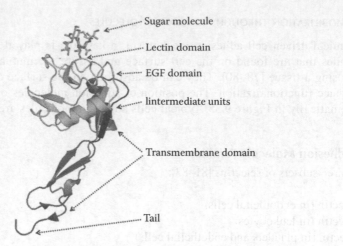

FIGURE 9.36 Strip model of a selectin adhesion molecule while binding a sugar molecule at the lectin domain.

Integrins [86,87] have two main functions:

- Attachment of the cell to the extracellular matrix (ECM)
- Signal transduction from the ECM to the cell

However, they are also involved in a wide range of other biological activities, including immune patrolling and cell migration. Integrins contain two distinct chains, called the α and β subunits [88,89]. In mammals, 18 different α and 8 different β subunits have been characterized. The α and β subunits each penetrates the plasma membrane and possesses small cytoplasmic domains. A schematic representation of the structure of an integrin and of its position through the cell membrane is shown in Figure 9.37.

There are dozens of types of integrins, each with a specific task. Most of them link to actin inside the cell, using adapter proteins like talin, but some link instead to intermediate filaments. On the outside of cells, different integrins have many different targets. Most cells have integrins that bind to

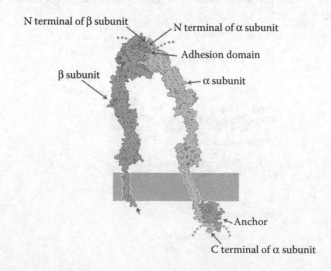

FIGURE 9.37 Schematic representation of the structure of an integrin and of its position through the cell membrane.

components of the ECM, like collagen, fibronectin, or laminin. Other integrins are used for special tasks, for instance, white blood cells have special integrins that allow them to attach to other cells as they search for infection, and tiny platelets in the blood have integrins that bind to fibrinogen, allowing them to assist with the formation of blood clots.

One important function of integrins on cells in tissue culture is their role in cell migration. Cells adhere to a substrate through their integrins. During movement, the cell makes new attachments to the substrate at its front and concurrently releases those at its rear. When released from the substrate, integrin molecules are taken back into the cell by endocytosis; they are transported through the cell to its front by the endocytic cycle where they are added back to the surface. In this way, they are cycled for reuse, enabling the cell to make fresh attachments at its leading front. It is not yet clear whether cell migration in tissue culture is an artifact of integrin processing, or whether such integrin-dependent cell migration also occurs in living organisms.

Cadherins play their main role in adhesion of similar cells within a tissue, forming adherens junctions to bind cells together. They are dependent on calcium ions to function, hence their name.

The cadherin superfamily includes cadherins, protocadherins, desmogleins, and desmocollins, besides a vast variety of rarer molecules [90,91]. All cadherins share cadherin repeats, which are the extracellular Ca^{2+} binding domains.

Each class of cadherins is designated with a prefix in general, indicating the type of tissue with which it is associated. It has been observed that cells containing a specific cadherin subtype tend to cluster together to the exclusion of other types, both in cell culture and during development [92]. For example, cells containing N-cadherin tend to cluster with other N-cadherin-expressing cells. In other cases, however, binding of different types of cadherin together has been observed [93,94].

9.7.1.2 Adhesion Molecule-Based Cell Immobilizations

Considering the properties of the different cell adhesion molecules, integrins are generally selected as the most suitable for covalent bonding of cells on an activated surface. This is due to the large set of targets that can be bonded to different integrins and to the role of integrin in cell motion within a culture, which allows cell cultures on chip to be developed starting from immobilized cells.

In general, covalent immobilization has to be used with care, due to the need of preserving cell viability from possible damaging effects of the bonding reaction. As a rule of thumb, gentle reactions have to be used that allow the immobilized cells to be sufficiently far from the functionalized surface. An effective solution to achieve this goal is cell immobilization on functionalized gold electrodes. The long alkanethyol chain linking the functionalization molecule to the gold surface allows a sufficient spacing between the surface and the cell to be preserved; moreover, a large variety of peptide groups can be bonded at the alkanethyol end. The fact that gold is a very good material for electrochemical electrodes (see Section 10.4.3) is also an important element, allowing electrochemical study of the immobilized cells. Depending on the application, cells are either immobilized on a large gold area, or, more frequently, an array of small gold electrodes is fabricated [95–97] so that each electrode can immobilize a single cell.

The most common functionalization molecule that is used in immobilizing cells via integrins covalent bonding to a functionalized gold electrode is arginylglycylaspartic (RGD) acid, a tripeptide composed of L-arginine, glycine, and L-aspartic acid [95,98], whose structure formula is presented in Figure 9.38a [99]. In the figure the open form of RGD is shown; however, a closed form is also possible, and several spacers can be attached to RGD to work as intermediates with the head of the gold-bonded alkanethyol chain as shown, for example, in Figure 9.38b, where a circular RGD form obtained after PEGylation, that is combination with polyethylene glycol (PEG), is shown [100].

A typical problem that has to be solved when using immobilization via integrin on gold electrodes is to avoid unspecific bonding with other proteins, that both reduce the cell bonding density and risks to create improper reactions with the cell membrane. Moreover, when cell culture is performed, nonspecific protein adsorption on the culture substrate can have an impact on cells motion. This problem can be solved by mixing RGD functionalization groups with

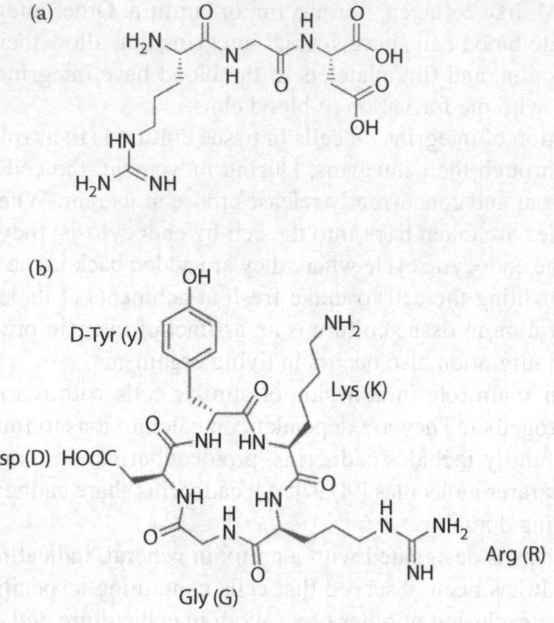

FIGURE 9.38 Structure formula of arginylglycylaspartic (RGD) acid (a) and of a cyclic RGD form (b).

oligo-(ethylene glycol) groups that greatly decreases nonspecific adsorption energy [98,101]. In addition, even better immobilization can be achieved by synergic interaction of the short amino acid sequence Pro-His-Ser-Arg-Asn (PHSRN) with the RGD in linking the integrin on the cell membrane. PHSRN is present in human fibronectin to enhance cell-adhesive function through integrins [102], and it can be used with the same role when adhesion to an artificial ECM is required.

The structure formula of PHSRN is reported in Figure 9.39, while scheme surface functionalization of a gold electrode through an alkanethiol monolayer and an RGD–PHSRN composite alternated with tri(ethylene glycol) groups in order to reduce nonspecific protein binding as shown in Figure 9.40 [101].

An alternative to the direct use of the specific properties of adhesion molecules, covalent immobilization of cells on a substrate can be obtained by functionalizing the substrate with adhesion molecules conjugated antibodies [103–105].

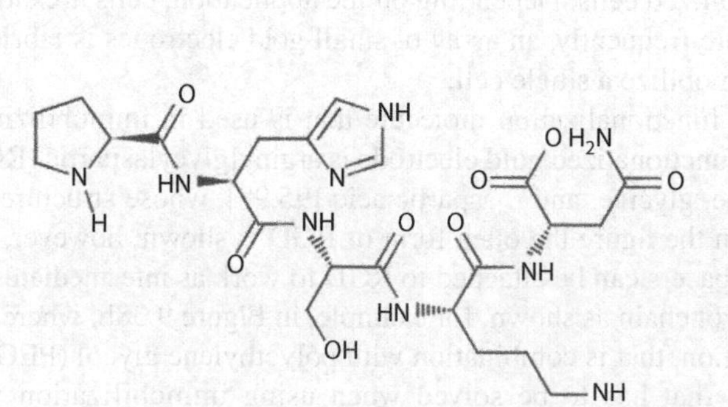

FIGURE 9.39 Structure formula of PHSRN.

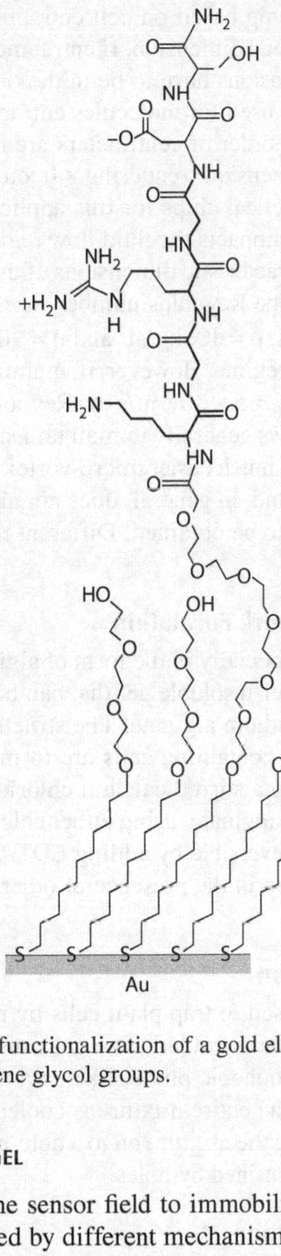

FIGURE 9.40 Scheme surface functionalization of a gold electrode through an alkanethiol monolayer and a peptide alternated with triethylene glycol groups.

9.7.2 IMMOBILIZATION IN GEL

A widely used technique in the sensor field to immobilize cells is to insert them in a gel matrix, where they remain immobilized by different mechanisms [106,107]. Mainly plant cell cultures are created in this way for their greater stability in a highly humid environment.

Cell trapping in continuous gel layers can be used in lab on chip, provided that the insertion of a gel-filled chamber in the chip is compatible with the overall chip fabrication process. Gel precursor can be patterned in different ways on polymeric chips, using, for example, soft lithography or ink-jet patterning (see Chapter 5). Drying and crosslinking can be completed after the patterning to obtain a gel with the suitable characteristics. If a silicon compatible technology is used conversely, including gel patterning during front-end fabrication is not easy, and frequently gel structures are created immediately before wafer bonding adopting a back-end machine like a modified wire bonding machine.

Much more diffused, however, is the use of gel beads immobilizing cells within them. The beads can be moved along in microfluidic circuits using gentle fluid drag so as to move through different chip areas where different tests can be performed. Moreover, the beads can be prepared separately from the chip and inserted in the chip in one of the final fabrication stages.

A relevant difference between lab on chip based on cell entrapping beads and those based on beads for molecule immobilization is the bead dimension. If entrapment of a certain number of cells per bead is required, the bead linear dimensions have to be in the order of millimeters, more than one thousand times greater than the beads used for molecules entrapment. This influences heavily the fluid structure dimension: ducts of the order of centimeters are required to correctly drive the beads. This not only impacts the chip dimension, rendering silicon-based technology completely unsuitable for this application, so that practical chips for this application are almost all produced with polymer-based technologies, but also impacts the fluid flow regime.

In a typical microfluidic circuit, the characteristic dimensions of ducts and reaction chambers are under the millimeter, and if we calculate the Reynolds number we obtain $\mathcal{R}_e$ (see Section 7.3.1.5) using $\ell_0 = 0.1\,\text{mm} = 10^{-4}$ m, $v_0 = 10^{-5}$ m/s, $\rho = 10^3$ kg/m^3 and $\eta = 10^{-3}$ Pa s; thus we get $\mathcal{R}_e = 10^{-3}$. This value characterizes microfluidic flow regime. However, if, maintaining the hypothesis to have a water solution, we set $\ell_0 = 1\,\text{cm} = 10^{-2}$ m, $v_0 = 5 \times 10^{-3}$ m/s the Reynolds number becomes $\mathcal{R}_e = 50$. Such a value for the Reynolds number allows generally to maintain stable laminar motion if a careful design of the circuit is done, but renders much easier micro-vortex formations in correspondence to discontinuities like angles or junctions and, in general, does not allow the Stokes approximation to be used if an accurate fluid motion has to be obtained. Different mechanisms cause cell entrapment in a gel matrix.

9.7.2.1 Gel Entrapment by Ionic Network Formation

Entrapment by ionic network formation, especially in the form of alginate beads, is the most widely used method for sensors. Alginate is a water-insoluble gel that can be created through the addition of aqueous calcium chloride to aqueous sodium alginate. The structure formula of Alginate gel is reported in Figure 9.41. Beads of alginate-containing cells are formed by dripping a cell suspension–sodium alginate solution mixture into a stirred calcium chloride solution. κ-Carragenan can also be used in a similar manner instead of alginate, using either calcium or potassium. The advantage of this method is that the gel can be reversible by adding EDTA. Moreover, syneresis, that is, expulsion of liquid from the gel, can happen in the presence of other calcium-chelating agent such as phosphates [108].

9.7.2.2 Gel Entrapment by Precipitation

Preparations of agar and agarose can be used to trap plant cells by precipitation. The polysaccharides form gel when a heated water solution is cooled. The gel can be dispersed into particles in the warm liquid state by mixing in a hydrophobic phase, like a natural or artificial oil. When the particles of the desired size are obtained, the entire mixture is cooled and this results in solidification. Solidification can be driven by pouring the mixture on to a hole-covered plate. In this way, both dimension and shape of the beads are determined by holes.

9.7.2.3 Gel Entrapment by Polymerization

Gel entrapment by polymerization is most commonly carried out using polyacrylamide. However, the toxicity of the initiator and cross-linking agents used in the polymerization has in some cases

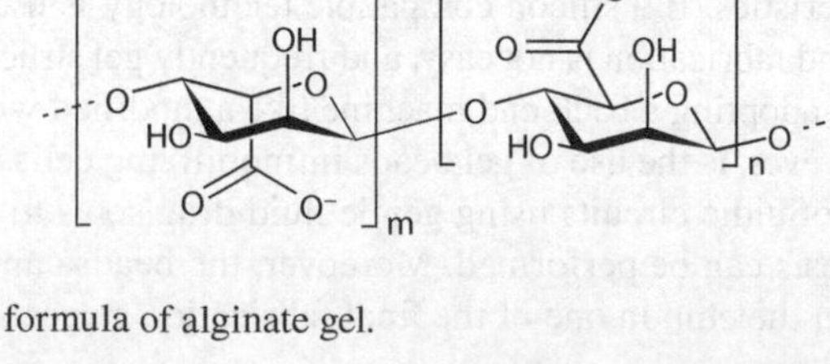

FIGURE 9.41 Structure formula of alginate gel.

caused a loss of cell viability. For this reason, entrapment by polymerization is generally performed by using inorganic precursors [5].

A typical entrapment protocol starts with mixing a cell suspension by Glycerol. In the second step, hydrochloric acid and sodium silicate solution is added to the mixture in order to promote the sol–gel process, causing a solid phase to be separated from the liquid phase and deposited at the bottom of the container [109]. During this process, glycerol particles during jellification form a sort of cavity enveloping the cells so that they have no contact with the chemically active matrix. This results in the fact that the process does not affect the cell membrane functionality and thus the cells viability.

9.7.3 Immobilization in Artificial Structures

On-chip cells immobilization via chemical bonds or gel absorption somehow mimic different natural mechanisms of cell adhesion and trapping, being under this point of view quite useful for study of natural evolution of many cell-related processes. However, chemical interaction of the cell membrane with the external matrix, especially when covalent bonds are created, has to be carefully controlled not to decrease cells viability.

A complete different approach for on-chip cell immobilization can be attempted, starting from the observation that in macroscopic cell cultures, a good cell adhesion directly on borosilicate glass or different types of inert polymers is obtained. Such an adhesion is mainly due to the electrostatic interaction between charged molecules on the cell membrane and the negative surface charges that are present in this material, so that the cell membrane never arrives in strict contact with the adhesion material. Adhesion analysis using microscopy [110,111] demonstrates that the minimum distance between the cell membrane rarely goes below 10 nm, a large distance with respect to the dimensions of the interacting molecules, which avoids formation of strong chemical bonds.

Glass and inert polymers are the main materials used in lab on chip fabrication near silicon; thus using this adhesion mechanism in lab on chip is quite attractive. Direct adhesion, however, results to be weaker with respect to chemical adhesion, especially if the cell culture is immersed in a liquid flow if no care is taken to maintain cells fixed on their place.

This is generally attained by building suitable obstacles arrays on chip where cells are trapped and protected both from vibrations, chemically induced forces and, in case, moving fluid drag. The simpler form of cell traps is that of the micro-well array, simply patterned on the chip with lithographic technologies [112,113]. Multi-well arrays on chip can be designed to trap a single cell per well allowing differentiated assays on different cells [114,115]. The well form can be shaped into different ways either to expose the cell in a way suitable for the executed assay [113] or even to induce on the cell membrane a controlled stress that is useful to study the cell behavior [116].

A different type of cell trap can be generated by exploiting a microfluidic flux and either suitable obstacles or a suitable shape of the ducts. An example of obstacle-based trap is shown in Figure 9.42 [117], where the cells are maintained inside the concave trap by the fluid flux. The fact that an incoming cell is captured or not by the trap is completely determined by the flow lines so that a careful design of the fluidic chip allows a good control of the trap working. An array of similar traps in a microfluidic duct can capture a large number of cells that are accessible one by one for assaying.

The design that is represented in Figure 9.42 is only one example of the many possible microfluidic structures that has been proposed to capture cells so as to provoke stable adhesion to the structure without the need of functionalized surfaces [118]. The fact that fluid channels can be shaped conveniently by using planar technologies makes such structure particularly suitable for a direct study of the adhesion strength [119,120]. In particular, a microfluidic structure that is able to exert a controlled stress on cells after the adhesion to the considered structure is created in this way and the phenomenon of cell detaching from the surface is studied in chip sections where different stress is exerted.

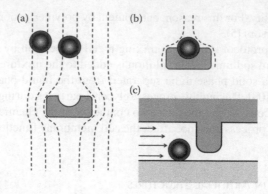

FIGURE 9.42 Cells traps based on fluid flow pressure: captured and noncaptured cells determined by flow lines (dashed lines in the figure) (a), flow pressure assuring cell trapping (b), vertical section of the trap along the duct axis (c).

REFERENCES

1. Goldberg S., Adsorption models incorporated into chemical equilibrium models, in *Chemical Equilibrium and Reaction Models*, Schwab A. P., Loeppert R. H., Goldberg S., editors, Soil Science Society of America; 1st edition (February 1995), ISBN-13:978-0891188179.

2. Schwartz, D. K., Mechanisms and kinetics of self-assembled monolayer formation. *Annual Review of Physical Chemistry*, vol. 52, pp. 107–37, 2001.

3. Elemans J. A. A. W., Lei S., De Feyter S., Molecular and supramolecular networks on surfaces: From two-dimensional crystal engineering to reactivity, *Angewandte Chemie International Edition*, vol. 48, pp. 7298–7332, 2009.

4. Birdi K. S., *Self-Assembly Monolayer Structures of Lipids and Macromolecules at Interfaces*, Springer; 1st edition (October 1, 1999), ISBN-13: 978-0306460999.

5. Banica F.-G., *Chemical Sensors and Biosensors: Fundamentals and Applications*, Wiley; 1st edition (October 4, 2012), ISBN-13: 978-0470710678.

6. Chow B. B. Y., Mosley D. W., Jacobson J. M., Perfecting imperfect "monolayers": Removal of siloxane multilayers by CO_2 Snow Treatment, *Langmuir*, vol. 21, pp. 4782–4785, 2005.

7. Schlecht C. A., Maurer J. A., Functionalization of glass substrates: Mechanistic insights into the surface reaction of trialkoxysilanes, *RSC Advances*, vol. 1, pp. 1446–1448, 2011.

8. Zammatteo N. et al., Comparison between different strategies of covalent attachment of DNA to glass surfaces to build DNA microarrays, *Analytical Biochemistry*, vol. 280, pp. 143–150, 2000.

9. Pil Pack S. et al., Direct immobilization of DNA oligomers onto the amine-functionalized glass surface for dna microarray fabrication through the activation-free reaction of oxanine, *Nucleic Acids Research*, vol. 35, pp. e110-1–e110-10, 2007.

10. Verné E., Vitale-Brovarone C., Bui E., Bianchi C. L., Boccaccini A. R., Surface functionalization of bioactive glasses, *Journal of Biomedical Materials Research Part A*, vol. 90A, pp. 981–992, 2009.

11. Mela P. et al., Monolayer-functionalized microfluidics devices for optical sensing of acidity, *Lab on a Chip*, vol. 5, pp. 163–170, 2005.

12. Mittal K. L. editor, *Polymer Surface Modification: Relevance to Adhesion*, Vol.5, CRC Press (16 March 2009), ISBN-13: 978-9004165908.

13. Uyama Y., Kato K., Ikada Y., *Surface Modification of Polymers by Grafting*, in Grafting, Characterization Techniques, Kinetic Modeling, Springer Advances in Polymer Science vol. 38, Springer; 1st edition (July1, 1998), ISBN-13: 978-3540640165.

14. Zhou J., Ellis A. V., Voelcker N. H., Recent developments in PDMS surface modification for microfluidic devices, *Electrophoresis*, vol. 31, pp. 2–16, 2010.

15. Xu Y., Takai M., Ishihara K., Phospholipid polymer biointerfaces for lab-on-a-chip devices, *Annals of Biomedical Engineering*, vol. 38, pp. 1938–1953, 2010.

16. Friedrich J., G. Kühn G., R. Mix R., Polymer surface modification with monofunctional groups of different type and density, in *Plasma Processes and Polymers*, d'Agostino R., Favia P., Oehr C., Wertheimer M. R. editors, Wiley-VCH; 1st edition (April 15, 2005), ISBN-13: 978-352740487.

17. Friedrich J. et al, Plasma-based introduction of monosort functional groups of different type and density onto polymer surfaces. part 1: Behaviour of polymers exposed to oxygen plasma, *Composite Interfaces*, vol. 10, pp. 139–171, 2003

18. Zanini S. et al., Plasma-induced graft-polymerization of polyethylene glycol acrylate on polypropylene films: Chemical characterization and evaluation of the protein adsorption, *Journal of Colloid and Interface Science*, vol. 341, pp. 53–58, 2010.

19. Svorcík V., Makajová Z., Kasálková-Slepicková N., Kolská Z., Bacáková L., Plasma-modified and polyethylene glycol-grafted polymers for potential tissue engineering applications, *Journal of Nanoscience and Nanotechnology*, vol. 12, pp. 6665–6671, 2012.

20. Yasuda, H., *Plasma Polymerization*, Academic Press, Inc.; 1st edition, 1985. ISBN-13: 978-0127687602.

21. Pu Q., Oyesanya O., Thompson B., Liu S., Alvarez J. C., On-chip micropatterning of plastic (cyclic olefin copolymer, COC) microfluidic channels for the fabrication of biomolecule microarrays using photografting methods, *Langmuir*, vol. 23, pp. 1577–1583, 2007.

22. Pourcelle V. et al., Light induced functionalization of pcl-peg block copolymers for the covalent immobilization of biomolecules, *Biomacromolecules*, vol. 10, pp. 966–974, 2009.

23. Groenbeck H., Curioni A., Andreoni W., Thiols and disulfides on the au(111) surface: The headgroup-gold interaction, *Journal of American Chemical Society*, vol. 122, pp. 3839–3842, 2000.

24. Kind M., Wöll C., Organic surfaces exposed by self-assembled organothiol monolayers: Preparation, characterization, and application, *Progress in Surface Science*, vol. 84, pp. 230–278, 2009.

25. Love J. C., Estroff L. A., Kriebel J. K., Nuzzo R. G., Whitesides G. M., Self-assembled monolayers of thiolates on metals as a form of nanotechnology, *Chemical Review*, vol. 105, pp. 1103–1169, 2005.

26. Kausaite-Minkstimiene A., Ramanaviciene A., Kirlyte J., Ramanavicius A., Comparative study of random and oriented antibody immobilization techniques on the binding capacity of immunosensor, *Analytical Chemistry*, vol. 82, pp. 6401–6408, 2010.

27. Liu G., Böcking T., Gooding J. J., Diazonium Salts: Stable monolayers on gold electrodes for sensing applications, *Journal of Electroanalytical Chemistry*, vol. 600, pp. 335–344, 2007.

28. Amendola V., Meneghetti M., Laser ablation synthesis in solution and size manipulation of noble metal nanoparticles, *Physical Chemistry Chemical Physics*, vol. 11, pp. 3805–3821, 2009.

29. Sperling R. A., Parak W. J., Surface modification, functionalization and bioconjugation of colloidal inorganic nanoparticles, *Philosophical Transactions of the Royal Society A*, vol. 368, pp. 1333–1383, 2010.

30. Grzelczak M., Vermant J., Furst E. M., Liz-Marzán L. M., Directed self-assembly of nanoparticles, *ACS Nano*, vol. 4, pp. 3591–3605, 2010.

31. Liu C., Tang T., Huang B., Preparation of macroporous functionalized polymer beads by a multistep polymerization and their application in zirconocene catalysts for ethylene polymerization, *Journal of Polymer Science Part A: Polymer Chemistry*, vol. 41, pp. 873–880, 2003.

32. Wood C. D., Cooper A. I., Synthesis of macroporous polymer beads by suspension polymerization using supercritical carbon dioxide as a pressure-adjustable porogen, *Macromolecules*, vol. 34, pp. 5–8, 2001.

33. Jiang K., Sposito A., Liu J., Raghavan S. R., DeVoe D. L., Microfluidic synthesis of macroporous polymer immunobeads, *Polymer* vol. 53, pp. 5469–5475, 2012.

34. Harris P. J. F., *Carbon Nanotube Science: Synthesis, Properties and Applications*, Cambridge University Press; 2nd edition (April 28, 2011), ISBN-13: 978-0521535854.

35. Philip Wong H.-S., Akinwande D., *Carbon Nanotube and Graphene Device Physics*, Cambridge University Press (February 14, 2011), ISBN-13:978-0521519052.

36. Inami N., Ambri Mohamed M., Shikoh E., Fujiwara A., Synthesis-condition dependence of carbon nanotube growth by alcohol catalytic chemical vapor deposition method, *Science and Technology of Advanced Materials*, vol. 8, pp. 292–295, 2007.

37. Ishigami N. et al., Crystal plane dependent growth of aligned single-walled carbon nanotubes on sapphire, *Journal of American Chemical Society*, vol. 130, pp. 9918–9924, 2009.

38. Naha S., Ishwar K. P., A model for catalytic growth of carbon nanotubes, *Journal of Physics D: Applied Physics*, vol. 41, pp. 065304–065309, 2008.

39. Banerjee S., Naha S., Ishwar K. P., Molecular simulation of the carbon nanotube growth mode during catalytic synthesis, *Applied Physics Letters*, vol. 92, pp. 233121–233124, 2008.

40. Ren Z. F. et al., Synthesis of large arrays of well-aligned carbon nanotubes on glass, *Science*, vol. 282, pp. 1105–1107, 1998.

41. Hata K., Futaba D. N., Mizuno K., Namai T., Yumura M., Iijima S., Water-assisted Highly efficient synthesis of impurity-free single-walled carbon nanotubes, *Science*, vol. 306, pp. 1362–1365, 2004.

42. Hou P.-X., Liu C., Cheng H.-M., Purification of carbon nanotubes, *Carbon*, vol. 46, pp. 2003–2025, 2008.

43. Ebbesen T. W., Ajayan P. M., Hiura H., Tanigaki K., Purification of nanotubes, *Nature*, vol. 367, pp. 519–526, 1994.
44. Hauquier F. et al., Carbon Nanotube-Functionalized Silicon Surfaces with Efficient Redox Communication, *Chemical Communications*, pp. 4536–4538, 2006.
45. Mueller A., Amsharov K. Y., Jansen M., Synthesis of End-Cap Precursor Molecules for (6, 6) Armchair and (9, 0) Zig-zag single-walled carbon nanotubes, *Tetrahedron Letters*, vol. 51, pp. 3221–3225, 2010.
46. Basiuk V. A., Basiuk E. V., Saniger-Blesa J.-M., Direct amidation of terminal carboxylic groups of armchair and zigzag single-walled carbon nanotubes: A theoretical study, *Nano Letters*, vol. 1, pp. 657–661, 2001.
47. Burghard M., Balasubramanian K., Chemically functionalized carbon nanotubes, *Small*, vol. 1, pp. 180–192, 2005.
48. Prodana M., Ionita D., Bojin D., Demetrescu I., Different methods to functionalization of multiwalled carbon nanotubes for hybrid nanoarchitectures, *Journal of Sustainable Energy*, vol. 3, pp. 62–66, 2012.
49. Chen J. et al., Solution. properties of single-walled carbon nanotubes, *Science*, vol. 282, pp. 95–98, 1998.
50. Yu, R. et al., Platinum deposition on carbon nanotubes via chemical modification, *Chemistry of Materials*, vol. 10, pp. 718–722, 1998.
51. Prodana M., Ionita D., Ungureanu C., Bojin D., Demetrescu I., Enhancing antibacterial effect of multi-walled carbon nanotubes using silver nanoparticles, *Digest Journal of Nanomaterials and Biostructures*, vol.6, pp. 549–556, 2011.
52. Pulikkathara M. X., Kuznetsov O. V., Khabashesku V. N., Sidewall covalent functionalization of single wall carbon nanotubes through reactions of fluoronanotubes with urea, guanidine, and thiourea, *Chemistry of Materials*, vol. 20, pp. 2685–2695, 2008.
53. Jaffe L. R., Quantum chemistry study of fullerene and carbon nanotube fluorination, *Journal of Physical Chemistry B*, vol. 107, pp. 10378–10388, 2003.
54. Balasubramanian K., Burghard M., Electrochemically functionalized carbon nanotubes for device applications, *Journal of Material Chemistry*, vol. 18, pp. 3071–3083, 2008.
55. Wei D., Kvarnström C., Lindfors T., Ivaska A., Electrochemical functionalization of single walled carbon nanotubes with polyaniline in ionic liquids, *Electrochemistry Communications*, vol. 9, pp. 206–210, 2007.
56. Moghaddam M. J., Taylor S., Gao M., Huang S. M., Dai L. M., McCall M. J., High efficient binding of DNA on the sidewalls and tips of carbon nanotubes using photochemistry, *Nano Letters*, vol. 4, pp. 89–93, 2004.
57. Girard-Lauriault P.-L., Illgen R., Ruiz J.-C., Wertheimer M. R., Unger W. E. S., Surface functionalization of graphite and carbon nanotubes by vacuum-ultraviolet photochemical reactions, *Applied Surface Science*, vol. 258, pp. 8448–8454, 2012.
58. Parekh B., Debies T., Knight P., Santhanam K. S. V., Takacs G. A., Surface functionalization of multiwalled carbon nanotubes with UV and vacuum UV photo-oxidation, *Journal of Adhesion Science and Technology*, vol. 20, pp. 1833–1846, 2006.
59. Parham P., The Immune System, Garland Science; 3rd edition (January 19, 2009), ISBN-13: 978-0815341468.
60. Baniukevic J., Kirlyte J., Ramanavicius A., Ramanaviciene A., *Application of Oriented and Random Antibody Immobilization Methods in Immunosensor Design*, Sensors and Actuators B: Chemical, Verificare Dati esatti, 2013.
61. Maschini M., *Aptamers in Bioanalysis*, Wiley-Interscience; 1st edition (March 23, 2009), ISBN-13:978-0470148303.
62. Hall B., Hesselberth J. R., Ellington A. D., Computational selection of nucleic acid biosensors via a slip structure model, *Biosensors and Bioelectronics*, vol. 22, pp. 1939–1947, 2007.
63. Han K., Liang Z., Zhou N., Design strategies for aptamer-based biosensors, *Sensors*, vol. 10, pp. 4541–4557, 2010.
64. Seitz O. et al., Control and stability of self-assembled monolayers under biosensing conditions, *Journal of Material Chemistry*, vol. 21, pp. 4384–4392, 2011.
65. Chrisey L. A., Lee G. U., O'Ferrall C. E., Covalent attachment of synthetic dna to self-assembled monolayer films, *Nucleic Acids Research*, vol. 24, (15), pp. 3031–3039, 1996.
66. Kim T., Chan K. C., Crooks R. M., Polymeric self-assembled monolayers. 4. chemical, electrochemical, and thermal stability of ω-functionalized, self-assembled diacetylenic and polydiacetylenic monolayers, *Journal of the American Chemical Society*, vol. 119, pp. 189–193, 1997.
67. Srisombat L.-O., Zhang S., Lee T. R., Thermal stability of mono-, bis-, and tris-chelating alkanethiol films assembled on gold nanoparticles and evaporated "flat" gold, *Langmuir*, vol. 26, pp. 41–46, 2010.

68. Schoenfisch M. H., Pemberton J. E., Air stability of alkanethiol self-assembled monolayers on silver and gold surfaces, *Journal of the American Chemical Society*, vol. 120, pp. 4502–4513, 1998.

69. Flynn N. T., Tran T. N. T., Cima M. J., Langer R., Long-term stability of self-assembled monolayers in biological media, *Langmuir*, vol. 19, pp. 10909–10915, 2003.

70. Maciel J., Martins M. C. L., Barbosa M. A., The Stability of self-assembled monolayers with time and under biological conditions, *Journal of Biomedical Materials Research Part A*, vol. 94A, pp. 833–843, 2010.

71. Calistri-Yeh M. et al., Thermal stability of self-assembled monolayers from alkylchlorosilanes, *Langmuir*, vol. 12, pp. 2747–2755, 1996.

72. Ramin M. A. et al., Functionalized hydrogen-bonding self-assembled monolayers grafted onto SiO_2 substrates, *Langmuir*, vol. 28, pp. 17672–17680, 2012.

73. Knoll W., Advincula R. C. editors, *Functional Polymer Films*, Wiley-VCH; 1st edition (June 7, 2011), ISBN-13: 978-3527321902.

74. Wong I., Ho C.-M., Surface molecular property modifications for poly(dimethylsiloxane) (PDMS) Based microfluidic devices, *Microfluidics Nanofluidics*, vol. 7, pp. 291–306, 2009.

75. Hellmich W. et al., Poly(oxyethylene) based surface coatings for poly(dimethylsiloxane) microchannels, *Langmuir*, vol. 21, pp. 7551–7557, 2005.

76. El-Ali J., Sorger P. K., Jensen K. F., Cells on chip, *Nature*, vol. 442, pp. 403.4011, 2006.

77. Ho C.-T., Liver-Cell Patterning Lab Chip: Mimicking the Morphology of Liver Lobule Tissue, *Lab on a Chip, inserire riferimento complete*, 2013.

78. Edelman G. M., Cells adhesion molecules, *Science*, vol. 219,pp. 450–457, 1983.

79. Katz A. M., Rosenthal D., Sauder D. N., Cell adhesion molecules, *International Journal of Dermatology*, vol. 30, pp. 153–160, 1991.

80. Beckerle M. C. editor, *Cell Adhesion*, Oxford University Press, USA (April 18, 2002), ISBN-13: 978-0199638710.

81. Gumbiner B. M., Cell adhesion: The molecular basis of tissue architecture and morphogenesis, *Cell*, vol. 84, pp. 345–357, 1996.

82. Tedder T. F., Steeber D. A., Chen A., Engel P., The selectins: Vascular adhesion molecules, *The FASEB Journal*, vol. 9, pp. 866–873, 1995.

83. Somers W. S., Tang J., Shaw G. D., Camphausen R. T., Insights into the molecular basis of leukocyte tethering and rolling revealed by structures of P- and E-selectin bound to SLe(X) and PSGL-1, *Cell*, vol.103, pp. 467–79, 2000.

84. Downing A. K., Knott V., Werner J. M., Cardy C. M., Campbell I. D., Handford P. A., Solution Structure of a Pair of Calcium-Binding Epidermal Growth Factor-Like Domains: Implications for the Marfan Syndrome and Other Genetic Disorders, *Cell*, vol. 85, pp. 597–605, 1996.

85. Wouters M. A., Rigoutsos I., Chu C. K., Feng L. L., Sparrow D. B., Dunwoodie S. L., Evolution of distinct EGF domains with specific functions, *Protein Science*, vol. 14, pp. 1091–1103, 2005.

86. Cheresh D. A., editor, *Integrins: Molecular and Biological Responses to the Extracellular Matrix*, Academic Press; 1st edition (October 10, 1994), ISBN-13: 978-0121711603.

87. Hynes R., Integrins: Bidirectional, allosteric signaling machines, *Cell*, vol. 110, pp. 673–87, 2002.

88. Humphries M. J., Integrin structure, *Biochemical Society Transactions*, vol. 28, pp. 311–339, 2000.

89. Xiong J. P. et al., Crystal Structure of the Extracellular Segment of Integrin Alpha Vbeta3, *Science*, vol. 294, pp. 339–45, 2001.

90. Hulpiau P., van Roy F., Molecular evolution of the cadherin superfamily, *The International Journal of Biochemistry & Cell Biology*, vol. 41, pp. 349–69, 2009.

91. Duguay D., Foty R., Steinberg M., Cadherin-Mediated Cell Adhesion and Tissue Segregation: Qualitative and quantitative determinants, *Developmental Biology*, vol. 253, pp. 309–323, 2003.

92. Bello S. M., Millo H., Rajebhosale M., Price S. R., Catenin-dependent cadherin function drives divisional segregation of spinal chord motor neurons, *Journal of Neuroscience*, vol. 32, pp. 490–505, 2012.

93. NiessenC. M., Gumbiner B. M., Cadherin-mediated cell sorting not determined by binding or adhesion specificity, *The Journal of Cell Biology*, vol. 156, pp. 389–399, 2002.

94. Volk T., Cohen O., Geiger, B., Formation of heterotypic adherens-type junctions between L-CAM Containing liver cells and a-CAM containing lens cells, *Cell*, vol. 50, pp. 987–994, 1997.

95. Yoon S.-H., Chang J., Linb L., Mofrad M. R. K., A biological breadboard platform for cell adhesion and detachment studies, *Lab on a Chip*, vol. 11, pp. 3555–3562, 2011.

96. Triroja N., Jaroenapibal P., Beresford R., *Gas-Assisted Focused Ion Beam Fabrication of Gold Nanoelectrode Arrays in Electron-Beam Evaporated Alumina Films for Microfluidic Electrochemical Sensors*, Sensors and Actuators B, Chemical, insert final citation, 2013.

97. Qingjun Liu et al., Impedance studies of bio-behavior and chemosensitivity of cancer cells by micro-electrode arrays, *Biosensors and Bioelectronics*, vol. 24, pp. 1305–1310, 2009.

98. Mrksich M., A surface chemistry approach to studying cell adhesion, *Chemical Society Reviews*, vol. 29, pp. 267–273, 2000.

99. Ruoslahti E., Pierschbacher M. D., Arg-gly-asp: Aversatile cell recognition signal, *Cell*, vol. 44, pp. 517–518, 1986.

100. Rangger C., Influence of pegylation and RGD loading on the targeting properties of radiolabeled liposomal nanoparticles, *International Journal of Nanomedicine*, vol. 2012, pp. 5889–5900, 2012.

101. Feng Y., Mrksich M., The synergy peptide PHSRN and the adhesion peptide RGD mediate cell adhesion through a common mechanism, *Biochemistry*, vol. 43, pp. 15811–15821, 2004.

102. Aota S., Nomizu M., Yamada K. M., The short amino acid sequence pro-his-ser-arg-asn in human fibronectin enhances cell-adhesive function, *Journal of Biological Chemistry*, vol. 269, pp. 24756–24761, 1994.

103. Suraniti E. et al., Real-time detection of lymphocytes binding on an antibody chip using SPR imaging, *Lab on a Chip*, vol. 7, pp. 1206–1208, 2007.

104. Roupioz Y. et al., Individual blood-cell capture and 2D organization on microarrays, *Small*, vol. 5, pp. 1493–1497, 2009.

105. Suo Z. et al., Antibody selection for immobilizing living bacteria, *Analytical Chemistry*, vol. 15; 81, pp. 7571–7578, 2009.

106. Nedovic V., Willaert R., editors, *Fundamentals of Cell Immobilisation Biotechnology*, Springer; Reprint of 2004 edition (December 3, 2010), ISBN-13: 978-9048165346.

107. Kühtreiber W. M., Lanza R. P., Chick W. L., editors, *Cell Encapsulation Technology and Therapeutics*, Birkhäuser; Reprint of 1999 edition (October 15, 2012), ISBN-13: 978-1461272052.

108. Williams P. D., Mavituna F. Immobilized plant cells. In: *Plant Biotechnology, in Comprehensive Biotechnology*. Second Supplement, Fowler M., Warren G., M. Moo-Young, editors, Pergamon; 2nd edition (September 9, 2011), ISBN-13: 978-0444533524, pp. 63–78.

109. Pena-Vazquez E., Maneiro E., Perez-Conde C., Microalgae fiber optic biosensors for herbicide monitoring using sol-gel technology, *Biosensors and Bioelectronics*, vol. 24, pp. 3538–3543, 2009.

110. Braun D., Fromherz P., Fluorescence interference-contrast microscopy of cell adhesion on oxidized silicon, *Applied Physics A: Material Science*, vol. 65, pp. 341–348, 1997.

111. Curtis A. S. G., The mechanism of adhesion of cells to glass: A study by interference reflection microscopy, *The Journal of Cell Biology*, vol. 20, pp. 199–215, 1964.

112. Sakai Y., Yoshiura Y., Nakazawa K., Embryoid body culture of mouse embryonic stem cells using microwell and micropatterned chips, *Journal of Bioscience and Bioengineering*, vol. 111, pp. 85–91, 2011.

113. Selimović S., Piraino F., Bae H., Rasponi M., Redaellic A., Khademhosseini A., Microfabricated polyester conical microwells for cell culture applications, *Lab on a Chip*, vol. 11, pp. 2325–2332, 2011.

114. Lindstrom S., Andersson-Svahn H., Miniaturization of biological assays—overview on microwell devices for single-cell analyses, *Biochimica et Biophysica Acta*, vol. 1810, pp. 308–316, 2011.

115. Liu C., Liu J., Gao D., Ding M., Lin J.-M., Fabrication of microwell arrays based on two-dimensional ordered polystyrene microspheres for high-throughput single-cell analysis, *Analytical Chemistry*, vol. 82, pp. 9418–9424, 20120.

116. Lew V., Nguyen D., Khine M., Shrink-induced single-cell plastic microwell array, *Journal of Laboratory Automation*, vol. 16, pp. 450–456, 2011.

117. Kobel S., Valero A., Latt J., Renaud P., Lutolf M., Optimization of microfluidic single cell trapping for long-term on-chip culture, *Lab on a Chip*, vol. 10, pp. 857–863, 2010.

118. Kim S. M., Leeb S. H., Suh K. Y., Cell research with physically modified microfluidic channels: A review, *Lab on a Chip*, vol. 8, pp. 1015–1023, 2008.

119. Lu H., Koo L. Y., Wang W. M., Lauffenburger D. A., Griffith L. G., Jensen K. F., Microfluidic shear devices for quantitative analysis of cell adhesion, *Analytical Chemistry*, vol. 76, pp. 5257–5264, 2004.

120. Rupprecht P. et al., A tapered channel microfluidic device for comprehensive cell adhesion analysis, using measurements of detachment kinetics and shear stress-dependent motion, *Biomicrofluidics*, vol. 6, pp. 014107–014119, 2012.

10 Electronic Detection

10.1 INTRODUCTION

The final target of a lab on chip is the individuation, quantification, and characterization of one or more target species. After sample insertion and processing, this is attained through the measurement of physical quantities that can be related to the amount of target molecules or to the target property to be studied. This operation is called detection. Available techniques for detection in the lab on chip can be divided essentially into two categories: electronic and optical detection.

We will define electronic detection as all detection techniques that generate an electronic signal as output of the detection process. In this case, the electronic signal is directly amplified by a low-noise electronic amplifier, digitalized by an analog-to-digital converter and processed by a signal processing algorithm to obtain the desired information. Quite frequently, the electronic detection chain is not embedded in the lab on chip because microelectronic circuits are fabricated with a different process flow, which is frequently not compatible with the lab on chip fabrication (see Chapters 4 and 5).

In cases of disposable labs on chip, this is further justified by the fact that the electronic detection chain is generally more expensive than the lab on chip itself and there is no need to dispose of it every time a lab on chip is used.

For these reasons, a lab on chip using electronics detection generally has a need to pass the electronic signal out of the chip via a suitable electronic interface. This is generally not a problem, considering that in this application very wide band signals are almost never present. A large number of standard and low-cost electronic interfaces exist that are widely used in consumer electronics. This is one of the advantages of electronic detection.

On the other hand, a rich set of optical techniques exists that can be used for detection in lab on chip applications. Optical detection allows an impressive accuracy and sensitivity, besides the fact that integrated optical circuits can be fabricated directly on the lab on chip in several situations. This allows complex optical devices such as resonators and interferometers to be built on the chip bursting the performances of optical detection techniques.

The main practical limit of optical detection is in the need to generate and detect suitable optical beams. In a case in which the optical beam generator and detectors are placed out of the chip, as is frequently the situation, the optical signal has to be injected into the chip and extracted from it to allow the assay to be carried out. Both free space and guided optics interfaces are not easy to be realized and limit the lab on chip resilience when it is designed for field use.

On the other hand, integration of optical sources and detectors on the chip itself requires hybrid integration techniques (see Section 6.3.1), increasing the chip cost and rendering difficult the realization of disposable chips.

In this chapter, after an introductory review of the parameters used to describe performances and the quality of detection systems, we will analyze electronic detection while optical detection will be considered in Chapter 11. A great variety of electronic techniques have been proposed [1,2]; in this chapter, we focus mainly on electrochemical detection, describing briefly detection techniques based on microcantilevers, calorimetric measures, and surface acoustic waves.

Electrochemical detection is mainly based on the electrical activity of target molecules. A molecule is electrically active if, in suitable conditions, it is either charged or it can lose or gain electrons; in other words, it either oxidizes or reduces.

Electrolyte solutions in an electrochemical cell are characterized by the phenomenon of the double-layer formation (see Section 7.5.2) that generates a well-defined cell behavior under an electrical point of view. Measurement of the electrical characteristics of the cell provides information on the solution and its electrochemical properties.

If reduction–oxidation processes, frequently called RedOx processes, happen in a suitable electrochemical cell, either the generated current or the voltage at the cell electrodes can be observed and used to detect the presence of the target or its characteristics.

The most common arrangement of electrochemical detection is realized by controlling the voltage that is applied to the cell and detecting the generated current; in this case, the measure is called voltammetry and its output is represented by the so-called voltammogram, which is a plot of current versus potential. Different types of voltammetry exist, depending on the way the voltage is varied in time and on the variation speed. In other cases, either the voltage or other variables are changed in time, for example, the sample if a solution flows continuously in a duct, and the current is observed versus time. In these cases, the detection technique is called amperometry.

Owing to the fact that metallization can be easily built in typical lab on chip arrangements, electrochemical cells can be realized directly on the chip with suitably shaped electrodes of selected materials and the needed electrical power can be directly provided by an external driver that is always needed for the power feeding of active labs on chip. The signal generated by electrochemical detection is an electrical signal; thus, no complex interface is to be realized, maintaining a potentially low cost and robust lab on chip design. The main disadvantage of electrochemical detection is the impossibility of detecting targets that are not electrically active besides a delicate calibration required by such systems.

Many biochemical reactions also produce heat when they happen spontaneously. Even if great quantities of energy are never released during biochemical reactions, due to their compatibility with the need to maintain the stable condition of living bodies, microcalorimeters have the ability to measure very small heat quantities so that heat measurements can also be used in labs on chip as detection methods.

Cantilever-based detection exploits microcantilevers to detect the target presence and activity. Generally, either owing to direct adhesion of the target to the cantilever surface or through suitable cantilever surface functionalization, a cantilever deformation is generated that can be detected with electronic means, for example, by observing a capacity change.

Finally, surface acoustic waves, whose generation and detection in integrated chips is used for a wide variety of applications, interact with target molecules, providing another possible detection technique.

10.2   DETECTION SYSTEM PARAMETERS

It is not easy to give an absolute measure of the quality and performances of a detection system due to the variety of parameters influencing the measure quality. In general, the detection system design consists of a trade-off between different performances in order to optimize the design for the intended use.

Let us assume that detection consists of the measure of a variable x. Even in this simple situation, there is a long list of possible detection performance parameters, including the following:

Operating range: It is the difference between the minimum and the maximum value of the parameter that can be measured; often, it is also called the detection dynamic range. The existence of a minimum measurable value is generally either due to the fact that measured values below the detection noise level cannot be distinguished or due to the so-called "inertia" of the detection system, which is the fact that the detection system itself practically does not react to very low values of the measured variable. The presence of a maximum measurable value is often caused by saturation phenomena that are always present in practical systems.

Resolution: It is the smallest possible variation of the measured variable that can be detected.

Sensitivity: It is the ratio between the variation of the signal at the detection system output and the variation of the measured variable. This is a constant value in linear detection systems, while if the relation between the output signal and the measured variable is not linear, the sensitivity depends on the average value of the measured variable. It is to underline that sometimes the definition of the sensitivity coincides with that of the resolution, so that care has to be taken in interpreting sensitivity data.

Accuracy: Theoretically, accuracy is defined as the maximum error that can affect the measure as a fraction of the maximum measurable value. In real detection systems, the measurement error is a random variable, so that the maximum possible error is theoretically infinite. Thus, in order to evaluate the accuracy, a limit error probability P_{lim} is defined and the maximum error Δx is defined so that $Pr\{|x - \langle x \rangle| > \Delta x\} \leq P_{lim}$. Where $\langle x \rangle$ is the average value of the measured variable.

Offset: It is the value of the detector output signal when the variable under measure is zero.

Linearity: This is the second derivative of the output detector signal with respect to the measured variable. If the linearity is zero at a certain point, the relation between the output signal and the measured variable around that point is linear so that if that relation is linear in a given interval, the linearity is zero at all points of that interval.

Detection bandwidth: If the variable to be measured depends on time, the detector bandwidth is the bandwidth where the detector output signal depends on the instantaneous value of the measured variables. If the signal frequency goes beyond the detection bandwidth, the detection mechanism is no more able to reproduce instantaneous values of the detected variable, but it integrates them over the detector response time. On the other hand, if the measured variable is too slow, selected detection systems could not be able to produce an output signal due to the inability to respond to a constant input. This is, for example, typical of an electronic system coupled with the output through a capacitor that is not able to transmit a continuous current.

Drift: It is the variation in time of the output signal obtained from the long-term measure of a constant target variable. The drift can be measured in different ways depending on the detection technique and on the time that is considered, standard deviation over a pre defined time, maximum fluctuation, and first derivative of the difference with the measurement at the initial instant are all ways used to measure the drift.

Selectivity: This is a quality parameter that is frequently used in lab on chip, where the detection system is sensible not only to the wanted variable but also to many other variables related, for example, to the presence of unwanted chemical species in the sample. In this case, the selectivity is the ratio of the output signal produced by a unitary value of the measured variable with the sum of the signals provoked by a unitary measure of all the interfering variables.

Repeatability: It is the standard deviation between average values of measurements performed on identical samples in identical environmental situations and in different instants.

Hysteresis: When a hysteresis cycle is present in the detection process, this is the maximum cycle width. If the hysteresis is zero, no cycle is present.

In general, the ideal sensor should be perfectly linear in all the interesting dynamic ranges with perfect repeatability and no drift and no hysteresis. In case of dynamic measurements, a measurement bandwidth sufficiently wide for all interesting cases is also desired, while the random noise should be at the attainable minimum, which is generally dictated by quantum mechanical considerations.

However, many deterministic deviations from the ideal sensors can be managed via a suitable signal processing without decreasing in practice the detector performances. Deterministic drift and bias can be directly compensated for and a complex linear response of the detector can be deconvolved from the output signal as far as is completely known.

In order to manage these problems, real-time calibration of the detection system can also be performed. This procedure consists of estimating the deterministic distortion of the measure either immediately before or after, or simultaneously with the detection process. A very simple example is the system calibration against the bias. This consists of starting the measure before the sample introduction, so as to evaluate the bias that has to be subtracted from the output signal when the sample is introduced in the system. A similar procedure can be applied for the deconvolution of the linear detection system response.

As far as random noise is considered, the only way to eliminate part of the purely random noise, that is, the noise component that is both uncorrelated with the measured signal output and has no autocorrelation, is to reduce to the minimum the detection system bandwidth so as to filter out all the noise power that does not directly affect the measurement bandwidth.

10.3 IMPEDANCE DETECTION

Although a large variety of electrochemical detection systems exists, the base for electrochemical detection is in any case the creation of an electrolytic cell. It is a cell where the sample solution is inserted in between two electrodes in order to create an electrical potential across the solution or to force a known electrical current to pass through the solution.

An electrolytic cell is simply obtained by standard SiO_2–Si lab on chip technologies by suitable metallization of the walls of a detection room. It is possible to both deposit metal on the room side walls and contact it with suitable contacts on the top of the chip or deposit metal layers on the room floor and on the part of the overlay wafer that will constitute the roof of the detection chamber. If more than three electrodes are required, different metal layers can be built on one of the detection room walls. Moreover, a second room where a reference solution is inserted for baseline determination can be built besides the detection room with the same technology when required, as is frequently the case for voltammetry.

Once the electrolytic room is built, the electrical circuit that is needed to bring the signal out from the chip can be built with standard processes inherited from microelectronics.

The electrochemical cell interaction with the target molecule depends essentially on the so-called electrode affinity with the molecule. The electrode affinity with the molecule represents, in general, the ability of the metal crystal constituting the electrode to interact with the molecule. Here, mainly two types of interactions are important: surface binding and electron exchange.

In Section 9.2, we have seen that several metals, gold, for example, have a strong affinity with a few biomolecules up to give rise in selected conditions to a spontaneous monolayer generation. This phenomenon can be greatly enhanced by suitable electrode surface activation as shown in Section 9.2. If the target molecule is absorbed on the electrode surface, the behavior of the cell is strongly influenced by the resulting interaction.

Another possible interaction between a macromolecule and a metal electrode is electron exchange. In order for electron exchange to be possible, the electron energy levels of the molecule and of the electrode metals have to be in a suitable relation. Electrons in metals have a set of energy levels distributed in continuous intervals, called electron energy bands, interrupted by forbidden energy intervals, called energy gaps [3,4]. Although the band structure is generally a complex structure due to the spatial anisotropy of the crystal, it is sufficient for our qualitative description to consider a simple, one-dimensional band structure as those shown in Figure 10.1. Since electrons are Fermi particles, they are distributed in the band structure so that every single spin state is occupied by a single electron following the Fermi distribution $F(\varepsilon)$ that is given by

$$F(\varepsilon) = \frac{1}{\exp[(\varepsilon - \varepsilon_F / \kappa_B T)] + 1} \tag{10.1}$$

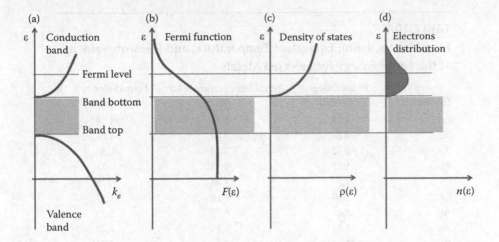

FIGURE 10.1 Energy distribution of conduction electrons in metals: (a) energy band profiles versus the electron moment in the crystal k_e (a one-dimensional crystal is imagined for simplicity), (b) Fermi distribution, (c) density of states in the conduction band, and (d) conduction electrons energy distribution.

where ε_F is the Fermi energy, or Fermi level, the fundamental parameter of the Fermi distribution. The Fermi distribution transits from one (complete level occupation), to zero (no level occupation), in a small energy interval around the Fermi energy that has the dimension of the thermal energy $\kappa_B T$, as shown in Figure 10.1.

Values of Fermi energies of pure metals are reported in Table 10.1, besides the velocity of electrons at the Fermi energy and the so-called Fermi temperature. The Fermi temperature is the temperature at which the average thermal energy is equal to the Fermi energy; it results is much higher than the room temperature in the range of 10^4 K. This means that at room temperature the interval around the Fermi energy, where there is partial occupation of electron levels, is very small with respect to the Fermi energy itself. Thus, in many applications, the energy of all conduction electrons in a metal can be approximated without great errors with the Fermi energy.

The final electron distribution in the metal energy bands is obtained by multiplying the Fermi distribution by the density of states in the band $\rho(\varepsilon)$ that can be demonstrated to be

$$\rho(\varepsilon) = \frac{8\sqrt{2}\,\pi\sqrt{m_e^3}}{h^3}\sqrt{\varepsilon - \varepsilon_c} \tag{10.2}$$

where m_e is the effective mass of the electron [3,4] and ε_c is the bottom energy of the conduction band.

In order for the metal to be a conductor, the Fermi level has to be inside the conduction band, generally at the bottom of it, as shown in Figure 10.1. In this condition, the density of electrons in the conduction band that is given by

$$n_e(\varepsilon) = \rho(\varepsilon)F(\varepsilon) \tag{10.3}$$

is sufficiently high to provide enough conduction band electrons, having the possibility to jump to free higher-level states giving rise to a macroscopic current. When a potential ψ is applied to the metal, the electrons are accelerated in such a way that their energy is increased by the product of the potential by the electron charge. This is equivalent to saying that the electron distribution is moved toward higher energies by adding the applied potential to the Fermi level.

TABLE 10.1
Fermi Levels, Fermi Equivalent Temperature, and Electron Velocity at the Fermi Energy for Selected Metals

Element	Fermi Energy (eV)	Fermi Temperature $\times 10^4$ (K)	Fermi Velocity $\times 10^6$ (m/s)
Li	4.74	5.51	1.29
Na	3.24	3.77	1.07
K	2.12	2.46	0.86
Rb	1.85	2.15	0.81
Cs	1.59	1.84	0.75
Cu	7.00	8.16	1.57
Ag	5.49	6.38	1.39
Au	5.53	6.42	1.40
Be	14.3	16.6	2.25
Mg	7.08	8.23	1.58
Ca	4.69	5.44	1.28
Sr	3.93	4.57	1.18
Ba	3.64	4.23	1.13
Nb	5.32	6.18	1.37
Fe	11.1	13.0	1.98
Mn	10.9	12.7	1.96
Zn	9.47	11.0	1.83
Cd	7.47	8.68	1.62
Hg	7.13	8.29	1.58
Al	11.7	13.6	2.03
Ga	10.4	12.1	1.92
In	8.63	10.0	1.74
Tl	8.15	9.46	1.69
Sn	10.2	11.8	1.90
Pb	9.47	11.0	1.83
Bi	9.90	11.5	1.87
Sb	10.9	12.7	1.96

Source: Data from Ziman J. M., *Principles of the Theory of Solids*, Cambridge University Press; 2nd edition (November 30, 1979), ISBN-13: 978-0521297332; Ashcroft N. W., Mermin N. D., *Solid State Physics*, Brooks Cole; 1st edition (January 2, 1976), ISBN-13: 978-0030839931.

Let us now imagine that a macromolecule is in contact with a metal electrode. We can assume that free electrons, that is, electrons near the Fermi level, are exchanged between the macromolecule and the electrode if they transit to a lower energy level due to the process. Let us focus on the donation of electrons from the metal to the macromolecule.

The possible energy levels of an electron in the metal, and while bonded to the molecule, are represented in Figure 10.2, where the relations between the electron energy levels at the metal surface and in an absorbed macromolecule are shown. Free electrons at the Fermi level have to overcome an extraction energy barrier to be extracted from the metal surface. This energy barrier can be greatly reduced by an effective absorption of the molecule on the metal surface, but generally cannot be completely eliminated. Moreover, owing to the highly stable nature of the metal structure, the Fermi level in the metal is generally lower than the excited electron levels in the molecules. Thus,

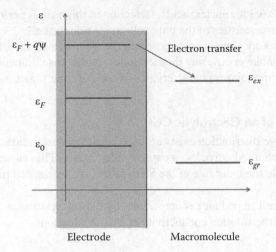

FIGURE 10.2   Electron energy levels inside an electrode and in an absorbed macromolecule affine with the electrode with and without the application of a potential ψ to the electrode.

spontaneous donations of electrons from the electrode to the macromolecule in practical cases do not happen.

However, if the energy gap

$$\Delta G = \varepsilon_{mol} - \varepsilon_F \qquad (10.3a)$$

is sufficiently small, it can be overcome by the application of a suitable potential of the electrode so as to cause the transition of an electron from the metal to the molecule. This causes a reduction process of the molecule. Similarly, an oxidation process can happen if an electron is donated by the molecule to the metal.

In order to obtain such effects, largely exploited in electrochemical detection, not only must the target molecule effectively absorb on the surface of the electrode so as to reduce the extraction energy, but also the Fermi level and the excited electron levels of the molecules have to be sufficiently near each other.

10.3.1   NON-FARADAIC IMPEDANCE DETECTION

Impedance is an important characteristic of an electrical system; thus, it is quite intuitive that measuring the impedance of an electrolytic cell gives a great deal of information, allowing the quantization of sample components and characterization of their properties.

Impedance detection methods are divided into two categories: Faradaic and non-Faradaic impedance detection. In the first case, an alternate current flow through the electrolytic cell is caused by the oxidation of a chemical species at one of the electrodes, the anode, and by the reduction of the complementary species at the other electrode, the cathode. Differently, in the case of non-Faradaic impedance detection, no chemical reaction happens in the sample solution during impedance detection.

If any affinity between the electrode and the target macromolecule is avoided, an electrical double layer is formed around the electrodes, as described in Section 7.5.2, without further interaction among the macromolecule and the electrodes. The double layer is constituted practically only by ions that have a much higher mobility with respect to macromolecules, even if the macromolecules generally acquire an electrical charge in an electrolyte solution, as detailed in Section 3.6.2 for proteins and in Section 3.6.3 for nucleic acids. Detection in this case is performed by testing the cell impedance to detect characteristics of the bulk solution inside the cell.

If the target molecules are somehow absorbed on the electrode surface, the double layer is heavily influenced by the monolayer covering the electrodes. In this case, impedance detection is mainly meant to determine the monolayer characteristics to quantify the target molecule or to investigate its characteristics.

10.3.1.1 Impedance of an Electrolytic Cell

Since a nonneutral charge distribution exists around the electrodes, besides the electrical resistance due to the presence of charged particles, a capacity also exists. This capacity is mainly generated by the Debye layer, while the main role of the Stern layer is to fix the cell inner potential to the zeta potential of the solution.

The real part of the cell impedance is constituted by the cell resistance. The cell resistance R_c is related to the inverse of the solution conductivity σ_s by the equation

$$R_s = \frac{L_c}{A\sigma_s} \tag{10.4}$$

where we assume a parallelepiped cell with length L_c and section A equal to the plane electrode area.

The conductivity can be evaluated, as shown in Section 9.3.2.2, through the Kohlrausch law that, in the case of simultaneous presence of several different charged particles and for a nonneutral solution, is written as

$$\sigma_s = \Lambda_m c_s - K c_s \sqrt{c_s} \tag{10.5}$$

where c_s is the sum of the concentrations of all the electrolytes and K the Kohlrausch experimental constant. In the limit of low concentrations, the molar solution conductivity is given by

$$\Lambda_m = \sum_j \Lambda_j \bar{c}_j = \sum_j \Lambda_j \frac{c_j}{c_s} \tag{10.6}$$

where Λ_j and $\bar{c}_j$ are the jth electrolyte molar conductivity and relative concentration, respectively.

The Debye layer capacity C_D can be evaluated by integrating the charge density of the layer in conditions of continuous applied voltage and dividing it by the voltage that appears at the cell extremes, which in this case is equal to the zeta voltage. In general, this is a complex task because the Poisson–Boltzmann equation can be solved in specific conditions only numerically. However, if the Debye–Hückel approximation (7.231) can be used, a simple expression is obtained:

$$C_D = A\varepsilon_0 \frac{\varepsilon_r}{\lambda_D} \tag{10.7}$$

where A is the plane electrode area and the Debye λ_D length is given by Equation 7.229. In the expression of the Debye length, in the hypothesis to have different ions in the solution, the ion concentration can be simply substituted by the ionic strength Y that depends on the concentration c_j and the normalized charge $z_j = Q_j/q$ of each charged molecule in the solution as

$$Y = \sum_j c_j z_j^2 \tag{10.8}$$

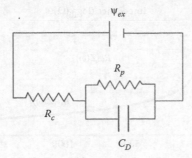

FIGURE 10.3 Electrical circuit equivalent of an electrolytic cell with electrodes without compatibility with the solutes: the resistances and the capacity are defined in the text; ψ_{ex} represents the external applied voltage.

Considering the fact that a small current is in every case flowing through the electrolytic cell due to the spurious currents and polarization effects [5], the whole reaction room can be modeled as shown in Figure 10.3. The overall cell impedance $Z(\omega)$ is thus provided by the equation

$$Z(\omega) = R_c + \frac{R_p}{1 + i R_p C_D \omega} \tag{10.9}$$

It is interesting to observe that Equation 10.9 has a complex dependence on the dielectric constant of the solution, which at low frequency can be considered constant with frequency, since the Debye length depends on this parameter. Substituting Equation 7.229 in Equation 10.7, we obtain the following expression for the capacity:

$$C_D = A \sqrt{\frac{2(Zq)^2 Y \varepsilon}{\kappa_B T}} \tag{10.10}$$

To obtain an order of magnitude estimation of the stationary values of this capacity, let us assume having a dielectric constant equal to that of water, so that $\varepsilon = 78 \ \varepsilon_0$; thus, we have $\lambda_D = 9.6\sqrt{(c^*/Z^2 c_0)}$ nm where $c^* = 1(\text{mmole/m}^3)$. Thus, for monovalent ions and a concentration of the order of $1(\text{mmole/m}^3)$, which is sufficiently low to use the low concentration approximation and neglecting K in Equation 10.5, we obtain $\lambda_D \sim 10$ nm and $C_D/A \sim 0.075$ F/m².

The plots of the real and imaginary parts of the impedance (10.9) for a parallelepiped cell with an electrode area of 10^{-6} m² and a length of $100\ \mu$m are plotted setting $R_s = 1$ MΩ and $R_p = 10$ MΩ, which are values typical of a diluted solution of monovalent ions in water and of a cell of the considered dimensions (see Table 11.2 for the cell resistance evaluation). The imaginary part of the impedance has a threshold frequency of the order of 300 Hz, as shown in Figure 10.4, corresponding to the characteristic time τ_c that is of the order of 3.4 ms. As a matter of fact, we get

$$\tau_c \approx \frac{1}{R_c C_D} = \frac{\varepsilon}{2\sigma_e} \frac{L_c}{\lambda_D} \tag{10.11}$$

The time τ_c can be interpreted as the time needed to form the double layer; as a matter of fact, every phenomenon with a characteristic time that is much longer experiments with the effect of a fully built-up double layer, while every phenomenon with a much shorter characteristic time sees the cell as a simple conductor, since the imaginary part of the impedance becomes negligible.

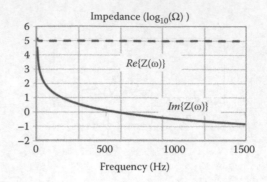

FIGURE 10.4 Real and imaginary parts of a microelectrolysis cell with a diluted solution of monovalent ions.

Intuition suggests that if charged particles with very different masses are present in the solution, the double layer built up should be longer for heavier particles. This fact is reflected by the dependence of the conductivity from the mobility of a charged particle, that is, from the ratio between its average velocity and the local electrical field.

In order to have a first idea of the dependence of the cell characteristic time from the charge carrier mass, we can assume that charge carriers move in the solution like rigid bodies in a viscous continuous environment. We know from Section 1.5.1 that this is a fairly good approximation for macromolecules, and from Section 7.5 that this approximation correctly reproduces the trend of experimental results for monovalent and bivalent ions, excluding hydrogen and hydroxyl ions, whose propagation mechanism in water is not the electrically induced drift [5].

Under this approximation, a simple conduction model can be made by assuming the Stokes expression for the viscous drag coefficient of the charge carriers, so as to obtain Equation 7.223, which compared with Equation 10.6 in the low concentration hypothesis provides the following expression for the molar conductivity of the jth charge carrier:

$$\Lambda_j \approx \frac{z_j q}{6\pi\eta R} \approx \frac{z_j q}{6\pi\eta \sqrt[3]{(3/4)(m_j/\rho_{eq})}} \tag{10.12}$$

where ρ_{eq} is a sort of equivalent density that was used to relate the radius of the spheres representing the charge carriers with their mass and, for an order of magnitude evaluation, is assumed to be the same for all the charge carriers. For diluted solutions, the molar conductivity depends on the inverse of the cubic root of the molecular mass.

Let us now consider a solution that is composed of a set of similar ions, for example, monovalent ions, and a target macromolecule. The double layer capacity changes mainly due to the fact that the zeta potential depends on the whole composition of the solution that is present in the cell, even if the double layer itself is mainly formed by ions. Thus, the new cell capacity is related in a complex manner to the presence of the target molecule. On the other end, the bulk solution resistance, dominating the real part of the cell impedance, is influenced by the contemporary presence of different types of charge carriers, so that, in low concentration conditions, where charge carrier interactions can be neglected, the overall conductivity is the sum of the conductivities due to each carrier type. This is equivalent to saying that the cell resistance is the parallel of the resistances that the cell would have if only one carrier was present.

It is important to underline that deviations from this simple rule are frequently observed if the concentrations of different species are not very low, due to different types of interactions between the solutes. This phenomenon is evident, for example, when proteins are dissolved in an ionic water solution. Strong interaction arises when increasing ion concentration between ions and proteins

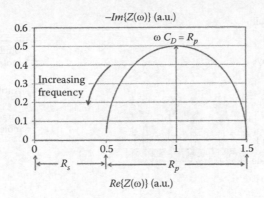

FIGURE 10.5 Shape of the Nyquist diagram for the circuit in Figure 10.3; a.u. indicates arbitrary units.

generating the phenomenon called "salting out" [6,7] and even protein–protein interaction is observed [8,9] if the protein concentration is not very small. In such conditions, naturally the conductivities of the single solutes cannot be added anymore and a more complex model of the molecule interaction is needed to evaluate the cell impedance.

The impedance of an electrolytic cell is frequently represented on the so-called Nyquist plot. This diagram relates real and imaginary parts of the cell impedance while the frequency changes from zero to the maximum frequency at which the measurement is done; an example of such a diagram is provided in Figure 10.5 for the equivalent circuit of Figure 10.3.

Direct impedance measurement can be used to determine the concentration of salts and macromolecules in a target solution [10,11]. The main problem affecting direct impedance detection is its lack of specificity. Unless a very clean sample is available, the nonspecific response of the detector renders it very hard to distinguish targets that have similar electrical responses.

The problem is overcome by impedance affinity detection. In this case, the target molecule is bound to the electrode with a specific chemical bond, so that nonspecific bonds are almost eliminated. Even if a macromolecule monolayer is quite thin, it greatly influences the capacity of the electrical double layer through a change of its dielectric or even causing a current due to the oxidation or reduction of the bound molecules. Thus, the presence of the monolayer and surface density can be detected through impedance detection [1]. The most used electrode metal in such systems is gold, due both to its chemical neutrality and its suitability for functionalization with organic molecules (see Section 9.2.1).

10.3.1.2 Non-Faradaic Impedance Affinity Detection

The most used configuration of a non-Faradaic detection system in a lab on chip is shown in Figure 10.6. Two plain gold electrodes are built at the sides of the detection room and functionalized with suitable binding molecules (generally thiols, see Section 9.2.1) and antibodies that specifically bind with the target molecule or suitable aptamers (see Section 9.2.4).

When the target solution starts to flow into the detection room, the functionalized surface starts to saturate with the target molecules. The surface saturation is generally achieved during a slow flow of the solution in the detection room so as to be able to process a quantity of the sample solution greater than the detection room volume, but in select cases it can also be achieved by simply inserting the sample into the reaction room and leaving it in a static condition.

The analysis of the dynamic saturation of a functionalized surface by a flowing sample has been carried out in Section 9.5.2 and the same results apply here, in particular regarding the relation between the target molecule concentration in the sample solution and its average surface density on the activated surface. After a suitable time, when equilibrium is reached and the electrode surface is saturated, a potential is applied to the electrode and the cell impedance is measured [11–13].

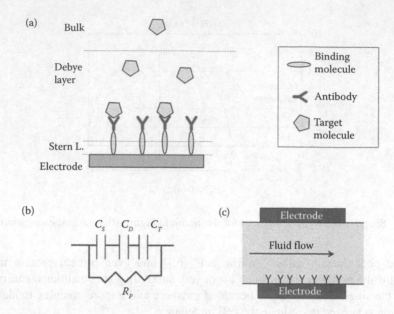

FIGURE 10.6 Scheme of the simplest arrangement of non-Faradaic affinity impedance detection: mono-layer formation near the electrode due to the affinity relationship between antibodies and target molecules (a), equivalent circuit of the double layer near the functionalized electrode (b), and possible sample solution flow arrangement (c).

In Figure 10.6, the equivalent circuit of the double layer near the functionalized electrode is shown. Besides an unavoidable parallel parasitic resistance R_p, the impedance is constituted by a series of three different capacities: the first is related to the Stern layer (C_S) as it is constituted both by ions that could absorb on the electrode surface and the monolayer that is built over the electrode; the second (C_D) is due to the Debye layer, also presenting in this case also a double contribution from ions and antibody monolayers; and the third (C_T) is caused by the target molecules captured by the antibodies. The estimation of the capacity C_T allows the detection of the target molecule. Once the monolayer density of the target molecules is determined, the concentration of the target molecules in the bulk solution can be deduced as shown in Section 9.5.2.

Since the determination of C_S and C_D with theoretical means or direct measurements on the detection room is very difficult, the detection is frequently realized using a reference room besides the main detection room. The reference room is fabricated exactly in the same way as the detection room but no sample solution is flown through it. It is statically filled with a solution with a content of salts and small molecules, possibly similar to that of the sample solution, so that the capacity measured in the reference room is equal to $C_S + C_D$ with the better possible approximation. This allows C_T to be obtained through a measure of the capacity difference between the two rooms.

The functionalization of gold electrodes with antibodies is very useful for protein assays, while for nucleic acid assays, functionalization with other nucleic acids is frequently used [14–16]. In the case of a DNA assay, for example, the DNA helices are frequently opened before the assay so as to obtain a single-stranded DNA sample that is inserted in the detection room where the electrode is functionalized with the complementary DNA chain. The chains that are bonded on the electrode surface combine with the single-stranded DNA sample allowing non-Faradaic impedance detection. The accuracy of detection is sufficiently high to detect single nucleotide differences between the bonded chains and the sample chains, constituting a powerful instrument for the analysis of short nucleic acid samples.

Another interesting variation of the non-Faradaic impedance detection is constituted by the use of functionalized nanoparticles that are inserted into the sample solution before injection into the

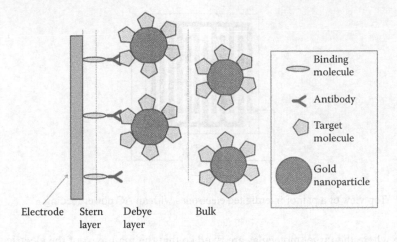

FIGURE 10.7   Scheme of the simplest arrangement of non-Faradaic affinity impedance detection using functionalized gold particles.

detection room [17,18]. Functionalized nanoparticles, generally made of gold, are coated by the target molecules so that when the sample travels through the detection room, they are fixed on the electrode surface. This creates a thin gold particle layer within or immediately out of the Debye length that can be detected by non-Faradaic impedance detection. A possible scheme of this detection technique is reported in Figure 10.7.

Nanoparticles can also be patterned directly in the electrode surface [19,20], obtaining a structure similar to that considered in Section 5.9.3 dealing with localized plasmon resonance. This process is used to increase the density of the monolayer coating the electrode so as to increase the maximum density of target molecules and the accuracy of the assay.

Sometimes, it is convenient to passivize the electrode with a dielectric thin film, like an SiO_2 or a PMMA film [21]. This operation could be required due to the type of target that can interact with the electrode material causing spurious reactions, mainly oxidation at the electrode surfaces, that have to be avoided if non-Faradaic detection has to be carried out. An insulating film covering the electrode is also needed if it is not possible to create the required monolayer directly on the electrode surface. In this case, a further capacity is placed in series to the capacities that are shown in Figure 10.6, that is, the dielectric layer capacity. The dielectric capacity does not have to be much greater than the capacities to be measured, so as not to decrease the detector accuracy; moreover, the dielectric thin film growth has to be very well controlled.

A different architecture for non-Faradaic impedance detection is the so-called planar architecture [22,23]. The principle scheme of a non-Faradaic impedance biosensor based on planar architecture is shown in Figure 10.8. The electrodes in this detection arrangement are placed on the side

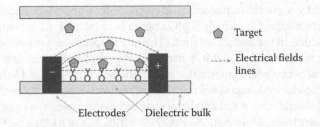

FIGURE 10.8   Principle principal scheme of a non-Faradaic impedance biosensor based on planar architecture.

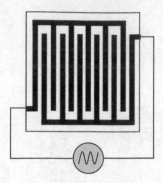

FIGURE 10.9   Top view of a pair of interdigited electrodes with an AC power feeding.

of the surface where the target molecules are fixed so that the main part of the electrical field force lines traverse the monolayer in a horizontal direction, maximizing the interaction with the monolayer itself. On the other hand, owing to the electrode geometry, the electrical field force lines also extend within the bulk of the solution in such a way that the impedance depends not only on the monolayer structure but also on the solution bulk properties.

This problem can be faced using two different complementary arrangements that are frequently contemporarily implemented in this type of systems. Since the electrical field extends through the bulk solution less and less while the electrodes are nearer and nearer, using very near electrodes is a possible way to limit the penetration of the field in the sample bulk. On the other hand, if the electrodes are very near, the surface where the functionalized surface can be fabricated reduces. In order to have a very small distance between electrodes and a large functionalized area, interdigitated electrodes can be used. The top view of a couple of interdigitated electrodes is shown in Figure 10.9. The electrode shape resembles the shape of two intersected combs, so that the distance between them is in any case very small, but the overall functionalized surface can be as big as needed, at the expenses of increasing the number of comb teeth.

The second way of eliminating the influence of the bulk solution on the impedance measure is to realize, in parallel to the detection room, a reference room where a solution as far as possible similar to the sample solution is inserted, but for the absence of the target molecule. When the impedance that is measured in the reference room is subtracted from the impedance measured in the detection room, the bulk solution effect is also eliminated, but the residual effect of the target molecules that are not captured by the functionalized surface. The last effect, however, is generally completely negligible if the system is correctly designed, so that the target molecules are almost all captured by the functionalized surface.

10.3.2   FARADAIC IMPEDANCE DETECTION

Different from non-Faradaic detection, in order to perform Faradaic impedance detection, the target has to be constituted by a couple of molecules giving rise to a reversible RedOx reaction that we call R and O. In practical cases, if a single RedOx target is to be assayed, a complementary RedOx molecule has to be added in the sample solution. The target species are captured by functionalized surfaces realized on the electrodes, and it is here that they undergo either reduction or oxidation, depending on the kind of considered molecules and on the potential sign and value. In order for this reaction to happen, the electrode metal not only has to be functionalized so as to capture the target molecule, but also it should have a suitable band structure so that electrons can be either acquired or transferred to the electrode. Moreover, the RedOx reaction has to happen only for the target molecules, that is, only for the molecule that is captured by the functionalized surface, so as to avoid nonspecific response of the detection system.

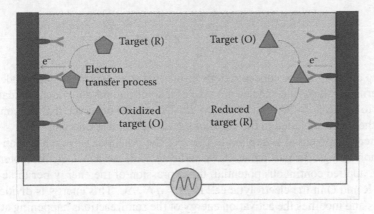

FIGURE 10.10 Principal scheme of a Faradaic cell for impedance detection.

The principal scheme of a Faradaic cell for impedance detection is presented in Figure 10.10. The sample solution is charged in the cell, and generally detection happens in static conditions. It is preferable for the better working of the detection system that the target molecules are present in the sample solution almost at the same concentration. The cell is biased with a continuous potential, assuring the equilibrium of the molecules in the sample solution, and an alternate potential is added for the impedance measurement [1,2].

Two main phenomena related to the RedOx reaction influence the impedance measurement: the reaction rate and the diffusion time of the species in the cell.

10.3.2.1 Reaction Rate Influence on Faradaic Impedance Detection

In order to study the influence of the reduction and oxidation rates, let us write the cathodic and anodic reactions as follows:

$$O(aq) + n_e\, e^- \to R(aq) \quad \text{(cathodic reduction)} \tag{10.13a}$$

$$R(aq) \to O(aq) + n_e\, e^- \quad \text{(anodic oxidation)} \tag{10.13b}$$

where n_e is the number of exchanged electrons. In almost all practical cases, reactions (10.13a) and (10.13b) are single-step reactions, so that a single activation free energy can be considered for them (see Section 1.2.4) that we indicate with ΔG_{red} and ΔG_{ox}, respectively, when referring to a mole of species.

The Arrhenius law (see Section 1.2.4) can be applied to express the unit reaction rates k_{red} and k_{ox} as a function of the temperature and of the rate coefficients v_{red} and v_{ox} by writing

$$k_{red} = v_{red}\, e^{-\frac{\Delta G_{red}}{R_g T}} \tag{10.14a}$$

$$k_{ox} = v_{ox}\, e^{-\frac{\Delta G_{ox}}{R_g T}} \tag{10.14b}$$

where $R_g = N_a\,\kappa_B$ is the perfect gas constant, N_a the Avogadro number, and κ_B the Boltzmann constant.

The real reaction rate can be obtained by the dynamic equation of a single-step reaction (Equation 1.45). Since the two partial reactions produce and burn the same species, the overall reaction rate is the difference of the rates of the two partial reactions so that it can be written as

$$\frac{\partial \bar{c}_o}{\partial t} = v_{ox}\, e^{-\frac{\Delta G_{ox}}{R_g T}}\, \bar{c}_R - v_{red}\, e^{-\frac{\Delta G_{red}}{R_g T}}\, \bar{c}_o \tag{10.15a}$$

$$\frac{\partial \overline{c}_R}{\partial t} = -v_{ox} \, e^{-\frac{\Delta G_{ox}}{R_g T}} \, \overline{c}_R + v_{red} \, e^{-\frac{\Delta G_{red}}{R_g T}} \, \overline{c}_o \tag{10.15b}$$

where $\overline{c}_o$ and $\overline{c}_R$ are the surface concentrations of the two species near the electrodes. Since in the absence of alternate voltage the species are stable in solution and no evident oxidation–reduction happens, it has to be $\Delta G_{red} \gg R_g T$ and $\Delta G_{ox} \gg R_g T$. It is to be observed that the continuous potential applied to the cell is included in the value of the activation free energies.

When an alternate potential is applied to the cell, the potential variation has an impact on the RedOx activation energy. In particular, if we indicate with $\Delta \psi = \psi - \psi_0$ the potential variation, where ψ_0 is the applied continuous potential, the expression of the energy per mole applied to the populations of R and O in the electrolytic cell is $\Delta \varepsilon = q \, N_a \, \Delta \psi$. This energy is divided between the two populations and modifies the activation energy of the semireactions happening at the electrodes so that the sum of the new activation energies $\Delta \overline{G}_{red}$ and $\Delta \overline{G}_{ox}$ can be expressed as

$$\Delta \overline{G}_{red} + \Delta \overline{G}_{ox} = \Delta G_{red} + \Delta G_{ox} - n_e \, q \, N_a \, \Delta \psi \tag{10.16}$$

It is not easy to evaluate theoretically the new activation energies individually; a detailed theory of RedOx reactions is needed, taking into account the reaction details at a molecular level by means of a quantum analysis of the implied phenomena. Several such theories do exist, of which the most diffused is probably the Marcus theory. It was elaborated initially as a classical theory of RedOx reactions and it has been successively extended to include a detailed quantum analysis. The interested reader is invited to refer to the rich literature on this subject [24–27].

Starting from Equation 10.16, a phenomenological parameter α is introduced so that

$$\Delta \overline{G}_{red} = \Delta G_{red} - \alpha \, n_e \, q \, N_a \, \Delta \psi \tag{10.17a}$$

$$\Delta \overline{G}_{ox} = \Delta G_{ox} - (1 - \alpha) n_e q N_a \Delta \psi \tag{10.17b}$$

with $0 \le \alpha \le 1$. From Equation 10.7, it is clear that the application of a potential difference unbalances the global reaction either in the reduction or in the oxidation sense, increasing one of the activation energies and decreasing the other. Very often in practical cases $\alpha \approx 0.5$, but counterexamples exist [25].

In order to determine the current that flows through the electrodes when an external potential difference is applied, we can use the following expression of the current density J in terms of the net number of flowing electrons per unit electrode area:

$$J = n_e \, q \, N_a \left(\frac{\partial \overline{c}_o}{\partial t} - \frac{\partial \overline{c}_R}{\partial t} \right) = n_e \, q \, N_a \left(k_{ox} \, \overline{c}_o \, e^{\frac{\alpha \, n_e \, q \, N_a \, \Delta \psi}{R_g T}} - k_{red} \, \overline{c}_R \, e^{\frac{(1-\alpha) \, n_e \, q \, N_a \, \Delta \psi}{R_g T}} \right) \tag{10.18}$$

where the activation energies in the presence of the potential difference are substituted into the rate Equations 10.15 to obtain the last term of Equation 10.18. The current density to voltage relation is shown in Figure 10.11 where expression of the current density is rewritten as follows:

$$J = J_0 \left(\hat{k}_{ox} \, \hat{c}_o \, e^{\frac{\alpha \, q \, n_e \, N_a \, \Delta \psi}{R_g T}} - \hat{k}_{red} \, \hat{c}_R \, e^{\frac{(1-\alpha) \, q \, n_e \, N_a \, \Delta \psi}{R_g T}} \right) \tag{10.19}$$

where

$$J_0 = n_e \, q \, N_a \, (\overline{c}_R + \overline{c}_0)(k_{ox} + k_{red}) \tag{10.20a}$$

$$\hat{c}_m = \frac{\overline{c}_m}{(\overline{c}_R + \overline{c}_0)} \quad m = R,O \tag{10.20b}$$

$$\hat{k}_m = \frac{k_m}{(k_{ox} + k_{red})} \quad m = ox, \, red \tag{10.20c}$$

and it is supposed that $\overline{C}_R = \overline{C}_0$ and $\alpha = 0.5$. From Figure 10.11, it is clear that in general the relationship between current density and voltage difference is strongly nonlinear, rendering the circuit impedance dependent on the applied voltage, unless the potential difference has a very small amplitude, so as to obtain a current variation approximately linear, as shown in Figure 10.12. Once this condition is satisfied, the continuous bias can be chosen in such a way as to obtain $\hat{k}_{red} \, \hat{c}_R = \hat{k}_{ox} \, \hat{c}_o$ so that the characteristic passes from the axis origin. This can be done simply by changing the continuous potential up to the elimination of the current in the absence of an alternate potential difference.

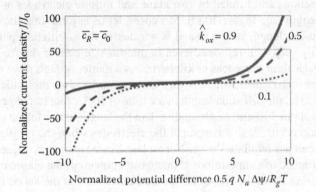

FIGURE 10.11 Current density versus normalized potential difference for an electrolytic cell for Faradaic impedance measure. The surface densities of the RedOx species on the electrodes surfaces are assumed to be equal and the value $\alpha = 0.5$ is adopted.

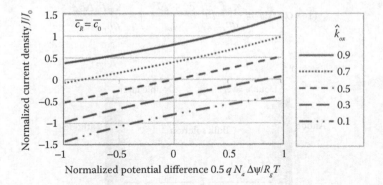

FIGURE 10.12 Current density versus normalized potential difference for an electrolytic cell for Faradaic impedance measure in the case of a small potential difference maintaining the system in a linear current–potential regime. The other conditions are the same as in Figure 10.11.

Once the cell is correctly biased and the potential difference amplitude selected is sufficiently small, Equation 10.18 can be approximated with a linear equation as

$$J = J_0 \left[\hat{k}_{ox} \hat{c}_o \, \alpha - \hat{k}_{red} \hat{c}_R (1 - \alpha) \right] \Delta\psi = R_{ct} \, \Delta\psi \qquad (10.21)$$

It is thus clear that in this condition the fact that electrons are not instantly released or acquired by the RedOx species can be modeled as a series resistance R_{ct} that has to be added to the equivalent circuit that represents the electrical phenomena happening on the electrodes. The expression of R_{ct} can be easily derived from Equation 10.19.

10.3.2.2 Mass Transport Influence on Faradaic Impedance Detection

While the species react on the electrodes, they detach from the metal surface and a concentration gradient is generated between the solution bulk and the R and O species near the electrodes. The concentration gradient generates a diffusion of the RedOx species toward the electrodes where they are fixed on the surface and aliment the electrical current.

However, diffusion is not an instantaneous process, so that the diffusion speed limits the electrical current in the cell. In this section, we will analyze the effect of diffusion on the cell impedance.

Let us assume that we can consider the cell as a one-dimensional system, that is, a space unlimited along the y and z directions and limited by two plane and infinite electrodes at $x = 0$ and at $x = L_c$, where L_c is the cell length (see Figure 10.13). Moreover, let us assume that the cell length is much greater than the diffusion length of the O and R species in the oscillating potential period. This assumption is generally very well respected even in micron-size cells if the frequency of the oscillating potential is greater than a few tens of kilohertz. As a matter of fact, if we consider a diffusion coefficient of the order of 10^{-9} m²/s, which is very large for an organic molecule (see Section 7.4.2), and a frequency of 10 kHz, the diffusion length in the time of 10^{-4} s, that is, the period of the potential oscillation, is equal to about 300 nm, much smaller than the length of any lab on chip detection room.

The two semireactions (10.13) that happen at the electrodes when the oscillating voltage difference is applied to the cell are regulated by the Nernst law. Since we have polarized the cell so that no current flows in the absence of a superimposed fluctuation potential, the biased cell reference potential is zero [5] and we can write the Nernst law at the cathode and at the anode (see Appendix 5) as

$$\alpha \, \Delta\psi = \frac{\kappa_B T}{q n_e} \ln\left(\frac{\overline{c}_R + \Delta\overline{c}_R}{\overline{c}_R} \right) \approx \frac{\kappa_B T}{q n_e} \frac{\Delta\overline{c}_R}{\overline{c}_R} \qquad (10.22a)$$

$$(1 - \alpha) \, \Delta\psi = \frac{\kappa_B T}{q n_e} \ln\left(\frac{\overline{c}_o + \Delta\overline{c}_o}{\overline{c}_o} \right) \approx \frac{\kappa_B T}{q n_e} \frac{\Delta\overline{c}_o}{\overline{c}_0} \qquad (10.22b)$$

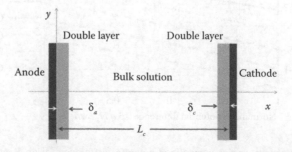

FIGURE 10.13 Geometry of the electrolytic cell used for the determination of the expression of the Warburg impedance.

where linearization is justified by the small oscillating voltage amplitude. Moreover, owing to the fact that the oscillating current density is proportional to the flux of the molecules multiplied by the charge, we also get

$$\Delta J = -q n_e \left[D_o \left(\frac{\partial c_o}{\partial x} \right)_{x=0} + D_R \left(\frac{\partial c_R}{\partial x} \right)_{x=L_c} \right] \tag{10.23}$$

where c_o and c_R are respectively the volume concentrations of the species O and R (not to be confused with the surface concentrations on the electrodes that are indicated with $\bar{c}_o$ and $\bar{c}_R$), while D_o and D_R represent the diffusion coefficients of the two species.

The mass transport through the cell is regulated by the diffusion equation, so that in our one-dimensional approximation we can write

$$\frac{\partial \Delta c_R}{\partial t} = D_R \frac{\partial^2 \Delta c_R}{\partial x^2} \tag{10.24a}$$

$$\frac{\partial \Delta c_o}{\partial t} = D_o \frac{\partial^2 \Delta c_o}{\partial x^2} \tag{10.24b}$$

By Fourier transforming Equations 10.24 and solving the resulting ordinary differential equation for the concentration fluctuations, we get

$$\Delta c_o = \Delta c_o(0)e^{-\sqrt{\frac{i\omega}{D_o}}x} \tag{10.25a}$$

$$\Delta c_R = \Delta c_R(L_c)e^{-\sqrt{\frac{i\omega}{D_R}}(L_c-x)} \tag{10.25b}$$

From Equations 10.25, we deduce that

$$\lim_{x\to\infty} \Delta c_o = \lim_{x\to-\infty} \Delta c_R = 0 \tag{10.26}$$

This is a correct conclusion in the hypothesis that the diffusion length is much shorter than the cell length, meaning that the bulk concentrations of the species O and R are practically unaffected by the oscillating voltage.

At this point, the impedance contribution $Z_W(\omega)$ of the mass transfer can be evaluated directly by setting

$$Z_W(\omega) = \frac{1}{A} \frac{\Delta \psi}{\Delta J} \tag{10.27}$$

which is the area of the cell section (and of the electrodes). The potential can be obtained by adding Equations 10.22 in their linearized form and replacing the surface concentrations with volume concentrations setting

$$c_R(L_c) = \bar{c}_R \delta_c \tag{10.28a}$$

$$c_o(0) = \bar{c}_o \delta_a \tag{10.28b}$$

where δ_c and δ_a are the cathode and anode distance at which an electron can be exchanged with the electrode. Evaluating the bulk concentrations and fluxes from Equations 10.25, we finally get

$$Z_W(\omega) = \frac{\kappa_B T}{q^2 n_e^2} \frac{1}{A} \frac{1}{\sqrt{i\omega}} \left(\frac{1}{c_o \sqrt{D_o}} + \frac{1}{c_R \sqrt{D_R}} \right)$$

$$= \frac{\kappa_B T}{q^2 n_e^2} \frac{1}{A} \frac{1-i}{\sqrt{\omega}} \left(\frac{1}{c_o \sqrt{D_o}} + \frac{1}{c_R \sqrt{D_R}} \right) \tag{10.29}$$

where c_o and c_R are the bulk concentrations of the RedOx species. This is called Warburg impedance and it represents the effect of the mass transport on the overall impedance of the electrolytic cell.

10.3.2.3 Faradaic Impedance Detection in Lab on Chip

After the analysis of the Faradaic impedance measure process and of the different elements constituting the electrolytic cell, it is possible to analyze the detection result.

Taking into account all the impedance contributions, the equivalent circuit of the cell can be represented as in Figure 10.14, where besides the resistance R_{ct} related to the RedOx reaction rate and the Warburg impedance, the overall cell capacity C_I and resistance R_s are also present. The bulk cell resistance can be evaluated using the Kohlrausch law (see Equations 10.5 and 10.6) while the overall cell capacity is mainly related to the ion double layer contribution (see Equation 10.10).

In the equivalent circuit, the capacity and the impedance related to the RedOx reaction are in parallel since the current can follow two alternative pathways: passing through the cell bulk and the capacity of the double layer or being generated by the RedOx reaction. The cell bulk resistance is instead in series to both the pathways due to the fact that it is experimented by both the current types.

The characteristic Nyquist diagram of a Faradaic impedance detection is reported in Figure 10.15; it is essentially constituted by the superposition of the Nyquist diagram of the cell with the Nyquist diagram due to the RedOx activity, which is also called the Faradaic diagram. The output of a Faradaic impedance detection is generally interpreted by fitting on experimental curves the expression of the overall impedance so as to obtain an estimate of the equivalent circuit parameters. Starting from these estimates, several characteristics of the sample solution can be deduced.

The bulk concentrations of the RedOx molecules can be estimated by the cell resistance. Once the bulk concentrations are known, the RedOx kinetic parameters can be estimated by the value of the RedOx resistance and the diffusion coefficients from the estimated values of the Warburg impedance [28,29].

The type of electrode functionalization is very important in Faradaic impedance measurements. Gold electrodes are most common and molecules are generally fixed to them using thiol chains (see Section 9.2.1). Both colloidal films [30] and different types of nucleic acid-based aptamers [31–33] have been used to improve the performances of such electrodes. Chemically modified carbohydrates can also be used as binding molecules [34], but the performances of such monolayers seem to be inferior with respect to antibodies and aptamer monolayers.

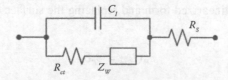

FIGURE 10.14   Equivalent circuit of the electrolytic cell for the Faradaic impedance detection.

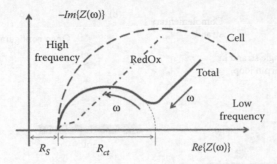

FIGURE 10.15   Characteristic Nyquist diagram of a Faradaic impedance detection.

Carbon nanotubes can also be used to fabricate electrodes for impedance detection, exploiting the high conductivity of selected nanotubes (see Section 9.2.2) and the excellent capability of these structures to accept monolayer formation on their surface [35–37].

The form of the electrodes is also important in determining the characteristics of the measurement. Interdigitated electrodes are used as in the case of non-Faradaic measurements to improve the electrode area, thus increasing the detected signal [38]. Arrays of detection rooms with electrode arrays can be used to perform parallel measurements [39] and several other particular electrode designs have been realized for different purposes [40].

An alternative type of Faradaic impedance detection is performed in biocatalytic sensors. In this case, a biological reaction happens in the sample solution due to the insertion of an enzyme coupling with a substrate that is dissolved in the sample. The reaction product is not soluble; thus, it precipitates on the electrodes while the reaction proceeds, changing the electrode characteristics while the precipitation layer increases its thickness. A suitable RedOx couple is also inserted into the sample before the assay so as to perform Faradaic impedance detection and reveal the electrode modification.

This principle has been exploited in the glucose bienzyme sensor whose mechanism is shown in Figure 10.16 [41]. Glucose oxidation catalyzed by glucose oxidase produces hydrogen peroxide. Hydrogen peroxidase oxidizes the peroxidase molecule forming an insoluble product that deposits on the lower electrode of the detection room. The thickness of the deposited film is proportional to the assay time and to the quantity of oxidized glucose and it is tested by inserting into the sample

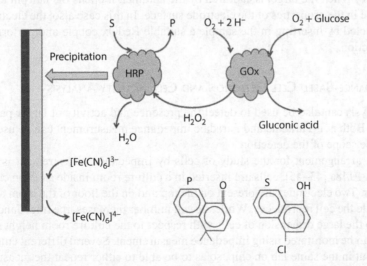

FIGURE 10.16   Mechanism of glucose detection via oxidation by glucose oxidase and Faradaic impedance detection.

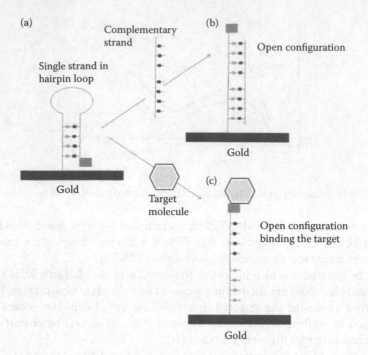

FIGURE 10.17 Single-stranded DNA aptamer fixed in a hairpin configuration on a gold surface: (a) fabricated monolayer, (b) open aptamer after the binding of the conjugate DNA strand, and (c) open aptamer after binding a target molecule with its arm termination.

solution an inorganic RedOx couple, such as $[Fe(CN)_6]^{3-}/[Fe(CN)_6]^{4-}$ and performing a Faradaic impedance detection.

Aptamers presenting a hairpin loop are also used in detection methods based on the revelation of changes in the electrode surface parameters. A scheme of the working of a hairpin loop aptamer is shown in Figure 10.17 [42] when the target is either a conjugated DNA strand or a different molecule that could be bonded using a specific receptor placed on the aptamer termination not absorbed in the metal surface. When the target is captured by the aptamer, it opens the hairpin loop generating a relevant change in the properties of the electrode surface. In this case also, the electrode modification can be detected by inserting in the sample a suitable RedOx couple and performing Faradaic impedance detection.

10.3.3 Impedance-Based Cell Detection and Cell Activity Analysis

Impedance analysis can also be used to detect the presence and activity of larger particles such as cells or viruses. Both non-Faradaic and Faradaic impedance measurement can be used in this case, depending on the scope of the detection.

The simplest arrangement for the study of cells by impedance measurement is schematically shown in Figure 10.18a [43–45]: cells are inserted in a culture room inside a lab on chip and adhere to the room floor. Two electrodes are present on the top and on the floor of the room and impedance is measured while the cell reproduces. While the cell number increases, the impedance changes significantly due to the large dimension of cells with respect to the culture room height so that the cell multiplication can be monitored using impedance measurement. Several different culture rooms are frequently present in the same lab on chip, so as to be able to either repeat the measure to increase accuracy or to test the cell population in different situations. Non-Faradaic impedance measurement is frequently used in this situation, but exceptions exist.

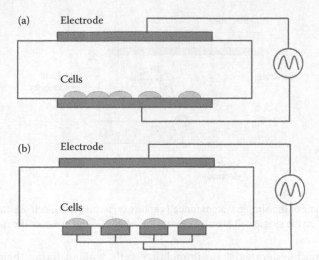

FIGURE 10.18 Schemes of cell culture chambers in a lab on chip for cell population (a) and single cell (b) impedance detection.

Owing to the cell dimension, single cell measurements can be performed if an electrode array is used to collect small electrodes prepared in such a way as to attach on their surface a single cell. This is not difficult to do by activating the electrode surface with monolayers that bind to the external membrane of the cell. Such an arrangement is schematically shown in Figure 10.18b. Several cell properties can be monitored in this way, such as cell adhesion to the electrode [46], cell mortality [47] and the properties of the interface between the cell and the electrode, for example, its thickness [48]. These measurements can be done by changing the environmental conditions such as temperature and the composition of the background solution. A prototype of a structure for impedentiometry cells analysis integrating eight wells for cells culture in a single chip is reported in Figure 10.19.

In different situations, the cells are not to be created in a culture room over the electrodes, but their presence is to be detected in a liquid sample and they have to be captured by electrodes while the sample flows in a microfluidic duct. This is the case of several bacteria or virus detection. In this case, it is possible to inject the sample in a detection room and to measure the impedance, but this method can be difficult if the sample contains several different species, especially if they have a strong electronic activity.

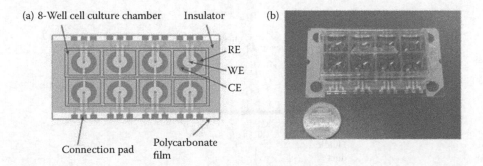

FIGURE 10.19 Example of cell culture array realized on a lab on chip for characterization via impedance measurement: lab on chip top view (a) and lab on chip photograph (b). (Reprinted from *Analytical Biochemistry*, vol. 341, Yeon J. H., Park J.-K., Cytotoxicity test based on electrochemical impedance measurement of HepG2 cultured in microfabricated cell chip, pp. 308–315, Copyright 2005, with permission from Elsevier.)

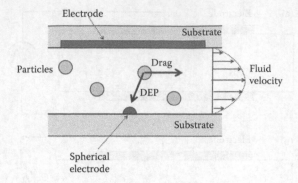

FIGURE 10.20   Scheme of the simple system for cell capture on a spherical electrode that is considered in the text. The forces acting on the single cell are also evidenced, where DEP represents the dielectrophoresis force.

In this case, a smart system exists to immobilize cells without fixing them to a solid surface that is based on the use of dielectrophoresis (see Section 7.5.5) [49,50]. In order to understand the principle and to evaluate the order of magnitude of the main involved parameters, let us consider the simple system that is represented in Figure 10.20. A fluid containing cells to be detected, for example, bacteria, flows through a microfluidic rectangular channel. The channel dimension along the y axis W is very wide with respect to the channel height h so that the channel can be considered an infinite slab for fluid dynamical calculations. A semispherical electrode is realized on the floor of the channel at the point $x = 0$ and $y = 0$ and a flat and wide electrode is realized on the channel roof.

Since the roof can be considered a perfect plane conductor, the electrical field force lines can be evaluated by applying the mirror theorem of electrostatics to solve the Poisson equation. We can thus imagine a symmetric virtual spherical electrode on the other side of the conducting plate, as shown in Figure 10.21, and solve the Poisson equation obtaining [51]

$$\psi(r) = \frac{b}{|r - 2hz|}\Delta\psi \tag{10.30}$$

where $\boldsymbol{u}_x$, $\boldsymbol{u}_y$, and $\boldsymbol{u}_z$ are the unit vectors associated with the reference system that is shown in Figure 10.21, r is the radial coordinate in a reference system having the center in the electrode center, that is

$$\boldsymbol{r} = x\boldsymbol{u}_x + y\boldsymbol{u}_y + z\boldsymbol{u}_z \tag{10.31}$$

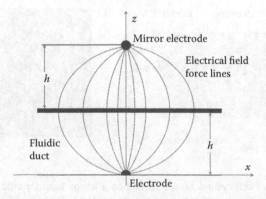

FIGURE 10.21   Reference system adopted for the analysis of the system in Figure 10.20 and scheme of the electrical field evaluation through the electromagnetic mirror theorem (the field force lines are shown in the plot).

and $\Delta\psi$ is the potential difference between the semispherical electrode and the conduction roof. The electrical field force lines constitute a sort of cage around the spherical electrode causing the dielectrophoresis force to act on the particle transiting through the channel, especially if they are in the vicinity of the electrode. In the very vicinity of the electrode, where $r \ll h$, the expression of the electrical field simplifies as follows:

$$E = -\nabla\psi \approx \frac{b}{r^2} \Delta\psi \, e_r \qquad (10.32)$$

where e_r is the unit radial vector. Inserting expression (10.32) of the electrical field into Equation 7.251 providing the electrophoresis force after transformation of the field gradient in spherical coordinates, we get the following expression of the dielectrophoresis force:

$$F_{DEP} = -8\pi \frac{\varepsilon_p - \varepsilon_L}{\varepsilon_p + 2\varepsilon_L} \frac{a^3 b^2}{r^5} \varepsilon_0 \varepsilon_p \Delta\psi^2 \, e_r \qquad (10.33)$$

where b is the electrode radius and a the particle radius. The dielectrophoresis force depends in a substantial way on the distance of the particle center from the electrode center. If we introduce the parameter $\Gamma = b/a$, that is, the ratio between the radii of the particle and of the electrode, we can rewrite Equation 10.33 as

$$F_{DEP} = -8\pi \frac{\varepsilon_p - \varepsilon_L}{\varepsilon_p + 2\varepsilon_L} \frac{\Gamma^2}{(1 + \Gamma)^5 \rho^5} \varepsilon_0 \varepsilon_p \Delta\psi^2 \, e_r \qquad (10.34)$$

where $\rho = r/(b + a)$, that is, the ratio between the effective distance from the particle and the electrode centers and its minimum value, which is obtained when the particle surface touches the electrode surface. If a particle such as a cell is considered, we have $\Gamma \sim 1$.

Assuming a Poiseuille flow in the duct, the average velocity of the flow is given by Equation 7.88. If the center of the particles is on the z axis, the drag velocity exerted by the fluid on the particles can thus be written as

$$v = 6\frac{Q}{Wh}\left[1 - \zeta \, (1 + \Gamma)\frac{a}{h}\right] \zeta \, (1 + \Gamma)\frac{a}{h} \approx 6\frac{Q}{Wh}\zeta \, (1 + \Gamma)\frac{a}{h} \qquad (10.35)$$

where Q is the flow rate and in the hypothesis that the particle is near the electrode we have $r \ll h$, implying $\rho(1 + \Gamma)(a/h) \ll 1$. In a first approximation, we can assume that the drag force F_D exerted by the fluid on the particle can be evaluated using the Stokes formula (see Section 7.4.2) so that

$$F_D = 6\pi\eta v = 36\pi\eta\frac{Q}{Wh}\zeta \, (1 + \Gamma)\frac{a^2}{h} \, x \qquad (10.36)$$

where $\zeta = r/(b + a)$. After passing over the electrode, the particle is dragged away from the electrode by the fluid flow and attracted toward the electrode by the dielectrophoresis force. The geometry of the forces involved in the system is shown in Figure 10.20.

The complete study of the particle motion, even with the great number of approximations we have introduced, cannot be determined in closed form by solving the motion equation. As a matter of fact, the combination of the dielectrophoresis and the drag force causes the particle to decelerate the motion along the x axis that brings it far from the electrode while it decreases its vertical coordinate due to the electrode attraction. It is however intuitive that, owing to the strong dependence of the dielectrophoresis force on the distance between the particle and the electrode, a sort of capturing range has to exist for the main problem parameters.

In order to determine at least approximately the capturing conditions, let us note that, while the particle drops toward the lower wall of the duct, a greater part of the dielectrophoresis force is opposite to the drag force and the particle motion along the x axis is more and more decelerated up to the moment in which it eventually inverts and the particle is attracted toward the electrode. The extreme case in which this happens occurs when the particle reaches the lower wall of the duct and the z coordinate of its center is equal to a. In this case, since we have assumed $\Gamma \sim 1$, we can imagine that the dielectrophoresis force is purely horizontal, that is, parallel to the drag force. Thus, the extreme capture condition is written as

$$\left| \frac{F_{DEP}}{F_D} \right| > 1 \tag{10.37}$$

Since the dielectrophoresis force decreases rapidly with the distance from the electrode, we can assume that if the distance from the electrode increases too much after the moment in which the particle travels vertically on top of the electrode, there can be no capture; thus, we can assume that the distance of the particle from the electrode decreases if capture happens after the moment in which the particle is vertically over the electrode. Exploiting this observation, as a worst-case condition, we can assume ρ as a constant, equal to the value it has when the centers are one on top of the other.

Substituting into Equation 10.37 the expressions (10.36) and (10.34) and observing that, in the above condition, $\zeta = \rho$, the maximum flow rate for which the capture condition (10.37) is realized is given by

$$\frac{Q_{Max}}{Wh} = \frac{2}{9} \frac{\varepsilon_p - \varepsilon_L}{\varepsilon_p + 2\varepsilon_L} \frac{\Gamma^2}{(1 + \Gamma)^6 \rho^6} h \frac{\varepsilon_0 \varepsilon_p}{\eta a^2} \Delta\psi^2 \tag{10.38}$$

The first observation is that in order for the flow rate to be positive, for the capture to be possible with some value of $\Delta\psi$, it has to be $\varepsilon_p > \varepsilon_L$. This is generally true for cells such as bacteria or human cells in salt water solution. This is due to the very high concentration of macromolecules in the cell interior and the effect of the membranes of the cell itself and of the organelles [52].

The plot of $v = Q_{Max}/Wh$, that is, the average fluid velocity in the duct, versus the value of ρ is plotted in Figure 10.22 assuming the parameter values in Table 10.2. Assuming the cell dielectric constant smaller than 100 is a very hypothesis, generally true for viruses. In the case of cells, the

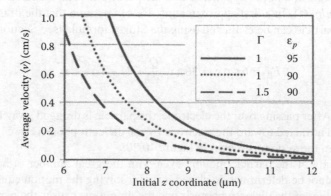

FIGURE 10.22 Maximum values of the average fluid velocity allowing cell capture by the electrode in the system of Figure 10.20.

TABLE 10.2
Parameters Used in the Example of Dielectrophoresis Capture of Cells

Duct Height	h	200 µm
Cell diameter	a	5 µm
Solvent viscosity	η	0.078 Pa s
Solvent relative dielectric constant	ε_L	78
Cell relative dielectric constant	ε_p	95
Voltage difference	$\Delta\psi$	20 V

value is generally quite higher; for example, the dielectric constant of *Escherichia coli* is around 400 [53]. It is evident that if the cells transit in the relative vicinity of the electrode, the velocity needed to avoid the capture is very high, out of the range of several lab on chip, thus confirming that cell capture over an electrode due to dielectrophoresis is possible with reasonable parameters values.

In practice, a further improvement of the capture capability of the electrode can be obtained by suitably designing the electrodes and channel geometry [54] and the interdigitated electrodes are used frequently [55].

Once the cell is captured by the electrode, different types of tests can be performed. Simple cell counting can be done by observing the measurement of the impedance of the electrodes of an array in front of a sudden voltage increase. Such an impedance is greatly affected by the presence of an electrode captured cell and by the fact that the cell lives or not [47]. A more complete impedance measure can be performed by adding a small alternate tension to the tension-causing cell capture by dielectrophoresis and measuring the induced current [56]. Complete impedance characterization can be used either to detect the level of activity inside the cell [57] or to detect the interaction of the cell membrane with suitable molecules that are patterned on the electrode surface [58].

10.3.4 IMPEDANCE MEASUREMENT TECHNIQUES

The impedance of an electrolytic cell provides a great deal of information on the substances that are present in the cell: the bulk resistance gives information on the conductivity of the bulk solution and the capacity provides information on the electrical double layer through the dielectric constant.

The last observation is particularly useful in case of target molecule fixing on the electrode, as we have also seen in the case of plasmon-based detection in Section 11.4.

In order to exploit this fact, the impedance of the cell has to be measured with great accuracy. Several methods exist to measure an unknown impedance, all based on some sort of electrical reference circuit, on a voltage generator and on a high-resolution amperometer [59,60].

The base method for the measurement of an unknown impedance is the so-called divider, whose circuit scheme is shown in Figure 10.23. The circuit converts the value of the unknown impedance in an electrical voltage that can be amplified and detected. Applying the Kirchhoff rules to the circuit and solving for the unknown impedance, we get

$$Z(\omega) = \frac{\psi_M}{\psi_M - \psi_0} Z_1$$

(10.39)

Repeating the measurement at different frequencies, an impedance–frequency curve or a Nyquist diagram can be obtained. Fitting one of those curves, more frequently the Nyquist diagram, with the cell impedance expression (10.9), the cell parameters can be obtained.

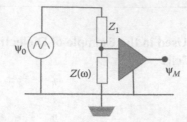

FIGURE 10.23 Circuit scheme of the voltage divider for impedance measurements.

The voltage divider is a very simple measurement circuit, and it is widely used when the measurement accuracy and sensitivity is not to be very high. However, several limitations arise when the measurement performances have to be pushed at the limit.

From Equation 10.39, it is evident that the accuracy in measuring $Z(\omega)$ critically depends on the accuracy with which Z_1 is known, since every error in the value of Z_1 directly reflects in a similar error in the value of $Z(\omega)$. As far as the driving voltage is concerned, it also has to be controlled with great accuracy in order to obtain an accurate measurement.

In addition, the voltage at the amplifier output ranges between ψ_M and $\psi_M Z/(Z + Z_1)$. This means that the amplifier has to be designed to amplify a signal intensity that is never zero. This limits the possible amplification range due to the intrinsic signal saturation and constitutes one of the limits of the voltage divider.

An impedance measurement method that overcomes this limitation is based on the Wheatstone bridge reference circuit, whose scheme is shown in Figure 10.24. The impedance under measure, in our case the electrolytic cell, is inserted in a bridge configuration with three known impedances. One or, more frequently, two of the known impedances can be changed by tracking their value with great precision. Several ways are available to realize such a configuration in an integrated electronic circuit or even directly on the lab on chip, if suitable materials and technologies are selected for its fabrication.

A known alternate voltage is applied to the points B and C of the bridge and the tension at the points A and D is amplified and measured. The bridge is operated by changing the known impedances to obtain a null measured voltage. This condition is generally called bridge balancing. When the bridge is balanced, it is easy to demonstrate with a direct application of Kirchhoff rules that

$$Z(\omega) = \frac{Z_1}{Z_2} Z_3 \tag{10.40}$$

As in the case of the voltage divider, by repeating the measurement at different frequencies and balancing every time the bridge, the Nyquist plot for the impedance under test can be obtained. This can be interpolated using Equation 10.9 to produce an estimation of the cell impedance parameters.

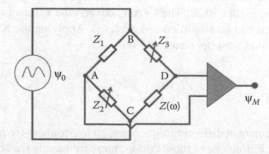

FIGURE 10.24 Scheme of a Wheatstone bridge for impedance measurements.

Since the Wheastone bridge is balanced before every measure, the average measured voltage is always zero, so that the low noise amplifier gain can be much higher than in the case of the divider without generating saturation at the output. This increases sensibly the measurement sensitivity in practical cases. Moreover, the driving voltage is not present in the expression of the measured impedance, so that it is not needed to control the driving voltage with great accuracy to obtain an accurate impedance measure.

From Equation 10.40, it is clear that the accuracy of the measurement is directly related to the accuracy with which the reference impedances are known. Moreover, by decomposing every reference impedance in its real and imaginary parts, it can be directly seen that the best accuracy is obtained in the case in which real and imaginary parts of all the impedances are known with an error of the same order of magnitude. As a matter of fact, if one of these parameters has an error much higher than the other, it is the worst-known parameter that mainly influences the final error on the measured impedance. Without carrying out all the computation with complex variables, this can be seen very simply also assuming having purely real or purely imaginary impedances.

The Wheatstone bridge sensitivity can be derived by considering what voltage is measured in correspondence of a small variation of the impedance under test. In an unbalanced situation, the application of the Kirchhoff rules to the bridge produces the following expression of the measured complex potential:

$$\psi_M = \psi_0 \left[\frac{Z_2}{Z_3 + Z_2} - \frac{Z_1}{Z_1 + Z} \right]$$ (10.41)

We can derive this expression with respect to the complex variable Z by using the rules of the derivation of functions of complex variable [61] attaining

$$\frac{d\psi_M}{dZ} = \frac{Z_1}{(Z_1 + Z)^2} \psi_0$$ (10.42)

If $|Z_1| \ll |Z|$, in order to balance the bridge $|Z_2| \ll |Z_3|$, it is also needed. In this condition, it is generally difficult to have the same accuracy in the knowledge of all the reference impedances, so obtain a measurement accuracy essentially determined by the impedances with the smaller real or imaginary part. In contrast, if $|Z_1| > |Z|$, the bridge sensitivity gets worse with at the increase of $|Z_1|$, as can be seen from Equation 10.18. Thus, it is very often that a Wheatstone bridge is designed so that the impedance Z_1 is approximately equal to the expected value of Z. In this case, Equation 10.42 simplifies greatly becoming

$$\frac{d\psi_M}{dZ} = \frac{\psi_0}{4Z}$$ (10.43)

Equation 10.43 can be used to obtain the sensitivity of the measure for the particular case under consideration. If we image, for example, that all the impedances are real, that is, they can be represented with resistances, the voltages can be continuous, since no frequency dependence is expected, so that we have the following expression for the relative resistance sensitivity:

$$\frac{dR}{R} = 4 \frac{d\psi_M}{\psi_0}$$ (10.44)

Owing to the high sensitivity attainable with the measure of ψ_M, great sensitivities can be attained using a Wheatstone bridge.

Measuring impedance by using the Wheatstone bridge and repeating the measure for different frequencies, that is, performing a frequency domain measure, is a very accurate procedure, but it is also long, requiring not only one measure for each frequency, but also requiring the bridge balancing to be repeated for each measure. When the measurement band is wide or a large number of points have to be obtained, this technique is not practical.

In these cases, a time domain measurement procedure can be used. The time domain measurement procedure is ideally based on the measure of the current flowing through the cell when an ideal tension step is applied at its extremes. In practice, it is carried out by changing the voltage at the cell extremes from zero to a constant voltage in a time much shorter than the inverse of the higher frequency at which the cell is expected to provide an electrical response.

An electrical potential step can be represented by means of the Heaviside function $\eta_H(t)$ that is equal to one for $t \geq 0$ and zero for $t < 0$ (see Section 7.4.3.2). Since impedance measurements imply the possibility to model the cell like a linear system, if we indicate the current flowing through the cell with $I(T)$, the time response to the step voltage of the cell can be modeled with a stationary linear operator that can be expressed as [62]

$$I(t) = \int_{-\infty}^{t} V_0 \eta_H(\tau) A(t - \tau) d\tau \tag{10.45}$$

The Fourier transform of the Heaviside function can be derived from its definition [62] getting

$$\mathfrak{F}\left\{\eta_H(t)\right\} = \pi \delta(\omega) + \frac{i}{\omega} \tag{10.46}$$

where the imaginary term comes from the Cauchy principal value of the related integral. By Fourier transforming both the terms (10.45), applying the convolution theorem, and neglecting the delta term in the origin that is generally filtered by the low-pass filter that avoids coupling of the measure instrument with continuous signals, we get

$$I(\omega) = \frac{V_0}{i\omega} A(\omega) d\tau \tag{10.47}$$

Thus, for the definition of impedance, we have

$$Z(\omega) = \frac{V_0}{i\omega I(\omega)} = \frac{1}{A(\omega)} \quad \omega > \omega_B \tag{10.48}$$

where ω_B is the low-frequency limit of the measuring instrument bandwidth.

The Fourier transform can be digitally executed in real time with great accuracy using fast Fourier transform algorithms [63] so that the time domain method is very effective in terms of measurement time and bandwidth, but has a smaller sensitivity with respect to the frequency domain method that uses a Wheatstone bridge arrangement. Moreover, the time domain method has the weakness of losing accuracy and sensitivity when the module of the impedance is very large. In this case, the module of $A(\omega)$ is very small and even small percentage errors reflect in large errors in the estimation of $Z(\omega)$.

10.4 VOLTAMMETRY DETECTION

Under the general name of voltammetry, a large set of electrochemical sensing methods are collected having in common the fact that a RedOx reaction happens in the electrolytic cell while voltage is varied and the resulting current is measured [64]. As in all Faradaic electrochemical procedures, the analyte has to be a RedOx species while the conjugate species can either be present in the cell before the test, or more frequently only be created during the test due to the applied voltage.

The voltammetry output is a current versus voltage plot, also called a voltammogram. Depending on the configuration of the measure, either the anode or the cathode currents are measured, or both of them in particular configurations. In order to clarify the voltammogram meaning, the cathode and the anode currents are represented with different signs on the plot. The IUPAC standard prescribes that the anode current is represented as positive and the cathode current as negative, while positive potential differences are represented on the positive potential axis. In the literature, however, another convention is also used that was introduced by the American Polarographic Society; it prescribes assigning the positive sign to the cathode current and representing potentials in the inverse sense on the ordinate axis, that is, positive on the left side and negative on the right side, so as to grow from right to left. Since both the conventions are used in practice, the way in which a voltammogram is built is to be clear before facing the voltammogram interpretation.

The Nernst equation (see Appendix A5) referring to the whole RedOx reaction in the case of an unpolarized cell is written in exponential form as

$$\frac{\overline{c}_o}{\overline{c}_R} = e^{\frac{q\, n_e}{\kappa_B T}(\psi - \psi_0)} \tag{10.49}$$

where ψ_0 is the so-called RedOx potential or formal potential of the reaction and $\overline{c}_R$, $\overline{c}_o$ are the surface concentrations of the two elements R and O of the RedOx couple near the surfaces of the electrodes. When there is no applied potential, the cell is at equilibrium. In the case in which $q n_e \psi_0 \ll \kappa_B T$, the RedOx elements have similar concentrations near the electrodes and, since we are at equilibrium, in the solution bulk. Conversely, if the formal potential is sufficiently high that $q n_e \psi_0 \gg \kappa_B T$, at equilibrium, one species only has an appreciable concentration in the solution, and no appreciable current flows in the cell. This is generally the starting situation of a voltammetry measure whose scope is to quantify the presence of a species in a solution or to study its redox characteristics.

Conversely, if $|q n_e \psi| \gg \kappa_B T$, the concentration of O near the cathode is negligible with respect to the concentration of R near the anode. Since in the typical voltammetry experiment O was the only species that was initially present in the solution, the opposite happens in the cell bulk, where the reduced species concentration is negligible with the oxidized one. Thus, the cathode current dominates the process and the cathode is called the working electrode, while the anode is called the counterelectrode.

The opposite happens for a positive applied potential much greater than the module of the formal potential; in this case, it is the surface concentration of R to be negligible besides the anode while almost only R is present in the solution bulk. Thus, the anode current drives the electrolytic process and the anode is called the working electrode.

A voltammetry detection exploits these dynamics to detect the current change occurring when the external potential is changed so as to pass from equilibrium, where a small current passes through the cell, to the working electrode current-driven regime, where the current passing through the cell is relevant.

In principle, the voltammetry electrolytic cell is a standard cell with a working electrode and a second electrode, both closing the RedOx reaction and providing the potential reference. This configuration, however, presents a few practical problems. On the one hand, the second electrode has to be suitably entered in the RedOx reaction; on the other hand, in order to be a good voltage reference, it should be completely neutral. This is to avoid errors in the acquisition of the reference potential that influences the whole measurement.

For this reason, a three electrode electrolytic cell is generally used. Both the cathode and the anode potentials are measured with respect to a third electrode that is constructed with a completely neutral metal and placed far from the electrodes where the RedOx reaction happens. In the case of lab on chip, this solution can be difficult to integrate in the chip, both for the restricted choice of metals with which the electrodes can be realized and for the small dimension of the cell. In this case, the reference electrode is frequently placed in a parallel reference chamber where a solution similar to that present in the detection room is present, but no voltage is applied and no reaction happens.

The electrode surface preparation is another important element in voltammetry detection. Functionalized electrodes can be used in particular cases to fix the target on the electrode, but commonly the electrodes are clean metal surfaces because the target molecules are attracted near the electrode by the electrical field that is present in the cell and by the concentration gradient that forms due to the reaction.

In many biochemical cases, the sample is ions reach so that an ion double layer is created around the electrodes. In this condition, the potential in the cell bulk is equal to the zeta potential relative to the particular solution and cell. This is not however the potential that molecules react in the electrodes experiment. Owing to both diffusion and electrostatic attraction, target molecules penetrate the Debye and the Stern layers to arrive in strict contact with the electrode, as it is necessary to generate an electron exchange. In this condition, the double-layer screen exists no more, justifying the fact that it is the potential applied at the cell electrodes to influence the electrochemical reaction instead of the zeta potential that is present in the solution bulk.

10.4.1 Step Voltammetry or Chronoamperometry

The simplest case of voltammetry is the so-called step voltammetry. This electrochemical technique is also called chronoamperometry because, differently from other voltammetry methods, the current versus time is measured instead of current versus voltage. We prefer to deal with this method besides other voltammetry methods because its analysis is carried out with typical voltammetry methods.

In the step voltammetry case, the cell is fed with a step potential, that is, with a potential passing from zero to the final value in a very small time with respect to the mass transport in the cell. In the absence of fluid mass motion or other active phenomena, mass transport in the cell is due to diffusion so that, to perform step voltammetry, the applied voltage pulse has to be much faster than diffusion of the target species in the cell. Representing the applied pulse as in Figure 10.25, we can write this condition in mathematical terms as

$$t_v \ll \frac{L_c^2}{D} \tag{10.50}$$

where L_c is the cell length and D is the smaller of the diffusion coefficients of the RedOx species. Assuming that small molecules are targeted with $D = 5 \times 10^{-10}$ (see Section 7.4.2) and considering

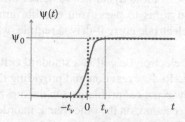

FIGURE 10.25 Voltage pulse used for step voltammetry.

an electrode distance equal to 50 µm, we get $t_v \ll 5s$, that is, a very easy condition to be fulfilled assuming, for example, that $t_v = 1$ ms.

Since the pulse rise time is not shorter than the electron transfer time, it is possible to assume that as soon as the voltage overcomes the formal reaction voltage, the molecules that are present on the electrode interface are instantly reduced and oxidized so that the current flowing through the cell rises at the same pace of the voltage pulse up to the moment when the electrode surface is completely depleted of RedOx molecules. In order to provide new RedOx molecule to the interface and maintain the reaction, new molecules have to diffuse from the bulk toward the electrodes. This is a slow process, however, with respect to the rise time of the applied pulse; thus, its time dynamics can be observed after the pulse end.

At the very beginning, new molecules are provided by the solution zones very near to the electrodes, so that the diffusion time is relatively short. While the reaction goes on, the solution is depleted of RedOx molecules in zones farther from the electrodes, the diffusion time increases and the current decreases. Thus, we have to expect a measured current pulse increasing at the beginning at the same pace of the applied voltage pulse and then decreasing at the slow pace related to the diffusion process.

In order to elaborate a simple model of this mechanism, let us consider both the voltage pulse rise and the electron transfer as instantaneous phenomena, so as to represent the applied voltage pulse with a Heaviside function, represented by the dotted line in Figure 10.25. Let us also consider a parallelepiped cell geometry with plane electrodes deposited on the opposite sides of the cell, so that the half-cell containing the working electrode can be represented as in Figure 10.26.

If the observation time is smaller than L_c^2/D, it is possible to assume that the solution bulk near the center of the cell is not sensibly depleted and that the RedOx molecules concentration maintains constancy in the cell if we get sufficiently far from the electrodes. In this condition, in order to study the evolution of the concentration of one of the RedOx species, we can consider a mathematically semi-infinite setting, a reference system with the origin in the electrode position, assuming that the concentration of the target molecule at infinity is constant and equal to the species concentration in the cell before the start of the voltammetry. This model is shown in Figure 10.26.

Considering the anode where the oxidation occurs, semireaction (10.13b), we now want to estimate the concentration of the species R. Under the assumed hypothesis and considering the electrodes as infinite planes, we have to solve the diffusion equation

$$\frac{\partial c_R}{\partial t} = D_R \frac{\partial^2 c_R}{\partial x^2} \tag{10.51}$$

with the following conditions:

$$\lim_{x \to \infty} c_R(x,t) = c_{R0} \tag{10.52a}$$

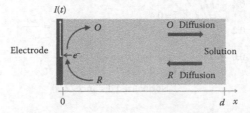

FIGURE 10.26 Scheme of half the step voltammetry cell for the evaluation of the mass transport effect.

$$c_R(0,t) = \frac{\bar{c}_R}{\delta} \tag{10.52b}$$

$$c_R(x,0) = c_{R0} \tag{10.52c}$$

where c_{R0} is the initial concentration of R, that is, in the cell bulk, $\bar{c}_R$ is the surface concentration on the anode, and δ is the very small distance from the electrode at which the oxidation can happen.

The solution of this equation can be obtained directly with the Green function method (see Section 7.4.3) getting

$$c_R(x,t) = \left(c_{R0} - \frac{\bar{c}_R}{\delta} \right) \text{erf} \left(\frac{x}{2\sqrt{Dt}} \right) + \frac{\bar{c}_R}{\delta} \tag{10.53}$$

If the axis origin $x = 0$ is set at the working electrode, we can set $\bar{c}_R = 0$ so that Equation 10.53 simplifies as

$$c_R(x,t) = c_{R0}\text{erf} \left(\frac{x}{2\sqrt{Dt}} \right) \tag{10.54}$$

The behavior of the concentration $c_R(x,t)$ in space and time is shown in Figure 10.27, assuming that the progressive depletion of the solution due to the anodic reaction is evident.

If a real instantaneous voltage pulse would be applied to the cell, we will observe a transitory current that is formed by two distinct terms: a Faradaic term due to the RedOx reaction and a non-Faradaic term due to the accumulation of charges near the electrodes due to the double-layer formation. In reality, we are using a pulse rise time that is, very fast with respect to diffusion times, but not fast with respect to the double layer formation time, that is, of the order of a few milliseconds. Thus, we can assume that the double layer will form at the same pace of the pulse rise so that the non-Faradaic current contribution is not observed.

The Faradaic current per unit electrode area $J(t)$ is due to electron exchange at electrodes and in our case, where the anode is the working electrode, it is proportional to the number of oxidized molecule for unit time, to the number of released electrons per molecules, and to the electron charge.

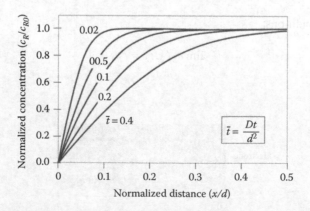

FIGURE 10.27 Concentration profiles at different times of the analyte, that is, also the driving electrolyte, in a step voltammetry cell.

The number of oxidized molecules for unit time at the anode is simply the flux of the concentration in the anode position, so that we can write the current as

$$J(t) = q \, n_e \, N_A \, k_{ox} \, D_R \left. \frac{\partial c_R(x,t)}{\partial x} \right)_{x=0} = q n_e N_A k_{ox} c_{R0} \sqrt{\frac{D_R}{\pi t}} \tag{10.55}$$

As expected by the slow diffusion dynamics, the current density decreases in time as the inverse of the square root of time, as shown in Figure 10.28, where the following definition of the limit voltammetry current is used:

$$J_0 = q n_e N_A k_{ox} c_{R0} \frac{L_c}{t_v} \tag{10.56}$$

where L_c is the cell length and t_v the voltage pulse rise time.

It is to be noted that Equation 10.55 diverges for $t = 0$. This is a consequence of the physical impossibility of having a perfectly instantaneous growth of the voltage pulse in the origin. Thus, if we observe the current density for times of the order of the voltage pulse rise time, it deviates slightly from Equation 10.55, manifesting a very short peak and tending to zero at the instant in which the voltage pulse is applied. In general, the short time dynamics is of no use in step voltammetry detection and the observed current is simply fitted with Equation 10.55 up to the instant t_v in which the voltage pulse arrives at the final value.

The current density depends on the target molecule concentration; thus, if the diffusion coefficient is known, step voltammetry can be used to quantify the target in the sample solution. Owing to the dependence of the current density on the diffusion coefficient, step voltammetry is also frequently used to estimate the diffusion coefficient of macromolecules using reference solutions whose concentration is well known.

Step voltammetry has been extensively used in lab on chip in several different configurations, for example, to detect specific DNA segments and to detect and drive the genes switch activity [65,66], to detect enzymes activity [67], and to detect the presence of a large number of organic and inorganic molecules [68,69]. Step voltammetry can also be applied in droplet systems using small electrodes for the characterization of electrochemical processes confined inside the droplets (see Section 8.6) [70].

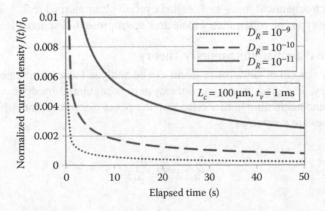

FIGURE 10.28 Time dependence of the measured current in step voltammetry. These curves are frequently called chronoamperometry plots.

10.4.2 VARIABLE POTENTIAL VOLTAMMETRY

Although step voltammetry is widely used, in a typical voltammetry measure, the voltage applied to the cell varies in time in a sufficiently slow manner to allow the charge distribution near the electrode to vary in pace with the applied potential. The measured current is then plot versus the applied voltage to represent the data and to interpret them [1,71].

The simpler voltammetry experiment with a varying potential is linear scan voltammetry [72,73]. In this case, the applied potential has the form

$$\psi(t) = \psi_m + \psi' t \quad 0 < t < t_F \tag{10.57}$$

where t_F is the measurement duration and ψ' is the scar rate. Another interesting case of variable potential voltammetry is the square wave voltammetry [74], where the applied potential is a square wave with period Λ so that

$$\psi(t) = \begin{cases} \psi_M & h\Lambda < t < \beta\Lambda + h\Lambda & \forall h \in \mathbb{Z} \\ \psi_m & \beta\Lambda + h\Lambda < t < (h+1)\Lambda & \forall h \in \mathbb{Z} \end{cases} \tag{10.58}$$

where $\psi_M > \psi_0$, $0 < \beta < 1$ is the square wave duty cycle and, as indicated, h is a generic integer number. Linear square wave voltammetry is a fairly well used combination of linear and square wave voltammetry [75]. In this case,

$$\psi(t) = \begin{cases} \psi_m + \psi' t & h\Lambda < t < \beta\Lambda + h\Lambda & \forall h \in \mathbb{Z} \\ \psi_m - \Delta\psi + \psi' t & \beta\Lambda + h\Lambda < t < (h+1)\Lambda & \forall h \in \mathbb{Z} \end{cases} \tag{10.59}$$

All the above examples of variable potential voltammetry are used in practice; however, the one most used and of variable potential is a triangular periodic wave, so that

$$\psi(t) = \begin{cases} \psi_m + \psi'(t - h\Lambda) & h\Lambda < t < 0.5\Lambda + h\Lambda & \forall h \in \mathbb{Z} \\ \psi_m + \psi' 0.5\Lambda - \psi'(t - 0.5\Lambda - h\Lambda) & 0.5\Lambda + h\Lambda < t < (h+1)\Lambda & \forall h \in \mathbb{Z} \end{cases} \tag{10.60}$$

This kind of electrochemical measure is called cyclic voltammetry [76,77]. The potential waves used in the different types of voltammetry measures are represented schematically in Figure 10.29.

10.4.2.1 Variable Potential Voltammetry Theory

Under a mathematical point of view, the problem can be analyzed using the same procedure adopted for step voltammetry. The mass transport in the system is regulated by diffusion, and assuming a parallelepiped cell and neglecting border effects on the plane electrodes, the diffusion equations for the two redox species are written as

$$\frac{\partial c_R}{\partial t} = D_R \frac{\partial^2 c_R}{\partial x^2} \tag{10.61a}$$

$$\frac{\partial c_o}{\partial t} = D_o \frac{\partial^2 c_o}{\partial x^2} \tag{10.61b}$$

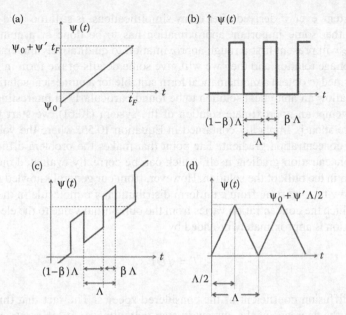

FIGURE 10.29 Selected potential dependence on time in different types of voltammetry: linear voltammetry (a), square wave voltammetry (b), linear square wave voltammetry (c), and cyclic voltammetry (d).

These equations have to be solved with boundary and initial conditions. In particular, we have the following set of conditions:

- The bulk concentrations at the initial instant have to coincide with the concentrations in the sample, that is

$$c_R(x,0) = c_{R0}, \quad c_o(x,0) = c_{o0} \tag{10.62}$$

- The bulk concentrations have to be maintained constant during the measurement, that is

$$\lim_{x \to \infty} c_R(x,t) = c_{R0}, \quad \lim_{x \to \infty} c_o(x,t) = c_{o0} \tag{10.63}$$

- Since the number of electrons absorbed at the anode has to be equal to the number of electrons released at the cathode, the flux of the species R and O has to be opposite to that at the working electrode; thus, it has to be

$$D_R \left. \frac{\partial c_R}{\partial x} \right)_{x=0} + D_o \left. \frac{\partial c_o}{\partial x} \right)_{x=0} = 0 \tag{10.64}$$

- The current has to be continuous at the working electrode; thus, the net number of electrons generated has to be equal to the net flux of one of the species. Thus,

$$D_o \left. \frac{\partial c_o}{\partial x} \right)_{x=0} = k_{red} c_o(0,t) - k_{ox} c_R(0,t) \tag{10.65}$$

The above system, even if derived after many simplifications, is still too hard to be solved analytically; thus, either some important approximation has to be done or a numerical solution is needed. First, we will present first a rough approximation to qualitatively understand the behavior of the current–voltage relation and then we will give some details of the form in which the system (10.61) is transformed to obtain a mathematical form suitable for a numerical solution. This transformation will also allow an analytical solution to be found particularly in interesting cases.

In order to attempt an approximate solution of the system (10.61), we start to notice that the current–voltage relation is implicitly contained in Equation 10.55, where the voltage contribution is merged in the concentration gradient. The point that makes the problem difficult to solve is to determine the concentration gradient itself, which can be correctly evaluated only by solving the diffusion problem in the bulk of the solution. However, from our general knowledge of the diffusion problems, we know that, starting from a uniform distribution of a molecule in the electrolytic cell, the distance in which the concentration varies from the bulk initial value to the electrode value after potential application is approximately provided by

$$l = \sqrt{Dt} \tag{10.66}$$

where D is the diffusion coefficient of the considered species. The fact that this distance grows with time causes the decrease of the current in step voltammetry experiments, which is just proportional to the inverse of δ. Starting from this consideration, considering both the equations, allowing evaluation of the flowing current from the cathode and the anode reactions, we can try the approximation

$$J(t) = qn_e N_A k_{ox} D_R \left. \frac{\partial c_R(x,t)}{\partial x} \right)_{x=0} \approx qn_e N_A k_{ox} D_R \frac{c_R(0,t) - c_{R\infty}}{\sqrt{D_R t}} \tag{10.67a}$$

$$J(t) = -qn_e N_A k_{red} D_o \left. \frac{\partial c_R(x,t)}{\partial x} \right)_{x=0} \approx -qn_e N_A k_{red} D_o \frac{c_o(0,t) - c_{o\infty}}{\sqrt{D_o t}} \tag{10.67b}$$

where $c_{R\infty}$ and $c_{o\infty}$ indicate concentration in the solution bulk. Let us now assume that the anode is the driving electrode, being $c_{o0} = 0$. Under this condition, we can assume $c_{R\infty} \approx c_{R0}$ and $c_{o\infty} \ll c_{R0}$. Moreover, since the cathode and anode currents have to be equal, we can write

$$k_{red} \sqrt{D_o} \left[c_o(0,t) - c_{o\infty} \right] \approx k_{red} \sqrt{D_o} \, c_o(0,t) = k_{ox} \sqrt{D_R} \, c_{R0} \tag{10.68}$$

Using the Nernst equation for the whole cell and substituting to surface concentrations with volume concentration, we get

$$\psi = \psi_0 + \frac{\kappa_B T}{q n_e} \log\left(\frac{k_{ox} D_R}{k_{red} D_o} \right) + \frac{\kappa_B T}{q n_e} log\left(1 - \frac{A_R}{J} \frac{c_{R0}}{\sqrt{D_R t}} \right)$$

$$= \psi_{1/2} + \frac{\kappa_B T}{q n_e} log\left(1 - \frac{A_R}{J} \frac{c_{R0}}{\sqrt{D_R t}} \right) \tag{10.69}$$

where we have assumed that the depth of the layers at which the reaction happens is equal at the anode and at the cathode and we have used the approximation in Equation 10.68 to express $c_o(0,t)$ as a function of c_{R0}. The following parameters have also been defined:

$$\psi_{1/2} = \psi_0 + \frac{\kappa_B T}{q n_e} \log\left(\frac{k_{ox} D_R}{k_{red} D_o}\right) \tag{10.70}$$

and

$$A_R = q n_e N_A k_{red} D_R \tag{10.71}$$

Inverting Equation 10.67, we get

$$J = \frac{A_R}{1 + e^{(q n_e / \kappa_B T)(\psi - \psi_{1/2})}} \frac{c_{R0}}{\sqrt{D_R t}} \tag{10.72}$$

The last step to obtain a current–voltage relation is to express the time as a function of the voltage exploiting the voltage wave shape. Considering as an example the simplest case, that is, the linear sweep voltammetry, we have from the equation

$$t = \frac{\psi - \psi_m}{\psi'} \tag{10.73}$$

so that we obtain

$$J = \frac{A_R}{1 + e^{(q n_e / \kappa_B T)(\psi - \psi_{1/2})}} \frac{c_{R0}}{\sqrt{D_R (\psi - \psi_m / \psi')}} \tag{10.74}$$

We cannot expect from Equation 10.74 a good quantitative reproduction of the shape of the current–voltage relation, essentially due to the coarse approximation of the concentration gradient we have used. In particular, we have to expect that, as is evident looking at Figure 10.27, the error that is implied in this approximation changes in time, thus influencing the relation shape. On the other hand, we have to expect that all the main qualitative elements of the characteristics have to be present in Equation 10.74.

The first element to verify is the dependence of the maximum value of the current density of the different parameters of the measure. Deriving Equation 10.74 and setting the derivatives to zero, we get the following expression of the maximum value J_M of the current density:

$$J_M = q n_e N_A k_{red} \sqrt{D_R} \sqrt{\psi'} \, c_{R0} f(n_e) \tag{10.75}$$

The function $f(n_e)$ is the solution of a transcendental equation and it can be evaluated numerically. The function $f(n_e)$ is plotted in Figure 10.30 versus n_e for the voltammetry parameters listed in Table 10.3. The deviation from the proportionality to the square root of n_e in this case and in all the ranges of physically acceptable parameters is not greater than 10%. Thus, we can write

$$J_M = F \sqrt{n_e^3} \, k_{red} \sqrt{D_R} \sqrt{\psi'} \, c_{R0} \tag{10.76}$$

where F is a constant. Equation 10.76 reflects the well-known empirical law for the maximum current of a linear voltammetry in case of a fast electron exchange reaction and it expresses correctly the dependence of the maximum current on the main parameters of the experiment [71]. It is not

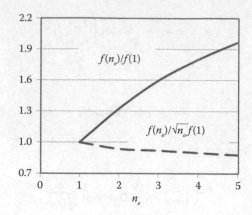

FIGURE 10.30 Plot of the function $f(n_e)$ introduced in the text and of $f(n_e)/\sqrt{n_e}$ for the parameters reported in Table 10.3.

surprising that approximation (10.74) works better for fast electron exchange, since the faster the exchange, the more the expression of the problem solution in the form of a product of a slow term (the square root) and of a fast term (the exponential term) is correct because the fast term can be considered an adiabatic evolution with respect to the slow term.

If a more accurate expression of the current–voltage characteristics has to be obtained, a numerical solution of the system (10.61) is required. This system can be solved directly using algorithms for the numerical integration of differential equations, but frequently numerical solutions are attained after transformation with the unilateral Laplace transform method. This procedure not only produces an integral equation that can be solved numerically with efficient algorithms, but also allows particular exact solutions to be discovered, which has quite a practical importance.

The first step is to transform Equation 10.65 by using the Nernst equation to divide the applied potential between the electrode partial reactions and using Equations 10.28 to relate the surface concentrations entering in the Nernst law with the volume concentrations at the electrode position.

TABLE 10.3
Parameters Used in the Example of Approximated Calculation of the Linear Voltammetry Maximum Current

Parameter	Value	Unit
δ_{an}	1	nm
k_{ox}	10^{-4}	s
D_R	10^{-10}	m²/s
n_e	1	
c_{o0}	1	m⁻³
$\kappa_B T$	4.14×10^{-21}	J
ψ_0	−3	V
$\psi_{1/2}$	0.5	V
ψ'	0.3	V/s
t_v	40	s
A	2.5×10^{-7}	m²

We obtain

$$D_o \frac{\partial c_o}{\partial x}\bigg)_{x=0} = k_{st}\, e^{-\alpha \frac{q\,n_e}{\kappa_B T}(\psi-\psi_0)} \left[c_o(0,t) - c_R(0,t) e^{\frac{q\,n_e}{\kappa_B T}(\psi-\psi_0)} \right] \tag{10.77}$$

where k_{st} is the reaction rate for $\psi = \psi_0$. The first exponential term at the second member can be divided into two terms: the first containing only the formal potential and the second containing only the applied potential. The term containing the formal potential, for the Nernst equation again, is equal to the ratio between the bulk concentrations of the redox species, but for the electron exchange efficiency term α. The second term is a known function, a sort of effective driving term of the process, and we can set

$$S(t) = e^{\frac{qn_e}{\kappa_B T}\psi(t)} \tag{10.78}$$

The same procedure can be applied to the second exponential term, so that Equation 10.77 can be rewritten as

$$D_o \frac{\partial c_o}{\partial x}\bigg)_{x=0} = \frac{k_{st}}{(c_{o0}/c_{R0})^\alpha\, S^\alpha(t)} \left[c_o(0,t) - c_R(0,t) S(t) \frac{c_{o0}}{c_{R0}} \right] \tag{10.79}$$

At this point, the derivative $\partial c_o/\partial x$ can be derived from Equation 10.61a by Laplace transforming with respect to time and integrating the resulting ordinary differential equation with the suitable conditions, as was already done in Section 10.3.1. The result can be substituted in Equation 10.79 after setting $x = 0$. A linear integral equation is thus obtained, which is equivalent to the initial differential problems with its initial and boundary conditions.

In order to approach a numerical solution of such an equation, it is generally supposed that the potential dependence on time is either linear or a periodic function that is composed of linear segments with the same absolute value of the potential rate ψ'. This is a fairly general assumption considering the potential shapes that are shown in Figure 10.29. Under this assumption, the integral equation is written in terms of nondimensional variables and parameter settings

$$\Gamma_D = \sqrt{\frac{D_o}{D_R}} \tag{10.80a}$$

$$\tau = \frac{q\,n_e}{\kappa_B T}\,\psi'\, t \tag{10.80b}$$

$$\chi(\tau) = \frac{1}{c_{o0}} \sqrt{\frac{\kappa_B T D}{\pi q n_e \psi'}}\, \frac{\partial c_o}{\partial x}\bigg)_{x=0} \tag{10.80c}$$

$$\Psi = \Gamma_D^\alpha\, k_{st} \sqrt{\frac{\kappa_B T}{\pi q n_e \psi' D_o}} \tag{10.80d}$$

Using these parameters, the integral equation is written as

$$\frac{\chi(\tau)}{\Psi}\left[\Gamma_D \frac{c_{o0}}{c_{R0}} S(\tau)\right]^{\alpha} = 1 - S(\tau) - \int_0^{\tau} \frac{\chi(w)}{\sqrt{\tau - w}}\, dw - \Gamma_D \frac{c_{o0}}{c_{R0}} S(\tau) \int_0^{\tau} \frac{\chi(w)}{\sqrt{\tau - w}}\, dw \qquad (10.81)$$

The integral that is present at the second member of Equation 10.69 is obtained by Laplace transform; thus, it has to be interpreted as a Cauchy principal value, that is

$$\int_0^{\tau} \frac{\chi(w)}{\sqrt{\tau - w}}\, d\tau = \lim_{z \to \tau} \int_0^{\tau} \frac{\chi(w)}{\sqrt{z - w}}\, dz \qquad (10.82)$$

Owing to the slow divergence of the term $1/\sqrt{x}$ with x, this limit converges in all the cases in which $\chi(\tau)$ is a regular function, that is, in all the relevant cases. However, the nature of the integral has to be always taken into account when operating on it, for example, to calculate its derivative with respect to τ.

It is to be noted that if Ψ is sufficiently large, the first member becomes negligible, and Equation 10.81 simplifies greatly as

$$\int_0^{\tau} \frac{\chi(w)}{\sqrt{\tau - w}}\, dw = \frac{1 - S(\tau)}{1 - \Gamma_D(c_{o0}/c_{R0})S(\tau)} \qquad (10.83)$$

This equation can be directly formulated as a function of the current flowing through the cell, since the current is related to the flux of the RedOx species at the driving electrode through Equation 10.55. It derives

$$\chi(\tau) = \frac{1}{c_{R0}}\sqrt{\frac{\kappa_B T}{\pi q^3 n_e^3 D_o \psi'}}\frac{J(\tau)}{N_A k_{st}} = \chi_0 J(\tau) \qquad (10.84)$$

Substituting Equation 10.71 into Equation 10.70 and returning to normal variables and parameters, it is obtained as

$$\int_0^t \frac{J(w)}{\sqrt{t - w}}\, dw = N_A\, k_{st}\, c_{R0}\sqrt{\frac{\pi q^3 n_e^3 D_o \psi'}{\kappa_B T}}\frac{1 - e^{(qn_e/\kappa_B T)\psi(t)}}{1 - \sqrt{(D_o/D_R)}(c_{o0}/c_{R0})e^{(qn_e/\kappa_B T)\psi(t)}} \qquad (10.85)$$

This is an integral form of the current voltage characteristic of voltammetry in this particular case and, when the approximation of large Ψ can be used, it can be adopted to interpolate experimental data. In particular, from the observed values of the current, the first member can be estimated and compared with the second member for data interpretation.

The large Ψ approximation is not infrequent in practice. It implies either a large reaction rate or a slow applied potential rate, since in both cases $S^{\alpha}(\tau)/\Psi$ is small with respect to the other terms of the equation. It is to be underlined that the case of a very fast reaction rate corresponds to the case of a completely reversible RedOx reaction, a case in which Equation 10.70 can be derived independently.

Since the approximation (10.72) holds in the case of fast electron exchange, it has to provide the dependence of the maximum current on the system parameters evidenced in Equation 10.76. This can be simply demonstrated on the ground of the expression of the factor appearing in front of the potential function at the first member. As a matter of fact, if we normalize the current with this factor and evaluate the maximum of the obtained normalization function, whatever this maximum is, the resulting current maximum results are proportional to the normalization factor. Thus, Equation 10.76 is obtained again.

In contrast, Ψ approaches zero for very small values of the large reaction rate, so that Equation 10.79 simplifies as

$$J(t) = k_{st} \sqrt{\frac{\kappa_B T}{\pi\, q\, n_e \psi' D_o}}\; e^{\frac{-2\alpha q n_e}{\kappa_B T}\psi(t)} \left(\frac{c_{o0}}{c_{RO}}\right)^{\alpha} \tag{10.86}$$

where we have again used Equation 10.71. This is an explicit voltage–current relationship, holding for slow reactions, in a case in which the RedOx reaction appears to be not reversible.

10.4.2.2 Linear Voltammetry

We have used the example of linear voltammetry to obtain explicit expression of the general voltammetry equation in the above paragraph: in general terms, the linear voltammetry current–potential curve can be obtained by numerically solving Equation 10.69, while explicit results can be obtained in the cases of fast electron exchange and slow electron exchange, corresponding to perfectly reversible and perfectly irreversible RedOx reactions.

The typical current–potential curve resulting from linear sweep voltammetry of a single RedOx couple is represented in Figure 10.31. This curve is calculated by using Equation 10.85 with the parameters in Table 10.3 and it is compared with the curve obtained by Equation 10.74. The profile obtained by Equation 10.74 fails to correctly reproduce the rising shape of the characteristics, while it reproduces the falloff part, mainly due to the increase of the diffusion characteristic length. The dependence of the current–voltage characteristics on the scan rate and on the electron exchange rate is shown in Figure 10.32.

In realistic sweep voltammetry experiments, besides the presence of an almost unavoidable spurious current, adding a linearly increasing plateau to the sweep voltammetry curve, several RedOx species are present in the sample. Some of them are part of the sample itself, for example, being different molecules that have to be quantified; others come from either imperfect purification or unwanted sample contamination. The resulting linear sweep voltammetry is not clean as shown in Figure 10.31. An example of the linear sweep voltammetry curve obtained by the RedOx reactions of two RedOx couples is reported in Figure 10.33 [78]. In this case, two voltammetry peaks are clearly visible due to the two possible RedOx reactions. This is due to the fact that the formal potential is a fingerprint of a RedOx couple and it is almost impossible to find different couples with the same formal potential, especially when complex molecules are considered. Thus, the formal

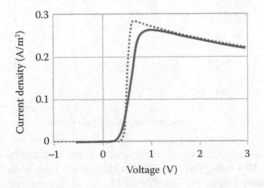

FIGURE 10.31 Typical current–potential curve resulting from linear sweep voltammetry of a single RedOx couple (continuous line) compared with the curve obtained by Equation 10.74 (dotted line).

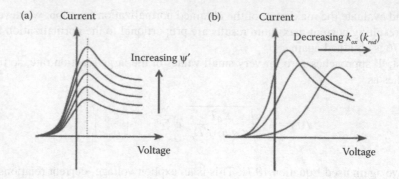

FIGURE 10.32 Dependence of the current–voltage characteristics on the scan rate (a) and on the electron exchange rate (b).

potential can be used as a fingerprint to recognize the different species that participate in the same voltammetry experiment.

The procedure to identify all the species that are present in a sample when the voltammetry peaks can be directly recognized can be described with the following steps:

- The contribution of the spurious current is eliminated by interpolating the straight curve, which is the base of the measured voltammetry characteristic.
- The different peaks are insulated and the formal potential is identified.
- The different molecules are identified through the formal potential.
- The measured curve is fitted with a theoretical curve obtained by a superposition of the curves relative to every single RedOx couple.
- The values of the maximum of each observed peak are estimated.
- Each species is quantified by using the property that the current maximum is proportional to the initial concentration of the analyte.

Cases are present, however, when the different voltammetry peaks cannot be easily separated. An extreme example is shown in Figure 10.34 where the voltammetry characteristic relative to a sample containing three different substances is shown [79] (the considered substances are pesticides

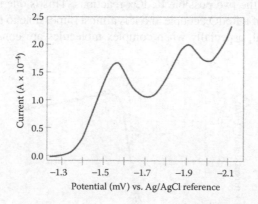

FIGURE 10.33 Example of the linear sweep voltammetry curve obtained by two RedOx couples: reductive cleavage of CCl_4 in DMF + n-Bu_4NBF_4 at 300 K with a glassy carbon electrode. Scan rate: 200 mV/s. (Reprinted from *Electrochimica Acta*, vol. 49, Prasad M. A., Sangaranarayanan M. V., Formulation of a simple analytical expression for irreversible electron transfer processes in linear sweep voltammetry and its experimental verification, pp. 2569–2579, Copyright 2004, with permission from Elsevier.)

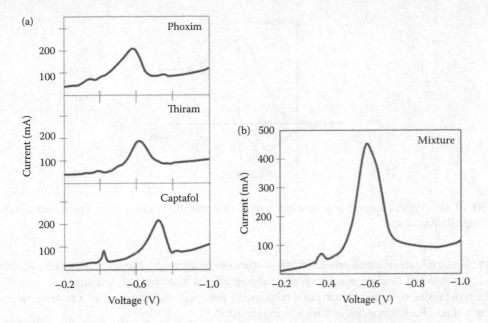

FIGURE 10.34 Example of a single peak voltammetry characteristic obtained by a sample containing three different substances; mixed sample voltammetry result (b) and voltammetry results for the individual components (a). (Data from Qiu P., Ni Y.-N., Kokot S. *Chinese Chemical Letters*, vol. 24, March pp. 246–248, 2013.)

used in fruit cultivation). The three substances reveal different formal potentials when tested separately, but the voltammetry when executed on a mixture of the three substances shows a single peak due to the small distances among the formal potentials. The first way to detect that a single peak like that is not due to a single RedOx reaction but due to the combination of several reactions is the fact that the peak shape is not fitted by the shape of a classical voltammetry. Frequently, this information is also known *a priori* by the knowledge of the sample.

If the elements constituting the sample are known, the knowledge of the individual voltammetry characteristics can be used to decompose the measured curve in the sum of individual contributions and to quantify the sample components. Several algorithms have been proposed to perform the individual peak separation, ranging from heuristic curve fitting [80] to genetic [81] and neural network-based [79] algorithms. A comparison of the selected techniques is reported in Reference [82].

Linear voltammetry has been used in lab on chip in different configurations [83–85]. In the lab on chip application, the case of plane electrodes is by far more common; in general, the effect of the electrode shape has been analyzed in the case of several possible electrode shapes. This is an interesting issue because the electrode shape influences the diffusion process, thus partially determining the shape of the descending tail of the voltammetry curve. This is, for example, an important point when nearby peaks have to be distinguished since the interference of a peak on the others depends on the shape of the peak tail. Spherical [86] and cylindrical [87] electrodes have been analyzed in detail and applied in practice in macroscopic voltammetry experiments.

10.4.2.3 Cyclic Voltammetry

Cyclic voltammetry is essentially similar to linear sweep voltammetry but for the fact that the excitation potential is constituted by a repeated series of periods composed of a linear rise of the potential up to a maximum followed by a linear decrease to again reach the initial potential.

This technique is designed to measure both the anode and the cathode currents during the two different phases of the potential wave period so as to acquire more information on the RedOx

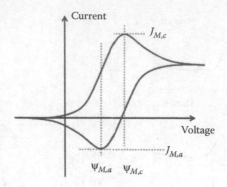

FIGURE 10.35   Typical shape of a cyclic voltammetry voltammogram obtained from a pure sample containing a single RedOx analyte.

analyte. The cycle repletion allows different measures to be averaged, reducing the error and obtaining a lower effect of random noise and other random effects affecting the measure.

The typical shape of the characteristic response of the cyclic voltammetry of a pure sample containing a single RedOx species is shown in Figure 10.35.

From the theoretical expression of the response of cyclic voltammetry in the case of a perfect reversible system, two simple relations can be derived, involving the coordinates of the two peaks of the voltammogram. As it is intuitive, for geometrically identical plane electrodes, the maximum values of the anode and the cathode currents have to be equal. Moreover, the separation between the peaks of the anode and cathode parts of the voltammogram depends only on the number of exchanged electrons and on the temperature since it can be written as

$$\Psi_{Ma} - \Psi_{Mc} = K_\psi \frac{\kappa_B T}{q} \frac{1}{n_e} \qquad (10.87)$$

where the constant K_ψ has a value of about 2.303. Thus, as the number of electrons exchanged in the reaction increases, the two peaks get nearer, and as the temperature increases, they get farther.

The above properties are in any case theoretical and they can be verified, at least approximately, in real voltammograms only after the elimination of the parasitic current, which introduces a linear bias of the measured curve, and of interferences by other side reactions, either due to other species that are present in the solution or due to spurious phenomena.

Examples of real cyclic voltammograms are shown in Figure 10.36 [88]. In the first part of the figure, the cyclic voltammogram of potassium ferrocyanide reduction is shown. The structural formula of potassium ferrocyanide is shown in Figure 10.37. It is an almost ideal voltammogram evidencing the parasitic current baseline. In the second part of the figure, the voltammogram of healthy human serum is shown. Here, the situation is completely different: several RedOx species are present in the sample, causing different peaks in the anodic voltammogram profile. The strong irreversible nature of the reaction in the cell is shown by the completely different shape of the anodic and the cathodic current characteristic.

An example of the use of cyclic voltammetry for the investigation of the activity of biomolecules, for example, enzymes, is provided in Reference [89], where the activity of the oxidoreductase enzymes is analyzed. Adsorption of oxidoreductase on a chemically modified electrode, a technique known as protein film voltammetry, allows direct electron transfer between the enzyme and the electrode, enabling electrochemically driven catalysis [90]. The electrode replaces the natural electron exchange partner of the enzyme, while confinement of the enzyme to the electrode surface overcomes the disadvantage of slow enzyme diffusion to the electrode surface. Ideally, the

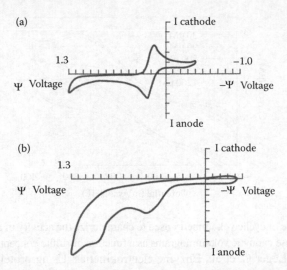

FIGURE 10.36 Example of real cyclic voltammograms. Potassium ferrocyanide in the range of −0.3 to 1.3 V at a rate of 100 mV/s versus Ag/AgCl reference electrode (a). Healthy human plasma in the range of −0.3 to 1.3 V at a rate of 100 mV/s versus Ag/AgCl reference electrode (b). (Data from Chevion S., Roberts M. A., Chevion M., *Free Radical Biology and Medicine*, vol. 28, pp. 860–870, 2000.)

enzyme retains its full native activity while being confined to the electrode. The characteristic of this method is that the catalytic activity of the enzyme can be investigated as a function of electrochemical potential. The operating potential of an enzyme relates to the minimal electrochemical driving force that must be provided for catalysis and is typically in the vicinity of the formal potential of the enzyme's physiological redox partner.

The superposition of different sulfite dehydrogenase cyclic voltammograms acquired in correspondence of different concentrations of sulfide is shown in Figure 10.38. At low sulfite concentrations (90 μM), the expected voltammogram shape was obtained, which depends on the specific chemical form of the enzyme. As the substrate concentration increased toward saturating levels (see Section 2.5), the voltammogram became distinctly peak-shaped, showing a strong current decrease as the catalytic potential is traversed. This property allows characterization of the enzyme activity.

Many proteins of various kinds present electrochemical activity and can be characterized through cyclic voltammetry [91,92]. Among them, metalloproteins have been extensively studied by voltammetry [93–95]. Cyclic voltammetry has also been used for the characterization of nucleic acids due to the RedOx characteristics of the nucleotides [96]. The interaction of specific sequences with selected substances can be analyzed by voltammetry [97] and the number of nucleobases that are present in a sample nucleic acid can be quantified by exploiting their different RedOx properties [98]. This property of the nucleobases is shown in Figure 10.39 [98], where the voltammogram

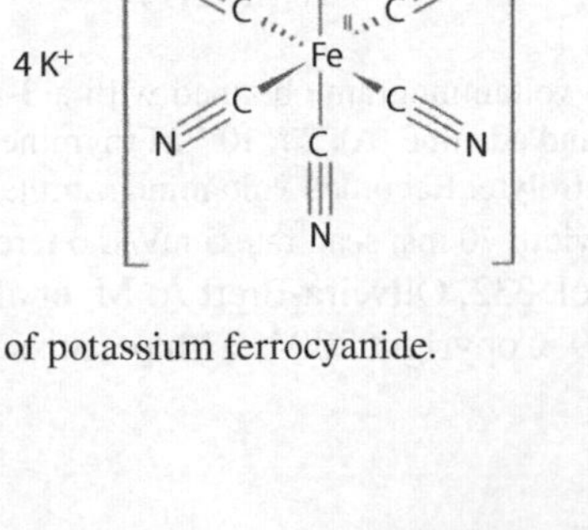

FIGURE 10.37 Structural formula of potassium ferrocyanide.

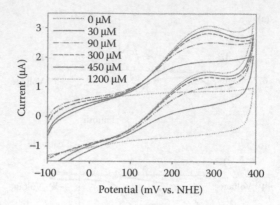

FIGURE 10.38 Example of cyclic voltammetry used to characterize the activity of an enzyme: superposition of the sulfite dehydrogenase catalytic voltammograms as a function of sulfite concentration. (Reprinted from *Biochemistry*, vol. 42, Leger C. et al., Enzyme electrokinetics: Using protein film voltammetry to investigate RedOx enzymes and their mechanisms, pp. 8653–8662, Copyright 2003, with permission from Elsevier.)

peaks of the DNA nucleobases are shown in a linear sweep voltammogram and in its version where the baseline has been eliminated. Clearly separated peaks can be individuated in Figure 10.39, allowing the nucleobases to be individuated on the ground of their electrochemical activity once they have been exposed to interaction with the electrode, for example, by using single-stranded, denatured DNA or RNA whose chain is completely linearized.

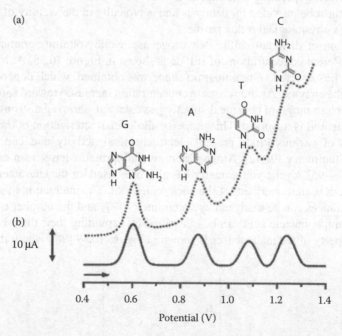

FIGURE 10.39 Differential pulse voltammogram obtained with a 3-mm-diameter GCE electrode for the mixture of 2×10^{-5} M guanine (G) and adenine (A), 2×10^{-4} M thymine (T) and cytosine (C) in a pH 7.4, 0.1 M phosphate buffer supporting electrolyte. Recorded voltammogram (a); baseline-corrected voltammogram (b). Pulse amplitude 50 mV; pulse width 70 ms; scan rate 5 mV/s, reference electrode Ag/AgCl. (Reprinted from *Analytical Biochemistry*, vol. 332, Oliveira-Brett A. M. et al., Voltammetric determination of all DNA nucleotides, pp. 321–329, Copyright 2004, with permission from Elsevier.)

Many of the above techniques have been transferred on lab on chip platforms, mainly based on polymeric materials [99,100]. Owing to the importance of the electrode structure and materials in voltammetry measurements, many proposals have been made for electrode technology both in polymer chips [101,102] and in silicon-based chips, frequently using CMOS structures [103,104]. CMOS-based electrode subsystems have the advantage of integrating the electronic front-end on the chip, avoiding transmission of the electronic signal out of the chip via electrical connection. This assures both a lower level of electronic noise, avoiding the low-power electrical signal attenuation along the connection with the external amplifier, and a lower chip cost.

Integrating CMOS circuitry over a lab on chip is, however, a challenging operation due to the need of not ruining the doped semiconductor structure through high-temperature processes following the CMOS fabrication (see Section 4.2.1). For this reason, the CMOS circuitry has to be fabricated frequently after the microfluidic structures, thus complicating the chip fabrication processes.

10.4.3 ELECTRODES FOR VOLTAMMETRY DETECTION

The selection of a suitable electrode material is a key issue in electrochemical detection. The electrode material has to be compatible with mass fabrication processes typical of lab on chip (see Chapters 4 and 5), so that not any material can be chosen; moreover, it has to guarantee good quality when used for electrochemical sensing.

First, the electrode has to allow the measurement in a substantial potential window for the relevant electrochemical reaction; moreover, the reaction potential, depending on both the target RedOx couple and the electrode, should be as low as possible. As a matter of fact, a very high reaction potential requires a high feeding voltage that is to be avoided for on-chip applications.

Last but not least, in the case in which particular properties are required from the electrode surface, surface modification has to be possible.

Taking into account these requirements, three main material families are used for electrochemical microelectrodes: carbon-based materials, metals, and metal oxides.

10.4.3.1 Carbon Electrodes for Lab on Chip

Carbon-based electrodes are probably the most used in standard electrochemical systems for their very good chemical inertia, wide potential range, and good conductivity. When lab on chip is considered, however, some widely used materials are found to be not compatible with microfabrication.

The most important example is highly ordered pyrolytic graphite, which requires pressure annealing at about 3000°C to assume its characteristic ordered structure.

The situation is different in the case of the so-called glassy carbon [1]. This material has a disordered structure containing micrographite structures and a high proportion of random generated fullerene-related structures. Glassy carbon is impermeable to almost all liquids and gases and has a quite wide potential window that runs from −1 V to about 1.5 V when measured with an Ag/AgCl reference electrode. Owing to its structure, glassy carbon can be manufactured using soft lithography (see Section 5.2) and patterned using imprinting techniques over polymers such as PDMS [105,106].

Boron-doped diamond is another carbon structure that can be used as an electrode in electrochemistry on chip because it can be deposited in thin films by CVD methods [107] either by direct doping during deposition or using on-site doping after the film fabrication [108]. Boron-doped diamond is a p-type semiconductor characterized by a large potential window ranging from −0.75 V to 2.35 V if a 0.5 M H_2SO_4 buffer is used. Moreover, the lower limit of the potential window can be lowered to −1 V by fluorination of the material. Among materials normally used in electrodes for electrochemistry, this is by far the one with the widest potential range. Oxygen plasma etching (see Section 4.7.3) allows one to transform a thick boron-doped diamond film into a nanostructured surface and patterning with metal nanoparticles can be used to achieve particular surface functionalities.

In the case of standard electrochemical sensors, carbon electrodes based on the above materials are frequently pretreated to remove absorbed impurities on the surface and to control the density of spurious oxygen defects that almost unavoidably are present on the electrode surface. Many pre-treatments suitable for macroscopic electrodes are not suitable for microfabricated lab on chip; on the other hand, clean room fabrication sensibly lowers the need for pretreatment due to the density of very small impurities to which the material is exposed during fabrication. Pretreatments that are compatible with microfabrication processes are chemical washings and ultrasound treatments, which can be operated on the whole substrate where several chips are fabricated. In order to remove excess oxygen groups on the surface, the electrode is heated in vacuum so as to provoke detachment and evaporation of oxygen atoms.

In selected applications, a high superficial density of oxygen ions has to be obtained, in order to enhance the electrochemical activity of the carbon electrode. In this case, electrochemical oxidation at 1–2 V in acid solution is beneficial if it does not disrupt other elements that are present on the substrate.

Besides carbon-based materials used in standard electrochemical electrodes, carbon nanotubes have been widely used to fabricate on-chip electrochemical electrodes [109,110]. Carbon nanotubes, either single-walled or multiwalled, can be fixed to traditional carbon or metal electrodes by drop casting of nanotube suspension on an underlying electrode. This method produces an uneven dispersion of nanotubes on the electrode surface, so that the nanotubes are oriented not only in different ways, but also in areas of great nanotube concentration, alternate with bare electrode areas. This characteristic sometimes renders measures difficult to interpret because the electrochemical reaction happens both at the bare electrode surface and on the nanotube structure with different characteristics.

The so-called nanotube forests have much better performances under this point of view [111,112]. They are regular nanotube structures deposited on dielectric surfaces such as oxidized silicon. As shown in Section 9.4.1, nanotube forests can be obtained by vapor deposition of carbon on a surface containing a regular pattern of catalytic metal nanoparticles.

The main advantage of nanotube electrodes is due to the very fast electron exchange rate happening when the RedOx reaction is activated by such electrodes. In the case of single-walled nanotubes, this is mainly due to defects on the nanotube surface that catalyze the electron exchange. When the metal particle used for nanotubes growth is left at the nanotube base, it can also catalyze the electrochemical reaction near the nanotube base. Sometimes, in the case of single-walled structures [113] and more frequently in multiwalled nanotubes [114], the discontinuity at the nanotube end seems to dominate the electron exchange due to the inherent change of the carbon–carbon bond arrangement. Because the electrochemical reaction speed is mainly catalyzed on specific nanotube sites such as wall defects and end points, the effectiveness of carbon nanotube patterned electrodes can also be optimized by optimizing the nanotube forest orientation and density [115].

Another nanostructured carbon material that has very interesting electrocatalytic properties is graphene [116]: graphene is a single sheet of sp^2-bonded carbon atoms forming a flat honeycomb structure as shown in Figure 10.40. Electrochemical catalysis happens due to oxygen defects that are

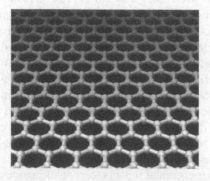

FIGURE 10.40   Schematic structure of a graphene sheet.

included in the graphene structure and at its borders as in the case of carbon nanotubes. For its own structure, graphene supports much higher defect densities, so it promises to be a very interesting material for electrochemical electrodes [117]. However, many aspects of the electrochemical effects on graphene are yet to be completely understood [118] and a practical application of such electrodes in lab on chip seems not to be a possibility in the near future.

10.4.3.2 Noble Metal Electrodes for Lab on Chip

Gold and platinum are the most popular electrodes for lab on chip applications. Besides their chemical stability, they are easily deposited with planar technologies on both silicon and silicon oxide.

Gold is particularly convenient due to its wide application in microelectronics and integrated optics, which allow well-established processes to be used when working with this material. Gold also allows surface functionalization via thiols (see Section 9.3.3), which is useful both for target immobilization on the electrode and for electrode functionalization with catalyzing molecules such as enzymes.

Under anodic polarization in aqueous solution, gold undergoes oxidation by forming a surface monolayer of gold oxide. This layer undergoes reductive dissolution under cathode polarization so that, when cyclic voltammetry of the gold electrode in water is performed, a sharp gold oxide dissolution peak is present, as shown in Figure 10.41a [119]. As a consequence, the gold electrode potential window has to exclude the zone where this peak appears. When the potential window has to be extended, this effect can be prevented by coating the gold surface with a monolayer of long alkanethiol chains that prevents water access to the electrode surface. When using gold electrodes, particular care has to be excercised to avoid the presence of chlorine ions. They form a soluble gold complex under anodic polarization.

Platinum shows a more complex behavior due to its property of absorbing hydrogen. The reduction of hydrogen ions on a platinum potential happens at a very low potential, so that it is practically present very near the equilibrium potential of the cell. Hydrogen atoms formed by reduction are then absorbed on the platinum surface to be oxidized under cathode polarization to H^+. This effect gives rise to the peak indicated with A in the platinum cyclic voltammogram reported in Figure 10.41b [119]. In addition, oxidation and reduction of absorbed oxygen on the platinum surface generates a second strong peak, indicated by B in Figure 10.41b, so that the voltage window of platinum is restricted to the interval that is shown in the figure.

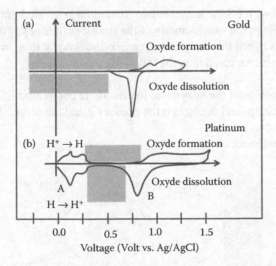

FIGURE 10.41 Cyclic voltammetry of gold (a) and platinum (b) electrodes in water. The voltage window for anode and cathode applications is evidenced in gray. (Bugg T. D. H., *Introduction to Enzyme and Coenzyme Chemistry*, 2012, 3rd edition. Copyright Wiley-VCH Verlag GmbH & Co. KGaA. Reproduced with permission.)

10.5   AMPEROMETRY DETECTION

In amperometry detection methods, an electrochemical process, generally happening at a constant potential, is used to monitor the variation of current with time. In this case, current variation is not due to a variable applied potential, but to other causes, such as variation in time in the composition of the sample that flows through the detection room.

First, we will consider enzyme amperometry detection, perhaps the most diffused amperometry detection method, based on enzyme-driven RedOx reactions, and then we will analyze hydrodynamic amperometry detection, which is electrochemical detection systems operating out of a flowing sample.

10.5.1   AMPEROMETRY ENZYMATIC DETECTION

Amperometry is a very effective detection method if it is coupled with enzyme-catalyzed RedOx reactions such as those driven by enzymes such as oxidase and dehydrogenase [1]. The first enzyme catalyzes the oxidation of RedOx sites in the substrate while the second enzyme catalyzes reactions where the substrate loses hydrogen atoms, resulting being oxidized in the process.

The most diffused types of enzyme amperometry detectors are based on the reaction that is illustrated in Figure 10.42. In a first step, electrons are transferred from the substrate S, that is, the analyte to be detected, to the enzyme active site E_o. As a result, the analyte is oxidized to the product P and the active side is reduced to its form E_R. The reduced enzyme active site interacts with the oxidized form of the detector mediator M_o being regenerated to the oxidized for while the mediator is reduced to the form M_R. In the last step, the reduced mediator transfers an electron to the electrode being regenerated in the oxidized form that enters again in the detection process.

The whole process can be described as a set of three parallel chemical reactions as follows:

$$S + E_o \leftrightarrows ES \to P + E_R \tag{10.88a}$$

$$E_R + \beta M_o \to E_o + \beta M_R \tag{10.88b}$$

$$M_R \to M_o + n_e \, e^- \, (\text{electrode reaction}) \tag{10.88c}$$

where we have indicated with ES the intermediate compound generated during the enzymatic reaction (see Section 2.5.1). From the stoichiometry of the reactions, it is easily deduced that the number of electrons exchanged between the analyte and the enzyme is equal to $n'_e = n_e \beta$. In correspondence to the above reaction chain, we can define the following reaction rates:

k_1 and k_{-1} for the formation of the enzymatic intermediate compound ES
k_2 for the enzymatic compound decay into the product P and the original form of the enzyme
k_M for the mediator reduction
k_e for the electrode semireaction

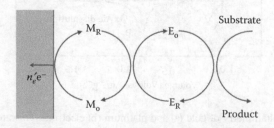

FIGURE 10.42   Schematics of the reaction in a mediated amperometry sensor.

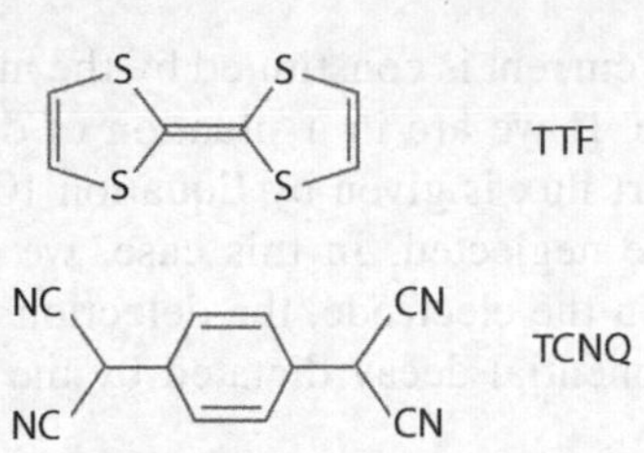

FIGURE 10.43   Structural formulas of TTF and TCNQ.

The whole process can be globally represented as an electron transmission from the analyte, which is also the enzyme substrate, to the electrode through the enzyme itself and the mediator.

Detection can be performed while the enzyme and the mediator are solved in a solution where the analyte is either diffused or injected from outside. In this case, RedOx reactions happen in solution and the reduced mediator reaches the electrode by diffusion. More frequently, in amperometry sensors, both the enzyme and the mediator are entrapped in a biocatalytic layer on the electrode so that the analyte arrives on the electrode either by diffusion or by hydrodynamic transport and the whole reaction chain happens on the electrode surface.

An alternative way of designing amperometry enzymatic sensors is to rely on direct electron exchange between the electrode and the oxidized enzyme [120]. This can be realized by fabricating the working electrode with an organic conducting salt. These compounds are constituted by the combination of an electron donor and an electron acceptor such as tetrathiafulvalene (TTF) and tetracyanoquinodimethane (TCNQ), respectively [121–123], whose structural formulas are shown in Figure 10.43. The TTF-TCNQ salt can be prepared for direct reaction in acetonitrile [124]; the product is a plane molecule with π orbitals so that electrons are delocalized both above and below the molecule plane.

Structurally, the solid salt consists of segregated stacks of anions and cations while relative stable bonding between different stacks is assured by the exchange of delocalized electrons. Owing to this structure, this salt behaves like a semiconductor having electrocatalytic properties toward various enzymes.

Amperometry sensors based on organic salt electrodes are quite promising but it is not completely clear if this technology is really promising for labs on chip. The organic salt electrode fabrication procedure is not easy to integrate with the complex lab on chip fabrication process, especially in case of silica on silicon devices. Thus, we will concentrate on the case of mediated amperometry detection.

10.5.1.1   Amperometry Enzymatic Detector Analysis

The dynamic analysis of an amperometry enzyme detector depends completely on the way the detector is realized, for example, on the fact that the enzyme and the mediator are solved or immobilized on the electrode. Since it is impossible to consider in detail all the possible cases, we will concentrate on the case in which both the enzyme and the mediator are fixed on the electrode functionalized surface and the analyte, which is also the enzyme substrate, reaches the electrode from the bulk of a microfluidic structure. Other situations can be analyzed with similar procedures, changing the diffusion and reaction terms as needed.

Moreover, we will assume that $n_e' = n_e = \beta = 1$. This will allow us to obtain simpler equations, concentrating on the dependence on the relevant design parameters. The extension to generic values of the number of exchanged electrons is trivial.

Since both the enzyme and the mediator regenerates at each process cycle, the whole process can be schematized as

$$S \rightarrow P + e^-$$

(10.89)

the ultimate limit to the observed current is constituted by the mass transport of the analyte from the solution bulk to the electrode. If we are in a situation of diffusion-driven transport from a steady solution, the mass transport flux is given by Equation 10.55, where generally the surface substrate concentration cannot be neglected. In this case, we have to expect that in the presence of a step potential applied on the electrode, the detection never reaches a steady state, but the observed current has an exponential decay dictated by the diffusion time as in the case of chronoamperometry.

The situation is different if we consider a sensor designed as in Figure 10.44, where the working electrode is fabricated on the floor of a slab duct where the sample flows continuously. In this case, since the analyte concentration is continuously replenished near the electrode by the flowing sample, we have to imagine that after a transient due to the potential switch-on, the detection arrives at a steady state if the microfluidic circuit is suitably designed.

The slab nature of the duct allows one to render diffusion of the substrate as efficiently as possible, also considering that in the presence of fluid flow Taylor dispersion happens, which is generally much more efficient with respect to simple molecular dispersion (see Section 7.4.5). Moreover, if the electrode is much shorter than the other linear dimensions of the problem, we can also assume that the bulk concentration in the flowing sample is not heavily modified by the electrode RedOx reaction, so that the substrate concentration is constant along the electrode and so is the current density. This assures that the flowing sample is not depleted by the RedOx reaction and that the electrode length is effectively used.

In order to fulfill this condition, we have to verify that the substrate amount that is consumed at the electrode in the unit time is much smaller than the substrate quantity flowing in the same time.

If we indicate the current coming from a unit electrode area with J, the flux Φ through an electrode length L_E is given by

$$\Psi = \frac{J}{q} w L_E \tag{10.90}$$

where n'_e is the number of electrons per elementary RedOx reaction at the electrode. The flux of the substrate through the duct is much greater than the flux of the substrate that is consumed by the electrode, so that

$$c_s \bar{v} N_A \ hw \gg \frac{J}{q} w L_E \tag{10.91}$$

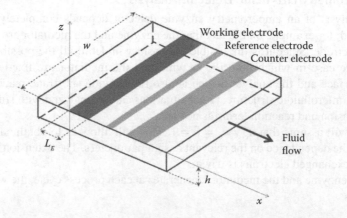

FIGURE 10.44 Principal scheme of the fluid part of an amperometry enzymatic sensor.

where $\bar{v}$ is the average flow velocity, N_A is the Avogadro number, and c_s is measured in mole/m³. We can derive from Equation 10.91 a limit velocity $\bar{v}_1$ defined as

$$\bar{v}_1 = \frac{J}{q}\frac{w}{h}L_E\frac{1}{c_s\,N_A} \qquad (10.92)$$

so that if the real average velocity through the duct is much greater than the limit velocity, our condition is satisfied. Assuming $c_s = 0.01$ mole/m³, $(J\,w\,L_E) = 5$ nA, $w = 2$ mm, $h = 80$ µm, and $n'_e = 1$, it is obtained $\bar{v}_1 \approx 0.8$ µm/s. An average fluid speed of the order of 40 µm/s can be easily attained in a square microfluidic channel with a section of 2 mm $\times$ 120 µm; thus, condition (10.91) can be easily attained with a suitable design of the fluid channel.

Thus, from now on, we will simply assume that the substrate concentration on the electrode surface $\bar{c}_s$ is proportional to the bulk concentration of the substrate c_S through the inverse of the depth of the electrode functionalization film, which we will indicate with δ. Thus, we have, neglecting diffusion in the slab, $\bar{c}_s = \delta c_S$.

Since we are assuming that the reaction chain (10.88) happens completely at the electrode interface and that the surface concentrations of the reagents have no relevant spatial dependence, we can write a set of rate equations as follows:

$$\frac{d\bar{c}_{es}}{dt} = k_1\,\bar{c}_s\,\bar{c}_{eo} - k_{-1}\,\bar{c}_{es} \qquad (10.93a)$$

$$\frac{d\bar{c}_P}{dt} = \frac{d\bar{c}_{er}}{dt} = k_2\,\bar{c}_{es} \qquad (10.93b)$$

$$\frac{d\bar{c}_{mr}}{dt} = \frac{d\bar{c}_{e0}}{dt} = k_m\,c_{mo}\,\bar{c}_{er} \qquad (10.93c)$$

besides the following mass balance equations for the enzyme and the mediator that assures that enzyme and mediator molecules are not created or destroyed:

$$\bar{c}_{et} = \bar{c}_{e0} + \bar{c}_{es} + \bar{c}_{er} \qquad (10.94a)$$

$$\bar{c}_{mt} = \bar{c}_{m0} + \bar{c}_{mr} \qquad (10.94b)$$

All the concentrations in Equations 10.93 and 10.94 are to be intended as surface concentrations at the electrode location and they are defined as follows:

$\bar{c}_{e0}$ is the oxidized enzyme concentration
$\bar{c}_{er}$ is the reduced enzyme concentration
$\bar{c}_{es}$ is the enzyme–substrate concentration
$\bar{c}_{mo}$ is the oxidized mediator concentration
$\bar{c}_{mr}$ is the reduced mediator concentration
$\bar{c}_{et}$ is the total enzyme molecule concentration, which is the surface concentration before the assay
$\bar{c}_{mt}$ is the total mediation molecule concentration, which is the surface concentration before the assay

Equation 10.93c regulates the mediation dynamic for the part depending on the interaction with the enzyme. The mediator, however, also reacts with the electrode. Since the detectors work more efficiently if the related reactions are fast, the mediator reduction at the electrode has to be a fast process, so that it can be assumed to be thermodynamically reversible. Under this condition, $\bar{c}_{mo}$ and $\bar{c}_{mr}$ are also related by the Nernst equation so that it can be written as

$$\psi = \psi_0 + \frac{\kappa_B T}{q} \ln\left(\frac{\bar{c}_{mo}}{\bar{c}_{mr}}\right) \tag{10.95}$$

Using the mediation mass conservation Equation 10.95b, we can write

$$\bar{c}_{mo} = \frac{\bar{c}_{mt}}{1 + e^{-(\kappa_B T/q)(\psi-\psi_0)}} \tag{10.96}$$

Using Equation 10.96, the last of the system rate equations, Equation 10.93c becomes

$$\frac{d\bar{c}_{e0}}{dt} = k_m \frac{\bar{c}_{mt}}{1 + e^{-(\kappa_B T/q)(\psi-\psi_0)}} \bar{c}_{er} \tag{10.97}$$

Equation 10.97 appears as a rate equation for enzyme regeneration because $\bar{c}_{mt}$ is a known parameter of the detector. The regeneration rate of the enzyme depends both on the applied potential and on the initial mediation density on the electrode surface. This is due to the fact that the enzyme needs to couple with an oxidized mediation molecule to regenerate so that the applied potential has to be sufficiently high to generate oxidation of mediation molecules in the reduced state and enough mediation molecules have to exist to fuel the reaction at a good pace.

If a constant potential is applied, which is sufficiently higher than the mediation formal potential, the exponential term at the denominator of Equation 10.97 can be neglected, so as to write

$$\frac{d\bar{c}_{e0}}{dt} = k_m \bar{c}_{mt} \bar{c}_{er} = k_{re1}\bar{c}_{er} \tag{10.98}$$

where k_{re1} is the so-called pseudo-first-order regeneration rate, depending both on the mediator reduction rate at the electrode and on the initial mediator density. When Equation 10.98 holds, the detector works in the so-called limiting regime, and it is the situation in which almost all the practical detectors work, due to the need to maximize the enzyme regeneration rate for an efficient detection.

Since we are at steady state, the concentrations have to be constant, which can be attained if all the fluxes in the reaction chain are the same so that they balance. Since the current is proportional to the substrate flux, leveraging the steady-state condition, we can write

$$J = qN_A (k_1 \bar{c}_s \bar{c}_{eo} - k_{-1} \bar{c}_{es}) \tag{10.99a}$$

$$J = q N_A k_2 \bar{c}_{es} \tag{10.99b}$$

$$J = q N_A k_{re1}\bar{c}_{er} \tag{10.99c}$$

Eliminating the concentrations from Equations 10.99, exploiting the enzyme mass conservation (10.94a), the definition of k_{rel}, the relation between the surface and the bulk substrate concentration and the definition of the Michaelis–Menten constant K_m (see Section 2.5.6.1, Equation 2.26), we get

$$J = \frac{q N_A \bar{c}_{et}}{(K_m / \delta c_S k_2) + (1/k_2) + (1/k_m \bar{c}_{mt})}$$ (10.100)

This equation provides the dependence of the observed current in steady state from the design constants and on the concentration of the analyte c_S. If the substrate concentration is very small with respect to the enzyme concentration on the electrode surface, which is a realistic case for the detection of a diluted analyte, we have

$$\frac{1}{k_2} + \frac{1}{k_m \bar{c}_{mt}} \ll \frac{K_m}{k_2 \delta c_S}$$ (10.101)

that is called the first-order kinetic condition for the detector. In this condition, we get

$$J = q N_A \, \bar{c}_{et} \frac{k_2}{K_m} \delta c_S$$ (10.102)

This is a linear relation between the observed current density and the concentration of the analyte, which is the desired detector characteristic.

It is worth noting that by increasing the analyte concentration this relation is not maintained, and the measured current depends on the kinetic term related to enzyme and mediator regeneration. Equation 10.100 is plotted versus the analyte concentration for different values of the enzyme total concentration considering the parameter values reported in Table 10.4. From the table, since the mediator enzyme layer is 50 nm thick, it is evident that it is not realized like a monolayer. In these cases, multilayer systems are realized, superimposing different monolayers with a repetition of linkers and active molecule layers using the techniques that are analyzed in Chapter 9.

The above procedure to analyze the dynamics of the enzymatic detection at the electrode is also needed to obtain an expression of the current in the simple configuration where the solution is standing in a detection room while the potential is applied. The stationary analysis of the electrode reaction can be used in this case because it is much faster than the diffusion in the cell, so that the adiabatic approximation can be used. In this case, Equation 10.55 is rewritten as

$$J(t) = q N_A k' \left(c_s - \frac{\bar{c}_s}{\delta} \right) \sqrt{\frac{D_S}{\pi t}}$$ (10.103)

where, assuming the electrode reduction is much faster than all the other reactions happening at the electrode,

---

TABLE 10.4

Example Parameter Values Used to Plot the Amperometry Current

K_m	0.35 (mole/m^2)
k_2	5×10^7 s^{-1}
L_E	0.5 mm
Δ	50 nm
$\bar{c}_{mt}$	1.2×10^{-9} mole/m^2
k_m	5×10^8 m^2/s/mole

$$k' = \frac{k_2\, k_m\,(k_1 - k_{-1})}{k_m\, k_2 + (k_1 - k_{-1})k_2 + (k_1 - k_{-1})k_m} \tag{10.104}$$

is the overall electrode rate. The relation between the current and the surface concentration of the analyte is written as

$$J = \frac{q\, N_A\, \bar{c}_{et}}{(K_m/\bar{c}_S\, k_2) + (1/k_2) + (1/k_m\, \bar{c}_{mt})} \tag{10.105}$$

Eliminating $\bar{c}_s$ from Equations 10.103 and 10.104, the direct relation between the current and the concentration of the analyte in the solution bulk can be found analyte in the solution bulk can be found. The obtained relation is plotted in Figure 10.45 for different values of the total enzyme concentration and considering parameter values in Table 10.4. If the linear approximation can be used for Equation 10.104, we obtain

$$J = q\, N_A\, k' \frac{c_s}{\left(1 + \bar{c}_{et}\, \delta\,(k_2/K_m)\right)} \sqrt{\frac{D_S}{\pi t}} \tag{10.106}$$

It is not surprising that, in a linear regime, the current depends on the inverse of the square root of time, as in the case of chronoamperometry, while it depends on a complex combination of the different rate parameters characterizing the electrode process, due to its complexity.

10.5.1.2 Mediator Selection

The key problem in designing an amperometry-mediated detector is the mediator selection. The first requirement that the mediator has to fulfill is the capacity to acquire electrons from the selected enzyme; thus, the mediator potential has to be higher than the potential of the enzyme. Extensive research has been carried out on an organic mediator, and standard formal potentials are tabled for a large variety of such compounds [124].

In addition, a suitable mediator has to be very stable and compatible with complex multilayer immobilization techniques so as to render possible the fabrication of a sufficiently thick enzyme–mediator layer. Alternatively, if the mediator is intended to be added to the sample, it has to be soluble in water in great quantities under the same conditions in which the analyte is solved and to have a high diffusion coefficient so as not to be the current limiting element. This last condition in particular limits the choice of mediators to be solved with the analyte to small molecules.

Another important characteristic of both immobilized and solved mediators is the independence of hydrogen ions, so as to avoid a pH-dependent electrode potential.

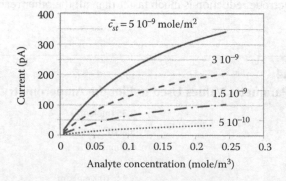

FIGURE 10.45 Amperometry current versus the analyte concentration for different values of the total enzyme concentration and considering parameter values in Table 10.4.

Since the detector is more efficient if the overall RedOx rate is high, the mediator has to be characterized by a high RedOx rate both in the interaction with the enzyme and in the reduction at the working electrode. A fast RedOx reaction also means that both reactions are reversible.

In addition, a mediator with a small formal potential, compatibly with the required RedOx activity, is preferable. In this case, the electrode can be polarized not far from the mediator potential, thus excluding a great number of possible spurious RedOx reactions happening at the electrode.

A common interference in mediated amperometry enzymatic detectors is due to oxygen, which is almost unavoidably present in water solutions [125]. It competes with the mediator in the electrode RedOx reaction, giving a biased current contribution. If this bias can be estimated, it can be deconvolved from the result; otherwise, this interference can be alleviated by increasing the mediator concentration as much as possible.

The first class of commonly used mediators is small inorganic molecules that have many of the properties characterizing a good mediator. The ferricyanide ion (see Figure 10.46) is one of these mediators; it undergoes a one-electron reduction to ferricyanide with no hydrogen ion participation. It can be trapped by electrostatic forces into a positively charged matrix or, more suitably, to lab on chip fabrication, patterned using several patterning methods. Inks usable with an inkjet printer (see Section 5.4.1) have been realized for patterning of such mediators. Moreover, the presence of carbon nanotubes in the electrode functionalization layer enhances the electron transfer rate [126]. Functional layers based on a ferricyanide ion generally show leakage, so they are mainly suitable for disposable lab on chips.

Inkjet technology can also be used to pattern mediators based on other Fe salts such as Fe_3O_4 and $Fe_3O_3MnO_2$. Even better results can be obtained with metal oxides of the platinum group, particularly IrO_2, for their low potential that allows the effect of spurious reactions on detection to minimize [127].

Several organic RedOx couples can work as mediators in amperometry enzymatic detectors. The first class of such compounds is the class of diquinones, such as benzoquinone, whose RedOx reaction is shown in Figure 10.47a. This reaction involves hydrogen ion exchange, so that the electrode potential is pH dependent. This fact generally obliges either to measure the pH of the sample before detection, or, when possible, to add a pH buffer. The same characteristic is shared by RedOx dyes, such as phanzine, phenoxazine, and phenothiazine. In this case, the mediator can show photo-induced instabilities, which are frequently not important in closed lab on chip. As an example, the RedOx reaction of phenazine methosulfate is shown in Figure 10.47b.

Another class of organic mediators is heteroatomic nonsaturated compounds whose ionic or radical forms are stabilized by charge delocalization over a conjugated π orbital system. As a result of such a structure, these compounds undergo hydrogen ion-independent RedOx reaction. Common examples are TCQN and TTF [128] (see Figure 10.43).

An important class of organic mediators is constituted by ferrocene derivatives. Ferrocene's, structural formula is shown in Figure 10.48 besides its RedOx reaction. Ferrocene is a charge transfer complex of iron and the cyclopentadienyl aromatic anion. The chemical bonding in this compound derives from the partial transfer of the delocalized electron from the π ligand of the anion to

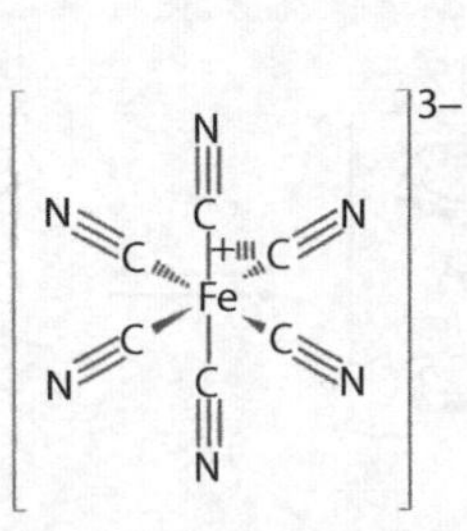

FIGURE 10.46   Structural formula of the ferricyanide ion.

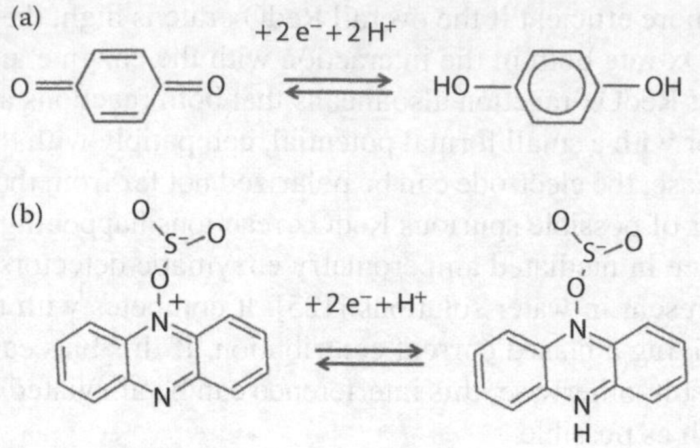

(a)

$$+2\,e^- + 2\,H^+$$

$$O = \langle \rangle = O \quad \rightleftarrows \quad HO - \langle \rangle - OH$$

(b)

$$+2\,e^- + H^+$$

FIGURE 10.47 RedOx reactions of selected organic mediators: benzoquinone (a) and phenazine methosulfate (b).

the empty orbitals of the iron ion. The electrochemical transformation between the reduced and oxidized species happens with a half-way potential ($\psi_{1/2}$, see Equation 10.70) of about 409 mV referred to as a standard hydrogen electrode. Solubility and formal potential can be adjusted, adding to the solution a suitable substituent on the ligand. Electron-attracting groups, for example, carboxylate or aromatic groups, increase the standard potential while electron-repelling groups, such as alkyls or amines, decrease it. Ferrocene itself is soluble in ether; its solubility can be tuned by hydrophobic or hydrophilic substituents.

The standard way to fabricate a ferrocene functionalized electrode requires a carbon electrode. Functionalization is obtained by the following process. In the first step, a water-insoluble compound of ferrocene, such as 1.1′-dimethyl ferrocene, is deposited on the electrode by evaporation of its solution in toluene. Then the enzyme is immobilized with a suitable linker on the obtained surface. Finally, the electrode is generally coated with a membrane. This procedure is not always easy to incorporate into a lab on chip fabrication process; however, ferrocene compounds can also be patterned on an already enzyme functionalized surface with inkjet printing or microcontact printing (see Section 5.2.1).

Ferrocene can also be fixed on carbon nanotubes [129] and nanoparticles [130] to be better incorporated in on-chip detection systems.

A last effective way of mediation in enzymatic sensors is to exploit polymers grafting-from to fix a mediation moiety to a polymer thin film that was deposited on the electrode [131,132]. The typical structure of this kind is shown in Figure 10.49. Electron transfer from the enzyme to the mediator is facilitated in such structures from the vicinity of the enzyme active site to the mediator itself, although direct contact is generally prevented by steric factors. The electrons can then be transmitted directly from the mediator to the electrode through a thin polymer layer, frequently constituted by a few monolayers of polymer chains. However, if the functionalization layer is thick in order to increase the generated current, electron transmission is needed through the polymer layer. This can be facilitated by different methods, more likely short- or long-range polymer chain motions. Thus,

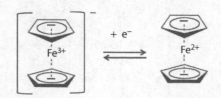

FIGURE 10.48 Ferrocene RedOx reaction.

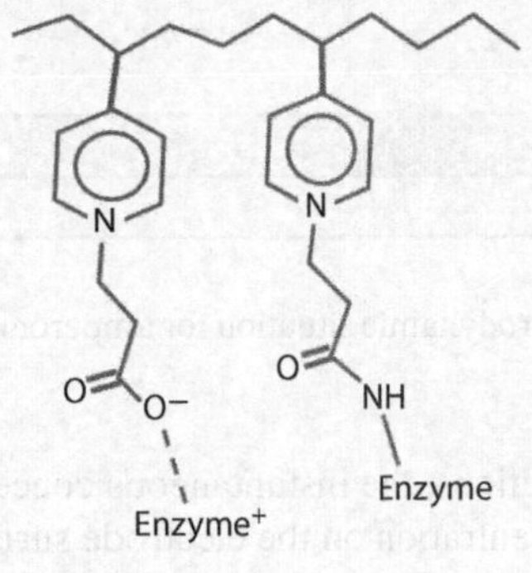

FIGURE 10.49 Mediation moieties attached to a polymer graft from.

the efficiency of electron transfer depends to a great extent on the flexibility of the linker chain between the mediator and the polymer surface.

Electron diffusion can also be limited by the mobility of the positive ion that is needed to maintain the electrical charge balance during electron migration to the electrode. Thus, the polymer somehow has the role of connecting electrically the enzyme with the electrode, like a sort of electrical wire. Thus, in this kind of structure, the enzyme is said to be wired to the electrode. Polysiloxane and polyethylene oxides have been proved to provide a very good flexibility of the linker chains.

10.5.2 Amperometry Detection with Integrated Capillary Electrophoresis

Owing to the need for a constant potential, amperometry detection is well suited for application in hydrodynamic conditions. The first example is the dynamic enzymatic assay we have shown in the previous section, where the continuous replenishment of the analyte on the electrode surface prevents current decrease due to the lengthening of diffusion time.

Since capillary electrophoresis (see Section 8.5.2.2) is an effective separation technique, well suited for application in labs on chip, the use of amperometry as a detection technique in capillary electrophoresis chips is an interesting possibility [133–135].

The sample flows under the electrode continuously after capillary electrophoresis separation. The electrode potential is maintained slightly greater than the formal potential of the analyte. When a species with a formal potential equal to or greater than that of the analyte travels below the electrode, a RedOx reaction is generated at the electrode and a current peak is seen on the amperometry diagram, as shown in the figure. If the electrophoresis bands of the different species that are contained in the sample are well separated, the peaks are well separated too, so that the analyte-related peak can be easily recognized. Naturally, in this configuration, species that are not electrochemically compatible with the electrode or species that do not cause RedOx reactions are not detected at all.

Owing to the hydrodynamic condition in which amperometry happens, the sample flows continuously under the electrode and the RedOx reaction products are continuously eliminated by the hydrodynamic flux. The detection is thus operated in a condition similar to electrolysis, and the Faraday law (A5.15) can be applied.

With reference to the scheme of Figure 10.50, let us define the instantaneous analyte concentration $\chi(t)$, which is the analyte concentration traveling under the electrode from the instant t to the instant $t + dt$. The standard electrophoresis distribution is proportional to $\chi(t)$ and the standard analyte concentration in the initial sample is given by the integral of $\chi(t)$ to all the time needed to move all the samples from the insertion room to the waste room by capillary electrophoresis.

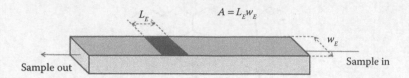

FIGURE 10.50 Schematic of the hydrodynamic situation for amperometry integrated with on-chip capillary electrophoresis.

In standard hydrodynamic conditions, the instantaneous concentration of the analyte $\chi(t)$ is proportional to the instantaneous concentration on the electrode surface $\bar{\chi}_{(t)}$ through the width δ of the thin layer near the electrode surface where the RedOx reaction happens so that

$$M = A \int_0^t \bar{\chi}(\tau)d\tau = A\delta \int_0^t \chi(\tau)d\tau \tag{10.107}$$

where A is the electrode area and M is the total mass of electrolyte freed at the electrode. Differentiating the Faraday law, we get

$$\chi(t) = \frac{m}{q\,n_e\,N_A\,A\delta} \tag{10.108}$$

where m is the analyte molecular mass, A is the electrode area, and $I(t)$ is the observed current. Typical amperometry diagrams for a capillary electrophoresis system, which is proportional to a plot of $\chi(t)$ versus time, are reported in Figure 10.51 [136] in case of carbohydrate detection and in Figure 10.52 [137] in case of DNA separation by weight.

Since the separation in all electrophoresis methods is obtained by applying an electrical field acting on charged molecules, one important point in designing an amperometry detection system to use with electrophoresis is to dealwith the interference between detection and the electrophoretic potential. This interference mainly depends on the system geometry and on the placing of electrophoresis and amperometry electrodes; thus, this is an important design characteristic.

Capillary electrophoresis happens in a capillary where analyte separation is attained while it flows through the duct. Three general configurations can be used to perform amperometry in a

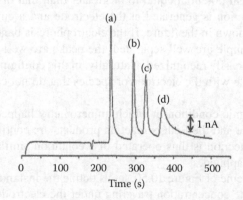

FIGURE 10.51 Example of amperometry result after capillary electrophoresis separation: electrophoresis plots for 100 µM sucrose (a), cellobiose (b), glucose (c), and 200 µM fructose (d). (Reprinted from *Talanta*, vol. 64, Lee H.-L., Chen S.-C., Microchip capillary electrophoresis with amperometric detection for several carbohydrates, pp. 210–216, Copyright 2004, with permission from Elsevier.)

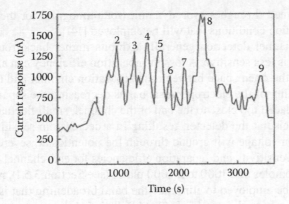

FIGURE 10.52   Example of amperometry result after capillary electrophoresis separation: electrophoresis plots of a mix of DNA strands up to a weight of 1500 base pairs. Separation channel length: 2 cm, separation voltage: 100 V, detection voltage: 0.7 V, buffer solution: 1X phosphate buffered saline (PBS), pH 7.4. The labels on the peaks indicate the fragment weight: (1) 100 base pairs (bp), (2) 200 bp, (3) 300 bp, (4) 400 bp, (5) 500 bp, (6) 600 bp, (7) 800 bp, (8) 1000 bp, and (9) 1500 bp. (Reprinted from *Current Applied Physics*, vol. 9, Supplement, Joo G.-S., Jha S. K., Kim Y.-S., A capillary electrophoresis microchip for amperometric detection of DNA, pp. e222–e224, Copyright 2009, with permission from Elsevier.)

capillary electrophoresis chip, which are shown in Figure 10.53: end-channel detection, in-channel detection, and off-channel detection.

End-channel detection is a commonly used configuration [138–140]. The working electrode is placed tens of micrometers from the end of the separation channel; at this distance, the separation voltage is effectively isolated from the working electrode. However, because the separation voltage is grounded within the detection reservoir, the working electrode is still influenced by the electric field. The separation field will cause a small but significant shift in potential of the working electrode [141]. Therefore, to determine the appropriate detection potential, a system biasing is required.

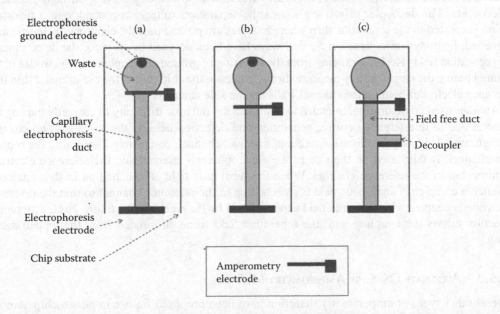

FIGURE 10.53   Different electrode architectures for amperometry and capillary electrophoresis detection: end-channel detection (a), in-channel detection (b), and off-channel detection (c).

Generally, it is performed through a hydrodynamic voltammogram for the compound of interest under the exact separation conditions that will be employed [141].

In addition, end-channel detection generally exhibits higher background currents than off-channel detection and is less sensitive. A loss in separation efficiency can also occur due to diffusion of the analyte in the open space between the separation channel and the working electrode. This causes a broadening of the electrophoresis bands decreasing the separation efficiency.

If the electrode is placed too close to the end of the channel, small fluctuations in the separation voltage can produce noise at the detector, resulting in a decrease in sensitivity. In the worst-case scenario, the separation voltage will ground through the potentiostat, severely damaging the electronics. The detection sensitivity and separation efficiencies for end-channel detection range from 1 micromole to 100 nanomoles and 1000 to 20,000 plates (see Section 3.5.1), respectively.

A method that can be employed to eliminate the band broadening that is characteristic of end-channel detection is in-channel detection [142–144]. This involves the placement of the working electrode directly within the separation channel. The analytes migrate over the electrode while still confined to the channel, thus eliminating the band broadening. The in-channel configuration helps eliminate some of the negative separation performance characteristics encountered with an end-channel configuration, especially with respect to the alignment of the working electrode at the end of the separation channel. This was demonstrated by comparing in-channel detection with end-channel detection using catechol as a model analyte. When compared to end-channel detection, in-channel amperometry detection exhibited a 4–6 increase in plate number while lowering the peak skew by a factor of 1.2–1.4. However, as with end-column detection, a potential shift occurs at the working electrode due to the electrophoresis field. This shift is a function of both the separation voltage and the distance of the electrode from the end of the separation channel. Therefore, to ensure that the optimum detection potential is chosen, hydrodynamic voltammetry must be performed for each analyte of interest. Both end-channel and in-channel detection exhibit similar separation performances in terms of plate height and peak symmetry in the same conditions.

Off-channel amperometry detection has also been employed to overcome the drawbacks of end-channel detection. Electrode placement in off-channel detection is similar to that in in-channel detection, but the separation voltage is isolated from the amperometry current through the use of a decoupler. The decoupler effectively shunts the separation voltage to ground, and a field-free region is created in the separation duct where analytes are pushed past the electrode by inertia and, if needed, hydrodynamic pressure. Several ways have been adopted to decouple the detection and the separation field [145,146], ranging from the insertion of ground electrophoresis electrodes in the channel before the amperometry measure through holes in the chip roof to the use of metal thin film reference electrodes both on the channel walls and on side channels.

Another used configuration, intended to eliminate the intrinsic difficulty in correctly biasing the detector due to interference between separation and detection field, is the so-called two-channel configuration [147,148]. In this configuration, a second channel, completely identical to the separation channel, is fabricated on the side of the electrophoresis channel and the reference electrode is immersed in the reference channel. When the separation field is switched on in the separation channel, a completely analogous field is switched on in the reference channel so that the reference electrode is coupled with the same field experimented by the working electrode. Thus, differential detection allows the coupling with the separation field to be eliminated from the amperometry result.

10.5.3 ALTERNATE ON-CHIP AMPEROMETRY METHODS

Several other types of amperometry detection have been proposed for use in lab on chip. Among them, pulse amperometry and amperometry adopting electrode arrays have been diffusely used to extend the reach of amperometry detection.

10.5.3.1 Pulsed Amperometry

Pulsed amperometry is most commonly used for analytes that tend to foul electrodes [49]. Analytes that foul electrodes reduce the signal with each analysis and necessitate cleaning of the electrode. In pulsed amperometry detection, a working potential is applied for a short time, usually a few hundred milliseconds, followed by higher or lower potentials that are used for cleaning the electrode. In the most common procedure, the detection electrode is first cleaned at a high positive potential, then reactivated at a negative potential dissolving the surface oxide, and finally used to oxidize the analyte at a moderate positive potential. The current is measured only while the working potential is applied; then sequential current measurements are electronically filtered by the detector to produce a smooth output.

Let us imagine that the current is measured along all the working voltage pulses for N consecutive pulses, and that the working potential pulse rises over the analyte potential in a short time with respect to the whole pulse duration, as represented in Figure 10.54, dashed line. Since the dependence of the current on the potential in the vicinity of the formal potential is exponential for the Nernst equation and the RedOx rate is much faster than the pulse duration, we can assume that the resulting current pulse is an almost squared pulse, as shown in Figure 10.54, continuous line where the current pulse maximum corresponds to the current I_m that would be measured in a constant potential amperometry detection.

The measured current is then given by

$$I(t) = \sum_{n=1}^{N} [I_m + i(t - nT)] H_{0,\tau}(t - nT) \tag{10.109}$$

where $i(t)$ represents all the noise and spurious contributions to the measure, $H_{a,b}(y)$ is the so-called rectangular function (see Section 7.4.3.2) that is defined as

$$H_{a,b}(y) = \begin{cases} 1 & y \in [a,b] \\ \\ 0 & \text{otherwise} \end{cases} \tag{10.110}$$

the period of the sampling is indicated with T, the voltage pulse duration with τ, and $\tau \ll T$.

If a continuous response has to be interpolated from the discontinuous functions (10.109), it is necessary that the electronic system processing the amperometry output filters the current signal with a bandwidth approximately equal to the inverse of the sampling period. Assuming a perfect

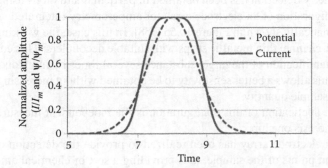

FIGURE 10.54 Example of potential and current pulses in pulsed amperometry.

bandpass filter, which is a squared frequency response in the wanted bandwidth and zero outside, the filter pulse response is given by [150,151]

$$h_T(t) = \frac{\sin(2\pi(t/T))}{2\pi(t/T)} \tag{10.111}$$

After filtering, we get

$$I(t) = \sum_{n=1}^{N} I_m \int_{-\infty}^{\infty} H_{0,\tau}(\theta - nT) h_T(\theta) d\theta + \sum_{n=1}^{N} \int_{-\infty}^{\infty} i(\theta - nT) H_{0,\tau}(\theta - nT) h_T(\theta) d\theta \tag{10.112}$$

The second sum represents no more than the filtered noise and spurious contribution terms, which we will call $i_F(t)$ and whose power is lowered by the elimination of all out-of-band contributions. In the first term, owing to the hypothesis $\tau \ll T$, we can approximate the square function $H_{0,z}$ $(\theta - nT)$ as a pulse of infinitesimal duration, which is a Dirac pulse. In this case, approximately applying the sampling theorem [150,151], we have

$$\sum_{n=1}^{N} I_m \int_{-\infty}^{\infty} H_{0,\tau}(\theta - nT) h_T(\theta) d\theta = \sum_{n=1}^{N} I_m h_T(t - nT) = I_m \tag{10.113}$$

Thus, far from the measurement interval extremes, we have

$$I(t) = I_m + i_F(t) \tag{10.114}$$

which is the same response that would provide a continuous potential amperometry after noise reduction by filtering.

Pulse amperometry is typically used to detect carbohydrates, for their property of fouling almost all types of electrochemical electrodes [152] frequently coupled with capillary electrophoresis for target separation [153,154], but several other substances that are difficult to quantify correctly with continuous amperometry have been successfully detected using pulsed amperometry [155–157].

10.5.3.2 Amperometry Detection Using Electrode Arrays

Enhanced amperometry detection has been obtained in particular situations using electrode arrays. A first possible configuration of an electrode array for amperometry integrated with capillary electrophoresis is schematically shown in Figure 10.55 [158]. In this case, the working electrode is constituted by many off-channel thin metallic strips with suitable decouplers. This configuration allows one to repeat the quantification of the target substance several times by individually addressing the single electrodes. This allows a better sensitivity to be obtained without increasing the measurement time or the needed sample quantity.

Another possible application of this configuration is the independent measure of different analytes after electrophoresis on chip.

A more complex electrode array has been realized to provide the detection of several analytes detection in different points of the sample, thus providing a sort of chemical ample imaging. Such electrode arrays are generally integrated with CMOS technology to provide a self-sufficient, portable microsystem [159,160].

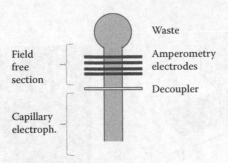

FIGURE 10.55 Possible scheme of multielectrode amperometry in a capillary electrophoresis chip with off-chip detection.

10.6 MECHANICAL DETECTION BASED ON MICROCANTILEVERS

Besides electrochemical methods, a large number of other detection methods exist that rely on the creation of an electrical detection signal, but do not exploit the electrochemical properties of the target molecule. These methods can be roughly classified into three categories:

- Mechanical methods
- Calorimetric methods
- Acoustic methods

Mechanical methods exploit mechanical interaction between the sample and micromechanical systems to create the electrical detection sample. Even if several different structures can be devised, by far the most diffused methods belonging to this category exploit a microcantilever to generate the sensing interaction.

Calorimeteric methods rely on detection of heat generated or absorbed by a chemical reaction selectively involving the analyte. Calorimeteric detection methods are very diffused in the field of inorganic species sensing, when they can be detected through strongly energetic reactions. This is almost never the case of biological species, so that calorimeter detection in the biological case has to rely on very high sensitivity. Nevertheless, it is an attractive detection method having the relative simplicity of a microcalorimeter with respect to the complex structures that have to be fabricated to carry out other kinds of detection.

Detection methods based on the use of acoustic waves are essentially a variation of mechanical methods, where the mechanical interaction is obtained through the high-frequency, low-amplitude density variations related to the propagation of acoustic waves through the sample. The fact that the technology for generation and processing of surface acoustic waves in integrated chips is well assessed in other application fields and that the acoustic properties of solutions are quite sensitive to the presence of selected analytes renders these detection methods attractive for gas sensors. The huge dumping experienced by surface acoustic waves due to the presence of a liquid environment makes them less suitable for labs on chip, and we will not detail their structure here. Rather, we will analyze cantilever-based detection in this section and calorimeter detection in Section 10.6.

A microcantilever is a submillimeter beam of solid material that is constrained on one of the short planar dimensions. Figure 10.56a shows a rectangular cantilever, but several designs have been used like U-shaped or V-shaped cantilevers, depending on the application. An electron microscope photograph of a microcantilever is shown in Figure 10.56b [161].

The most commonly used technology for microcantilever fabrication is surface MEMs technology (see Section 4.2) allowing cantilevers made by silicon, polysilicon, silicon nitride, and other silicon-based materials to be fabricated on a silicon wafer [162–164]. Polymer microcantilevers

(a)

(b)

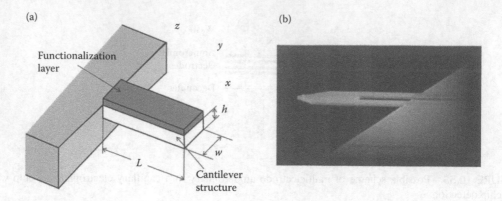

Functionalization layer

z

y

x

h

L

w

Cantilever structure

FIGURE 10.56 Scheme of a square microcantilever (a) and microcantilever electron microscope photo (b). (Reprinted from *Sensors and Actuators B: Chemical*, vol. 99, Kooser A. et al., Gas sensing using embedded piezoresistive microcantilever sensors, pp. 474–479, Copyright 2004, with permission from Elsevier.)

have also been fabricated by using micromolding (see Section 5.5) using different polymers [165,166].

Detection based on the use of microcantilevers exploits configuration in which the presence of the analyte in the sample creates a stress on the cantilever structure that can be detected in several ways. Cantilever sensors exist that detect cantilever deformation mainly with electrical and optical methods.

Optical detection relies on the fact that cantilever deformation provokes a deviation of a beam that is reflected by the cantilever surface [167,168]. This deviation can be detected with a simple imaging system, such as a CCD, or by interference-based systems. Optical detection, however, requires the use of free space optics and a method of deflection measurement that is difficult to integrate within a lab on chip. Moreover, if optical detection using free space optics has to be used in a lab on chip, attenuation or fluorescence spectroscopy (see Section 11.3) is simpler and more flexible. Thus, measurement of the microcantilever deformation by optical means is not diffused in lab on chip applications even if optical detection systems using integrated optical means have also been proposed [169].

Electronic detection is mainly based on the measure of the change of the electrical properties of suitable cantilever structures in consequence of a cantilever deformation. This is a detection method more suitable for lab on chip applications and we will consider it in this section.

Cantilever-based detectors can be divided into two main groups: static and dynamic. In static detectors, the analyte presence generates a static deformation of the cantilever, which passes from an equilibrium configuration in the absence of an analyte to a different equilibrium configuration in the presence of the analyte. In the case of dynamic systems, the cantilever is left to oscillate around its equilibrium position at its main resonance frequency in the analyte's absence. The analyte's presence changes the cantilever resonance frequency and this change is detected by the system.

10.6.1 Static Cantilever-Based Detection

Deformation in static cantilever detectors is due to the change of the surface free Gibbs energy due to the analyte's presence. For this reason, static cantilever detectors are essentially based on the functionalization of the upper cantilever surface in order to generate selective capture of the target. When the target is captured on the cantilever surface, the change of the structure of the surface due to the absorption process causes a change in the free energy, implying a positive or negative tensile stress in the beam. Moreover, if charged targets are captured, their charges either attract or repel depending on the sign so as to generate stress in the monolayer and, as a consequence, in the

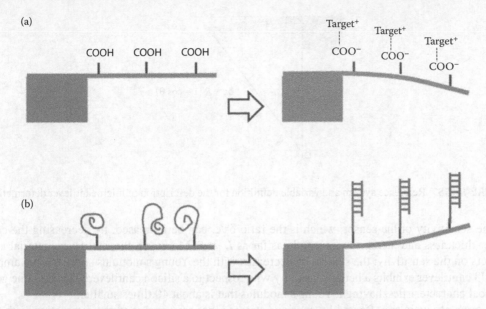

FIGURE 10.57 Tensile stress in a microcantilever due to surface immobilization of target molecules: electrostatic immobilization (a) and supercoiling state change due to hybridization in DNA recognition (b).

cantilever. Last but not least, the creation of a monolayer generally implies a change in the entropy of the analyte molecule population that also contributes to the free energy of the surface.

Two examples of these phenomena are reported in Figure 10.57a and b. In Figure 10.57a, it is shown as the immobilization due to electrostatic attraction between the functionalization molecules on the cantilever surface, and the target creates an electrostatically charged layer that, due to electrostatic repulsion, generates a cantilever bend. In Figure 10.57b, a DNA cantilever sensor is considered. In this case, the functionalized molecules are single-stranded DNA fragments that are synthetized so as to be complementary to the single-stranded target. In the absence of the target, the functionalizing strands assume a random coiling on the cantilever surface, generating a configuration where the cantilever stress is zero and the affinity and repulsive forces among different strands balance. When the target links to the surface, the two stranded composite of the target and the functionalizing DNA assume a linear configuration vertical to the cantilever plane. In this way, bond energy is minimized. This situation, however, almost cancels the previously present interaction between nearby strands, thus modifying the surface free energy and causing a cantilever deformation.

To analyze cantilever deformation let us consider the reference system and variable definition reported in Figure 10.58. As we have seen in Chapter 8, as far as the deformation δz of a square beam is much smaller than the beam dimensions, the solution of the elastic equations for the structure equilibrium allows the following relation between the deformation radius R and the constant tensile stress ς

$$\frac{1}{R} = 6\frac{(1-\nu)}{\varepsilon h^2}\varsigma \qquad (10.115)$$

where ν is the Poisson ratio, ε the Young's modulus of the cantilever material, and h the cantilever thickness. Adding the hypothesis that the cantilever length L is much smaller than the deformation radius R, which is always satisfied by practical cantilevers, we can obtain from Equation 10.115 the expression of the cantilever extreme displacement δx as

$$\delta z = 3\frac{(1-\nu)}{\varepsilon}\left(\frac{L}{h}\right)^2\varsigma \qquad (10.116)$$

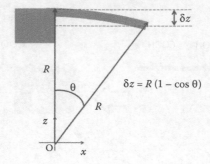

FIGURE 10.58   Reference system and variable definition for the description of microcantilever deformation.

The sensitivity of the sensor, which is the ratio $\delta z/\varsigma$, can be increased, by decreasing the cantilever thickness and increasing its length, as far as $L \ll R$. Moreover, the cantilever material also impacts on the sensitivity: the sensitivity decreases with the Young's modulus so that, for example, an SU8 cantilever exhibits a better sensitivity with respect to a silicon cantilever with the same geometrical characteristics, having a Young's modulus that is about 40 times smaller.

Microcantilevers are affected by spurious stresses that are not due to the interaction with the analyte. Thermal drift can cause stress due to thermal expansion or compression, nonspecific interactions and other elements can also introduce unwanted deformations. For this reason, generally two cantilevers are built one after the other. The first cantilever is activated so as to generate specific interaction with the target while the other remains neutral, so as to undergo only nonspecific interactions and environmental caused deformations. A differential measure carried out using both cantilevers is much more reliable than a measure performed using only the working cantilever.

This is one of the reasons why cantilevers are frequently fabricated in arrays: this configuration allows one to share one reference cantilever among several tests carried out by more working cantilevers specifically designed for different targets [168,170].

10.6.2   Dynamic Cantilever-Based Detection

A cantilever vibrating at its resonance frequency can be an extremely sensitive mass sensor, being able in selected cases to perform even single molecule detection. In Section 8.2.3.1, we have seen that the deformation of many simple sensors can be evaluated by substituting the real distributed pressure acting on the sensor surface with an equivalent concentrated force acting on the point of maximum deformation of the structure. While the deformation happens in the elastic regime, the relation between the applied force and the displacement of every point of the structure is linear and if the equivalent force application point is considered, the proportionality constant is called structure equivalent spring.

The equivalent spring of the most used structure in lab on chip detectors can be evaluated solving the elastic equations from the structure deformation and selected results are reported in Table 8.6.

This means that if the structure is perturbed by a small perturbation while in an equilibrium position, it starts to oscillate with a frequency related to the equivalent spring from the relation

$$f_0 = \frac{1}{2\pi} \sqrt{\frac{k}{\xi M}} \qquad (10.117)$$

where M is the cantilever mass. Ideally, the parameter ξ should be equal to one. In practical cases, where the beam is not one-dimensional, the structure of transversal modes both in the horizontal and in the vertical dimension cannot be completely neglected if a very accurate estimation of the resonance frequency has to be carried out. Owing to the fact, however, that this influence is quite small, it can be taken into account by the phenomenological parameter ξ that in practice is near to unit. Values of ξ can be obtained either by realistic cantilever simulations in different environments [171,172] or by measurement on fabricated structures.

Two different cantilever configurations are used in dynamic detectors: one side constrained and two sides constrained cantilevers, whose structures are presented in Figure 10.59. The spring constant for the two structures is given by

$$k = \frac{w\varepsilon}{4}\left(\frac{h}{L}\right)^3 \tag{10.118a}$$

$$k = 16\varepsilon w\left(\frac{h}{L}\right)^3 \tag{10.118b}$$

for the one side constrained and two sides constrained cantilevers, respectively. If we consider two cantilevers made from the same material, and of the same mass and dimensions, Equations 10.118 show that the two side constrained cantilever has a greater spring constant and thus a higher resonance frequency.

If a change in the cantilever mass is caused by fixing of the analyte on the cantilever surface, the resonance frequency changes according to Equation 10.117, so that

$$\Delta M = \frac{k}{4\pi^2\xi}\left(\frac{1}{f_0'^2} - \frac{1}{f_0^2}\right) \approx \frac{k}{2\pi^2\xi}\frac{\Delta f}{f_0^3} \tag{10.119}$$

where $f_0' = f_0 - \Delta f$ is the new resonance frequency of the loaded cantilever and the approximation holds if the frequency variation is much smaller with respect to the unloaded cantilever resonance frequency. From Equation 10.119, it is clear that in order to accurately measure the mass difference, the frequency difference between the loaded and the unloaded cantilever has to be accurately measured.

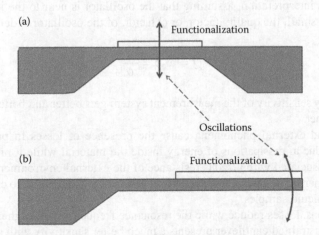

FIGURE 10.59 Scheme of one-side-constrained (b) and two-side-constrained (a) microcantilever for dynamic detection.

Using the equivalent spring constant, the motion of the cantilever extreme (or center in the double side constrained case) can be described like a dumped oscillator so that

$$\frac{\partial^2}{\partial t^2} \delta z + \alpha \frac{\partial}{\partial t} \delta z + \omega_0^2 \delta z = 0 \tag{10.120}$$

where α is the dumping constant, taking into account the energy losses, and ω_0 is the unperturbed resonance angular frequency. Assuming that the displacement at $t = 0$ is equal to A, Fourier transforming Equation 10.120 and solving for δz, we get

$$\delta z = \frac{A}{(\omega_0^2 - \omega^2) + i\alpha\omega} \tag{10.121}$$

This is a typical dumped oscillator linewidth, having the maximum in correspondence of the resonance frequency, and a linewidth that depends on the dumping constant, that is, on the losses. In particular, if we assume that the system is in a small losses regime, that is, $\omega_0^2 \gg \alpha^2$, the angular frequency ω_F at which the square module of the resonance line is half the maximum value is simply given by

$$\omega_F = \frac{\alpha}{2} \tag{10.122}$$

The sensitivity of the frequency detection can be assumed to be proportional to the linewidth of the corresponding oscillator, that is, it gets better if the losses decrease.

Equation 10.122 also has another interesting interpretation. The square module of the resonance line provides for the Fourier transform energy theorem [150] the energy spectral density of the system. Thus, we can define the time constant of the dumped oscillator as the full width at half maximum (FWHM) of the energy spectral density as

$$\tau = 2\frac{\omega_F}{2\pi} = \frac{1}{\alpha} \tag{10.123}$$

and interpret it as the time needed to dissipate half the energy stored in the elastic vibrations. As a consequence of this interpretation, assuming that the oscillator is near to the ideal behavior if the dissipated energy is small, the quality factor, or Q factor, of the oscillator is defined as

$$Q = \omega_0 \tau = \frac{\omega_0}{\alpha} \tag{10.124}$$

so that the frequency sensitivity of the measurement system gets better and better while the Q factor gets higher and higher.

Both internal and external phenomena cause the presence of losses in practical cantilevers. Internal losses are due to dissipations of energy inside the material while it moves while external losses are mainly associated with viscous resistance of the external environment. Thus, cantilevers operating while immersed in gases have much better sensitivity with respect to cantilevers operating while immersed in liquid samples.

In many conditions, losses reduce while the resonance frequency gets higher, justifying the fact that the two side constrained cantilever presents a much better sensitivity with respect to the single side constrained system. The sensitivity of single side constrained cantilevers working in a gas environment is in the range of 10^{-12} g, while the sensitivity decreases up to two orders of magnitude for systems working in a liquid environment [173,174]. Two side constrained oscillators working in a gas environment can be constructed with very small masses so as to reach a resonance frequency of the order of 100 MHz and a sensitivity of 10^{-18} g, which makes possible the individuation of single macromolecules [175].

10.6.3 PIEZO-RESISTIVE CANTILEVER DISPLACEMENT MEASURE

The most diffused method to measure the stable deformation or the resonance frequency deviation of a microcantilever is to fabricate on the cantilever surface, generally under the functionalized layer, a piezoresistor [162,174,175].

The piezoresistive effect consists of the change of electrical resistivity of a semiconductor or a metal when mechanical stress is applied. In contrast to the piezoelectric effect (see Section 8.2.2.5), the piezoresistive effect only causes a change in electrical resistance, not in electric potential. Different causes generate a piezoresistive effect in metals and semiconductors. In the case of metals, the resistance changes simply due to a change of the resistor shape. Considering a simple beam resistor that undergoes compressive stress, change its length slightly. Owing to Ohm's second law, the beam resistance change ΔR can be expressed as

$$\Delta R = r\frac{\Delta L}{A} = r\frac{(1 + 2\nu)\varsigma}{A} \tag{10.125}$$

where r is the specific resistance, ΔL the resistor length variation, A the resistance cross-section area, ς the suitable component of the stress tensor, and ν the metal Poisson ratio. Owing to the small values of compressibility of metals, the piezoresistive effect of metals is quite small and difficult to be used in practical applications.

The situation in semiconductors is quite different. In semiconductors such as silicon or germanium, the main cause of piezoresistance is not the resistor shape change but the fact that change in atomic distance variation causes a variation of the profile of the bands [176], rendering either easier or more difficult to electrons and holes to move along the crystal. Under a mathematical point of view, this fact reflects in a dependence of the charge carrier mobility on the applied stress that gives a much stronger effect with respect to the simple shape change. Let us consider the case of a heavily doped semiconductor, when a single charge carrier exists: either holes or electrons. The resistivity or a beam resistor can be written as

$$r = \frac{1}{q\mu\rho} \tag{10.126}$$

where q is the electron charge, ρ the charge carrier density, and μ the mobility of the carriers. A perturbation of bands causes a change both in the carrier density and in the carrier mobility, thus causing a change in resistivity.

In order to consider the crystal structure of the semiconductor, we can introduce tensor representation for the stress and the resistivity (see Section 8.2.2.5). In this general situation, we can introduce a tensor piezoresistance factor $\Pi_{i,j,k,h}$ where the first indexes (i, j) represent the current propagation direction and the second indexes (k, h) the stress direction. The piezoresistance tensor is thus defined as

$$\Pi_{i,j,k,h} = \frac{\partial R_{i,j}}{\partial \varsigma_{k,h}} = \frac{r_{i,j}}{A}\frac{\partial L}{\partial \varsigma_{k,h}} - r_{i,j}\frac{L}{A^2}\frac{\partial A}{\partial \varsigma_{k,h}} + \frac{L}{A}\frac{\partial r_{i,j}}{\partial \varsigma_{k,h}} \tag{10.127}$$

where the third factor is generally dominant in heavily doped semiconductors.

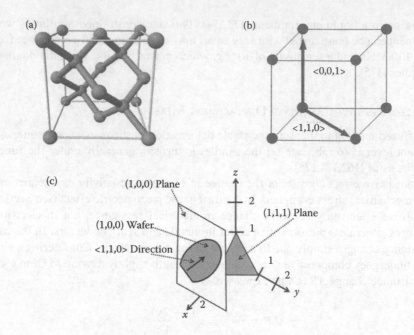

FIGURE 10.60 Silicon crystal structure (a), crystal directions in the cubic silicon cell (b), and reference system adopted in the text with respect to the main crystal planes where the position of a (1,0,0) wafer is evidenced (c).

This expression can be simplified a bit if a silicon wafer is considered taking into account both the wafer type (see Section 4.3.2) and the symmetries of the silicon cell, which is shown in Figure 10.60a, and of the stress tensor. In particular, let us take as a reference a (1,0,0) wafer and let us assume the reference system in Figure 10.60b. In this case, the piezoresistance tensor has only two independent elements and the expression of the resistance variation becomes

$$\Delta R = \frac{1}{q\mu\rho}\frac{L}{A}\left(\Pi_L\varsigma_L + \Pi_T\varsigma_{T1} + \varsigma_{T2}\right) \tag{10.128}$$

where Π_L and Π_T are the longitudinal and transversal piezoresistance coefficients, respectively, ς_L is the stress component in the current propagation direction, while ς_{T1} and ς_{T2} are the two independent stress components in the plane orthogonal to the current propagation direction.

Values of the piezoresistance coefficients in silicon for a (1,0,0) wafer in different situations are reported in Table 10.5 [176]. In particular, tensile strain in (100) silicon increases the mobility for

TABLE 10.5

Values of the Piezoresistance Coefficients in Silicon for a (1,0,0) Wafer in Different Situations

Current Propagation Direction	Carrier	Π_L ($\times 10^{-11}$ Pa^{-1})	Π_T ($\times 10^{-11}$ Pa^{-1})
<1,1,0>	Electrons	−31.6	−17.7
	Holes	71.8	−66.3
<1,0,0>	Electrons	−102	53.4
	Holes	6.6	1.1

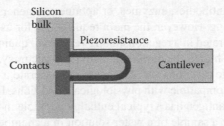

FIGURE 10.61 Possible architecture of a piezoresistor fabricated on top of a lightly doped silicon cantilever: top view.

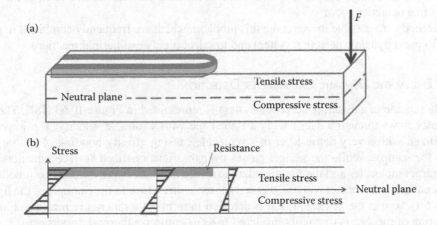

FIGURE 10.62 Scheme of a cantilever with an embedded piezoresistance (a) and stress distribution along the structure due to a bend of the cantilever.

electrons in the <110> direction, while compressive strain in (100) silicon increases the mobility for holes in the <110> direction. The piezoresistance coefficients reported in the table are about two orders of magnitude greater than those caused in metals by the bare geometric effect and allow piezoresistance to be used as a method to detect stress in microcantilevers.

The fabrication of a piezoresistance on top of a lightly doped silicon microcantilever is simply obtained by creating a strongly doped, wire-like region below the cantilever surface; a possible shape of the resistor is shown in Figure 10.61 [177–179]. As shown in the figure, the piezoresistor is built only in the initial part of the cantilever, where the stress is higher. Prolonging it to the whole cantilever length would decrease the percentage resistance variation and, consequently, the cantilever sensitivity. Naturally, the resistor cannot be too short, due to the fact that the resistor end and the connections to the pads must be negligible in determining the whole resistance, being not affected by the stress. Thus, the optimum resistor length can be determining, depending on the structure characteristics [180]. The resistor length is almost aligned only with the cantilever direction so that a cantilever bend produces an internal stress in the resistor, as shown in Figure 10.62, and a consequent resistance change. The resistance change can be measured with great accuracy by a Wheatstone bridge, as detailed in Section 10.2.4.

10.7 CALORIMETRIC DETECTION

Calorimetric detection essentially relies on the possibility of quantifying the product of a chemical exothermal reaction through the measurement of the produced heat. Since the heat quantity is proportional to the quantity of the generated reaction product, it can be used to quantify either the product, or more frequently, the reactant.

The possibility of using antibodies, enzymes, or aptamers to generate highly selective reactions renders this method interesting. However, the main requirement for use of calorimetric detection is that the quantity of heat generated in a reaction among very small quantities of reactants, as happens in lab on chip, is sufficiently high to be detectable with good accuracy.

In general, macromolecule reactions are not deemed to generate a large amount of heat, due to the fact that they have to be compatible with physiological conditions. Even the strong bonding of an IgG antibody to the specific antigen has a typical enthalpy per mole in the order of 150 kJ/mole (see Section 3.7.1). If we consider a sample of a water solution in a chamber of 1 mm ×1 mm × 100 μm containing 0.01 mole/m^3 of a target and its conjugated antibody and assume $\Delta H = 150$ kJ/mole, using data for water, we obtain a temperature rise of about 4×10^{-4} K, which is very difficult to determine with accuracy. This is the main element limiting calorimeter detection if the target is stationary in a detection room.

Two methods are possible to overcome this problem, which are frequently combined in practical systems: to use a dynamic detection system and to select highly exothermal reactions.

10.7.1 ENZYMATIC DYNAMIC CALORIMETER DETECTION

A possible scheme of a dynamic detection system is represented in Figure 10.63 [181]. The sample continuously flows through a duct having a slab shape with a suitable velocity. The lower wall is functionalized with a very dense layer of a molecule causing affinity bonding of the target molecules in the sample. While the sample passes over the functionalized surface, reactions happen between target molecules and the functionalized surface and heat is generated. The functionalized surface is put in direct contact with the thermal sensor, a thermistor in the example of the figure (see Section 6.6.1), so that the generated heat is detected in terms of temperature increase. Finally, the active section of the duct is thermally insulated so as to minimize thermal dispersion.

The dynamic system that is represented in Figure 10.63 has to be designed with care due to the different elements that can influence the measure. Part of the heat can be transported from the fluid flux far from the thermistor. This effect increases while increasing the fluid velocity, so that minimizing it would require a very low velocity in the duct. The velocity cannot be too low, however, due to the need to replace the exhausted sample with a fresh one in a time not so long to cause dissipation of the heat produced on the functionalized surface. Thus, an accurate system simulation is needed both to select an optimum speed in the duct and to compensate the residual effect correctly in the phase of measured data processing. Moreover, owing to the fact that the system is necessarily open in correspondence of the duct input–output, thermal insulation cannot be perfect, and heat dispersion also has to be estimated and compensated to obtain an accurate measure.

While dynamic systems present little advantage if the analyte is permanently fixed to the functionalized surface via aptamers or antibodies, they are very effective if the calorimeter surface is functionalized with enzymes. As a matter of fact, after capture of the analyte and its transformation in the product, the enzyme releases the product molecule, being ready to operate on another analyte

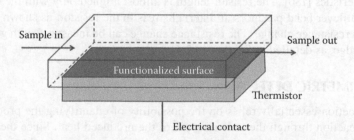

FIGURE 10.63 Principal scheme of dynamic calorimeter detection based on a thermistor.

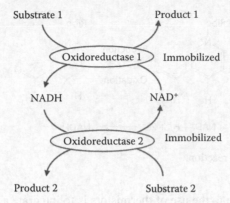

FIGURE 10.64 Double enzymatic reaction leveraging the NAD reduction used in a lab on chip calorimeter detection.

molecule. Moreover, enzymatic reactions are among the more exothermic in the biological field. Thus, enzyme-based calorimeter detectors are very effective.

As an example, let us consider the case in which a RedOx reaction happens on the functionalized surface through a couple of enzymes of the oxidoreductase type [1] mediated by the nicotinamide adenine dinucleotide (NAD⁺) reduction/oxidation. Both the enzymes are immobilized on the functionalized surface, NAD, or one of the substrates is the analyte and the other substances are added to the sample as needed [1]. The reaction scheme is shown in Figure 10.64 while the structural formula of NADH is shown in Figure 10.65. The RedOx reaction NAD⁺ ⇌ NADH, whose scheme is reported in Figure 10.66, is at the center of the reaction cycle. This is a very fast and exothermic reaction, since the role of NADH in organic systems is mainly to move electrons from one molecule to the other, having a standard enthalpy equal to 225 kJ/mole. Moreover, the enzymes are continuously regenerated, so as to be able to provoke a temperature increase sufficiently high to be detected with great accuracy.

10.7.2   On-Chip Calorimeters

10.7.2.1   Thermopile-Based Microcalorimeters

The use of thermistors is widely diffused for temperature difference measurements due to their sensitivity and the possibility of integrating thermistors in the fabrication process of several types

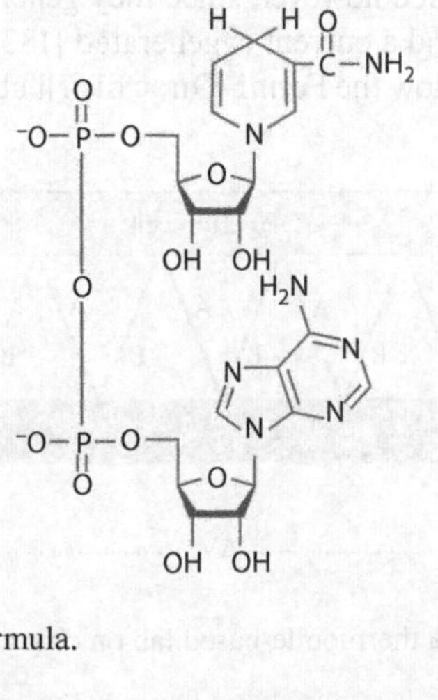

FIGURE 10.65   NADH structural formula.

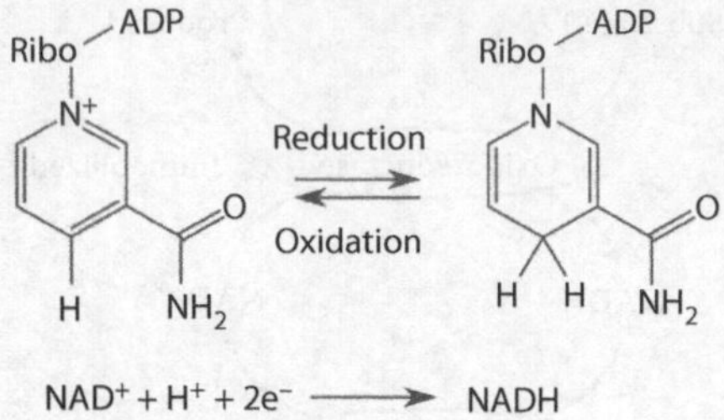

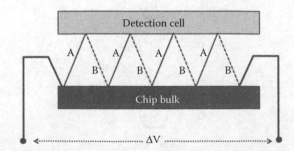

FIGURE 10.66 NAD$^+$ RedOx reaction.

of lab on chip. An alternative to the use of thermistors is to integrate a thermopile with the detection room.

Heat thermopile calorimeters are structures that transfer the heat produced by chemical reactions happening in the detection room to a jacket through a heat vessel that allows heat quantity measure. The temperature of the jacket is kept constant so that it is to a good approximation unaffected by the heat exchange with the reaction cell. The jacket is therefore designed to function as a heat source/ sink of virtually infinite heat capacity. In the lab on chip case, owing to the very small quantity of heat produced, the jacket simply coincides with the bulk of the chip that is in thermal contact through the package with the external environment.

In a lab on chip detection system, the heat transfer vessel is constituted by a series of cascaded identical thermocouple junctions fabricated on the reaction the cell and connecting its outside wall to the chip bulk. The principal scheme of a thermopile is presented in Figure 10.67, where the two conductors constituting the thermocouple junction are indicated as A and B. The determination of the heat flow relies on the Seebeck effect, an electrothermal effect such as the Peltier effect we considered in Section 6.6.2.

The Seebeck effect consists of the conversion of a temperature difference between the junctions of a thermocouple in an electrical current if the electrical continuity is maintained or in a voltage difference if the continuity is broken at one of the junctions as in Figure 10.67 so that the overall current is zero.

Under a fundamental point of view, the Seebeck effect is due to the fact that the distribution of the electron energies in a conductor depends on the temperature: increasing temperatures at one extreme of a conductor bar causes the average electron energy to increase at that extreme, thus generating a small potential difference at the bar ends. This is a small effect that cannot cause a current flow in a circuit constituted by a single conductor, due to the balance of the potential along the circuit. If different conductors are joined however, since they generate different potentials, the overall potential is not null in the circuit and a current is generated [182,183]. This mechanism is shown in Figure 10.68: electrons energies follow the Fermi–Dirac distribution, so that they are more energetic

FIGURE 10.67 Principal scheme of a thermopile-based lab on chip calorimeter.

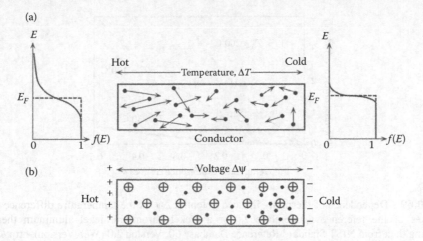

FIGURE 10.68 Qualitative explanation of the Seebeck effect in a conductor. (a) Schematic representation of a conductor wire with electrons represented with black dots. Electron energies follow Fermi–Dirac distributions, represented on the side of (a), where E_F represents the Fermi level. In (b), both reticle atoms, represented with ⊕, and electrons are shown evidencing the uneven distribution of electrons in the wire.

on the hot side of the conductor. The difference in the energy distribution causes an uneven diffusion of electrons, resulting in a higher density on the cold side, while atoms at reticle nodes do not change their average position. The wire side where the electron distribution is higher is determined from the energy dependence of the electron parameters such as density of states and scattering cross section, which is different from conductor to conductor, so that the Seebeck potential can be either positive or negative. The uneven electron distribution causes the Seebeck potential.

The Seebeck effect can be described locally with the presence of a microscopic electromotive force that locally adds to the externally imposed potential difference in determining the current density. This electromotive force is locally proportional to the temperature gradient through the Seebeck coefficient, which in the more general case is a temperature-dependent tensor. Thus, we can write in coordinate form the following relation:

$$J_i = \sigma_{i,h} \left(-\frac{\partial \psi}{\partial x_h} + S_{h,k} \frac{\partial T}{\partial x_k} \right)$$ (10.129)

where $\sigma_{i,h}$ is the conductivity tensor of the material and $S_{h,k}$ is the Seebeck coefficient tensor. Owing to the above-discussed explanation of the Seebeck effect, the tensor $S_{h,k}$ can be written as the difference of two Seebeck tensors related to the two materials constituting the thermocouple as

$$S_{h,k} = S_{h,k}^{(1)} - S_{h,k}^{(2)}$$ (10.130)

Equation 10.129 is quite important, representing the fact that the Seebeck-induced current is generated along the bulk of the material where a temperature difference exists, not only at the two thermocouple junctions. This means that the junction realization, besides introducing a concentrate resistance in the circuit due to the imperfect adaptation of the materials constituting the thermocouple, has no impact in the generated current. In contrast, it is the nature of the material constituting the thermocouple elements that is important, and local contamination in the thermocouple branches can impact the thermocouple working.

In a microscopic thermopile, the electrical continuity of each element is disrupted at one end, so that no electrical current passes through the system. In this case, the potential difference that

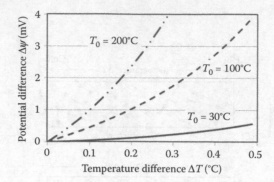

FIGURE 10.69 Dependence of thermally induced potential $\Delta\psi$ on the temperature difference ΔT for different values of the reference temperature T_0 for a nickel–chromium/nickel–aluminum thermocouple. (Interpolating data from NIST Standard Reference Database 60, Version 2.0 (Web Version), http://srdata.nist.gov/its90/main/its90_main_page.html, last accessed on June 11, 2013.)

is observed at the open circuit extremes is simply the sum of the potential differences that can be observed at the extremes of each thermocouple. Considering a one-dimensional model for each thermocouple, setting $J_i = 0$ and assuming that they are in identical conditions, we get

$$\Delta\psi = N \int_{T_0}^{T_0+\Delta T} S(T)dT = N \int_{T_0}^{T_0+\Delta T} \left[S^{(1)}(T) - S^{(2)}(T) \right] dT \tag{10.131}$$

where N is the thermocouple number and $S(T)$ is the relevant element of the Seebeck tensor. The dependence of $\Delta\psi$ on the temperature difference ΔT for different values of the reference temperature T_0 is plotted in Figure 10.69 for an example thermocouple [184]. From the figure it is clear that if a precise temperature evaluation has to be performed, it is generally not possible to assume a temperature-independent Seebeck coefficient. In practical applications, the integral (10.130) is approximated as a polynomial and the coefficients are tabled for each couple of conducting materials [184,185].

Example values of the Seebeck coefficients of different metals are reported in Table 10.6 while examples of potential differences for thermocouples of selected materials with P_t are reported in Table 10.7.

10.7.2.2 Calorimeter Implementation

An on-chip calorimeter is essentially constituted by a calorimeter room and a heat-sensing element. The main point of the calorimeter room is that it has to allow the sample to enter and, if required, to exit while limiting as far as possible thermal contact of the sampling inside the chamber with the external environment. Moreover, the thermal capacity of the calorimeter chamber needs to be as small as possible in order to avoid the absorption of a relevant part of the produced heat with a small temperature change.

The above requirements summarize the need to build the calorimeter chamber from a strongly insulating material maintaining the mass as low as possible. A common solution is to use a membrane-limited calorimeter chamber as shown in Figure 10.70. The chip is built out of silicon by using wafer bonding. The fluid circuit assuring either calorimeter chamber charging or continuous flow of the sample is realized in the lower wafer while the calorimeter chamber is contained between two membranes fabricated in the lower and in the upper wafer. The whole silicon structure is passivized by thermal oxide so as to obtain a thermal insulating surface. Both a control element, as a heater, if needed, and the thermal measurement element can be integrated in the upper membrane, thus

TABLE 10.6

Seebeck Coefficient for Selected Conductors

for a Heat Sink Temperature of 0°C and 27°C

Metal	S (µV/K)	
	@ 0°C	@ 27°C
Na		−5
K		−12.5
Al	−1.6	−1.8
Mg	−1.3	
Pb	−1.15	−1.3
Pd	−9	−9.99
Pt	−4.45	−5.28
Mo	4.71	5.57
Li	14	
Cu	1.70	1.84
Ag	1.38	1.51
Au	1.79	1.94

TABLE 10.7

Potential Differences for Thermocouples of

Selected Materials with Pt Are Reported

with a Low Temperature of 0°C and a High

Temperature of Either 100°C or 200°C

Material	$\Delta\psi$ (mV)	
	@ 100°C	@ 200°C
Elements		
Copper	0.76	1.83
Gold	0.78	1.84
Aluminum	0.42	1.06
Molybdenum	1.45	3.19
Nickel	−1.48	−3.10
Palladium	−0.57	−1.23
Silver	0.74	1.77
Tungsten	1.12	2.62
Iron	1.89	3.54
Composites		
Alumel	−1.29	−2.17
Chromel	2.81	5.96
Constantan	−3.51	−7.45

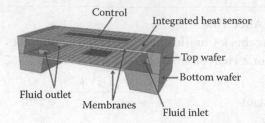

FIGURE 10.70 Principal scheme of a membrane-based microcalorimeter chamber for flow through calorimetry.

decoupling the process on the two wafers with a simplification of the process flow [186]. A similar two-membrane structure can be built by closing the calorimeter chamber with an epitaxial silicon layer, as shown in Figure 10.71 [187].

The thermal insulation of the system can be improved while decreasing the calorimeter wall thermal capacity by excavating an air trench on the side of the calorimeter chamber, as shown in Figure 10.71. In this case, the membrane closing on top of the chamber has to be designed as a floating membrane, a design that is also well consolidated in microvalves (see Section 8.2).

Dimensions of on-chip calorimeter chambers are influenced by the dimensions of membranes (see Section 8.2), being generally from 1 mm × 1 mm to 100 μm × 100 μm.

In the simpler on-chip calorimeter, the sensing element is simply a monolithic thermistor that is built in strict contact with the calorimeter chamber, generally in an excavation on top of the upper membrane, so as to be in strict contact with the chamber content. The working principle of silicon integrated thermistors is based on the fact that by doping the silicon or polysilicon resistors with different dopant densities and species, it is possible to obtain one material with positive resistance temperature coefficient (TCR) or one with negative TCR. The value of the resistance is measured with a Wheatstone bridge that is balanced by a careful choice of TCRs so that the measured voltage is zero at the environmental temperature. In this way, the Wheatstone bridge can be used to measure small temperature differences with great accuracy.

While the integrated thermistor solution allows a very good calorimeter performance, with low noise and high sensitivity, it is strongly dependent on the adopted materials, and thus on the adopted fabrication processes. This is the reason why a thermopile-based solution is frequently used.

The main advantages of integrated thermopiles are

- An output signal without offset and offset drift, because there cannot be any output signal without input power
- No interference from physical or chemical signals except light, which can easily be shielded
- No need for bias

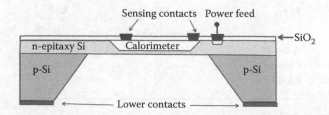

FIGURE 10.71 Principal scheme of a membrane-based microcalorimeter chamber where the upper membrane is realized via an epitaxy deposition of doped silicon.

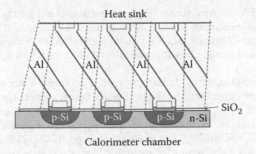

FIGURE 10.72   Design of an integrated thermopile fabricated on a silicon platform.

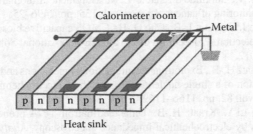

FIGURE 10.73   Alternative design of an integrated thermopile fabricated on a silicon platform.

- Very simple readout; only a voltage has to be measured
- Seebeck's coefficient is quite large in silicon
- The fabrication process is fully compatible with both standard and bipolar CMOS process and with micromachining

The more frequently used design of an integrated thermopile fabricated on a silicon platform is shown in Figure 10.72 [188]. The two elements of the thermopile are heavily p-doped silicon channels connected by aluminum metals. The arrangement is near to the ideal arrangement of Figure 10.67: each couple has an extreme on the top of the calorimeter chamber and the other extreme in contact with the heat sink. An alternative structure is provided in Figure 10.73, using alternated strips of highly p- and n-doped silicon [189]. Since the membrane is frequently rounded, a round arrangement is usual for the thermocouples set [190].

REFERENCES

1. Banica F.-G., *Chemical Sensors and Biosensors: Fundamentals and Applications*, Wiley; 1st edition (October 4, 2012), ISBN-13: 978-0470710678.
2. Yoon J.-Y., *Introduction to Biosensors: From Electric Circuits to Immunosensors*, Springer; 1st edition (October 29, 2012), ISBN-13: 978-1441960214.
3. Ziman J. M., *Principles of the Theory of Solids*, Cambridge University Press; 2nd edition (November 30, 1979), ISBN-13: 978-0521297332.
4. Ashcroft N. W., Mermin N. D., *Solid State Physics*, Brooks Cole; 1st edition (January 2, 1976), ISBN-13: 978-0030839931.
5. Hamann C. H., Hamnett A., Vielstich W., *Electrochemistry*, Wiley-VCH; 2nd edition (April 9, 2007), ISBN-13: 978-3527310692.
6. Chang R., *Physical Chemistry for the Biosciences*, University Science Books; 1st edition (January 30, 2005), ISBN-13: 978-1891389337.

7. Arakawa T., Timasheff S. N., Mechanism of protein salting in and salting out by divalent cation salts: Balance between hydration and salt binding, *Biochemistry*, vol. 23, pp. 5912–5923, 1984.

8. Dumetz A. C., Snellinger-O'Brien A. M., Kaler E. W., Lenhoff A. M., Patterns of protein–protein interactions in salt solutions and implications for protein crystallization, *Proteins Science*, vol. 16, pp. 1867–1877, 2007.

9. Sugiyama M., Gasperino D., Derby J. J., Barocas V. H., Protein-salt-water solution phase diagram determination by a combined experimental-computational scheme, *Crystal Growth and Design*, vol. 8, pp. 4208–4214, 2008.

10. Narakathu B. B., Bejcek B. E., Atashbar M. Z., *Impedance Based Electrochemical Biosensors*, Proceedings of IEEE SENSORS 2009 Conference, vol. 1, pp. 1212–1216, 2009.

11. Feng W. et al., Electrochemical sensor for multiplex biomarkers detection, *Clinical Cancer Research*, vol. 15, pp. 09-0050-OF1–09-0050-OF7, 2009.

12. Chikkaveeraiah H. V., Bhirde A. A., Morgan N. Y., Eden H. S., Chen X., Electrochemical immunosensors for detection of cancer protein biomarkers, *Nano*, vol. 6, pp. 6546–6561, 2012.

13. Rusling J. F., Kumar C. V., Gutkinde S., Patele V., Measurement of biomarker proteins for point-of-care early detection and monitoring of cancer, *Analyst*, vol. 135, pp. 2496–2511, 2010.

14. Lee K.-H., Choi S., Lee J. O., Yoon J.-B., Cho G.-H., CMOS capacitive biosensor with enhanced sensitivity for label-free dna detection, Proceedings of 2012 IEEE International Solid-State Circuits Conference, vol. 1, pp. 120–122, 2012.

15. Li C., Li X., Liu X., Kraatz H.-B., Exploiting the interaction of metal ions and peptide nucleic acids – DNA duplexes for the detection of a single nucleotide mismatch by electrochemical impedance spectroscopy, *Analytical Chemistry*, vol. 82, pp. 1166–1169, 2010.

16. Wang Y., Li C., Li X., Li Y., Kraatz H.-B., Unlabeled hairpin-DNA probe for the detection of single-nucleotide mismatches by electrochemical impedance spectroscopy, *Analytical Chemistry*, vol. 80, pp. 2255–2260, 2008.

17. Liu G., Liu J., Davis T. P., Gooding J. J., Electrochemical impedance immunosensor based on gold nanoparticles and aryl diazonium salt functionalized gold electrodes for the detection of antibody, *Biosensors and Bioelectronics*, vol. 26, pp. 3660–3665, 2011.

18. Chen A., Chatterjee C., Nanomaterials based electrochemical sensors for biomedical applications, *Chemical Society Reviews*, vol. 42, pp. 5425–5438, 2013.

19. Li C.-Z., Liu Y., Luong J. H. T., Impedance sensing of DNA binding drugs using gold substrates modified with gold nanoparticles, *Analytical Chemistry*, vol. 77, pp. 478–485, 2005.

20. Zhang K., Ma H., Zhang L., Zhang Y., Fabrication of a sensitive impedance biosensor of dna hybridization based on gold nanoparticles modified gold electrode, *Electroanalysis*, vol. 20, pp. 2127–2133, 2008.

21. Berggren C., Bjarnason B., Johansson G., Capacitive biosensors, *Electroanalysis*, vol. 13, pp. 173–180, 2001.

22. Lisdat F., Schäfer D., The use of electrochemical impedance spectroscopy for biosensing, *Analytical and Bioanalytical Chemistry*, vol. 391, pp. 1555–1567, 2008.

23. Hong. J., AC frequency characteristics of coplanar impedance sensors as design parameters, *Lab on a Chip*, vol. 5, pp. 270–279, 2005.

24. Marcus R. A., Electron transfer reactions in chemistry theory and experiment, *Pure & Applied Chemistry*, vol. 69, pp. 13–29, 1997.

25. Miller C. J., Heterogeneous electron transfer kinetics at metal electrodes, in *Physical Electrochemistry: Science and Technology*, Rubinstein I. editor, CRC Press; 1st edition (March 30, 1995), ISBN-13: 978-0824794521.

26. Zare H. R., Eslami M., Namazian M., Coote M. L., Experimental and Theoretical studies of redox reactions of o-chloranil in aqueous solution, *Journal of Physical Chemistry B*, vol. 113, pp. 8080–8085, 2009.

27. Lee W. T., Masel R. I., Ab initio calculations of the transition state energy and position for the reaction $H + C_2H_5R \rightarrow HH + C_2H_4R$, with $R = H, CH_3, NH_2, CN, CF_3, C_5H_6$: Comparison to Marcus' theory, Miller's theory, and Bockris' model, *Journal of Physical Chemistry*, vol. 100, pp. 10945–10951, 1996.

28. Luo X., Davis J. J., Electrical biosensors and the label free detection of protein disease biomarkers, *Chemical Society Reviews*, vol. 42, pp. 5944–5962, 2013.

29. Qureshi A., Gurbuz Y., Kallempudia S., Niazi J. H., Label-free rna aptamer-based capacitive biosensor for the detection of c-reactive protein, *Physical Chemistry, Chemical Physics*, vol. 12, pp. 9176–9182, 2010.

30. Chen H., Jiang J.-H., Huang Y., Deng T., Li J.-S., Shen G.-L., Yu R.-Q., An electrochemical impedance immunosensor with signal amplification based on au-colloid labeled antibody complex, *Sensors and Actuators B: Chemical*, vol. 117, pp. 211–218, 2006.

31. Liu Y., Tuleouva N., Ramanculov E., Revzin A., Aptamer-based electrochemical biosensor for interferon gamma detection, *Analytical Chemistry*, vol. 82, pp. 8131–8136, 2010.

32. Rodriguez M. C., Kawde A.-N., Wang J., Aptamer biosensor for label-free impedance spectroscopy detection of proteins based on recognition-induced switching of the surface charge, *Chemical Communications*, vol. 0, pp. 4267–4269, 2005.

33. White R. J. et al., Wash-free, *electrochemical platform for the quantitative, multiplexed detection of specific antibodies*, *Analytical Chemistry*, vol. 84, pp. 1098–1103, 2012.

34. Zhang Y. et al., Carbohydrate – protein interactions by "Clicked" carbohydrate self-assembled monolayers, *Analytical Chemistry*, vol. 78, pp. 2001–2008, 2006.

35. Rohrbach F., Karadeniz H., Erdem A., Famulok M., Mayer G., Label-free impedimetric aptasensor for lysozyme detection based on carbon nanotube-modified screen-printed electrodes, *Analytical Biochemistry*, vol. 421, pp. 454–459, 2012.

36. Lee C.-S., Baker S. E., Marcus M. S., Yang W., Eriksson M. A., Hamers R. J., Electrically addressable biomolecular functionalization of carbon nanotube and carbon nanofiber electrodes, *Nano Letters*, vol. 4, pp.1713–1716, 2004.

37. Shenggao W., Integrated carbon nanotubes electrodes in microfluidic chip via MWPCVD, *Plasma Science and Technology*, vol. 12, pp. 556–560, 2010.

38. Berdat D., Rodríguez A. C. M., Herrera F., Gijs M. A. M., Label-free detection of DNA with interdigitated micro-electrodes in a fluidic cell, *Lab on a Chip*, vol. 8, pp. 302–308, 2008.

39. Steude A., Schmidt S., Robitzki A. A., Pänke O., An electrode array for electrochemical immuno-sensing using the example of impedimetric tenascin c detection, *Lab on a Chip*, vol. 11, pp. 2884–2892, 2011.

40. Odijk M., Olthuis W., van den Berg A., *Improved Conversion Rates in Drug Screening Applications Using Miniaturized Electrochemical Cells with Frit Channels*, Analytical Chemistry, vol. 84, pp. 9176–9183, 2012.

41. Katz E., Probing biomolecular interactions at conductive and semiconductive surfaces by impedance spectroscopy: Route to impedimetric immunosensors, dna sensors and enzyme biosensors, *Electroanalysis*, vol. 15, pp. 913–947, 2003.

42. Xu D., Xu D., Yu X., Liu Z., He W., Ma Z., Label-free electrochemical detection for aptamer-based array electrodes, *Analytical Chemistry*, vol. 77, pp. 5107–5113, 2005.

43. Yeon J. H., Park J.-K., Cytotoxicity test based on electrochemical impedance measurement of HepG2 cultured in microfabricated cell chip, *Analytical Biochemistry*, vol. 341, pp. 308–315, 2005.

44. Daza P., Olmo A., Cañete D., Yúfera A., Monitoring living cell assays with bio-impedance sensors, *Sensors and Actuators B: Chemical*, vol. 176, pp. 605–610, 2013.

45. López Rodriguez M. L., Madrid R. E., Giacomelli C. E., Evaluation of impedance spectroscopy as a transduction method for bacterial biosensors, *IEEE Latin America Transactions*, vol. 11, pp. 196–200, 2013.

46. Qiu Y., Liao R., Zhang X., Real-time monitoring primary cardiomyocyte adhesion based on electrochemical impedance spectroscopy and electrical cell – substrate impedance sensing, *Analytical Chemistry*, vol. 80, pp. 990–996, 2008.

47. Luong J. H. T., Habibi-Rezaei M., Meghrous J., Xiao C., Male K. B., Kamen A., Monitoring motility, spreading, and mortality of adherent insect cells using an impedance sensor, *Analytical Chemistry*, vol. 73, pp. 1844–1848, 2001.

48. Seriburi P., McGuire S., Shastry A., Böhringer K. F., Meldrum D. R., Measurement of the cell – substrate separation and the projected area of an individual adherent cell using electric cell – substrate impedance sensing, *Analytical Chemistry*, vol. 80, pp. 3677–3683, 2008.

49. Syed L. U., Liu J., Price A. K., Li Y. F., Culbertson C. T., Li J., Dielectrophoretic capture of e. coli cells at micropatterned nanoelectrode arrays, *Electrophoresis*, vol. 32, pp. 2358–2365, 2011.

50. Lagally E. T., Lee S.-H., Soh T. H., Integrated microsystem for dielectrophoretic cell concentration and genetic detection, *Lab on a Chip*, vol. 5, pp. 1053–1058, 2005.

51. Jonassen N., Electrostatics, Springer; 2nd edition (August 31, 2002), ISBN-13: 978–1402071614.

52. Prodan E., Prodan C., Miller Jr J. H., The dielectric response of spherical live cells in suspension: An analytic solution, *Biophysical Journal*, vol. 95, pp. 4174–4182, 2008.

53. Asami K., Hanai T., Koizumi N., Dielectric analysis of escherichia coli suspensions in the light of the theory of interfacial polarization, *Biophysical Journal*, vol. 31, pp. 215–228, 1980.

54. Jones P. V., Staton J. R., Hayes M. A., Blood cell capture in a sawtooth dielectrophoretic microchannel, *Analytical and Bioanalytical Chemistry*, vol. 401, pp. 2103–2111, 2011.

55. Yang L., Banada P. P., Bhunia A. K., Bashir R., Effects of dielectrophoresis on growth, viability and immuno-reactivity of listeria monocytogenes, *Journal of Biological Engineering*, vol. 2, 2008.

56. Suehiro J., Hamada R., Noutomi D., Shutou M., Hara M., Selective detection of viable bacteria using dielectrophoretic impedance measurement method, *Journal of Electrostatics*, vol. 57, pp. 157–168, 2003.

57. Gómez-Sjöberg R., Morisette D. T., Bashir R., Impedance microbiology-on-a-chip: Microfluidic bioprocessor for rapid detection of bacterial metabolism, *Journal of Microelectromechanical Systems*, vol. 14, pp. 829–838, 2005.

58. Borghol N. et al., Electrochemical monitoring of chlorhexidine digluconate effect on polyelectrolyte immobilized bacteria and kinetic cell adhesion, *Journal of Biotechnology*, vol. 151, pp. 114–121, 2011.

59. Callegaro L., *Electrical Impedance: Principles, Measurement, and Applications*, Taylor & Francis; 1st edition (December 20, 2012), ISBN-13: 978-1439849101.

60. Lvovich V. F., *Impedance Spectroscopy: Applications to Electrochemical and Dielectric Phenomena*, Wiley; 1st edition (July 3, 2012), ISBN-13: 978-0470627785.

61. Sarason D., *Complex Function Theory, American Mathematical Society*; 2nd edition (December 20, 2007), ISBN-13: 978-0821844281.

62. Friedlander F. G., Joshi M., *Introduction to the Theory of Distributions*, Cambridge University Press; 2nd edition (January 28, 1999), ISBN-13: 978-0521649711.

63. Brigham O., *The Fast Fourier Transform: An Introduction to Its Theory and Application*, Prentice Hall; 1st edition (November 1973), ISBN-13: 978-0133074963.

64. Compton R. G., Banks C. E., *Understanding Voltammetry*, Imperial College Press; 2nd edition (January 31, 2011), ISBN-13: 978-1848165861.

65. Komarova E., Aldissi M., Bogomolova A., Direct electrochemical sensor for fast reagent-free DNA detection, *Biosensors and Bioelectronics*, vol. 21, pp. 182–189, 2005.

66. Yang Y., Liu G., Liu H., Li D., Fan C., Liu D., An electrochemically actuated reversible DNA switch, *Nano Letters*, vol. 1 pp. 1393–1397, 2010.

67. Inoue K. Y. et al., Electrochemical monitoring of hydrogen peroxide released from leucocytes on horseradish peroxidase redox polymer coated electrode chip, *Biosensors and Bioelectronics*, vol. 25, pp. 1723–1728, 2010.

68. Chuang M.-C., Lai H.-Y., Ho J.-A. A., Chen Y.-Y., Multifunctional microelectrode array (mMEA) chip for neural-electrical and neural-chemical interfaces: Characterization of comb interdigitated electrode towards dopamine detection, *Biosensors and Bioelectronics*, vol. 41, pp. 602–607, 2013.

69. Mason A., Huang Y., Yang C., Zhang J., Amperometric readout and electrode array chip for bioelectrochemical sensors, *Proceedings of IEEE International Symposium on Circuits and Systems*, 2007, pp. 3562–3565, 2007.

70. Liu H., Crooks R. M., Highly reproducible chronoamperometric analysis in microdroplets., *Lab on a Chip*, vol. 13, pp. 1364–1370, 2013.

71. Compton R. G, Banks C. E., Understanding Voltammetry, World Scientific Publishing Company; (September 10, 2007), ISBN-13: 978-9812706256.

72. Keller H. E., Reinmuth W. H., Potential scan voltammetry with finite diffusion. unified theory, *Analytical Chemistry*, vol. 44, pp. 434–442, 1972.

73. M. Seralathan M., Osteryoung R. A., Osteryoung J. G., General equivalence of linear scan and staircase voltammetry, *Journal of Electroanalytical Chemistry and Interfacial Electrochemistry*, vol. 222, pp. 69–100, 1987.

74. Osteryoung J. G., Osteryoung R. A., Square wave voltammetry, *Analytical Chemistry*, vol. 57, pp. 101A–110A, 1987.

75. Oldham K. B., Gavaghan D. J., Bond A. M., A full analytic treatment of reversible linear-scan voltammetry with square-wave modulation, *Journal of Physical Chemistry B*, vol. 106, pp. 152–157, 2002.

76. Nicholson R. S., Theory and application of cyclic voltammetry for measurement of electrode reaction kinetic, *Analytical Chemistry*, vol. 37, pp. 1351–1355, 1965.

77. Raoof J.-B., Ojani R., Nematollahi D., Kiani A., Digital simulation of the cyclic voltammetry study of the catechols electrooxidation in the presence of some nitrogen and carbon nucleophiles, *International Journal of Electrochemical Science*, vol. 4, pp. 810–819, 2009.

78. Prasad M. A., Sangaranarayanan M. V., Formulation of a simple analytical expression for irreversible electron transfer processes in linear sweep voltammetry and its experimental verification, *Electrochimica Acta*, vol. 49, pp. 2569–2579, 2004.

79. Qiu P., Ni Y.-N., Kokot S., Application of artificial neural networks to the determination of pesticides by linear sweep stripping voltammetry, *Chinese Chemical Letters*, vol. 24, March, pp. 246–248, 2013.

80. Polo-Corpa M. J., Salcedo-Sanz S., Pérez-Bellido A. M., López-Espí P., Benavente R., Pérez E., Curve fitting using heuristics and bio-inspired optimization algorithms for experimental data processing in chemistry, *Chemometrics and Intelligent Laboratory Systems*, vol. 96, pp. 34–42, 2009.

81. Górski Ł., Jakubowska M., Baś B., Kubiak W. W., Application of genetic algorithm for baseline optimization in standard addition voltammetry, *Journal of Electroanalytical Chemistry*, vol. 684, pp. 38–46, 2012.

82. Jakubowska M., Hybrid signal processing in voltammetric determination of chromium(VI), *Journal of Hazardous Materials*, vol. 176, pp. 540–548, 2010.

83. Nyholm L., Electrochemical techniques for lab-on-a-chip applications, *Analyst*, vol. 130, pp. 599–605, 2005.

84. Wang J., Polsky R., Tian B., Chatrathi M. P., Voltammetry on microfluidic chip platforms, *Analytical Chemistry*, vol. 72, pp. 5285–5289, 2005.

85. Ge R. et al., Evaluation of a microfluidic device for the electrochemical determination of halide content in ionic liquids, *Analytical Chemistry*, vol. 81, pp. 1628–1637, 2009.

86. Galvez J., Park S.-M., A unified treatment for potentiostatic voltammetry at spherical and planar electrodes, *Journal of Electroanalytical Chemistry and Interfacial Electrochemistry*, vol. 259, pp. 21–37, 1989.

87. Murphy M. M., Stojek Z., O'Dea J. J., Osteryoung J. G., Pulse voltammetry at cylindrical electrodes: Oxidation of anthracene, *Electrochimica Acta*, vol. 36, pp. 1475–1484, 1991.

88. Chevion S., Roberts M. A., Chevion M., The use of cyclic voltammetry for the evaluation of antioxidant capacity, *Free Radical Biology and Medicine*, vol. 28, 15 pp. 860–870, 2000.

89. Rapson T. D., Kappler U., Bernhardt P. V., Direct catalytic electrochemistry of sulfite dehydrogenase: Mechanistic insights and contrasts with related mo enzymes, *Biochimica et Biophysica Acta— Bioenergetics*, vol. 1777, pp. 1319–1325, 2008.

90. Leger C., Elliott S. J., Hoke K. R., Jeuken L. J. C., Jones A. K., Armstrong F. A., Enzyme electrokinetics: Using protein film voltammetry to investigate redox enzymes and their mechanisms, *Biochemistry*, vol. 42, pp. 8653–8662, 2003.

91. Hu N., Direct electrochemistry of redox proteins or enzymes at various film electrodes and their possible applications in monitoring some pollutants, *Pure and Applied Chemistry*, vol. 73, pp. 1979–1991, 2001.

92. Mazzei F. et al., Soft-landed protein voltammetry: A tool for redox protein characterization, *Analytical Chemistry*, vol. 80, pp. 5937–5944, 2008.

93. Armstrong F. A., Heering H. A., Hirst J., Reaction of complex metalloproteins studied by protein-film voltammetry, *Chemical Society Review*, vol. 26, pp. 169–179, 1997.

94. Davis J. J., O Hill H. A., Bond A. M., The application of electrochemical scanning probe microscopy to the interpretation of metalloprotein voltammetry, *Coordination Chemistry Reviews*, vol. 200–202, pp. 411–442, 2000.

95. Jensen P. S., Engelbrekt C., Sørensen K. H., Zhang J., Chia Q., Ulstrup J., Au-biocompatible metallic nanostructures in metalloprotein electrochemistry and electrocatalysis, *Journal of Material Chemistry*, vol. 22, pp. 13877–13882, 2012.

96. Rawson F. J., Jackson S. K., Hart, J. P., Voltammetric behaviour of DNA and its derivatives using screen printed carbon electrodes and its possible application in genotoxicity screening, *Analytical Letters*, vol. 43, pp. 1790–1800, 2010.

97. Zhao G.-C., Zhu J.-J., Zhang J.-J., Chen H.-Y., Voltammetric studies of the interaction of methylene blue with DNA by means of b-cyclodextrin, *Analytica Chimica Acta*, vol. 394, pp. 337–344, 1999.

98. Oliveira-Brett A. M., Piedade J. A. P., Silva L. A., Diculescu V. C., Voltammetric determination of all DNA nucleotides, *Analytical Biochemistry*, vol. 332, pp. 321–329, 2004.

99. Odijk M. et al., A microfluidic chip for electrochemical conversions in drug metabolism studies, *Lab on a Chip*, vol. 9, pp. 1687–1693, 2009.

100. Yoo S. J. et al., Microfluidic chip-based electrochemical immunoassay for hippuric acid, *Analyst*, vol. 134, pp. 2462–2467, 2009.

101. Illa X., Ordeig O., Snakenborg D., Romano-Rodríguez A., Comptonc R. G., Kutterb J. P., A cyclo olefin polymer microfluidic chip with integrated gold microelectrodes for aqueous and non-aqueous electrochemistry, *Lab on a Chip*, vol. 10, pp. 1254–1261, 2010.

102. Sasso L. et al., Doped overoxidized polypyrrole microelectrodes as sensors for the detection of dopamine released from cell populations, *Analyst*, vol. 138, pp. 3651–3659, 2013.

103. Levine P. M., Gong P., Levicky R., Shepard K. L., Active CMOS sensor array for electrochemical biomolecular detection, *Journal of Solid-State Circuits*, vol. 43, pp. 1859–1871, 2008.

104. Sungkil H., LaFratta C. N., Agarwal V., Xin Y., Walt D. R., Sonkusale S., CMOS microelectrode array for electrochemical lab-on-a-chip applications, *Sensors Journal*, vol. 9, pp. 609–615, 2008.

105. Schueller O. J. A., Brittain S. T., Marzolin C., Whitesides G. M., Fabrication and characterization of glassy carbon MEMS, *Chemistry of Materials*, vol. 9, pp. 1399–1406, 1997.

106. Schueller O. J. A., Brittain S. T., Whitesides G. M., Fabrication of glassy carbon microstructures by soft lithography, *Sensors and Actuators A, Physical*, vol. 72, pp. 125–139, 1999.

107. Trava-Airoldi V. J. et al., Development of chemical vapor deposition diamond burrs using hot filament, *Review of Scientific Instruments*, vol. 67, pp. 1993–1997, 1996.

108. Vadali V. S. S., Srikanth P., Sampath K., Vijay B. K., A brief review on the *in situ* synthesis of boron-doped diamond thin films, *International Journal of Electrochemistry*, vol. 2012, Article ID 218393, 2012.

109. Crevillén A. G., Pumer M., Gonzàlez M. C., Escarpa A., Towards lab-on-a-chip approaches in real analytical domains based on microfluidic chips/electrochemical multi-walled carbon nanotube platforms, *Lab on a Chip*, vol. 9, pp. 346–353, 2009.

110. Okuno J., Maehashi K., Matsumoto K., Kerman K., Takamura Y., Tamiya E., Single-walled carbon nanotube-arrayed microelectrode chip for electrochemical analysis, *Electrochemistry Communications*, vol. 9, pp. 13–18, 2007.

111. Malhotra R., Patel V., Vaqué J. P., Gutkind J. S., Rusling J. F., Ultrasensitive electrochemical immunosensor for oral cancer biomarker il-6 using carbon nanotube forest electrodes and multilabel amplification, *Analytical Chemistry*, vol. 82, pp. 3118–3123, 2010.

112. Kihara T. et al., Direct electron transfer to hydrogenase for catalytic hydrogen production using a single-walled carbon nanotube forest, *International Journal of Hydrogen Energy*, vol. 36, pp. 7523–7529, 2011.

113. Yu X., Chattopadhyay D., Galeska I., Papadimitrakopoulos F., Rusling J. F., Peroxidase activity of enzymes bound to the ends of single-wall carbon nanotube forest electrodes, *Electrochemistry Communications*, vol. 5, pp. 408–411, 2003.

114. Taurino I., Carrara S., Giorcelli M., Tagliaferro, De Micheli G., Comparing sensitivities of differently oriented multi-walled carbon nanotubes integrated on silicon wafer for electrochemical biosensors, *Sensors and Actuators B: Chemical*, vol. 160, pp. 327–333, 2011.

115. Lamberti F., Ferraro D., Giomo M., Elvassore N., Enhancement of heterogeneous electron transfer dynamics tuning single-walled carbon nanotube forest height and density, *Electrochimica Acta*, vol. 97, pp. 304–312, 2013.

116. Geim A. K., Novoselov K. S., The rise of graphene, *Nature Materials*, vol. 6, 183–191, 2007.

117. Brownson D. A. C., Fostera C. W., Banks C. E., The electrochemical performance of graphene modified electrodes: An analytical perspective, *Analyst*, vol. 137, pp. 1815–1823, 2012.

118. Brownson D. A. C., Munro L. J., Kampourisa D. K., Banks C. E., Electrochemistry of graphene: Not such a beneficial electrode material?, *RSC Advances*, vol. 1, pp. 978–988, 2011.

119. Armstrong N. R., Lin A. W. C., Fujihira M., Kuwana T., Electrochemical and surface characteristics of tin oxide and indium oxide electrodes, *Analytical Chemistry*, vol. 48, pp. 741–750, 1976.

120. Bugg T. D. H., *Introduction to Enzyme and Coenzyme Chemistry*, Wiley; 3rd edition (August 13, 2012), ISBN-13: 978-1119995944.

121. Čenas N. K., Kulys J. J., Biocatalytic oxidation of glucose on the conductive charge transfer complexes, *Bioelectrochemistry and Bioenergetics*, vol. 8, pp. 103–113, 1981.

122. Kalys J. J., Enzyme electrodes based on organic metals, *Biosensors*, vol. 2, pp. 3–13, 1986.

123. Bartlett P. N., *Conducting Organic Salt Electrodes*, in Biosensors: A Practical Approach, Cass A. E. G. editor, Oxford University Press, USA; (August 30, 1990), ISBN-13: 978-0199630479.

124. Fultz M. L., Durst R. A., Mediator compounds for the electrochemical study of biological RedOx systems—a compilation, *Analytica Chimica Acta*, vol. 140, pp. 1–18, 1982.

125. Martens N., Hindle A., Hall E. A. H., An assessment of mediators as oxidants for glucose oxidase in the presence of oxygen, *Biosensors and Bioelectronics*, vol. 10, pp. 393–403, 1995.

126. Guang L., Hui X., Wenjun H., You W., Yesi W., Rabindra P., A pyrrole quinoline quinone glucose dehydrogenase biosensor based on screen-printed carbon paste electrodes modified by carbon nanotubes, *Measurement Science and Technology*, vol. 19, pp. 065203–065203, 2008.

127. Kotziana P., Brazdilovà P., Kalcherb K., Handlíř K., Vytřas K., Oxides of platinum metal group as potential catalysts in carbonaceous amperometric biosensors based on oxidases, *Sensors and Actuators B*, vol. 124, pp., 297–302, 2007.

128. Canevet D., Sallé M., Zhang G., Zhang D., Zhub D., Tetrathiafulvalene (TTF) derivatives: Key building-blocks for switchable processes, *Chemical Communications*, pp. 2245–2269, 2009.

129. Qiu J.-D., Deng M.-D., Liang R.-P., Xiong M., Ferrocene-modified multiwalled carbon nanotubes as building block for construction of reagentless enzyme-based biosensors, *Sensors and Actuators B: Chemical*, vol. 135, pp. 181–187, 2008.

130. Chen M., Diao G., Electrochemical study of mono-6-thio-beta-cyclodextrin/ferrocene capped on gold nanoparticles: Characterization and application to the design of glucose amperometric biosensor, *Talanta*, vol. 80, 815–820, 2009.

131. Heller A., Electrical wiring of redox enzymes, *Account of Chemical Research*, vol. 23, pp. 128–134, 1990.

132. Karan H. I., *Enzyme Biosensors Containing Polymeric Electron Transfer Systems*, in: Biosensors and Modern Biospecific Analytical Techniques, Gorton L. Editor, Elsevier Science; 1st edition (June 1, 2005), ISBN-13: 978-0444507150, pp. 131–178.

133. Ghanim M. H., Abdullah M. Z., Integrating amperometric detection with electrophoresis microchip devices for biochemical assays: Recent developments, *Talanta*, vol. 85, pp. 28–34, 2011.

134. Floris A., Lenk S. S., Staijen E., Kohlheyer D., Eijkelb J., van den Bergb A., A prefilled, ready-to-use electrophoresis based lab-on-a-chip device for monitoring lithium in blood, *Lab on a Chip*, vol. 10, pp. 1799–1806, 2010.

135. Fernández-la-Villa A., Bertrand-Serrador V., Pozo-Ayusoa D. F., Castaño-Álvarez M., Fast and reliable urine analysis using a portable platform based on microfluidic electrophoresis chips with electrochemical detection, *Analytical Methods*, vol. 5, pp. 1494–1501, 2013.

136. Lee H.-L., Chen S.-C., Microchip capillary electrophoresis with amperometric detection for several carbohydrates, *Talanta*, vol. 64, pp. 210–216, 2004.

137. Joo G.-S., Jha S. K., Kim Y.-S., A capillary electrophoresis microchip for amperometric detection of DNA, *Current Applied Physics*, vol. 9, Supplement, pp. e222–e224, 2009.

138. Wu Y., Lin J. M., Su R., Qu F., Cai Z., An end-channel amperometric detector for microchip capillary electrophoresis, *Talanta*, vol. 64, pp. 338–344, 2004.

139. Wu Y.-Y., Feng Q., Lin J.-M., Microchip capillary electrophoresis with an end-channel amperometric detector and its preliminary application, *Chinese Journal of Chemistry*, vol. 23, pp. 155–159, 2005.

140. Tomazelli Coltro W. K. et al., Electrophoresis microchip fabricated by a direct-printing process with end-channel amperometric detection, *Electrophoresis*, vol. 25, pp. 3832–3839, 2004.

141. Wallenborg S. R., Nyholm L., Lunte S. C. E., End-column amperometric detection in capillary electrophoresis: Influence of separation-related parameters on the observed half-wave potential for dopamine and catechol, *Analytical Chemisty*, vol. 71, pp. 544–549, 1999.

142. Gunasekara D. B., Hulvey M. K., Lunte S. M., In-channel amperometric detection for microchip electrophoresis using a wireless isolated potentiostat, *Electrophoresis*, vol. 32, pp. 832–837, 2011.

143. Hebert N. E., Kuhr W. G., Brazill S. A., A microchip electrophoresis device with integrated electrochemical detection: A direct comparison of constant potential amperometry and sinusoidal voltammetry, *Analytical Chemistry*, vol. 75, pp. 3301–3307, 2003.

144. Vázquez M., Frankenfeld C., Tomazelli Coltro W. K., Diamonda D., Lunte S. M., Dual contactless conductivity and amperometric detection on hybrid PDMS/glass electrophoresis microchips, *Analyst*, vol. 135, pp. 96–103, 2010.

145. Chen D.-C., Hsu F.-L., Zhan D.-Z., Chen C.-H., Palladium film decoupler for amperometric detection in electrophoresis chips, *Analytical Chemistry*, vol. 73, pp. 758–762, 2001.

146. Lin K.-W., Huang Y.-K., Su H.-L., Hsieh Y.-Z., In-channel simplified decoupler with renewable electrochemical detection for microchip capillary electrophoresis, *Analytica Chimica Acta*, vol. 619, pp. 115–121, 2008.

147. Chen C., Hahn J. H., Dual-channel method for interference-free in-channel amperometric detection in microchip capillary electrophoresis, *Analytical Chemistry*, vol. 79, pp. 7182–7186, 2007.

148. Chen C., Teng W., Hahn J. H., Nanoband electrode for high-performance in-channel amperometric detection in dual-channel microchip capillary electrophoresis, *Electrophoresis*, vol. 32, pp. 793–956, 2011.

149. Manica D. P., Mitsumori Y., Ewing A. G., Characterization of electrode fouling and surface regeneration for a platinum electrode on an electrophoresis microchip, *Analytical Chemistry*, vol. 75, pp. 4572–4577, 2003.

150. Roberts M. J., Signals and Systems: Analysis of Signals through Linear Systems, McGraw-Hill Science/ Engineering/Math; 1st edition (June 18, 2003), ISBN-13: 978-0072930443.

151. Brandt A., Noise and Vibration Analysis: Signal Analysis and Experimental Procedures, Wiley; 1st edition (February 14, 2011), ISBN-13: 978-0470746448.

152. Fanguya J. C., Henry C. S., Pulsed amperometric detection of carbohydrates on an electrophoretic microchip, *Analyst*, vol. 127, pp. 1021–1023, 2007.

153. García C. D., Henry C. S., Enhanced determination of glucose by microchip electrophoresis with pulsed amperometric detection, *Analytica Chimica Acta*, vol. 508, pp. 1–9, 2004.

154. García C. D., Henry C. S., Coupling capillary electrophoresis and pulsed electrochemical detection, *Electroanalysis*, vol. 17, pp. 1125–1131, 2005.

155. Islam K., Jha S. K., Chand R. Han D., Kim Y.-S., Fast detection of triazine herbicides on a microfluidic chip using capillary electrophoresis pulse amperometric detection, *Journal of Microelectronic Engineering*, vol. 97, pp. 391–395, 2012.

156. García C. D., Henry C. S., Direct detection of renal function markers using microchip ce with pulsed electrochemical detection, *Analyst*, vol. 129, pp. 579–584, 2004.

157. Hompesch R. W., García C. D., Weiss D. J., Vivancod J. M., Henry C. S., Analysis of natural flavonoids by microchip-micellar electrokinetic chromatography with pulsed amperometric detection, *Analyst*, vol. 130, pp. 694–700, 2004.

158. Holcomb R. E., Kralya J. R., Henry C. S., Electrode array detector for microchip capillary electrophoresis, *Analyst*, vol. 134, pp. 486–492, 2009.

159. Mason A., Lansing M. I., Huang Y., Yang C., Zhang J., *Amperometric Readout and Electrode Array Chip for Bioelectrochemical Sensors*, Proceedings of IEEE International Symposium on Circuits and Systems, ISCAS 2007, New Orleans, LA, pp. 3562–3565, 2007.

160. Hasegawa J., Uno S., Nakazato K., Amperometric electrochemical sensor array for on-chip simultaneous imaging: Circuit and microelectrode design considerations, *Japanese Journal of Applied Physics*, vol. 50, pp. 153–162, 2011.

161. Kooser A., Gunter, R. L., Delinger W. D., Porter T. L., Eastman M. P., Gas sensing using embedded piezoresistive microcantilever sensors, *Sensors and Actuators B: Chemical*, vol. 99, pp. 474–479, 2004.

162. Yang S. M., Chang C., A piezoresistive bridge-microcantilever biosensor by cmos process for surface stress measurement, *Sensors and Actuators B: Chemical*, vol. 145, pp. 405–410, 2010.

163. Fernandez R. E., Chadha A., Bhattacharya E., Stolyarova S., Nemirovsky Y., *MEMS Composite Porous Silicon/Polysilicon Cantilever Sensor for Enhanced Triglycerides Biosensing*, Proceedings of IEEE Sensors 2008, pp. 1468–1471, 2008.

164. Youzheng Z., Wang Z., Qi Z., Wenzhou R., Liu L., A front-side released single crystalline silicon piezoresistive microcantilever sensor, *Sensors Journal*, vol. 9, pp. 246–254, 2009.

165. Kale N. S., Nag S., Pinto R., Ramgopal Rao V., Fabrication and characterization of a polymeric microcantilever with an encapsulated hotwire CVD polysilicon piezoresistor, *Journal of Microelectromechanical Systems*, vol. 18, pp. 79–87, 2009.

166. Liu Y., Schweizer L. M., Wang W., Reuben R. L., Schweizer M., Shu W., Label-free and real-time monitoring of yeast cell growth by the bending of polymer microcantilever biosensors, *Sensors and Actuators B: Chemical*, vol. 178, pp. 621–626, 2013.

167. Battiston F. L. et al., A chemical sensor based on microfabricated cantilever array with simultaneous resonance-frequency and bending readout, *Sensors and Actuators B: Chemical*, vol. 77, pp. 122–131, 2001.

168. Wu L., Zhou X.-R., Wu S.-Q., Wang P., Zhang Q.-C., Wu X.-P., Preparation of a novel microcantilever array biochemical sensor, *Chinese Journal of Analytical Chemistry*, vol. 40, pp. 493–497, 2012.

169. Zinoviev K., Dominguez C., Plaza J. A., Busto V. J. C., Lechuga L. M., A novel optical waveguide microcantilever sensor for the detection of nanomechanical forces, *Journal of Lightwave Technology*, vol. 24, pp. 2132–2138, 2006.

170. McKendry R. et al., Multiple label-free biodetection and quantitative dna-binding assays on a nanomechanical cantilever array, *Proceedings of the National Academy of Science of United States of America*, vol. 99, pp. 9783–9788, 2002.

171. Afshari M., Jalili N., Towards non-linear modeling of molecular interactions arising from adsorbed biological species on the microcantilever surface, *International Journal of Non-Linear Mechanics*, vol. 42, pp. 588–595, 2007.

172. Dufour I., Fadel L., Resonant microcantilever type chemical sensors: Analytical modeling in view of optimization, *Sensors and Actuators B: Chemical*, vol. 91, pp. 353–361, 2003.

173. Khanafer K., Alamiri A., Pop I., Fluid–structure interaction analysis of flow and heat transfer characteristics around a flexible microcantilever in a fluidic cell, *International Journal of Heat and Mass Transfer*, vol. 53, pp. 1646–1653, 2010.

174. Gunter R. L., Zhine R., Delinger W. G., Manygoats K., Kooser A., Porter T. L., Investigation of DNA sensing using piezoresistive microcantilever probes, *Sensors Journal*, vol. 4, pp. 430–433, 2004.

175. Tuantranont A., Lomas T., Jaruwongrungsee K., Jomphoak A., Wisitsoraat A., Symmetrical PolyMUMPs-based piezoresistive microcantilever sensors with on-chip temperature compensation for microfluidics applications, *Sensors Journal*, vol. 8, pp. 543–547, 2008.

176. Barlian A. A., Park W.-T., Mallon Jr J. R., Rastegar A. J., Pruitt B. L., Semiconductor piezoresistance for microsystems, Proceedings of Institute of Electrical and Electronic Engineering, vol. 97, pp. 513–552, 2009.

177. Quist A., Chand A., Ramachandran S., Cohena D., Lal R., Piezoresistive cantilever based nanoflow and viscosity sensor for microchannels, *Lab on a Chip*, vol. 6, pp. 1450–1454, 2006.

178. Lee J. et al., Suspended microchannel resonators with piezoresistive sensors, *Lab on a Chip*, vol. 11, pp. 645–651, 2011.

179. Polesel-Maris J., et al. Piezoresistive cantilever array for life sciences applications, *Journal of Physics*, vol. 61, pp. 955–959, 2007.

180. Park S.-J., Doll J. C., Pruitt B. L., Piezoresistive cantilever performance—part i: Analytical model for sensitivity, *Journal of Microelectromechanical Systems*, vol. 19, pp. 137–148, 2010.

181. Xie B., Ramanathan K., Danielsson B., Mini/Micro thermal biosensors and other related devices for bio-chemical/clinical analysis and monitoring, *TrAC Trends in Analytical Chemistry*, vol. 19, pp. 340–349, 2000.

182. Goldsmid H. J., Introduction to Thermoelectricity, Springer; 1st edition (October 28, 2009), ISBN-13: 978–3642007156.

183. MacDonald D. K. C., Thermoelectricity: An Introduction to the Principles, Dover Publications; (October 27, 2006), ISBN-13: 978-0486453040.

184. Burns G. W., Scroger M. G., Strouse G. F., Croarkin M. C., Guthrie W. F., Temperature-electromotive force reference functions and tables for the letter-designated thermocouple types based on the ITS-90. *Natl. Inst. Stand. Technol. Monograph*, vol. 175, p. 630, 1993.

185. NIST Standard Reference Database 60, Version 2.0 (Web Version), http://srdata.nist.gov/its90/main/its90_main_page.html, last accessed on June 11, 2013.

186. Adrega T., van Herwaarden A. W., Chip calorimeter for thermal characterization of bio-chemical solutions, *Sensors and Actuators A: Physical*, vol. 167, pp. 354–358, 2011.

187. van Herwaarden A. W., Overview of calorimeter chips for various applications, *Thermochimica Acta*, vol. 432, pp. 192–201, 2005.

188. Bataillard P., Steffgen E., Haemmerli S., Manz A., Widmer H. M., An integrated silicon thermopile as biosensor for the thermal monitoring of glucose, urea and penicillin, *Biosensors and Bioelectronics*, vol. 8, pp. 89–98, 1993.

189. Allison S. C., Smith R. L., Howard D. W., González C., Collins S. D., A bulk micromachined silicon thermopile with high sensitivity, *Sensors and Actuators A: Physical*, vol. 104, pp. 32–39, 2003.

190. Wonhee L., Warren F., Blake W. A., Roukes M. L., High-sensitivity microfluidic calorimeters for biological and chemical applications, Proceedings of the Academy of Science of United States of America, vol. 106, pp. 15225–15230, 2009.

11 Optical Detection

11.1 INTRODUCTION

In this chapter we analyze the optical detection techniques, while techniques generating an electronic detection signal are reviewed in Chapter 10.

Optical detection systems can be divided into free optics and integrated optical systems. Free optical techniques use free propagation optics to test the optical response of the target inside a detection chamber of the lab on chip. In this case, a transparent window is generally created on the surface of the lab on chip and it is inserted into an external device integrating one or more optical sources, generally lasers, and one or more optical detectors. The sources illuminate the sample inside the lab on chip and the detectors collect the output light and analyze it to provide the detection result. In the case of integrated optical detection, an integrated optics circuit is realized inside the lab on chip. Sources and detectors can be either integrated onto the lab on chip too, using either monolithic or hybrid technologies (see Section 6.3.1), or placed in an external equipment where the lab on chip has to be inserted. In both cases, sources and detectors have to be coupled with the integrated optical circuits and, if the external solution is chosen, the chip has also to integrate an optical interface between the on-chip waveguides and the external system (see Section 6.5.4).

Another important classification of optical detection methods can be done by distinguishing labeled and unlabeled methods. In labeled methods, the optical response is generated by the presence of an optically active molecule, called label that emits photons in the presence of the target molecule. ELISA assays are among the most common assays using optical labeling. No label is present in unlabeled detection, where an optical property of the sample solution like the refraction index is directly measured in order to quantify the presence of the target. Labeled methods are very sensible and accurate, but require costly reagents and a complex assay procedure. Moreover, as in the case of functionalized surfaces, the reagents have to be frequently inserted into the lab on chip during fabrication, implying severe requirements in terms of stability. Such requirements are much relaxed if unlabeled detection is adopted.

Here, we will treat mainly unlabeled detection systems, since labeled detection is not different from detection carried out in macroscopic assays considered in Chapter 3.

A last type of optical detection can be used in the case of application of lab on chip to cell study: direct optical imaging. As a matter of fact, cell dimension allows optical microscope observation so that they can be observed using an optical microscope through a transparent window in the chip. This is mainly a laboratory technique, but it can be very useful when lab on chip is used for laboratory cell study due to their stability, ease of use, and reproducible results. Finally, direct observation detection methods exist, simply based on the observation of some optical property of the lab on chip surface that changes due to the assay result. Frequently, this is done through a dye changing its color in the assay room and visible from the outside of the lab on chip. This kind of detection is naturally not strictly quantitative, but it is very simple and it can be useful for field use lab on chips whose scope is the identification of the presence of a given substance.

A scheme of the classification of optical detection techniques for lab on chip is reported in Figure 11.1.

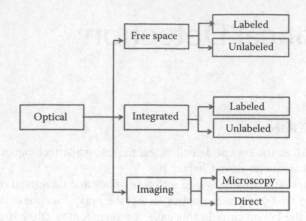

FIGURE 11.1   Classification of optical detection technique for lab on chip.

11.2   ELEMENTS OF OPTICS

The most fundamental theory of matter we have is the so-called standard theory, based on the quantum field description of matter and energy [1,2]. This is a quantum-relativistic theory, where matter and energy are effectively the same entity and seamless transformation of matter into energy and vice versa happens. In such circumstances, the approach of describing the motion of a particle through a motion equation providing motion description starting from the energy characteristics of the system cannot be adopted. As a matter of fact, particles appear and disappear, while they transform one into the other and into energy.

System dynamics is described by the so-called quantum field approach. The quantum field is essentially a collective description of the whole energy that is present in the system: each particular form that such energy assumes, for example, a particular set of particle with a particular quantum state of each particle, is no more than a specific quantum state of the field. While the field evolves through different quantum states the particles are transformed one into the other, while particles are created and destructed.

Such a complex matter representation is never needed in analyzing lab on chip systems, since it is required only when huge amounts of energy, that is, velocities near to light speed, are present. It is evident that fluids, molecular populations and material probes, never reach these conditions, with light being an exception. As a matter of fact, light travels at light speed by definition so that we have to expect that phenomena related to quantum field theory are intrinsic to any analysis of light interaction with matter.

As a matter of fact, the simpler conceivable quantum field is just the electromagnetic field and the particles associated with the electromagnetic fields are photons. Photons are really created when they are emitted and destroyed when they are absorbed, while the photon energy and number depend on the state of the corresponding electromagnetic field. This means that we can analyze the phenomena related to light both by considering the light field as a field defined by the electrical and magnetic vectors and as a photon population, provided that a correct quantum description is adopted for both.

In addition, when we consider light as a field we will stay on the classical form of the Maxwell equations, without the need of adopting a covariant version of the electromagnetic field equations [3] that would be needed in case we need to change a reference system with respect to the laboratory reference.

A detailed analysis of the optical field quantization and of the rigorous definition of photon is completely out of the scope of this book and it can be found in dedicated electrodynamics and field theory books [4,5]; we simply limit ourselves to remember a few key relations holding when classical coherent light is considered, that is, almost always the situation in lab on chip detection. These will allow us to use either the wave or the photon representation depending on the convenience.

11.2.1 Light Description by Waves and Photons

Dynamics of the classical electromagnetic field in vacuum is governed by the Maxwell equations that read in intrinsic notation:

$$\mu_0 \nabla \cdot H = 0 \tag{11.1a}$$

$$\nabla \times E + \mu_0 \frac{\partial H}{\partial t} = 0 \tag{11.1b}$$

$$\varepsilon_0 \nabla \cdot E = \rho_{el} \tag{11.1c}$$

$$\nabla \times H + \varepsilon_0 \frac{\partial E}{\partial t} = J \tag{11.1d}$$

where the electromagnetic field is described by the electrical field E and by the magnetic field H and charges and currents are sources of such fields. The dielectric and the magnetic constants of vacuum are given by $\varepsilon_0 \approx 8.854 \times 10^{-12}$ F/m and $\mu_0 = 4\pi \times 10^{-7}$ $V \cdot s/(A \cdot m)$. It is to be observed that the magnetic constant, also called vacuum permeability, has an exact value, since the definition of the magnetic unit of measure is to be derived from the setting of this value. Moreover, the measurement units of the fields and the corresponding values of the electromagnetic constants depend on the adopted measurement systems not only due to the different choice of the reference quantities, but also due to the different values conventionally assigned to the magnetic permeability. From now on, we use consistently the International System of Units (SI), conversion rules for the electromagnetic quantities in different measurement unit systems are summarized in every basic book on electromagnetism. A general set of boundary conditions can be found for the electromagnetic fields across the surface between different zones where they have to be solved [3,11]. In particular, tangential components of the electrical field and normal components of the magnetic fields have to be continuous across the surface. Conversely, the difference between normal components of the electrical field is related to the surface density of electrical charge while the difference between tangential components of the magnetic fields to the surface density of electrical current.

If no charge or current is present in the portion of space where we have to solve the Maxwell equations and if we have initial and boundary conditions in terms of values of the electrical and magnetic fields, the Maxwell equation simplifies sensibly and separate equations can be obtained for the two fields. In particular, taking the curl of Equation 11.1b we obtain

$$\nabla \times \nabla \times E + \mu_0 \frac{\partial}{\partial t} \nabla \times H = 0 \tag{11.2}$$

Using the identity

$$\nabla \times \nabla \times A = \nabla(\nabla \cdot A) - \nabla^2 A \tag{11.3}$$

where A is a generic vector, and Equations 11.1d and 11.1a we obtain the governing equation for the electrical field, that is, the so-called homogeneous wave equation:

$$\nabla^2 E - \frac{1}{c_0^2} \frac{\partial E}{\partial t} = 0 \tag{11.4}$$

where $c_0 = 1/\sqrt{\varepsilon_0 \mu_0} = 299,792,458$ m/s is the speed of light in vacuum. It is interesting to observe that this is an exact value, because the length of the meter is conventionally defined from this constant and the international standard for time.

Starting from Equation 11.1d and following a similar procedure we also obtain

$$\nabla^2 H - \frac{1}{c_0^2}\frac{\partial H}{\partial t} = 0 \tag{11.5}$$

which is the wave equation for the magnetic field.

Once Equation 11.4 is solved with suitable boundary and initial conditions the magnetic field can be univocally determined by a simple integration with respect to time starting from Equation 11.1b. Naturally in a completely similar way, Equation 11.5 for the magnetic field can be solved with suitable boundary and initial conditions and the electrical field can be deduced after that from other Maxwell's equations.

The conclusion is that, if a purely propagating electromagnetic field is considered, far from the field sources, electrical and magnetic fields are not independent and one of them is sufficient to describe the propagating field. Conventionally, optical fields are described by the electrical field E. Moreover, from Equations 11.1d and 11.1b it is immediately seen that in a purely propagating electromagnetic field the electrical and the magnetic fields are always orthogonal to one another.

Since Equation 11.4 is a linear homogeneous equation we can solve it by individuating the eigenfunctions of the corresponding differential operator by variable separation. Assuming that each component of the electrical field is a product of four functions, each of which depends on a single variable and finally using the superposition principle to write the overall solution we obtain

$$E(r,t) = \int\limits_{-\infty}^{\infty}\int e(k,\omega)e^{i(k\cdot r-\omega t)}dV\,d\omega + \int\limits_{-\infty}^{\infty}\int e^*(k,\omega)e^{i(k\cdot r+\omega t)}dV\,d\omega \tag{11.6}$$

where dV indicates the volume integral and the vector k and the scalar ω are the separation constants.

A similar expression of the general solution of the wave equation in vacuum can be obtained by Fourier transforming the equation with respect to the space variables and taking into account that if the field has to have a finite energy it must be

$$\lim_{x,y,z\to\infty} E = \lim_{x,y,z\to\infty} H = 0 \tag{11.7}$$

Equation 11.6 can be physically interpreted as the sum of a set of progressive waves plus the superposition of a continuous set of regressive waves. As a matter of fact, the time dependence of the solution is completely contained in the exponential terms so that the wavefront advances toward positive values of the product $k \cdot r$ if the exponent is of the form $k \cdot r - \omega t$, while it recedes toward negative values of $k \cdot r$ if the exponent is of the form $k \cdot r + \omega t$.

The single component wave can be written as

$$E(r,t) = e(k,\omega)e^{i(k\cdot r\pm\omega t)} \tag{11.8}$$

where it always happens that

$$e(k,\omega) \cdot k = 0 \tag{11.9}$$

as a consequence of the variable separation procedure. Since from the exponent of Equation 11.8 we can interpret the vector k as the vector indicating the wave propagation direction, we can conclude that electromagnetic waves are always a superposition of transversal waves, that is, waves where the fluctuating quantity is orthogonal to the propagation direction. No electromagnetic transversal wave exists in vacuum.

The nature of such elementary waves is clearer if we change the reference system, assuming a new reference where the (x, y) plane is orthogonal to the vector k, as shown in Figure 11.2a. In this case, dropping the indices for the variables in the new reference without ambiguity, we find that the vector k is parallel to the z-axis unit vector while the electrical field is always comprised in the (x, y) plane. The vector k is thus the wave propagation vector and it is constant in space and time. This means that the points reached by a wavefront in a given instant form a plane individuated by the equation $k \cdot r = \pm \omega t$ and the elementary waves can be called plane waves.

After the reference change of Figure 11.2a the elementary plane wave can be written as

$$E(z,t) = e(k,\omega)e^{i(kz\pm\omega t)} = E_0(a_x e^{i\varphi_x} x + a_y e^{i\varphi_y} y)e^{i(kz\pm\omega t)} \tag{11.10}$$

where we have dropped the dependence of the wave amplitude on (k, ω) and we have written it as the product of a real constant E_0 and of a unitary complex vector $a = (a_x e^{i\varphi_x} x + a_y e^{i\varphi_y} y)$ that always belong to the (x, y) plane. As expected, the electrical field depends on z only, due to the fact that the wavefront is a plane and the propagation happens along the z-axis.

Plane waves are quite important beyond the fact that they are the elementary component of every propagating electromagnetic wave. As a matter of fact, if we are sufficiently far from the wave source and we consider a small area of the wavefront, almost every electromagnetic wave can be approximated as a plane wave, where the plane wavefront is the tangent plane to the real wavefront in the considered point. Thus, it is quite frequent while analyzing the interaction of matter with light in small volumes, like in lab on chip, to simply approximate the wavefront of the incoming light with a plane so to drop the volume integral from Equation 11.7. A similar approximation not always can be done with respect to the angular frequency ω. As a matter of fact, even if lasers produce light waves with a very narrow frequency distribution, approximating it to a single frequency wave frequently brings to incorrect results.

A brief discussion regarding the physical dimensions of the components of a plane wave is useful at this point. The individual plane wave is an elementary component of field (11.7); thus in general it has to be measured in V s/m^4 since after the double integral in Equation 11.6 the electrical field has to be measured in V/m. If the structure of the integral expressing the field is changed, either with a variable change or with an approximation, the measurement unit of the components of the individual plane wave has to be determined accordingly. For example, if a multi-wavelength plane wave is considered, the volume integral is dropped by Equation 11.6 so that the components of the individual plane wave have to be measured in V s/m. This is a quite frequent situation, thus it is commonly stated that the plane-wave components have these physical dimensions; however, the specific situation has always to be checked.

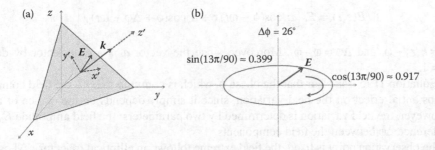

FIGURE 11.2 Wavefront of a generic plane wave and reference system where the propagation takes place along the z' axis (a) and polarization ellipse of the electromagnetic wave (b).

Let us now consider only the progressive component of the wave, that is, let us take the minus sign in the exponent of Equation 11.10, and let us analyze the dependence of the electrical field from time and space. Focusing on the progressive wave and neglecting the regressive components means that we will obtain complex values for the electrical field.The real part of this complex numbers represents the effective field value, while the imaginary part can be neglected since it would be cancelled by the regressive part of the wave if the complete expression would be considered. Progressive only waves and complex electromagnetic fields are frequently used as a trick to simplify expressions, with the implicit assumption that only the real part of the obtained equations has physical significance.

Substituting expression (11.10) of the plane wave in the Maxwell Equation 11.1 we obtain

$$k \times E - \omega \mu_0 H = 0 \tag{11.11a}$$

$$k \times H - \omega \varepsilon_0 E = 0 \tag{11.11b}$$

From these equations we obtain that the three vectors (k, E, H) are in the same relationship of the unit vectors of a Cartesian reference system in space. Moreover, a simple relationship exists between the intensities E and H of the fields

$$H = \sqrt{\frac{\varepsilon_0}{\mu_0}} E \tag{11.12}$$

since the energy density $\mathcal{E}$ of the electromagnetic field is the sum of the electrical and the magnetic energy densities, in the case of plane waves we get

$$\mathcal{E} = \frac{\varepsilon_0}{2}|E|^2 + \frac{\mu_0}{2}|H|^2 = \varepsilon_0 E_0^2 \tag{11.13}$$

The electromagnetic energy density is thus simply related to the square modulus of the complex electrical field associated with the progressive wave. Moreover, if we want to evaluate the energy flux transported by the wave we have simply to divide the energy density for the wave velocity.

Looking at the dependence of a plane wave on space, we can immediately see that the space period of the wave, that is, the wavelength λ, can be immediately related to the module of the propagation vector and to the wave frequency ν as

$$\lambda = \frac{2\pi}{k} = 2\pi \frac{c_0}{\omega} = \frac{c_0}{\nu} \tag{11.14}$$

Another important characteristic of a plane wave is related to the dependence of the electrical field on time in the points of a specific wavefront. Let us fix a value z_0, and write the physical value of the electrical field taking the real part of its complex expression (11.10):

$$E(z,t) = E_0 \left[a_x \cos(\phi - \omega t)x + a_y \cos(\phi + \Delta\varphi - \omega t)y \right] \tag{11.15}$$

where $\phi = k\, z_0 + \varphi_x$ and $\Delta\varphi = \varphi_y - \varphi_x$. Moreover, since the vector a is a unit vector by definition $a_x^2 + a_y^2 = 1$.

From Equation 11.15 it is clear that the phase ϕ, which is common to both the field components, has no substantial effect on the field variation, since it simply depends on the choice of the time origin. However, the field variation is determined by two parameters: the field amplitude E_0 and the phase difference $\Delta\varphi$ between the field components.

Once the observation point is fixed, the field extreme follows an elliptical trajectory, whose extension is determined by E_0 and whose form by $\Delta\varphi$. If we normalize this ellipse setting $E_0 = 1$, we obtain the so-called field polarization, and as a consequence vector a is called the field polarization vector.

The general elliptical field polarization can degenerate in a linear polarization if $\Delta\varphi = 0$ and if $\Delta\varphi = \pi$, when the field extreme trajectory is a segment, or in a circular polarization if $\Delta\varphi = \pi/2$ and if $\Delta\varphi = -\pi/2$, when the ellipse axes have the same length and the field extreme trajectory is a circle. These different situations are represented in Figure 11.2b. Since each polarization vector can be expressed as a linear combination with suitable coefficients of either linear or circular polarization vectors, any possible polarization can be decomposed into linear components or in circular components.

The plane wave (11.10) is also called coherent wave, this means that its frequency and its polarization are exactly defined. This property can also be expressed saying that the wave is monochromatic and polarized. If several coherent waves are superimposed, the coherent characteristic is lost. As an example, in Figure 11.3 the trajectories of the electrical field resulting from the superposition of two plane waves with the same wavefront energy and polarization and with frequencies ω and $3\omega/2$ are shown.This is, for example, the case of the superposition of a red light with a frequency of 480 THz and a violet light with a frequency of 720 THz. Different trajectories correspond to different values of the relative phase of the two fields.If we superimpose a great number of waves with different frequencies the electrical field trajectories gets more and more complex changing greatly in correspondence of a small change in the parameters of the component waves.

Moreover, random fluctuations generally takes place in the parameters of the waves emitted by a real source due to several phenomena like small changes in the environmental temperature, small vibrations, and so on. In this condition the trajectories of the electrical fields not only are very complex, but also have a random behavior and the resulting light is called unpolarized light.

A depolarization effect also happens when plane waves with different wavefronts are superimposed to obtain an overall curve wavefront. In this case, the trajectories of the field in general are not plane curves and if fluctuations exist, their shape becomes a random component too.

When electromagnetic radiation interacts with matter it gives rise to a wide variety of phenomena depending on the wavelength range of the considered wave. For this reason different frequency bands of the electromagnetic spectrum take different names as shown in Figure 11.4. In many cases the different parts of the electromagnetic spectrum are characterized in terms of wavelength bandwidth more than in terms of frequency bandwidth. The wavelength range $\Delta\lambda$ of a part of the electromagnetic spectrum can be easily related to the corresponding frequency range $\Delta\nu$ using Equation 11.14 so to get

$$\Delta\lambda = c_0 \frac{\Delta\nu}{\nu_1 \nu_2} \qquad (11.16)$$

where ν_1 and ν_2 are the extremes of the frequency range, so that $\Delta\nu = \nu_2 - \nu_1$.

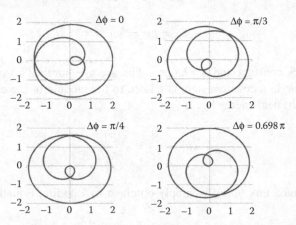

FIGURE 11.3 Trajectories of the electrical field resulting from the superposition of two plane waves with the same wavefront, the same energy and the same polarization having angular frequencies of ω and $3\omega/2$; different trajectories corresponds to different values of the relative phase of the two fields, which is indicated by $\Delta\phi$.

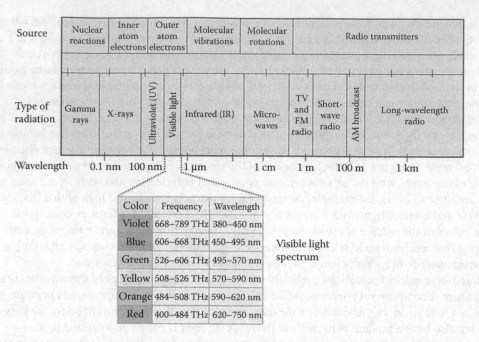

FIGURE 11.4 Electromagnetic spectrum with a detailed view of the visible light wavelength band.

The electromagnetic field quantization proceeds on the same trace of the classical analysis we have done up to now [4,5]. The field is decomposed in coherent waves that are the result of the variable separation solution of the wave equation. Since each single variable equation is similar to the equation of a harmonic oscillator, they are individually quantized as independent harmonic oscillators. This procedure thus associates to each coherent classical wave a quantum coherent state of the field and each generic field state can be decomposed in a superposition of coherent fields.

The particles associated with each coherent state are photons of a well-defined energy that are the energy quanta of the electromagnetic field. Thus, a generic field state presents a population of photons of different energy. The photon energy $\mathcal{E}_\nu$ is simply related to the photon frequency ν by the relation

$$\mathcal{E}_\nu = h\nu = \hbar\omega \tag{11.17}$$

Where h is the Planck constant and $\hbar = h/(2\pi)$. The average number $\langle n \rangle$ of photons in the unit volume that are present in a coherent state is related to the module of the electrical field through expression (11.13) of the field energy by

$$\langle n \rangle = \frac{\mathcal{E}}{\mathcal{E}_\nu} = \frac{\varepsilon_0 E_0^2}{h\nu} \tag{11.18}$$

while the average photon flux $\langle \Phi(n) \rangle$ is simply obtained by dividing Equation 11.18 for the light speed so that

$$\langle \Phi(n) \rangle = \sqrt{\frac{\varepsilon_0}{\mu_0}} \frac{E_0^2}{h\nu} \tag{11.19}$$

Since the photon number and the photon flux are quantum variables and coherent states are not eigenstates of these variables, Equations 11.18 and 11.19 provide average values, and the number of photons measured in a certain instant or the photons flux are random variables whose distributions $p(n)$ and $p(\Phi)$ can be evaluated starting from the properties of the quantum harmonic oscillator. They come out to be Poisson variables whose distribution can be expressed, for example, in the case of photons number, as

$$p(n) = e^{-\langle n \rangle} \frac{\langle n \rangle^n}{n!} \tag{11.20}$$

Owing to the properties of the Poisson distribution, the photon number variance is equal to its average $\langle n \rangle$ so that increasing the field energy, the variance increases too. The Poisson distribution is plotted in Figure 11.5 for different values of the average.

As a particle, the photon is a boson with spin equal to 1. Differently from other bosons, the photon has only two eigenstates of the spin, corresponding to the spin aligned along the x- and the y-axis if the photon propagates along the z-axis. This fact is directly related to the fact that electromagnetic waves can only be transversal and the spin state of a photon in a coherent state is the quantum analogous of the classical wave polarization. Since the two components of the electrical field are commuting operators, coherent states with a well-defined photon spin do exist, being the equivalent of linearly polarized classical states.

At the end of this very brief summary of possible representations of electromagnetic waves in vacuum, it is to be observed that since energy and frequency are different ways to express the same photon quantum variable, a photon with a perfectly defined frequency should be emitted at a completely undefined time for the energy–time indetermination principle [6]. Thus, real coherent sources emit a light field that are only approximately coherent. From the indetermination principle, if the uncertainty on the emission moment is equal to τ, a time that is generally related to the decay time of some quantum system, the minimum spectrum width $\Delta \nu$ of the emitted radiation is given by

$$\Delta \nu = \frac{1}{4\pi\tau} \tag{11.21}$$

Real sources, however, generally emit fields with a much greater spectral width, due to a plethora of other phenomena generating spectrum widening.

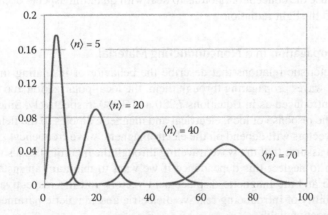

FIGURE 11.5 Plot of the Poisson distribution with different average values.

11.2.2 CLASSICAL DESCRIPTION OF INTERACTION OF LIGHT WITH MATTER

Even if light propagation in empty space allows the main characteristic of the field to be analyzed, in practical applications light interacts with matter either while propagating through a material or while being absorbed by molecules or other atomic scale systems.

If we look at light propagation in a material under a microscopic point of view, propagation is constituted by a huge number of absorption and emission of photons by the molecules constituting the material. The result of this process is macroscopically described with a set of propagative phenomena such as attenuation, dispersion, scattering, and so on. Even if it is possible to analyze these phenomena starting from a quantum representation of the field [4] this is not generally needed to obtain a satisfactory theory from applications. With exclusion of specific cases, like the photoelectric effect [5], a classical approach can be adopted, where the medium supporting the field propagation is considered a continuous medium whose properties are described by constitutive relations obtained by averaging the microscopic behavior.

In particular it is assumed that the light propagation through a continuous medium is still regulated by the Maxwell equations. The experimental results obtained by propagating electromagnetic waves through the great majority of materials can be represented by multiplying the dielectric constant and the magnetic permeability of vacuum by the relative dielectric constant ε_r and the relative magnetic permeability μ_r that contains the medium response to the electromagnetic field propagation. The product $\varepsilon = \varepsilon_0 \varepsilon_r$ is called medium dielectric constant and the product $\mu = \mu_0 \mu_r$ is called medium magnetic permeability.

If the considered medium is not homogeneous the relative electromagnetic parameters depend on position, while if it is not isotropous they will be tensors of order 3 to take into account the dependence on the wave propagation direction. Finally, in case in which the electromagnetic wave energy is sufficient to change the medium properties, the relative parameters will depend on the electromagnetic field itself and the Maxwell equations will become nonlinear.

The values of the material characteristic constants in a continuous medium are derived in a classical framework by considering an elementary part of the material, that is, a material volume much smaller than the characteristic length of variation of the intensity of the electromagnetic field, but much greater than the molecules constituting the material, and studying the behavior of distributed changes and magnetic momenta as they react to the presence of the external field. This procedure is somehow similar to the procedure that has been carried out in Chapter 7 to study fluid motion assuming the fluid as a continuous medium.

The classical approach, however, cannot be used in the case in which the details of the interaction between light and atomic scale systems, like macromolecules, are important. This happens in many detection systems adopted in lab on chip, like transmission and fluorescence spectroscopy. In these cases we will use the concept of photons to deal with quantum aspects of interaction between macromolecules and the light radiation.

11.2.2.1 Light Propagation in a Nonconducting Material

To introduce characteristic relations that describe the behavior of insulating material in front of the electromagnetic waves propagating through them, the local polarization and magnetic moment vectors have to be introduced as in Equations 7.220 and 7.260, respectively. Since these vectors in general depend on the response of local electrical and magnetic dipoles to the field, the polarization and magnetization vectors will depend on the electromagnetic wave frequency.

Thus, we have to assume that the wave traveling through the medium has a sufficiently compact frequency spectrum to neglect this dependence if we want to maintain an instantaneous relation between the electric and the magnetic displacement vectors and the respective fields that corresponds to the possibility of introducing relative dielectric and magnetic parameters that are independent of the propagating field.

From now on we will maintain this approximation, so that we simply indicate the dependence of the material parameters from frequency as a dependence of the central frequency of the wave, assuming them to be constant in the frequency interval where the wave spectrum is contained.

As far as the external field is not so high to induce substantial modification of the microscopic structure of the material the relation between the polarization vector and the electrical field, as the relation between the magnetization vector and the magnetic field, can be assumed to be linear. If the material is also homogeneous and isotropic, the linear relation reduces to a simple proportionality through a constant, ε for the electrical field and μ for the magnetic field.

If the local values of the electrical and the magnetic field is sufficiently high to induce a modification of the material optical characteristics, the dependence of the polarization and of the magnetization vectors on the respective fields will be no more linear. This means that the wave propagation equation that will result will not be linear and optical nonlinear effects will be generated [7,8]. While optical nonlinearities are important in selected optical detection systems used in macroscopic assays [9,10] nonlinear optical phenomena are not common in labs on chip and we will not analyze them here.

The decomposition of the generic electromagnetic wave in plane waves remains unchanged when propagation happens in a linear, isotropous, and homogeneous dielectric medium, but for the fact that the wave velocity c is now expressed as

$$c = \sqrt{\frac{1}{\varepsilon_r \varepsilon_0 \mu_r \mu_0}} = \frac{c_0}{\sqrt{\varepsilon_r \mu_r}} = \frac{c_0}{n} \tag{11.22}$$

where $n = \sqrt{\varepsilon_r \mu_r}$ is the medium refractive index. Since $\varepsilon_r > 1$ and considering diamagnetic media $\mu_r \sim 1$, the refraction index results to be greater than 1 and the light velocity in an insulating medium is smaller than the light speed in vacuum. A wide refractive indexes list, comprising many typical materials used in lab on chip applications, is reported in Table 11.1.

The wave vector intensity in a dielectric medium is given by an extension of Equation 1.14, that is, $k = 2\pi/\lambda = \omega/(2\pi c)$. As a consequence, the speed of light in a dielectric medium can also be written as $c = \omega/(2\pi k)$.

Since the medium constants depend on frequency, the refraction index depends on frequency too, inducing a frequency dependence of the speed of light. This phenomenon is called dispersion. In particular, if a wave is composed of a superposition of different coherent waves and its spectrum is sufficiently wide so that the dependence of n on the frequency cannot be neglected, the wave shape changes during propagation due to the fact that different coherent components travel at different velocities. This causes, for example, pulses to broaden while traveling through dispersive media [11]. It is interesting to evaluate in this situation the velocity c_G of the center of mass of a light pulse obtained by superposition of multiple frequencies. This velocity is called group velocity and it is the effective velocity at which electromagnetic energy is transported by the pulse. It results in [11]

$$\frac{1}{c_G} = \left. \frac{\partial k}{\partial \omega} \right)_{\omega_0} \tag{11.23}$$

where ω_0 is the angular frequency of the pulse spectrum of the center of mass.

The dependence of pure SiO_2 refractive index from the wavelength in the IR region is plotted in Figure 11.6 for three different temperatures, so evidencing the refractive index dependence on temperature. The dependence of the refraction index in the IR region is also shown in Figure 11.7 for three polymers [12].

Since the refractive index represents the macroscopic effect of interaction between the material molecules and the light, it depends on the material density also and, in general, it increases increasing

TABLE 11.1
Refractive Indexes List at a Wavelength of 589.29 nm, Corresponding to the Yellow Light Emitted by Standard Low-Pressure Sodium Lamps

Material	Refraction Index
Air at Standard Conditions	1.000277
Gasses at 0°C and 101.325 kPa	
Air	1.000293
Carbon dioxide	1.00045
Helium	1.000036
Hydrogen	1.000132
Liquids at 20°C	
Benzene	1.501
Carbon disulfide	1.628
Carbon tetrachloride	1.461
Ethyl alcohol (ethanol)	1.361
Water	1.3330
Sugar Solution, 25%	1.3723
Sugar Solution, 50%	1.4200
Sugar Solution, 75%	1.4774
Acetone	1.36
Ethanol	1.36
Glycerol	1.4729
Solids at 300°K	
Diamond	2.419
Fused Quartz	1.458
Sodium Chloride	1.544
PMMA	1.4893–1.4899
PETg	1.57
PDMS	1.43
SU8	1.59
PET	1.5750
Crown glass (pure)	1.50–1.54
Flint glass (pure)	1.60–1.62
Crown glass (doped)	1.485–1.755
Flint glass (doped)	1.523–1.925
Sapphire	1.762–1.778
Polycarbonate	1.584–1.586
Gallium(III) phosphide	3.5
Gallium(III) arsenide	3.927
Zinc Oxide	2.4
Germanium	4.01
Silicon	3.96

Note: In the case of crystals the average value of the refraction indices along the different crystal planes is reported.

the density. An example is reported in Figure 11.8, where experimental dependence of the refraction indexes of borosilicate glasses on density is reported [13]. For the same reason, the refraction index of a solution depends on the solute concentration [14] as it is shown in Figure 11.9, where the refraction index of an ethanol/glycerol solution in water is shown versus the concentrations of the two solutes [15]. This is a property frequently used for optical measurement of solutes concentration.

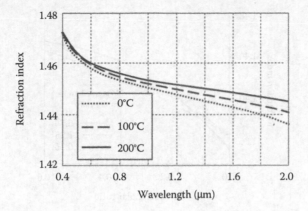

FIGURE 11.6 Dependence of pure SiO_2 refractive index on the wavelength in the IR region.

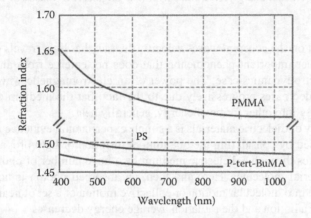

FIGURE 11.7 Dependence of the refractive index of three polymers on the wavelength in the IR region. Poly-tert-butylmethacrylate (P-tert-BuMA), polystyrene (PS), and polymethyl-methacrylate (PMMA) are considered. (Data from Hass R. et al. Industrial applications of photon density wave spectroscopy for in-line particle sizing, *Applied Optics*, vol. 52, pp. 1423–1431, 2013.)

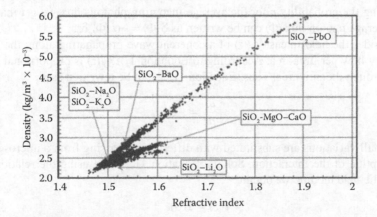

FIGURE 11.8 Experimental determination of the dependence of the refraction indexes of borosilicate glasses on density. (The figure is put in public domain by its author for any use [13].)

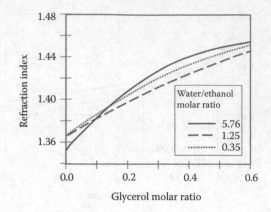

FIGURE 11.9 Refraction index of an ethanol/glycerol solution in water is shown versus the concentrations of the two solutes. (Data from Moreira R., Chenlo F., LeGall D., Kinematic viscosity and refractive index of aqueous solutions of ethanol and glycerol, *Industrial and Engineering Chemical Research*, vol. 48, pp. 2157–2161, 2009.)

Besides the impact on the coherent waves velocity, the fact that light travels through a dielectric medium causes another important phenomenon that does not emerge from an extension of static properties to the electrodynamics case. The power of an electromagnetic wave traveling through a dielectric medium decreases progressively due to the fact that the medium converts part of the electromagnetic energy into other forms of energy, generally heat.

While this property of dielectric materials is a simple experimental evidence in a classical framework, it can be justified by considering the quantum description of light propagation. As a matter of fact, light propagates through a dielectric medium by a huge number of photons absorption and emission by the material molecules. Here and then, an absorbed photon is not reemitted, but its energy is transformed into molecular motion or collective motion of a set of nearby molecules. That photon is lost for the radiation and the radiation average energy decreases.

This simple quantum description of the light attenuation in matter is the start for a phenomenological derivation of a very general attenuation law. Let us consider a very thin layer of material, so thin that the probability that a photon is absorbed and reemitted more than one time passing through the layer is negligible. Under this hypothesis it is possible to assume that the probability p that a photon traversing the layer is absorbed is proportional to the number of molecules M that it encounters. The number of molecules is proportional to the density of the material to the layer thickness δz so that, multiplying the probability p for the average incoming photons flux we get that the variation $\delta \langle \Phi \rangle$ of the average photon flux $\langle \Phi \rangle$ can be written as $\delta \langle \Phi \rangle = -\alpha \langle \Phi \rangle \, \delta z$.

Let us consider the field intensity $I(z)$ of a coherent wave propagating along the z-axis, that is, the field energy flow per unit area. According to Equation 11.13 $I(z)$ is proportional to the average photon flux through the unit area. Thus, Equation 11.22 can be rewritten as

$$\frac{dI}{dz} = -\alpha I \tag{11.24}$$

where very small variations are substituted with differentials passing from a microscopic to a continuous description of the interaction. Solving Equation 11.24 and using the relation between the intensity and the field module we obtain

$$I(z) = I(0)e^{-\alpha z} \tag{11.25a}$$

$$|E(z)| = |E(0)| e^{-\frac{\alpha}{2} z} \tag{11.25b}$$

The coefficient α is called material absorption coefficient and, as the refraction index, it depends on the frequency, but not on the field intensity, at least as far as linear interaction of the field with the material is maintained.

Up to now we have considered absorption as the only form of attenuation, but in selected cases absorption and attenuation are not exactly the same thing. When a collimated beam of light passes through a substance, the beam will lose intensity due to two processes: the light is absorbed and scattered. Scattering is the process causing part of the incoming light to change propagation direction, generally due to defects and irregularities in the traversed material [11]. In this case, a more general attenuation coefficient is defined, that is, the sum of an absorption term and of a scattering term.

If the traversed substance is a solution where absorption from the solvent is negligible so that absorption is due almost only to the solute, Equation 11.25 has a specific form frequently used in the analysis of biochemical assays. In this case, the number of molecules causing absorption in the thin solution layer is simply proportional to the solvent concentration and the absorption coefficient can be written as

$$\alpha = \epsilon(\omega)c_s \tag{11.26}$$

where $\epsilon(\omega)$ is the absorbance of the solute molecules and c_s is the solute concentration. When Equation 11.26 is used for the absorption coefficient, the attenuation law is also called Beer–Lambert law.

To insert attenuation in an empirical way in the expression of a plane wave, complex values of the propagation vector module k and of the refraction index n_c are defined as

$$n_c = n + i \frac{c_0}{4\pi\nu}\alpha \tag{11.27a}$$

$$k = \frac{n_c\omega}{2\pi c_0} = \left(n + i \frac{c_0}{4\pi\nu}\alpha\right)\frac{\omega}{2\pi c_0} \tag{11.27b}$$

Where Equation 11.27b is obtained as an extension of Equation 11.14 to the case of an attenuating dielectric material.

Using this expression, the plane wave (11.10), when propagation in a dielectric material is considered, can be written as

$$E(z,t) = E_0 a e^{i(kz-\omega t)} = E_0 a e^{i\omega\left(\frac{n_c}{c_0}z-t\right)} = E_0 a e^{-\frac{\alpha}{2}z} e^{i\omega\left(\frac{n}{c_0}z-t\right)} \tag{11.28}$$

11.2.2.2 Light Propagation in an Electrolyte Solution

Up to now we have considered propagation of an electromagnetic wave in the absence of charges and currents. If the wave propagates in a conducting medium, like a neutral electrolyte, for example, this hypothesis has to be dropped. The presence of an electrical and magnetic field generates charge motion in the electrolyte rendering wave propagation more complex.

In general, external field-induced charge motion generates emission of electromagnetic waves, so that the wave propagating through the conducting material is the superposition of the external wave and of an internally generated wave. However, if the induced charge speed is not very high the internally generated electromagnetic field can be neglected in a first approximation. It is the case of an electrolyte where a laser beam propagates, due to the fact that ions have a much higher mass with respect to electrons and accelerating them to high speed is much more difficult.

Since generally electrolyte solutions using water as solvent are diamagnetic materials whose magnetic constant differs for no more than 10 parts in a million from the value in void [16], we will assume that the magnetic constant of the solution will be equal to μ_0.

With these hypotheses, the presence of ions in the solution has to be represented in the Maxwell equations through a conductivity term that relates currents with the electrical field, which in our hypothesis coincides with the external wave field. This conductivity σ_s will depend on the concentration and nature of the ions that are present.

If we consider a diluted solution of a single ion, the solution conductivity can be related to the ion concentration c_s through the Kohlrauschlaw [17]:

$$\sigma_s = \Lambda_m c_s - K c_s \sqrt{c_s} \qquad (11.28a)$$

The conductivity is the sum of a term that is proportional to the concentration and a nonlinear correction that vanishes for very low concentration values. This is why the term Λ_m is called limit molar conductivity, in the sense that it is the leading term for the concentration tending to zero.

More frequently, however, a conductive solution is obtained dissolved in water or in another solvent a salt, so that both cations and anions are contemporarily present. Let us consider a strong electrolyte, that is, a salt that completely dissolves in solution, and a sufficiently diluted solution allowing linear approximation of Equation 11.28 to be used for the cations and anions separately. In this case Equation 11.28 can be used to evaluate the dependence of the conductivity on the salt concentration if the limit conductivity Λ_m is evaluated as

$$\Lambda_m = \Lambda_0^+ \, \overline{c}_+ + \Lambda_0^- \, \overline{c}_- \qquad (11.29)$$

where $\overline{c}_+$ and $\overline{c}_-$ are the moles of cation and anion that are obtained by dissolving a single mole of the salt and Λ_0^+ and Λ_0^- are the limit molar conductivities of cations and anions, respectively. Values of $\Lambda_0^\pm$ for common ions are reported in Table 11.2. The Kohlrausch law can be used also for weak electrolytes, that is, salts that do not completely dissociate in water, if the dissociation constant of the salt is known. In this case, the product between the dissociation constant and the concentration has to be used in Equation 11.28. If the salt concentration is not sufficiently low to allow linear approximation of Equations 11.28 and 11.29 loses its validity since simple addition of conductivities is no more possible.

Repeating the derivation of the wave equation starting from Maxwell equations in the case of propagation through a conducting solution, due to the high frequency of the light waves we can neglect the charge term, but not the current term. The whole electrolyte being neutral, we can assume that the relevant ion gradients do not form, while currents play a nonnegligible role. Setting

$$\boldsymbol{J} = \sigma_s \boldsymbol{E} \qquad (11.30)$$

TABLE 11.2
Values of the Limit Molar Conductivity for Common Ions

Cations	Λ_0^+ (mS m²/mol)	Anions	Λ_0^- (mS m²/mol)
H^+	34.96	OH^-	19.91
Li^+	3.869	Cl^-	7.634
Na^+	5.011	Br^-	7.84
K^+	7.350	I^-	7.68
Mg^{2+}	10.612	SO_4^{2-}	15.96
Ca^{2+}	11.900	NO_3^{-}	7.14
Ba^{2+}	12.728	$CH_3CO_2^-$	4.09

In Equation 11.1d and substituting the void dielectric constant with the dielectric constant of the material we get the following wave equation:

$$\nabla^2 E = \frac{1}{c^2}\frac{\partial^2 E}{\partial t^2} + \frac{\sigma_s}{\varepsilon c^2}\frac{\partial E}{\partial t} \tag{11.31}$$

This is still a linear homogeneous equation that can be solved using the variable separation technique. Plane coherent waves are found also in this case as particular solutions of the equation and substituting expression (11.8) of a progressive coherent wave into Equation 11.31 we get the following dispersion relation providing the propagation constant as a function of the angular frequency:

$$k^2 = \frac{\omega^2}{c^2} + i\frac{\sigma_s}{\varepsilon c^2}\omega = n^2\frac{\omega^2}{c_0^2}\left(1 + i\frac{\sigma_s}{\varepsilon\omega}\right) \approx n^2\frac{\omega^2}{c_0^2}\left(1 + i\frac{\sigma_s}{2\varepsilon\omega}\right)^2 \tag{11.32}$$

where we have taken into account that for a typical electrolyte solution $\sigma_s/\varepsilon\,\omega \ll 1$ at optical frequencies. Considering, for example, $\omega = 3 10^{15}$ rad/s, corresponding to blue light, and a solution of 10^{-3} moles of electrolyte with $\varepsilon = 1.6 \times 10^{-11}$ F/m and $\sigma_s = 10^{-5}$ S/m, we obtain $\sigma_s/\varepsilon\,\omega = 2.2 \times 10^{-7}$.

From Equation 11.32 and the definition of the complex refraction index we obtain

$$k = \frac{n_c\omega}{c_0} = \sqrt{\varepsilon_c}\,\frac{\omega}{c_0} \tag{11.33}$$

where we have defined a complex dielectric constant so that $n_c^2 = \mu_0\varepsilon_c \approx \varepsilon_c$. Combining this equation with Equation 11.32 we get

$$n_c = n\left(1 + i\frac{\sigma_s}{2\varepsilon\omega}\right) = n + i\frac{\sigma_s}{2n\omega} \tag{11.34}$$

This equation is directly comparable with the general definition (11.27) of the complex refraction index obtaining the following expression of the attenuation α_s caused by the presence of the electrolyte in the solution:

$$\alpha = \sigma_s/(2nc_0).$$

The presence of an electrolyte-induced attenuation can be easily interpreted by fact that part of the wave energy is converted into mechanical energy of the motion of ions and subsequently into thermal energy by the viscosity of the environmental fluid, thus being lost for the electromagnetic wave. This is a simple example of evaluation from the molecular mechanisms of the value of the attenuation coefficient. It is to be noted that the attenuation depends on the wave frequency through the refraction index. Moreover, evaluating the value of α_s in the previous numerical example, the distance that the wave has to travel to be reduced by a factor 1/e results to be equal to about 70 cm. This is an important result, indicating that in the distance scale typical of lab on chip, visible light can traverse even moderately concentrated electrolytes without undergoing great attenuation.

11.2.3 QUANTUM DESCRIPTION OF INTERACTION OF LIGHT WITH MATTER

Up to now, we have described the interaction of light with matter modeled as a continuous medium. If we want to use light to explore the properties of a specific macromolecule, however, we have to pass from a macroscopic to a microscopic description of light–matter interaction [3,11].

Since all the charged particles constituting atoms and molecules are constrained by mutual attraction–repulsion forces, the overall energy of a bonded atomic system can be described by a discrete set of equilibrium states corresponding to a set of discrete energy levels. The energy levels are frequently represented on the so-called energy levels plot as shown in Figure 11.10. Molecular degrees of freedom can be classified as electronic, vibrational, and rotational, depending on the physical variables they refer to. Electronic degrees of freedom generate far away energy levels; in between adjacent electronic levels rotational and vibrational levels form a sort of discrete energy band that characterize, as shown in Figure 11.10, the molecular energy spectrum.

In the case of a simple molecule, the energy states can be directly related in the energy diagram to one of the molecule dynamic variables. An example is presented in Figure 11.11, where the energy levels related to the first two electronic energies of the hydrogen molecule H_2 are related to the average distance between the two hydrogen atoms. In this representation it is possible to note, as intuitive, that increasing vibrational energy the average distance between the atoms increases up to a moment in which the molecule is no more stable and the atoms return in a standalone state.

Even if the nonrelativistic quantum mechanical analysis of the molecule itself states that each energy level is a stable state, molecules occupying an energy level different from the so-called ground state, that is, the minimum energy level, tends to relax on the ground state somehow releasing the excess energy. This phenomenon is partially due to the fact that the single molecule belonging to a material is not insulated, it interacts with other molecular systems with forces much lower that the molecular cohesion forces, but that are sufficient to alter the complete stability of high-energy states. Even in the case of a completely insulated molecule however, high-energy states would not be ideally stable. This is essentially due to a completely quantum-relativistic effect, that is, the interaction with virtual photons that are present even in a complete void space. This effect is related to the fact that the quantization of the field, as suggested in the previous section, under a mathematical point of view reduces to the quantization of an infinite system of harmonic oscillators. Each harmonic oscillator exhibits a zero-point energy that is always present and that causes interaction of insulated molecules with the void itself. We are not going to investigate this complex phenomenon further, interested readers can start from one of the many texts on quantum field theory detailing the physical and mathematical framework of interaction with virtual particles [1,3].

As a consequence of these phenomena a spontaneous decay time is associated with each excited state of the molecule, which indicates the time needed for a population of a great number of molecules in the excited state to reduce their number of a factor $1/e$ due to decay. The fact that decay exists has an important consequence. Owing to the energy–time indetermination principle the decay

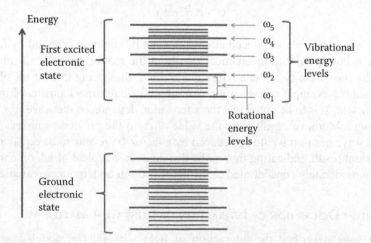

FIGURE 11.10 Example of molecular energy levels scheme where electronic, vibrational, and rotational levels are evidenced.

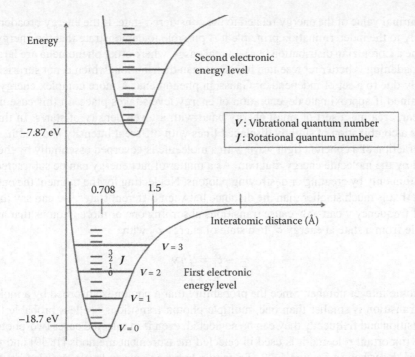

FIGURE 11.11 Energy levels of the hydrogen molecule H_2 in the interatomic distance/energy plane. Energy values are referred to the value of two hydrogen standalone atoms so that they appear to be negative.

time and the energy cannot be contemporarily known exactly. Assuming simple exponential decay from the energy state, which is by far the most common case, this implies that the uncertainty on the value of the state energy cannot be smaller than $\Delta \mathcal{E}_{min}$ where

$$\Delta \mathcal{E}_{min} = \frac{h}{4\pi\tau} \tag{11.35}$$

and τ is the $1/e$ decay time. Equation 11.35 implies that the energy levels are not infinitely sharp lines in the energy diagram, but small continuous bands of energy centered on the theoretical energy value of the level.

In real cases, the broadening of energy levels is much greater than the minimum value provided by Equation 11.35 due to several phenomena. For example, interactions between the nearby molecules in the material create a small alteration of the molecular state so that a small dependence of the energy level exists on the molecule environmental situation. This causes the fact that the energy of a certain level is a bit different from molecule to molecule and from time to time, so that if we observe a molecule population for a certain time, the energy of each level is distributed in a small band around the theoretical value. Another effect creating a broadening of a molecular energy level is the molecular thermal motion. As a matter of fact, in order to measure the energy of a quantum level we have to probe it in some way. Imagine to observe photons emitted by a molecule in a certain level, their energy is equal to the energy of the level only in the reference system where the molecule center of mass is constant. Since we observe the emission in the laboratory reference system, the photon frequency, and then energy, is affected by the Doppler effect [11] due to the molecule center of mass velocity. This is nothing else than the thermal molecular velocity, that is, a random variable. Thus, this phenomenon also creates broadening of energy levels.

As a consequence of the above analysis we can associate with each molecular energy level a decay time and a broadening, which is a probability that the molecular energy is $\mathcal{E} = \mathcal{E}_0 + \Delta \mathcal{E}$, where

$\mathcal{E}_0$ is the nominal value of the energy related to the considered state. If the energy broadening would be due solely to the indetermination principle it is possible to demonstrate that the energy broadening would be a Lorentzian distribution [3,4]. In real cases, where other phenomena are largely prevalent, the broadening is better represented by a Gaussian distribution, which is not surprising since it is essentially due to a set of independent Gaussian phenomena. A more complex energy linewidth can be obtained if approximate degeneration of energy levels takes place. In this case more levels are very near, creating a sort of small energy band with a given density of states. In this case the linewidth is a combination of slightly displaced lines with different intensity and width.

The interaction of a coherent light wave with a molecule is governed essentially by the wave frequency and by the molecule energy diagram. As a matter of fact energy can be subtracted or added to the radiation only by creating or destroying photons. Neglecting for the moment the energy levels broadening that is much smaller than the distance between different states, we can say that a coherent wave of frequency ν can only cause transitions absorbing one or more photons that are exciting the molecule from a state at energy $\mathcal{E}_1$ to a state of energy $\mathcal{E}_2$ with

$$\mathcal{E}_2 - \mathcal{E}_1 = jh\nu \tag{11.36}$$

where j is some integer number. Since the probability that a photon is absorbed by a molecule with a suitable transition is smaller than one, multiple photon transitions are less probable than single photon transition and frequently they can be neglected, even if in selected cases two-photon absorption has an important role and it is used in selected measurement methods [18,19] and fabrication processes, as described in Section 5.4.2. Transition between energy levels can also be determined by reasons different from emission or absorption of photons. All the transitions that are not related to interaction with the light field are called nonradiative and they can be caused, for example, by transmitting energy to the solution contained or to the solute by collisions. In this case, the transmitted energy macroscopically increases the solution or the container temperature.

Let us now consider the case in which a macromolecule solution presents a molecular transition that is resonant with a coherent light beam traversing the solution while the solute being completely inactive under an optical point of view. This means that Equation 11.36 is fulfilled with $j = 1$ by a couple of energy levels of the molecule. Let us also assume that the energy difference between couples of other energy levels is so far from the photon energy that optical transitions only involve levels of energy $\mathcal{E}_1$ and $\mathcal{E}_2$ and that thermally generated photons are much less than the external beam photons at the operating frequency, as it is true for near IR, visible, and UV frequencies at room temperature. The interaction of light and matter under these assumptions can cause three possible phenomena:

Spontaneous Emission: A molecule in the state $\mathcal{E}_2$ decays in the state $\mathcal{E}_1$, also called ground state, emitting a photon at frequency $\nu = (\mathcal{E}_2 - \mathcal{E}_1)/h$, that is, the frequency of the external light beam. This phenomenon would take place also if the external beam would not be present, thus we have to assume that the probability A that a molecule will decay in the unit time does not depend on the external beam. For the same reason, the spontaneous emitted photons will have the frequency, but not the polarization and the propagation direction of the external beam, since it comes from a completely independent phenomenon.

Absorption: A molecule in the state $\mathcal{E}_1$ is promoted to the state $\mathcal{E}_2$ absorbing a photon. This is a basic phenomenon causing the absorption of radiation that we have phenomenologically inserted into the classical electromagnetic theory through the coefficient α. The probability that absorption happens in unit time and per unit photon density is indicated by B_{12}. Moreover, it is intuitive that the absorption probability is also proportional to the photons density spectrum $\langle n(\omega) \rangle$. It is to note that $\langle n(\omega) \rangle$ is measured in s/m^3 since it is a photon number per unit volume and unit frequency.

Stimulated Emission: A molecule in the state $\mathcal{E}_2$ decays in the state $\mathcal{E}_1$ while also absorbing a photon and emits two photons at the same energy and with the same polarization and propagation direction. The complete coherence between the absorbed photon and the two emitted photons is due to the interdependence of stimulated emission and the presence of the external field and it can be completely demonstrated by a prime principle quantum description of the phenomenon. The probability that stimulated emission happens in unit time and per unit photon density is indicated by B_{21}. Moreover, it is intuitive that the stimulated emission probability is proportional to the photons density $\langle n(\omega) \rangle$ as well.

The three possible interactions between the external light beam and the molecule are shown in Figure 11.12. The three coefficients A, B_{21}, and B_{12} are called Einstein coefficients and they can be calculated from the knowledge of molecular orbitals using the rules of quantum mechanics. In the original Einstein work, since the calculation was carried out in terms of field energy density instead of photon density, the original Einstein coefficients where for sake of precision $B_{12}^{*} = B_{12}/h\nu$ and similarly for B_{21}. The coefficients B_{12} and B_{12} are measured in $s^{-1}\ m^{-3}$, due to the fact that we are working with photon and molecule densities, while the original Einstein coefficients are measured in $J^{-1}\ s^{-1}\ m^{-3}$, due to the fact that the photon density is substituted by the energy density.

If a population of N molecules is present in the volume traversed by the beam and no other energy state is occupied, but for $\mathcal{E}_1$ and $\mathcal{E}_2$, the three fundamental processes we have described can be used to evaluate the number of molecules that are in each state once the average number of photons is known. In particular, we can write the following set of equations, called rate equations, for the molecular populations of the two energy levels N_1 and N_2:

$$\frac{dN_1}{dt} = A N_2 + B_{21} \langle n \rangle N_2 - B_{12} \langle n \rangle N_1 \tag{11.37a}$$

$$\frac{dN_2}{dt} = -\frac{dN_1}{dt} = -A N_2 - B_{21} \langle n \rangle N_2 + B_{12} \langle n \rangle N_1 \tag{11.37b}$$

$$N = N_1 + N_2 \tag{11.37c}$$

where the last equation reflects the conservation of the number of molecules. Equations 11.37 are called rate equations and they are the governing equation that we will use to analyze interaction of a quantized electromagnetic field with molecular systems. While we have not underlined it up to now, Equations 11.37 imply an important approximation: they neglect quantum coherence between the populations of the considered energy levels. The populations N_1 and N_2 represents the average number of molecules in a state, directly related to the probability that a random molecule is found

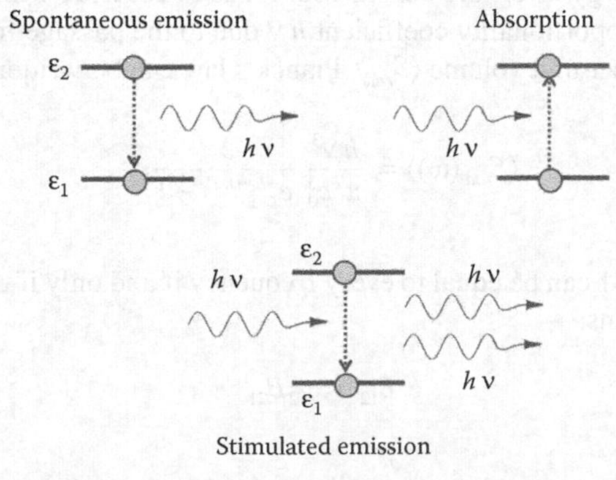

FIGURE 11.12   Possible interactions with coherent light beams and a resonant couple of molecular levels.

in that state. However, statistical correlation generally exists between the populations that are completely neglected in Equations 11.37. To obtain a more correct model the density matrix formalism has to be used, thus obtaining a more general set of governing equations that are called optical Bloch equations [4].

The Bloch equations reduce to the rate equations in two important cases: for incoherent light, for example, when a lamp light or sunlight is considered, and when a coherent light source like a laser is considered, with a line broadening dominated by interaction between the laser material molecules. This is the case of almost all solid state lasers, which is the most important case for lab on chip.

On the contrary, when the laser line broadening is dominated by the Doppler effect, that is, by thermal molecules motion, the correlation effect is important and rate equations can be used only for qualitative phenomena description, while the complete Bloch equations have to be used to attain quantitative result. In practice this is the case of gas lasers that are rarely used in lab on chip applications.

A set of important conclusions can be obtained if we consider the stationary case, that is, the case in which the derivatives of the populations are zero. In this case, the rate equations are simply a set of algebraic linear equations that can be solved expressing the average number of photons as a function of the populations as

$$\langle n \rangle = \frac{A}{(N_1/N_2)B_{12} - B_{21}} \tag{11.38}$$

This equation is in particular valid if no external light beam is present and the only photons that are present are those generated by thermal transitions of the molecules in the state of high energy and subsequent photon spontaneous emission. In this case we know from statistical mechanics that Boltzmann distribution can be applied, so that

$$\frac{N_1}{N_2} = \frac{g_1 \, e^{-\mathcal{E}_1/\kappa T}}{g_2 \, e^{-\mathcal{E}_2/\kappa T}} = \frac{g_1}{g_2} e^{-h\nu/\kappa T} \tag{11.39}$$

where g_1 and g_2 are the number of different quantum number combinations providing the same energy, that is, the energy states degeneration. Substituting in Equation 11.38 we have

$$\langle n \rangle = \frac{A}{(g_1/g_2)e^{-h\nu/\kappa T}B_{12} - B_{21}} \tag{11.40}$$

Equation 11.40 is no more than the spectral density of the thermal radiation emitted by our molecules in case only two energy levels are considered. It has to coincide with Planck's law of blackbody emission, but for a proportionality coefficient $h\nu$ due to the passage from the average photon density $\langle n \rangle$ to light energy per unit volume $\langle \mathcal{E}_{rad} \rangle$. Planck's law can be written as [4]

$$\langle \mathcal{E}_{rad}(\omega) \rangle = \frac{h\nu^3}{\pi^2 c_0^3} \frac{1}{e^{-h\nu/\kappa T} - 1} \tag{11.41}$$

Equations 11.40 and 11.41 can be equal to every frequency if and only if the Einstein coefficients satisfy the following relations:

$$g_1 B_{12} = g_2 B_{21} \tag{11.42a}$$

$$\frac{\nu^2}{\pi^2 c_0^3} B_{12} = A \tag{11.42b}$$

It is to be noted that, due to the fact that Equation 11.41 is an energy spectral density per unit volume it is measured in J s/m^3 as it happens for $\langle n \rangle$, which being a number of photons per unit frequency and unit volume is measured in s/m^3.

Thus the three Einstein coefficients are not independent, but once one of them in known it is possible to deduce the other two. Relations (11.42) are completely confirmed by a prime principle calculation of Einstein coefficients from quantum mechanical rules and it is one of the bases of molecules light interaction study.

Our scope is now to analyze the optical excitation of the molecule population as an example of using the optical rate equations. Let us imagine that at the instant $t = 0$ all the molecules are in the ground state, which means neglecting thermal excitation, and that at that instant the light beam is turned on. Moreover, in order to simplify the analysis, let us assume that we have no degenerate levels, so that $g_1 = g_2 = 1$. In this condition we have that $B_{12} = B_{21}$ so that we can drop the indices and consider a single B coefficient. Substituting Equation 11.37c into Equation 11.37a brings to a simple ordinary differential equation whose solution is

$$N_2(t) = N \frac{\langle n \rangle}{n_s + 2\langle n \rangle} (1 - e^{-(A + 2B\langle n \rangle)t}) \tag{11.43a}$$

$$N_1(t) = N - N_2(t) = N \left[\frac{n_s + \langle n \rangle}{n_s + 2\langle n \rangle} + \frac{\langle n \rangle}{n_s + 2\langle n \rangle} e^{-(A + 2B\langle n \rangle)t} \right] \tag{11.43b}$$

where the saturation photons density n_s is given by

$$n_s = \frac{v^2}{\pi^2 c_0^3} \tag{11.44}$$

After a transient the molecular populations reach a steady state that is given by

$$N_2(t) = N \frac{\langle n \rangle}{n_s + 2\langle n \rangle} \tag{11.45a}$$

$$N_1(t) = N - N_2(t) = N \frac{n_s + \langle n \rangle}{n_s + 2\langle n \rangle} \tag{11.45b}$$

whose value is shown in Figure 11.13. At low light energy, for $\langle n \rangle \ll n_s$, the population of the high-energy state increases almost linearly increasing the light energy, but when the light beam is near the saturation energy the high-energy level population increases slowly and slowly up to reach a limit value of half the overall number of molecules that cannot be overcome, whatever the light beam energy. This justifies the name of n_s.

Owing to its importance, it is interesting to evaluate the values of the saturation energy corresponding to a typical laser beam wavelength band in the visible and near-IR region. Multiplying n_s by $h \nu$ to obtain an energy density per unit frequency bandwidth, dividing by c_0 to obtain an energy flux and multiplying by the radiation spectral width $\Delta \nu$, we obtain the threshold light intensity I_s measured in W/m^2 that is given by

$$I_s = \frac{h}{\pi^2 c_0^2} \int_{\nu_0 - \Delta\nu}^{\nu_0 + \Delta\nu} \nu^3 d\nu \approx \frac{2h\nu_0^3}{\pi^2 c_0^2} \Delta\nu \tag{11.46}$$

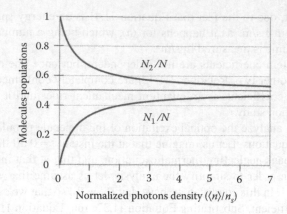

FIGURE 11.13 Molecular saturation population on the ground and the excited levels versus the normalized light beam average photon density.

If we put $\nu = 4 \times 10^{14}$ Hz and $\Delta\nu = 10^{10}$ Hz, which is the typical value of a broadband natural source, we get $I_s = 1.8 \times 10^5$ W/m². The most powerful conventional sources have an intensity at least two orders of magnitude smaller than that, thus we have to expect that the linear behavior of molecule excitation is well respected. The situation is different in case of lasers, for which the spectral width is much smaller (lasers with $\Delta\nu \sim 10^5$ Hz does exist) and having a much higher power. In these cases nonlinear behavior is really observed, even if in this case a two-level model neglecting quantum coherence between the populations in the two energy levels is at its validity limits. To obtain accurate quantitative results a more accurate analysis based on the concept of density matrix, the quantum operator corresponding to the energy distribution of the molecules, have to be carried out [3,4].

11.2.4 Light Detection

After being generated and interacting with the sample, light has to be detected to measure its characteristics and infer the properties of the observed sample. Light detection in general consists in the focusing of the incoming light beam on the detector surface by a suitable set of lenses and in its conversion in an electrical current by a suitable device. We do not analyze in detail the focusing optics since it is generally quite close to an ideal performance, we simply assume that the light emerging from the sample is focused in a Gaussian beam [11] (see Section 5.7.2.2) on the detector surface. If this is a relevant issue, we will consider a power loss related to light collection, which is unavoidable in selected cases.

Detection, on the other hand, is a key step in determining the performances of the whole assay. Optical detection is frequently placed outside the lab on chip itself, both due to the difficulty in integrating on board of a low-cost chip the components needed for detection, which are frequently realized either using III–V alloys like GaAs and InP or even by micromechanical technologies, and due to the fact that lab on chip are frequently disposable components. However even if placed outside the chip, even the detection system has to undergo the same low-cost constrain of the chip itself, so that costly macroscopic components like monochromators or photon counters are rarely used in lab on chip applications, while either integrated or micromechanical components are preferred.

11.2.4.1 Structure of an Optical Detector

The general block scheme of an optical detector is shown in Figure 11.14. The incoming light beam is firstly focused on the detector by an optical system composed of one or more lenses. Since nonlinear propagation is almost never important in the considered cases the field $E_F(x, y, t)$ at the output of the focusing system can be written as

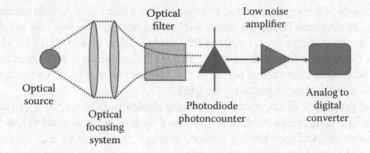

FIGURE 11.14 Block scheme of a typical optical detection system.

$$E_{F,i}(x,y) = \int_{S_O} F_{i,j}(\xi,\zeta)\Big[\bar{E}_j(x-\xi,y-\zeta,t) + \vartheta_j(x-\xi,y-\zeta,t)\Big]dx\,dy \qquad (11.47)$$

where $\bar{E}_j$ is the signal field, that is, the field coming from the assay cell, $\vartheta_j(x, y, t)$ the optical noise field, that is, generally due to the background black-body emission, and $F_{i,j}(x, y)$ is the spatial filter function representing the focusing system. The incoming field is assumed to have a plane wavefront parallel to the (x, y) plane and S_O is the conventional plane where the spatial filtering function is defined. Approximation (11.47) is valid if the focusing system extension along the propagation direction is much smaller than the distance between the sampler and the detection plane, as generally happens.

If optical aberrations are important, the whole expression of the spatial filter function has to be retained; in general, the only practically important factor is related to the fact that part of the radiation coming from the assay cell is not captured by the optical system. This effect can be expressed by a focusing loss that we call A_F, so that Equation 11.47 can be sensibly simplified as

$$E_{F,i}(x,y) = A_F\Big[E_j(x,y,t) + \vartheta_j(x,y,t)\Big] \qquad (11.48)$$

in order not to introduce false elements in the assay, the attenuation A_F has to be independent of wavelength in the considered range.

After focusing the signal is filtered by an optical filter whose role is to eliminate out-of-band optical noise and insulate the optical bandwidth under observation. In a spectrometer, whose role is to determine the frequency spectrum of the incoming light, this is a narrowband tunable filter that is tuned across the optical signal bandwidth to measure the power in every frequency slice.

After filtering the optical field $E(x, y, t)$ is given by

$$E_i(x,y) = \int_{S_O} H_{i,j}(\tau)E_{F,j}(x,y,t-\tau)dx\,dy \qquad (11.49)$$

In particular, if the filter is polarization independent we have $H_{i,j}(t) = H(t)\delta_{i,j}$, while, for example, if the filter has to detect only the x polarization of the incoming field we have $H_{1,1}(t) = H(t)$ while

$$H_{i,j}(t) = 0 \quad \text{for} \quad i \neq 1 \quad \text{and} \quad j \neq 1.$$

After filtering, the light beam is detected by a component that transforms light in an electrical current at the device output [20–22]. The most common device used in lab on chip applications is a photodiode or a photodiode array. Photodiodes are commonly used for light detection from ultraviolet light with a wavelength smaller than 200 nm to IR light beyond 1700 nm. Photodiodes are basically constituted of an inverse polarized P–N junction with an intrinsic intermediate layer which is called a PIN junction, and hence the name PIN photodiodes. The junction is fabricated using semiconductors materials like silicon carbide (SiC) for UV light, Si and GaAs for visible light and III–V alloys like GaAsP and InGaAsP covering all the IR bandwidth. An avalanche multiplication mechanism can be present in the active region of the photodiode junction to enhance the sensitivity, obtaining the so-called avalanche photodiodes (APD).

The types and properties of commonly used photodiodes in lab on chip applications are summarized in Table 11.3. The presented data are obtained by looking at normal values for standalone commercial photodiodes and they tend to indicate average performances and not records attained by prototypes. The bandwidth refers to the inverse of the biggest between the rise and the fall time, thus indicating practically the fastest signal that the photodiode is able to detect with minimal distortion. This factor can be important in real-time measurements of fast varying fields. No APD is listed, due to the fact that they are rarely used in lab on chip applications.

The selected photodiodes have a relatively large sensitive area, required to design an effective focusing optics. The consequence is that the photodiode junction capacity is relatively high (in the order of 500 pF generally) and the response time is no higher than 10–50 MHz. This is not a problem even in real-time measurements, due to the typical flow velocity of samples in labs on chip. A bandwidth of 10 MHz, for example, with a rise time of 100 ns, allows a measurement time of the order of a few microseconds, which is practically an instant measure for a sample moving at a speed of the order of mm/s. Much faster photodiodes are designed for other applications at the expense of the sensitive area and of noise parameters, but they are generally not used in lab on chip systems.

If a very low light intensity has to be detected in a very small time, a photon counter can be adopted. In macroscopic assays carried out in clean rooms, photon counters maintained at liquid helium temperature can be used to count even single photons, but this complex technology is not well suited for labs on chip that are used either in field or in the lab as low-cost assay vehicles, thus we will not describe in more detail photon counting techniques.

In any case one or more electrons are generated for each detected photons, so that the main component of the current at the detector output, which is called photocurrent, is proportional to the average number of photons incident on the detector surface. However, several phenomena generate biases and noise during detection.

- Electrons are emitted due to reasons different from photon absorption, so constituting a random current that exists also in the absence of incoming light and that creates both a bias and

TABLE 11.3
Types and Properties of Commonly Used Photodiodes

Material	Spectral Range	Peak Wavelength (nm)	Responsivity (A/W)	Active Area (mm²)	Bandwidth (MHz)	Inverse Bias (V)	Dark Current Variance (nA)
GaP	UV	150	0.012	4	8	10	9
SiC	UV	250	0.15	4	9	5	8
Si	Blue	480	0.25	5	5	10	7
Si	Green	560	0.45	7.7	10	16	4
Si	Near IR	800	0.55	1	100	15	0.5
GaAs	Near IR	800	0.6	2	60	10	10
InGaAs	Near IR	1300	0.8	3	80	15	30
InGaAs	Near IR	1500	0.95	3	70	15	70

Note: Data are extrapolated as typical room temperature performances of real products.

a noise in optical detection. This current is generally called detector dark current. The dark current can be considered a Gaussian process with an average value different from zero.

- Since the incident number of electrons is a random variable even in the case of perfect coherent quantum state, the number of electrons generated by incident photons is a random variable too, whose average is the signal component and whose random part is the so-called shot noise. We have already seen that the distribution of the photon number in a quantum coherent state is a Poisson distribution, so that the shot noise is a Poisson process. If the photon number is sufficiently high, more than 100 as a reference, the Poisson distribution can be approximated with a Gaussian distribution with the variance numerically equal to the average value.
- When avalanche gain is present inside the detector, the avalanche gain is a random variable itself, due to the fact that multiplication is a statistical phenomenon. The related noise component is called multiplication noise. Owing to the gain generation by cascading of individual independent phenomena, the multiplication noise can be considered a Gaussian process too.

After detection, the electrical signal is amplified by a low-noise analog amplifier up to a power suitable to drive the following electronic processing elements, then it is generally sampled to obtain a digital signal that is suitable for subsequent signal processing. The low-power signal amplification introduces another noise source, that is, the amplifier thermal noise, that depends on the design and performances of the electronic amplifier [23].

Thus, the current $J_R(t)$ at the input of the sampler, assuming propagation in air before detection, can be expressed as

$$J_R(t) = R_F \frac{\varepsilon_0}{\mu_0} \left| \int_{S_F} E_i(x,y,t) dx\, dy \right|^2 + N_S(t) + \bar{J}_B + N_B(t) + N_T(t) \qquad (11.50)$$

where

S_F is the detector surface, which is assumed to be a plane surface orthogonal to the propagation direction

R_F the photodiode responsively, that is, the current generated by an input power of 1 Watt

$N_S(t)$ the shot noise, that is, a process equal to the quantum-related variation of the photon number

$\bar{J}_B$ the average of the detector dark current

$N_B(t)$ the variation of the dark current

$N_T(t)$ is the amplifier thermal noise

The photodiode responsivity can be expressed directly as a function of frequency and of the photodiode quantum efficiency χ, which is the probability that an absorbed photon generates an output current corresponding to a single exited electron obtaining

$$R_F = \frac{q}{h\nu} \chi \qquad (11.51)$$

Various phenomena contribute to the fact that $\chi < 1$, for example, the probability that the photon energy is thermally dissipated or the fact that a small number of generated electrons give rise to spurious currents that are not detected at the photodiode output. In any case χ the quantum efficiency of PIN photodiodes is generally quite near one. The ideal responsivity value corresponding to a quantum efficiency equal to 1 is compared in Figure 11.15 with the responsivity values listed in Table 11.4 evidencing the corresponding quantum efficiency values.

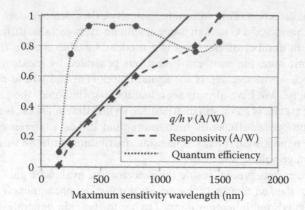

FIGURE 11.15 Ideal responsivity corresponding to a quantum efficiency equal to one compared with the responsivity values listed in Table 11.5 evidencing the corresponding quantum efficiency values.

11.2.4.2 Optical Detector Performances

The main global quality parameters of the detector are the signal-to-noise ratio SN, and the signal-to-background ratio SB [24]. The signal-to-background ratio is defined as

$$SB = \frac{\langle J_R(t)\rangle - \langle J_B(t)\rangle}{\langle J_B(t)\rangle} \qquad (11.52)$$

where $J_B(t)$ is the current detected in the absence of signal coming from the assay cell, for example, due to the switch-off of the optical source. Since $\langle J_B(t)\rangle$ is a deterministic value, whose slow fluctuations are mainly due to temperature and mechanical vibrations, the detector can be biased to compensate for this effect. In a correctly biased detector SB is very high, different from infinity only due to residual effects, and the background effect can be neglected.

The signal-to-noise ratio, neglecting the background influence, is defined as

$$SN = \frac{\langle J_R(t)\rangle^2}{\langle J_R^2(t)\rangle - \langle J_R(t)\rangle^2} \qquad (11.53)$$

Let us imagine that the assay requires to identify the presence of a peak in the detected signal and to quantify its intensity with a prescribed accuracy, let us say one part out of 10^a, where a is

---

TABLE 11.4
Values of Parameters Used in Evaluating Numerical Performances of Optical Detectors

Amplifier bandwidth	B_R	140 kHz
Optical power	W_S	0.1 mW
Optical receiver attenuation	A_s	0.7
Photodiode bandwidth	B_P	50 nm
Noise equivalent factor	$NEF = 2\sqrt{\kappa T\,F_a/\mathcal{R}_a}$	6 pA/$\sqrt{\text{Hz}}$

Note: The amplifier thermal noise is expressed as noise equivalent factor (NEF) as it is defined in the table. This is a parameter frequently found in optical detectors specifications.

the detection accuracy, that approximately coincides with the number of significant digits in the performed measurement.

Let us consider Equation 11.51 as the sum of a deterministic pulse $J_s(t)$ carrying the signal to be detected and a Gaussian stationary noise $n(t)$; denoting J_{sM} the peak pulse, it is detected with an accuracy of one part out of 10^a with a probability P_e if the probability that the noise sample at the instant in which the pulse is maximum is less that $J_{SM}/10^a$ with a probability $(1 - P_e)$. This means

$$\frac{1}{\sqrt{2\pi\sigma_n^2}} \int_{J_{SM}/10^a}^{\infty} e^{-\frac{x^2}{2\sigma_n^2}} \, dx = erfc\left(\frac{\sqrt{SN}}{\sqrt{2}\,10^a}\right) \le P_e \tag{11.54}$$

Thus it is clear that the value of SN in the instant in which the input signal is maximum directly determine the accuracy of the measurement. Moreover, it is also clear that a certain accuracy can be required only within a given probability, due to the random nature of the noise.

If $J_{SM}/10^a \gg \sigma_n$, as it has to be in practical cases, an upper limit of the signal-to-noise ratio required to obtain a certain accuracy with a required probability can be obtained using the asymptotic approximation of the error function written as

$$erf\left(\frac{\sqrt{SN}}{\sqrt{2}\,10^a}\right) \simeq \sqrt{\frac{2}{\pi}} \frac{10^a}{\sqrt{SN}} e^{-\frac{SN/2}{10^{(2a)}}} < e^{-\frac{SN/2}{10^{(2a)}}} \tag{11.55}$$

inserting the upper bound (11.55) into Equation 11.54 we obtain

$$\log_{10} SN \le 2a + \log_{10}(-\ln P_e) + \log_{10} 2 < 2\,(a+1) \tag{11.56}$$

where the right limitation holds for values of the probability P_e greater than 10^{-25} that are completely reasonable in this case. As a matter of fact we have

$$\left[\log_{10}(-\ln P_e) + \log_{10} 2\right] \sim 1 \tag{11.57}$$

For $P_e \ll 1$ as shown in Figure 11.16. This means that in a very first approximation the logarithm of the signal-to-noise ratio is simply related to the number of significant digits of the performed measure.

Equation 11.56 also indicates the order of magnitude the signal-to-noise ratio must have in order to assure a high accuracy measure of the average value of the detected optical power, that is, the

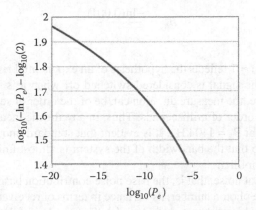

FIGURE 11.16 Factor $\left[\log_{10}(-\ln P_e) + \log_{10} 2\right]$ appearing in Equation 11.55 versus the probability P_e.

average number of detected photons in the observation interval. To have three digits of accuracy we have to reach a signal-to-noise ratio of the order of 10^8. This could seem a huge number, but we will see that such values are well within the reach of optical detection systems.

The expression of SN can be evaluated by analyzing each term of Equation 11.50. In doing that we will assume that the detector is ideally biased so that SB can be considered infinite. Under this condition we immediately deduce

$$\langle J_R(t) \rangle = R_F \frac{\varepsilon_0}{\mu_0} \left| \int_{S_F} E_i(x,y,t)\,dx\,dy \right|^2 = R_F A_R W_S \tag{11.58}$$

where W_S is the signal optical power and A_R represents the cumulated effect of the optical receiver losses. Such losses are due, for example, to radiation that is not captured by the focusing system, by the fact that the propagation vector is not perfectly orthogonal to the detection plane and to radiation falling out of the detector active area. The average value of the thermal background has been eliminated due to the assumption of ideal detector biasing.

As far as $\langle J_R^2(t) \rangle$ is concerned, different noise terms are statistically independent and Gaussian processes, but for the shot noise, which is a Poisson process. In the case in which the average number of detected photons is very high, as it is almost always the case, the Poisson distribution can be approximated with a Gaussian distribution with a small error, so that we will consider all the noise process as Gaussian processes. Assuming that the signal bandwidth is much smaller than the frequency interval in which the power spectral densities of such processes undergo sensible variations we will evaluate the variance of such processes simply by multiplying the detector overall bandwidth by a constant power spectral density.

Last, but not least, we will neglect the black-body background, assuming operation at room temperature. As a matter of fact in this condition it is easy to verify from the Planck distribution that the black-body radiation power is negligible with respect to all other noise components.

Thus, we can write

$$\langle J_R^2(t) \rangle - \langle J_R(t) \rangle^2 = (S_s^2 + S_T^2 + S_D^2)B_R \tag{11.59}$$

where B_R is the receiver bandwidth, essentially determined by the front-end amplifier bandwidth, S_s^2, S_T^2 and S_D^2 are the shot noise, amplifier thermal noise, and dark current noise spectral densities, respectively. The electrical bandwidth is directly related to the measure duration t_m by the relation

$$B_R \approx \frac{-\ln(0.001)}{t_m} \tag{11.60}$$

where the factor $-\ln(0.001) \approx 7$ reflects the hypothesis of an exponential rise and decay of the signal and the assumption that the signal is considered switched off when it is 0.1% of its maximum. In the case of a static measure, the measure duration can be of the order of seconds, while in real-time measures t_m can be of the order of milliseconds. Thus, in a real-time measurement it is reasonable to assume $t_m = 50$ μs so that $B_R = 140$ kHz. It is evident that standard photodiodes have a detection bandwidth much larger, so that the bandwidth of the system is almost uniquely determined by the design of the low-noise amplifier.

Considering first the shot noise, that is, the base noise contribution basically reflecting the quantum indetermination of the photon number, its variance in terms of received photons in the unit time is equal to the average number of detected photons $\langle n \rangle$. The number of detected photons in the unit time is related to the detected optical power by the equation

$$\langle n \rangle = \frac{A_R W_S}{h\nu} \tag{11.61}$$

This is the photon number variance, to obtain the electron number variance we have to multiply by the square of the electron charge q. Using the definition of the photodiode responsivity (11.51) we get

$$S_s^2 = q^2 n = \frac{q}{\chi} R_F A_R W_S \tag{11.62}$$

The variance $\bar{J}_D^2$ of the dark current in the sensitivity bandwidth is a characteristic of the photo-diode and reference values are reported in Table 11.3. This value is generally measured immediately after the photodiode, thus

$$S_D^2 = \bar{J}_D^2 / B_P \tag{11.63}$$

where B_P is the photodiode sensitivity bandwidth.

The thermal noise introduced from the low-noise amplifier depends on the amplifier design [23,25] and mainly on the required saturation power and bandwidth. Since in lab on chip applications high power or large bandwidth are not required, we can represent the excess thermal noise due to the amplification process with a simple frequency independent noise factor F_a so that we can write

$$S_T^2 = 4 \frac{\kappa T}{\mathcal{R}_a} F_a \tag{11.64}$$

where κ is the Boltzmann constant, T the absolute temperature, and $\mathcal{R}_a$ the amplifier load resistance. Equation 11.64 does not explicitly indicate the contribution of the so-called $1/f$ noise, an electrical noise whose spectrum increases with the inverse of frequency at low frequencies. Such a noise has to be minimized by a suitable amplifier design and further suppressed by setting a minimum pass frequency in the amplifier pass band, so as to eliminate very low frequencies. If this is not possible due to the fact that the signal has a nonnegligible continuous wave component, an artificial modulation has to be superimposed on to the signal, for example, by a slow modulation of the light source. In any case, due to the low-pass bands used in the considered applications, a $1/f$ noise residue is frequently present and it justifies the high value of the amplifier noise factor in this case.

Collecting the different terms we get

$$SN = \frac{R_F^2 A_R^2 W_S^2}{\left[(q/\chi) R_F A_R W_S + (\bar{J}_D^2 / B_P) + 4(\kappa T / \mathcal{R}_a) F_a \right] B_R} \tag{11.65}$$

Almost all the parameters in Equation 11.65 depends on the spectral zone where the detection is performed, out of the amplifier parameters. A comparison of the different terms at the denominator of Equation 11.65 can be done considering the values of the parameters reported in Figure 11.15 and Table 11.4. The first result is that in normal conditions the dark current contribution is completely negligible with respect to the other noise terms due to the very small value of the ratio between the signal bandwidth and the photodiode sensitivity bandwidth. The term $S_D^2 B_R$ is never above 10^{-21} W in our example, while the other terms are of the order of 10^{-18} W.

Owing to the fact that in lab on chip application the optical received power is frequently at least in the order of 10^{-5} W, the shot noise is not negligible with respect to the electronic thermal noise and it is to be taken into consideration when analyzing the receiver performances. When the received power is higher than a few milliwatts it is the major noise contribution. This is a very different situation

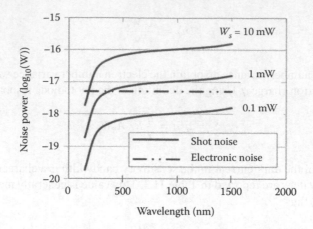

FIGURE 11.17 Comparison between shot noise and electrical noise power for different wavelength ranges and signal power.

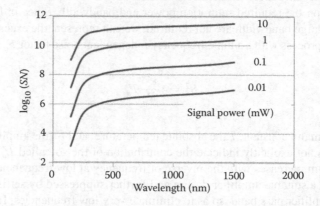

FIGURE 11.18 Signal-to-noise ratio for different wavelengths and signal powers.

with respect to high-speed detectors, like those used in telecommunications or for resolution of very short laser pulses. In this case the received power is much lower, for example, of the order of nW, and the electronic noise dominate the detector performances. Electronic and the shot noise power are reported versus wavelength in Figure 11.17 for different values of the signal power.

Values of the signal-to-noise ratio versus the central detected wavelength and for different values of the signal power are reported in Figure 11.18. Figure 11.18 confirms the fact that a very good accuracy can be obtained by optical detection using a photodiode without selecting extremely performing components.

11.2.5 INTEGRATED OPTICAL CIRCUITS

Free-space light propagation is suitable to describe many lab on chip-related applications, like the external detection systems based on absorption and fluorescence spectroscopy; however, if light has to propagate inside the chip through planar optical structures, integrated optics has to be adopted [26,27].

Integrated optical circuits can perform complex functionalities like guiding light along determined paths in the lab on chip, integrate resonators, and other components directly beside microfluidic structures and even directly integrate with fluid structure, for example, using fluidic channels as waveguide core.

However, almost only near-IR light and low-frequency visible light can be processed in integrated optical circuits, due to the characteristics of glass, silicon, and the main polymers used to fabricate optical waveguides.

11.2.5.1 Optical Propagation in Integrated Dielectric Waveguides

The base component of integrated optical circuit is the dielectric waveguide, whose scheme is reported in Figure 11.19, a more detailed version of Figure 4.5 that we used to illustrate waveguide fabrication processes in Chapter 4. The waveguide is constituted by a dielectric core surrounded by different dielectric cladding zones with smaller refraction index. The core can have in principle whatever section, but really fabricated waveguides are almost only rectangular, but for the so-called diffused waveguides where the core is obtained by diffusing a dopant in the cladding material so that the core section results to have the typical diffusion shape. Moreover, in practical integrated waveguides fabricated with glass, silicon, or suitable polymers the diffraction index difference between the different parts of the waveguide section are small, of the order at maximum of 4.5% and frequently much smaller, in the order of 0.5% in this condition the so-called weakly guiding approximation can be adopted, which we will always assume to be satisfied in this section.

In principle, the dielectric in each cladding zone can have a different refraction index; in practice the fabrication procedure determines the real index distribution so that different types of dielectric waveguides are generated by different fabrication processes. The sections of common waveguides are reported in Figure 11.20 besides their conventional names. In particular:

- A buried waveguide is formed with a high-index guiding core buried in a low-index surrounding medium.
- A strip-loaded waveguide is formed by loading a planar waveguide, which already provides optical confinement in the x direction, with a dielectric strip of index $n_3 < n_1$ to facilitate optical confinement in the y direction.
- A ridge waveguide has a structure that looks like a strip waveguide, but the strip, or the ridge, on top of its planar structure has a high index and is actually the guiding core.
- A rib waveguide has a structure similar to that of a strip or ridge waveguide, but the strip has the same index as the high index planar layer beneath it and is part of the guiding core.
- A diffused waveguide is formed by creating a high-index region in a substrate through diffusion of dopants. Owing to the diffusion process, the core boundaries in the substrate are not sharply defined.

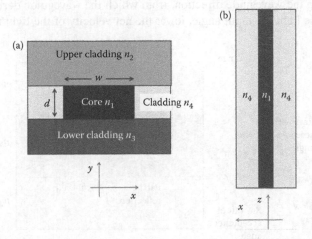

FIGURE 11.19 Basic structure of an integrated dielectric waveguide: Section (a) and top view below the upper cladding (b).

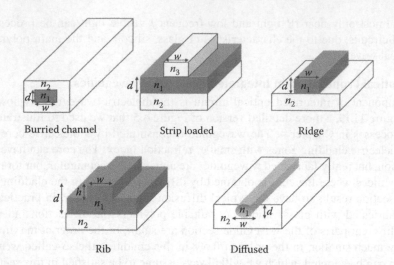

Burried channel   Strip loaded   Ridge

Rib   Diffused

FIGURE 11.20 Different types of dielectric integrated waveguides. The field propagates in the z direction.

Under a qualitative point of view, the working of a dielectric waveguide can be understood by a simple ray-based model, whose main element is depicted in Figure 11.21. Since the core has the highest refraction index, a total refraction angle θ_R can be defined at each core-cladding interface that is provided by

$$\theta_R = \arcsin\left(\frac{n_2}{n_1}\right) \tag{11.66}$$

If for simplicity we image a square waveguide with uniform cladding index equal to n_2, as depicted in Figure 11.21, whenever a light ray enters the structure from the front facet with an angle smaller than θ_R with respect to both the (x, z) and the (y, z) planes it experiences total reflection each time it encounters a core-cladding boundary, while if at least one of the above angles is greater than the total refraction angle the light ray experiences a loss every time it is reflected at the core boundary and after a small number of reflections is practically completely extinguished.

This behavior is evidence for the fact that there is a category of input light rays that are guided by the core following the waveguide direction, from which the waveguide derives its name. It also results that higher the light ray input angle, lower the net velocity of the light ray along the z-axis,

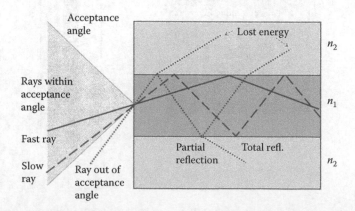

FIGURE 11.21 Elements of a simple ray model for light propagation in an optical dielectric waveguide.

due to the greater number of total reflections it undergoes to travel the same distance. This is a hint of the waveguide modal dispersion.

Electromagnetic field propagation in the structure can be analyzed by solving the electrical field wave equation with suitable boundary and initial conditions. Assuming unlimited external cladding, the boundary conditions prescribe that the electrical field and its normal derivative are continuous at the interface between different dielectrics.

The general solution of the wave equation in such a structure is extremely difficult, as it is evident if we consider the case of an initial condition consisting of a traveling wave with a wave vector having the direction $(1, 1, 1)$ that is transversal to the guide structure in the reference system of Figure 11.19. Such a general solution however is not required here since the waveguide aim is guiding the light along its axis with small losses. On the ground of the qualitative ray analysis it is reasonable to assume that the wave vector forms an angle smaller than $\pi/2$ with the waveguide axis and that the initial condition represents a traveling wave propagating along the axis itself. Under these hypothesis the wave equation (11.6) can be formally solved with the variable separation method. As we know this procedure allows the structure modes to be determined. In determining the waveguide modes it is convenient to divide them into three categories based on the characteristics of the longitudinal field components as follows:

- A transverse electric and magnetic mode, or TEM mode, has $E_z = 0$ and $H_z = 0$. Dielectric waveguides do not support TEM modes.
- A transverse electric mode, or TE mode, has $E_z = 0$ and $H_z \neq 0$.
- A transverse magnetic mode, or TM mode, has $E_z \neq 0$ and $H_z = 0$.
- A hybrid mode, or H mode, has $E_z \neq 0$ and $H_z \neq 0$.

In the case of TE and TM modes, if we use the electrical field and the magnetic field wave equation, respectively, to solve the problem, we can eliminate the z spatial coordinate. This means that variable separation produces two spatial equations in the variables x and y. These are harmonic oscillation equations that, after the imposition of boundary conditions, produces sinusoidal solutions in the core and exponential solutions in the cladding. To satisfy the boundary conditions, the wave number in the considered direction cannot be arbitrary, but it can assume only discrete values, allowing the derivative continuity to be attained. A set of solutions of the x equation for a TE mode is represented in Figure 11.22.

Owing to their structure, TE and TM modes can be tagged with two indices, which represent the values of the x and y components of the wave vector so to have $\text{TE}_{i,j}$ and $\text{TM}_{i,j}$ modes. In the case of hybrid modes on the contrary whatever field is considered we have to solve an equation with three spatial variables thus obtaining a final solution with three indexes that is tagged $\text{H}_{j,j,k}$.

Owing to the guiding structure, the propagation constant of a specific mode depends on the wavelength in a nonlinear way, which is called the waveguide dispersion relation. An example of the dielectric waveguide dispersion relation is represented in Figure 11.23. From the figure it is evident that the $(k - v)$ plane is divided into three regions. In the lower part of the plane there is a region characterized

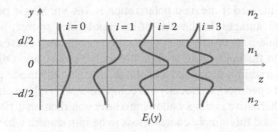

FIGURE 11.22 A few solutions of the x spatial equation for a TE mode in a symmetric buried waveguide.

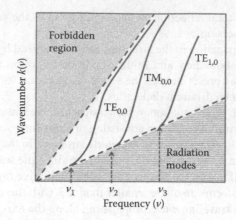

FIGURE 11.23 Qualitative example of the dielectric waveguide dispersion relation.

by a wavenumber–frequency combination that does not allow light to be guided by the waveguide; light modes corresponding to these wavenumbers are rapidly attenuated by radiating energy out of the waveguide core, corresponding to the rays out of the acceptance angle that were encountered in the ray waveguide model. In the upper part of the plane there is the so-called forbidden region, which is a region where light with the wave vector parallel to the waveguide axis simply does not propagate.

In between the forbidden and the radiative region there is the region where the dispersion relations of the guided modes are contained. From Figure 11.23 it can be noted that every mode has a lower possible propagation frequency, that is, minimal frequency at which such mode can propagate. This is called the cutoff frequency. This means that if the light frequency is in between the first and the second mode cutoff frequencies, the only mode that can propagate is the first waveguide mode and the waveguide is called single mode at that frequency.

Generally, integrated waveguides are designed so to work in single mode regime in order to avoid modal dispersion. As a matter of fact, different modes propagate with a frequency-dependent velocity $c(\nu)$ that is given by

$$c(\nu) = k(\nu)\nu \tag{11.67}$$

so that they have quite different propagation velocities even at the same frequency. This means that a light pulse constituted by a superposition of different modes broadens rapidly while propagating through the waveguide due to the fact that the constituting modes propagate at different velocities. This phenomenon is called modal dispersion to distinguish it from normal dispersion that causes the broadening of a pulse in a medium in which the wave number depends on the frequency due to the fact that different frequency components propagate at different speeds.

Single mode operation also guarantees single polarization operation. As a matter of fact, in an asymmetric waveguide the modes corresponding to orthogonal polarizations have different cutoff frequencies. Single polarization propagation is often desirable, due to the fact that a better control of detection is frequently obtained if the field polarization is known. Single polarization propagation, however, has a few disadvantages. In the case of an unpolarized source, like a lamp for example, the fact that the waveguide selects only one polarization component causes the power propagating through the waveguide to fluctuate in time while the source polarization distribution changes. If a laser is used, whose polarization is defined and stable, aligning the mode polarization to the laser polarization is a difficult operation, frequently not compatible with lab on chip operative conditions.

If a laser is used, an alternative is simply allowing a laser polarization different from the mode one. If stable coupling is realized this simply causes a loss to be introduced, which cannot be a problem.

If we consider a fixed shape of the waveguide the modes have the same form, independently of the waveguide dimensions and the wavelength, provided that all the parameters are suitably normalized. Thus, for each waveguide type a set of nondimensional parameters are defined so as to provide universal design plots for that type of waveguide. As an example we will consider the buried waveguide that is represented in Figure 11.19 setting $n_4 = n_2$. This is a frequent condition, occurring when the core is obtained by deposition and etching while lateral and upper cladding are fabricated by deposition of the same material up to completely cover the underlying core.

In this case, the following normalized parameters are defined to summarize the material and geometric properties of the waveguide:

$$n_{eff} = k(\nu)\frac{c_0}{2\pi\nu} \quad \text{effective index} \tag{11.68a}$$

$$b = \frac{n_{eff}^2 - n_3^2}{n_1^2 - n_3^2} \quad \text{normalized index} \tag{11.68b}$$

$$V = \frac{2\pi\sqrt{d\,w}}{\lambda_0}\sqrt{n_1^2 - n_3^2} \quad \text{normalized frequency} \tag{11.68c}$$

$$a = \frac{n_3^2 - n_2^2}{n_1^2 - n_3^2} \quad \text{normalized asymmetry} \tag{11.68d}$$

where λ_0 is the propagating light wavelength in vacuum and both the refraction indexes and the waveguide geometrical dimensions are defined in Figure 11.19. An example of design plot for such a waveguide is reported in Figure 11.24, where the dispersion curves of the first two guided modes are reported in terms of normalized index versus the normalized frequency for two values of the asymmetry.

To provide an example let us assume that we are realizing a silica waveguide intended for near-IR single mode propagation. The material index of refraction and the waveguide thickness are dictated by the technology process, so that the free design parameter is the waveguide width that has to be chosen in order to obtain a single mode waveguide at the desired wavelength.

From the data in Table 11.5 we can evaluate the asymmetry, which in this case is equal to 10. From Figure 11.24 we can read the cutoff normalized frequencies for the first two modes with the assigned asymmetry as a function of the waveguide width. After converting the normalized

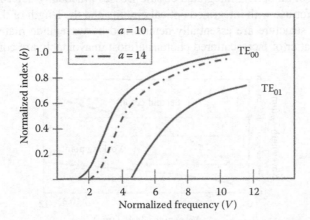

FIGURE 11.24 Example of design plot for the waveguide is considered in the text: the dispersion curves of the first two guided modes are reported in terms of normalized index versus the normalized frequency for two values of the asymmetry.

TABLE 11.5

Data for the Example of Design of Single Mode Waveguide in the Near Infrared Carried Out in the Text

Wavelength	λ_0	1.55 μm
Substrate refraction index	n_3	1.570
Core refraction index	n_1	1.550
Cladding refraction index	n_2	1.568
Cladding-core index variation		0.64%
	$\delta_c = 2\dfrac{n_1 - n_2}{n_2 + n_1}$	
Substrate-core index variation		0.06%
	$\delta_s = 2\dfrac{n_1 - n_3}{n_3 + n_1}$	
Waveguide thickness	d	2 μm

frequency in vacuum light wavelength using Equation 11.68c we obtain the plot of Figure 11.25. In Figure 11.25 the working point of the waveguide at the desired wavelength can be individuated so to obtain single mode operation. In this example, the working point corresponds to a waveguide width of 6 μm and to a normalized frequency equal to 1.057.

After the working point identification it is possible to evaluate the waveguide effective index from Figure 11.24 (n_{eff} = 1.56989 in our case) and from the effective index definition the wavenumber at the considered wavelength, which in our case results $k = 1.012 \times 10^6$.

A last observation has to be done before closing the general discussion on modes propagation in dielectric integrated waveguides. Besides integrated waveguides, another type of optical dielectric waveguides is widely used: optical fibers. Optical fibers have a huge diffusion for many applications: millions of kilometers of fibers are installed in telecommunication systems, millions of fiber optic sensors are deployed in the field for a variety of applications, comprising biosensing. An optical fiber is simply a dielectric waveguide with a circular symmetry, as shown in Figure 11.26. The analyses we have carried out up to now for integrated waveguides completely apply in the fiber optic case. In the fiber optic case multimode optical fibers are widely used in several applications.

11.2.5.2 Optical Dielectric Waveguide Attenuation

The determination of the attenuation experiences by light traversing a dielectric waveguide is a key element in the design of an optical integrated circuit. Losses practically determine the wavelength range that is suitable for use with integrated optical circuits and the length of the circuit itself.

Losses in guiding structure are essentially determined by waveguide material absorption and by scattering. As a matter of fact, scattered photons almost unavoidably are coupled with radiation

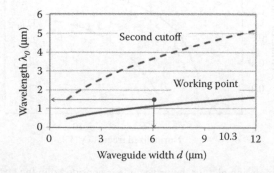

FIGURE 11.25 Cutoff wavelength of the first and the second mode of the waveguide of the example in the text versus the waveguide width and working point determination for single mode at 1.5 μm.

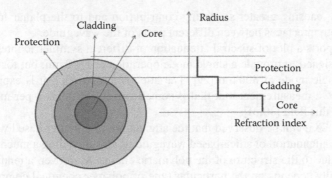

FIGURE 11.26 Transversal section of an optical fiber.

modes so to be lost by the propagation mode. The main scattering source, the so-called Rayleigh scattering [11], creates a loss plateau continuously decreasing with wavelength. As far as absorption is concerned, both glass and the high majority of relevant polymers have high absorption peaks both in far IR and in the UV region, causing the overall loss versus wavelength curve to have a very wide minimum in the near IR region that for a few polymers extends in the visible range too. Moreover, the vast majority of polymers become chemically unstable in the UV region, making losses almost impossible to be measured.

In the near-infrared and visible regions the waveguide absorption presents a set of peaks corresponding to the resonant absorption by material and impurity transitions whose energy is located in this region. Probably, the most important of these peaks is due to water [26,28]. Three main absorption peaks due to the presence of OH ions generated by water impurities in the waveguide material are present in the near-IR spectrum, at 950, 1244, and 1383 nm, practically defining wavelength ranges of quite high attenuation that cannot be practically used for integrated optical circuits.

The different elements constituted the overall loss of a dielectric optical waveguides are evidenced in Figure 11.27, where the attenuation of a low glass optical fiber for telecommunication applications is reported evidencing its main components. The considered fiber is designed to work single mode at 1300 and 1550 µm and the attenuation at 1550 mm is so low that the travelling wave intensity is attenuated only by a factor 0.89 after 1 km of fiber propagation.

For a great number of factors attenuations in integrated wavelengths are not so low, even if sufficiently low propagation can be attained for lab on chip applications. This is due both to lack of

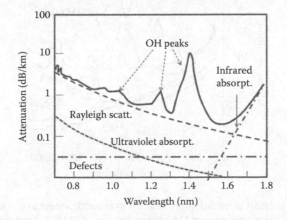

FIGURE 11.27 Loss profile of a very low loss glass optical fiber allowing single mode propagation at 1300 and 1550 nm. The different components contributing to fiber loss are evidenced. The propagation loss A of a fiber piece 1 km long, is measured in dB/km, that is, $A = -10 \, \alpha L \, \log_{10}(e)$, with $L = 1$ km.

circular symmetry, causing greater scattering contribution and to the planar fabrication process, creating less smooth interfaces between different parts of the waveguide.

Figure 11.28 reports a plot of spectral attenuation of different symmetric integrated waveguides ($n_2 = n_3$, $d = w$) designed to provide a single mode operation at 1550 nm, but for the PMMA waveguides that are single mode at 800 nm [29]. The attenuation coefficient is expressed as 10 times the logarithm of α, a measurement unit that is sometimes called decibel per meter (dB/m) and is frequently used in this field [30,31].

From Figure 11.28 it can be observed that the attenuation of polymer-based waveguide is higher with respect to the attenuation of silica-based waveguides, also including a much greater number of resonance peaks, due to the structure of the polymeric chains. Moreover, attenuation of polymeric waveguides critically depends on the particular type of polymer chemical composition and on the polymerization process used for fabrication. In the example reported in the figure two PMMA waveguides present sensibly different attenuations due to the different density and type of the side groups in the two PMMA types used. Two curves are also reported for silica waveguide, corresponding to different index differences between the core and the cladding, also called index contrast. Higher the index contrast, smaller the waveguide section and higher the propagation loss. This is mainly due to the higher scattering contribution.

Besides propagation losses bending losses are also important in integrated optical circuits. Every curve in the layout of an integrated waveguide is a perturbation of the ideal straight waveguide shape and provokes excitation of unguided modes and a consequent electromagnetic power emission from the waveguide. While in case of a curvature radius of the same order of the waveguide width or smaller almost all the optical energy is lost, if the curvature radius is much larger than the waveguide width a curve in the waveguide layout can be represented as a concentrated loss that adds to the propagation loss. This is called bending loss.

The bending losses essentially depend on two key parameters [32,33]: the bend curvature radius r and the curve angle, which is the angle θ between the two straight waveguides before and after the curve (see Figure 11.29). As intuitive the overall loss depends exponentially on the curvature angle with a good approximation in case of circular curves so that a bending loss coefficient $\alpha_B(r)$ can be defined starting from the overall bending loss A_B as

$$A_B = e^{-\alpha_B(r)\theta} \tag{11.69}$$

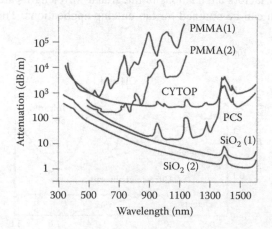

FIGURE 11.28 Plot of spectral attenuation of different symmetric integrated waveguides ($n_2 = n_3$, $d = w$) designed to provide single mode operation at 1550 nm or, in case of PMMA waveguides, at 800 nm. Two different PMMA compositions are considered in the plot and, in case of silica waveguides, two different index contrast: 0.3% for SiO_2 (2) and 0.6% for SiO_2 (1). CYTOP is a fluorinated polymer [107] and PCS is a preceramic polymer polycarbosilane [32]. The propagation loss A, is measured in dB/m, that is, $A = -10 \, \alpha \, \log_{10}(e)$.

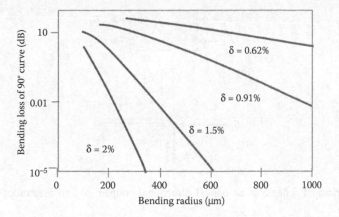

FIGURE 11.29 Example of the bending loss of a silicon core symmetric waveguide versus the bending radius for the fundamental mode of the waveguide at 1.55 μm. The core refraction index is 3.24. Different index contrast ratios δ are considered and the waveguides dimensions are designed for each contrast ratio to obtain the desired working conditions. The bending loss of a 90° curve A_B, is measured in dB, that is, $A_B = -10\,\alpha_B(\pi/2)\,\log_{10}(e)$. (Razavi B., *Design of Integrated Circuits for Optical Communications*, 2012, 2nd edition. Copyright Wiley-VCH Verlag GmbH & Co. KGaA. Reproduced with permission.)

As an example, the bending loss of a silicon core symmetric waveguide versus the bending radius is shown in Figure 11.29 for the fundamental mode of the waveguide at 1.55 μm. Different index contrast ratios are considered and the waveguide dimensions are designed for each contrast ratio to obtain the desired working conditions. The core refraction index is 3.24.

From the figure it is evident that the bending loss rapidly increases with decreasing the waveguide index contrast ratio, mainly due to the fact that the waveguide dimensions increases in order to maintain the same operative conditions. This fact, besides the propagation losses increase with the contrast ratio, determines the contrast ratio optimization criterion. Thus, high contract ratios are used in very compact, integrated circuits, where many curves with small curvature ratios are present, at the expenses of a higher propagation loss. On the contrary, if curves are either not present or can be designed with a curvature radius sufficiently high, a small index contrast ratio can be selected, so to minimize propagation losses.

Another concentrated loss arises from the coupling of the integrated waveguide with whatever external optical systems, either in free space through an optical focusing system or via a fiber optics. Different coupling techniques are discussed in Section 6.5.4.

Typical parameters for different types of silica symmetric waveguides are reported in Table 11.6, where the bending radius is defined as the radius at which the bending loss of a 90° curve is 0.1

TABLE 11.6

Typical Parameters for Different Types of Silica Symmetric Waveguides

	δ = 0.3%	δ = 0.45%	δ = 0.75%	δ = 1.5%
Core size (μm)	8	7	6	4.5
Propagation loss (dB/m)	1	2	4	7
Bending radius (mm)	25	15	5	2
Coupling loss (dB)	0.05	0.1	0.4	2.0

Note: The bending radius is defined as the radius at which the bending loss of a 90° curve is 0.1 times the propagation loss through the curve. The propagation loss a is measured in dB/m, a measurement unit defined as $A = -10\,\alpha\,\log_{10}(e)$.

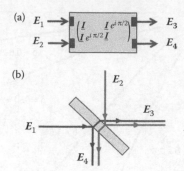

FIGURE 11.30 Principal scheme of an optical directional coupler (a) and macroscopic realization via a beam splitter (b).

times the propagation loss through the curve and the coupling loss refers to coupling with a single mode optical fiber via a V groove and a fiber taper.

11.2.5.3 Integrated Optics Components

Starting from the waveguide as a base building block several different optical components can be realized using integrated optics based on silica, silicon, or polymers. It is clearly impossible to review even briefly all the integrated optical components that have been realized for sensors applications. Here, we rapidly review few common components to provide examples that will be useful in the discussion of specific detection systems used in lab on chip.

Several integrated optics components need the realization of optical directional couplers. A directional coupler is a component having two input and two output guides, frequently called input and output ports, as shown in Figure 11.30. We assume that the structure is realized so that the input and output single mode waveguides are identical and that the optical traveling waves traversing the device enters from ports 1 and 2 and exit from ports 3 and 4. If we indicate with E_j the electrical field that is present at the ith coupler port, an ideal directional coupler is characterized by the following input–output relation:

$$\begin{pmatrix} E_3 \\ E_4 \end{pmatrix} = \frac{1}{\sqrt{2}} \begin{pmatrix} \underline{I} & \underline{I} e^{i\pi/2} \\ \underline{I} e^{i\pi/2} & \underline{I} \end{pmatrix} \begin{pmatrix} E_1 \\ E_2 \end{pmatrix} \tag{11.70}$$

where $\underline{I}$ represents the unit 3×3 matrix. Equation 11.70 implies that if the electrical field is present only at one input port, the incoming optical power is divided equally between the output ports. It is interesting to note that this is not only a directional coupler property, but also an alternative definition since imposing to a two input–two output linear device to fulfill this property directly brings to Equation 11.70.

The most diffused macroscopic directional coupler is the beam splitter, see Figure 11.30b. The beam splitter is a thin optical glass plate that is placed between two orthogonal light beams at an angle of $\pi/4$ with respect to the beam wave vectors. If the plate is fabricated with the suitable thickness it provokes a phase change of $-\pi/2$ in the beam traversing it, while the beam reflected experiences a phase change of π. Thus, superimposing the beams at the output we obtain exactly the directional coupler characteristics.

Highly performing directional couplers can be fabricated using integrated optics by adopting the so-called mode tails coupling. The scheme of an integrated optics directional coupler is reported in Figure 11.31. Two waveguides are fabricated so that they run parallel for a length L. If the distance between the waveguides axes Δ is sufficiently small, the exponential tails of the mode propagating in one of the waveguide penetrates in the core of the other guide and they results to be coupled.

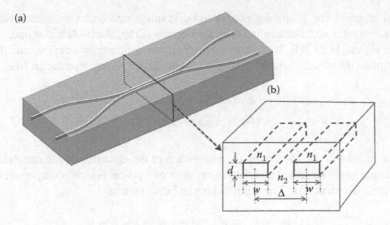

FIGURE 11.31 Integrated optics directional coupler: complete view (a), vertical section of the coupling zone (b).

Indicating the input and output waveguides as in Figure 11.30 the relation between the input and the output fields can be written through the so-called scattering matrix $\underline{S}$ as

$$\begin{pmatrix} E_3 \\ F_4 \end{pmatrix} = \underline{S} \begin{pmatrix} E_1 \\ E_2 \end{pmatrix} = \begin{pmatrix} \underline{S}_{13} & \underline{S}_{23} \\ \underline{S}_{14} & \underline{S}_{24} \end{pmatrix} \begin{pmatrix} E_1 \\ E_2 \end{pmatrix} \tag{11.71}$$

where $\underline{S}_{ij}$ are in general 3×3 complex matrixes depending on the structure parameters. By suitably selecting the design parameters Δ and L, it is possible to obtain, but for an overall component loss that is different from zero.

Besides directional couplers based on mode tail coupling, Y branch single port couplers and splitter can be built. The scheme of a Y branch splitter is reported in Figure 11.32. Working with single mode waveguides, far from the branching section, the modes in the exiting waveguides have to be equal for the symmetry of the structure, so that the electrical field at the output ports has the same power. As far as their phase is concerned, it is easy to demonstrate that, in order to satisfy the energy conservation principle, that is, to avoid that energy is created by the splitter, the output fields have to be transmitted with a phase difference equal to $\pi/4$. As a matter of fact the output fields are perfectly coherent and the overall output power has to be evaluated as the power of the sum of the fields. This is equal to the input power if and only if the fields have a phase difference of $\pi/4$.

This means that a directional coupler can also be fabricated by the sequence of a Y coupler and a Y splitter. Couplers fabricated via Y splitters/couplers produces generally devices with higher losses, but more compact, which can be an important advantage in selected applications.

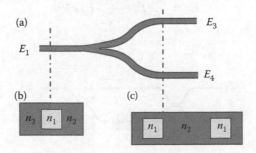

FIGURE 11.32 Scheme of a Y splitter: Top view below the upper cladding (a), input waveguide section (b) and output waveguides section (c).

Directional couplers are the base elements to build integrated optics interferometers. The most common interferometer architecture in integrated optics is the Mach–Zehnder one, schematically represented in Figure 11.33 [11]. It is a two input port, two output ports device, much like a directional coupler, thus it has to be represented by a scattering matrix representation like

$$\begin{pmatrix} E_3 \\ E_4 \end{pmatrix} = \begin{pmatrix} \underline{S}_{13} & \underline{S}_{23} \\ \underline{S}_{14} & \underline{S}_{24} \end{pmatrix} \begin{pmatrix} E_1 \\ E_2 \end{pmatrix} \qquad (11.72)$$

To evaluate, at least in the ideal case, the expression of the elements of the scattering matrix, let us assume a single mode structure and the propagation of a single Fourier component of the field in a perfectly symmetric structure. The input fields can be written as

$$E_1 = E_2 = E_j \, e^{i(kz - \omega t)} \, \boldsymbol{p} \quad (j = 1, 2) \qquad (11.73)$$

where $\boldsymbol{p}$ is the common polarization vector of the input fields. After combining the two fields propagate along the interferometer arms that have the same length, but for the presence along one of them of a variable length section introducing an optical path difference equal to l among the branches. The variable length section can be realized using different techniques. Thermal expansion can be exploited by integrating a heater over one of the arms; electro optics effect can be used in electro optics materials like lithium niobate (LiNbO$_3$) [34] and, in many lab on chip application, the composition of a sample to be analyzed that is placed along one interferometer branch can provide an optical path difference.

In front of the output coupler the fields have the following expression:

$$E_5 = \frac{E_1}{\sqrt{2}} e^{i(kz + kL - \omega t)} \, \boldsymbol{p} + \frac{E_2}{\sqrt{2}} e^{i(kz + kL + kl - \omega t + \pi/2)} \boldsymbol{p} \qquad (11.74a)$$

$$E_6 = \frac{E_1}{\sqrt{2}} e^{i(kz + kL + kl - \omega t + \pi/2)} \boldsymbol{p} + \frac{E_2}{\sqrt{2}} e^{i(kz + kL - \omega t)} \, \boldsymbol{p} \qquad (11.74b)$$

After the output coupler the fields,

$$E_3 = \frac{1}{\sqrt{2}} E_5 + \frac{1}{\sqrt{2}} E_6 \, e^{i\pi/2} \qquad (11.75a)$$

$$E_4 = \frac{1}{\sqrt{2}} E_6 + \frac{1}{\sqrt{2}} E_5 \, e^{i\pi/2} \qquad (11.75b)$$

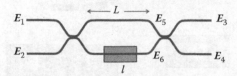

FIGURE 11.33 Principal scheme of an integrated optics Mach–Zehnder interferometer: the position of a possible device for the control of the optical path difference is indicated.

Inserting Equation 11.74a,b into Equation 11.75a,b and putting in evidence the oscillatory tem and the phase common to all the fields we get

$$E_3 = [E_1 \cos(kl) + E_2 \sin(kl)] \, \boldsymbol{p} \tag{11.76a}$$

$$E_4 = [-E_1 \sin(kl) + E_2 \cos(kl)] \, \boldsymbol{p} \tag{11.76b}$$

Thus obtaining

$$\underline{S} = \begin{pmatrix} \cos(kl/2)\underline{I} & \sin(kl/2)\underline{I} \\ -\sin(kl/2)\underline{I} & \cos(kl/2)\underline{I} \end{pmatrix} \tag{11.77}$$

Once l is fixed, the wavelengths for which the optical path difference kl is a multiple of 2π are called interferometer resonance wavelengths.

The interferometry behavior is evident when an optical field is injected only at the first port. In this case, the field that is present at the output ports depends on the optical path difference that if the waveguides on the interferometer arms have the same effective index,

$$\delta = kl = \pi \, n_{eff} \, \frac{l}{\lambda_0} \tag{11.78}$$

where n_{eff} is the effective waveguide refraction index. If the path difference l is chosen in such a way that $\delta = 2j\pi$ with j integer, the fields propagating on the two interferometer arms interfere constructively on output 3 and destructively on output 4 so that the field exits from port 3. Differently, if the path difference is selected in such a way that $\delta = \pi/2 + 2\, j\pi$ the field exits from port 4.

Mach–Zehnder interferometers find a variety of applications: switching [35–37] and modulation [38,39], where the path difference is actively controlled, filtering [40,41], where an equivalent path difference is created by the frequency difference between the resonance interferometer wavelength and the wavelength of the input light and sensing [42,43], where the path difference is the variable to be determined by measuring the optical power at the output of the interferometer arms. We consider mainly this last case in the following.

Where a Mach–Zehnder interferometer is used for sensing, the measured quantity is the intensity I_4 at one of the interferometer outputs divided by the input intensity I_1 so to obtain the following interferometer characteristics:

$$\frac{I_4}{I_1} = \frac{|E_4|^2}{|E_1|^2} = \cos^2\left(\pi n_{eff} \frac{l}{\lambda_0}\right) = \frac{1}{2} + \frac{1}{2}\cos\left(2\pi n_{eff} \frac{l}{\lambda_0}\right) \tag{11.79}$$

This characteristic is generally biased so that in the absence of the sample under test the interferometer is frequently biased at the middle of the linear part of its characteristics, as shown in Figure 11.34. Even if the interferometer characteristic is not linear, its deterministic behavior can be compensated as far as it is sufficiently near an ideal linear characteristic.

A common integrated optics component used for sensors and many other applications is based on ring resonators. The scheme of a ring resonator is reported in Figure 11.35 [44,45]. In the version of the figure the device has one input and one output, thus it can be represented with the relation

$$E_{out}(\nu) = S(\nu)E_{in}(\nu) \tag{11.80}$$

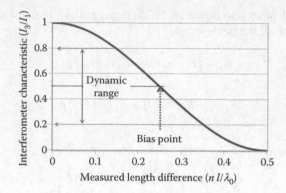

FIGURE 11.34 Sensing characteristic of a Mach–Zehnder interferometer, bias point, and dynamic range.

where the scattering matrix reduces to a scalar transfer function due to the assumption that all the waveguides are single mode so that the polarization vector is fixed in all the system sections.

To determine the ideal behavior of the system, let us imagine that we insert a continuous wave signal at the first port whose wavelength in vacuum is λ.

When the field traverses the coupler connecting the straight waveguide with the ring we have that part of the power will pass from the waveguide to the ring and part of the optical power recirculating in the ring will pass back in the waveguide. In a perfect directional coupler the power splitting ratio will be exactly 1/2, but it is not surprising that this splitting ratio can be changed by adjusting the coupler parameters, in particular, the distance between the straight waveguide and the ring. Thus, we will assume that the coupler ratio is given by ζ, that is, to be less or almost equal to 1. Once the coupling parameter is given in a specific direction, the coupler parameter in the other direction is necessarily the same, due to the system symmetry.

A field component entering the ring through the first coupler performs a full ring round before presenting again at the input coupler location. To exit from the output port it has to undergo another half-ring round and pass through the exit coupler causing attenuation and phase shift. The full round attenuation a is due to propagation and bending losses, so that we can write

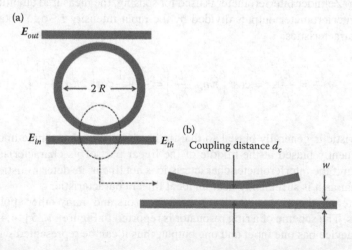

FIGURE 11.35 Scheme of a ring resonator interferometer: Top view below the upper cladding (a) and particular of the coupling section (b).

$$a = e^{-2\pi(\alpha R + \alpha_B)} \tag{11.81}$$

while the phase shift due to propagation through the ring length can be written as

$$\varphi = 2\pi n_{eff}\frac{R}{\lambda} = 2\pi n_{eff}\, R\,\frac{v}{c_0} \tag{11.82}$$

In both cases R is the ring radius, α is the waveguide propagation loss, α_B the bending loss, and n_{eff} is the ring wavelength effective index. The wavelength, frequency, and speed of light in vacuum are indicated as λ, v, and c_0, respectively.

Perfect resonance happens in the resonator when all the contributions propagating through the ring positively interfere at the output port. This condition is realized at the wavelengths $j\lambda_j = \pi n_{eff}R$, since this relation means that half the ring circumference hosts j times the whole wavelengths. Thus, we have to expect a periodic characteristic function, typical of optical resonators.

In a steady-state condition, the light traveling through the ring is constituted by the superposition of infinite contributions. The first-order contribution is given by the field that travels half a ring length. It is given by

$$E_1 = \zeta^2\, a\, E_{in}\, e^{i\left(\pi n_{eff} R \frac{v}{c_0} + \pi\right)} \tag{11.83}$$

Analogously, the jth contribution is given by the field that traveled $2j + 1$ times half the ring length before coupling back in the input waveguide. Adding all contributions, the output field E_{out} can be represented as

$$E_{out} = E_{in}\sum_{0=1}^{\infty}\zeta^{2(2j+1)}a^{2j+1}e^{i(2j+1)\left(\pi n_{eff} R\frac{v}{c_0} + \pi\right)}$$
$$= -\frac{\zeta^2 a E_{in}\, e^{i\left(\pi n_{eff} R\,(v/c_0)\right)}}{1 + \zeta^4 a^2 e^{2\pi i n_{eff} R(v/c_0)}}E_{in} \tag{11.84}$$

As in the case of the Mach–Zehnder interferometer what is observed is the ratio between the input and the output optical intensity such that

$$\frac{I_{out}}{I_{in}} = \left|\frac{E_{out}}{E_{in}}\right|^2 = \frac{\zeta^4 a^2}{2\zeta^4 a^2\cos(2\pi n_{eff}(v/c_0)R) + \zeta^8 a^4 + 1} \tag{11.85}$$

The plot of the ring resonator normalized characteristic is presented in Figure 11.36. The first observation is that the characteristic is not exactly proportional to $(a\zeta^2)$ so that dependence remains after normalization, the plot is provided for $(a\zeta^2) = 0.6$ and naturally, smaller the lost factor, lower the peaks.

The characteristic is composed by a periodic series of resonance peaks as it was qualitatively foreseen occurring at the resonance frequencies corresponding to the wavelength in vacuum λ_j whose expression is given by

$$\frac{1}{n_{eff}R}j = \frac{1}{\lambda_j} \tag{11.86}$$

The ring length is the design parameter fixing the position of the resonance peaks. The distance between the adjacent peaks is called free spectral range and it is an important characteristic of all

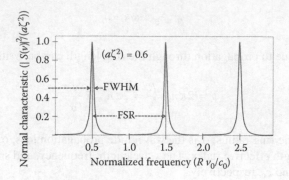

FIGURE 11.36 Characteristic of a ring resonator for $(a\zeta^2) = 0.6$. The full-width at half-maximum (FWHM) and the free spectral range (FSR) are indicated.

interferometers since it indicates the possible frequency range of an optical signal that do not cover two resonance peaks. From Equation 11.86 and assuming as in all practical applications

$$\Delta\lambda_{FSR} = \lambda_{j+1} - \lambda_j \ll \lambda_0 \tag{11.87}$$

we have

$$\Delta\lambda_{FSR} \approx \frac{\lambda_j^2}{2\pi n_{eff} R} \tag{11.88}$$

It is evident that the free spectral range depends on the working wavelength when it is expressed as a wavelength interval. As a matter of fact, it is uniform on the frequency axis. Moreover, a great ring has a small FSR, so that the limit to the ring length is given by the fact that if the ring is longer than the threshold, the free spectral range becomes too small in the considered wavelength range and with practical ring losses it no longer behaves as a resonator. The peak width is generally reported as full-width at half-maximum (FWHM), that is, at half the peak height, and provides a good approximation:

$$\Delta\lambda_{FWHM} = 2\frac{\lambda_j^2}{\pi n_{eff} R} \arcsin\left(\frac{1 - a(1 - \zeta^2)}{2\sqrt{a(1 - \zeta^2)}}\right) \tag{11.89}$$

where the dependence of $\Delta\lambda_{FWHM}$ from the wavelength is also intrinsic in the values of the attenuation and coupling coefficient that are generally wavelength dependent. The FHWM decreases with the ring length too, at the same pace of the FSR.

The plot of the FWHM is provided in Figure 11.37 as a function of a and ζ. The resonance width gets smaller, which is better, decreasing the total ring loss and increasing the coupling of the input waveguide with the ring. Since essentially the coupling between the input waveguide with the ring increases decreasing the distance between the two, called d_c in Figure 11.35, obtaining a sufficiently small value of d_c is one of the technology challenges posed by the realization of efficient ring resonators.

A third integrated optics component we would like to review for its importance in biosensors is thewaveguide Bragg grating [11,46,47]. A waveguide Bragg grating is obtained by applying a periodic perturbation to the effective index of a straight waveguide either through the perturbation of the cladding index or through the perturbation of the core index or both. The grating is obtained when the number of periods of the perturbation is very high so to neglect border effects with respect to the bulk perturbation effect. A schematic of possible Bragg grating structures is presented in Figure 11.38.

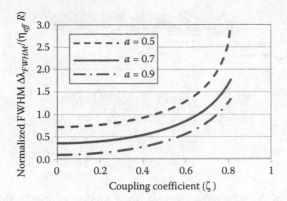

FIGURE 11.37 Normalized wavelength FWHM of a ring resonator versus the ring loss and the coupling parameter.

The working principle of a Bragg grating rely on the fact that at each effective index discontinuity the propagating mode is partially reflected and partially transmitted. Thus, in every waveguide section, the transmitted field is the sum of N transmitted contributions and the reflected field is the sum of N reflected contributions, where N is the number of gratings periods. The situation is similar to that encountered in the case of the ring resonator. Taking into account all the contributions it is possible to evaluate the grating characteristics in terms of transmitted and reflected field as a function of the input field.

Bragg gratings can be realized with different behavior of the effective index fluctuations along the grating and also introducing a slow grating period fluctuation, called apodization [48,49]. Both these techniques are meant to shape suitably the grating characteristics. Apodization, in particular, is often used to decrease the characteristic lateral peaks when a strong suppression of the reflected optical signal out of the grating bandwidth is required. For the simple analysis we will concentrate on purely periodic gratings with an effective index dependence on the axial coordinate z provided by

$$n_{eff}(z) = \bar{n}_{eff} + \delta n \left[1 + \cos\left(2\pi \frac{z}{\Lambda} \right) \right] \tag{11.90}$$

as shown in Figure 11.39.

The key parameters of the grating are the grating period Λ and the effective index difference δn. Frequently, the grating period is also expressed through the so-called Bragg wavelength, or resonance wavelength, which is given by

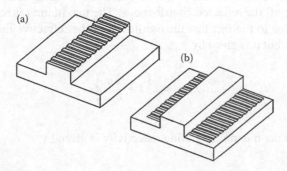

FIGURE 11.38 Integrated optics waveguide Bragg grating: corrugated core (a) and corrugated cladding (b). A ridge waveguide is assumed as grating base as an example.

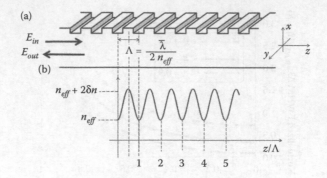

FIGURE 11.39 Scheme of the idealized waveguide Bragg grating we use for the characteristic function evaluation; waveguide core with definition of the grating period Λ and of the base resonance frequency $\bar{\lambda}$ (a) and effective index dependence on the waveguide axis (b).

$$\bar{\lambda} = 2\bar{n}_{eff}\Lambda \tag{11.91}$$

Assuming that the Bragg grating is very long, that is, $L_c \gg \delta n \bar{\lambda}$, the characteristic function of the grating is found to be [46]

$$\frac{I_{out}}{I_{in}} = \left|\frac{E_{out}}{E_{in}}\right|^2 = \frac{\sinh^2\left(L_c\sqrt{K^2(\nu) - R^2(\nu)}\right)}{\cosh^2\left(L_c\sqrt{K^2(\nu) - R^2(\nu)}\right) - (R^2(\nu)/K^2(\nu))} \tag{11.92}$$

where

$$K(\nu) = \frac{\pi}{c_0}\delta n\nu \tag{11.93}$$

$$R(\nu) = 2\frac{\pi}{c_0}\delta n\nu + 2\pi\bar{n}_{eff}\frac{\nu - \bar{\nu}}{c_0} \tag{11.94}$$

and $c_0/\bar{\nu} = \bar{\lambda}$ From Equation 11.92 it is seen that the grating reflects effectively only a set of wavelength around the Bragg wavelength, that is, the wavelengths for which almost constructive interference takes place among all the reflected contributions. The maximum reflectivity is not exactly at the Bragg wavelength due to the fact that the oscillation of the refractive index given in Equation 11.90 has no zero mean, but it is given by

$$\lambda_{max} = \bar{\lambda}\left(1 + \frac{\delta n}{n_{eff}}\right) \tag{11.95}$$

and the relative value of the maximum grating reflectivity is given by

$$\left.\frac{I_{out}}{I_{in}}\right|_{MAX} = \tanh^2(KL_c) \tag{11.96}$$

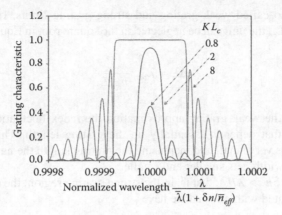

FIGURE 11.40 Waveguide grating characteristic function for different values of the parameter KL_c.

The width of the grating reflection wavelength band can also be derived by Equation 11.92 evaluating the distance between the first points where the characteristic is zero on the left and on the right-hand side of the maximum. It is obtained as

$$\Delta\lambda = \lambda_{max} \frac{\delta n}{\bar{n}_{eff}} \sqrt{1 + \left(\frac{\bar{\lambda}}{\delta n L_c}\right)^2} \qquad (11.97)$$

A plot of the considered waveguide Bragg grating characteristic is provided in Figure 11.40 versus the input wavelength for different values of the product $K L_c$.

The grating characteristic reflects the fact that only a set of wavelength around the maximum are effectively reflected, showing however lateral peaks beside the main passband. Lateral peaks are higher and higher while the characteristic is flatter and flatter in the passband, that is, while the ratio $K L_c$ increases. Since once the optical desired characteristics of the grating are selected, the ratio $K L_c$ is mainly determined by the grating length, it has to be selected on the ground of a tradeoff between flatness and side peak height.

The bandwidth of the grating as it is given by Equation 11.97 depends both on the grating length L_c and on the index fluctuation δn. An example of dependence of the grating bandwidth on the effective index variation is shown in Figure 11.41. Two distinct limit regions are present in the figure,

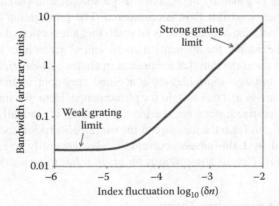

FIGURE 11.41 Example of dependence of the passband of a waveguide Bragg grating versus the effective index variation for a fixed grating length.

corresponding to the so-called weak grating and strong grating limits. If the index variation is small, that is, $\delta n \ll \bar{\lambda}/L_c$, the unit can be neglected in the square root in Equation 11.97 and we have

$$\Delta\lambda \approx \lambda_{max} \frac{\bar{\lambda}}{\bar{n}_{eff} L_c} \tag{11.98}$$

This means that in the weak grating approximation the index fluctuation disappears from the bandwidth expression that depends essentially on the grating length. This reflects the fact that every single reflection is very small and increasing the grating length the number of reflections also increases and the bandwidth gets smaller and smaller.

On the contrary, for $\delta n \gg \bar{\lambda}/L_c$, that is, in the strong grating region, the square root in Equation 11.97 can be approximated with one and we have

$$\Delta\lambda = \lambda_{max} \frac{\delta n}{\bar{n}_{eff}} \tag{11.99}$$

In this extreme condition, the bandwidth does not depend on the grating length, due to the fact that wavelengths that are near the grating resonance does not penetrate up to the grating end due to strong reflections at each discontinuity and the number of effective reflections practically does not depend on the length of the grating.

11.3 LAB-ON-CHIP SPECTROSCOPY

11.3.1 Absorption Spectroscopy

From the analysis of the interaction between a biological solution of target molecules and an optical radiation it is clear that the attenuation a light beam experiences while traveling through the solution is composed by essentially three phenomena, each of which contributes to the overall attenuation to a specific attenuation coefficient:

- Absorption of photons by solvent molecules or ions
- Ion current generated by the optical field
- Absorption of photons by target molecules

The first phenomenon is generally negligible when a solvent transparent to the light frequency is used, for example, water if visible light is considered. The propagation distance into the lab on chip chamber where the solution is contained is so small that attenuation of a transparent media can be neglected: just for an example, the attenuation coefficient of green light traversing 1 mm of pure water is about 0.9999. As far as the ions that are present in almost all biological solutions to guarantee proper pH and solubility of target molecules are concerned, they contribute with sensible absorption only if they have energy levels that can sustain the phenomenon. Here, for simplicity, we will assume that this situation is not realized, but since the ion contribution is generally known, a possible ion absorption can be eliminated from the measure of the overall absorption coefficient easily.

Absorption generated by light-induced currents is also generally negligible, as estimated in Section 11.3.2.2, so that if relevant absorption is observed it has to be ascribed to target molecules themselves.

11.3.1.1 Absorption Spectroscopy Theory

Let us now imagine that we model the macromolecule with a two-level energy system, that is, only the ground level and one excited energy level are able to absorb photons of the propagating light beam. To develop a useful expression of the observed light attenuation as a function of the target molecule energy levels we have to remove the approximation that the level themselves correspond to perfectly individuated energy values. To do that let us introduce an energy level line $F_j(v)$ $j = 1, 2$, where the dependence of the energy level linewidth on energy has been cast in terms of frequency v, simply dividing the energy by the Planck's constant h. In correspondence to the level lines we can define a transition line as

$$F(v) = \int F_1(\xi) F_2(v - \xi) d\xi \tag{11.100}$$

If the line functions $F_j(v)$ are normalized so that their integral to the whole frequency axis is one, $F(v)$ is also normalized in the same way. The physical meaning of $F(v)$ is quite clear: it represents the fraction of transitions whose frequency is in the infinitesimal range $(v, v + dv)$.

Assuming to be at steady state, from the rate equations (11.37) and the relations among the Einstein coefficients, assuming absence of level degenerations, we obtain

$$A N_2 = B \langle n \rangle (N_2 - N_1) \tag{11.101}$$

where N_2 and N_1 are here intended as molecules per unit volume.

If we consider a traveling wave passing through the solution we have to assume that both the populations and the average photon number depends on the position along the wave propagation axis, which we call z. With this interpretation, the first term of Equation 11.101 represents the number of photons scattered out of the beam by stimulated emission, while the second term is the number of absorbed photons minus the number of photons returned to the beam by stimulated emission. It is clear that both expressions are equal to the photons the beam loses in the unit time. Thus, we have

$$\frac{d\langle n \rangle}{dt} = -B\langle n \rangle F(v) (N_2 - N_1) \tag{11.102}$$

where we have introduced on a phenomenological ground the transition line considering its physical meaning. Exploiting Equations 11.45 and indicating with N the target molecules density we have

$$\frac{d\langle n \rangle}{dt} = -B \, F(v) N \frac{n_s}{n_s + 2\langle n \rangle} \langle n \rangle \tag{11.103}$$

Since $\langle n \rangle$ and n_s are photon densities we can transform them in an energy density by multiplying by hv and in an intensity by further dividing by c_0. The molecule density can be converted in the molecules into concentration c_m divided by the Avogadro number N_A. A last transformation of Equation 11.103 can be done observing that if we consider wavefront traveling through our solution and we call W the average energy density in the volume contained in an infinitesimal slab of solution around the wave front we can write

$$hv \frac{d\langle n \rangle}{dt} = \frac{dW}{dt} = \frac{dW}{dz}\frac{dz}{dt} = c_0 \frac{dW}{dz} = \frac{dI}{dz} \tag{11.104}$$

Finally, Equation 11.103 can be rewritten in terms of macroscopic light intensity $I(z)$, that is, the average flow of energy through a unit area of a wavefront, as

$$\frac{1}{I(z)}\left(1 + \frac{2I(z)}{I_s}\right)\frac{dI(z)}{dz} = -\frac{BF(v)N_A}{c_0} c_m \tag{11.105}$$

We have seen that light propagation is in linear regime if $I(z) \ll I_s$, a condition that is fulfilled in almost all cases where labs on chip are adopted, even if lasers are used. In this case, Equation 11.105 simplifies as

$$\frac{dI(z)}{dz} = -\frac{BF(\nu)N_A}{c_0} c_m I(z) \tag{11.106}$$

This equation coincides with Equation 11.24 that we have empirically introduced to take into account light attenuation and provides a microscopic expression of the attenuation coefficient, which as per the Beer–Lambert law is proportional to the target molecule concentration.

Besides confirming with a microscopic analysis the classical analysis of attenuation by a molecule solution, Equation 11.106 constitutes the base for a much diffused molecule detection and quantization method called attenuation spectroscopy. From Equation 11.106 the solute absorbance $\epsilon(\nu)$ has the expression

$$\epsilon(\nu) = \frac{BF(\nu)N_A}{c_0} \tag{11.107}$$

which depends on the molecule energy transition levels. In particular, $\epsilon(\nu)$ presents two different frequency-dependent terms: the coefficient B and the transition line $F(\nu)$. The transition line has the form of a pulse, frequently with an approximated Gaussian shape, as seen in the discussion of the energy level broadening causes. The coefficient B can be written as the product between the frequency and a term slowly varying with frequency so as to be almost constant within the range of a single transition line, but being substantially different from transition to transition [3]. Adopting for the slow-varying term the expression of the original Einstein coefficient we can write

$$\epsilon(\nu) = \frac{h\nu B^*(\nu)F(\nu)N_A}{c_0} \tag{11.108}$$

Thus, we conclude that every molecule is characterized by a unique profile of the attenuation that is composed of a set of attenuation peaks whose shape is provided by the corresponding transition line multiplied by the light frequency. An example of absorption spectrum of a biological macromolecule is provided in Figure 11.42 [50]. Here, the absorption spectrum of a myoglobin excited state is shown in the visible spectrum region; in the figure the absorption peaks are named with the names of the corresponding transitions. As usual in absorption spectrograms, the absorption A' is simply given by $A' = 1 - A$, where A is the attenuation experienced by the beam traveling through the sample cell.

An example of the capability of the absorbance spectrum to identify a target molecule via even small changes of the energy level values is provided in Figure 11.43 [51], where the absorbance spectrum $\epsilon(\nu)$ (see Equation 11.26) of a very heavy hemoglobin molecule coming from an annelid called *Glossoscolex paulistus* is shown versus the pH of the water solution where the molecule is solved.

The set of absorption peaks can be used to recognize the presence of a target molecule in a solution. Once the specific peak set is identified, the concentration can be estimated by estimating the peak intensity using the Beer–Lambert law. This assay detection method is called absorption spectroscopy. Besides the base technique consisting of a direct measurement of the spectral behavior of attenuation, several modified techniques exist, based, for example, on real-time spectroscopy [52,53].

11.3.1.2 Absorption Spectroscopy Implementation in Lab on Chip

A direct way of using absorption spectroscopy to quantify a molecule present after sample purification in a lab on chip is represented in Figure 11.44 [54]. The assay chamber in the lab on chip is

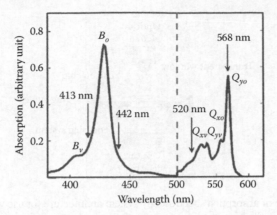

FIGURE 11.42 Absorption spectrum of a myoglobin excited state is shown in the visible spectrum region. (Reproduced from *Biophysical Journal*, vol. 78, Engler N. et al. Protein dynamics in an intermediate state of myoglobin: optical absorption, resonance raman spectroscopy, and x-ray structure analysis, pp. 2081–2092, Copyright 2000, with permission from Elsevier.)

accessible by external light both on top and on bottom through transparent windows that are frequently simply obtained by using a transparent material like glass or PMMA for chip fabrication. The lab on chip package presents a plug slide allowing insertion into an external device after sample loading. The external device contains the optical source and the optical detector that are needed to perform absorption measurements. As a final step, raw absorption measurements are processed by suitable algorithms to extract the required data.

Even if the scheme of Figure 11.44 is simple and can be fabricated as a compact equipment, at least as far as IR spectroscopy is concerned, performing absorption spectroscopy via a lab on chip opens the possibility to use integrated optical cavities like microrings to enhance the detection performances via two variations of plain absorption spectroscopy: cavity ring down (CRD) spectroscopy and cavity enhances absorption (CEA) spectroscopy.

CRD spectroscopy is an absorption technique in which the sensitivity is primarily improved by increasing the absorption path length using a high-performance optical cavity [55]. In conventional CRD spectroscopy light from a pulsed laser is coupled into the cavity and the light inside the cavity experiences many reflections therby increasing the path through the absorbing medium: absorption

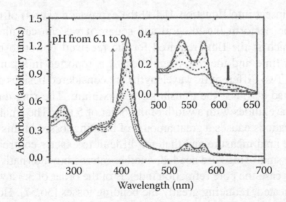

FIGURE 11.43 Absorbance spectrum $\epsilon(v)$ of a very heavy hemoglobin molecule coming from an annelid called *Glossoscolex paulistus* is shown versus the pH of the water solution where the molecule is solved. (Reproduced from *Biophysical Journal*, vol. 94, Santiago P. S. et al. Dynamic light scattering and optical absorption spectroscopy study of pH and temperature stabilities of the extracellular hemoglobin of glossoscolex paulistus, pp. 2228–2240, Copyright 2008, with permission from Elsevier.)

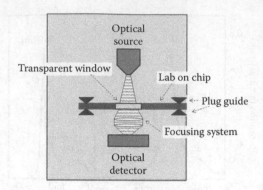

FIGURE 11.44 Example of absorption spectroscopy system architecture for use with lab on chips.

path lengths up to 10 km can be reached. The light exiting the cavity is detected and the decay rate of the light intensity is determined, which is a direct measure for the total cavity loss.

This can easily be seen by considering the cavity as a filter that processes the input light pulse. Moreover, if the polarization of light is the same for all considered signals and it does not change while traveling through the absorbent solution, we can drop the polarization vector from the electrical field expression and work with scalar fields. While this approximation is not always valid in macroscopic spectroscopy, this is true in integrated optics circuits.

If the pulse duration is much shorter than the inverse of the cavity resonation bandwidth it can be considered as a Dirac pulse of amplitude E_{in}, so that the signal E_{out} out of the cavity is given by

$$E_{out}(t) = E_{in} \int_{-\infty}^{\infty} S(\nu)e^{2\pi i \nu t} d\nu \qquad (11.109)$$

where $S(\nu)$ is the resonator characteristic function. This means that the observed response corresponds to a field that is the Fourier transform of the cavity characteristic function. Since the cavity characteristic function is a pulse in frequency whose width depends on the cavity loss and increases while it increases, its Fourier transform is a decay function whose characteristic decay time is approximately inversely proportional to the frequency pulse width, thus depending mainly on the cavity loss.

In particular, if we insert into Equation 11.109 the expression (11.84) of the characteristic function of a ring resonator, perform the integral and square it we can calculate the halving time of the obtained pulse, which is the time required for the received power to become half. The relation between the decay time and the ring overall loss A is reported in Figure 11.45 for a ring with $n_{eff} = 1.52$ and $\zeta = 0.75$. Two different IR wavelengths are considered besides different ring radii. The decay time τ is evaluated at $1/e$ of the transmission maximum. The ring data correspond to silica rings fabricated with waveguides with a width of the order of 5 μm. The small dimension of the ring needed for some applications causes a great amount of bending losses in this kind of rings that have to be eliminated by the final measure and that are difficult to exactly control in a realistic ring fabrication process. When small rings are needed, another interesting alternative is to fabricate silicon core rings. Since in this case the core refraction index is of the order of 3.3 a very high index contrast waveguide can be fabricated, reducing greatly the bending losses [56,57]. However, in this case the core dimension to obtain the single mode operation at the same wavelength has to be much smaller than that of silica waveguides, thus increasing the coupling losses and, in case of labs on chip, the fabrication complexity of the optical connection between the chip and the external environment [58–60].

From the figure we see that the decay time in the IRspectral region are quite low, in the order of picoseconds or even smaller. Increasing the ring length the ring passband decreases thereby

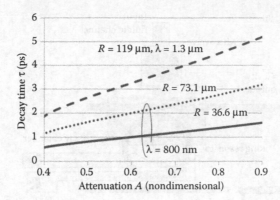

FIGURE 11.45 Relation between the decay time and the ring overall loss A for a ring with $n_{eff} = 1.52$ and $\zeta = 0.75$. Two different IR wavelengths are considered besides different ring radii. The decay time τ is evaluated at $1/e$ of the transmission maximum.

increasing the decay time, while decreasing the attenuation the passband increases and the decay time decreases. This means that such a detection technique requires an optical detection system that is able to detect real-time shapes of very fast pulses, quite different from detection systems we analyzed in Section 11.3.3.

In this case, an accurate detection of the decay time is performed by repeating the measure a great number of times using subsequent pulses and averaging the results so as to decrease the effect of the noise.

An absorption spectrum is obtained by this technique by scanning the laser wavelength and the cavity resonance peak and determining the decay time of the light intensity at each wavelength. It is important to observe that the CRD measurement is independent of the intensity of light, which has not to be controlled with great accuracy.

Cavity-enhanced absorption (CEA) spectroscopy is another absorption spectrometry technique using a high-quality optical cavity. Light is coupled into the cavity when the light frequency coincides with the frequency of one of the cavity resonances and the signal exiting from the cavity is measured and timeintegrated.

Since we are measuring the cavity response to a resonant wavelength, the response intensity will depend inversely on the attenuation, so that the attenuation spectrum can be measured in correspondence with all the cavity modes. Moreover, if the cavity can be tuned, for example, by changing the cavity length somehow, the light and the cavity can be synchronously tuned so as to have a continuous attenuation spectrum. This can be done in integrated ring cavities, for example, by inserting heaters along the ring path so as to change the ring length exploiting thermal expansion of the material [61,62].

CRD and CEA spectroscopies are frequently adopted in lab on chip when absorption spectroscopy has to be performed and the system is not designed for field use, so that a relatively complex optical transmission and detection system can be incorporated in the equipment hosting the disposable lab on chip [63–65]. This is due mainly on the ease to fabricate and control high-performance ring cavities by integrated optics. CRD requires very short pulse lasers that are complex equipment, so that the lab on chip when used for CRD is mainly a part of a more complex equipment. On the contrary, CEA is a much simpler technique that can be implemented in a more compact equipment, where laser tunability is obtained either by directly tunable semiconductor lasers or by laser arrays. Thus, CEA is generally considered more suitable for lab on chip applications, having over other absorption spectroscopy techniques the advantage of a greater sensibility.

A possible scheme of a lab on chip for CEA applications is shown in Figure 11.46. The top view of the detection system is shown in part (a): a detection chamber is fed via a microfluidic channel

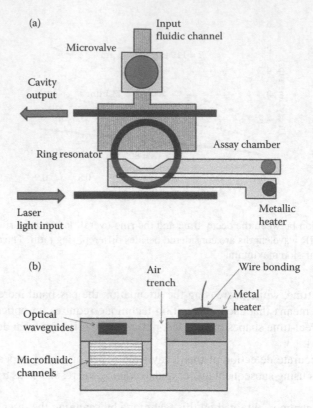

FIGURE 11.46 Scheme of a possible implementation of a lab on chip implementing CEA through a microring resonator: top view (a) and vertical section (b).

with the sample solution. The feeding channel and the detection chamber are divided by a microvalve that opens when the external pressure has to fill the chamber and closes before the assay begins. The feeding solution based on a microvalve is only one of the many possibilities, assuring insulation of the assay chamber from the rest of the microfluidic circuit both before the assay, during a possible sample purification phase, and during the assay.

The assay chamber is fabricated below half the circumference of a ring resonator, whose structure is indicated with thick black lines in the figure. The ring resonator and the assay chamber are coupled through the exponential tail of the optical mode propagating in the lower cladding of the ring waveguides. To create a sufficient coupling the interface between the assay chamber and the ring waveguide has to be designed as thin as possible and the refraction index of the lateral and upper cladding has to be designed in such a way that the more is sufficiently extended in the assay chamber direction. To enhance coupling it is also possible to insert in the sample a suitable neutral chemical component to bias its refraction index.

The ring resonator is tuned by a metallic heater that is well divided by the reaction chamber, not to provoke heating of the sample with possible problems for the assay accuracy. If this risk is not present, due to the fact that molecules in the sample are quite heat resistant, the assay chamber and the heater can both cover all the resonator area thus improving both the optical coupling and the tunability of the resonator.

The vertical section of the detection system is represented schematically in Figure 11.46b. It is imagined that the optical waveguides are built on the upper wafer and the fluidic circuit on the lower wafer before wafer bonding. This solution allows clear process separation between the two parts of the chip and the possibility to realize, if advantageous, the fluidic part using a polymer substrate and the optical part using a glass or glass on silicon substrate. To obtain a better thermal insulation between the assay chamber and the heater an air trench is excavated between them. The trench is not to interrupt optical waveguides however, thus it cannot extend over all the thermal boundary between the assay chamber and the heater. The valve closing the assay chamber can be fabricated in several different ways (see Section 8.2). If a horizontal membrane valve is selected, the membrane could be built in the upper wafer, closing a channel in the lower wafer.

Since ring tunability is a key factor in assuring wide range spectroscopy via CEA, it is interesting to understand the order of magnitude of thermal tuning for ring resonators built on glass or silicon core waveguide. As far as polymer waveguides are concerned, thermal tuning is more difficult due to the intrinsic instability of many polymers versus wide thermal cycles. In this case other tuning methods have to be adopted, for example, incorporating materials whose refraction index can be changed with applied tension [66] or using electro-optic effect [67], or a particular attention has to be paid in the choice of polymers that are stable in the considered temperature range [68].

The thermal expansion coefficient of silica is about 8.5×10^{-6} K^{-1}. Let us consider a silica optical ring with a radius of 73 μm, whose resonance is of the order of 800 nm that is heated on half the circumference. Heating to a temperature gradient of 100 K results in a percentage increase of the ring length of 0.085% corresponding to a tuning range of 0.68 nm, which corresponds to a frequency of 319 GHz. This is a small tuning range and an increase of a different order of magnitude is needed to allow practical CEA.

Several possible solutions can be adopted. The easier is to integrate on the chip several different rings, covering contiguous spectral ranges, and distribute the optical signal either among different chip inputs using an external optical system, or inside the chip among different rings adopting an optical switch. This is a practical solution in this case, since CEA is generally not used for lab on chip designed for field operation, but it is considered a lab solution. Another possible solution is to combine thermal tuning with some nonthermal tuning mechanism in order to increase the tuning range.

An effective way to obtain discontinuous but very wide thermal tuning of an integrated optics ring resonator is to couple two different rings as it is shown in Figure 11.47. If the free spectral range of the two rings is accurately designed, as shown in Figure 11.48, only one of the passband characteristics of the rings superimposes, thereby both eliminating the resonator periodic characteristics and obtaining a sharper resonator characteristic due to the product of the ring characteristics [69–71]. This effect is called the Vernier effect.

Moreover, as shown in Figure 11.48, even a small tuning of one or both the rings can change the order of the superimposing peaks in the ring characteristics, so causing a very wide resonator characteristic tuning. If both rings are tuned the tuning characteristic of the device exhibits larger continuous tuning regions and smaller forbidden regions.

Owing to the fact that Vernier effect is better designed if the free spectral range is not too small, double-ring resonators are frequently fabricated starting with silicon core waveguides. As a matter of fact, the high index contrast that is typical of these waveguides assures the possibility of designing small radius rings.

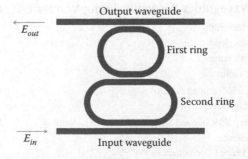

FIGURE 11.47 Scheme of a double-ring resonator designed to generate the Vernier effect.

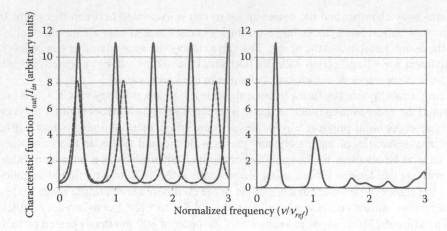

FIGURE 11.48 Scheme of working of the Vernier effect. Plot of the characteristic functions of the two resonators (a) and the resulting characteristic function (b).

An example of design parameters for a silicon waveguide double-ring resonator is reported in Table 11.7. Here the rings are built with small waveguides [69] so as to obtain small ring radii. It is assumed that the larger ring is heated over all its length while the smaller ring is not heated. The required temperature difference jumps from superposition of the peaks at 1.300 μm to the superposition of the peaks at 1.31724 μm is only 46.44°C so that up to a bandwidth of 51.72 nm can be run with a thermal heating of about 140°C. The forbidden region in divided into three bands that depends on the intrinsic resonator losses. The design parameters reported in Table 11.7 are obtained using the simple description of the working of a ring resonator presented in this section, and a more detailed description of the optical propagation in the structure is needed to obtain a detailed design. On the other hand, no attempt has been made to optimize the design for a specific need, and much more optimized designs can be obtained once the detailed requirements are fixed.

Other arrangements of rings [45,72,73] and of combinations of Mach–Zehnder interferometers and rings have been proposed [74,75], so as to cover a wide area of applications.

11.3.2 FLUORESCENCE SPECTROSCOPY

Fluorescence refers to the ability of several organic and inorganic components to emit electromagnetic radiation when illuminated with an external source of different wavelengths. The emitted

---

TABLE 11.7

Design Parameter for an Example of Two Ring Silicon Core Waveguides Resonator Using Vernier Effect

Waveguides width	200 nm
Waveguides depth	40 nm
Wavelength range	1.3 μm
First ring radius	7.88 μm
First ring FSR (around 1.3 μm)	10.35 nm
Second ring radius	4.73 μm
Second ring FSR (around 1.3 μm)	17.24 nm
FSR Difference	6.89 nm
Silicon Thermal Coefficient	$3°K^{-1}$
Required ΔT for first step	46.44°K

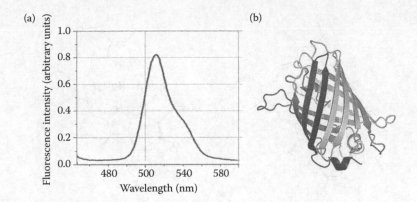

(a) (b)

FIGURE 11.49 Fluorescence spectrum in the green spectrum range (a) and stereographic strip representation (b) of the GFP protein.

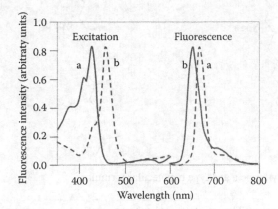

FIGURE 11.50 Fluorescence excitation spectra and the fluorescence emission spectra of chlorophyll type a and type b.

wavelength is always longer than the illumination one, revealing the fact that electromagnetic radiation is partially absorbed by the material and partially emitted by lower energy photons.

A specific fluorescent molecule exhibits frequently several possible excitation wavelengths, while the fluorescence wavelength, even with some exceptions, is independent of the used excitation wavelength.

An example of fluorescence spectrum in the visible and near IR spectral range is reported in Figure 11.49, where fluorescence of a protein called green fluorescence protein (GFP) [76] is reported beside the stereographic GFP representation. The fluorescence spectrum is an important characteristic distinguishing even very similar molecules, being related, as we will see soon, to the detailed distribution of the so-called fluorescence energy levels of the molecule.

An example of the fluorescence capacity of distinguishing similar molecules is provided in Figure 11.50, where the fluorescence excitation spectra and the fluorescence emission spectra of chlorophyll type a and type b are shown. The fluorescence excitation spectra represent the set of wavelength at which fluorescence is obtained weighted with the total amount of fluorescence emitted when the molecule is excited at the considered wavelength. The molecular formulas of the two considered chlorophyll types [77,78] are reported in Figure 11.51.

11.3.2.1 Fluorescence Spectroscopy Theory

Generally speaking, fluorescence is observed when the excitation radiation provokes the transition to a high-energy molecular state that does not relax directly in the ground state by emission of a

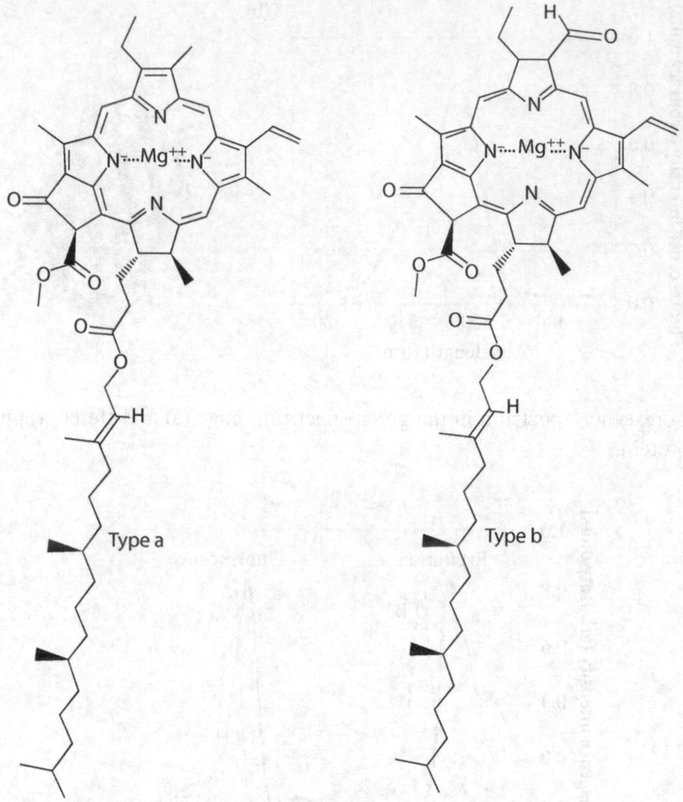

FIGURE 11.51 Chlorophyll type a and type b molecular formulas.

photon of the same frequency. The excited state relaxes to the ground state in two phases: in a first phase the molecule losses energy by nonradiative ways, as by collisions with other molecules or with the solvent, until it reaches an intermediate state; in the second phase, a lower energy photon is emitted to relax from the intermediate state to the ground state. In a few cases, further nonradiative relaxation can be needed after phase two to reach the ground state.

The most common fluorescence type takes place when the absorbed photon causes the transition of the molecules between energy states with different electronic quantum number, as shown in Figure 11.52, where it is assumed that transition between s_0 and s_1 electronic states happens. Since the electronic state s_1 is split by rotational and vibrational states in many nearby levels, the molecule relaxes in the first phase with a great number of small decays between vibrational and rotational states without changing the electron quantum numbers. When the molecule is arrived at the border of the $s1$ states it emits a photon to cross the energy gap between states s_0 and s_1 so as to be able to reach the ground state with another set of small energy steps.

A simple physical model of fluorescence can be set up assuming the three-level scheme of Figure 11.53. Similar schemes in the framework of fluorescence are often called Jablonski diagrams. The exciting photon provokes a transition between the ground state and the state with energy $\mathcal{E}_2$, fluorescence is observed due to radiative decay of molecules from state 2 to state 1, then a fast nonradiative transition provokes the final decay of molecules to the ground state. To differentiate radiative and nonradiative decays we will introduce nonradiative decay rates, indicating with $D_{i,j}$ the rate of nonradiative decay through the transition $i \rightarrow j$.

In the model of Figure 11.53, due to the assumption that fluorescence is observed from the transition $2 \rightarrow 1$, we can simplify greatly the general form of the rate equations. In particular, the following approximations can be done:

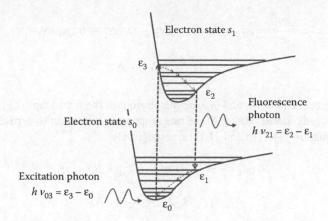

FIGURE 11.52 Example of fluorescent emission due to the excitation between states with different electron quantum numbers.

- We consider only a thin layer of material so that attenuation and spatial dynamics of the considered variables can be neglected.
- We assume that the solvent is transparent with negligible attenuation at all the considered wavelengths and that its refraction index is equal to 1, water often satisfy this approximations, but in proximity of its absorption peaks [79].
- Spontaneous emission on the transition $1 \rightarrow 0$ is neglected; this implies that no photon is present at frequency $\nu_{0,1}$ so that the stimulated emission at this frequency can be neglected as well.
- Nonradiative decay and stimulated emission in the transition $2 \rightarrow 0$ are neglected with respect to decay through the intermediate state 1. A rate of spontaneous emission is in any case required for physical consistence of the model.

Moreover, proceeding as in the case of interaction of light with a two-level system it is possible to demonstrate that

$$B_{2,1} = B_{1,2} \tag{11.110}$$

so that we can simplify the notation setting $B_1 = B_{2,1} = B_{1,2}$ and $B_0 = B_{2,0}$.

Using these approximations we get the following rate equations for the molecule populations:

$$\frac{dN_0}{dt} = A_{2,0}N_2 + D_{1,0}N_1 - B_2\langle n_p\rangle N_0 \tag{11.111a}$$

$$\frac{dN_2}{dt} = B_2\langle n_p\rangle N_0 + B_1\langle n_f\rangle N_1 - A_{2,1}N_2 - B_1\langle n_f\rangle N_2 \tag{11.111b}$$

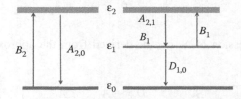

FIGURE 11.53 Energy diagram of the simple fluorescence model considered in this section.

$$\frac{dN_1}{dt} = A_{2,1}N_2 + B_1\langle n_f\rangle N_2 - D_{1,0}N_1 - B_1\langle n_f\rangle N_1 \tag{11.111c}$$

$$N_0 + N_1 + N_2 = N \tag{11.111d}$$

where $\langle n_f\rangle$ are fluorescence photons and $\langle n_p\rangle$ are the photons at the wavelength of the external source.

Searching for a steady-state solution of the rate equations we can set to zero the time derivatives and obtain from Equations 11.111c and 11.111a, respectively.

$$N_2(A_{2,1} + B_1\langle n_f\rangle) = N_1(D_{1,0} + B_1\langle n_f\rangle) \tag{11.112a}$$

$$A_{2,0}N_2 + D_{1,0}N_1 = B_2\langle n_p\rangle N_0 \tag{11.112b}$$

From Equation 11.112a we see that the parameter $\vartheta = D_{1,0}/A_{2,1}$ is important in determining the behavior of target molecules. As a matter of fact, Equation 11.112a tells us that if $\vartheta < 1$ there is no condition in which $N_1 < N_2$ while if $\vartheta > 1$ the molecule population in the higher energy state can be greater than that in the lower one. In this last condition, which is called population inversion [3,4], stimulated emission overcomes spontaneous emission at the fluorescence frequency v_f so that every spontaneous emitted photon is amplified several times by stimulated emission and the radiation is constituted by bunches of coherent photons. In this condition, also called super-luminescence, a small light beam at frequency v_f inserted into the system is amplified by spontaneous emission, so that the system works like an optical amplifier [80]. Moreover, if the system is inserted into an optical cavity, for example, placing it between two mirrors, spontaneous oscillations arise and the system works like a laser [81].

Super-luminescence is to be avoided if luminescence has to be used for quantitative assays, so that if $\vartheta > 1$ for the target molecule, the external light source intensity has to be maintained sufficiently weak to avoid population inversion.

Equations 11.112a and 11.112b are easily solved for the molecule populations obtaining

$$N_2 - N_1 = \frac{A_{2,1}(\vartheta - 1)\langle n_p\rangle N}{D_{1,0}(A_{2,0} + A_{2,1}) + (D_{1,0} + A_{2,0})B_1\langle n_f\rangle} \tag{11.113}$$

where it is set $N_0 \approx N$, which is an approximation fully satisfied in all practical situations. The general structure of Equation 11.113 is the same already encountered in Equation 11.45, but for the fact that due to the three-level structure of the considered system, the difference $N_2 - N_1$ can be either positive or negative. This means that for high values of the external source, intensity nonlinear phenomena related to saturation of the population difference occur. However, in order to stimulate this nonlinear behavior in practical experiments, extremely powerful lasers have to be used, which are not suitable for fluorescence spectroscopy. Thus, in almost all the cases we are dealing with, the saturation term at the denominator of Equation 11.113 can be neglected and we can write

$$N_2 - N_1 = \frac{(\vartheta - 1)}{\vartheta}\frac{\langle n_p\rangle N}{A_{2,0} + A_{2,1}} \tag{11.114}$$

as a consequence the expression of N_2 can be derived from the approximation $N_0 \approx N$ and from Equation 11.111d as

$$N_2 = \left[\frac{B_2}{(A_{2,0} + D_{1,0})} + \frac{D_{1,0} - A_{2,1}}{A_{2,0} + D_{1,0}}\frac{A_{2,1}}{A_{2,0} + A_{2,1}}\right]\langle n_p\rangle\, N \tag{11.115}$$

Besides the rate equation for the molecule populations we can write the equations for the photon densities as a function of the external source intensity and of the emission and absorption phenomena occurring in the material. Since we have assumed that in any case the population at states 1 and 2 are orders of magnitude smaller than the ground state population, we can set

$$\langle n_p \rangle \approx \frac{I_0}{h \nu_p c_0} \tag{11.116}$$

where I_0 is the intensity of the external light source. Considering the radiation at the fluorescence frequency we can follow the same method adopted to derive Equation 11.103 to obtain

$$A_{21} N_2 - \frac{I_f}{h \nu_f c_0} = B_1 \langle n_f \rangle (N_2 - N_1) \tag{11.117}$$

where I_f is the peak intensity of fluorescence radiation that leaves the sample due to irradiation. Both terms represent the variation rate of the photons at fluorescence frequency, which at the steady state has to be equal to zero. Thus setting to zero the first member of Equation 11.117, using Equations 11.115 and 11.1116 and passing from frequencies to wavelengths we can write

$$I_f = \frac{1}{2} \frac{\lambda_p}{\lambda_f} \xi(\lambda_f, \lambda_p) c_n I_0 \tag{11.118}$$

where the target molecules concentration in c_n moles/m^3 is given by $c_n = N/N_A$ N_A being the Avogadro number. The fluorescence efficiency $\xi(\lambda_f, \lambda_p)$ at given fluorescence and excitation wavelengths is given by

$$\xi(\lambda_f, \lambda_p) = \left(\frac{B_2}{A_{2,0} + D_{1,0}} + \frac{D_{1,0} - A_{2,1}}{A_{2,0} + D_{1,0}} \frac{A_{2,1}}{A_{2,0} + A_{2,1}} \right) N_A \tag{11.119}$$

The fluorescence intensity, in the assumed conditions where saturation is neglected, is proportional both to the target molecule concentration and to the excitation intensity. Moreover, the ratio between the external and fluorescence wavelengths reflects the fact that the fluorescence is composed of less energetic photons with respect to the external source.

Equation 11.118 indicates the fact that quantitative fluorescence detection is a mean to evaluate the concentration of a target molecule in a solution. This is a powerful technique, since the fluorescence wavelength is specific of a radiative transition of the target molecule and it is quite difficult to find molecules having the same fluorescence spectrum. For this reason, fluorescence spectroscopy allows assaying solutions where many different molecules are present.

Moreover, from the analysis we have carried out, it is evident that if several higher energy levels are present, but only a single fluorescent transition, the fluorescence wavelength does not depend on the excitation wavelength. This is an important property allowing accurate assays without a careful control of the excitation wavelength. Unfortunately, this property does not hold if several competing fluorescent levels are present. In this case the excitation wavelength is an important factor in selecting their activation and weight. In this case, the form of the fluorescence linewidth and even the fluorescent wavelength can change by changing the excitation wavelength.

The above discussion is based on a quite simplified model of fluorescence, and several important phenomena are neglected. However, it is suitable for fluorescence analysis in lab on chip conditions.

The first important point that is neglected in the above analysis is the polarization of the emitted fluorescence photons. While in the case of atomic fluorescence the polarization of spontaneously emitted photons is a random process, this is not true in the case of molecules [82,83]. Transitions involving vibrational and rotational levels are not isotropic in space and the polarization statistic of emitted photons is not uniform. This phenomenon is widely exploited in polarization fluorescence spectroscopy [84,85]. In this case, the target molecules are embedded into a solid matrix in such a way to cause a prevalent and stable orientation of their structure. This creates an inhomogeneous distribution of the fluorescence polarization providing several information on the molecular structure. In lab on chip, however, molecules are embedded into a liquid solution, usually a diluted solution, in order to maintain suitable fluid-dynamic properties.

When in a diluted solution molecules are free to rotate and no prevalent orientation is present so that the observed polarization statistic is uniform even for highly asymmetric macromolecules. Neglecting polarization effects in lab on chips using a solution sample is thus generally possible. When a molecule monolayer is constituted the macromolecules are aligned with an ordered and stable orientation, thus in this case polarization effects could be observed. These effects however are not reproduced by our simple model and a much more detailed theory is needed.

A second effect taking place in the presence of concentrated solution of different kinds of molecules is the so-called Förster resonance energy transfer (FRET) [86,87]. FRET is based on the interaction between two nearby molecules provoking different fluorescence emissions immediately after the first molecule is excited by the external light source. The interaction mechanism is shown in Figure 11.54. After absorption of the exciting photons happening in a time of a few attoseconds (1) and nonradiative decay typical of fluorescence (2) the donor molecule transfers the energy that would cause fluorescence to an acceptor molecule with a relaxation time comparable to that of fluorescence, which is in the order of nanoseconds (3). Fluorescence at the expected frequency thus is not observed, instead the acceptor molecule starts another fluorescence process causing fluorescence at a lower frequency (4).

Energy transfer in FRET happens via the exchange of a virtual photon, that is, a photon with a very low lifetime created by the ground-level fluctuations of the electromagnetic field due to the energy–time indetermination principle [1,2,88]. Thus, no external radiation is involved in the process.

Since the virtual photon has a very short lifetime, the process probability is extremely dependent on the molecule distance and decay very fast when this distance increases. In lab on chip the sample solutions have to maintain low viscosity and possible Newtonian behavior to be processed by fluid

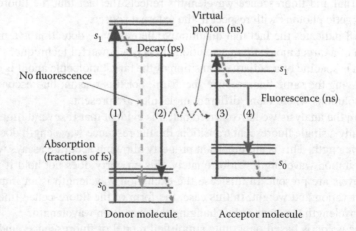

FIGURE 11.54 Schematic energy level diagram for FRET interaction between fluorescent molecules in the same solution.

systems like filters and mixers. This implies that highly concentrated solutions are generally not used, so that FRET is practically not present in lab on chips.

11.3.2.2 Fluorescence Spectroscopy Implementation in Lab on Chip

A main difference between absorption spectroscopy and fluorescence spectroscopy is the possibility of using detection while the target molecules are bonded to a suitably functionalized surface. A macromolecule monolayer is a very thin structure, generally of the order of few nanometers. Such a thin layer generally is not sufficiently dense to provoke sensible absorption in propagating light, even if it is generated in the cladding of a standard integrated waveguide very close to the core. As a matter of fact the tail of the propagating mode of a silica or polymer core waveguide has a decay length of the order of a micron, thus a nanometer layer practically does not influence both attenuation and effective mode index.

The situation is quite different if very small silicon waveguides are fabricated. The high silicon refraction index allows IR single mode waveguides with a width of less than 100 nm to be fabricated if a suitable cladding refraction index is selected. In this case the cladding tail of the mode has a decay length of the order of 10 nm and a monolayer could be visible through attenuation or refraction index. Such waveguides however are very difficult to be fabricated, requiring sub-micron step lithography or electron beam lithography, see Sections 4.5 and 4.6. Typical fluid structures are not easy to be integrated within such small optical waveguides, coupling of light in and out of such chips is very complex and, last but not least, such complex technologies are very expensive unless a very large-scale production in terms of billion pieces is required.

The situation is completely different if we consider fluorescence spectroscopy. Emission at the fluorescence wavelength happens only by the target molecules, thus attaching the molecules to the surface of the detection room via a dense monolayer can be useful to increase their number with respect to a small quantity of diluted solution.

If we consider static detection, without real-time needs, an observation time of 1 s corresponds to an equivalent detection bandwidth of the order of 1 Hz. It can be obtained while eliminating the electronic low-frequency $1/f$ noise by modulating at higher frequency the external light source and then averaging at digital level to reach the wanted observation time. Assuming the parameters of Table 11.4 and repeating the sensitivity evaluation of Section 11.33 we obtain a signal-to-noise ratio of 10^8, corresponding approximately to a fluorescence measurement with an accuracy of one part out of a thousand, with a detected light power of 571 nW at a wavelength of 800 nm that goes down to 222 nW, if we consider a top-performance electronic amplifier instead of a standard one. This is a very high sensitivity, allowing accurate measurements of fluorescence emission by macromolecule monolayers.

For this reason, fluorescence spectroscopy on chip is frequently carried out by suitably functionalizing a surface of the detection room when this does not imply reliability problems [89–91].

A detection setup like those shown in Figure 11.54 can be used for fluorescence spectroscopy. In this case, the fluorescence emission is divided from the exciting light in front of the receiver by a suitable optical filter that is tuned over all the desired bandwidth to obtain the fluorescence spectrum. Since fluorescence is essentially generated by spontaneous emission, it is emitted uniformly in all spatial directions. In this case, the optical detector is located below the lab on chip plane, thus it is able to collect generally less than half the emitted radiation. In particular, if we call Ω_D the acceptance solid angle at the input of the optical system in front of the detector the detected intensity has to be multiplied by $\Omega_D/4\pi$ Moreover, it is to take into account that the excitation light intensity I_0 reported in Equation 11.118 is the intensity of the light effectively interacting with the sample in the lab on chip. In whatever arrangement it is a fraction of the light emitted by the exciting light source. This fraction depends both on the acceptance angle of the optical system focusing the light beam on the chip detection chamber window and on the various attenuation and scattering terms. Calling A_E the effective fraction of the emitted light interacting with the sample and I_E the intensity emitted by the external light source and I_D the detected fluorescence intensity, Equation 11.118 can be rewritten in the one considered and in similar cases as

$$I_D = \frac{1}{2} \frac{\lambda_p}{\lambda_f} \xi c_n \frac{\Omega_D}{4\pi} A_E I_E = \xi_M c_n I_E \qquad (11.120)$$

where the macroscopic measure efficiency ξ_M has been introduced, which is the main calibration parameter of the fluorescence spectrometer.

The measurement scheme of Figure 11.54 can be integrated onto a chip by using a combination of monolithic and hybrid integration. A possible scheme of such a devise is presented in Figure 11.55 [92]. The first fabrication step is to build a photodiode into the silicon substrate by standard fabrication processes. To obtain the photodiode active junction-doped silicon has to be used, thus sequential fabrication steps have to be designed in such a way not to destroy the photodiode junction. This is a critical aspect of the fabrication process since it means avoiding high-temperature processes, for example, when performing wafer bonding to close the upper microfluidic circuit terminating with the detection room.

Alternatively, the circuit can be constructed on a glass or silicon wafer without fabricating the photodiode. After ending the circuit fabrication the wafer is thinned and a similar wafer containing all the photodiodes is bonded on the back. This technique allows more freedom in designing the fabrication processes, but requires a complex wafer alignment for photodiodes mounting and could have problems due to the mechanical stability versus temperature changes and stresses of the resulting three-bonded wafer structures.

On top of the photodiode a multilayer filter is fabricated in order to reflect the exciting wavelength and to transmit the fluorescence wavelength [93]. The filter can be realized either with several silica layers with different refraction indexes caused by different doping or by layers of different materials. In any case the multiplayer filter exploits the combination of multiple reflection taking place at each interface between different materials to cause constructive interference at the filter output at the transmitted wavelength and destructive interference at the filtered wavelength. Several variations of this basic design have been proposed to obtain either tunable or more efficient filters [94,95]; moreover, such filters can be fabricated also with polymeric layers [96] in the case in which a polymeric substrate is used and the photodiodes are added only at the end of the process by wafer bonding.

On top of the multilayer filter a thin CVD oxide layer is deposited where the microfluidic circuit terminating with the detection chamber is fabricated. The detection chamber floor can be functionalized before wafer bonding in order to create a monolayer of the target molecules if needed. The microfluidic circuit is close by bonding either a glass wafer or a suitable polymer substrate. The

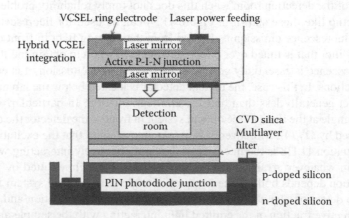

FIGURE 11.55 Vertical section of the on-chip fluorescence spectrometer based on monolithic integration of a photodiode, filtering by a multilayer filter and hybrid integration of a VCSEL.

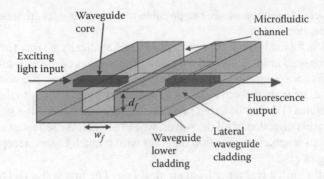

FIGURE 11.56 Example of a possible scheme of fluorescence spectrometer on chip where light is managed through optical waveguides.

closing substrate is micromachined after bonding and thinning to create the structure for the hybrid integration of a VCSEL laser [97] (see Section 6.3.1) that is meant to provide the excitation beam (see Section 6.3.1). Specific design of photodiodes and VCSEL lasers for this application have been considered [98] and this kind of integrated fluorescence detection system is a powerful tool for on-chip assays.

An alternative way of bringing exciting light to the sample and collect the fluorescence is by an optical waveguide, that is, horizontally on the chip plane instead of vertically to it. An example of a possible scheme is reported in Figure 11.56 [99,100], where only the microfluidic channels where the sample either is still during measures or continuously flowing and the waveguides are shown. The optical source and the detection photodiodes can be either added by hybrid integration after front-end fabrication or maintained external to the chip, in the equipment hosting the chip itself. The last solution is particularly suitable when the chip is meant to be disposable, so that more expensive components have to be maintained outside.

Advantages of the scheme of Figure 11.56 are the possibility of realizing it completely using polymers, especially if hybrid integration of optically active components is not needed, and the simpler fabrication process. Disadvantages reside in the greater difficulty in hybrid integration of active components due to the need of edge-emitting lasers and edge-sensitive photodiodes and the fact that, in the absence of hybrid integration, coupling between the inner waveguides and external source and detector is needed.

Moreover, the measurement efficiency is necessarily lower in this scheme, due to the fact that only the fluorescence light coupled with the propagating mode of the output waveguide is transmitted up to the receiver. Different systems can be used to alleviate this problem. The captured fluorescence is greatly increased by terminating the output waveguide with a suitable taper near the detection room. A taper, whose scheme is represented in Figure 11.57 [101,102], is a structure

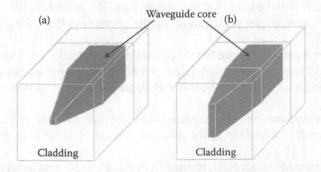

FIGURE 11.57 Type of integrated waveguide tapers: 3D taper (a) and 2D taper (b).

that reduces the waveguide section as near as possible to a point in a length much greater than the waveguide original section width.

If the tapering is sufficiently slow the optical mode adiabatically adapts to the section change and small excess propagation losses are added due to the section change. In an ideal taper, when the propagating optical wave arrives to the terminal point it behaves as the power emitted from a point source, thus it exits from the waveguide as a spherical wave. Owing to the reciprocal nature of the Maxwell equations [11], that is, to the fact that they are still valid if the sign of time changes, inverting the propagation direction of all the waves, when the taper is used as an antenna to intercept outside radiation, it has a spherical radiation diagram with a much higher acceptance with respect to the original waveguide.

Two elements distinguish a real taper from an ideal one. The first is the fact that the taper is not immersed into the material where the wave is propagating, but it is surrounded by the material constituting the core of the original waveguide. This fact, causing light reflection, decreases greatly the acceptance. Thus, some sort of refraction index adaptation has to be performed between the solution in the detection chamber and the waveguide cladding. This is not so difficult since water refraction index in the near IR and visible spectrum is about 1.33 and the presence of ions tends to increase the index further nearing it to the index of glass and many polymers in the same range. The adaptation can be performed adding to the sample a passive refraction index adaptation component [103]. Alternative to index adaptation a micromachining exposing the very point of the taper directly into the sample solution naturally solve the problem, creating an optical antenna directly in the solution.

Moreover, even if three-dimensional tapers like that shown in Figure 11.57a can be built, the fabrication process is complex, requiring 3D micromachining of the waveguide core. For this reason much more frequently two-dimensional tapers are realized, as those presented in Figure 11.57b. In this case the fact that the waveguide depth does not decrease along the taper width creates a further acceptance reduction. In any case, a tapered waveguide behaves much better than a simple waveguide interrupted in correspondence of a specific section.

Another alternative is to mix the designs of Figures 11.55 and 11.56 using a planar waveguide to couple the external source light to the detection room and an integrated photo-detector that extends all over the chip to detect fluorescence [104]. As an alternative to photodiodes or photodiodes arrays, CCD [105] can be used if fluorescence is to be observed in other spectral ranges.

Fluorescence polarization spectroscopy [106,107] can be applied in a lab on chip environment only if an ordered and stable molecule configuration is attained. This can be done by blocking the target molecules on a functionalized surface. In this case polarization anisotropy is observed in the emitted fluorescence giving information on the internal structure of the molecule.

The first step to perform fluorescence spectroscopy is to use polarized light as excitation, with the possibility of changing the light polarization. In principle, this can be performed using a laser source associated with a polarizer and an attenuator. The laser source produces a perfectly polarized light, generally a linearly polarized light parallel to some axis of the laser cavity. For example in edge-emitting semiconductor lasers the emitted light is polarized along the plane of the laser active waveguide and perpendicular to the waveguide axes. The polarizer allows the light polarization to be converted into whatever polarization and the attenuator allows the light amplitude to be accurately controlled.

At the receiver the fluorescence light has to be examined in polarization. This can be done either by using another polarizer to analyze the output polarization or splitting the output light with a beam splitter and using a half-wavelength plate to evaluate the intensity of two orthogonal polarization components.

These optical arrangements are easily implemented using micro-optics, so that polarization fluorescence spectroscopy can be realized by the scheme in Figure 11.44 by an extension of the macroscopic setup [108].

An interesting integrated arrangement, starting from this idea and from hybrid integration of light sources and detectors on top and bottom of the microfluidic chip is shown in Figure 11.58 [109].

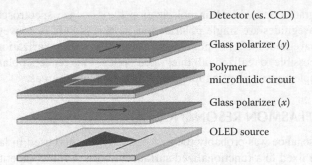

Detector (es. CCD)

Glass polarizer (*y*)

Polymer
microfluidic circuit

Glass polarizer (*x*)

OLED source

FIGURE 11.58   Principal scheme of a hybrid integrated on-chip polarization fluorescence spectrometer.

The chip is obtained by bonding five different wafers. The central wafer, realized either in a compatible polymer-like PDMS and PMMA or on a glass substrate, is thinned and bonded on the upper and lower faces with two glass substrates. The glass substrates are treated so as to filter orthogonal linear polarizations. This allows the exciting light component to be eliminated before reaching the detector.

On top of the obtained wafer the detector is integrated by bonding or hybrid integration. It can be a CCD or a photodiodes array, depending on the wavelength that has to be observed. The source is integrated at the bottom of the system. Organic light-emitting diodes (OLED) [110,111] seem to be particularly suitable for this use, due to their ability to emit many wavelengths in the visible and near-IR range and for their structure. The structure of an OLED is schematically shown in Figure 11.59. The active layer is constituted by an organic semiconductor substance, either a solid constituted by small molecules or a suitable polymer. It is excited by means of an electrical current injected through a metallic electrode on one hand and an ITO electrode on the other, so as to maintain a side of the device transparent. On the ITO side, the anode is insulated by means of a transparent protection layer, either glass or a polymer like PMMA. Bonding this protection layer to the glass polarizer on the bottom of the device is a simple operation and assures an effective integrated source for polarization fluorescence spectroscopy. The availability of several wavelengths is realized by creating a matrix of OLEDs that alternates OLEDs at different wavelengths that can be activated separately.The device is compatible with use of low-cost materials and mass industrial production if the stresses that accumulate at the interface of the bonded layers are kept under control.

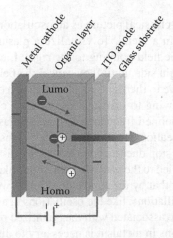

Metal cathode

Organic layer

ITO anode

Glass substrate

Lumo

Homo

FIGURE 11.59   Principal scheme of a single-cell organic light-emitting diode (OLED).

The use of integrated optics for this polarization fluorescence spectroscopy is instead quite difficult. Optical waveguides are single polarization, so that if light is conveyed to the sample or extracted through waveguides it is not possible to change the light polarization; in addition, polarizers are almost impossible to realize with integrated optics. This renders polarization fluorescence not suitable to be implemented adopting integrated detectors and sources.

11.4 SURFACE PLASMON RESONANCE

Surface plasmon resonance was probably the first detection method used in lab on chip where the target molecules are fixed to a functionalized surface and it is still a competitive technique, especially in lab on chip meant for use in a laboratory environment.

Plasmons are essentially collective oscillations of the population of free electrons that is present in a metal. They can couple with electromagnetic waves near a metal dielectric surface to obtain light waves propagating in strong vicinity to the surface itself. The observation of such electromagnetic waves, probing the surface properties, is a powerful method not only in surface analysis, but also to detect the characteristics of molecular monolayer that forms over a suitably activated surface.

11.4.1 Plasmons: Definition and Properties

A first step to discuss plasmon-based detection in labs on chip is to introduce under a physical point of view plasma resonances in conductors and understand their properties and the way in which they can be excited and observed.

11.4.1.1 Bulk Plasmons

The base for the description of bulk plasmons in metals is the crystal band theory [112,113]. The metal bonds are created by the fact that metal atoms share electrons on macroscopic distances, ideally over all the space occupied by the crystal. These electrons move through the electrical potential created by the metal ions fixed at the crystal nodes following the quantum mechanical rules.

The result of a quantum mechanical analysis of the electrons motion is that in many phenomena involving electrons, like conductivity and specific heat, the electron–electron interaction can be neglected. Under this approximation, the relation between energy and momentum is regulated in many practical cases by an almost parabolic rule, but for the fact that the electron mass has to be corrected by a factor taking into account the fact that they move in the crystal. The corrected mass is generally called electron effective mass. Thus, allowing the electron mass to have a corrected value, a sort of perfect electron gas exists in the crystal somehow similar to the free electron gas embedded into a plasma.

Plasmons can be described in a classical picture as an oscillation of the free electron density with respect to the fixed positive ions in a metal. To visualize a plasma oscillation, imagine a cube of metal placed in an external electric field pointing to the right. Electrons will move to the left side, uncovering positive ions on the right side, until they cancel the field inside the metal. If the electric field is removed, the electrons move to the right, repelled by each other and attracted to the positive ions left bare on the right side. Owing to inertia of electrons, a collective oscillation is started in the electron population at a well-defined frequency, called the plasma frequency. Owing to various dissipative phenomena like heat creation due to collisions with ions or electromagnetic energy emission, this oscillation is dumped to stop due to complete energy dissipation.

Second quantization can be applied to the plasmon field, much like we have sketched for the electromagnetic field, taking into account that by the simple description we have provided plasmons are not traveling waves, but stationary oscillations, like the oscillations in a resonant cavity. By second quantization a particle population can be associated with the quantized plasmaoscillation called plasmons.

In analyzing plasmon oscillations in metals it is necessary to distinguish two possible situations: the so-called cold and hot electron cases. In the first case, plasma oscillations have an energy much greater than the thermal energy of electrons so that thermal motion can be neglected. In the second case, the thermal energy is comparable to the plasmon energy and thermal motion has to be taken into account. The cold electrons approximation is generally valid for metals in standard conditions, even if hot electrons have a role in a few observed phenomena [114].

In the cold electrons approximation, and assuming an infinite crystal and infinite ions mass, it is possible to demonstrate that plasmon oscillations have a resonance at the so-called plasmon frequency f_{pl}, which is given by

$$f_{pl} = \frac{1}{2\pi} \sqrt{\frac{\rho_e \, q^2}{m^* \varepsilon_0}} \qquad (11.121)$$

where m^* is the electrons effective mass, q is the electron charge, and ρ_e is the electron density. If we substitute the effective mass with the free electron mass we can derive an order of magnitude of the plasmon resonance frequency, which is $f_{pl} \approx 8.98 \sqrt{\rho_e}$ The order of magnitude of the electron density in metals is 5×10^{28} m^{-3}, thus we obtain $f_{pl} \approx 10^{15}$ Hz. An electromagnetic wave with this frequency in void has a wavelength in the UV range. A summary of electron density, electron effective mass, and plasma resonance frequency for selected metals is provided in Table 11.8.

Plasmons play a great role in the optical properties of metals. Light of frequency below the plasma frequency is reflected by the metal surface, because the electrons in the metal screen the electric field of the light. Light of frequency above the plasma frequency is transmitted, because the electrons cannot respond fast enough to screen it. Some metals, such as copper and gold, have electronic transitions between different electronic bands with energy in the visible range, whereby specific light energies are absorbed, yielding their distinct color.

11.4.1.2 Surface Plasmons

Like bulk plasmons, surface plasmons are coherent electron oscillations: in this case the oscillations generate at the interface between a conductor and a dielectric, for example, at the surface between air and a metal. Surface plasmons have lower energy than bulk plasmons, due to their nature of surface waves.

Like bulk plasmons, surface plasmons can couple with photons, creating the so-called polariton, called in this case, surface polaritons. Polaritons represent in a quantum quasi-particle model the interaction between the electromagnetic field and the electron gas.

As a matter of fact the presence of the electromagnetic field creates a collective excitation of the electron population that exists only in the presence of an electromagnetic field. On the other hand, the electron population density fluctuations generate emission of electromagnetic waves, thus influencing the external electrical field. Thus, the light wave and the electron gas perturbation are correlated

TABLE 11.8

Electron Density, Relative Effective Electron Mass, and Plasma Frequency for Selected Metals at Standard Conditions

	ρ_e m^{-3} ($\times 10^{28}$)	m^*/m_e	f_{pl} Hz ($\times 10^{15}$)
Li	4.70	2.18	1.31
Na	2.65	1.26	1.30
Cu	8.45	1.38	2.22
Au	5.90	1.14	2.04
Al	18.06	1.15	3.56
Pb	13.20	2.10	2.25

Note: The free electron mass is indicated with m_e

and depend on one another. By applying the second quantization process to the wave-like interaction between them, polaritons are obtained. Polaritons are bonded surface electromagnetic and electron waves that propagate on the separation surface between the two media up to the moment when their energy is dissipated in heat production and in the emission of electromagnetic waves.

For our purposes we will describe surface plasmons adopting a classical approach, where surface electromagnetic waves are coupled with nonpropagating surface electron oscillations. To approach such a theory we have to search the conditions required for a classical electromagnetic surface wave at the interface between a conductor and a dielectric medium to propagate [115–118].

Surface electromagnetic waves are obtained if the electromagnetic wave vector is parallel to the surface, that is, to the x-axis in the reference geometry of Figure 11.60, and has the main part of the electromagnetic energy concentrated near the surface. Moreover, the fields have to vanish far from the interface. Since we have to cope with a conductor, where free charges exist, the wave equation for the electrical field writes similar to Equation 11.31. In this case, however, approximation (11.33) is not generally feasible, thus it is more effective to work in terms of complex dielectric constant than in terms of refraction index.

In terms of complex dielectric constant, the wave equation writes in the same way both in the dielectric medium and in the conducting medium as

$$\nabla^2 \mathbf{E} - \varepsilon_0 \varepsilon_j(\omega) \frac{\partial \mathbf{E}}{\partial t} = 0 \quad (j = 1,2) \tag{11.122}$$

where index 1 indicates the conductor and 2 the dielectric material. This equation has to be solved with the electromagnetic boundary conditions [11] that can be written as

$$\boldsymbol{\tau} \times (\mathbf{E}_2 - \mathbf{E}_1) = 0 \tag{11.123a}$$

$$\boldsymbol{\tau} \cdot (\mathbf{D}_2 - \mathbf{D}_1) = \rho_s \tag{11.123b}$$

Where τ is the unit vector normal to the surface as in Figure 11.60. The first condition requires the continuity of the electrical field component tangent to the surface, that is, the x component, while the second condition requires continuity of the vertical components of the electrical displacement vector. The tangential component of the electrical displacement has instead a discontinuity that equals the surface charge density induced by the field. This surface density, due to the oscillations of the electromagnetic field, also oscillates along the z direction and it is to expect that if the oscillation of electrons is strongly dumped, it dissipates all the electromagnetic energy preventing the electromagnetic wave propagation, while if it can propagate it allows propagation of the surface electromagnetic wave.

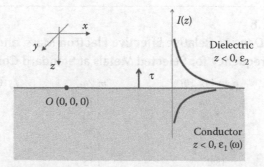

FIGURE 11.60 Reference geometry for electromagnetic surface wave analysis. The unit vector normal to the interface τ and the intensity $I(z)$ of the electromagnetic surface wave are evidenced.

Before facing the solution of the wave equation in the case of surface electromagnetic waves, the very general expression of the complex dielectric constants of the two media can be simplified in case we consider high-frequency waves, essentially in the visible or in the UV range.

In case of the dielectric material, the dielectric constant is purely real and positive, and its wavelength dependence can be neglected if the wave frequency range is suitably restricted. In the case of the conducting material, the dielectric constant can be written as [112,113]

$$\varepsilon_1(\omega) = \varepsilon_{r1}(\omega) + i\frac{\sigma(\omega)}{\varepsilon_0\omega} \tag{11.124}$$

In principle, both $\varepsilon_{r1}(\omega)$ and the conductivity $\sigma(\omega)$ are complex numbers; thus, the imaginary part of $\varepsilon_{r1}(\omega)$ and the real part of $\sigma(\omega)$ contribute to the imaginary part of $\varepsilon_1(\omega)$ being important in phenomena such as dissipation, absorption, and dispersion. On the other hand, the real part of $\varepsilon_{r1}(\omega)$ plus the imaginary part of $\sigma(\omega)$ contribute to the real part of $\varepsilon_1(\omega)$ determining, for example, the index of refraction and the electromagnetic phase velocity.

The situation simplifies if we consider frequencies much higher than the electrons mean collision time.These frequencies correspond typically to the visible light and ultra violet ranges for normal metals. If we consider the fact that the dielectric characteristics of the metal, that is, $\varepsilon_{r1}(\omega)$, mainly depends on the electronic clouds of the ions at crystal nodes, at visible light frequencies these bounded electrons have too high inertia to follow the field oscillation, so that we can assume $\varepsilon_{r1}(\omega) \approx 1$ Conduction electrons on the contrary determine the conductivity. Owing to the high electromagnetic frequency, conduction electrons do not form a net current in the conductor, but oscillate rapidly around the random motion due to thermal energy. These oscillations are represented by a purely imaginary conductivity.

The net result is that the complex dielectric constant results to be purely real, and with the following form:

$$\varepsilon_1(\omega) = 1 - \frac{\sigma_0}{\varepsilon_0\omega^2\tau} - 1 - \left(\frac{2\pi f_{pl}}{\omega}\right)^2 \tag{11.125}$$

the expression where the plasma frequency is evaluated using a pure free electron theory, the so-called Drude [112,113] theory, and replacing the electron mass with its effective mass in the considered crystal.

Let us now insert in the wave equation a test solution representing a single frequency surface wave, propagating along the x-axis and vanishing exponentially for $z \rightarrow \pm\infty$. This means to select a target solution of the form

$$\boldsymbol{E}_j = E_0\,\boldsymbol{p}_j(\omega)e^{i(kx-\omega t)}\,e^{-\alpha_j(\omega)|z|} \tag{11.126}$$

Where $\boldsymbol{p}(\omega)$ is the polarization vector that, in principle, can depend on the wave frequency and, as usual, the physical form of the electromagnetic field is obtained by the real part of Equation 11.126. Substituting into the wave equation and imposing the conditions at the interface we get

$$p_{j,x}(\omega) = 1 \tag{11.127a}$$

$$p_{j,y}(\omega) = 0 \tag{11.127b}$$

$$p_{j,z}(\omega) = \frac{ik}{\sqrt{(k^2 - \varepsilon_j(\omega^2/c_0^2))}} \tag{11.127c}$$

$$\alpha_j(\omega) = \sqrt{\left(k^2 - \varepsilon_j \frac{\omega^2}{c_0^2}\right)} > 0 \tag{11.127d}$$

Moreover, the continuity of the tangential component of the electrical field generates the additional constrain

$$-\varepsilon_2 \sqrt{\left(k^2 - \varepsilon_1(\omega) \frac{\omega^2}{c_0^2}\right)} = \varepsilon_1(\omega) \sqrt{\left(k^2 - \varepsilon_2 \frac{\omega^2}{c_0^2}\right)} \tag{11.128}$$

This condition can be fulfilled only if $\varepsilon_1(\omega) < 0$.

A last set of constrain can be obtained by the boundary conditions on the magnetic fields that writes [11]

$$\boldsymbol{\tau} \times (\boldsymbol{H}_2 - \boldsymbol{H}_1) = \boldsymbol{J}_s \tag{11.129a}$$

$$\boldsymbol{\tau} \cdot (\boldsymbol{B}_2 - \boldsymbol{B}_1) = 0 \tag{11.129b}$$

where $\boldsymbol{J}_s$ is the current per unit area at the interface. In our case, due to the hypothesis of high electromagnetic frequencies, no net current density is generated at the interface, thus the tangential component of the magnetic field is continuous at the interface. The magnetic field corresponding to the surface wave can be evaluated by the Maxwell equation (11.1d) once the electrical field is known and the currents are set to zero.

Imposing the boundary condition (11.129d) we get

$$\frac{\alpha_1(\omega)}{\varepsilon_1(\omega)} = \frac{\alpha_2(\omega)}{\varepsilon_2} \tag{11.130}$$

Since all the other boundary conditions are not explicitly considered to be automatically satisfied once we have imposed the constrains (11.127d), (11.128), and (11.130) we have all the elements that are needed to evaluate the dispersion relation of the electromagnetic surface wave.

As already done in Equation 11.33 we can introduce the complex wave vector that, taking into account the vector direction and the magnetic coefficient, is defined as $\boldsymbol{k}_c = \sqrt{\varepsilon_r \mu_r} \boldsymbol{k} = n_c \boldsymbol{k}$ where the complex refraction index is defined in Equation 11.27. Thus the complex wave vector squared module writes

$$\left| \boldsymbol{k}_c \right|^2 = n_c^2(\omega) \frac{\omega^2}{c_0^2} = \varepsilon_r \mu_r \frac{\omega^2}{c_0^2} \tag{11.131}$$

This is a completely general equation for electromagnetic wave propagation in homogeneous and isotropic materials. Applying this equation to our case gives

$$k^2 + \alpha_2^2 = \varepsilon_2 \frac{\omega^2}{c_0^2} \tag{11.132a}$$

$$k^2 + \alpha_1^2 = \varepsilon_1(\omega) \frac{\omega^2}{c_0^2} \tag{11.132b}$$

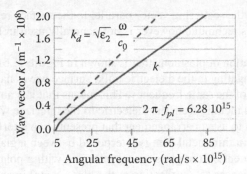

FIGURE 11.61 Dispersion relation for surface plasmons compared with the ideal dispersion relation in the dielectric medium.

Eliminating α_2 through relation (11.130) and solving for k and α_1 we obtain

$$k^2 = \frac{\omega^2}{c_0^2} \frac{\varepsilon_2\varepsilon_1(\omega)}{\varepsilon_2 + \varepsilon_1(\omega)} \tag{11.133}$$

This is the dispersion relation of the electromagnetic surface wave. Since $\varepsilon_1(\omega) < 0$ in order to have a real value of k, assuring a propagating surface wave, from Equation 11.133 we get $|\varepsilon_1(\omega)| > \varepsilon_2$. Combining the fact that $\varepsilon_1(\omega)$ has to be negative with the condition $|\varepsilon_1(\omega)| > \varepsilon_2$ and with Equation 11.125 we get

$$2\pi f_{pl} < \omega < \frac{2\pi f_{pl}}{\sqrt{\varepsilon_2 - 1}} \tag{11.134}$$

We obtain in this way the important results that surface electromagnetic wavelength can propagate at the interface between a conductor and an insulator only if the frequency of the wave is in a well-defined interval around the plasma resonance wavelength. This behavior can be physically interpreted considering the fact that the propagating wave excites a transversal surface plasma oscillation due to the presence of the electrical field immediately below the conductor interface. This oscillation does not propagate, as it is demonstrated by the fact that no electron-related wave vector appears in the dispersion relation. To allow propagation of the electromagnetic wave, the plasma oscillation must not be dumped by the inertia of the electron gas. We know that this happens only in the immediate vicinity of the plasma frequency, thus it is to expect that the surface wave propagates only in proximity of the plasma frequency.

A plot of the dispersion relation of Equation 11.133 where expression (11.125) and the approximation $\varepsilon_2 \approx 1$ are adopted is reported in Figure 11.61.

Another important characteristic of surface waves is their exponential decay with the distance from the conducting surface in the dielectric material. The decay rate can be directly deduced from Equation 11.127d. Substituting data relative to silver and glass, for example, we obtain a typical decay length of 24 nm at $\lambda_0 = 600$ nm. As expected surface waves are localized in a very small layer on top of the conductor surface, thus they are suitable for the investigation of surface-related phenomena, in lab on chip mainly molecular monolayers, which are localized in layers of thickness of few nanometers or less.

11.4.1.3 Surface Plasmon Excitation

Surface plasmons can be excited by both electrons and photons. Excitation by electrons is created by firing electrons into the bulk of a metal. As the electrons scatter, energy is transferred into the bulk plasma. The component of the scattering vector parallel to the surface results in the formation of a surface plasmon [116]. This technique however is not generally used in lab on chip, where optical excitation is adopted.

Since the dispersion relation of plasmons that is shown in Figure 11.61 lies below the dispersion characteristic of light propagating in the dielectric bulk, surface waves have longer wavelength with respect to bulk light waves of the same frequency. This means that it is not possible to excite surface wave simply by bulk waves inciting from the dielectric to the interface with the conductor.

A first possible means is to use an arrangement that presents two interfaces, as shown, for example, in Figure 11.62, where a thin metal film is interposed between a glass substrate and air. If we consider a plane wave incident on the glass–metal interface with a polarization that is parallel to the incident plane, it experiences total reflection at the glass–metal interface while a surface wave can form on the other interface, at the metal–air interface, due to coupling with the evanescent wave. This is the wave that forms in the low refractive index medium, metal in this case, when total reflection takes place at the interface.The purely imaginary wave vector of the evanescent wave is directed orthogonally to the surface so that it is attenuates exponentially in the metal [11].

However, if the electrical field of the evanescent wave is not yet zero on the second dielectric–metal interface there is the possibility that this excitation will create a surface plasma wave on the other interface. This happens when the evanescent wave dispersion relation and the plasma wave vectors are matched and the polarization of the evanescent wave field matches the polarization of the plasma wave field.

The second condition is fulfilled if the electrical field of the wave incident on the metal film is linear and parallel to the plane of incidence. The second condition writes, taken into account expression (11.133) of the plasma wave and of the wave vector of the evanescent wave (see Figure 11.62) as

$$\frac{\omega}{c_0}\sqrt{\frac{\varepsilon_1(\omega)}{1+\varepsilon_1(\omega)}} = \frac{\omega}{c_0}\frac{1}{\sqrt{\varepsilon_2}\sin\theta_0} \qquad (11.135)$$

where the dielectric constant of air is assumed, with a very good approximation, equal to 1. This relation can be satisfied due to the fact that the air dielectric constant is smaller than that of glass for a particular value of the incidence angle, that is, the incidence angle causing excitation of plasma waves on the metal air surface.

Owing to the need for creating a coupling between a surface wave on the opposite interface and the evanescent wave in the metal, the metal film has to be very thin, of the order of tens of nanometers, but similar films can be deposited with several different deposition technologies, as shown in Chapter 4.

In practice, this principle is implemented by using a prism for the coupling of the volume light wave with the dielectric metal interface. The prism can be positioned against a thin metal film, to reproduce exactly the configuration discussed above, in the so-called Kretschmann configuration,

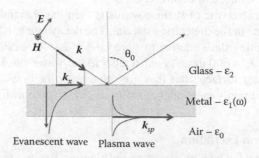

FIGURE 11.62 Basic arrangement for surface plasma wave generation by a double metal–dielectric interface.

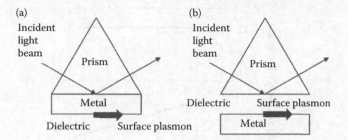

FIGURE 11.63 Coupling of light photons with surface plasmons via a prism: Kretschmann configuration (a) and Otto configuration (b).

or very close to a metal surface, in the Otto configuration, as shown in Figure 11.63. In this second case, total reflection occurs at the glass–air interface and the evanescent wave decay exponentially in the thin air layer between the glass interface and the metal surface. The coupling condition can be deduced with the same method adopted for the first configuration, but it is the air layer that has to be very thin, while the metal surface can be the surface of a bulk crystal.

In both cases a correct choice of the incident angle and of the polarization of the incident wave creates excitation of surface plasmons at the air–metal interface. The creation of surface plasmons implies transfer of electromagnetic energy from the incident wave to the surface plasmon, so that it can be detected by observing a decrease in the energy reflected by the metal surface inside. Optimum excitation is performed theoretically when all the incident energy is coupled with the surface wave and no reflection is observed through the prism. Once the metal characteristics are given, the optimum coupling condition depends both on the incident angle and on the thickness of the metal film. Optimum thickness and incidence angle can be evaluated by solving the Maxwell equations in the glass–metal–air system so as to obtain the fields and maximizing the surface wave power.

An example of the behavior of reflectivity in optical surface plasmon excitation through a prism in Kretschmann configuration is reported in Figure 11.64 versus the coupling angle and for different film thickness at a wavelength of 546 nm. The real and imaginary parts of the relative dielectric constant of silver are shown versus the film thickness at the considered frequency in Figure 11.65. In the Maxwell equations solution has been taken into account that in order to obtain accurate quantitative results the dependence of the relative dielectric constant on the film thickness has to be considered [119,120]. Moreover, a more complex model of the dielectric constant has to be used with respect to that provided by Equation 11.125 that also takes into account the small imaginary part of the dielectric constant of the metal [112,113]. However, the good approximation of Equation 11.124

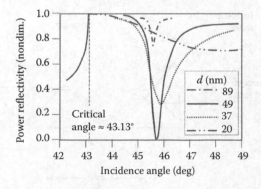

FIGURE 11.64 Behavior of power reflectivity of the metal surface in surface plasmon excitation through a prism in Kretschmann configuration. The considered metal is silver and the metal film thickness is indicated by d.

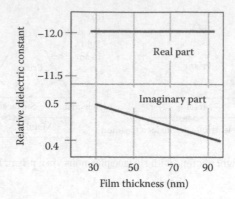

FIGURE 11.65 Dielectric constant of a silver thin film versus the film thickness at standard conditions.

is confirmed by the fact that the ratio between the imaginary and the real part of the dielectric constant is in any case smaller than 4%.

Instead of having two different surfaces and exploiting the evanescent wave to couple the incident wave to the surface wave, a grating can be adopted to match the incident bulk wave with the plasma wave by remaining on the same metal surface. The scheme of this coupling mechanism is reported in Figure 11.66.

The theory of surface plasmon excitation via a grating is based on the Bloch theorem [112,113], a very general theorem dealing with wave interaction with a periodic refractive index or, which is the same in quantum mechanics, particle wave–functions interaction with a periodic potential. If we apply the Bloch theorem to our case, a Bragg grating can be viewed as a one-dimensional periodic index variation.

In this case, the Bloch theorem simply states that surface electromagnetic waves can be coupled whenever their wave vectors k_1 and k_2, both directed in the same direction along the grating axis, are in the following relation:

$$k_1 = k_2 + \frac{2\pi}{L} j \qquad (11.136)$$

where L is the grating period and j is whatever integer number. This relation is indeed quite intuitive since it states that the periodicity of the grating can compensate mismatch between the wave vectors

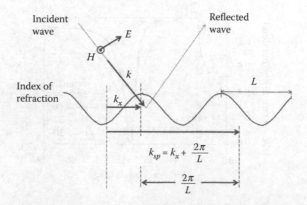

FIGURE 11.66 Surface plasma wave excitation through a bulk light wave and a grating for wave vector adaptation.

by the mechanism of reflections that is typical of the grating. In particular, one wave can be coupled with the other directly (with $j = 0$), through one reflection at the grating nodes (with $j = 1$), through two reflections, and so on. Since reflections occur due to index variations with a period equal to L, only a mismatch that is a multiple of $1/L$ can be compensated.

Since the impossibility of directly exciting a surface plasma wave at a conductor surface by an incident light wave depends on the mismatch between the components of the wave vector parallel to the surface of the incident wave and of the plasma wave, a grating with a suitable period can be used to match these two different vectors.

11.4.2 Surface Plasmon Immunoassay Detection

The most direct way of using plasma surface resonance to detect antigen–antibody binding is represented in Figure 11.67 [121–123]. Different assay protocols can be used exploiting surface plasmon resonance.

In a dynamic assay protocol the target solution continuously flow through the assay chamber. Let us assume that the lab on chip is fabricated out of a transparent material such as glass or a polymer like PMMA or PDMS. The assay reaction of the lab on chip is metallized with a gold film on the bottom. The gold film is activated via thiols (see Section 11.21) binding the specific antibody that has to react with the target molecule. A semispherical prism with the same refraction index of the lab on chip material is fixed to the bottom of the lab on chip and the system is used to excite surface plasmon on the functionalized gold surface.

Then a reference system characterization via the determination of the reflectivity at different incident angles is carried out. During the assay the angle at which maximum coupling is observed is tracked while the target solution first and the solute then flows through the assay chamber. The qualitative behavior of the observed reflectivity versus time is shown in Figure 11.68.

Different zones are evident in the plot of Figure 11.68, corresponding to different phases in the assay. At the beginning, the angle is at its baseline value, corresponding to no-binding target molecule. While target molecules flow through the reaction chamber they bind to the antibodies and the maximum coupling angle changes to reach a stationary value corresponding to the equilibrium percentage of binding antibodies. After the end of the target solution, the simple solvent is flown through the chamber. In correspondence to the solvent, target molecules starts to detach from the surface to reach eventually the situation in which no antibody binds a target molecule. At this point, after a transitory period, the angle returns equal to the baseline.

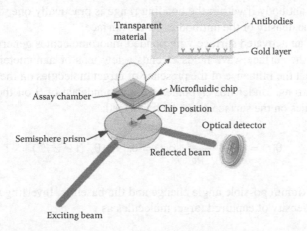

FIGURE 11.67 Surface plasma resonance exploitation for the monitoring of an immunoassay. Surface plasmons are excited with a semispherical prism in Kretschmann configuration.

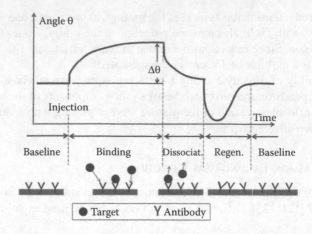

FIGURE 11.68 Reflectivity versus time in an immunoassay detected using flow surface plasmon resonance.

Immediately after the injection of the target solution the angle changes due to the binding of target molecules to antibodies, while the surface is saturated with target molecules more evidently and the angle changes to a stationary value. When the solute starts to flow, the target molecules start to detach from the surface to reach equilibrium between the bonded and the solute phase. Owing to the fact that the solution is continuously renewed with the new solvent the equilibrium is never reached and eventually all the target molecules leave the surface. At this point, the functionalized surface has to undergo a transition period to regain its equilibrium ordered structure: after this time the angle returns to its baseline value.

If we consider the probability that a target molecule will bind to a free antibody when it arrives near the antibody location constant in time, that is, independent of the surface saturation status and of the test solution concentration, it is not difficult to demonstrate that the increase in the number of bonded target molecules follows an exponential rule that can be written as

$$\rho(t) = \rho_0(1 - e^{-t/\tau}) \tag{11.137}$$

where ρ_0 is the saturation density and τ is the saturation characteristic time. Both the parameters can be experimentally determined on the ground of the characteristics of the fabricated system and used for assay calibration. In particular, in almost all practical cases, the probability that a target molecule binds to an antibody if within the bonding range is practically one, thus the density ρ_0 is simply provided by the density of the antibodies on the surface.

Since the depth of an activated surface with bonded macromolecules generally does not exceed few nanometers and the surface wave fields extends a few tens of nanometers into the dielectric layer, it is to expect that the influence of the presence of target molecules on the maximum coupling angle θ will not be strong. Under this hypothesis the dependence of θ on the average density of bonded target molecules on the surface ρ can be linearized:

$$\theta(t) = \theta_0 + \left(\frac{\Delta\theta_M}{\rho_0}\right)\rho(t) = \theta_0 + \Delta\theta_M(1 - e^{-t/\tau}) \tag{11.138}$$

where $\Delta\theta_M$ is the maximum possible angle change and the baseline. Inverting this function we can evaluate the average density of captured target molecules as

$$\rho(t) = \frac{\theta(t) - \theta_0}{\Delta\theta_M}\rho_0 \tag{11.139}$$

Once the surface density $\rho(t)$ has been determined it is needed to correlate it with the concentration in the target sample. Considering the details of the fluid dynamics motion is quite complex, since blocking the target molecules on the functionalized surface creates a transversal concentration gradient with the consequent Taylor dispersion in the transverse direction (see Section 7.4.5). However, it is to be taken into account that the target of the design is to bind to the functionalized surface all the target molecules, thus the system has to be designed so that Taylor dispersion is so effective to bring all the molecules near the bottom of the assay room.

To have this result it is needed that the characteristic time needed by the molecules to diffuse through the greater linear dimension of the assay room section is much smaller than the time needed to traverse it in the longitudinal direction. Assuming the molecular diffusion coefficient to be negligible with respect to the Taylor diffusion coefficient as in Section 7.4.5, the diffusion time across the assay room is much smaller than the time for the room crossing if

$$\frac{D_T}{L_x^2} \gg \frac{v}{L_z} \tag{11.140}$$

where L_x, L_y, L_z are the width, the depth, and the length of the assay room, respectively, and v is the average fluid velocity in the z direction. Using Equation 7.212 correct for a rectangular duct we get

$$v \gg \frac{128 D}{L_z} \left(\frac{L_y}{L_x} \right)^2 \tag{11.141}$$

where, D is the diffusion coefficient of the target molecules. If we assume $L_x = 100~\mu m$, $L_y = 10~\mu m$, $L_z = 2$ mm and a diffusion coefficient $D = 10^{-11}$ we get $v \gg 1.28 \times 10^{-2}~\mu m/s$. This condition is almost always realized, thus Taylor dispersion in practical cases is sufficiently efficient to maintain the target molecule concentration almost constant in the assay room.

The above conclusion allows us to evaluate the concentration of molecules in the assay solution versus the density of molecules bonded to the functionalized surface with a simple one-dimensional model. If the antibodies concentration on the functionalized surface is sufficiently high we can assume

$$c_m L_x L_y v\, t_a \ll \rho_0 L_z L_x \tag{11.142}$$

where v is the fluid average velocity in the assay room and t_a is the binding phase duration. This means that the number of antibodies bonded to the surface is much higher than the maximum number of target molecules in the solution passing through the assay room so that we can assume that almost all the target molecules are bonded to the surface at the end of the target solution flow. Thus, we have

$$c_m \approx \rho(t_a) \frac{L_z}{L_y v t_a} \tag{11.143}$$

Frequently, a calibration constant is added empirically to the second term of Equation 11.143 to take into account both the limits of the one-dimensional approximation and other practical deviations from the ideal assay conditions.

If condition (11.142) is not fulfilled the dynamics of the bonding in the assay room has to be studied in detail to determine the relationship between the density of the saturated antibodies, that is, the measured maximum coupling angle, and the concentration of the target molecule in the flowing solution.

In a one-dimensional model this can be done by considering that the antigen–antibody reaction is a single-step reaction that is almost unidirectional (see Section 3.7.1) and very fast. Thus, we can write the fluid–chemical equations in the reaction room as

$$\frac{\partial \hat{c}_m}{\partial t} + v \frac{\partial \hat{c}_m}{\partial z} = K \hat{c}_m \hat{c}_a \tag{11.144a}$$

$$\frac{\partial \hat{c}_a}{\partial t} = -K \hat{c}_m \hat{c}_a \tag{11.144b}$$

$$\hat{c}_b + \hat{c}_a = \hat{c}_0 \tag{11.144c}$$

where K is the antigen–antibody reaction constant, $\hat{c}_m = c_m L_x L_y$ the linear concentration of target molecules in the flowing solution, $\hat{c}_a = \rho_a L_x$ the linear density of unsaturated antibodies, and $\hat{c}_b = \rho L_x$ is the linear density of saturated antibodies. The surface density of unsaturated antibodies ρ_a is provided by $\rho_a = (\rho_0 - \rho)$ while $\hat{c}_0 = \rho_0 L_x$.

The above equation system is not easy to be solved, even in the simplest fluid dynamic conditions in which v can be considered a constant. As a matter of fact, after solving Equation 11.13b, substituting into Equation 11.144a and changing variable to work in the reference system of the moving fluid we get

$$\frac{\partial \hat{c}_m}{\partial \zeta} = K \hat{c}_m e^{-K \int \hat{c}_m \, dt} \tag{11.145}$$

where ζ is the spatial coordinate in the moving reference frame. This is an equation that is difficult to solve analytically, but it can be solved numerically to find the wanted relation between the concentration of the target molecule in the sample solution and the observed surface concentration of bonded molecules.

The dynamic immunoassay, where the sample solution flows through the assay chamber while the assay is performed has an important advantage with respect to a static configuration. In a static configuration the assay chamber is filled, the stationary situation is expected and the measurement is performed. The quantity of the sample solution is then directly related to the volume of the assay chamber, that is, a microfluidic circuit is never big. This can be an advantage if the quantity of sample solution is very small, but limits the assay sensitivity. On the contrary, in a dynamic solution any quantity of sample solution can be processes up to the moment in which the available antibodies are all saturated and no more target molecule can be captured on the surface. This explains why creating very dense patterns on functionalized surfaces is very important.

The sensitivity of surface plasmons resonant assays is very good, relying on the capability of measuring with a great accuracy optical intensities and incident angles and on the possibility to use relatively high-quantity samples to saturate high-density antibodies functionalized surfaces. Sensitivity up to femtomoles per liter have been attained [124] in experiments where particular care has been adopted in avoiding spurious reflections of the incident light beam and unwanted metal-induced fluorescence quenching.

An important extension of lab on chip testing a sample solution in a single assay room is constituted by labs on chip using the possibility of illuminating simultaneously several parallel assay rooms disposed to form an array. Using such a device different measurements can be performed in parallel. A possible use of such a device is to test the surface plasmon resonance simultaneously with different surface concentrations of antibodies [125]. This procedure is important for the determination of the equilibrium constant of the antibodies binding to the target molecule.

In this application a static assay is performed by filling each chamber of the array with the same target solution, waiting for equilibrium and measuring the maximum coupling angle. The quantity of bonded target molecules is detected in each case and a first estimation of the equilibrium constant is done on the ground of the knowledge of the concentration of both the target molecule and of the surface antibodies. An accurate estimation is then obtained by interpolating the results coming from all the chambers of the array. A similar system can be used to simply monitoring the antigen–antibody binding events in different array chambers [122].

Grating coupling is also used in alternative to coupling through a prism [126,127]. It is more difficult to implement, but it requires much less real estate and has the potential to be integrated into small systems, where compact laser sources and detectors are used.

11.4.3 Localized Plasmon Resonance Detection

A completely different type of plasma wave is excited in surfaces where conducting nanoparticles are patterned so that they cannot exchange electrons. In this case, due to the small particle dimensions, much smaller than the light wavelength, electrons within the same particle move practically in the same way when the particle interacts with an electromagnetic wave, thus no plasma wave can be excited on the single particle. On the other hand, plasma waves can be excited in the particle population involving several particles, each of which plays the role of an oscillating dipole [128–130], as shown in Figure 11.69. In the case of localized plasmons electrons oscillated over all the particle volume, but the peak of the electrical field remains in strict proximity of the particle surface; that is why these different types of plasma oscillations are also called as localized surface plasmons.

11.4.3.1 Localized Plasmons and Scattering from Nanoparticles

Even a classical model of localized surface plasmons is much harder than that of simple surface plasmons, due to the complex scattering pattern created in general by a light beam incident on a microscopic particle.

Two different phenomena influence the dependence of the intensity of the light reflected by a pattern of metal nanoparticles on the incidence angle: light scattering from single particles and localized plasma resonance excitation. Thus, if an accurate theoretical prediction of the scattering wave intensity and angle dependence is known the effect of coupling with localized plasma oscillations can be detected.

Another way of detecting localized plasma oscillations, relying in any case on the knowledge of the scattering pattern, is based on the observation of the beam reflected by the surface. Conventionally, the ratio between the incident and the reflected intensity, I_0 and I_r respectively, is written as

$$\frac{I_R}{I_0} = \frac{S_P}{S_B} (K_\lambda + K_E) \tag{11.146}$$

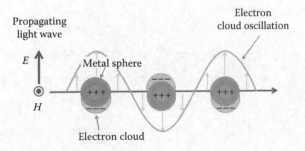

FIGURE 11.69 Working principle of localized surface plasmons on a surface patterned with metal nanoparticles.

where S_B is the light beam wave-front area and the area of the particle section as seen from the light incident direction. The scattering and extinction efficiencies thus are ratios between the effective scattering and extinction cross-section and the particle geometric cross-section. Extinction is due to material absorption and, when localized plasma resonance is excited, due to energy transfer to localized plasmons. Thus, if it is known for the measurement configuration and I_0 and I_r are measured, K_E can be deduced simply.

In the limit of an insulated particle that is much smaller than the light wavelength, practically smaller than 1 part out of 10 parts of the wavelength, the particle shape has almost no importance, due to the complete inability of the incident light to detect it. In this case, scattering is well described by the Rayleigh scattering law coming from a solution of the Maxwell equations where the field is always constant in all the particle volume [131,132]. Considering a plane wave with wave front parallel to the (x, y) plane, the Rayleigh scattering law forecasts a scattered intensity profile having a rotational symmetry with respect to the incident light propagation direction, the z-axis in this case. The scattering profile can be represented on the (x, y) plane as a function of the angle θ that the observation direction forms with the z-axis (see Figure 11.70) as follows:

$$\frac{I(r,\theta)}{I_0} = \frac{(1 + \cos^2\theta)}{2r^2}\left(\frac{2\pi}{\lambda}\right)^4\left(\frac{n^2 - 1}{n^2 + 2}\right)\left(\frac{d}{2}\right)^6 \qquad (11.147)$$

where the environmental refraction index is assumed to be equal to 1 and

r is the distance of the measurement point from the scattering particle;

I_0 the incident wave intensity;

λ the incident wavelength;

n the particle refraction index; and

d is the particle average linear dimension.

The Raleigh scattering profile is shown in Figure 11.70. Besides the famous dependence on the fourth power of wavelength, having a main impact on the color of earth and sky [133], an important feature of the Rayleigh scattering law is the fact that the scattering pattern is symmetrical with respect to the plane parallel to the incident wave planes, so that forward and backward scattering have the same intensity.

If the nanoparticle environment has a different refraction index it has to be taken into account in Equation 11.146, but it does not influence the shape of the scattered light wavefront or the dependence of the scattered light in the wavelength and on the particle dimension, but only the scattered intensity. This means that Rayleigh scattering can be used per se as a way to measure particle dimension and refraction index via the so-called Rayleigh scattering spectroscopy.

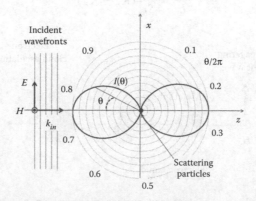

FIGURE 11.70 Rayleigh scattering profile for an insulated particle.

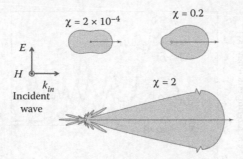

FIGURE 11.71 Mie scattering patterns for gold particles with different dimensional ratio at $\lambda = 500$ µm. The scattering patterns, that have rotational symmetry around the incident light beam axis, are evaluated using the Mie solution of the Maxwell equations for a free spherical particle. The environment refraction index is considered to be equal to 1.

If the Rayleigh hypothesis is true the scattering of the particle pattern can be evaluated by assuming each particle as insulated and taking into account the substrate reflectivity besides superposition of the light scattered by each particle. Considering coherent superposition between the waves scattered by different particles due to their dimension smaller than the light wavelength we have to add the electrical field and then square the result to obtain the final scattered intensity. Exploiting Equation 11.147 we get

$$K_\lambda = \rho^2 A^2 \frac{S_B}{S_P} \int_0^{2\pi} \frac{I(R,\theta)}{I_0} d\theta = \frac{3\pi}{2R^2} \rho^2 A^2 \frac{S_B}{S_P} \left(\frac{2\pi}{\lambda}\right)^4 \left(\frac{n^2-1}{n^2+2}\right) \left(\frac{d}{2}\right)^6 \tag{11.148}$$

where ρ is the surface particle density, A the chip area, and R the detector distance from the chip.

This relatively simple approach however is not possible in several practical cases; for example, if we work with visible light at 500 nm, the particle linear dimension has to be below 50 nm in order to generate Rayleigh scattering and if detection is operated in the UV range at 300 nm, particles smaller than 30 nm are needed.

When the particle linear dimensions are nearer the light wavelength the situation becomes more complex. In this case the scattered pattern depends on the particle shape and position with respect to the incidence direction besides the other factors that are present in the Rayleigh formula. In case of spherical or cylindrical particles the scattered wave can be exactly determined through the Mie solution of the Maxwell equations, that even if much complex of the Rayleigh one can be used to study coupling of electromagnetic waves with surfaces patterned with metal nanoparticles.

Mie scattering from a sphere, while reduces to Rayleigh scattering for a vanishing sphere radius, becomes more and more asymmetric while the sphere radius increases up to the light wavelength, as is shown in Figure 11.71. In the figure the particle dimensional ratio χ is defined as the ratio between the particle diameter and the light wavelength.

While the dimension of the sphere increases, the pronounced dependence of Rayleigh scattering from the light wavelength attenuates. Moreover it appears as a dependence of the scattering efficiency on the particle absorption, that is, the complex part of the refraction index, that is not present in the Rayleigh scattering equation. This effect is shown in Figure 11.72, where the scattering efficiency K_λ, is plotted versus particles dimensional ratio χ for different particle attenuations, expressed and imaginary part of the refraction index.

11.4.3.2 Detection through Localized Plasma Resonance Measurement
When the scattering efficiency is known, the extinction efficiency can be evaluated by the measure of the reflected intensity. The extinction efficiency can be expressed with a simple equation

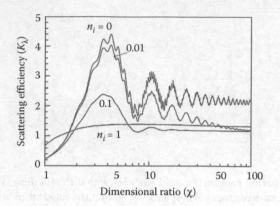

FIGURE 11.72 Scattering efficiency for spherical particles with different dimensional ratios and different attenuation coefficients. The environment refraction index is considered to be equal to 1 and n_i represents the particle complex part of the refraction index at the considered frequency.

starting from the Mie solution of the Maxwell equations in the case of a spherical particle with a radius much smaller than the wavelength. In this case, the position of the particle with respect to the incident wave vector is not important due to the spherical symmetry and the field can be assumed uniform in all the particle volume so to obtain [134]

$$K_E = 9 \frac{\omega}{c_0} \sqrt{\varepsilon_2^3} \, V_p \rho \frac{\varepsilon_{1,I}(\omega)}{\left[2\varepsilon_2 + \varepsilon_{1,R}(\omega)\right]^2 + \varepsilon_{1,I}^2(\omega)} \frac{S_B}{S_P} \tag{11.149}$$

where ε_2 is the dielectric constant of the medium embedding the nanoparticles, V_p is the spherical nanoparticle volume, and the nanoparticles material dielectric constant is provided by

$$\varepsilon_1(\omega) = \varepsilon_{1,R}(\omega) + i \, \varepsilon_{1,I}(\omega) \tag{11.150}$$

being $\varepsilon_{1,R}(\omega)$ and $\varepsilon_{1,I}(\omega)$ its real and imaginary parts, respectively. The surface plasmon absorption band appears when

$$2\varepsilon_2 \approx -\varepsilon_{1,R}(\omega) \tag{11.151}$$

Where Equation 11.149 has a maximum and the amplitude of such a maximum is directly related to ε_2. This shows the possibility to measure the value of the dielectric constant of the medium surrounding the conducting nanoparticles by detection of the localized plasmon resonance, which is the principle on which the use of this phenomenon for detection in labs on chip rely.

Owing to the fact that Equation 11.149 is rigorously valid only in the limit of vanishing nanoparticle radius, it does not contain the dependence of the extinction maximum position on the particle dimension. Moreover, if the particle dimension is not completely negligible with respect to the light wavelength, a strong dependence of the position and shape of the extinction peak is also revealed. An example of dependence of the extinction spectrum on the particle size is shown in Figure 11.73, where the extinction efficiency of a single spherical silver particle is plotted versus the incident light wavelength for two different particle radius R_p.

The dependence on the particle shape is shown in Figure 11.74 where the extinction efficiency is reported for an oblate ellipsoid, that is, an ellipsoid with rotational symmetry around the minor axis, versus the wavelength for different ratios between the minor and major axes. All the ellipsoids have the same volume, equal to that of a sphere with a radius of 80 nm and data are averaged over the light incident direction so to simulate a surface with randomly distributed nanoparticles. Both

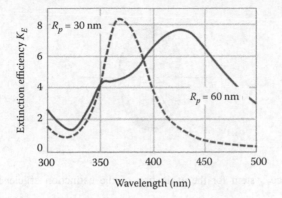

FIGURE 11.73 Accurate electrodynamics simulation of the extinction efficiency of a single spherical silver particle versus the incident light wavelength for two different particle radius R_p.

Figures 11.73 and 11.74 are obtained by an accurate electromagnetic simulation of the scattering from a single particle using the solution of the Maxwell equations with suitable boundary conditions.

Another important fact that is implicit in the presence of nonspherical particles is the dependence of the position of the localized plasma resonance on the polarization of the incident light. The most common situation is that the polarization of the incident light is randomly placed with respect to the particles, so that the result is averaged with respect to the particle position with respect to the incident polarization.

The extinction efficiency of a single oblate ellipsoid can be evaluated analytically using an extension of the Mie theory, called the Gans theory [129], so to obtain results in good agreement with accurate simulations and experience [135]. In particular, the following expression is obtained [136] for a randomly disposed single particle and a linear polarization of the incident light. The particle is a prolate ellipsoid and the reference system is chosen as in Figure 11.75, with the origin at the particle center and the x axis parallel to the particle major axis:

$$K_E = \frac{\omega}{3c_0} \sqrt{\varepsilon_2^3}\, V_p \rho\, \frac{S_B}{S_P} \sum_{j=1}^{3} \frac{\left((1/P_j^2) \right) \varepsilon_{1,I}(\omega)}{\left[(1 - P_j/P_j)\, \varepsilon_2 + \varepsilon_{1,R}(\omega) \right]^2 + \varepsilon_{1,I}^2(\omega)} \tag{11.152}$$

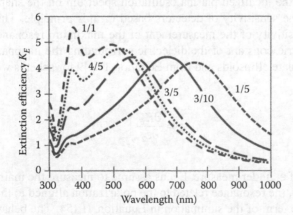

FIGURE 11.74 Accurate electrodynamics simulation of the extinction efficiency of ellipsoids with rotational symmetry with respect to the minor axis (oblate ellipsoids). All the ellipsoids have the same volume, equal to that of a sphere with a radius of 80 nm. Data are averaged over the light incident direction so as to simulate a surface with randomly distributed nanoparticles.

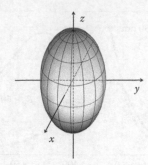

FIGURE 11.75 Reference system for the evaluation of the extinction efficiency of a prolate ellipsoid nanoparticle.

where the so-called depolarization factors P_j, representing the effect of the random particle position, are given by

$$P_3 = \frac{1-\phi^2}{\phi^2}\left[\frac{1}{2\phi}\ln\left(\frac{1+\phi}{1-\phi}\right)-1\right] \tag{11.153a}$$

$$P_2 = P_1 = \frac{1-P_3}{2} \tag{11.153b}$$

the factor ϕ being related to the ratio between the major and minor axes of the ellipsoid δ as

$$\phi = \sqrt{1-\left(\frac{1}{\delta}\right)^2} \tag{11.154}$$

The extinction spectrum resulting from Equation 11.152 has two peaks, ne corresponding to the transverse plasmon peak from the contributions of the x- and y-axis to the sum, and the other corresponding to the longitudinal plasmon peak from the z-axis contribution. This is also evident from Figure 11.74.

The dependence of the localized plasma oscillation spectrum on the shape of particles can be exploited to improve the sensitivity of detectors based on this principle. This can be understood by considering the sensitivity of the measurement of the maximum resonance wavelength versus a change in the dielectric constant of the dielectric surrounding the nanoparticles. Starting from Equation 11.152 for prolate ellipsoids and from Equation 11.149 for spheres we can define the measurement sensitivity as

$$s = \frac{\partial K_E}{\partial \varepsilon_2}\bigg)_{\hat{\varepsilon}_2} \tag{11.155}$$

where $\hat{\varepsilon}_2$ is the value of ε_2 under measure. Let us assume to measure the main resonance peak of a prolate ellipsoid, that is, the resonance related to the polarization aligned to the ellipsoid main axis, so to consider only one term of the summation in Equation 11.154. The behavior of the sensitivity normalized to its amplitude versus the ellipsoid shape parameter δ is represented in Figure 11.76 in the case of silver having $\varepsilon_{1,I} \approx 0.3$ and $\varepsilon_{1,R}(\omega) \approx -12$ at 500 nm and assuming $\varepsilon_2 \approx 1$ The sensitivity for a prolate ellipsoid with the major axis 10 times longer than the minor one is about 128 times the sensitivity associated with a sphere. This means that it is quite advantageous to use metal

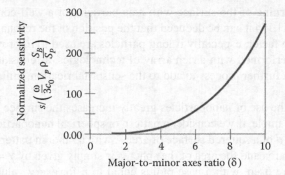

FIGURE 11.76 Normalized sensitivity of localized plasmon detection versus the ratio between main and secondary axes of the metal prolate ellipsoids used as nanoparticles for surface patterning.

nanorods instead of metal spheres to pattern the surface that is used for the measure. Nanorods have been fabricated and patterned on dielectric surfaces in different ways: almost all the patterning techniques have been used like nanoimprint lithography [137], evaporation [138], and self-assembly procedures [139] among many others.

Once the surface is patterned with nanoparticles and the nanoparticles are suitably functionalized so as to be able to capture the target molecules, a localized plasma resonance assay is carried out with a base assembly that is not different from the equivalent assay based on surface plasmons (see Figure 11.77) [140–142]. This base arrangement has been varied in several ways with the start of either improving the assay performance or to render the assay equipment smaller or easier to use. Among other systems a cavity has been used to enhance localized plasmon resonance [143] the effect of a static magnetic field has been studied [144] and nanoparticles with a complex structure, like several layers, have been adopted [145].

Beyond the different improvement that can be done to the base localized plasmon sensing equipment, the fact that the detection sensitivity seems to increase monotonically with the aspect ratio of the nanoparticles brings to explore the possibility to use the so-called nanowires. Metal nanowires are structures whose section has linear dimensions much smaller than the wavelength, but whose length is longer than the wavelength itself. If nanowires are adopted, however, the theory of localized plasmon is not yet valid, since a sort of one-dimensional plasma waves can propagate along the length of such structures [146,147]. The general structure of a nanowire-based sensor is similar to that of other types of plasmon-based sensors with its specific characteristics [148,149].

A last important comment is needed on the comparison between sensors based on surface plasmons and localized surface plasmons. Under a technology point of view the adoption of localized

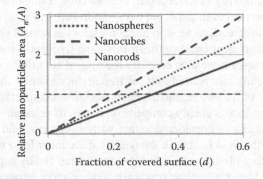

FIGURE 11.77 Ratio between the nanoparticles area A_n and the whole surface area A versus the patterned area fraction d for different kinds of nanoparticles.

plasmon requires patterning of the surface with nanoparticles of a well-controlled dimension and shape. From Equation 11.154 it can be deduced that the position of the resonance peak is quite sensitive to the particle form factor, especially if long particles are used to improve sensitivity.

Patterning can be performed with a rich array of technologies, as considered in Chapters 4 and 5, but in any case it is a further process to add to the sensor fabrication, influencing both yields and fabrication cost.

On the other hand, the use of nanoparticles greatly increases the surface that can be functionalized on the chip. For example, if we consider a pattern of spherical nanoparticles with a radius equal to r covering a fraction d of a squared surface of area A with a random pattern, for $d < 0.63$ the ratio χ between the covered area and the area of the spheres is simply given by $\chi = 4\,d$, while if perfectly cylindrical nanorods are used, with a base radius equal to r, for every value of d we have $\chi = \pi\,d$ and if we use nanocubes we have $\chi = 5\,d$. As it is evident from Figure 11.77, as d is greater than very small values, the area available for functionalization is much greater in nanoparticle patterned surfaces with respect to flat surfaces.

This property allows more compact lab on chip to be realized by maintaining the density of functionalizing elements on the surface constant.

As far as a sensitivity comparison is concerned it greatly depends on the measurement apparatus structure and on the type of measurement that is performed. In principle, sensitivity of the surface plasmon resonance-based detection can be evaluated by obtaining the maximum absorption angle from Equation 11.135 and calculating the derivative with respect to the angle in the maximum absorption angle position. We simply get

$$\left.\frac{\partial\theta}{\partial\varepsilon_2}\right)_{\hat{\varepsilon}_2} \approx \frac{1}{2\cos\theta\sqrt{\hat{\varepsilon}_2}} \tag{11.156}$$

This means that, if an angle of $0.05°$ can be measured, that is, a standard performance for angle measurements in laboratory, and the reference value of the environmental dielectric constant is $\varepsilon_2 = 1.1$, surface plasmon resonance through a thin film allows to measure a dielectric constant difference of about 5×10^{-4}, while an accurate measurement system is set up, it is theoretically possible to arrive to measure a dielectric constant difference of 5×10^{-5}.

If we consider practical parameters and evaluate under the same conditions the accuracy of a measurement system based on extinction measure through localized plasmon resonance through Equation 11.155 we get a result more than one order of magnitude worse. Thus, the theoretical sensitivity of the pure plasmonic part of the detection is at least an order of magnitude better for the case of surface plasmons on thin metallic films [150].

However, to obtain an overall sensitivity of the measure we have to superimpose the plasmonic sensitivity to the optical sensitivity of the receiver, besides considering many other elements that are not considered in our theoretical evaluation, but have importance in a practical measurement device. In case of real-time measurements, as seen in Section 11.3.4 the optical sensitivity plays an important role, due to the measurement bandwidth. In this case frequently the difference between the two methods greatly decreases if we also consider the optical sensitivity, and if we also add many practical problems, frequently also related to the different dimension of the chips necessary for the two assays, the sensitivity of the two methods becomes almost comparable. In this case, detection by localized plasmon resonance is clearly competitive, due to its other advantages.

If a static measurement can be considered, either with a very low fluid velocity in the detection chamber or even leaving the fluid to stay in the detection chamber for a while in order to saturate the activated surface, surface plasmons on thin films are instead clearly superior as far as sensitivity is concerned. In practice, however, the dynamic case is much more frequent.

Reference sensitivities that can be obtained through surface and localized plasmon resonance are reported in Table 11.9. Sensitivity is reported in refractive index units (RIU), that is, in terms of

TABLE 11.9
Reference Sensitivities for Surface and Localized Plasmon Resonance Detection (SPR and LSPR, Respectively)

Method	Target	Optical Detector	Sensitivity (Assay)	Sensitivity (Molar)
SPR	Proteins	Direct Detection	10^{-5}–10^{-8} RIU	1 nM
SPR	Proteins	Coherent Detection	10^{-7}–10^{-8} RIU	1 nM
SPR	DNA/RNA	Direct Detection	10^{-5}–10^{-8} RIU	10 pM
LSPR	Proteins	Direct Detection	10^{-5}–10^{-7} RIU	10 nm

Note: Sensitivity is reported in refractive index units (RIU), that is, in terms of the minimum refraction index change the system can detect and in terms of molarity of a typical solution causing such a refraction index change.

the minimum refraction index change the system can detect and in terms of molarity of a typical solution causing such a refraction index change.

Data are obtained by a synthesis of the specific cases presented in technical literature, by excluding cases where the detection system is specifically designed for very high sensitivity, for example, adopting photon counting instead of photodiodes [3,4], freezing the detector with liquid gas to reduce thermal electronic noise and the like. In these cases, detection systems can reach molecule counting sensitivity [129,151], on the edge of 100 molecules or less. However, such systems are specifically designed for research application and the lab on chip is not the key element of the system, but a particular part of a very complex measurement setup.

The only particular case is that of the adoption of coherent detection, in contrast with direct detection that we have described in Section 11.3.4 [11]. This technique consists, in general, in coupling the incoming optical beam at the receiver with a local laser with the same central wavelength to exploit the amplification effect due to positive interference. Even if one laser is needed at the receiver, whose wavelength has to be actively controlled to match that of the incoming beam, very compact and low-cost coherent detectors have been developed for other applications and this can grow up to become a standard technique.

11.5 LAB-ON-CHIP INTERFEROMETRY

The main target of plasma resonance-based detection is to reveal the density of molecules that are bonded to a suitably functionalized surface through the detection of the consequent change in the refraction index, or the dielectric constant, which is its square in the purely paramagnetic case if $\mu_0 = 1$.

Plasmon resonance detection is a very sensible detection method, at the limit that molecule counting can be performed. On the other hand, it has some practical problems that make it essentially a laboratory method. The first, and probably more important problem, is related to the long-term stability of functionalized surfaces under temperature changes and mechanical vibrations (see Section 11.2.4). In laboratory environment, where the lab on chip can be stored under controlled conditions, even at low temperature if needed, this is not a problem. On the contrary, this is a blocking problem for field applications and when the lab on chip has to be distributed and stored under standard industrial conditions.

A second limitation of plasmon resonance-based detection is its difficulty to be integrated on chip. The need of a three-dimensional optical arrangement and of accurate angle or extinction measure renders very difficult monolithic integration of this kind of system.

An interferometry detection system, based on the measurement of refraction index change in a sample solution can overcome both these limitations: it can be monolithically integrated by means of integrated optics interferometers and, due to its use of a sample solution, without the need of functionalized surfaces is much more robust to environmental condition changes.

The price to pay is generally a reduction in detection sensitivity with respect to plasmon detection adopting accurate angle or extinction measurements. This is mainly due to the fact that the sample solution in the typical arrangement cannot flow in the detection room by depositing the target molecule, but it has to be charged there so to execute the detection in static conditions. This limits the refraction index change magnitude if diluted solutions have to be assayed.

One of the most used configurations for an integrated interferometry detection is that based on an integrated Mach–Zehnder interferometer [152,153], whose principal scheme is presented in Figure 11.78. The solution to be analyzed is inserted in a detection room that is built below the sensing arm of a Mach–Zehnder monolithic interferometer. The solution refraction index, depending on the target molecule concentration, contribute to determine the effective index of the sensing branch of the interferometer, thus influencing the light fly time.

A heater is fabricated for calibration on the reference branch of the Mach–Zehnder so that in correspondence to a target concentration equal to zero the input light is completely conveyed toward one of the interferometer output ports. When the target concentration changes the observation of the light power on both the interferometer ports allows the target concentration to be determined.

Mach–Zehnder interferometers in near IR are fabricated in SiO_2–Si technology in large volumes for different applications [154,155] and are well-established components. Polymer-based interferometers have also been proposed for biosensing that well integrate with other elements of lab on chip using polymeric materials [156,157].

If we consider single mode propagation in the sensing arm of the interferometer, the waveguide effective index depends on the refraction indexes of the core and cladding materials, so that if the evanescent wave propagating in the lower cladding has nonnegligible field values in correspondence of the detection room points it depends on the refraction index of the solution injected in such a chamber.

Since the refraction index of a diluted solution depends on the concentrations of the solutes, as shown in Section 11.3.2.1, we can write

$$n_{eff} = n_{e0} + \frac{\partial n_{eff}}{\partial n_s} \sum_{j=1}^{N} \frac{\partial n_s}{\partial c_j} c_j \tag{11.157}$$

where n_{e0} is the effective index in the absence of solutes, n_s the effective cladding refraction index that takes into account both the detection room and the solid part of the cladding, N the solutes number and c_j is the concentration of the jth solute.

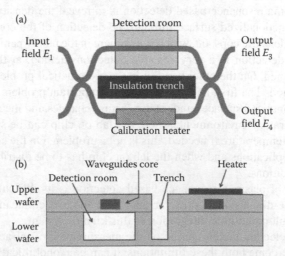

FIGURE 11.78 Scheme of an integrated Mach–Zehnder interferometry detection system: top view (a) and section in the middle of the interferometer branches (b).

If the index $j = 1$ indicates the target molecule we can rearrange Equation 11.157 collecting in a single term n_{eN} the effect of all the other solutes and write

$$n_{eff} = n_{e0} + \frac{\partial n_{eff}}{\partial n_s}\left(n_{e0} + \frac{\partial n_s}{\partial c_1}c_1\right) \tag{11.158}$$

The transfer function of the Mach–Zehnder interferometer is provided by Equation 11.79 where the optical path difference is caused by an effective index difference and the arms' physical lengths are equal. If we have input light at input port 1 only and we measure the intensity at output ports 3 and 4 we get

$$\frac{I_3}{I_1} = \sin^2\left(\pi\Delta n_e \frac{L}{\lambda_0}\right) \tag{11.159a}$$

$$\frac{I_4}{I_1} = \cos^2\left(\pi\Delta n_e \frac{L}{\lambda_0}\right) \tag{11.159b}$$

where L is the physical length of the interferometer arms and Δn_e is the effective index difference. The most effective way to measure a difference in the refraction index using the Mach–Zehnder interferometer is to detect the difference between the light intensity at ports 4 and 3 that is practically measured through the arrangement of two serialized photodiodes at the output of the interferometer, as shown in Figure 11.79. Thus, the normalized current $C(t)$ at the sensor output can be written as

$$c(t) = A\left(\frac{I_4}{I_1} - \frac{I_3}{I_1}\right) + A\mu = A\left[\cos^2\left(\pi\Delta n_e \frac{L}{\lambda_0}\right) - \sin^2\left(\pi\Delta n_e \frac{L}{\lambda_0}\right)\right] + A\mu$$

$$= A\sin\left(2\pi\Delta n_e \frac{L}{\lambda_0}\right) + A\mu \tag{11.160}$$

where A is an amplitude depending on the characteristics of the detection circuit, like photodiodes responsivity, amplifier gain, and so on and μ is a global noise term (see Section 11.3.4). This photodiode arrangement is called differential receiver and it has advantages over the simpler method of measuring one intensity only.

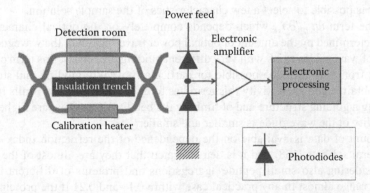

FIGURE 11.79 Scheme of a balanced optical receiver at the end of a Mach–Zehnder interferometer for biosensing.

From Equation 11.160 a calibration curve can be derived for the measure of the index difference Δn_e and from Equation 11.158 it can be related to the concentration of the target molecule.

In many practical cases the index difference is small due to the evanescence wave coupling realized in the interferometer and we can expand Equation 11.160 at first order obtaining

$$\frac{c(t)}{A} = 2\pi\Delta n_e \frac{L}{\lambda_0} + \mu = 2\pi \frac{L}{\lambda_0} \frac{\partial n_{eff}}{\partial n_s} \frac{\partial n_s}{\partial c_1} c_1 + 2\pi \frac{L}{\lambda_0} \frac{\partial n_{eff}}{\partial n_s} n_{e0} + \mu \tag{11.161}$$

Equation 11.161 can be used for a very accurate measure of c_1 if the material characteristics are known and if the term n_{e0} is also known. It is relevant that, differently from the impact of noise that can be reduced increasing the optical power or improving the photodiodes quality, any error on the value of n_{e0} is directly reflected on an error on the estimate of c_1. This is the reason why, if it is possible, a reference cell is often placed below the reference arm of the interferometer, possibly far from the heater, where a solution that is identical to the assayed sample is placed, but without the target molecule. In this way, Equation 11.161 becomes

$$\frac{c(t)}{A} = 2\pi\Delta n_e \frac{L}{\lambda_0} + \mu = 2\pi \frac{L}{\lambda_0} \frac{\partial n_{eff}}{\partial n_s} \frac{\partial n_s}{\partial c_1} c_1 + \mu \tag{11.162}$$

eliminating the need of subtracting the term n_{e0} from the assay result.

The pure assay resolution can be obtained from Equation 11.160 by eliminating the noise term and deriving with respect to c_1. It is obtained as

$$\frac{1}{c_{10}} \frac{\partial C}{\partial c_1}\bigg)_{\bar{c}_1} = 2\pi \frac{L}{\lambda_0} A \cos\left(2\pi \frac{L}{\lambda_0} \frac{\partial n_{eff}}{\partial n_s} \frac{\partial n_s}{\partial c_1} c_{10} \right) \frac{\partial n_{eff}}{\partial n_s} \frac{\partial n_s}{\partial c_1} \tag{11.163}$$

where c_{10} is the measurement nominal value. The first observation is that the relative sensitivity is higher for small values of the target molecule concentration, as clear from the cosine term in Equation 11.163. This is due to the fact that for small values of the concentration the characteristic of the interferometer is almost linear. The maximum sensitivity depends critically from the factor $(\partial n_{eff}/\partial n_s)(\partial n_s/\partial c_1)$.

The first term is maximized by constructing weakly guiding interferometers, where the evanescent wave prolongs into the cladding zone and minimizing the thickness of the solid film dividing the waveguide core from the detection chamber. For this purpose, sometimes the detection chamber is also built on the side of the interferometer waveguide instead of below it. The second term can be maximized if it is possible to select a few characteristics of the sample solution.

Intuitively the term $\partial n_{eff}/\partial n_s$, which depends completely on the optical characteristics of the waveguide, is determined by the amount of optical power traveling out of the waveguide core. Since a large variety of waveguides exist, with very different guiding properties, this term can span a wide range of values from 0.15 to 0.005 possible for particularly weakly guiding and strongly guiding structures. To obtain a good sensitivity this term has to be large, within the limits imposed by the need of realizing a guiding structure and of limiting the bending losses that are higher and higher if the guiding ability of the waveguide is smaller and smaller.

A great amount of data is available on the dependence of the refraction index of solutions of proteins in several solvents [158] and it is demonstrated that they are almost of the same order of magnitude considering also small peptide aggregations and proteins of different types [159]. In particular, they range almost in any practical case within 0.14 and 0.21 if the protein concentration is measured in g/mL. Similar data are provided for a few substances in Table 11.10. Data for nucleic acids are also available [160].

TABLE 11.10

Index of Refraction Dependence on the Solute Concentration for Selected Solutions

Solute	Solvent	
Proteins	Water and NaCl	0.14–0.22
Sodium Chloride	Water	0.15
Propan-1-ol	Water	0.083
Sucrose	Water	0.17
Glucose	Water	0.12

Note: Concentration is measured in g/mL

Total assay sensitivities of the order of 10^{-7} RIUs can be practically achieved using Mach–Zehnder interferometry with evanescent wave coupling, which are of the same order of magnitude of the sensitivity of localized plasmon-based systems, while a bit lower of the best sensitivities of surface plasmon-based systems.

Besides the scheme represented in Figure 11.79 and its variations with the detection chamber besides the waveguide, several other detection arrangements based on Mach–Zehnder interferometers have been proposed. Many of them are based on immobilizing target molecules on a functionalized surface in a dynamic configuration similar to that used for plasmon-based detection. In this case, even if generally a smaller assay sensitivity is reached, the detection system can be completely integrated into the lab on chip.

REFERENCES

1. Itzycson C., Zuber J.-B., *Quantum Field Theory*, Dover Publications (February 24, 2006), ISBN-13: 978-0486445687.
2. Mandl F., Shaw G., *Quantum Field Theory*, Wiley; 2nd edition (May 17, 2010), ISBN-13: 978-0471496847.
3. Muller-Kirsten H. J. W., *Electrodynamics*, World Scientific Publishing Company; 2nd edition (April 8, 2011), ISBN-13: 978-9814340748.
4. Loudon R., *The Quantum Theory of Light*, Oxford University Press, USA; 3rd edition (November 23, 2000), ISBN-13: 978-0198501763.
5. Agarwal G. S., *Quantum Optics*, Cambridge University Press (December 28, 2012), ISBN-13: 978-1107006409.
6. Strange P., *Relativistic Quantum Mechanics*, Cambridge University Press; First Edition (November 13, 1998), ISBN-13: 978-0521565837.
7. Boyd R. W., *Nonlinear Optics*, Academic Press; 3rd edition (April 11, 2008),ISBN-13: 978-0123694706.
8. Powers P. E., *Fundamentals of Nonlinear Optics*, CRC Press; 1st edition (May 25, 2011), ISBN-13: 978-1420093513.
9. *Applications of Raman Spectroscopy to Biology: From Basic Studies to Disease Diagnosis*, Ghomi M. Editor, IOS Press; 1st edition (March 15, 2012), ISBN-13: 978-1607509998.
10. Borman S. A., Nonlinear raman spectroscopy, *Analytical Chemistry*, vol. 54, pp. 1021A–1026A, 1982.
11. Born M., Wolf E., *Principles of Optics*, Cambridge University Press; 7th edition (October 13, 1999), ISBN-13: 978-0521642224.
12. Hass R., Münzberg M., Bressel L., Reich O., Industrial applications of Photon density wave spectroscopy for in-line particle sizing, *Applied Optics*, vol. 52, pp. 1423–1431, 2013.
13. Fluegel A., *Statistical Calculation and Development of Glass Properties*, http://glassproperties.com/, last accessed on March 24, 2013.
14. Li W. B., Segrè P. N., Gammon R. W., Sengers J. V., Lamvik M., Determination of the temperature and concentration dependence of the refractive index of a liquid mixture, *Journal of Chemical Physics*, vol. 101, pp. 5058–5064, 1994.

15. Moreira R., Chenlo F., LeGall D., Kinematic viscosity and refractive index of aqueous solutions of ethanol and glycerol, *Industrial and Engineering Chemical Research*, vol. 48, pp. 2157–2161, 2009.

16. Arrighini G. P., Maestro M., Moccia R., Magnetic properties of polyatomic molecules: Magnetic susceptibility of H_2O, NH_3, CH_4, H_2O_2. *Journal of Chemical Physics*, vol. 49, pp. 882–889, 1968.

17. Write M. R., *An Introduction to Aqueous Electrolyte Solutions*, Wiley; 1st edition (June 5, 2007), ISBN-13: 978-0470842942.

18. Hayat A., Ginzburg P., Orenstein M., Observation of two-photon emission from semiconductors, *Nature Photonics*, vol. 2, pp. 238–241, 2008.

19. Drobizhev M., Makarov N. S., Tillo S. E., Hughes T. E., Rebane A., Two-photon absorption properties of fluorescent proteins, *Nature Methods*, vol. 8, pp. 393–399, 2011.

20. Hobbs P. C. D., *Building Electro-Optical Systems: Making It all Work*, Wiley; 2nd edition (August 3, 2009), ISBN-13: 978-0470402290.

21. Donati S., *Photodetectors: Devices, Circuits and Applications*, Prentice Hall; 1st edition (November 13, 1999), ISBN-13: 978-0130203373.

22. Johnson M., *Photodetection and Measurement: Maximizing Performance in Optical Systems*, McGraw-Hill Professional; 1st edition (August 1, 2003), ISBN-13: 978-0071409445.

23. Graeme J., *Photodiode Amplifiers: OP AMP Solutions*, McGraw-Hill Professional; 1st edition (December 1, 1995), ISBN-13: 978-0070242470.

24. Van Trees H. L., *Detection, Estimation, and Modulation Theory*, Wiley-Interscience; 1st edition (September 27, 2001), ISBN-13: 978-0471095170.

25. Schneider K., Zimmermann H., *Highly Sensitive Optical Receivers*, Springer; 2006 edition (September 14, 2006), ISBN-13: 978-3540296133.

26. Hunsperger R. G., *Integrated Optics*, Springer; Softcover reprint of hardcover 6th ed. 2009 edition (October 29, 2010), ISBN-13: 978-1441928023.

27. Ebeling K. J., *Integrated Optoelectronics: Waveguide Optics, Photonics, Semiconductors*, Springer; reprint of first edition (December 8, 2011), ISBN-13: 978-3642781681.

28. GoureJ. P., Verrier I., *Optical Fibre Devices*, Taylor & Francis; 1st edition (December 1, 2001), ISBN-13: 978-0750308113.

29. Holden H. T., The developing technologies of integrated optical waveguides in printed circuits, *Circuit World*, vol. 29, pp. 42–50, 2003.

30. Okamoto Y., Teng H., Synthesis and properties of amorphous perfluorinated polymers, *Chemistry Today*, vol. 27, pp. 46–48, 2009.

31. Zhu S., Ding S., Xi H., Wang R., Low-temperature fabrication of porous SiC ceramics by preceramic polymer reaction bonding, *Materials Letters*, vol. 59, pp. 595–597, 2005.

32. Heiblum M. Harris J. H., Analysis of curved optical waveguides by conformal transformation, *Journal of Quantum Electronics*, vol. 11, pp. 75–83, 1972.

33. Bienstman P., Six E., Roelens M., Vanwolleghem M., Baets R., Calculation of bending losses in dielectric waveguides using eigenmode expansion and perfectly matched layers, *Photonics Technology Letters*, vol. 14, 2002.

34. Razavi B., *Design of Integrated Circuits for Optical Communications*, Wiley; 2nd edition (August 21, 2012), ISBN-13: 978-1118336946. Interferometers, *Photonics Technology Letters*, vol. 15, pp. 810–812, 2003.

35. Lee, M.-H.; Min Y.-H.; Ju J. J.; Do J. N.; Park S. K., Polymeric electrooptic 2×2 switch consisting of bifurcation optical active waveguides and a Mach–Zehnder interferometer, *Journal of Selected Topics in Quantum Electronics*, vol. 7, pp. 812–818, 2001.

36. DeGui S. et al., Limitation factor analysis for silicon-on-insulator waveguide Mach–Zehnder interference-based electro-optic switch, *Journal of Lightwave Technology*, vol. 29, pp. 2592–2600, 2011.

37. Noguchi K., *Lithium Niobate Modulators*, in *Broadband Optical Modulators*, Chen A., Murphy E. J. Editors, pp. 151–173, CRC Press; 1st edition (November 16, 2011), ISBN-13: 978-1439825068.

38. Wooten E. L. et al., A review of lithium niobate modulators for fiber-optic communications systems, *Journal on Selected Topics in Quantum Electronics*, vol. 6, pp. 69–82, 2000.

39. Mizuno T., Kitoh T., Oguma M., Inoue y., Shibata T., Takahashi H., Uniform wavelength spacing Mach–Zehnder interferometer using phase-generating couplers, *Journal of Lightwave Technology*, vol. 24, pp. 3217, 3226, 2006.

40. Kuznetsov M., Cascaded coupler Mach–Zehnder channel dropping filters for wavelength-division- multiplexed optical systems, *Journal of Lightwave Technology*, vol. 12, pp. 226–230, 1994.

41. Xu Z., Mazumder P., Bio-sensing by Mach–Zehnder interferometer comprising doubly-corrugated spoofed surface plasmon polariton (DC-SSPP) waveguide, *Transaction on Terahertz Science and Technology*, vol. 2, pp. 460–466, 2012.

42. La Notte M., Passaro V. M. N., Ultra high sensitivity chemical photonic sensing by Mach–Zehnder interferometer enhanced Vernier-effect, *Sensors and Actuators B: Chemical*, vol. 176, pp. 994–1007, 2013.

43. Bruck R., E. Melnik E., P. Muellner P., R. Hainberger R., M. Lämmerhofer M., Integrated polymer-based Mach–Zehnder interferometer label-free streptavidin biosensor compatible with injection molding, *Biosensors and Bioelectronics*, vol. 26, 15 pp. 3832–3837, 2011.

44. Chin M. K., Ho S. T., Design and modeling of waveguide-coupled single-mode microring resonators, *Journal of Lightwave Technology*, vol. 15, pp.1433–1446, 1998.

45. Griffel G., Synthesis of optical filters using ring resonator arrays, *Photonics Technology Letters*, vol. 12, pp. 810–812, 2000.

46. Erdogan T., Fiber grating spectra, *Journal of Lightwave Technology*, vol. 15, pp. 1277–1294, 1997.

47. Kocabas A., Aydinli A., Polymeric waveguide bragg grating filter using soft lithography, *Optics Express*, vol. 14, pp. 10228–10232, 2006.

48. Wiesmann D., David C., Germann R., Emi D., and Bona G. L., Apodized surface-corrugated gratings with varying duty cycles, *Photonics Technology Letters*, vol. 12, pp. 639–641, 2000.

49. Greiner C., Mossberg T. W., Iazikov D., Bandpass engineering of lithographically inscribed channel-waveguide bragg gratings, *Optics Letters*, vol. 29, pp. 806–808, 2004.

50. Engler N. et al., Protein dynamics in an intermediate state of myoglobin: Optical absorption, resonance raman spectroscopy, and x-ray structure analysis, *Biophysical Journal*, vol. 78, pp. 2081–2092, 2000.

51. Santiago P. S.vol. et al., Dynamic light scattering and optical absorption spectroscopy study of ph and temperature stabilities of the extracellular hemoglobin of glossoscolex paulistus, *Biophysical Journal*, vol. 94, pp. 2228–2240, 2008.

52. Sych Y., Engelbrecht R., Schmauss B., Kozlov D., Seeger T., Leipertz A., Broadband time-domain absorption spectroscopy with a ns-pulse supercontinuum source, *Optics Express*, vol. 18, pp. 22762–22771, 2010.

53. A. Wirth A., Santra R., Goulielmakis E., Real time tracing of valence-shell electronic coherences with attosecond transient absorption spectroscopy, *Chemical Physics*, vol. 414, pp. 149–159, 2013.

54. Adams M. L., Quake S., Scherer A., *On-Chip Absorption and Fluorescence Spectroscopy with Polydimethylsiloxane (PDMS) Microfluidic Flow Channels*, Proceedings of 2nd Annual International IEEE-EMBS Special Topic Conference on Microtechnologies in Medicine & Biology pp. 369–373, 2002.

55. O'Keefe A., Deacon D. A. G., Cavity ring-down optical spectrometer for absorption measurements using pulsed laser sources, *Review of Scientific Instruments*, vol. 59, pp. 2544–2550, 1988.

56. Bogaerts W. et al., Silicon-on-insulator spectral filters fabricated with cmos technology, *Journal on Selected Topics in Quantum Electronics*, vol. 16, pp. 33–44, 2010.

57. Claes T., Molera J. G., De Vos K., Schachtb E., Baets R., Bienstman P., Label-free biosensing with a slot-waveguide-based ring resonator in silicon on insulator, *Photonics Journal*, vol. 1, pp. 197–204, 2009.

58. Kurczveil G., Pintus P., Heck M. J. R., Peters J. D., Bowers. J. E., Characterization of insertion loss and back reflection in passive hybrid silicon tapers, *Photonics Journal*, vol. 5, pp. 6600410, 2013.

59. Krishnamoorthy A. V., Optical proximity communication with passively aligned silicon photonic chips, *Journal of Quantum Electronics*, vol. 45, pp. 409–414, 2009.

60. Barkai A. et al., Double-Stage taper for coupling between soi waveguides and single-mode fiber, *Journal of Lightwave Technology*, vol. 26, pp. 3860–3865, 2008.

61. Rostami A., Rostami G., All-optical implementation of tunable low-pass, high-pass, and bandpass optical filters using ring resonators, *Journal of Lightwave Technology*, vol. 23, pp. 446–460, 2005.

62. Fang Q. et al., High efficiency ring-resonator filter with nisi heater, *Photonics Technology Letters*, vol. 24, pp. 350–352, 2012.

63. Nitkowski A., Chen L., Lipson M., Cavity-enhanced on-chip absorption spectroscopy using microring resonators, *Optics Express*, vol. 16,pp. 11930–11936, 2008.

64. Neil S. R., Rushworth C. M., Vallance C., Mackenzie S. R., Broadband cavity-enhanced absorption spectroscopy for real time, in situ spectral analysis of microfluidic droplets, *Lab on a Chip*. vol. 11, pp. 3953–3955, 2011.

65. Gupta R., Goddard N. J., A novel leaky waveguide grating (LWG) device for evanescent wave broadband absorption spectroscopy in microfluidic flow cells, *Analyst*, vol. 138, pp. 1803–1811, 2013.

66. Maune B., Lawson R., Gunn C., Scherer A., Dalton L., Electrically tunable ring resonators incorporating nematic liquid crystals as cladding layers, *Applied Physics Letters*, vol. 83, pp. 4689–4691, 2003.

67. Dalton L. R. et al., From molecules to opto-chips: Organic electro-optic materials, *Journal of Materials Chemistry*, vol. 9, pp. 1905–1920, 1999.

68. Oh M.-C., Integrated photonic devices incorporating low-loss fluorinated polymer materials, *Polymers*, vol. 3, pp. 975–997, 2011.

69. Claes T., Bogaerts W., Bienstman P., Experimental characterization of a silicon photonic biosensor consisting of two cascaded ring resonators based on the Vernier-effect and introduction of a curve fitting method for an improved detection limit. *Optics Express*, vol. 18, pp. 22747–22761, 2010.

70. Saeung P., Yupapin P. P., Vernier effect of multiple-ring resonator filters modeling by a graphical approach, *Optical Engineering*, vol. 46, pp. 075005–075009, 2007.

71. Passaro V. M. N., Troia B., De Leonardis F., A generalized approach for design of photonic gas sensors based on Vernier-effect in mid-IR, *Sensors and Actuators B: Chemical*, vol. 168, 2012.

72. Iqbal M. et al., Label-free biosensor arrays based on silicon ring resonators and high-speed optical scanning instrumentation, *Journal of Selected Topics in Quantum Electronics*, vol. 16, pp. 654–661, 2010.

73. Mario L.Y., Lim D. C. S., Chin M.-K., Proposal for an ultranarrow passband using two coupled rings, *Photonics Technology Letters*, vol. 19, pp. 1688–1690, 2007.

74. Zhang X.-Y., *Tunable Optical Ring Resonator Integrated With Asymmetric Mach–Zehnder Interferometer*, vol. 28, pp. 2512–2520, 2010.

75. Rasras M.S. et al., Demonstration of a tunable microwave-photonic notch filter using low-loss silicon ring resonators, *Journal of Lightwave Technology*, vol. 27, pp. 2105–2110, 2009.

76. Prendergast F., Mann K., Chemical and physical properties of aequorin and the green fluorescent protein isolated from aequorea forskålea, *Biochemistry*, vol. 17, pp. 3448–3453, 1978.

77. Ian F., Absolute configuration and the structure of chlorophyll. *Nature*, vol. 216, pp. 151–152, 1967.

78. Gitelson A. A., Buschmann C., Lichtenthaler H.K., The chlorophyll fluorescence ratio F735/F700 as an accurate measure of the chlorophyll content in plants. *Remote Sensing of Environment*, vol. 69, pp. 296–300, 1999.

79. Bertie J. E., Lan Z., . Infrared intensities of liquids XX: The intensity of the OH stretching band of liquid water revisited, and the best current values of the optical constants of H_2O (l) at 25°C between 15,000 and 1 cm^{-1}. *Applied Spectroscopy*, vol. 50, pp. 1047–1057, 1996.

80. Premarathne M., Agrawal G. P., *Light Propagation in Gain Media: Optical Amplifiers*, Cambridge University Press first edition (March 14, 2011), ISBN-13: 978-0521493482.

81. Siegman A. E., Lasers, University Science Books; First Edition (May 1, 1986), ISBN-13: 978-0935702118.

82. Weber G., Polarization of the fluorescence of macromolecules. 1. Theory and experimental method, *Biochemical Journal*, vol. 51, pp. 145–155, 1992.

83. Belford G. G., Belford R. L., Weber G., Dynamics of fluorescence polarization in macromolecules, *Proceedings of the National Academy of Science of U S A.*, vol. 69, pp. 1392–1393, 1972.

84. Loman A., Gregor I., Stutz C., Mund M., Enderlein J., Measuring rotational diffusion of macromolecules by fluorescence correlation spectroscopy, *Photochemical & Photobiological Sciences*, vol. 9, pp. 627–636, 2010.

85. Ito S., Kanno K., Ohmori S., Onogi Y., Yamamoto M., Fluorescence polarization method for studying molecular orientation of mono- and multilayered polyimide films prepared by the Langmuir-Blodgett technique, *Macromolecules*, vol. 24, pp 659–665, 1991.

86. Zheng J. *Spectroscopy-Based Quantitative Fluorescence Resonance Energy Transfer Analysis*. In *Ion Channels: Methods and Protocols*. Methods in Molecular Biology, Volume 337, Stockand J. D., Shapiro M. S., Totowa N. J. Editors, Humana Press, first edition (2006), ISBN-13: 978-1597450959.

87. Andrews D. L., A Unified theory of radiative and radiationless molecular energy transfer. *Chemical Physics*, vol. 135, pp. 195–201, 1989.

88. Andrews D. L., Bradshaw D. S., Virtual photons, dipole fields and energy transfer: A quantum electrodynamical approach. *European Journal of Physics*, vol. 25, pp. 845–58, 2004.

89. Du J. et al., Highly sensitive and selective chip-based fluorescent sensor for mercuric ion: Development and comparison of turn-on and turn-off systems, *Analytical Chemistry*, vol. 84, pp. 8060–8066, 2012.

90. Huang S., Chen Y., Ultrasensitive fluorescence detection of single protein molecules manipulated electrically on au nanowire, *Nano Letters*, vol. 8, pp. 2829–2833, 2008.

91. Kim J.-M. et al., A Polydiacetylene-based fluorescent sensor chip, *Journal of American Chemical Society*, vol. 127, pp. 17580–17581, 2005.

92. Hübner J. et al., Integrated optical measurement system for fluorescence spectroscopy in microfluidic channels, *Review of Scientific Instruments*, vol. 72, pp. 229–233, 2001.

93. Mcleod H. A., *Thin-Film Optical Filters*, CRC Press; 4th edition (March 16, 2010), ISBN-13: 978-14200 73027.

94. Lerose D. et al., CMOS-integrated geometrically tunable optical filters, *Applied Optics*, vol. 52, pp. 1655–1662, 2013.

95. Ohtera Y., Yamada H., Multichannel bandpass filters utilizing multilayer photonic crystal, *Optics Letters*, vol. 38, pp. 1235–1237, 2013.

96. Sharma N., V.K. Sharma V. K., K.N. Tripathi, K-resin based multilayer polymeric mode filter for integrated optics, Optik - International Journal for Light and Electron Optics, vol. 122, pp. 1719–1722, 2011.

97. *VCSELs: Fundamentals, Technology and Applications of Vertical-Cavity Surface-Emitting Lasers*, Michalzik L. Editor, Springer; 2012 edition (June 30, 2012), ISBN-13: 978-3642249853.

98. Porta P. A., Summers H. D., Vertical-cavity semiconductor devices for generation and detection of fluorescence emission on a single chip, *Applied Physics Letters*, vol. 85, pp. 1889–1891, 2004.

99. Sheridan A. K., Stewart G., Ur-Reyman H., Suyal N., Uttamchandani D., In-plane integration of polymer microfluidic channels with optical waveguides–a preliminary investigation, *Sensors Journal*, vol. 9, pp. 1627-1632, 2009.

100. Rudenko M. I., Kühn S., Lunt, E. I., Deamer D. W., Hawkins A. R., Schmidt H., Ultrasensitive Qβ phage analysis using fluorescence correlation spectroscopy on an optofluidic chip, *Biosensors and Bioelectronics* vol. 24, pp. 3258–3263, 2009.

101. Lee C.-T., Wu M.-L., Sheu L.-G., Fan P.-L., Hsu J.-M., Design and analysis of completely adiabatic tapered waveguides by conformal mapping, *Journal of Lightwave Technology*, vol. 15, pp. 403–410, 1997.

102. Campbel J. C., Tapered waveguides for guided wave optics, *Applied Optics*, vol. 18, pp. 900–902, 1979.

103. Staudt T., Lang M. C., Medda R., Engelhardt J., Hell S. W., 2,2′-thiodiethanol: A new water soluble mounting medium for high resolution optical microscopy. *Microscopy Research and Technique*, vol. 70, pp. 1–9, 2008.

104. Schmidt O., Bassler M., Kiesel P., Knollenberg C., Johnson N., Fluorescence spectrometer-on-a-fluidic-chip, *Lab on a Chip*, vol. 7, pp. 626–629, 2007.

105. *Charge-Transfer Devices in Spectroscopy*, Sweedler J. V., Ratzlaff K. L., Denton B. M., Editors, Wiley-VCH; 1st edition (February 1994), ISBN-13: 978-0471185581.

106. Manna T. L., Krull U. J., Fluorescence polarization spectroscopy in protein analysis, *Analyst*, vol. 128, pp. 313–317, 2003.

107. Pu Y., Wang W., Dorshow R. B., Das B. B., Alfano R., Review of ultrafast fluorescence polarization spectroscopy, *Applied Optics*, vol. 52, pp. 917–929, 2013.

108. Tach T., Kaji N., Tokeshi M., Baba Y., Microchip-based homogeneous immunoassay using fluorescence polarization spectroscopy, *Lab on a Chip*, vol. 9, pp. 966–971, 2009.

109. Banerjee A., Pais A., Papautsky I., Klotzkin D., A polarization isolation method for high-sensitivity, low-cost on-chip fluorescence detection for microfluidic lab-on-a-chip, *Sensors Journal*, vol. 8, pp. 621–627, 2008.

110. Müllen K., Scherf U., editors, *Organic Light Emitting Devices: Synthesis, Properties and Applications*, Wiley-VCH; 1st edition (March 7, 2006), ISBN-13: 978-3527312184.

111. Yersin H. editor, *Highly Efficient OLEDs with Phosphorescent Materials,* Wiley-VCH; 1st edition (November 28, 2007), ISBN-13: 978-3527405947.

112. Ziman J. M., *Principles of the Theory of Solids*, Cambridge University Press; 2nd edition (November 30, 1979), ISBN-13: 978-0521297332.

113. Ashcroft N. W., Mermin N. D., *Solid State Physics*, Brooks Cole; 1st edition (January 2, 1976), ISBN-13: 978-0030839931.

114. Lee Y. K., Jung C. H., Park J. Seo H., Somorjai G. A., Park J. Y., Surface plasmon-driven hot electron flow probed with metal-semiconductor nanodiodes, *Nano Letters*, vol. 11, pp. 4251–4255, 2011.

115. Pitarke J. M., Silkin V. M., Chulkov E. V., Echenique P. M., Theory of surface plasmons and surface-plasmon polaritons, *Reports on Progress in Physics*, vol. 70, pp. 1–87, 2007.

116. Raether H., *Surface Plasmons on Smooth and Rough Surfaces and on Gratings*, Springer, first edition (31 Dec 1988), ISBN-13: 978-3540173632.

117. Sarid D., Challener W., *Modern Introduction to Surface Plasmons: Theory, Mathematica Modeling, and Applications*, Cambridge University Press, first edition (May 6, 2010), ISBN-13: 978-0521767170.

118. Zeng S. et al. Size dependence of au NP-enhanced surface plasmon resonance based on differential phase measurement. *Sensors and Actuators B: Chemical*, vol. 176, pp. 1128–1134, 2012.

119. Levesque L., *Propagation of Electromagnetic Waves in Thin Dielectric and Metallic Films*, in *Electromagnetic Waves*, Zhurbenko V. Editor, InTech press first edition (2011), ISBN-13: 978-953-307-304-0, Available from: http://www.intechopen.com/books, last accessed April 24, 2013.

120. Stenzel O., *The Physics of Thin Film Optical Spectra: An Introduction*, Springer reprint of 2005 edition (November 19, 2010), ISBN-13: 978-3642062124.

121. Anker J. N. et al., Biosensing with plasmonic nanosensors, *Nature Materials* vol. 7, pp. 442 – 453, 2008.

122. Luo Y., Yua F., Zare R. N., Microfluidic device for immunoassays based on surface plasmon resonance imaging, *Lab on a Chip*, vol. 8, pp. 694–700, 2008.

123. Matveeva E., Gryczynski Z., Gryczynski I., Malicka J., Lakowicz J. R., Myoglobin immunoassay utilizing directional surface plasmon-coupled emission, *Analytical Chemistry*, vol. 76, pp 6287–6292, 2004.

124. Yu F., Persson B., Löfås S., Knoll W., Surface plasmon fluorescence immunoassay of free prostate-specific antigen in human plasma at the femtomolar level, *Analytical Chemistry*, vol. 76, pp. 6765–6770, 2004.

125. Ouellel E. et al., Parallel microfluidic surface plasmon resonance imaging arrays, *Lab on a Chip*, vol. 10, pp. 581–588, 2010.

126. Romanato F., Lee K. H., Kang H. K., Ruffato G., Wong C. C., Sensitivity enhancement in grating coupled surface plasmon resonance by azimuthal control, *Optics Express*, vol. 17, pp. 12145–12154, 2009.

127. Yuk J. S., Guignon E. F., Lynes M. A., Highly sensitive grating coupler-based surface plasmon-coupled emission (SPCE) biosensor for immunoassay, *Analyst* vol. 138, pp. 2576–2582, 2013.

128. Chen H., Shao L., Lia Q., Wang J., Gold nanorods and their plasmonic properties, *Chemical Society Reviews*, vol. 42, pp. 2679–2724, 2013.

129. Ringe E., Sharma B., Henry A.-I., Marks D. L., Van Duyne R. P., Single nanoparticle plasmonics, *Physical Chemistry, Chemical Physics*, vol. 15, pp. 4110–412, 2013.

130. Henry A.-I., Bingham J. M., Ringe E., Marks L. D., Schatz G. C. Van Duyne R. P., *Correlated Structure and Optical Property Studies of Plasmonic Nanoparticles*, vol 115, pp. 9291–9305, 2011.

131. Bohren C. F., Huffman D. R., *Absorption and Scattering of Light by Small Particles*, Wiley-VCH, first edition, (1998), ISBN-13: 978-0471293408.

132. Berne B. J., Pecora R., *Dynamic Light Scattering: With Applications to Chemistry, Biology, and Physics*, Dover Publications; Unabridged edition (August 14, 2000), ISBN-13: 978-0486411552.

133. Lynch D. K., Livingston W. C., *Color and Light in Nature*, Cambridge University Press; 2nd edition (June 18, 2001), ISBN-13: 978-0521772846.

134. Kreibig U., Vollmer M., *Optical Properties of Metal Clusters*, Springer; first edition (July 7, 1995), ISBN-13: 978-3540578369.

135. Kelly K. L., Coronado E., Zhao L. L., Schatz G. C., The Optical properties of metal nanoparticles: The influence of size, shape, and dielectric environment, *Journal of Physical Chemistry B*, vol. 107, pp. 668–677, 2003.

136. Hong Y., Huh Y.-M., Yoon D. S., Yang J., Nanobiosensors based on localized surface plasmon resonance for biomarker detection, *Journal of Nanomaterials*, vol. 2012, Article ID 759830, 13 pages, 2012.

137. Tomioka T., Kubo S., Nagase K., Hoga M., Nakagawa M., Fabrication of au nanorod and nanogap split-ring structures by reactive-monolayer-assisted thermal nanoimprint lithography involving electrodeposition, *Journal of Vacuum Science & Technology B: Microelectronics and Nanometer Structures*, vol. 30, pp. 06FB02–06FB02-7, 2012.

138. Losic D., Shapter J. G., Mitchell J. G., Voelcker N. H., Fabrication of gold nanorod arrays by templating from porous alumina, *Nanotechnology*, vol. 16, pp. 2275–2281, 2005.

139. Ahmed S., Ryan K. M., Self-assembly of vertically aligned nanorod supercrystals using highly oriented pyrolytic graphite, *Nano Letters*, vol. 7, pp. 2480–2485, 2007.

140. Szunerits S., Boukherroub R., Sensing using localised surface plasmon resonance sensors, *Chemical Communications*, vol. 48, pp. 8999–9010, 2012.

141. Mayer M. K. et al., A label-free immunoassay based upon localized surface plasmon resonance of gold nanorods, *Nano* vol. 2, pp. 687–692, 2008.

142. Stuart D. A., Haes A. J., Yonzon C. R., Hicks E. M., Van Duyne R. P., Biological applications of localised surface plasmonic phenomenae, IEE-Proceedings-Nanobiotechnology, vol. 152, pp. 13–35, 2005.

143. Ameling R., Langguth L., Hentschel M., Mesch M., Braun, P. V., Giessen H., Cavity-enhanced localized plasmon resonance sensing, *Applied Physics Letters*, vol. 97, pp. 253116–253116-3, 2010.

144. Du G.-X., Saito S., Takahashi M., Magnetic field effect on the localized plasmon resonance in patterned noble metal nanostructures, *IEEE Transaction on Magnetic*, vol. 47, pp. 3167–3169, 2011.

145. Changhong L., Mi C. C., Li B. Q., The plasmon resonance of a multilayered gold nanoshell and its potential bioapplications, *IEEE transaction on Nanotechnology*, vol. 10, pp. 797–805, 2011.

146. Nagao T., Yaginuma S., Inaoka T., Sakurai T., One-dimensional plasmons in an atomic scale metal wire, *Physical Review Letters*, vol. 97, pp. 116802–1, 116802–4, 2006.

147. Kukushkin I. V., Smet J. H., Kovalkii V. A., Gubarev S. I., von Klitzing K., Wegsheider W., Spectrum of one-dimensional plasmons in a single strip of two dimensional electrons, *Physical Review B*, vol. 72, pp. 161317–1, 161317–4, 2005.

148. Aravamudhan S., Kumar A., Mohapatra S., Bhansali S., *Sensitive estimation of total cholesterol in blood using Au nanowires based micro-fluidic platform*, Biosensors and Bioelectronics, vol. 22, pp. 2289–2294, 2007.

149. Byun K. M., Shuler M. L., Sung June K., Soon Joon Y., Donghyun K., Sensitivity enhancement of surface plasmon resonance imaging using periodic metallic nanowires, *Journal of Lightwave Technology*, vol. 26, pp. 1472–1478, 2008.

150. Svedendahl M., Chen S., Dmitriev A., Käll M., Refractometric sensing using propagating versus localized surface plasmons: A direct comparison, *Nano Letters*, vol. 9, pp. 4428–4433, 2009.

151. Mayer K. M.,Hao F., Lee S., Nordlander p., Hafner J. H., A single molecule immunoassay by localized surface plasmon resonance, *Nanotechnology*, vol. 21, pp. 255503–255508, 2010.

152. Crespi A. et al., Three-dimensional Mach–Zehnder interferometer in a microfluidic chip for spatially-resolved label-free detection, *Lab on a Chip*, vol. 10, pp. 1167–1173, 2010.

153. Briani M., Germani G., Iannone E., Moroni M., Natalini R., Design and optimization of reaction chamber and detection system in dynamic labs on chip for proteins detection, *Transactions on Biomedical Engineering*, vol. 60, pp. 2161–2166, 2013.

154. Yaffe H. H., Henry C. H., Kazarinov R. F., Milbrodt M. A., Polarization-independent silica-on-silicon Mach–Zehnder interferometers, *Journal of Lightwave Technology*, vol. 12, pp. 64–67, 1994.

155. Lanker M., Hunziker W., Melchior H., Tunable wavelength-selection switch and multiplexer/demultiplexer based on asymmetric silica-on-silicon Mach–Zehnder interferometer, *Electronics Letters*, vol. 34, pp. 266–267, 1998.

156. Lapsley M. I., Chiang K., Zheng Y. B., Ding X., Maoa X., Huang T. J., A single-layer, planar, optofluidic Mach–Zehnder interferometer for label-free detection, *Labs on a Chip*, vol. 11, pp. 1795–1800, 2011.

157. Esinenco D., Psoma S. D., Kusko M., Schneider A., Muller R., SU-8 micro-biosensor based on Mach–Zehnder interferometer, *Review of Advanced Materials Science*, vol. 10, pp. 295–299, 2005.

158. Hand D. B., The refractivity of protein solutions, *Journal of Biological Chemistry*, vol. 108, pp. 703–707, 1935.

159. Zhao H., Brown P. H., Schuck P., On the distribution of protein refractive index increments, *Biophysical Journal*, vol. 100, pp. 2309–2317, 2011.

160. Takao Y., Noritada K., Yukihiro O., Manabu T., Yasuhiro H., Yoshinobu B., *Label-Free Detection of DNA using Diffracted Laser in Nanowall Array Structures*, Proceedings of 15th International Conference on Miniaturized Systems for Chemistry and Life Sciences, Seattle, Washington, USA, pp. 54–57, 2011.

12 Building Blocks for Genetics

12.1 INTRODUCTION

The individuation, quantization, and functional analysis of specific substances from a biological sample are the tasks of the majority of lab on chip. A particular class of lab on chip however exists, with a different task: assays of nucleic acids. In its nature, a whole DNA is constituted by a sequence of code words constructed from an alphabet of four symbols, the nucleobases. Decoding such a code and studying how it works is of paramount importance both for the study of processes going on in healthy living bodies and to analyze diseases and the way they can be overcome.

DNA assays range from quantification of the DNA presence to sequencing, that is, the determination of the DNA code structure for particular beings, to the study of the interaction of DNA with other macromolecules, mainly RNA and proteins.

In this chapter, we focus on DNA assays, but several presented methods can be applied for RNA analysis too. Bibliography is also presented regarding RNA assaying for further reference.

DNA assaying can be operated with different techniques that are summarized in Section 3.8 using macroscopic laboratory equipment, but even the most advanced sequencing methods are long and complex operations. Moreover, sequencing techniques are not able to operate on a whole DNA molecule so that single fragments have to be sequenced and the obtained sequences have to be joined so as to reconstruct the whole DNA sequence. Joining subsequences is a complex and error-prone operation even if a gene only has to be sequenced, for example, in order to detect a wrong sequence in the gene expression.

For all the above reasons, DNA sequencing is a costly operation [1,2] whose use is limited today to research and specific diagnostic applications. The possibility to perform on-chip DNA sequencing and assaying could completely change this paradigm, allowing widespread application of genetic techniques in general medicine.

On-chip DNA assaying however poses a few different problems with respect to the case of lab on chip used for analytical biochemistry.

First, DNA is not available as directly dissolved in a biological fluid, but like intracellular proteins, it is present only inside cells. DNA, in particular, is present inside the cell nucleus, that is, the inner part of the cell. In order to access the DNA, cell lysis on chip has to be performed. Many macroscopic lysis methods require strong mechanical action (see Section 3.2.1), being not suitable for on-chip implementation. Lysis has to be operated with a microfabricated system without moving parts, leveraging either chemical or electrical methods, or both.

After lysis, DNA has to be extracted from the cell lysate, that is, a dense solution containing both a large number of different macromolecules and more complex parts generated by the destruction of organelles and membranes. Virtually no assay can be performed on the lysate directly, while its fluid properties render quite difficult to process it through fluid dynamic systems such as filters. The DNA has to be extracted from the lysate by dissolving it in a suitable solvent or by bonding it to microparticles through surface immobilization to render possible further processing.

Since the quantity of extracted DNA is generally small, DNA amplification through polymerase chain reaction (PCR) is generally required (see Section 3.3). Here, thermal cycles are required, besides the availability of suitable primers to generate the new DNA molecules. The chip thus has to be charged with a solution containing the primers before use and an accurate temperature control has to be present in various parts of the chip to drive the PCR process.

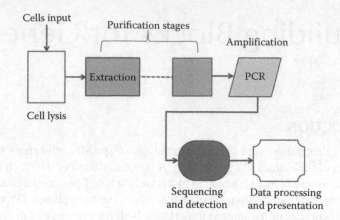

FIGURE 12.1 Functional scheme of a chip for DNA sequencing: extraction is here considered the first purification step.

After PCR, a sequencing method has to be implemented on the chip. Several methods are possible with characteristics suitable for miniaturization (see Section 3.8). In any case, however, it is a multistep biochemical process implying frequent optical detection and the use of several chemical reagents and in several cases selected nucleic acids primers.

Chips for DNA sequencing and assaying thus tend to be even more complex with respect to chip for analytical biochemistry, requiring an increased attention to back-end techniques typical of lab on chip such as chemical reagent insertion in the chip and local temperature control.

If we collect the considered steps, the functional scheme of a chip for DNA sequencing can be represented as in Figure 12.1. In the course of this chapter, we will analyze in some detail the implementation of the functional blocks that are represented in the figure.

12.2 ON-CHIP DNA PURIFICATION

The first step of any DNA-based analysis is the DNA purification, that is, the extraction of the DNA from the cell nucleus and its processing up to the production of the wanted DNA solution or DNA immobilization on the surface of a suitable vessel.

While the first step is almost independent of the type of processing implemented in the lab on chip, depending mainly on the cell type, the second step of the process is strictly related to the type of method selected for DNA analysis.

12.2.1 CELL LYSIS

Different methods have been proposed for on-chip cell lysis [3]; in general, they can be classified into four main categories:

- Mechanical lysis employs cellular contact forces to crush or burst the cells.
- Thermal lysis uses high temperatures to disrupt the cell membrane.
- Chemical lysis uses a chemical buffer or enzymes to break down the cell membrane.
- Electrical lysis induces cell membrane porosity with a low-strength electric field to ease complete lysis operated with other methods or perform a complete lysis of cells with a stronger field.

Such a variety of possible methods is justified by the wide array of situations in which cell lysis on chip is required. The main factors influencing the choice of the lysis method are the dimension of the cells to be disrupted, the sample dimension, and the cell. The largest among the cells have linear dimensions of the order of 50 mm, with a maximum length of the order of 100 μm. The smallest cells have linear dimensions of the order of 1 μm. This great dimension range strongly influences the structure of the chip part where lysis is performed. The sample dimension influences how important it is not to lose cells in the processing either because they are not disrupted or because after disruption the DNA results in any case not to be accessible to extraction. Finally, the cell toughness determines the required strength of the disruption forces. For example, *Escherichia coli*, blood cells, and brain tissue cells are relatively easy to disrupt and mild lysis methods can be used. More difficult samples, for example, yeast, fungi, and animal connective tissue, often require increased mechanical power or more aggressive chemical treatments in macroscopic lysis systems. An equivalent disruption force can be exerted on chip by using aggressive chemical reactions and strong electrical fields, but in these cases, care has to be paid to preserve the integrity of the DNA for further on-chip processing.

The most difficult samples, for example, spores, are disrupted in biochemical labs by strong mechanical forces combined with chemical or enzymatic methods. Disruption on chip of such cells is very difficult if integrity of intracellular molecules has to be preserved.

12.2.1.1 Mechanical Lysis

Cell lysis occurs when the cell membrane is disrupted allowing the contents of the cytoplasm to be released. The most conceptually simple method to achieve lysis is to use a mechanical force to tear or puncture the membrane.

One method for mechanical lysis is to force the cell through a filter with openings too small for a whole cell to pass through, thus shearing the cell membrane. This causes the cell to rupture and the contents to spill out [4]. The same effect can be obtained by using the shear stress caused in a T junction if the cells to be leased are carried out by the central flow whose width is reduced traveling after the junction [5]. The scheme of such a system is reported in Figure 12.2 while the main hydrodynamic variables of the system are evaluated in Section 8.7.

In order to avoid the use of high hydraulic pressures and to reduce the system dimension, such method can be improved by realizing on the filter walls sharp nanoscale barbs acting like "microknives" on the cell membrane [6,7]. Such structures can be fabricated with different shapes, such as nanoblades of nanowires, and interposed to the fluid flow where cells are contained as shown in Figure 12.3. Nanoblades can also be inserted in a system designed for cell lysis by squeezing thereby improving the amount of lysis compared to filtering cells through a similar sized filter with smooth walls.

Another basic method is simply to burst the cells by deforming the cell to the point that the membrane bursts [8]. A strong deformation of the cell membrane can be obtained by different means, such as crushing the cells against a polymeric membrane [5]. In this case, the fluid channel through

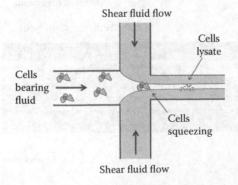

FIGURE 12.2   Example of on-chip mechanical cell lysing by shear stress in a T junction.

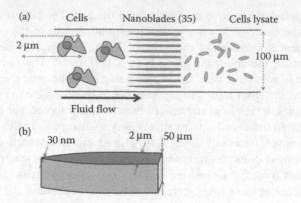

FIGURE 12.3 Example of on-chip mechanical cell lysing by the use of nanoblades. Duct structure with a nanoblade obstacle (a) and nanoblade structure (b).

which the cells flow is shaped to have a curved cross section on one side while the other side is a flat membrane separating the fluid channel from an actuator like those used in membrane-based valves (see Section 8.2) as shown in Figure 12.4a. The actuator forces the membrane to expand into the fluid channel and crush any cells trapped there. This basic design is used in a chip that can pull cell-containing fluid from a reservoir, seal the cell solution into a chamber with valves, and lyse the cells by crushing them with the membrane before sending the lysed solution to the outlet. As the pressure on the cells is slowly increased from ambient, the cells flatten out as they are compressed and deformed. Once pressure approaches a threshold dependent on the fluid system parameters, the cells begin to split open and spill their internal cellular structures.

Sonication (see Section 3.2.1.4) is another form of mechanical cell lysis that differs from the physical contact methods employing ultrasonic agitation to create pressure waves with enough energy to disrupt the cell, causing it to lyse. This method is used in widely diffused macroscopic equipment and it can be extended to on-chip lysis [9–11]. The most diffused method to generate ultrasound waves into the cell containing fluid is to use a piezoelectric actuator placed in contact

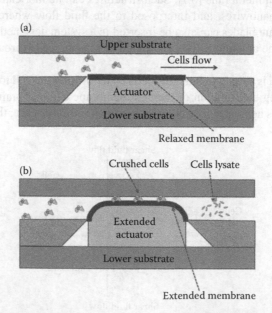

FIGURE 12.4 On-chip cell lysis using an actuated membrane. Cell flow with a relaxed membrane (a), and cell crush when the membrane is activated (b).

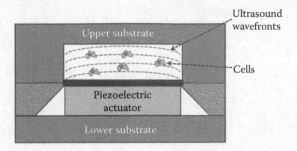

FIGURE 12.5   Principle scheme of a sonication-based on-chip cell lysis system incorporating a piezoelectric actuator.

with a chamber where the cells are suspended in a static liquid as shown in Figure 12.5; however, other configurations can be devised.

Sonication lysis can also be enhanced by the presence of sharp obstacles such as nanowires or nanoblades to combine two different lysis methods [12].

12.2.1.2   Thermal lysis

Thermal lysis is one of the more well-established lysis techniques in nucleic acid preparation, and is common in laboratory settings (see Section 3.2.1.6). This lysis method is, however, more difficult to integrate on a lab on chip, due both to the need of integrating heaters, which are not always needed for other on-chip processes, and for the required power, which could imply a relatively high feeding voltage of the chip, not compatible with portable devices.

Thermal lysis is frequently used on chip in conjunction with PCR-based assays [13]. The most common method to induce a heating of the cells is to store the cells in a chamber where a micro-heater is fabricated (see Section 6.6.3) [13,14]. This system is effective for single samples, but cannot be used as part of a continuous-flow assay or with downstream analysis techniques that require a sample free of protein and other cellular contaminants.

The simple heater system can be improved by allowing use in continuous-flow systems by moving the cells via an electrokinetic effect through a large duct where temperature is controlled by an integrated heater so as to obtain cell lysis to a final chamber where PCR is performed. Microelectrodes deposited on the lower glass substrate control the flow of cellular material through the chip while two sets of microheaters and microtemperature sensors control and monitor the temperature of the lysis [15].

An alternative method for heating the cells is to use a heating coil wrapped around the cell lysis chamber, thus avoiding the fabrication of an integrated heater [16]. A last possibility to heat the cell containing liquid without the need of an integrated microheater is to use a laser source that can be either integrated using hybrid techniques on the device or hosted in an external equipment. Gold nanorods have been built into the lysis chamber to convert in the optimum way the radiation energy of an 880 nm laser into heat demonstrating that an optimum rod aspect ratio exists [17] to generate effective lysis.

12.2.1.3   Chemical Lysis

In chemical lysis, buffers or other lytic agents are employed to break down the cell membrane. The wide range of sample cell types and target molecules accounts for the variety of chemicals used in lysis protocols [3].

Ammonium chloride, which is the main component of the lysis buffer known as red blood cell (RBC) buffer, acts on erythrocytes only and is ineffective in lysing nonerythrocytic mammalian cells. Nonionic and ionic detergents disrupt cell membranes by solubilizing membrane proteins and lipids and creating pores. Triton X (see Figure 12.6a), a nonionic detergent, acts more slowly and is

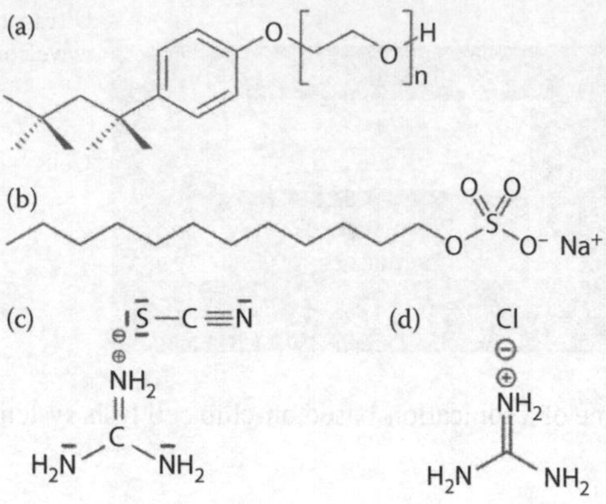

(a)

(b)

(c)   (d)

FIGURE 12.6 Structural formulas of triton X 100 (a), sodium dodecyl sulfate (b), guanidinium thiocyanate, (c) and guanidinium chloride (d).

primarily used in sample preparations for downstream assays requiring protein structure and function to be maintained. Sodium dodecyl sulfate (SDS, see Figure 12.6b), an ionic detergent, acts more quickly to totally denature proteins, and is primarily used in protein assays such as determination of molecular weight. SDS is also used in sample preparations for nucleic acid, as SDS denatures DNAse and RNAse enzymes [18]. As detergents act on cell membranes, they are incapable of bacterial lysis without a pretreatment to destroy the cell wall, and often follow an enzymatic degradation step such as treatment with lysozyme.

Chaotropic salts are commonly used in nucleic acid preparations. At high concentrations, guanidinium thiocyanate and guanidinium chloride (see Figure 12.6c and d) lyse cell membranes by disrupting protein intermolecular forces. They denature RNAses as well as membrane proteins, and so are valuable in nucleic acid extraction. The high salt concentration also allows the salt bridge that forms to extract RNA in silica environments (see Section 3.2.2.2). In principle, almost all the macroscopic techniques can be extended in a microfluidic environment if cells suspended in a suitable solution are mixed in a lysis chamber with a lysis buffer.

An effective way to join chemical lysis with fluid dynamic filtering to obtain a first separation stage embedded in the lysis system is presented in Figure 12.7 [19]. A sample containing the cells is injected into a fluid channel where it meets another solution containing a chemical lysing agent.

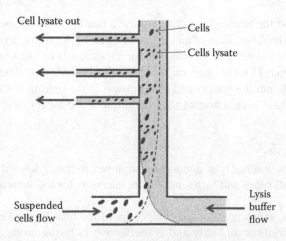

FIGURE 12.7 Example of microfluidic system architecture joining chemical lysis with fluid dynamic filtering.

After the two fluids join, they flow down a long channel that gives the lysing agent time to diffuse into the cell sample and disrupt the cell membranes. The fluid then comes to a fluid dynamic filtering when macromolecules coming from the cell lysate are divided by remaining cells and the bigger cell fragments. This device illustrates the ability of chemical lysis techniques to operate in a continuous-flow mode, which will enable high-throughput devices.

Different mixing configurations can be used to enhance the lysis efficiency and to obtain smaller devices [20–22].

Chemical cell lysis can also be operated by fixing cells before lysis in suitable blocking structures. Cells can be trapped in suitable polymers such as hydrogels [23] or in artificial traps such as microwells [24] or in different types of traps [25].

12.2.1.4 Electrical Lysis

Exposure of cells to strong electric fields can compromise cell membranes sufficiently to induce cell lysis. As cells are exposed to high-intensity pulsed electric fields, membranes are destabilized and become transiently permeable to macromolecules.

Electrically induced lysis can be attained by applying a constant voltage to a couple of electrodes at the extremes of a microfluidic channel where the cell containing buffer flows or by using a pulsed electrical excitation. As the electric field strength and, in case of pulsed systems, the pulse length reach a critical value, the cell is lysed by dielectric breakdown of the cell membrane [26,27]. Though the exact mechanism of increased permeability and lysis by electric fields is not fully understood, it has been shown that cell lysis occurs due to an electrical effect, and not as a result of Joule heating or electrolysis of the solution.

In case of both constant excitation and pulsed applied voltage, the critical electric field value is the most important parameter for lysis. It varies between types of bacteria and mammalian cells due to deviations in cell shape and radius, though this relationship has been mathematically determined and is well understood [28]. In general, cell membrane lysis is induced in both cases when the average potential of the membrane is of the order of 1–1.5 V, which means the application of electrical fields of the order of 10–50 kV/cm. Moreover, if pure electrical lysis is desired, hydrolysis of the buffer solution has to be avoided, so that the applied field does not have to overcome the hydrolysis threshold. Finally, energy loss due to Joule heating has to be minimized as the applied electrical energy has to be efficiently used for lysis.

Electrical on-chip lysis using a constant applied voltage has been implemented in several lab on chip prototypes [29,30] with different electrode geometry and fluid constants. This is a simple method in terms of chip fabrication and it is quite suitable for flow systems, thus allowing a good throughput compared to other on-chip cell lysis systems. The electrode material and design is a fundamental element in such systems, both to obtain effective lysis and to limit the great number of spurious effects that could arise by the application of a strong electrical field [31].

A very simple approach for a practical evaluation of the system parameters in this case is to associate to the critical electric field a critical electromagnetic energy that has to be reached to attain effective lysis. If the lysis channel is considered from an electromagnetic point of view, a system contained between parallel infinite conducting plates and a distance equal to d, the electrical field can be written as

$$E = \frac{\Delta\psi}{d} \tag{12.1}$$

where $\Delta\psi$ is the applied voltage. Evaluating the electrical field energy density and integrating it over the volume occupied by a cell, we obtain the following expression of the electromagnetic energy ε_E in the cell volume

$$\varepsilon_E = \frac{2}{3}\pi\varepsilon\,\Delta\psi^2\,\frac{R^3}{d^2} \tag{12.2}$$

where ε is the buffer dielectric constant and R the equivalent cell radius. However, accurate simulation [32] of the system using the Laplace equation for the evaluation of a realistic distribution of the electrical field and the Poisson–Boltzmann equation to define the charge distribution on the surface of a cell, which is considered as a dielectric particle, shows that the comparison of Equation 12.2 with a threshold energy simply provides an indication of the order of magnitude of the required applied potential. More accurate phenomenological expressions can be introduced from the study of simulation results that can be used to guide the system design.

In the case in which pulsed excitation is used, the lysis dynamics is even more complex than in the case of continuous excitation [33], and more parameters have to be controlled to design an efficient lysis system. Pulse length and duty cycle must also be set within critical parameters in case a pulsed excitation is used, with minimum DC square pulse thresholds as low as 4.5 ms for many bacterial cells.

Different architectures have been considered to obtain efficient lysis by pulsed electrical action. Both lysis of cells immobilized in traps or in microwells [34] and lysis of cells suspended in liquid buffer [35] have been demonstrated and electrical action has been coupled for synergic effect both with chemical and thermal action [36–38]. An important design factor in on-chip pulsed electrical cell lysis is the electrode design. As a matter of fact, a good electrode design allows both the spurious energy loss by Joule heating to be minimized and an effective concentration of the electromagnetic energy in the zone where the cells are present, thus minimizing the voltage that is required to obtain a good lysis process.

An alternative way to obtain cell lysis is by applying a voltage to obtain local hydroxide electrogeneration [39]. Lysis is consequently obtained by a high local value of the buffer pH. In a suitable arrangement of the microfluidic chip, the lysate can be separated by the residual cells and possible big cell fragments by a filter and residual OH⁻ ions can be neutralized by anodic H⁺ ion generation, so as to return to an almost neutral buffer situation. A possible chip arrangement [39] is shown in Figure 12.8. The chip is constituted by a couple of chambers separated by a filter constituted by a set of microducts with a too small diameter to accommodate cells. Hydroxide generation is obtained in the first chamber where the cathode is located; due to the hydrodynamic pressure, the lysate passes through the microducts in the second room where hydrogen ions neutralize the residue hydroxyl ions to obtain a finale lysate solution of the desired pH.

The limit of this architecture is constituted by the fact that the filter dividing the two chambers is clogged by residual cells so that the chip operation cannot be prolonged too much in time, but a

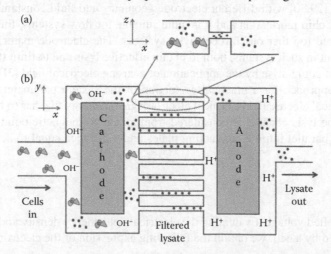

FIGURE 12.8 Example of chip design for a system operating cell lysis via electrostimulated local generation of hydroxide ions: top view of the chip under the upper substrate (a) and chip section in correspondence of the lysate filter (b).

more complex fluid arrangement based on periodic fluid dynamic wash of residual cells from the first chamber can be devised to overcome this limitation.

The use of high pH buffer, even if only for a transitory process, could denature macromolecules, thus impairing successive assay or sequencing. In case of DNA, alkaline conditions induced by sodium hydroxide are used in macroscopic assays to recover plasmid DNA arriving up to a pH of the order of 12.0 so that if the quantity of generated hydroxide is well controlled, this problem does not exist. In case of proteins or RNA with a complex tertiary structure on the contrary, unfolding often occurs at elevated pH. However, a number of proteins have been shown to refold to their native conformation when returned to normal pH, after a brief exposure to high pH values [40,41]; thus, if a similar protein has to be extracted, this method can be safely used.

The main advantage of the electrical lysis based on local hydroxide generation on standard electrical lysis by electroporation is the quite low voltage at which the process can be generated that for carefully designed chips can reach values of 2.5–5 V that are compatible with consumer electronics standards.

12.2.1.5 Comparison of On-Chip Lysis Techniques

The design considerations that are important for an on-chip cell lysis element and the different techniques that are described in this section are compared in Table 12.1 [3,33]. The table gives an overview of the four major lysis categories, with the understanding that there could be specific devices or applications within those categories that do not agree with the generalized statement applied to the group as a whole.

Knowing the typical fabrication techniques to create a cell lysis device will help understand what capabilities are required for manufacturing and how easily it could be produced in conjunction with later chip components. Information on the required controls will aid in determining if the device will work in the desired application environment. The lysis time is included in the table to help

TABLE 12.1
Summary and Comparison of Different On-Chip Cell Lysing Techniques

Method	Fabrication	Controls	Active Fluidic Elements	Lysis Time	Notes
Chemical	Polymers and silicon. Soft lithography and micromolding possible	Temperature and flow	Valves	0.5–3 min	Different chemistry for different cells and for different targets
Electrical	Silicon or glass preferred, electrode deposition. Electroplating with polymers	Voltage/current	–	10 ms–20 min	Frequently integrated with electrophoresis. Lysis time depends on geometry, electrodes, and applied voltage. Not all proteins can be used if electrogeneration of hydroxide is used
Mechanical	Polymers, glass, and silicon. Silicon preferred with nanoblades. Microfabrication, DRIE for nanoblades	Flow control	Pumps, actuators for membranes, ultrasonic generation	30 s–10 min	More involved fabrication and device operation. Very adaptable to different cells and targets
Thermal	Silicon preferred if microheaters are used	Temperature and flow	–	2–5 min	Increasing pressure allows the use of high temperature, avoiding buffer boiling so as to speed up the lysis

construct a picture of the time required for the system to operate. Finally, additional comments for consideration are included that might be specific to that cell lysis technique.

The type of cell lysis component can be chosen depending on what constraints are imposed by the microfluidic system. For example, if a system is being designed to be highly portable, it might be important to choose a cell lysis component that does not require excessive external controls, so a chemical system might be a good choice.

12.2.2 Nucleic Acid Extraction

Once cells or samples have been lysed and nucleic acid is freed from the cell, sensing systems require the nucleic acid to be purified, concentrated, and frequently amplified before they can be assayed. Thus, a number of nucleic acid extraction techniques have been developed for application in lab on chip [42].

Microfluidic nucleic acid extraction techniques can be categorized in terms of the basic mechanism that gives rise to the nucleic acid separation:

- Silica-based surface affinity
- Electrostatic interaction
- Nanoporous membrane filtration
- Functionalized microparticles

12.2.2.1 Silica-Based Surface Affinity Extraction

Micro-solid-phase extraction is widely used in genetic analysis macroscopic laboratory systems (see Section 3.2.2) and it is also widely used in lab on chip for its compatibility with lab on chip materials and microfluidic structure [43,44]. An example of nucleic acid extraction section of a lab on chip is represented in Figure 12.9.

Nucleic acid is able to bind with silica or glass fibers in high-ionic-strength solutions due to decreases in the electrostatic repulsion. After washing with a nonpolar solvent, DNA is eluted with a low-ionic-strength buffer. Thus, three different repositories are present on the chip of Figure 12.9: a sample repository where the cell lysate is stored, a high-pH buffer repository, and a low-pH buffer repository. In a first phase, the sample and the high pH buffer are pumped together in the fluid circuit while valve 1 is open and valve 2 is closed. While traveling through the duct filled with porous silica, DNA molecules are absorbed in the silica pores and the high pH buffer is accumulated in the waste. In a second phase, after closing valve 1 and opening valve 2, the low pH buffer is pumped through the silica so as to elute the DNA. The obtained purified solution is accumulated in the suitable repository for further processing.

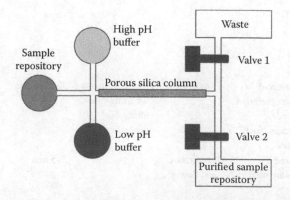

FIGURE 12.9 Example of chip design for DNA extraction from cell lysate through absorption in silica gel matrix.

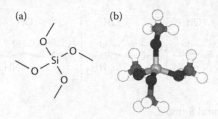

FIGURE 12.10 Structural formula (a) and stereographic representation (b) of the tetramethylorthosilicate molecule.

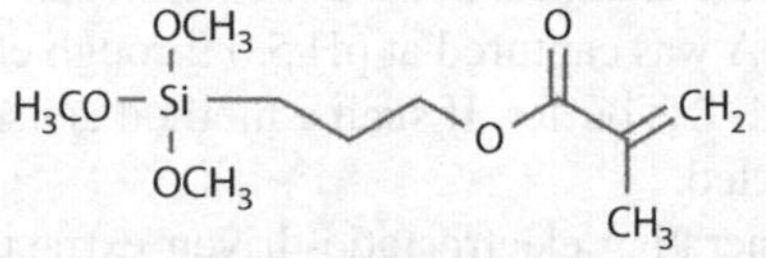

FIGURE 12.11 Trimethoxysilylpropyl methacrylate (TMSPM) monomer structure formula.

A microdevice containing only a nanogram of silica resin has been shown to be effective for the adsorption and desorption of DNA in a chaotropic salt solution. A sol–gel matrix and hybrid sol–gel/silica bead matrices within microchannels have also been successfully used [45]. Comparing the extraction efficiency of the three different immobilization techniques, hybrid sol–gel/silica bead matrices were found to be the most effective, showing ≈90% extraction efficiency from the λ-DNA experiment.

Considering the insertion of the hybrid sol–gel/silica matrix into the microfluidic channels, however, it is found that it exhibits bonding and shrinkage problems between the microchannel wall and the matrix. Owing to these problems, the surface area, which is critical in the binding process with DNA, decreased and the purity of the eluted DNA sample also decreased. To compensate for these problems, tetramethylorthosilicate (TMOS)-based sol–gel matrices with micropores were developed and used to extract the DNA. Tetramethylorthosilicate consists of four methyl groups attached to the SiO_4^{4-} group, as shown in Figure 12.10.

Photopolymerized silica-based column can also be embedded into lab on chips using a sol–gel solution of trimethoxysilylpropyl methacrylate (TMSPM) monomers, whose structure formula is presented in Figure 12.11. Photopolymerization can be obtained after the introduction of the initiator solution in the fluid duct by UV exposure of the interested zone of the chip.

The key points in implementing effective extraction using this technique are the design of the microfluidic channel, the buffer choice, and the silica matrix insertion technology. Optimization can be carried out both from a fluidic and a chemical point of view, selecting optimized buffer to work with specific silica structures [43,46].

12.2.2.2 Electrostatic Interaction-Based Extraction

A variety of nucleic acid extraction techniques based on electrostatic interactions between DNA and modified surfaces have been demonstrated. The most basic rely on an amine surface coating. Amine groups below neutral pH have a positive charge, causing negatively charged DNA to bind. Above neutral pH, this effect decreases so as to become very weak [47,48]. Isolation of DNA from cell lysate and elution in a suitable buffer can thus be controlled through the buffer pH change.

From a pure extraction point of view, this is an easy-to-implement and effective method; however, it can affect the DNA amplification step due to the high pH required for elution [26,27]. To overcome this pH problem associated with typical electrostatic methods, a chitosan surface-coated microfluidic duct can be used [49]. Chitosan, whose structural formula is reported in Figure 12.12, is a linear polysaccharide composed of randomly distributed β-(1-4)-linked D-glucosamine and

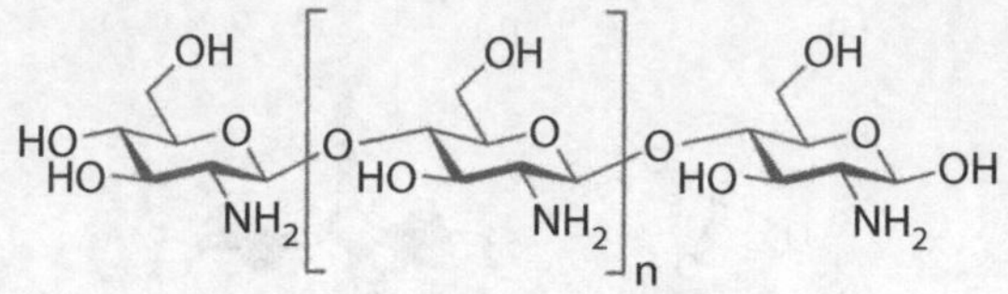

FIGURE 12.12 Chitosan structural formula.

N-acetyl-D-glucosamine (acetylated unit). It is made by treating shrimp and other crustacean shells with the alkali sodium hydroxide. Chitosan has a cationic charge at pH 5 and is easily neutralized at pH 9. High-density microfluidic channels coated with chitosan were fabricated and tested with lysed whole-blood samples. DNA was captured at pH 5.0 through electrostatic interactions with the chitosan and eluted using pH 9.1 Tris buffer. If such a method is used, no problem with subsequent PCR amplification will be detected.

Another possible way of generating electrostatic-driven extraction is creating a polycarbonate (PC) surface with positively charged carbonyl/carboxyl functional groups by an UV driver on-site polymerization reaction on the duct walls before closing the chip with the upper substrate. The buffer selection is very important to also obtain good immobilization in this case, but very good results can be achieved without any apparent problem in the case of subsequent amplification [50].

12.2.2.3 Nanoporous Membrane Filtration-Based Extraction

Filtration by nanoporous membrane is a combination of sieving and electrostatic interaction-based extraction. Different types of membrane can be used, the choice being mainly constrained by the compatibility with the adopted fabrication process flow. Aluminum oxide can be obtained as a nanoporous membrane working effectively for DNA separation [51]. In this case, the membrane can be directly built on a wall of the lysis chamber and the extracted DNA can be collected on the membrane surface opposite to the lysis chamber by washing, for example, with a suitable buffer after lysis completion. Under high-salt conditions, the DNA collection rate increases due to strengthened interactions between DNA, the surface, and the aggregation of the DNA itself. During elution, higher pH and anionic solutions allow higher extraction efficiencies.

The DNA extraction efficiency depends on the pore size and homogeneity of the membrane [52] and a membrane optimization can be carried out if the pores are artificially patterned, for example, excavating them in a horizontal membrane micromachined on the lab on chip (see Section 4.2). Pores with a diameter of the order of 100 nm can be obtained by using high-resolution lithography both on silicon membranes and on SU8 deposited on polymer substrate [53] so as to obtain efficient and regular membranes.

12.2.2.4 Functionalized Microparticle-Based Extraction

Nanoparticles with DNA adsorbent surfaces have been extensively used for DNA extraction. Magnetic particles coated with silica or functionalized carboxyl groups have been used to extract DNA from biological samples [17,54,55]. Magnetic nanoparticle coated either with amino group or with silica gel can be used to selectively bind DNA while magnetophoresis (see Section 7.6.2) can be used to extract the nanoparticles from the lysate and move them to a reservoir where a suitable buffer is present. Here, the DNA can be released in the buffer due to its chemical action.

An alternative technique to cause DNA release in the final buffer without any chemical action on the target DNA is to increase the buffer chamber temperature so as to weaken the forces binding the DNA to the nanoparticles. This technique is particularly suited when PCR amplification is performed immediately after the extraction so that integrated heaters have to be fabricated on chip too perform amplification.

Magnetic nanoparticles can also be coated with sequence-specific probes [56] such as complementary DNA sequences or specific aptamers. Using this technique, it is possible to extract species-specific DNA, but a few extra steps are required to functionalize the magnetic particles and more time is needed to effectively hybridize the target and the probe.

A drawback to using magnetic particles in microfluidic systems is that appropriate micromanipulating systems need to be implemented to control the magnetic field. Microfabricated coils can be realized on chip (see Section 8.2.2.1), but their fabrication constrains the lab on chip process flow and dimensions.

12.2.2.5 Comparison among On-Chip DNA Extraction Methods

A brief summary of different aspects of the considered on-chip extraction technologies is reported in Table 12.2. In the table, the extraction efficiency indicates what percentage of input nucleic acid has been extracted. Integration difficulty compares the ability of each extraction technique to be integrated on the same chip with other microfluidic components such as lysis or analysis systems.

Each of the different techniques has some clear advantages over the others, so that each specific device will use a specific technique depending on the application requirements. For example, physical filtration is more suitable for use in disposable components while microfabricated columns and extraction techniques based on magnetic particle control require expensive fabrication processes that limit disposability, but may be more useful for repeated use and have a smaller footprint.

12.2.2.6 RNA Extraction

Almost all on-chip extraction procedures are designed for DNA, due to both the great interest in DNA processing related, for example, to genetic research, drug discovery, and clinical applications, and the stability problems related to the treatment of RNA on chip. RNA has a life time of the order of minutes once extracted from its natural environment and several RNA enzymes exist in the cell, causing even faster RNA degradation once freed [57]. Last but not least, small RNA is difficult to insulate from similar RNAs that can be present in the cell.

Typically different techniques are used to extract RNA from lysates obtained from different kinds of cells.

The mRNA of eukaryotic cells is generally characterized by the so-called 3′ poly(A) tail. This is a long sequence of adenine nucleotides, often several hundred, added to the 3′ end of the mRNA. This tail promotes export from the nucleus and translation, and protects the mRNA from degradation. The presence of this very particular characteristic can be exploited to extract mRNA linking it to oligo-dTs. These molecules are often coated on the surface of paramagnetic beads that, once the mRNA is captured, can be moved through the microfluidic circuit using magnetic fields. This technique, which is used both on chip and in standard experimental setup, has a low efficiency, but the quantity of extracted mRNA is generally sufficient for the required use [58].

Magnetic particles with activated surface suitable to capture RNA molecules can also be used to detect viral RNA, for example, with the goal of virus identification. A possible coating molecule

TABLE 12.2
Summary and Comparison of Different on On-Chip DNA Extraction Techniques

Technique	Fabrication Difficulty	On-Chip Integration	Efficiency	Speed
Solid-phase extraction	Medium	Difficult	Around 90%	15–20 min
Electrostatic	Medium	Difficult	60–80%	25–30 min
Physical filtration	Low	Possible with care	Around 90%	5–10 min
Magnetic particles	High	Easy	Around 80%	10 min

Source: Data from Kim J., Johnson M., Hill P., Gale B. K., *Integrative Biology*, vol. 1, pp. 574–586, 2009.

for this kind of extraction is streptavidin. In this case, the target RNA has to be biotinylated before capture by the activated surface so as to exploit the strong avidin–biotin interaction (see Section 9.5.1) [59].

The main challenge related to the use of magnetic beads is the complexity of system fabrication and use: magnetic beads have to be separately fabricated and, in case coated, inserted during the fabrication stage into the lab on chip where a suitable magnetic system has to be built to move them. Finally, magnetic perturbations have to be avoided during use to assure a repeatable assay.

A more robust extraction system for mRNA from eukaryotic cells can be obtained by packing a microfluidic system with a UV-initiated methacrylate-based porous polymer monolith. This structure can be casted into the capillary constituting a microfluidic circuit and provides a large surface area, good adhesion, and stability within a microfluidic channel. In addition, the surface of a PPM is easy to modify with various amide-terminated functional groups [60].

All the above-cited mRNA extraction techniques exploit the poly(A) tails of the target molecules; thus, they cannot be used for rRNA and for RNA from prokaryote cells. In order to extract these kinds of RNA, different immobilization methods are required. An example is the use of photoactivated PC solid-phase reversible immobilization, which has been already considered analyzing DNA immobilization [61].

12.3 ON-CHIP PCR AMPLIFICATION

After nucleic acid extraction from cell lysate, PCR is generally performed to increase the number of molecules that are available for the subsequent assay.

12.3.1 STATIONARY PCR AMPLIFICATION

On-chip PCR can be performed using a protocol similar to the macroscopic equivalent describer in Section 3.3 and shown in Figure 3.6. The on-chip PCR procedure steps can be briefly described as follows [62,63]:

- *Sample injection*: The sample is injected in the PCR chamber besides the other composites that are required by amplification. Mixing can either happen in the chamber itself or in a previous mixer, so as to inject in the PCR chamber the whole solution that will provoke DNA amplification.
- *Hot start*: This is a means to reduce nonspecific amplifications during the start phase of the PCR by adding to the system specialized enzymes that inhibit the amplification action at ambient temperature (Section 3.3). Such substances dissociate or deactivate after exposure at high temperature. Thus, an initialization step is needed by heating the reaction components to the denaturation temperature (e.g., 95°C) before adding the polymerase. Even if hot start is not required in principle for PCR to work, it is very frequently used when amplification is performed on chip. Miniaturization causes a great reduction of the volume-to-surface ratio of the PCR chamber, thus increasing the impact of nonspecific interactions of the polymerase enzyme that very frequently happens near the chamber surface. For this reason, limiting nonspecific activity of the polymerase enzyme is a key point in on-chip PCR.
- *Denaturation step*: This step is the first regular cycling event and consists of heating the reaction to 94°C–98°C for 20–30 s. It causes disruption of the hydrogen bonds generating the helix–turn–helix tertiary structure of the DNA (see Section 2.5.1) and yielding single-stranded DNA molecules.
- *Annealing step*: The reaction temperature is lowered to 50°C–65°C for 20–40 s, allowing annealing of the primers to the single-stranded DNA template. Typically, the annealing temperature is about 3°C–5°C below the melting temperature of the primers used. Stable

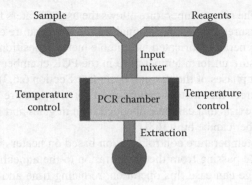

FIGURE 12.13   Principle structure of on-chip stationary PCR subsystem.

DNA–DNA hydrogen bonds are only formed when the primer sequence very closely matches the template sequence. The polymerase binds to the primer–template hybrid and begins DNA formation.

- *Extension/elongation step*: At this step, the DNA polymerase synthesizes a new DNA strand complementary to the DNA template strand by adding dNTPs that are complementary to the template in 5′–3′ direction, condensing the 5′-phosphate group of the dNTPs with the 3′-hydroxyl group at the end of the nascent, called extending, DNA strand. The extension time depends both on the DNA polymerase used and on the length of the DNA fragment to be amplified. As a rule of thumb, at its optimum temperature, the DNA polymerase will polymerize a thousand bases per minute.
- *Amplified sample extraction*: After PCR, the amplified sample is extracted from the amplification sample, by a filtering operation, and sent to different sections of the chip for further processing such as quantification or sequencing.

During the amplification process, the sample and the PRC reagents are still in the reaction chamber, from which the name of stationary PCR, and essentially sustain a series of thermal cycles. Thus, the on-chip PCR section can be represented as in Figure 12.13. Here, we can individuate three main elements: the PCR chamber itself, the injection section, operating both mixing and real injection in the PCR chamber, and the extraction system.

12.3.1.1   On-Chip PCR Temperature Control

Precise temperature control is required in all the PCR steps to optimize the PCR efficiency; moreover, temperature uniformity in the PCR chamber and a fast transient between different phases of the thermal cycle are also important elements. Thus, the temperature control system has to be carefully designed. It is possible to realize three on-chip thermal cycling methods with suitable accuracy:

- External heating and chip temperature control
- Use of integrated heater and thermistors
- Use of discrete or integrated Peltier junctions

In the first example of on-chip PCR, the chip heating was achieved by an external heater, for example, a lamp, and the on-board temperature was measured with a discrete temperature sensor, for example, a thermistor (see Section 6.6.1) [64,65]. This system is only suitable for chips that have to be used in laboratories, but it has the advantage of allowing a careful temperature control by well-established laboratory systems.

If the thermal cycling system has to be integrated on board of the chip, a first fabrication technology is based on the use of integrated heaters and thermistors. The fact that the temperature of all the

PCR cycles is higher than the room temperature allows the use of heaters for temperature regulation and suitable thermistors assures the feedback signal for the temperature control loop [66,67].

Integrated heaters are generally fabricated by suitable metal depositions and can be shaped in an optimized way so as to assure uniform temperature in the PCR chamber and a good control of the transient between different phases of the thermal cycle (see Section 6.6.3).

Both integrated or discrete thermistors can be used for temperature measurement, since very small discrete thermistors exists that can be embedded both in glass and in many passive polymers with which the PCR chamber can be built [68].

The main problem of a temperature control solution based on heaters is only related to the need of cooling the system while passing from the denaturation to the annealing step. A careful design of the chip external package can ease this operation, reducing time and maintaining temperature uniformity, but this remains a long transient step, requiring even minutes. In order to avoid such problems, both reducing efficiency and increasing duration, forced chip ventilation has been proposed [66]. Even if a very small fan is required so that energy consumption is rarely an issue, this solution is suitable only for selected applications.

Both heating and cooling can be obtained by using a Peltier junction (see Section 6.6.2) so that this is the most suitable solution for PCR chips, but for the high cost of a small Peltier of the required characteristics with respect to a microfluidic chip, especially when disposable chips are considered. Thermal cycling control by Peltier junctions is frequently used in PCR chips [15,62,69].

Thermal insulation of the PCR chamber is also important to assure accurate thermal cycle control. Most DNA assays such as temperature gradient electrophoresis are highly temperature sensitive and require precise temperature control. When these elements are integrated in the same chip with PCR, very effective temperature insulation between different chip parts has to be performed. The same problem arises when different PCR chambers are integrated on the same chip to form a PCR array [70–72] especially if different targets are amplified. In the last case, optimum temperature for thermal cycling can be different in each chamber.

Besides thermal insulation among different parts of the chip, a carefully designed thermal contact of the PCR chamber with the external chip package is also important. In case only heaters are used, a good thermal contact is required to accelerate as much as possible the cooling transient between denaturation and annealing steps. A good thermal contact is paid in term of required energy during the heating phase and an intrinsically worst insulation among different chip parts. On the contrary, if coolers are used, as in the Peltier case, the PCR chamber bulk can be insulated from the external environment.

Insulation among different parts of the same chip is generally achieved in silicon-based chips by excavating deep air trenches in between different chip zones [73,74,75], thus exploiting the very good insulation characteristic of air. This solution is suitable for the PCR chips due to the fact that horizontal dimensions of trenches are not very small so that the required aspect ratio can be reached without the use of complex processes such as deep RIE (see Section 4.7.3). However, trenches on the lower wafer can create problems if wafer bonding is required or if further lithography is needed. Resist spinning is not possible if deep and wide trenches are present on the wafer and alternative techniques have to be used for resist deposition.

Alternative techniques for horizontal insulation are possible in case polymers are used for the chip realization. A first possibility is the use of porous layers containing a large quantity of air thus assuring a good thermal insulation. This effect can be obtained, for example, by using parylene-cross-linking structure to achieve air gap thermal isolation [76].

When a good thermal contact has to be achieved with the chip package to favor the PCR chamber, cooling this can be achieved by thinning the wafer support below the PCR chamber with techniques similar those used for membrane fabrication (see Section 4.2). The resulting structure is schematically reported in Figure 12.14. If required, a conducting actuator such as a metallized membrane can be fabricated. It can be brought in contact with the PCR chamber floor when cooling is required and detached when a good thermal insulation is needed.

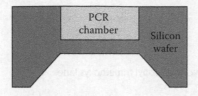

FIGURE 12.14 Scheme of wafer back-thinning to create a thermal contact between the PCR chamber and the external environment.

12.3.1.2 Bubble Formation and Evaporation Prevention

Owing to the high temperature reached in the PCR chamber, air bubble formation and possible evaporation of sample components can be relevant problems and have to be actively prevented by a suitable chip design.

Air bubbles form when the air molecules that are almost always dissolved in the sample injected into the PCR chamber aggregate. Bubble generation not only causes large temperature difference in the sample, but can also expel the sample from the PCR chamber if it is maintained open during the amplification.

For bubble formation, a superheated liquid and a set of nucleation sites acting as catalyzers are required. Several methods have been used to prevent bubble formation, almost all acting in different ways on these two elements.

The chamber shape and depth is important in preventing bubble formation. The deeper the chamber, the more probable the bubble formation maintaining the same injection system [77] while a polygonal chamber seems to be less prone to bubble formation with respect to a circular chamber [78,79]. The surface treatment of the PCR chamber, in particular the wetting properties of the chamber surface, have sizeable effect on the bubble formation. When the chamber surface is highly hydrophilic, the sample can flow into it smoothly and rapidly with minimal probability of bubble formation [77,79,80]. Moreover, under pressurization, the gas solubility will increase and the dissolved gases and bubbles cannot grow. Thus, an insulating sealing of the PCR chamber and an inner high pressure is beneficial from this point of view [69,72,81].

Finally, degasification of the PCR sample can eliminate noncondensable gases before loading into the PCR chamber and consequently decrease the risk of bubble formation; however, this operation in some cases is incompatible with the specific lab on chip application that is considered.

Sample evaporation is often problematic because on-chip PCR volumes are usually very small. As denaturation temperatures approach 100°C, the sample evaporation is so rapid that the sample would dry quickly under standard atmospheric pressure. To avoid evaporation, a mineral oil cover layer is frequently used as a vapor barrier [82–84]. The mineral oil is a suitable liquid cover because it has a boiling point far above 100°C and a density slightly below 10^3 kg/m³. However, it is difficult to apply this technique in highly integrated PCR systems, where the sample is injected via a microfluidic circuit. In this case, the only way to create the oil layer would be to insert oil after the sample and before the PCR from a suitable reservoir and with a different fluidic circuit. This is in principle not impossible but implies a great complication in the circuit design.

Another approach is using a chamber closing valve to resist the internal pressure generated during PCR. It is known that the evaporation rate decreases with the increase of the gas pressure around a liquid. Different types of valves have been used, for example, membrane-based valves [85], hydrogel valves [63], and other types of mechanical valves [86] while microporous membranes have also been used for this scope [62]. The key property of the valves used in PCR systems is the low residual loss in the closed state and their resistance to thermal cycles typical of PCR.

In addition, sample evaporation is also affected by the PCR chip substrate. For example, the water diffusion/vapor loss property of PDMS could lead to the sample evaporation and thus suitable techniques should be considered to reduce the sample loss at elevated temperatures [87,88].

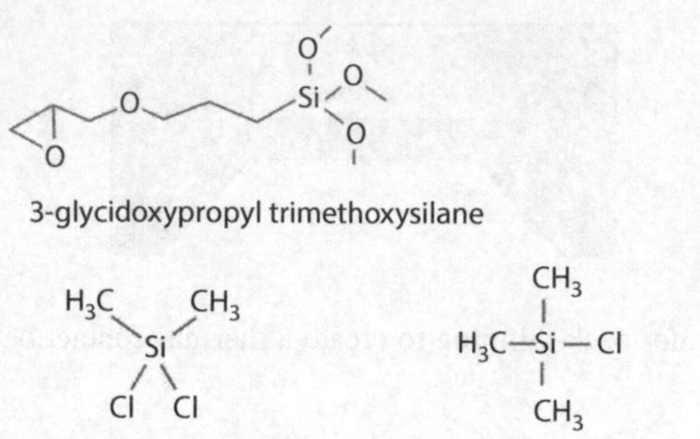

3-glycidoxypropyl trimethoxysilane

Dichlorodimethylsilane   Trimethylchlorosilane

FIGURE 12.15 Molecular formulas of silanizing agents used for passivation of the inner walls of on-chip PCR chambers.

12.3.1.3 PCR Chamber Fabrication Material

The material constituting the PCR chamber influences greatly the PCR efficiency and its reproducibility. Several material characteristics are relevant: thermal capacity of the material determines the amount of heat that is needed to reach the high temperature needed in PCR while its thermal conductivity is an important element for the PCR chamber insulation.

Surface characteristics are also very important, for example, if the surface of the PCR chamber results to be hydrophobic, as in the case of many polymers such as SU8 and other resins, it will be difficult to insert the water-based sample into the PCR chamber without using a high pressure and injecting a relevant air quantity too [77].

Perhaps, the most important surface property of the PCR chamber material is its chemical affinity with elements that are present in the sample. The PCR efficiency is often limited by interactions between the chip surface and the biomolecules in the PCR solution at the high temperature reached during the process, primarily due to the increase of the surface-to-volume ratio in a microscale environment. This means that a suitable treatment of the PCR chamber surface is generally required.

The treatment processes can be classified as static treatments and dynamic treatments. A static treatment involves the precoating of the chip surface, during fabrication of PCR chip or immediately before use, with a passivation substance. Several different substances have been used, including SiO_2 [13,78], bovine serum albumin (BSA) [69,89,90], polyethylene glycol (PEG) [91,92], or silanizing agents such as 3-glycidoxypropyl trimethoxysilane [93], dichlorodimethylsilane [94], or trimethylchlorosilane [95]. Molecular formulas of these compounds are presented in Figure 12.15.

The SiO_2 precoating is a reproducible and inexpensive standard MEMS process and can be accomplished in a batch fashion. BSA and other agents are used due to their simplicity but the reproducibility of the surface functionalization process and its resistance to repeated thermal solicitations in multiple use chips is not clear.

Diacrylated PEG (DAPEG) can be grafted into PDMS polymer for polyelectrolyte multilayers (PEM) deposition, and that the surface characteristic of PDMS polymer shifts from hydrophobic to hydrophilic after oxygen plasma treatment. The oxygen plasma activation on the surface of PDMS can be performed at the same time with the bonding processes (see Section 4.9.3), and thus it is a standard MEMS process with high reproducibility and low costs. Silanization is also a commonly used process to prevent on-chip adsorption of biomolecules, but it is difficult to scale on volumes and its reproducibility is problematic.

12.3.2 CONTINUOUS-FLOW AND DROPLET-BASED PCR AMPLIFICATION

PCR chips mimic macroscopic PCR procedures, using well-consolidated protocols. However, they do not completely exploit the possibilities that are intrinsic in process miniaturization, for example, including elements, such as microvalves, that are not easy to be realized and often limit the footprint reduction. In addition, specific injection and extraction systems have to be designed in order to inject the sample and the other components in the PCR chamber and extract them after the amplification.

Moreover, stationary PCR chips lack the possibility to change the PCR speed since it is fixed by the chip design and by the used reagent. In particular, when different samples are amplified in PCR arrays, different velocities are obtained.

A better exploitation of miniaturization characteristics has been attempted by alternative PCR approaches such as those based on continuous sample flow and PCR inside droplets.

12.3.2.1 Continuous-Flow PCR Amplification

Several problems intrinsic in stationary PCR chips are overcome by adopting continuous-flow PCR. In this case, nucleic acid amplification occurs as the sample is continuously pumped through a microfluidic channel during each temperature cycle [96–99].

There are two main architectures allowing continuous-flow PCR to be realized that are schematically shown in Figure 12.16: the linear and the spiral architecture. In a linear continuous-flow PCR, three heaters are created on the chip, generally through the deposition of metal thin films. The first electrode is heated at the denaturation temperature, the second to the extension temperature, and the third to the annealing temperature. The sample is injected into a microchannel passing below the heaters in sequence as shown in Figure 12.16a. Thus, thermal cycling is realized while the sample flows in the duct and the duration of different cycles is regulated by the average flow speed.

In the spiral architecture, the sample flows in a spiral channel that is excavated below three heaters shaped as complementary circular sectors, as shown in Figure 12.16b. Also, in this case, the sample flow directly realizes thermal cycling and the duration of different cycles is regulated by the average flow speed.

The interesting properties of the dynamic PCR approach can be summarized as follows:

- The temperature transition times depend only on the sample flow rate and the time needed for the sample to reach a thermal equilibrium.
- The heat inertia of PCR system is decreased to a minimum because only the sample's thermal mass needs to be taken into consideration.
- The reaction volume can range from several microliters to several tens of microliters.

However, continuous-flow PCR poses several problems during thermal cycling. Gas bubbles are easily generated in microchannels and the rate at which the PCR solution travels between different

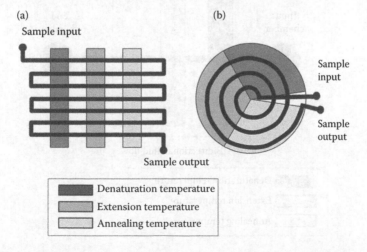

FIGURE 12.16 Linear (a) and spiral (b) architectures for continuous-flow on-chip PCR.

temperature zones is difficult to regulate. This causes the fact that the potential flexibility of continuous-flow systems is rarely fully exploited in practical systems.

The pressure-driven flow of the sample through a long microchannel often requires a relatively high-pressure micropump, if not an external pressure source, thus limiting the compatibility of such solution with strongly miniaturized lab on chip. Moreover, the presence of temperature transients and relatively high pressure creates a hyperbolic velocity profile in the ducts also influencing the PCR process [100]. An alternative to the use of a pressure-driven flow is to use electroosmosis (see Section 7.5.4) to move the sample through the chip. In this case, the velocity profile is with a good approximation constant along the channel section and it is possible to regulate the flow velocity within a certain range simply by changing the applied potential [100,101]. The chip design is, however, quite complex in this case, especially when the mix of the sample and the reagents have to happen on chip. In this case, either electroosmosis have to be used to generate the flow through the input mixer or a mixed electroosmosis-pressure regime has to be used.

The creation of a smooth temperature gradient in between nearby heaters also affects linear continuous-flow PCR systems. This gradient can be made steeper by reducing the heaters distance, but a lower limit to this distance exists if temperature cross-talk among different PCR cycles has to be avoided.

In the presence of a smooth temperature gradient in between adjacent cycles, a melted single-stranded DNA sample is very likely to form double strands with the template strands or their complementary fragments when passing the extension zone, which compromises the PCR efficiency. A first way to circumvent this problem is to use the spiral arrangement by maintaining the microchannel in the external part of the circle, including the PCR device. The double-stranded formation is drastically reduced in this case, at the expense of a greater chip footprint and an increased difficulty in performing parallel PCR on different samples using spiral architecture.

An alternative solution, also allowing simple parallel PCR operation on multiple samples, is the so-called oscillatory PCR approach [102,103]. Potentially oscillatory PCR combines the cycling flexibility of the stationary PCR with quick temperature transitions also providing the possibility of performing high-throughput PCR amplifications in a parallel format. The principle scheme of an oscillatory PCR chip is presented in Figure 12.17. Three heaters are deposited on the top of the chip to define three chip zones where the temperature of the PCR cycles is maintained. The sample is mixed with the reagents and injected in an injection chamber on one side of the chip. From the injection chamber, the sample is pushed through a duct passing below the heater so as to experiment the first thermal cycle, to reach an end chamber. Once the sample is completely transferred in the

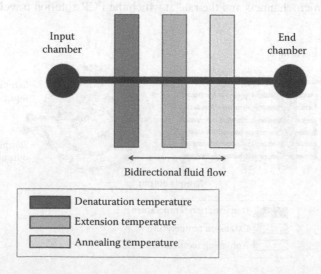

FIGURE 12.17 Scheme of an oscillatory PCR chip.

end chamber, the pressure through the system is inverted and the sample passes again into the input chamber by traversing the different temperature zones. Periodic repetition of this operation generates PCR thermal cycles.

The main problem of the oscillating technique resides in the need of using two pumps to generate pressure in two directions, or a bidirectional pump. This is not a problem when the pressure source can be external to the chip, but renders full integration of this PCR method difficult, especially when other fluidic or analytic building blocks have to be integrated too.

12.3.2.2 On-Chip Droplet-Based PCR

Droplet technology can be useful in designing on-chip PCR from several points of view [102,104,105].

Droplet creates highly reproducible, insulated small volumes, where PCR can be carried out without contamination due to the fact that the environmental liquid is immiscible with water and generally cannot dissolve the greater majority of biological macromolecules. For example, while designing a reusable PCR chip with traditional methods requires to somehow wash the chip after each PCR process, a droplet-based chip can be easily made reusable by simply eliminating the droplets where PCR happened from the chip. Similarly, different samples can be amplified in different droplets without using the cross-talk limiting techniques that are often required in traditional arrays. Last but not least, the fact that correctly generated droplets are naturally insulated (see Section 8.7) allows PCR chamber closure valves to be eliminated; thus greatly simplifying the fluidic structure of the chip.

Droplets can be fixed in a specific point or moved along the chip as required by using electrowetting (see Section 7.5.6) or other techniques, thus opening the possibility to operate either stationary PCR or a dynamic one. Moreover, integration with other droplet-based building blocks is generally easier with respect to other on-chip PCR technologies.

12.4 ON-CHIP NUCLEIC ACID ASSAYS

The simple assay that can be done on nucleic acids is the quantification of their presence by electrophoresis. This separation and quantification technique also allows supercoiling to be identified since similar molecules with a different coiling structure have different electrophoresis mobility (see Section 3.6.3). Electrophoresis can be performed on chip both by simply miniaturizing the macroscopic electrophoresis geometry and using different techniques exploiting the properties of the microscopic environment of a lab on chip as discussed in Section 8.5.2.

In the case of nucleic acids however, electrophoresis quantification has clear limitations. The nucleobases have similar molecular weights, and nucleic acids with the same supercoiling and the same number of bases are very difficult to be separated using electrophoresis.

Other quantification methods are frequently used in the case of nucleic acids such as fluorescence observation that results to be much more selective, being generally based on the labeling of DNA-specific molecules with suitable dyes. An interesting method for quantization in the case of very diluted molecules is based on nanofluidics, that is, on small fluid channels that are able to transmit a molecule a time, thus allowing practically a direct molecule counting.

Beyond simple quantification, the main DNA assay is the sequencing, the assay whose scope is to determine the DNA sequence, but other assays also exist that have an important role in determining the functionality and modification of DNA sections.

An important class of DNA assays has the task to study DNA interaction with proteins (see Section 2.6). A large range of proteins bind to DNA [106,107] and are involved in DNA replication, folding, and gene control. One very important group of control proteins are the transcription factors, which bind adjacent to specific genes along the DNA controlling the activity of the corresponding genes. Another level of control is modification of the DNA itself. Methylation of the base cytosine may control whether genes are switched on or off and is important for genomic imprinting. This type of modification, in addition to histone acetylation, is one of the most important epigenetic modifications of DNA, that is, modifications to the genome that do not involve changes in the sequence.

The fact that present technologies allow very small form factor elements to be used in lab on chip fabrication makes these assays category very interesting. Using nanoscale circuits and in particular nanofluidic manipulation, there is a potential to access the DNA on the length scale of the control factors and thereby directly read out the epigenetic factors that control the expression of the genes along the DNA.

A large number of DNA assays are also devoted to determine genetic variations, which is to compare a target DNA with a reference to determine the differences between them. Genetic variations are interesting because of their medical implications: they are the underlying factor for many diseases, and they may determine susceptibility to certain medications. Single nucleotide polymorphisms (SNPs), that is, variations in single bases, are very important in this context [108].

Whatever system is used, complete sequencing of DNA fragments is a very complex operation. Moving the whole sequencing chain from the lab on a chip would require to integrate on board of the chip several steps such as lysis and extraction, PCR, identification of bases, and finally quantization.

Even if we imagine to feed the sequencing chip with an already purified solution obtained by a separated lysis and purification system, integrating the whole base identification and quantization system in a single chip is a very difficult task.

Thus, besides lab on chip implementing the whole sequencing process, a great number of lab on chips have been proposed to integrate parts of the process with the aim of either generating a multichip integrated system or simply to ease the design of macroscopic sequencing machines.

12.4.1 COMPLETE SEQUENCING INTEGRATION

A great effort has been initiated to integrate the Sanger sequencing method (see Section 3.8.1.1) on a single chip, mainly with the goal of speeding the process and obtaining high reproducibility. Owing to the complexity of the procedure and to the high number of required reagents, it is generally impossible to obtain small chips with a simple structure; nevertheless important results have been obtained [109–111].

Frequently, the sequencing chip occupies a complete wafer area and requires superposition of wafers of different materials to achieve optimized fabrication of its parts. An example is the chip presented in Reference [111]. Both Sanger sequencing and fluorescence quantification after capillary electrophoresis separation are integrated on the chip, which cover the complete area of a 10 cm radius glass wafer. The chip fabrication requires the bonding of three wafers and a fourth featureless PDMS membrane constituting the membrane of valves and pumps. The situation is represented in Figure 12.18.

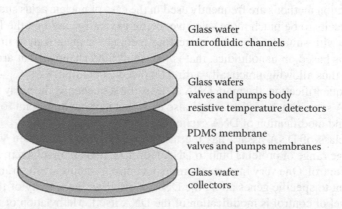

Glass wafer
microfluidic channels

Glass wafers
valves and pumps body
resistive temperature detectors

PDMS membrane
valves and pumps membranes

Glass wafer
collectors

FIGURE 12.18 Three layer superposition and role of each wafer in the chip for Sanger sequencing presented in Reference [111].

Pneumatic actuators for membrane-based valves and pumps are integrated on chip (see Sections 8.2.2 and 8.3.1), while capillary electrophoresis is adopted to separate different segments for nucleobase identification by fluorescence detection. The fluorescence detection system is completely external to the chip and interacts with the samples inside the chip through the transparent chip surface. Finally, temperature stabilization is achieved through resistive temperature detectors that are realized on the second glass wafer by thin film metal deposition.

Similar systems are quite complex; they occupy a relatively large area to be lab on chip and their use outside of a laboratory seems impossible due to the need of external detection. Nevertheless, performing Sanger sequencing by such systems can be substantially simple and more reproducible with respect to standard macroscopic methods while miniaturization of the different parts allows faster operation and use of low-volume samples. Last but not least, the main cost of Sanger sequencing is constituted by the cost of the reagents, whose volume is drastically reduced with the use of integrated sequencers.

Variations of the Sanger methods have also been introduced to better exploit the properties of miniaturized systems. Sequencing by denaturation is an interesting variation of the Sanger method that can be exploited both in macroscopic systems and in lab on chip [112,113].

Sequencing by denaturation is performed on amplified templates separated spatially by fixing them on a solid surface. First, a standard Sanger sequencing reaction is performed where fluorescently labeled dideoxyNTPs are randomly incorporated as the polymerase synthesizes the complementary strand from the amplified target template resulting in fragments of different lengths, each labeled with a fluorescent molecule corresponding to its ending base type. Because the melting temperature of a short DNA fragment is lower than a short DNA fragment with one additional base, the Sanger fragments are denatured sequentially from the shortest to the longest by gradually increasing the sequencing chamber temperature. By monitoring the decrease in fluorescence on the surface during this process, the signal can be analyzed to determine the base sequence of the target DNA template.

The fact that the sequencing reaction happens while the strands are fixed on a surface allows, besides standard microfluidic arrangements, an alternative way to move the sample among the different chambers of the sequencing chip: the use of superparamagnetic beads [113] (see Section 7.6.3). Once the DNA strands have been fixed on the surface of the beads, the use of a magnetic field generated by an artificial magnet can drive the beads through the chip without a bulk movement of the solution.

The use of magnets fed with variable current is not generally suitable for strong miniaturization, but in the case of sequencing chips, strong miniaturization is difficult for a variety of reasons; it can be a powerful technique.

Pyrosequencing has also been considered for integration in a lab on chip [114,115] (see Section 3.8.2.2). Generally, functionalized beads are also used in pyrosequencing chips and the DNA strands are fixed to the beads as a first step of the process. After this first step, all the sequencing process happens in a sequencing room where temperature is strictly controlled and two inlets are present: one for the bead containing solution and the other to apply a pressure from outside, generally through a micropump. The principle structure of the scheme of the whole process happening in the pyrosequencing room is presented in Figure 12.19. The chamber is divided into two parts by a filter that is able to transfer the solution that is present in the external part into the internal part and vice versa, but not to pass through the DNA-coated beads. Since the beads have a radius of several microns, the filter can be realized with simple mechanical means, by opening small passages in the separation layer between distinct chambers.

The different steps happening in the pyrosequencing room are schematically shown in Figure 12.20. In a first step (Figure 12.20a), beads carrying the DNA template are captured in the pyrosequencing chamber; after that, the pyrosequencing mixture containing one of the four nucleotides (see Section 3.8.2.2) is delivered into the chamber (Figure 12.20b) and the reaction is monitored in real time by observing the emit fluorescence under a suitable external excitation (Figure 12.20c).

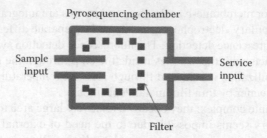

FIGURE 12.19 Principle scheme of a planar integrated sequencing chamber for pyrosequence process.

It is important that the quantity of nucleotide solution that is injected into the chamber is very well controlled in this phase and the injection fluidic circuit has to be carefully designed. After a short time, for example, 1 min, the reaction is terminated by washing the pyrosequencing chamber by a suitable buffer and applying external pressure (Figure 12.20d). After the washing step, a new reaction cycle is started with a mix containing one of the four nucleotides. At the end of a whole sequencing assay, the chip can be regenerated by washing with water and applying pressure from the outlet (Figure 12.20e). When the chamber is washed, another sample can be assayed.

While the whole sequencing assay is performed in the reaction chamber, nevertheless the sequence of different injections and washing operations is quite complex and a good temperature and volume control has to be realized if repeatability is to be assured. The simpler way of doing this is to locate a few microfluidic functions out of the chip. Microfluidic pumps and fluorescence detection are performed frequently using external equipment that is integrated into the system hosting the pyrosequencing chip.

In the same way, if the chip is to be reused several times, the reagents have to be supplied via an external source.

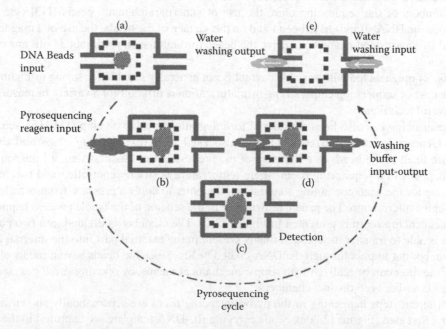

FIGURE 12.20 Steps of the pyrosequence assay on chip. Sample injection (a), pyrosequence reagent injection (b), reaction real-time monitoring (c), reagent elimination by washing (d), and full-chamber washing (e). (From Russom A., *Analytical Chemistry*, vol. 77, pp. 7505–7511, 2005.)

If the whole process and microfluidic control has to be integrated upon the same chip, a complex set of fluid functions such as valves, pumps, fluid flow control, and temperature control all have to be integrated. This is all but impossible, and there is not to expect an extremely miniaturized chip, as in the case of Sanger sequencing.

Droplet-based microfluidics has also been successfully adopted to perform full on-chip pyrosequencing [116,117]. Droplets can be used both to strictly control the sample and the reagents volumes, as it is needed in several steps in pyrosequencing, and to move the sample through the different lab on chip stages using electrowetting (see Section 7.5.6). This is a particularly useful technique when the whole sequencing processing that starts from cell lysing has to be integrated since it requires neither complex fluid flow control structures such as valves and pumps nor magnetic fields, whose source is difficult to integrate onto the chip.

Besides pyrosequencing, other sequencing by synthesis techniques have also been considered for integration in a lab on chip [118], leading to similar design and technology elements.

12.4.2   Lab-on-Chip Integrating Sequencing Subsystems

Integrating on a single lab on chip, the whole sequencing process is a very complex task; moreover, the obtained chips are not very small, frequently occupying a whole wafer. In this condition, a valid solution to exploit lab on chip potentialities in the sequencing area is to integrate on a lab on chip a subsystem that can be used in the sequencing process.

Such labs on chip can either be used to replace traditional subsystems in macroscopic sequencing equipment or they can be assembled together using hybrid integration on a multichip sequencing board (see Section 6.3). The last possibility is quite attractive as an evolution from single chip to multichip systems allowing complex operations to be performed by leveraging integration advantages even if simple integration on a single chip is not possible or not advantageous. In this case, however, stable and efficient microfluidic interconnections have to be realized among different chips that are part of the system. Moreover, fluidic interconnections should not to be too complex to fabricate or too costly from a testing point of view, so as not to ruin the cost advantage of integrated technologies.

The microfluidic interconnection problem is still not completely solved at the industrial level, but a great number of possibilities have been explored and industrial standardization seems not too far leveraging on today's technologies (see Section 6.5.3).

Besides lysis, extraction, and PCR, which are logically separated functions in the majority of sequencing procedures, thus naturally suitable to be integrated in separated chips, quantification and detection are also functions that can be integrated in stand-alone chips.

Fluorescence detection is frequently used in sequencing protocols, requiring laser sources and optical detectors. Integrated optics allows infrared laser sources and wide band high-accuracy photodiodes to be integrated in fluorescence detection chips (see Sections 6.3 and 11.3.2.2) [119]. A fluorescence integrated optical chip is more complex and costly with respect to a lab on chip, but it is not a disposable system and it can be integrated besides disposable lab on chip as a stable component of the sequencing systems. Alternative techniques can also be used for the realization of optical detectors by directly integrating them on top of the lab on chip, like the use of organic LEDs [11,120] or amorphous silicon thin films [121]. In this case, fluorescence detection can be carried out using an external laser and an integrated detector.

Electrochemical detection is a valid alternative to fluorescence detection in sequencing systems. This technique does not require optical interfaces and it is intrinsically more suitable for integration in lab on chips (see Sections 10.4 and 10.5). Both voltammetry [122] and potentiometric detection [123] have been proposed for this application.

Quantification of the results obtained after the sequencing reaction is another function that can be frequently integrated on a stand-alone chip. Electrophoresis is by far the most used quantification method in nucleic acid sequencing and both miniaturized electrophoresis and capillary electrophoresis can be used, besides capillary electrophoresis variations that exploit many parallel capillaries to obtain faster separation of the sequencing products [124].

REFERENCES

1. *DNA Sequencing Costs: Data from the NHGRI Genome Sequencing Program (GSP)*, National Human Genome Research Institute, http://www.genome.gov/sequencingcosts/, last accessed May 20, 2013.
2. Mardis E. A decade's perspective on DNA sequencing technology, *Nature*, vol. 470, pp. 198–203, 2011.
3. Kim J., Johnson M., Hill P., Gale B. K., Microfluidic sample preparation: Cell lysis and nucleic acid purification, *Integrative Biology*, vol. 1, pp. 574–586, 2009.
4. Xu C.-X., Yin X.-F., Continuous cell introduction and rapid dynamic lysis for high-throughput single-cell analysis on microfluidic chips with hydrodynamic focusing, *Journal of Chromatography A*, vol. 1218, pp. 726–732, 2011.
5. Kim Y. C., Kang J. H., Park S.-J., Yoon E.-S., Park J.-K., Microfluidic biomechanical device for compressive cell stimulation and lysis, *Sensors and Actuators B: Chemical*, vol. 128, pp. 108–116, 2007.
6. Yun S. S., et al., Handheld mechanical cell lysis chip with ultra-sharp silicon nano-blade arrays for rapid intracellular protein extraction, *Lab on a Chip*, vol. 10, pp. 1442–1446, 2009.
7. Kim J., Hong J. W., Kim D. P., Shinb J. H., Park I., Nanowire-integrated microfluidic devices for facile and reagent-free mechanical cell lysis, *Lab on a Chip*, vol. 12, pp. 2914–2921, 2012.
8. Takamatsu H., Takeya R., Naito S., Sumimoto H., On the mechanism of cell lysis by deformation, *Journal of Biomechanics*, vol. 38, pp. 117–124, 2005.
9. Marentis T. C., Kusler B., Yaralioglu G. G., Liu S., Hæggström E. O., Khuri-Yakub B. T., Microfluidic sonicator for real-time disruption of eukaryotic cells and bacterial spores for DNA analysis, *Ultrasound in Medicine & Biology*, vol. 31, pp. 1265–1277, 2005.
10. Deng C. X., Sieling F., Pan H., Cui J., Ultrasound-induced cell membrane porosity, *Ultrasound in Medicine & Biology*, vol. 30, pp. 519–526, 2004.
11. Feril Jr L. B. et al., Enhancement of ultrasound-induced apoptosis and cell lysis by echo-contrast agents, *Ultrasound in Medicine & Biology*, vol. 29, pp. 331–337, 2003.
12. Khanna P. et al., Nanocrystalline diamond microspikes increase the efficiency of ultrasonic cell lysis in a microfluidic lab-on-a-chip, *Diamond and Related Materials*, vol. 18, pp. 606–610, 2009.
13. Ke C., Kelleher A.-M., Berney H., Sheehan M., Mathewson A., Single step cell lysis/pcr detection of escherichia coli in an independently controllable silicon microreactor, *Sensors and Actuators B: Chemical*, vol. 120, pp. 538–544, 2007.
14. Marshall L. A., Wu L. L., Babikian S., Bachman M., Santiago J. G., Integrated printed circuit board device for cell lysis and nucleic acid extraction, *Analytical Chemistry*, vol. 84, pp. 9640–9645, 2012.
15. Lee C. Y., Lee G. B., Lin J. L., Huang F. C., Liao C. S., Integrated microfluidic systems for cell lysis, mixing/pumping and DNA amplification, *Journal of Micromechanics and Microengineering*, vol. 15, pp. 1215–1223, 2005.
16. Baek S.-K., Mina J., Park J. H., Wireless induction heating in a microfluidic device for cell lysis, *Lab on a Chip*, vol. 10, pp. 909–917, 2010.
17. Cheong K. H. et al., Gold nanoparticles for one step DNA extraction and real-time pcr of pathogens in a single chamber, *Lab on a Chip*, vol. 8, pp. 810–813, 2008.
18. Pang Z., Al-Mahrouki A., Berezovski M., Krylov, S. N., Selection of surfactants for cell lysis in chemical cytometry to study protein-DNA interactions. *Electrophoresis*, vol. 27, pp. 1489–1494, 2006.
19. Schilling E. A., Kamholz A. E., Yager P., Cell lysis and protein extraction in a microfluidic device with detection by a fluorogenic enzyme assay, *Analytical Chemistry*, vol. 74, pp. 1798–1804, 2002.
20. Sethu P., Anahtar P., Moldawer L. L., Tompkins R. G., Toner M., Continuous flow microfluidic device for rapid erythrocyte lysis, *Analytical Chemistry*, vol. 76, pp. 6247–6253, 2004.
21. SooHoo J. R., Herr J. K., Ramsey M., Walker G. M., Microfluidic cytometer for the characterization of cell lysis, *Analytical Chemistry*, vol. 84, pp. 2195–2201, 2012.
22. Johansson L., Johansson S., Nikolajeff F., Thorslund S., Effective mixing of laminar flows at a density interface by an integrated ultrasonic transducer, *Lab on a Chip*, vol. 9, pp. 297–304, 2009.
23. Heo J., Thomas K. J., Seong G. H., Crooks R. M., A microfluidic bioreactor based on hydrogel-entrapped e. coli: Cell viability, lysis, and intracellular enzyme reactions, *Analytical Chemistry*, vol. 75, pp. 22–26, 2003.
24. Jen C.-P., Hsiao J.-H., Maslov N. A., Single-cell chemical lysis on microfluidic chips with arrays of microwells, *Sensors*, vol. 12, pp. 347–358, 2012.

25. Bontoux N. et al., Integrating whole transcriptome assays on a lab-on-a-chip for single cell gene profiling, *Lab on a Chip*, vol. 8, pp. 443–450, 2008.

26. Hamilton W. A., Sale J. H., Effects of high electric fields on microorganism ii. mechanism of action of the lethal effect, *Biochimica et Biophysica Acta*, vol. 148, pp. 789–800, 1967.

27. Vorobien E., Lebovka N., *Pulsed-Electrical-Fields-Induced Effects in Plant Tissues: Fundamental Aspects and Perspectives of Application*, in Electrotechnologies for Extraction from Food Plants and Biomaterials, Vorobien E., Lebovka N. editors, Springer; of 2008 edition (December 6, 2010), ISBN-13: 978-1441927194, pp. 39–83.

28. Isheger H. H., Potel J., Niemann E. G., Electric field effects on bacteria and yeast cells, *Radiation and Environmental Biophysics*, vol. 22, pp. 149–162, 1983.

29. Wang H. Y., Banada P. P., Bhunia A. K., Lu C., Rapid electrical lysis of bacterial cells in a microfluidic device, *Methods in Molecular Biology*, vol. 385, pp. 23–35, 2007.

30. Hargis A. D., Alarie J. P., Ramsey J. M., Characterization of cell lysis events on a microfluidic device for high-throughput single cell analysis, *Electrophoresis*, vol. 32, pp. 3172–3179, 2011.

31. Mernier G., Martinez-Duarte R., Lehal R., Radtke F., Renaud P., Very high throughput electrical cell lysis and extraction of intracellular compounds using 3d carbon electrodes in lab-on-a-chip devices, *Micromachines*, vol. 3, pp. 574–581, 2012.

32. Morshed B. I., Shams M., Mussivand T., Analysis of electric fields inside microchannels and single cell electrical lysis with a microfluidic device, *Micromachines*, vol. 4, pp. 243–256, 2013.

33. Morshed B. I., Shams M., Mussivand T., Electrical lysis: Dynamics revisited and advances in on-chip operation, *Critical Reviews in Biomedical Engineering*, vol. 41, pp. 37–50, 2013.

34. Bao N., Lu C. A., Microfluidic device for physical trapping and electrical lysis of bacterial cells, *Applied Physics Letters*, vol. 92, pp. 214103–214106, 2008.

35. Rosa C., Tilley P. A., Fox J. D., Kaler K. V., Microfluidic device for dielectrophoresis manipulation and electrodisruption of respiratory pathogen bordetella pertussis, *IEEE Transactions on Biomedical Engineering*, vol. 55, pp. 2426–2432, 2008.

36. Gao J., Yina X.-F. Fang Z.-L., Integration of single cell injection, cell lysis, separation and detection of intracellular constituents on a microfluidic chip, *Lab on a Chip*, vol. 4, pp. 47–52, 2004.

37. Tanner Nevill J., Cooper R., Dueck M., Breslauera D. N., Lee L. P., Integrated microfluidic cell culture and lysis on a chip, *Lab on a Chip*, vol. 7, pp. 1689–1695, 2007.

38. Vulto P., Dame G., Maier U., Makohliso S., Podszun S., Zahna P., Urban G. A. A micro fluidic approach for high efficiency extraction of low molecular weight RNA. *Lab on a Chip*, vol. 10, pp. 610–616, 2010.

39. Di Carlo D., Ionescu-Zanetti C., Zhang Y., Hung P., Lee L. P., On-chip cell lysis by local hydroxide generation, *Lab on a Chip*, vol. 5, pp. 171–178, 2005.

40. Jaspard E., Role of protein-solvent interactions in refolding: Effects of cosolvent additives on the renaturation of porcine pancreatic elastase at various pHs. *Archives of Biochemistry and Biophysics*, vol. 375, pp. 220–228, 2000.

41. Kristinsson H., Hultin H., Effect of low and high ph treatment on the functional properties of cod muscle proteins, *Journal of Agricultural and Food Chemistry*, vol. 51, pp. 5103–5110, 2003.

42. Price C. W., Leslie D. C., Landers J. P., Nucleic acid extraction techniques and application to the microchip, *Lab on a Chip*, vol. 9, pp. 2484–2494, 2009.

43. Breadmore M. C. et al., Microchip-based purification of DNA from biological samples, *Analytical Chemistry*, vol. 75, pp. 1880–1886, 2003.

44. Bhattacharyya A., Klapperich C. M., Thermoplastic microfluidic device for on-chip purification of nucleic acids for disposable diagnostics, *Analytical Chemistry*, vol. 78, pp. 788–792, 2006.

45. Wu Q., Microchip-based macroporous silica sol – gel monolith for efficient isolation of DNA from clinical samples, *Analytical Chemistry*, vol. 78, pp. 5704–5710, 2006.

46. Breadmore M. C. et al., Toward a microchip-based solid-phase extraction method for isolation of nucleic acids, *Electrophoresis*, vol. 23, pp. 727–733, 2002.

47. Lee J.-G., Cheong K. H., Huh N., Kim S., Choi J. W., Ko C., Microchip-based one step dna extraction and real-time PCR in one chamber for rapid pathogen identification, *Lab on a Chip*, vol. 6, pp. 886–895, 2006.

48. Lui C., Cady N. C., Batt C. A., Nucleic acid-based detection of bacterial pathogens using integrated microfluidic platform systems, *Sensors*, vol. 9, pp. 3713–3744, 2009.

49. Cao W., Easley C. J., Ferrance J. P., Landers J. P., Chitosan as a polymer for pH-induced DNA capture in a totally aqueous system, *Analytical Chemistry*, vol. 78, pp. 7222–7228, 2006.

50. Kim J., Voelkerding K. V., Gale B. K., Multi-DNA extraction chip based on an aluminum oxide membrane integrated into a PDMS microfluidic structure, Proceedings of 3rd IEEE-EMBS Special Topic Conference on Microtechnology in Medicine and Biology, pp. 5–7, 2005.

51. Elgort M. G., Herrmann M. G., Erali M., Durtschi J. D., Voelkerding K. V., Smith R. E., Extraction and amplification of genomic DNA from human blood on nanoporous aluminum oxide membranes, *Clinical Chemistry*, vol. 50, pp. 1817–1819, 2004.

52. Kim J., Gale, B. K., A PCR reactor with an integrated alumina isolation membrane, *Lab on a Chip*, vol. 8, pp. 1516–1523, 2008.

53. Kim J., Voelkerding K. V., Gale B. K., Patterning of a nanoporous membrane for multi-sample DNA extraction, *Journal of Micromechanics and Microengineering*, vol. 16, pp. 33–39, 2006.

54. Bandyopadhyay A., Chatterjee S., Sarkar K., Rapid isolation of genomic DNA from e. coli XL1 blue strain approaching bare magnetic nanoparticles, *Current Science*, vol. 101, pp. 210–214, 2011.

55. Saiyed Z. M., Ramchand C. N., Telang S. D., Isolation of genomic DNA using magnetic nanoparticles as a solid-phase support, *Journal of Physics. Condensed Matter*, vol. 20, pp. 204153–204159, 2008.

56. Yeung S. W., Hsing I. M., Manipulation and extraction of genomic DNA from cell lysate by functionalized magnetic particles for lab on a chip applications, *Biosensors and Bioelectronics*, vol. 21, pp. 989–997, 2006.

57. Rio D. C., Ares M. Jr., Hannon G. J., Nilsen T. W., RNA: A Laboratory Manual, Cold Spring Harbor Laboratory Press, 1st edition (November, 2010), ISBN-13: 978-0879698911.

58. Jiang G., Harrison D. J., mRNA isolation in a microfluidic device for eventual integration of cDNA library construction, *Analyst*, vol. 125, pp. 2176–2179, 2000.

59. Zaytseva N. V., Montagna R. A., Baeumner A. J., Microfluidic biosensor for the serotype-specific detection of dengue virus RNA, *Analytical Chemistry*, vol. 77, pp. 7520–7527, 2005.

60. Satterfield B. C., Stern S., Caplan M. R., Hukari K. W., West J. A. A., Microfluidic purification and pre-concentration of mRNA by flow-through polymeric monolith, *Analytical Chemistry*, vol. 77, pp. 6230–6235, 2007.

61. Witek M. A., Hupert M. L., Park D. S.-W., Fears K., Murphy m. C., Soper S. A., 96-well polycarbonate-based microfluidic titer plate for high-throughput purification of DNA and RNA, *Analytical Chemistry*, vol. 80, pp. 3483–3491, 2008.

62. Khandurina J., McKnight T. E., Jacobson S. C., Waters L. C., Foote R. S., Ramsey J. M., Integrated system for rapid PCR-based DNA analysis in microfluidic devices, *Analytical Chemistry*, vol. 72, pp. 2995–3000, 2000.

63. Wang J., Chen Z., Corstjens P. L. A. M., Mauka M. G., Bau H. H., A disposable microfluidic cassette for DNA amplification and detection, *Lab on a Chip*, vol. 6, pp. 46–53, 2006.

64. Shin Y. S. et al., PDMS-based micro PCR chip with parylene coating, *Journal of Micromechanics and Microengineering*, vol. 13, pp. 768–774, 2003.

65. Cheng J., Shoffner M. A., Hvichia G. E., Kricka L. J., Wilding P., Chip PCR. II. Investigation of different PCR amplification systems in microfabricated silicon–glass chips, *Nucleic Acids Research*, vol. 24, pp. 380–385, 1996.

66. Yoon D. S., et al., Precise temperature control and rapid thermal cycling in a micromachined DNA polymerase chain reaction chip, *Journal of Micromechanics and Microengineering*, vol. 12 pp. 813–823, 2002.

67. El-Ali J., Perch-Nielsen I. R., Poulsen C. R., Bang D. D., Telleman P., Wolff A., Simulation and experimental validation of a SU-8 based PCR thermocycler chip with integrated heaters and temperature sensor, *Sensors and Actuators A: Physical*, vol. 110, pp. 3–10, 2004.

68. Michalski L., Eckersdorf K., Kucharski J., McGhee J., Temperature Measurement, Wiley, 2nd edition (December 15, 2001), ISBN-13: 978-0471867791.

69. Cady N. C., Stelick S., Kunnavakkam M. V., Batt C., A real-time PCR detection of listeria monocytogenes using an integrated microfluidics platform. *Sensors and Actuators B: Chemical*, vol. 107, pp. 332–341, 2005.

70. Ramalingam N. et al., Real-time PCR array chip with capillary-driven sample loading and reactor sealing for point-of-care applications, *Biomedical Microdevices*, vol. 11, pp. 1007–1020, 2009.

71. Panaro N. J., Lou X. J., Fortina P., Kricka L. J., Wilding P., Micropillar array chip for integrated white blood cell isolation and PCR, *Biomolecular Engineering*, vol. 21, pp. 157–162, 2005.

72. Matsubara Y., Kerman K., Kobayashi M., Yamamura S., Morita Y., Tamiya E., Microchamber array based DNA quantification and specific sequence detection from a single copy via PCR in nanoliter volumes, *Biosensors and Bioelectronics*, vol. 20, pp. 1482–1490, 2005.

73. Werno J., Kersjes R., Mokwa W., Vogt H., Reduction of heat loss of silicon membranes by the use of trench etching techniques, *Sensors and Actuators A: Physical*, vol. 42, pp. 578–581, 1994.

74. Op de Beeck M. et al., *Design and Fabrication of A Biomedical Lab on Chip System for SNP Detection in DNA*, Proceedings of 2010 IEEE International Electron Devices Meeting (IEDM), San Francisco, CA, pp. 36.3.1–36.3.4, 2010.

75. Lee D.-S. et al., Bulk-micromachined submicroliter-volume PCR chip with very rapid thermal response and low power consumption, *Lab on a Chip*, vol. 4, pp. 401–407, 2004.

76. Shih C. Y., Chen Y., Tai Y. C., Parylene-strengthened thermal isolation technology for microfluidic system-on-chip applications, *Sensors and Actuators A: Physical*, vol. 126, pp. 270–276, 2006.

77. Gong H. et al., Microfluidic handling of PCR solution and DNA amplification on a reaction chamber array biochip, *Biomedical Microdevices*, vol. 8, pp. 167–176, 2006.

78. Cho Y. K. et al. Clinical evaluation of microscale chip-based PCR system for rapid detection of hepatitis b virus. *Biosensing Bioelectronics*, vol. 21, pp. 2161–2169, 2006.

79. Niu Z. Q., Chen W. Y., Shao S. Y., Jia X. Y., Zhang W. P., DNA amplification on a PDMS-glass hybrid microchip, *Journal of Micromechanics and Microengineering*, vol. 16, pp. 425–433, 2006.

80. Toriello N. M., Liu C. N., Mathies R. A., Multichannel reverse transcription-polymerase chain reaction microdevice for rapid gene expression and biomarker analysis, *Analytical Chemistry*, vol. 78, pp. 7997–8003, 2006.

81. Nakayama T. et al. Circumventing air bubbles in microfluidic systems and quantitative continuous-flow PCR applications, *Analytical and Bioanalytical Chemistry*, vol. 386, pp. 1327–1333, 2006.

82. Guttenberg Z. et al. Planar chip device for PCR and hybridization with surface acoustic wave pump, *Lab on a Chip*, vol. 5, pp. 308–317, 2005.

83. Neuzil P., Pipper J., Hsieh T. M., Disposable real-time MicroPCR device: Lab-on-a-chip at a low cost, *Molecular BioSystems*, vol. 2, pp. 292–298, 2006.

84. Neuzil P., Zhang C. Y., Pipper J., Oh S., Zhuo L., Ultra-fast miniaturized real-time PCR: 40 cycles in less than six minutes, *Nucleic Acids Research*, vol. 34, pp. e77, 2006.

85. Liu C. N., Toriello N. M., Mathies R. A., Multichannel PCR-CE microdevice for genetic analysis, *Analytical Chemistry*, vol. 78, pp. 5474–5479, 2006.

86. Lagally E. T., Simpson P. C., Mathies R. A., Monolithic integrated microfluidic DNA amplification and capillary electrophoresis analysis system, *Sensors and Actuators B: Chemical*, vol. 63, pp. 138–146, 2000.

87. Pilarski P. M., Adamia S., Backhouse C. J., An adaptable microvalving system for on-chip polymerase chain reactions, *Journal of Immunological Methods*, vol. 305, pp. 48–58, 2005.

88. Prakash A. R., Adamia S., Sieben V., Pilarski P., Pilarski L. M., Backhouse C. J., Small volume PCR in PDMS biochips with integrated fluid control and vapour barrier, *Sensors and Actuators B: Chemical*, vol. 113, pp. 398–409, 2006.

89. Zou Z. Q., Chen X., Jin Q H., Yang M. S., Zhao J. L., A novel miniaturized PCR multi-reactor array fabricated using flip-chip bonding techniques, *Journal of Micromechanics and Microengineering*, vol. 15, pp. 1476–1481, 2005.

90. Zhang L. H., Dang F. Q., Kaji N., Baba Y., Fast extraction, amplification and analysis of genes from human blood, *Journal of Chromatography A*, vol. 1106, pp. 175–180, 2006.

91. Morrison T. et al. Nanoliter high throughput quantitative PCR, *Nucleic Acids Research*, vol. 34, pp. e123, 2006.

92. Kartalov E. P., Quake S. R., Microfluidic device reads up to four consecutive base pairs in DNA sequencing-by-synthesis, *Nucleic Acids Research*, vol. 32, pp. 2873–2879, 2004.

93. Consolandi C. et al., Polymerase chain reaction of 2-kb cyanobacterial gene and human anti-a1-chymotrypsin gene from genomic DNA on in-check single-use microfabricated silicon chip, *Analytical Biochemistry*, vol. 353, pp. 191–197, 2006.

94. Poulsen C. R., El-Ali J., Perch-Nielsen I. R., Bang D. D., Telleman P., Wolff A., Detection of a putative virulence cadF gene of campylobacter jejuni obtained from different sources using a microfabricated PCR chip, *Journal of Rapid Methods and Automation in Microbiology*, vol. 13, pp. 111–126, 2005.

95. Prakash R., Kaler K. V. I. S., An integrated genetic analysis microfluidic platform with valves and a PCR chip reusability method to avoid contamination, *Microfluidics and Nanofluidics*, vol. 3, pp. 177–187, 2007.

96. Kim J. A., Lee J. Y., Seong S., Cha S. H., Lee S. H., Kim J. J., Park T. H., Fabrication and characterization of a PDMS-glass hybrid continuous-flow PCR chip, *Biochemical Engineering Journal*, vol. 29, pp. 91–97, 2006.

97. Wang W., Li Z. X., Guo Z. Y., Numerical simulation of micro flow-through PCR chip, *Microscale Thermal Engineering*, vol. 9, pp. 281–293, 2005.

98. Zhang C. S., Xu J. L., Wang J. Q., Wang H. P., Continuous flow polymerase chain reaction microfluidics by using spiral capillary channel embedded on copper, *Analytical Letters*, vol. 40, pp. 497–511, 2007.

99. Chabert M., Dorfman K. D., de Cremoux P., Roeraade J., Viovy J.-L., Automated microdroplet platform for sample manipulation and polymerase chain reaction, *Analytical Chemistry*, vol. 78, pp. 7722–7728, 2006.

100. Chen J. F. et al., Electrokinetically synchronized polymerase chain reaction microchip fabricated in poly-carbonate, *Analytical Chemistry*, vol. 77, pp. 658–666, 2005.

101. Gui L., Ren C. L., Numerical simulation of heat transfer and electrokinetic flow in an electroosmosis-based continuous-flow PCR chip, *Analytical Chemistry*, vol. 78, pp. 6215–6222, 2006.

102. Wang W., Li Z. X., Luo R., Lü S. H., Xu A. D., Yang Y. J., Droplet-based micro oscillating-flow PCR chip, *Journal of Micromechanics and Microengineering*, vol. 15, pp. 1369–1377, 2005.

103. Cheng J. Y., Hsieh C. J., Chuang Y. C., Hsieh J. R., Performing microchannel temperature cycling reactions using reciprocating reagent shuttling along a radial temperature gradient, *Analyst*, vol. 130, pp. 931–940, 2005.

104. Beer N. R. et al., On-chip, real-time, single-copy polymerase chain reaction in picoliter droplets, *Analytical Chemistry*, vol. 79, pp. 8471–8475, 2007.

105. Griffith E. J., Akella S., Goldberg M. K., Performance characterization of a reconfigurable planar-array digital microfluidic system, *Transactions on Computer-Aided Design of Integrated Circuits and Systems*, vol. 25, pp. 340–352, 2006.

106. Micklos D. A., DNA Science: A First Course, Cold Spring Harbor; 2nd edition (September 30, 2010), ISBN-13: 978-1936113170.

107. Russell P., Genetics. Benjamin Cummings; 1st edition (2001), ISBN-10 0805345531.

108. Chicurel M. Faster, better, cheaper genotyping, *Nature*, vol. 412, pp. 580–582, 2001.

109. Aborn J. H. et al., A 768-lane microfabricated system for high-throughput DNA sequencing, *Lab on a Chip*, vol. 5, pp. 669–674, 2005.

110. Ahmadiana A., Svahna A., Massively parallel sequencing platforms using lab on a chip technologies, *Lab on a Chip*, vol. 11, pp. 2653–2655, 2011.

111. Blazej R. G., Kumaresan P., Mathies R. A., Microfabricated bioprocessor for integrated nanoliter-scale sanger DNA sequencing, *Proceedings of the National Academy of Science of the United States of America*, vol. 103, pp. 7240–7245, 2006.

112. Chen Y.-J., Huang X., DNA sequencing by denaturation: Principle and thermodynamic simulations, *Analytical Biochemistry*, vol. 384, pp. 170–179, 2009.

113. Chen Y.-J., Roller E. E., Huang X., DNA sequencing by denaturation: Experimental proof of concept with an integrated fluidic device, *Lab on a Chip.*, vol. 10, pp. 1153–1159, 2010.

114. Russom A., Tooke N., Andersson H., Stemme G., Pyrosequencing in a microfluidic flow-through device, *Analytical Chemistry*, vol. 77, pp. 7505–7511, 2005.

115. Huang H., Wu H., Xiao P., Zhou G., Single-nucleotide polymorphism typing based on pyrosequencing chemistry and acryl-modified glass chip, *Electrophoresis*, vol. 30, pp. 991–998, 2009.

116. Boles D. J. et al., Droplet-based pyrosequencing using digital microfluidics, *Analytical Chemistry*, vol. 83, pp. 8439–8447, 2011.

117. Fair R. B. et al., Chemical and biological applications of digital-microfluidics devices, *IEEE Design & Test of Computers*, vol. 24, pp. 10–24, 2007.

118. Seo T. S. et al., Four-color DNA sequencing by synthesis on a chip using photocleavable fluorescent nucleotides, *Proceedings of the National Academy of Science of United States of America*, vol. 102, pp. 5926–5931, 2005.

119. Banerjee A., Pais A., Papautsky I., Klotzkin D., A polarization isolation method for high-sensitivity, low-cost on-chip fluorescence detection for microfluidic lab-on-a-chip, *Sensors Journal*, vol. 8, pp. 621–627, 2008.

120. Organic Light Emitting Devices: Synthesis, Properties and Applications, Müllen K., Scherf U., editors, Wiley-VCH; 1st edition (March 7, 2006), ISBN-13: 978-3527312184.

121. Fixe F., Chu V., Prazeres D. M. F., Conde J. P., An on-chip thin film photodetector for the quantification of DNA probes and targets in microarrays, *Nucleic Acids Research*, vol. 32, pp. e70, 2004.

122. Oliveira-Brett A. M., Piedade J. A. P., Silva L. A., Diculescu V. C., Voltammetric determination of all DNA nucleotides, *Analytical Biochemistry*, vol. 332, 15 pp. 321–329, 2004.

123. Gabig-Ciminska M. et al., Electric chips for rapid detection and quantification of nucleic acids, *Biosensors and Bioelectronics*, vol. 19, pp. 537–546, 2004.

124. Liu S. et al., Automated parallel DNA sequencing on multiple channel microchips, *Proceedings of the Academy of Science of United States of America*, vol. 97, pp. 5369–5374, 2000.

125. Cady N. C., Stelick S., Kunnavakkam M. V., Batt C. A., Real-time PCR detection of listeria mono-cytogenes using an integrated microfluidics platform, *Sensors and Actuators B Chemical*, vol. 107, pp. 332–341, 2005.

Appendix 1: Convention for Organic Formulas and Molecules Stereographic Representation

A1.1 BIOMOLECULES CHEMICAL EQUATIONS

Molecular formulas are widely used in inorganic chemistry but rarely in organic and biological chemistry, since they simply count the number of each sort of atom present in the molecule and tell nothing about the way they are joined together.

Different conventions have been defined in order to code in chemical formulas the type of bonds that are present in the considered molecule and their spatial orientation.

In this appendix, we will review briefly the main conventions for writing organic formulas.

Some of these conventions are quite articulated and count a lot of particular forms to indicate particular structures and spatial dispositions.

We will not provide details regarding the exceptions and conventions of the selected classes of molecules, but simply review the general rules.

For a more detailed explanation we direct the reader to specific references such as [1] and [2].

We would also like to state that a chemical formula, also when a stereographic convention is used, generally does not give any indication on the name of the considered compound.

Naming conventions are quite articulated and the most basic of them are reviewed in Chapters 1 and 2 when dealing with particular classes of biochemical species.

However, they are only few of the articulated rules needed to create unique and somehow explicative names for all the complex array of organic components.

The only available source for all the relevant naming conventions is to access the original International Union of Pure and Applied Chemistry (IUPAC) documents directly on the IUPAC home site (www.iupac.org) or through IUPAC original publications whose list is reported in the IUPAC site [3].

In general, all formulas that are not simple molecule formulas are called structural formulas.

Nevertheless, there are various and quite different types of structural formulae that convey a different amount of information on the real structure of organic molecules.

A1.1.1 DISPLAYED FORMULAS

The first, and simpler, types of structural formulas are the so-called displayed formulas.

A displayed formula shows all the bonds in the molecule as individual lines. You need to remember that each line represents a pair of shared electrons.

For example, in Figure A1.1 a model of methane is represented (cf. Section 1.3.1) together with its displayed formula. Notice that the way the methane is drawn contains no information about the actual shape of the molecule.

This lack of information can lead to problems in cases in which the specific spatial position of the atoms is important.

For example, consider the simple molecule with the molecular formula CH_2Cl_2. It is possible to draw two different displayed formulas, as shown in Figure A1.2. However, they do not correspond to the presence of spatial isomers, due to the angles at which the Cl atoms are bonded to the central

(a)   (b)

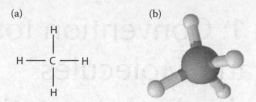

FIGURE A1.1   Methane displayed formula (a) and balls and sticks stereographic model (b).

carbon: the two different display formulas simply represent spatial rotations of the same molecule (as well as evident from stereographic models).

For anything other than the most simple molecules, drawing a fully displayed formula is too complicated (also simple biological molecules can have 50–70 atoms).

The most common feature of all biochemical components are the carbon–hydrogen bonds. Display formulas are simplified by synthesizing with a simple molecular expression the CH groups.

For example, ethanoic acid would be shown in a fully displayed form and a simplified form as

$$
\underset{\underset{H}{|}}{\overset{\overset{H}{|}}{H-C}}-C\underset{O-H}{\overset{O}{\diagup}} \qquad\qquad CH_3-C\underset{OH}{\overset{O}{\diagup}} \tag{A1.1}
$$

An even more simplified way to write display formulas is to set all the different groups one after the other as if they would for a chain.

In this way, ethanoic acid (frequently called acetic acid) can be represented as CH_3COOH, showing the two groups forming the molecule one after the other.

This representation is used only when there is no ambiguity on how the bonds work; as it happens, for example, in long C chains in saturated hydrocarbons.

Naturally, more simplifications are introduced in representing a display formula, more ambiguity arises due to lack of spatial information.

For example, we have seen in Chapter 1 that in long carbon chains of saturated hydrocarbons and of all the derived components (where a CH bond is substituted by some radical) rotation along the chain axis is possible, and this influences possible hydrogen or van der Waals bonds that can completely change the chain spatial form.

When there are side chains, as it is almost always true for biomolecules, a convention has to be added to the writing style of display formulas so as to not create so much ambiguity as to render this instrument useless.

(a)   (b)

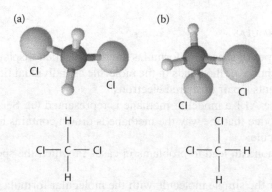

FIGURE A1.2   Chlorine display formulas and the relative stereographic models showing the absence of spatial isomeric structure. The display formula in (a) is nothing more that the representation of a spatial rotation of the structure represented by the apparently different display formula in (b).

As a matter of fact, the possibility of rotation of side chains and C–C bonds around the bond axis renders really difficult to recognize that some display formulas represent the same molecule. For example, both the formulas below represent the same molecule, that is, 2-methylbutane.

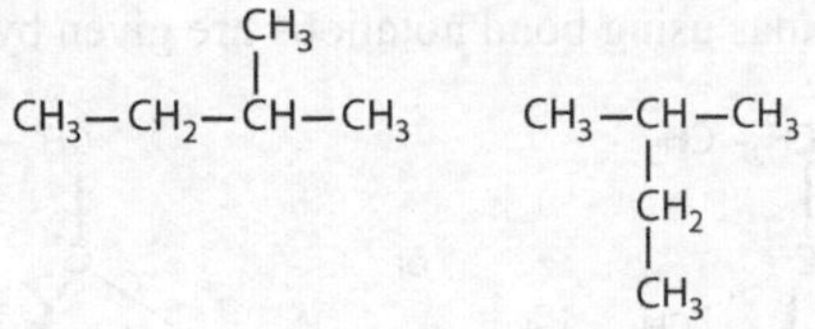

$$CH_3-CH_2-\overset{\overset{\displaystyle CH_3}{|}}{CH}-CH_3 \qquad CH_3-\overset{\overset{\displaystyle }{|}}{CH}-CH_3 \qquad (A1.2)$$

$$\underset{\overset{|}{CH_3}}{\overset{|}{CH_2}}$$

Owing to the bond angles, the only difference between the two diagrams is that some of the bonds are rotated around the axis and turned around a bit.

To avoid such problems, the convention is that the formula is always written looking for the longest possible chain of carbon atoms, and it is drawn horizontally. Any side chain spreads from the main chain; from the side it is more suitable graphically.

As a matter of fact, due to the possibility of rotating bonds, this creates no ambiguity. For example, both the formulas reported in Equation A1.2 obviously represent the same molecule, since they differ only by rotation of bonds.

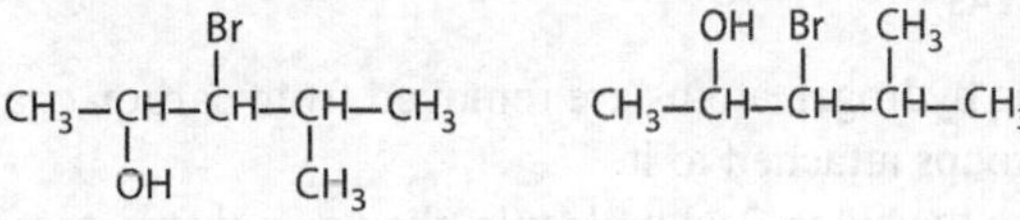

$$CH_3-\overset{\overset{\displaystyle Br}{|}}{CH}-\overset{}{CH}-\overset{\overset{\displaystyle }{|}}{CH}-CH_3 \qquad CH_3-\overset{\overset{\displaystyle OH}{|}}{CH}-\overset{\overset{\displaystyle Br}{|}}{CH}-\overset{\overset{\displaystyle CH_3}{|}}{CH}-CH_3 \qquad (A1.3)$$

$$\underset{OH}{} \quad \underset{CH_3}{}$$

A1.1.2 THREE-DIMENSIONAL STRUCTURE FORMULAS

As we have seen in Section A1.1.1, only a correct representation of the spatial position of the atoms in an organic molecule renders a structural formula easy to read and remove ambiguity completely.

A first step to do that is to adopt a convention for representing spatial position of the bonds in the formula.

The conventional symbols are reported in Figure A1.3.

For example, you might want to show the 3-D arrangement of the groups around the carbon which has the −OH group in butan-2-ol. Butan-2-ol has the full displayed formula:

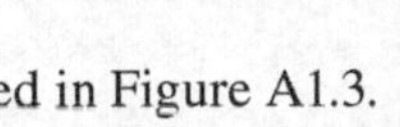

$$CH_3-\overset{\overset{\displaystyle }{|}}{CH}-CH_2-CH_3 \qquad (A1.4)$$

$$\underset{OH}{}$$

Full line bond	————————	Bond lies in the plane of the paper or of the screen if seen electronically
Dashed bond	– – – – – –	Bond extends backwards, away from the viewer into the paper or into the screen
Wedged bond	◢	Bond protundes forwards, towards the viewer out of the paper or out of the screen

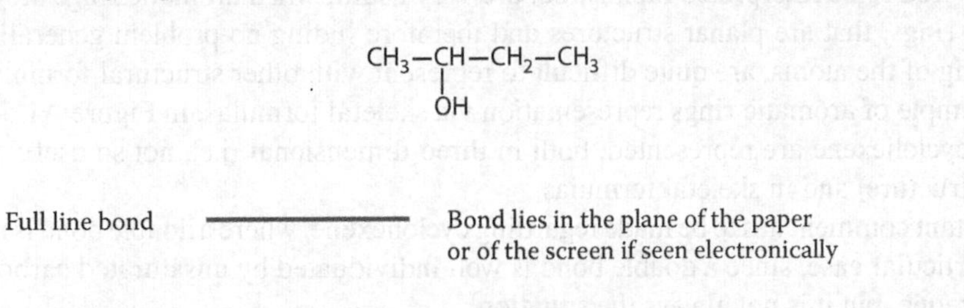

FIGURE A1.3 Conventional symbols used for bonds in three-dimensional structural formulas.

If conventional bond notations are used, there are several possible ways to draw the spatial structure of the molecule; all correspondent to a particular angle of view. They differ for a three-dimensional rotation of the reference system and, with bonds orientation, it is much easier to recognize it with respect to what happens using displayed formulas.

Two possible structure formulas using bond notations are given by

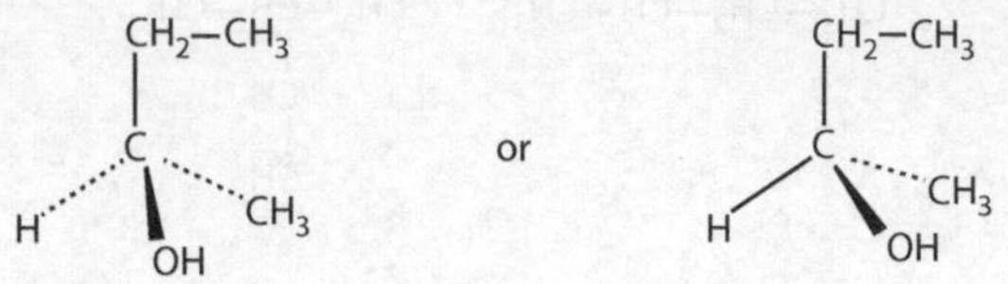

$$
\begin{array}{ccc}
\begin{array}{c}
CH_2-CH_3 \\
| \\
C \\
H \quad \quad CH_3 \\
OH
\end{array}
& \text{or} &
\begin{array}{c}
CH_2-CH_3 \\
| \\
C \\
H \quad \quad CH_3 \\
OH
\end{array}
\end{array}
\qquad (A1.5)
$$

Notice that no attempt was made to show the whole molecule in three dimensions in the structural formula diagrams. The CH_2CH_3 group was left in a simple form.

Three-dimensional formulas are useful to show particular parts of the molecules, where orientation is really a key point, but becomes difficult to read if too complex.

The trick of leaving the most common and simple groups indicated in molecular style is currently used to simplify three-dimensional formulas.

A1.1.3 SKELETAL FORMULAS

In a skeletal formula, all the hydrogen atoms are removed from carbon chains, leaving just a carbon skeleton with functional groups attached to it.

For example, considering the butan-2-ol molecule, the normal structural formula and the skeletal formula look similar to the one in Figure A1.4.

In a skeletal diagram of this sort

- There is a carbon atom at each junction between bonds in a chain and at the end of each bond (unless there is something else already there—like the –OH group in the example).
- There are enough hydrogen atoms attached to each carbon to make the total number of bonds on that carbon up to 4.

Skeletal formulas are not so much used for simple chains, since in long molecules skilled observation is required to be interpreted rapidly, but are very useful when aromatic rings are considered.

Aromatic rings, that are planar structures and therefore hiding no problem generally regarding spatial placing of the atoms, are quite difficult to represent with other structural formulas.

As an example of aromatic rings representation via skeletal formulas, in Figure A1.5 both cyclohexane and cyclohexene are represented, both in three-dimensional (i.e., not so useful in this case for a plane structure) and in skeletal formulas.

An important comment has to be made regarding cyclohexene, where a double bond is represented.

In this particular case, since a double bond is well individuated by unsaturated carbon atoms, its position is unique, but it is not always the situation.

Quantum resonance frequently happens in aromatic rings with the effect of delocalizing electrons shared in double bonds all around a part or even the whole ring.

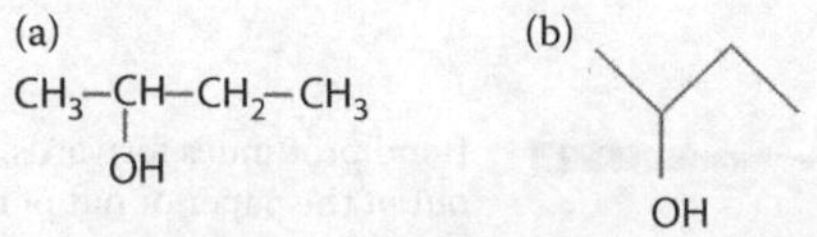

(a)
$$CH_3-CH-CH_2-CH_3$$
$$| $$
$$OH$$

(b)

FIGURE A1.4 Displayed (a) and skeletal (b) formula of butan-2-ol.

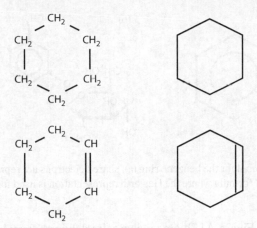

FIGURE A1.5 Three-dimensional and skeletal formula of cyclohexane (a) and cyclohexene (b).

This effect is maximum in the case of the benzene ring, where the double bond electrons are shared by all the carbon atoms of the ring so as to form a unique molecular orbital catching six atoms.

The schematic representation of molecular orbitals of the electrons shared in the double benzene bonds with the corresponding energy is shown in Figure A1.6, and the delocalization of these electrons over all the ring structure in the lower energy state is evident.

This is why in the case of the benzene ring double bonds are not indicated but a special skeletal symbol is used, which is presented in Figure A1.7a.

A last important convention regarding skeletal formulas is needed when it is necessary to understand which of the groups that bonded to a carbon ring are under the ring plane and which are above.

This characteristic sometimes differentiates isomers having quite different characteristics as in the case of carbohydrates.

In this case, the representation used in Figure A1.7b is used, that is called Haworth representation. In Haworth representation of a carbon ring, the approximate plane of the ring is perpendicular to the plane of the paper, with the heavy line on the ring projecting toward the reader.

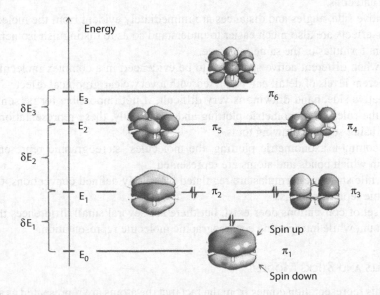

FIGURE A1.6 Schematic representation of molecular orbitals of the electrons shared in the double benzene bonds with corresponding energy.

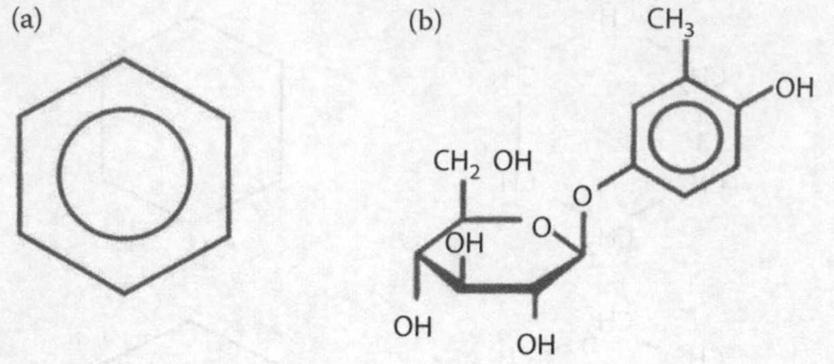

FIGURE A1.7 Skeletal symbol for the benzene ring (a): shared electrons are represented as a circle inside the hexagon; example of skeletal formula where the Haworth representation is used for one of the carbon rings (b).

Thus, the two rings in Figure A1.7b are on approximately orthogonal planes, with the benzene ring on the paper plane and the other ring on a plane orthogonal to paper.

Moreover, the groups that bonded to the orthogonal rings are above or below the ring plane depending on the position above or below the ring representation.

A1.2   BIOMOLECULES STEREOGRAPHIC MODELS

Whichever conventional formula is used, it does not represent real angles and bonds and bond lengths: this information, if needed, have to be reported at the side of the formula.

However, formula conventions are defined so as to be easily inserted in the text and to be drawn by hand.

With the diffusion of chemical calculation and drawing tools, another quite different set of conventions has been introduced, aimed to obtain a real three-dimensional representation of organic molecules.

The idea on the basis of the stereographic representation conventions is to represent the real spatial configuration of the molecule using an orthogonal axonometric representation with the same measurement unit on the three axis.

This approach, imitating the results obtained by the material models of organic molecules, has naturally pros and cons.

On the positive side, angles and distances are immediately evident from the molecule representation, rotation effects are also much easier to understand so as to distinguish isomeric forms from simply different formulas of the same molecule.

Moreover, when different active sites have to be evidenced in a complex molecule, representations with different levels of detail can be mixed with a very clear graphical effect.

On the negative side, hand drawing is very difficult, if not impossible for persons who are not familiar with the rules of axonometric plotting and, practically, these representations can be produced only by using suitable drawing tools.

Having in common axonometric plotting, the molecules' stereographic representations differ from the way in which bonds and atoms are represented.

However, while structure formulas are regulated by strictly defined conventions, this is not true for stereographic representations.

A de facto set of conventions does exist, but there are several small differences that have to be taken into account while interpreting a stereographic molecule representation.

A.1.2.1   BALLS AND STICKS MODEL

The name of this representation comes from the fact that the atoms are represented as solid balls and the bonds as sticks connecting those balls.

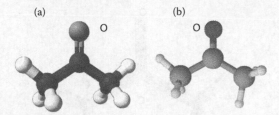

FIGURE A1.8 Acetone molecule balls and sticks representation with explicit double bonds (a) and with implicit double bonds (b).

Since on the length scale we are considering whatever nucleus is a point, sticks are drawn from nucleus to nucleus and the bond length is by definition the average distance among nuclei in the considered bond.

Owing to this way of representing bonds, angles between bonds are uniquely defined as the angle between the corresponding sticks.

As far as multiple bonds are considered, in some kinds of representations they are explicitly reported, whereas in others they are not marked, leaving their individuation to the valence analysis of the atoms comprised in the molecule.

An example of the two kinds of representations is reported in Figure A1.8, for the acetone molecule.

The two approaches have both strengths and weaknesses. By indicating explicitly double bonds renders the representation more immediate, but introduces a certain degree of inaccuracy in cases in which the molecule is generally in a hybrid state between quantum states where the double bonds are located in different positions.

In this book we have explicitly indicated double bonds in Chapter 1 to enable the reader to familiarize with this representation, then we have dropped this convention, leaving them implicit as in the case of the oxygen in Figure A1.8b.

As far as atoms are concerned, they are represented with balls of different colors (in color pictures) or of different gray tones (in gray scale pictures). In this last case, to avoid confusion, the main atoms of the molecules are generally tagged with its symbol, as done for the oxygen atom in Figure A1.8.

The atom radius is generally considered the radius of a sphere with a volume equivalent to the volume that cannot be penetrated due to the presence of the atom.

This definition is sufficiently vague to allow several interpretations, but the most consolidated in biochemistry applications is to adopt as radius of the atoms the van der Waals radius (see definition in Section 1.6) as it reflects quite well the volume that results, which is not penetrable by the weak forces dominating biochemical phenomena.

However, this is not a standard and somehow the spheres radius is simply chosen to render the plot as clear as possible. This effect is evident from Figure A1.8, where in part (b) the above convention is used, while in part (a) the spheres radii are changed so to avoid too small hydrogen atoms that can confuse with the stick representing the bond.

A1.2.2 STICK MODEL

The stick model is simply constituted by balls and sticks representations without balls. The sticks representing the bonds are generally two colored, depending on the atoms they bind.

This representation is useful where there are many atoms and the presence of balls will create confusion by covering, due to the three-dimensional effect of the axonometric representation, part of the molecule.

However, this convention practically requires colors if adopted as it is, since it is not possible to distinguish the atoms but for the different colors reported on the sticks.

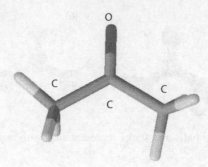

FIGURE A1.9   Gray scale stick representation of the acetone molecule.

Sometimes, to adapt this representation to gray scale representation, the atoms are represented in their position with their symbol, as reported for example in Figure A1.9 where this convention is used for the acetone molecule.

In this representation, both in the color version and in the gray scale version, double bonds are implicit, to maintain the simple appearance of the representation in case of great molecules.

A1.2.3   VOLUME MODEL

In this representation, atoms are represented by the equivalent volume they occupy, taking into account shared electrons.

As in the case of the sticks and balls representation, there are several ways to interpret this prescription, also depending on the kind of phenomena under analysis.

In biochemistry, the radius of the atoms is assumed to be coincident with their van der Waals equilibrium distance, thereby reflecting the fact that we are mainly interested in weak forces interactions.

The volume representation of the acetone molecule is compared with its sticks and balls representation in Figure A1.10.

It is important to note that the volume representation does not evidence bonds, but it permits to evidence atoms volumes superposition and the molecular surface defined on the ground of van der Waals radii, that are quite important, as we have seen in Section 1.6, for many statistical mechanical models of biochemical phenomena.

A1.2.4   MIXED BALLS AND STICKS AND VOLUME MODEL

It is possible that in some applications it is needed both to evidence the molecule dimension through a volume representation and the bond angles and length through a sticks and balls representation or through a sticks representation only.

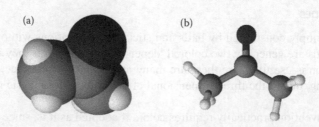

(a)   (b)

FIGURE A1.10   Volume (a) and sticks and balls (b) models of the acetone molecule.

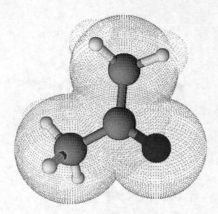

FIGURE A1.11   Mixed volume plus sticks and balls model of the acetone molecule.

In this case, to the sticks or sticks and bond representation a sort of cloud of points is added to represent the volume that would be occupied by the volume representation.

An example is reported in Figure A1.11.

A1.2.5   STRIPS MODEL

Although stereographic models are quite clear in representing the spatial shape of organic molecules, several times they also have the advantage of being produced by suitable computer tools, so as to be also graphically precise. In the case of very complex molecules such as proteins or RNA they become too complex very soon and tend to hide the main features of the molecule shape.

This is true while different levels of molecule organization emerge due to a first layer of covalent bonds superimposed to successive levels of structure introduced by weak forces, such as hydrogen or van der Waals bonds (see Sections 2.3.2 and 2.3.3).

Just to make an example, a section of a protein α-helix in balls and sticks representations is plotted, both seen from the side and from the top. It is apparent that, even if containing a lot of information, the representation is quite complex and tends to catch the attention more on particulars than on the complete structure shape.

To easily trace the main characteristics of the structure, nonconventional elements are frequently added to the standard representation, as the helix form in the side view in Figure A1.12, that both synthesize all the radicals of the helix backbone (whose explicit representation would render the scheme confused) and underline the helix shape.

(a)   (b)

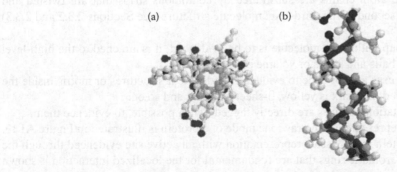

FIGURE A1.12   Section of α protein α-helix in balls and sticks representation seen from the top (a) and from the side (b).

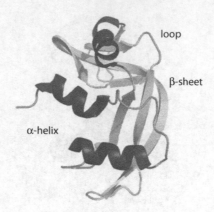

FIGURE A1.13 Strips model of a protein in gray scale representation with the main secondary structure elements suitably tagged.

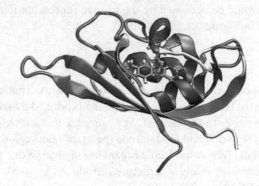

FIGURE A1.14 Strips model of a protein in gray scale representation with an active site evidenced through the sticks model to show the aromatic rings that are fundamental for the localized interaction.

If the high-level structure of the molecule is to be evidenced, generally more synthetic representations are used.

In this field there is even less standardization than in the field of stereographic representations and every author has its preferred style. In this book the strips style is generally used, that is one of the most diffused for biological applications.

In the strips style, the atom chains are substituted by continuous strips that are twisted and modeled so to render the second or the third-level molecule structure (see Sections 2.3.2 and 2.3.3) depending on the need.

If some particular group within the molecule is to be evidenced, it is attached to the high-level representation with local balls and sticks or volume plot.

These representations uses a color code to evidence the different structures or motifs inside the molecule like α-helix is red, 3_{10} helix is yellow, β-sheet is green, and so on.

In gray tones representation, motives are directly tagged, when possible, to evidence them.

An example of strips representation in gray tone mode of a protein is illustrated in Figure A1.13. The strips model of a protein in gray scale representation with an active site evidenced through the sticks model to show the aromatic rings that are fundamental for the localized interaction is shown in Figure A1.14, to present an example of mixed representation.

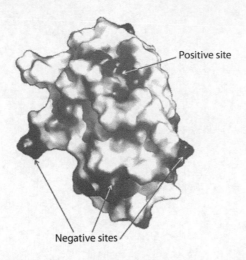

FIGURE A1.15 Example of surface representation in gray scale of a protein where areas of superficial charge accumulation are evidenced.

A1.2.6 SURFACE MODEL

In some applications, it is not the molecule spatial structure that has to be evidenced, but its surface, generally in order to better evidence active sites and surface characteristics.

In this case, the so-called surface model is used.

The molecule is represented in volume model and then the outer surface is interpolated so as to obtain a continuous profile. It is to note that in the convention where the volume model representation is obtained by considering the van der Waals atomic distances, this construction coincides with the surface definition, that is generally given in statistical mechanics models of macromolecule solutions (Section 1.6), and thus it is very useful in this field.

An example of surface representation in gray scale of a protein is reported in Figure A1.15.

REFERENCES

1. Stoker H. S. *General, Organic, and Biological Chemistry*, Brooks Cole; 5th edition (December 15, 2008), ISBN-13: 978-0547152813.
2. Raymond K. W., *General, Organic, and Biological Chemistry, An Integrated Approach*, Wiley; 1st edition (August 12, 2005), ISBN-13: 978-0471447078.
3. List of official IUPC books on Chemical conventions for naming, formulas and reactions: http://www.iupac.org/nc/home/publications/iupac-books/books-by-title.html (accessed last time March 12, 2012).

Appendix 2: Building Blocks of Proteins

In Chapter 2, we have seen that proteins are composed of a polypeptide chain, a biopolymer whose monomers are extracted by a limited set of small biomolecules: the 20 amino acids. They can be divided into two categories: amino acids with hydrophobic side groups, with hydrophilic side group and with neither hydrophobic nor hydrophilic side groups.

Here, we list structure and selected properties of those molecules that can be considered the building blocks of proteins. Structures are reported in Figures A2.1 through A2.20, properties in Tables A2.1, A2.2, and A2.3. All properties are at 279 K, if temperature dependent.

As far as amino acids coding is concerned, the three-letter codes convention is used throughout this book; however, a correspondence between three-letter codes and one-letter codes is reported in Table A2.4 for reference.

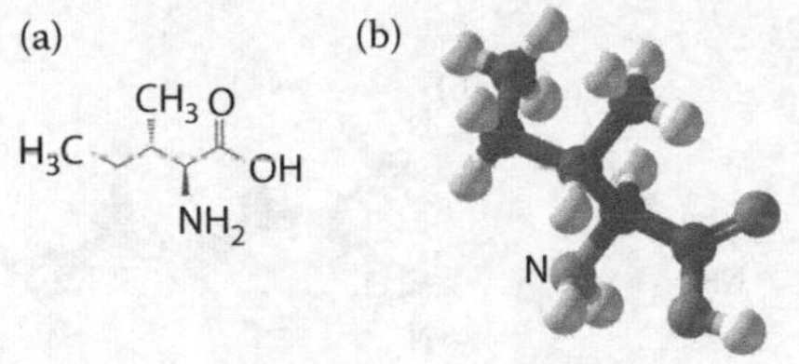

FIGURE A2.1 Isoleucine structure formula (a) and stereographic representation (b).

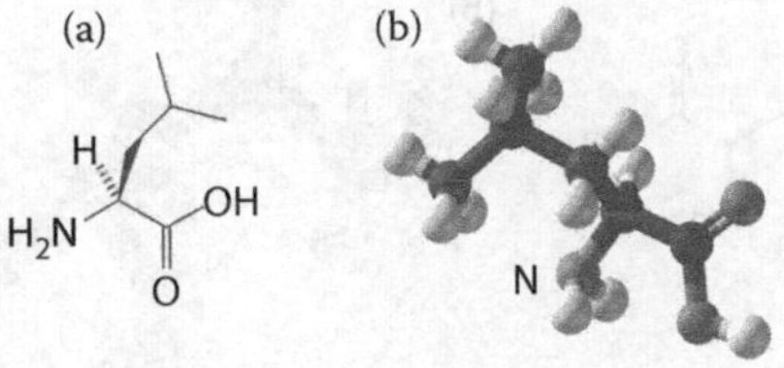

FIGURE A2.2 Leucine structure formula (a) and stereographic representation (b).

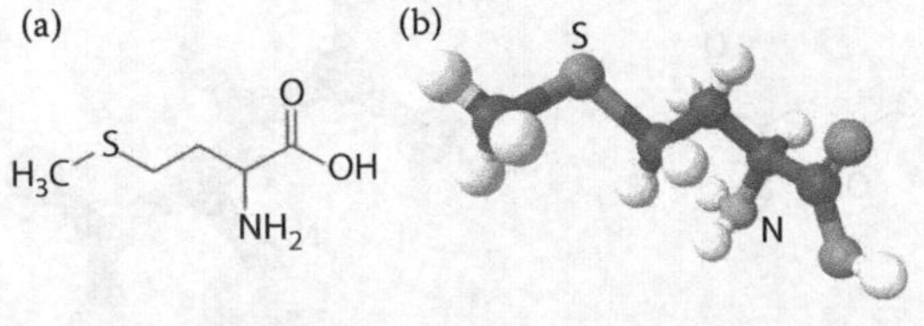

FIGURE A2.3 Methionine structure formula (a) and stereographic representation (b).

(a)   (b)

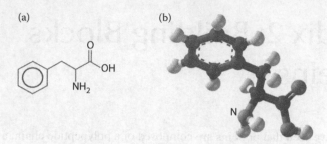

FIGURE A2.4   Phenylalanine structure formula (a) and stereographic representation (b).

(a)   (b)

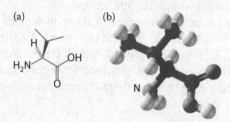

FIGURE A2.5   Valine structure formula (a) and stereographic representation (b).

(a)   (b)

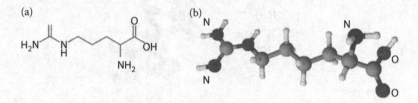

FIGURE A2.6   Arginine structure formula (a) and stereographic representation (b).

(a)   (b)

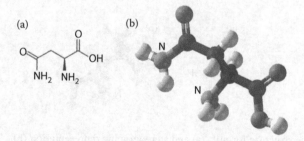

FIGURE A2.7   Asparagine structure formula (a) and stereographic representation (b).

(a)   (b)

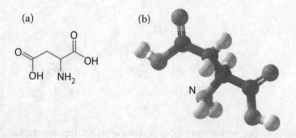

FIGURE A2.8   Aspartic acid structure formula (a) and stereographic representation (b).

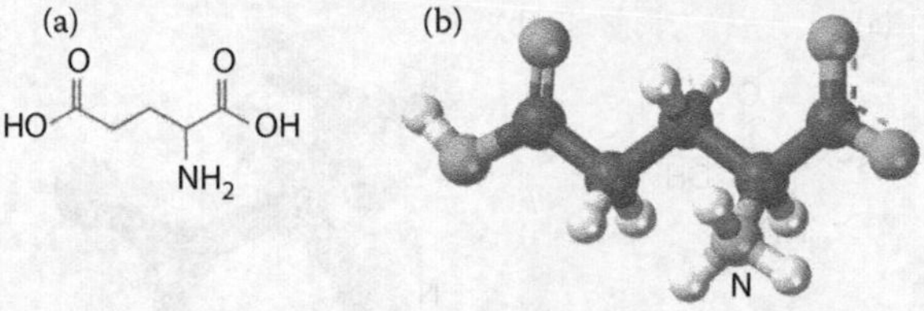

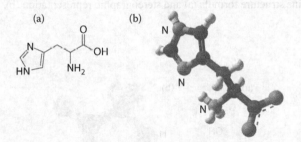

FIGURE A2.9　Glutamic acid structure formula (a) and stereographic representation (b).

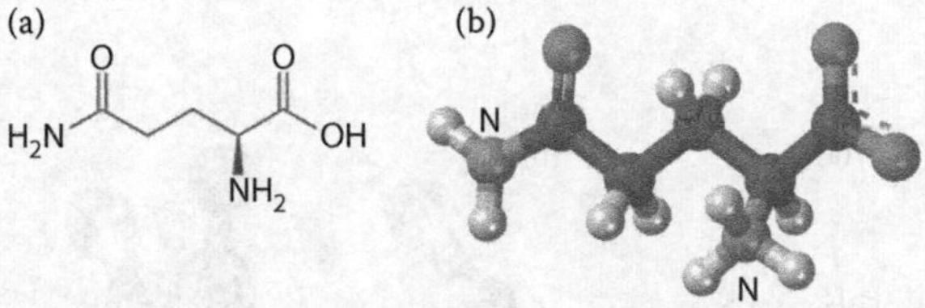

FIGURE A2.10　Glutamine structure formula (a) and stereographic representation (b).

FIGURE A2.11　Histidine structure formula (a) and stereographic representation (b).

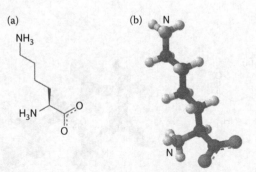

FIGURE A2.12　Lysine structure formula (a) and stereographic representation (b).

(a)   (b)

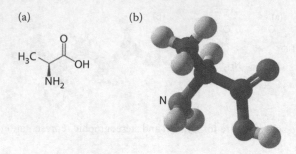

FIGURE A2.13   Alanine structure formula (a) and stereographic representation (b).

(a)   (b)

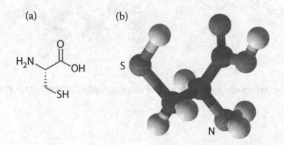

FIGURE A2.14   Cysteine structure formula (a) and stereographic representation (b).

(a)   (b)

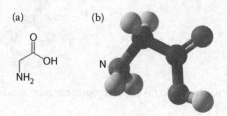

FIGURE A2.15   Glycine structure formula (a) and stereographic representation (b).

(a)   (b)

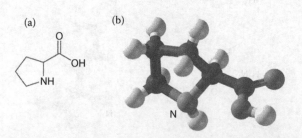

FIGURE A2.16   Proline structure formula (a) and stereographic representation (b).

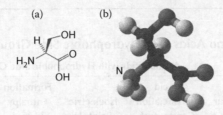

FIGURE A2.17 Serine structure formula (a) and stereographic representation (b).

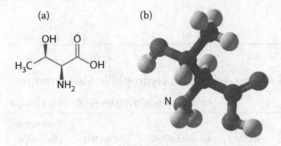

FIGURE A2.18 Threonine structure formula (a) and stereographic representation (b).

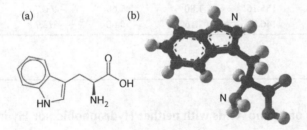

FIGURE A2.19 Tryptophan structure formula (a) and stereographic representation (b).

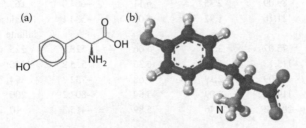

FIGURE A2.20 Tyrosine structure formula (a) and stereographic representation (b).

TABLE A2.1
Selected Properties of Amino Acids with Hydrophobic Side Groups

				Amino Acids with Hydrophobic Side Groups			
Name	Acronym	Molar Mass g	Acid Dissociation Constant pK_1	Isoelectric PointpH	Formation Enthalpy kJ/mol	Water Solubility g/L	Notes
Isoleucine	ile	131.18	2.32	6.05	−637.8	32.1	Chiral—nonpolar
Leucine	leu	131.18	2.33	6.01	−637.4	24	Chiral—nonpolar
Methionine	met	149.21	2.13	5.74	−577.5	48	Chiral—nonpolar
Phenylalanine	phe	165.19	2.20	5.49	−466.9	27	Chiral—nonpolar
Valine	val	117.15	2.39	6.00	−617.9	85	Chiral—nonpolar

TABLE 2.2
Selected Properties of Amino Acids with Hydrophilic Side Groups

				Amino Acids with Hydrophilic Side Groups			
Name	Acronym	Molar Mass g	Acid Dissociation Constant pK_1	Isoelectric Point pH	Formation Enthalpy kJ/mol	Water Solubility g/L	Notes
Arginine	arg	174.20	1.82	10.76	−623.5	148.7	Polar
Asparagine	asn	132.12	2.14	5.41	−789.4	22	Polar
Aspartic acid	asp	133.10	1.99	2.85	−973.3	4	Chiral
Glutamic acid	glu	147.13	2.10	3.15	−1009.7	11.1	Polar, chiral
Glutamine	gln	146.15	2.17	5.65	−826.4	26	Polar, chiral
Histidine	his	155.16	1.80	7.60	−466.7	38.2	Polar, chiral
Lysine	lys	146.16	2.16	9.60	−678.7	300	Polar, chiral

TABLE 2.3
Selected Properties of Amino Acids with neither Hydrophobic nor Hydrophilic Side Groups

				Amino Acids with neither Hydrophobic nor Hydrophilic Side Groups			
Name	Acronym	Molar Mass g	Acid Dissociation Constant pK_1	Isoelectric Point pH	Formation Enthalpy kJ/mol	Water Solubility g/L	Notes
Alanine	ala	89.09	2.35	6.11	−604.0	165.5	Nonpolar, chiral
Cysteine	cys	121.16	1.92	5.05	−534.1	Practically infinite	Polar, chiral
Glycine	gly	75.07	2.35	6.06	−528.5	225	Nonpolar, nonchiral
Proline	pro	115.13	1.95	6.30	−515.2	1500	Nonpolar, chiral
Serine	ser	105.09	2.19	5.68	−732.7	364	Polar, chiral
Threonine	thr	119.12	2.09	5.60	−807.2	200	Polar, chiral
Tryptophan	trp	204.23	2.46	5.89	−415.3	10	Polar (small dipole), chiral
Tyrosine	tyr	181.19	2.20	5.64	−685.1	0.38	Polar, chiral

TABLE A2.4
Three and One Letter Codes for Amino Acids

Amino Acid Name	Amino Acids Three-Letter Code	Amino Acids One-Letter Code
Alanine	Ala	A
Arginine	Arg	R
Asparagine	Asn	N
Aspartic acid	Asp	D
Cysteine	Cys	C
Glutamine	Gln	Q
Glutamic acid	Glu	E
Glycine	Gly	G
Histidine	His	H
Isoleucine	Ile	I
Leucine	Leu	L
Lysine	Lys	K
Methionine	Met	M
Phenylalanine	Phe	F
Proline	Pro	P
Serine	Ser	S
Threonine	Thr	T
Tryptophan	Trp	W
Tyrosine	Tyr	Y
Valine	Val	V

Appendix 3: Conventions for Mathematical Notations

A3.1 EUCLIDEAN TENSORS REPRESENTATION AND CALCULUS

In this appendix we will limit ourselves to introduce a formal and a coordinate representation for tensor algebra and calculus in Euclidean spaces, where covariant and contravariant versions of a vector are identical having the same coordinates [1].

In this book the need of using generalized Riemann varieties never arises, thus we will not enter into the complication of dealing with this general formalism.

We will use both an abstract notation, where vectors and tensors are represented with single symbols, and a coordinate notation, where the equations are represented through vector and tensor coordinates.

Owing to the linear transformation laws of vector coordinates from a Euclidean reference system to the other, relations among vector and tensor coordinates are invariant when a linear coordinate transformation is performed, so that they are as general as equations written in abstract notation.

To represent vector equations through the vector coordinates we will adopt the Einstein notation [1]. Thus, we represent vectors with bold letters, while we indicate the set of their coordinates with the vector name with a floating index.

As an example, the position vector will be $\mathbf{x}$, with coordinates x_1, x_2, and x_3, while the set of coordinates will be indicated with x_j. Index indicated in small Latin letters will always run from 1 to 3, when we will need indexes that will run over different intervals we will use either Greek letters or capital Latin letters.

A tensor of order two (that is often called a dyad in fluid dynamics literature) will be indicated in abstract notation with a bold letter with an underline (like $\underline{\mathbf{a}}$) and its coordinates with two indices like $a_{i,j}$ where in this case, due to the indices convention, both i and j will run from 1 to 3.

Higher-order tensors in abstract notation will be indicated with multiple underlines and the corresponding coordinates with multiple indices (e.g., a third-order tensor will be indicated with a and its coordinates with $a_{i,j,k}$).

The implicit summation rule will be used on repeated indices in equations, so that the inner product between the vector a and the second-order tensor $\underline{b}$, that is indicated in abstract notation with $\underline{b} \cdot a$ is indicated using the coordinates with $b_{j,i} a_i$ intending that the coordinates with index i has to be summated, so that

$$c_j = b_{j,i} a_i \underline{\underline{\mathrm{def}}} \sum_{i=1}^{3} b_{j,i} a_i \tag{A3.1}$$

In the cases where a repeated index will be present, but summation is not implied, this will be evident from the presence at the first member of the repeated index. In any case, to eliminate any possible misunderstanding, it will also be indicated explicitly as

$$c_{ji} = b_{j,i} a_i \; (\Sigma_i) \tag{A3.2}$$

As far as the external product between a and $\underline{b}$ is concerned, that is a third-order tensor and is indicated in abstract notation like $\underline{c} = \underline{b} \otimes a$, it will be indicated using the components like $c_{j,i,k} = b_{j,i} a_k$ where the absence of any summation is implied by the fact that there are no repeated indices.

The index notation is very useful to express inner product between complex tensors (also called indexes contraction), since the result depends on the indexes over which the contraction is operated.

For example, if we introduce two second-order tensors $\underline{a}$ and $\underline{b}$, the inner product between them cannot be uniquely defined, since different second-order tensors can be obtained from them by summing indexes of $\underline{a}$ and $\underline{b}$.

However, the difference is clearly visible if the index notation is used. For example, we can define the two tensors $\underline{c}$ and $\underline{c}'$ by using two different contraction operations

$$c_{i,j} = a_{i,k}b_{k,j} \tag{A3.3a}$$

$$c'_{i,j} = a_{i,k}b_{j,k} \tag{A3.3b}$$

In this simple case, the ambiguity could be solved also in abstract notation by introducing the transpose operation, but the situation gets increasingly complex if the tensor orders increase and more complex operators to reorder tensor indices should be introduced to represent correctly contraction in abstract notation.

Thus, generally, index contraction is represented directly in index notation.

Another particular case is that of function depending on a vector that is on all the vector coordinates. For example, if we have the scalar function $\mathcal{F}$ that depends on the vector $\boldsymbol{a}$, it will be indicated in abstract notation as $\mathcal{F}(\boldsymbol{a})$. In index notation, the vector $\boldsymbol{a}$ will be indicated with its generic coordinates, so that the function will be written as $\mathcal{F}(a_i)$. If a single a_1 coordinate would be indicated, the index should have a precise value, like $\mathcal{F}(a_1)$. It is possible that a function depends only on one vector coordinate, but it is not specified a priori on what coordinate.

In this case, however, the function also will depend on a vector index, that will be the same of the coordinate that appears as a variable.

To manage this case, the notation where the same index is repeated both in the function symbol and in a function vector variable, for example, $\mathcal{F}_i(a_i)$, will be interpreted as a set of functions (three in this case) each of which depends on a single coordinate of the vector a that is indicated by the same index reported in the function symbol.

This also means that the repeated index summation rule has not to be applied if an index is repeated in the function symbol and in one of the variables, since no summation is implied in $\mathcal{F}_i(a_i)$.

A3.1.1 DERIVATIVE AND DIFFERENTIAL OPERATORS

Applying the notation we have introduced to derivation operators, the derivative of a vector with respect to a generic coordinate can be indicated both in abstract and in coordinate notations as

$$b = \frac{\partial a}{\partial x_1} \tag{A3.4a}$$

$$b_j = \frac{\partial a_j}{\partial x_1} \tag{A3.4b}$$

In Euclidean spaces, we have no need of introducing the concept of covariant derivative that is needed in generic curve spaces [1].

A second-order tensor can be constructed by arranging the derivatives of the components of a vector with respect to the components of another vector (e.g., all the coordinates, that are the components of the position vector).

This tensor can be represented both in abstract notation and in coordinate notation as follows:

$$\underline{b} = \frac{\partial a}{\partial x} \tag{A3.5a}$$

$$b_{j,k} = \frac{\partial a_j}{\partial x_k} \tag{A3.5b}$$

The simpler differential operator that can be introduced is the gradient (grad()), that is the sum of the derivatives of the coordinates of a vector by the coordinate with the same index.

The gradient is traditionally represented in abstract notation by introducing the differential vector Del (∇), whose coordinates are the formal derivative operators with respect to the three coordinates, so that

$$\nabla_j = \frac{\partial}{\partial x_j} \tag{A3.6}$$

This notation is quite useful since the Del operator transforms exactly as a vector against Euclidean coordinate transformations, so that it can be used in abstract notation of differential equations exactly like a vector.

The gradient of a function of the coordinates is formally constructed by starting from the Del operator as the product of Del by the considered function, resulting in a vector. Thus, in abstract notation and in coordinates notation

$$grad(f(x)) = \nabla f(x) \tag{A3.7a}$$

$$grad_j(f(x)) = \nabla_j f(x) = \frac{\partial f(x)}{\partial x_j} \tag{A3.7b}$$

The scalar product of the Del by itself is a second-order differential operator, called generally Laplacian (∇^2), that is constituted by the sum of the second-order derivatives with respect to the coordinates. The Laplacian of a vector is thus a vector, while the Laplacian of a scalar is a scalar.

To make an example of Laplacian use in the coordinate notation, the Laplacian of a second-order tensor $\underline{a}$ is indicated in formal and in coordinate notation as

$$\frac{\partial^2 a_{i,j}}{\partial x_1^{\,2}} + \frac{\partial^2 a_{i,j}}{\partial x_2^{\,2}} + \frac{\partial^2 a_{i,j}}{\partial x_3^{\,2}} = \frac{\partial}{\partial x_k} \frac{\partial}{\partial x_k} a_{i,j} \tag{A3.8}$$

where the implicit summation convention is used in the last expression on the repeated index k.

Using the Del operator the divergence vector operator can be introduced (div()), obtained by the scalar product of Del by the considered vector. Since it is a scalar product, the divergence is a scalar and it is expressed in our notations as follows:

$$div(a) = \nabla \cdot a = \frac{\partial a_i}{\partial x_i} \tag{A3.9}$$

where the implicit summation rule is again used in the coordinate notation part of the equation.

A3.1.2 THE LEVI CIVITA SYMBOL AND THE CURL OPERATOR

Introducing vector cross product and the curl() operator in this purely linear notation is a bit more involved process, due to the fact that the vector cross product is a quadratic form in the coordinates of the two vectors that are multiplied.

In particular, indicating with $a \times b$ the cross product between the vectors a and b, its coordinates are provided in general by the equations

$$(a \times b)_1 = a_2 b_3 - a_3 b_2 \tag{A3.10a}$$

$$(a \times b)_2 = a_3 b_1 - a_1 b_3 \tag{A3.10b}$$

$$(a \times b)_3 = a_1 b_2 - a_2 b_1 \tag{A3.10c}$$

To express the vector product in the coordinate notation, the Levi Civita symbol [1] has to be introduced. Its introduction not only enables us to use a uniform coordinate notation also when the cross product is involved, but also allows more insight into the role of the cross product in a general tensor theory in Euclidean spaces.

The Levi Civita symbol $\epsilon_{i,j,k}$ is defined as follows:

$$\begin{cases} \epsilon_{1,2,3} = \epsilon_{2,3,1} = \epsilon_{3,1,2} = 1 \\ \epsilon_{3,2,1} = \epsilon_{2,1,3} = \epsilon_{1,3,2} = -1 \\ \text{All other components} = 0 \end{cases} \tag{A3.11}$$

The Levi Civita symbol is not a tensor, since it has the same components in all the reference systems, so that it does not follow the reference system transformation rules for tensors.

For its definition $\epsilon_{i,j,k}$ is antisymmetric in any pair of indices. Simple consequences of the structure of $\epsilon_{i,j,k}$ are

$$\epsilon_{i,i,k} = \epsilon_{i,k,k} = \epsilon_{i,k,i} = 0 \tag{A3.12}$$

and, if $s_{i,j}$ is a symmetric tensor

$$\epsilon_{i,j,k} s_{i,j} = 0 \tag{A3.13}$$

The introduction of the Levi Civita symbol allows the cross product between tensors to be easily represented in index notation as

$$(a \times b)_i = \epsilon_{i,j,k} a_j b_k \tag{A3.14}$$

due to the specific reference frame transformation property of the Levi Civita symbol, the cross product between the vectors a and b in a different reference system (where the vector coordinates are indicated with an apex) writes

$$(a \times b)'_i = \epsilon_{i,j,k} a'_j b'_k = \epsilon_{i,j,k} T_{j,n} a_n T_{k,m} b_m \tag{A3.15}$$

where $T_{j,n}$ are the components of the reference frame transformation operator.

From Equation A3.15 it is evident that the coordinates $T_{j,n} a_n T_{k,m} b_m$ are simply the coordinates in the new reference system of the external product between the vectors a and b, due to the properties of the transformation operator in a Euclidean space between Cartesian coordinate systems.

Thus we can say that, in every reference system, the cross product between two vectors can be obtained by contracting through the Levi Civita symbol the tensor obtained by the external products of the two involved vectors, whose coordinates have to be evaluated in the considered reference system.

A particular application of the definition of the vector cross product is given by the definition of the curl() differential operator, whose abstract notation definition can be written as

$$curl(a) = \nabla \times a \tag{A3.16a}$$

so that index notation is defined as

$$curl_i(a) = \epsilon_{i,j,k} \nabla_j a_k = \epsilon_{i,j,k} \frac{\partial a_k}{\partial x_j} a_k \tag{A3.16b}$$

From the properties of the Levi Civita symbol two useful identities well known in the classical vector calculus can be demonstrated easily

$$curl_i(grad(f(x))) = (\nabla \times \nabla f(x))_i = \epsilon_{i,j,k} \frac{\partial}{\partial x_j} \frac{\partial}{\partial x_k} f(x) = 0 \tag{A3.17}$$

$$div(curl(a(x))) = (\nabla \cdot \nabla \times a(x)) = \frac{\partial}{\partial x_i} \epsilon_{i,j,k} \frac{\partial}{\partial x_j} a_k(x) = 0 \tag{A3.18}$$

Finally, an important relation can be found between the Levi Civita symbol and the Kronecker symbol $\delta_{n,m}$ (that is one if the indices are equal and zero otherwise). In particular, the following equality holds:

$$\epsilon_{i,j,k} \epsilon_{i,n,m} = \delta_{j,n} \delta_{k,m} - \delta_{j,m} \delta_{k,n} \tag{A3.19}$$

A3.2   HILBERT SPACES AND EIGENVALUE PROBLEMS

In this book we will make a limited use of the concept of Hilbert space, always related to functional spaces of function that are square integrable in some domain of the independent variables.

This notation will be used mainly in conjunction of eigenvalues problems for differential operators that are used in fluid dynamics or in optics.

To indicate members of a functional Hilbert space and the operations among them in a compact way we will use the Dirac Bra–Ket notation [2].

Thus, if x_i is a set of independent variables and $f(x_i)$ is a function of those variables, being a member of a functional Hilbert space, we will indicate it also as a Ket vector $|f$ when the nature of element of the Hilbert space has to be put in evidence.

Using this notation, the complex conjugate of $f(x_i)$ will be indicated as a Bra vector $|f$. Naturally, if we are considering real-valued functions, the Bra and the Ket vectors coincide.

The norm of $f(x_i)$, which is formally the scalar product between the function and its complex conjugate in the Hilbert space, will be indicated with the Bra-Ket product notation, that is

$$\langle f|f \rangle = \int f(x_i) f^*(x_i) dD \tag{A3.20}$$

where D is the domain where the Hilbert space is defined.

Similarly, the scalar product between two functions $f(x_i)$ and $g(x_i)$ will be indicated as

$$\langle g|f \rangle = \int f(x_i)g^*(x_i)dD \tag{A3.21}$$

So that $\langle g|f \rangle = \langle f|g \rangle^*$.

A.3.2.1 COMPLETE SETS, OPERATORS, AND EIGENVALUE PROBLEMS

Linear operators are generally indicated with bold letters with a hat like $\hat{A}$ unless a more specific symbol exists for the specific operator (e.g., $\partial/\partial x$ or ∇).

If the set of orthonormal functions $|\varphi_n\rangle$ constitutes a complete set in the considered space, the following completeness property can be derived

$$\sum_n |\varphi_n\rangle\langle\varphi_m| = \hat{1}$$

where $\hat{1}$ (often simply indicated as 1) is the unitary operator.

Every member of the space can be written as a superposition of the functions of this set like

$$|f\rangle = \sum_n f_n |\varphi_n\rangle \tag{A3.22}$$

Also operators can be expressed through its representation in the $|\varphi_n\rangle$ base. This expression of a linear operator in the Dirac notation writes

$$\hat{A} = \sum_{n,m} A_{n,m} |\varphi_n\rangle\langle\varphi_m| \tag{A3.23}$$

where

$$A_{n,m} = \langle\varphi_n|\hat{A}|\varphi_m\rangle \tag{A3.24}$$

That notation allows to derive directly the components of the function obtained by applying a linear operator to a given function, resulting, for the orthonormal property of the set $|\varphi_n\rangle$

$$\hat{A}|f\rangle = \sum_n A_{n,m} f_m |\varphi_n\rangle \tag{A3.25}$$

The general eigenvalue problem for an operator $\hat{A}$ can be expressed in the Dirac notation like

$$\hat{A}|\psi_n\rangle = k_n |\psi_n\rangle \tag{A3.26}$$

A base constituted by the orthonormal set of eigenfunctions of a certain operator can be used to solve the general linear problem related to that operator.

In particular, let us consider the equation

$$\hat{A}|f\rangle = |g\rangle \tag{A3.27}$$

where $|g\rangle$ is a known function and $|f\rangle$ is the unknown. If the eigenvalue problem for $\hat{A}$ is solved by solving Equation A3.26 we can develop both the functions and the operator using the representation of the operator eigenfunctions and substitute this representation into Equation A3.27.

Using the completeness of the eigenfunctions set it is readily obtained as

$$\sum_n \hat{A} f_n |\psi_n\rangle = \sum_n g_n |\psi_n\rangle \tag{A3.28}$$

Owing to the orthonormal property of the eigenfunctions the sums have to be equal term by term as it is demonstrated by multiplying Equation A3.28 on the left by $\langle\psi_m|$ and saturating m.

Exploiting Equation A3.26 it is thus obtained as

$$k_n f_n = g_n \tag{A3.29}$$

So that the formal solution of Equation A3.27 can be written as

$$|f\rangle = \sum_n \frac{g_n}{k_n} |\psi_n\rangle = \sum_n \frac{\psi_n|g}{k_n} |\psi_n\rangle \tag{A3.30}$$

REFERENCES

1. De U. C., *Tensor Calculus*, Alpha Science Intl Ltd; 2nd edition (December 30, 2007), ISBN-13: 978-1842654484.
2. Van Eijndhoven S. J. L., *A Mathematical Introduction to Dirac's Formalism*, Elsevier Science Ltd (December 1986), ISBN-13: 978-0444701275.

Appendix 4: Time-Scale Separation Method

A4.1 DESCRIPTION OF THE TIME-SCALE SEPARATION METHOD

The problem of solving the diffusion equation when a concentration-dependent term appears at the second member is very difficult and it is the subject of a deep mathematical analysis because of the great number of applications.

A very wide and detailed review of analytical and semi-analytical methods designed to face this problem is reported in [1], while an analysis of this problem in the framework of a general analysis of diffusion problems is reported in the classic work [2].

However, a general analytical method of solution to this problem does not exist and a simulation algorithm has to be used [3,4].

Here, we want to introduce an approximate solution method that is useful in diffusion–chemical problems under a set of approximations that are well fulfilled in practically important problems related to lab on chip design.

We will not present a rigorous mathematical analysis of this approximation, which is beyond the scope of this book, but we will present a physical demonstration.

A4.1.1 HYPOTHESES

Consider the equation

$$D\nabla^2 c - \mathcal{F}(t, c) = \frac{\partial c}{\partial t} \tag{A4.1}$$

where $\mathcal{F}(t, c)$ (is an analytical function of its variables in any limited domain of the space (c, t). Equation A4.1 has to be solved in a regular domain of the space (x, y, z) whose border is a regular surface, which is a surface with analytical parametric equations in any part of the border, under both initial and boundary conditions. We call regular domain a domain whose border is a regular surface, that is, a surface with analytical parametric equations in any part of the border. It can also be not limited, that is half-lines can exist starting from suitable inner points and completely belonging to $\mathbb{D}_r$.

Let us also consider the following associated equations:

$$-\mathcal{F}(t, c) = \frac{\partial c}{\partial t} \tag{A4.2}$$

that is generally called associated chemical equation and

$$D\nabla^2 c = \frac{\partial c}{\partial t} \tag{A4.3}$$

that is the associated diffusion equation.

We will indicate with $Q(c_0, t)$ a solution of Equation A4.2 with the initial condition c_0 and with $c_s(r, t)$ is a solution of Equation A4.3 under the initial and boundary conditions of the initial problem.

Let us also assume that the function $Q(c_0, t)$ is sensibly different from zero in an interval [0, T_{chem}] with $T_{chem} \ll l^2/D$ where l is the smaller characteristic length of the problem. This can be expressed rigorously in the Fourier space by asserting that the spectrum of $Q(c_0, t)$ is band limited in a bandwidth Ω defined as

$$B_Q \equiv [2\pi/T_{chem} - \Omega_Q, 2\pi/T_{chem} + \Omega_Q] \tag{A4.4}$$

while $c_s(r, t)$ is also band limited in a bandwidth B_s defined as

$$B_s \equiv [0, \Omega_s] \tag{A4.5}$$

being $\Omega_s \sim 2\pi \, D/l^2$.

Since l^2/D is the characteristic time of the diffusion in the considered system, we can say that the chemical reaction arrives to a stationary status in a very short time with respect to the time needed to have sensible diffusion.

The above condition can also be enunciated by saying that the derivative $\partial c_s/\partial t$ is a small parameter with respect to the other time derivatives that are present in the problem and the problem solution can be approximately developed at the first order in this parameter.

A4.1.2 THESIS

Under the above conditions, the solution of Equation A4.1 can be written as the first order in $\partial c_s/\partial t$ as

$$c(r, t) = Q(c_s(r, t), t) \tag{A4.6}$$

A4.2 TIME-SCALE SEPARATION METHOD VALIDATION

A4.2.1 SUFFICIENT CONDITION

The first step consists of expressing the solution of Equation A4.1 through an identity as a function of a fast term plus a mixed one, that is, a term with bandwidth B_Q and a term with both large and small frequencies.

It can be done by writing

$$c(r,t) = \int \frac{dQ(c_s(r,t), t)}{dt} dt = \int \left[\frac{\partial Q}{\partial t} + \frac{\partial Q}{\partial c_s} \frac{\partial c_s}{\partial t} \right] dt \tag{A4.7}$$

Since $c(r,t)$ is assumed to be a solution of Equation 3.1, let us substitute it into this equation, obtaining

$$\frac{\partial Q}{\partial t} + \frac{\partial Q}{\partial c_s} \frac{\partial c_s}{\partial t} = D\nabla^2 \int \left[\frac{\partial Q}{\partial t} + \frac{\partial Q}{\partial c_s} \frac{\partial c_s}{\partial t} \right] dt - \mathcal{F}(t,c) \tag{A4.8}$$

Owing to the definition of Q, the first and the last term simplifies so as to obtain

$$\frac{\partial Q}{\partial c_s}\frac{\partial c_s}{\partial t} = D\nabla^2 \int \left[\frac{\partial Q}{\partial t} + \frac{\partial Q}{\partial c_s}\frac{\partial c_s}{\partial t} \right] dt \qquad (A4.9)$$

Let us now express also the first term of Equation 3.8 as an integral, by deriving and integrating it with respect to time. At this point, since the integration extremes are generic, the two integrands have to be equal, getting

$$\frac{\partial Q}{\partial c_s}\frac{\partial^2 c_s}{\partial t^2} + \frac{\partial^2 Q}{\partial c_s^2}\left(\frac{\partial c_s}{\partial t}\right)^2 + \frac{\partial Q}{\partial t \partial c_s}\frac{\partial c_s}{\partial t} = D\nabla^2 \left[\frac{\partial Q}{\partial t} + \frac{\partial Q}{\partial c_s}\frac{\partial c_s}{\partial t} \right] \qquad (A4.10)$$

The term $\partial Q/\partial c_s$ has to be evaluated by maintaining c_s as an independent variable. Thus it does not depend on the space variables, that are comprised within the expression of c_s. Thus, we obtain

$$\frac{\partial Q}{\partial c_s}\frac{\partial^2 c_s}{\partial t^2} + \frac{\partial^2 Q}{\partial c_s^2}\left(\frac{\partial c_s}{\partial t}\right)^2 + \frac{\partial Q}{\partial t \partial c_s}\frac{\partial c_s}{\partial t} = D\frac{\partial Q}{\partial t \partial c_s}\nabla^2 c_s + D\frac{\partial Q}{\partial c_s}\nabla^2 \frac{\partial c_s}{\partial t} \qquad (A4.11)$$

Assuming that c_s is a solution of the diffusion equation with the correct problem conditions we have

$$\frac{\partial c_s}{\partial t} = \nabla^2 c_s \qquad (A4.12)$$

And, by deriving in time, we also get

$$\frac{\partial^2 c_s}{\partial t^2} = \nabla^2 \frac{\partial c_s}{\partial t} \qquad (A4.13)$$

Simplifying the corresponding terms, Equation A4.11 reduces at

$$\frac{\partial^2 Q}{\partial c_s^2}\left(\frac{\partial c_s}{\partial t}\right)^2 = 0 \qquad (A4.14)$$

This is a term of second order in the time derivative of the diffusion term. Thus, our approximation can be neglected and it is demonstrated that, if c_s is a solution of the associated diffusion equation, then $Q(c_s(r, t), t)$ is a solution of Equation 3.1 as the first order in the small derivative of the diffusion term.

A4.2.2 NECESSARY CONDITION

The proof of the necessity of the condition is obtained by the fact that the first-order development with respect to a small parameter is unique and also the solution of equations of type (A4.1) is unique [2] with the assigned conditions.

A4.2.3   COMMENTS ON THE SCALE SEPARATION METHOD

Equation A4.6 is exact in the case of a linear dependence of $Q(c_0, t)$ from the initial condition c_0 as it is demonstrated using the integrating factor method in Section 7.4.5. In this case, the second derivative $Q(c_0, t)$ of with respect to the initial condition is exactly zero and Equation A4.14 is exactly fulfilled.

Naturally, besides the base assumption regarding the slow dependence of the diffusion equation solution from time with respect to the chemical equation solution, the condition $\partial^2 Q/\partial c_s^2 \ll (\partial Q/\partial c_s), (\partial^2 Q/\partial c_s^2)$ is another condition in which Equation A4.6 is a good approximation of the solution of Equation A4.1.

REFERENCES

1. Smoller J., *Shock Waves and Reaction–Diffusion Equations*, Springer; 2nd edition (October 14, 1994), ISBN-13: 978-0387942599.
2. Crank J., *The Mathematics of Diffusion*, Oxford University Press, USA; 2nd edition (March 13, 1980), ISBN-13: 978-0198534112.
3. Smith G. D., *Numerical Solution of Partial Differential Equations: Finite Difference Methods*, Oxford University Press, USA; 3rd edition (January 16, 1986), ISBN-13: 978-0198596509.
4. Johnson C., *Numerical Solution of Partial Differential Equations by the Finite Element Method*, Dover Publications (January 15, 2009), ISBN-13: 978-0486469003.

Appendix 5: Elements of Bio-Electrochemistry

Electrochemistry is a wide branch of chemistry dealing with chemical processes in which molecules lose or acquire electrons. These processes can happen during chemical reactions when the molecules come in contact or in electrochemical cells, where electron exchange takes place near electrodes [1,2].

A few among the most used methods in analytical chemistry are electrochemical methods and they are widely used in lab on chip design for detection, quantification, and characterization of target molecules.

In this appendix, we recall a few concepts of electrochemistry that will be used in Chapter 10 to describe and analyze electrochemical methods used in lab on chip.

The general scheme of an electrochemical cell is reported in Figure A5.1: the cell is a container in which the two species constituting a RedOx couple are present in specific concentrations. If needed, in order to avoid direct reaction of the two species in solution, they are divided either by a permeable membrane or are directly contained in two different containers joined by a salt bridge to allow ions exchange between them. This is a common arrangement where the cell is meant to produce energy, like a battery, while in analytical systems the two species are generally hosted in the same container.

Three conducting electrodes are immersed in the sample: the cathode, the anode, and a reference electrode. The cathode is an electrode that during the working of the cell will lose electrons, whereas the anode will acquire them. In principle, since the potential difference between the anode and the cathode is the driving force of the processes taking place in the cell, two electrodes will be sufficient. In practice, however, due to the electrochemical processes taking place at the electrodes, both the necessary reactions and the unavoidable spurious reactions due to electrode surface defects and potential contamination, it is difficult to measure a stable potential difference using the anode and the cathode only. This problem is overcome by using a third electrode providing a potential reference to the cell. Since the reference electrode is built using an inert material, which is not involved in RedOx reactions during the cell working, this stabilizes the potential reference measure.

In dealing with electrochemistry, a particular formula is used to represent RedOx reactions, which is useful to introduce here. If we want to represent the following RedOx reaction:

$$A + B' \rightleftarrows A' + B \tag{A5.1}$$

where the species A oxidized while B is reduced, the reaction is represented in Figure A5.2a, where the direction of the arrow indicates the principal reaction direction and n_e is the number of exchanged electrons that is frequently neglected in the graphic formalism if it is not explicitly needed. Enzymes are frequently involved in biochemical RedOx processes to obtain the process catalysis. In this case, the enzyme is indicated at the center of the representation graph, as reported in Figure A5.2b.

A similar representation is adopted for a semi-reaction taking place near an electrode in an electrolytic cell. If we consider the oxidation

$$A \rightarrow A' + n_e\, e^- \tag{A5.2}$$

it can be represented as in Figure A5.3a, where the continuous surface represents the electrode, the anode in this case. When an enzyme is involved in the electrode semi-reaction the representation is

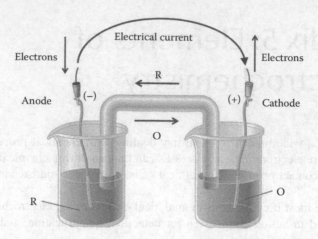

FIGURE A5.1 Principle scheme of an electrochemical cell where the passage of the reduced and oxidized species from one electrode to the other is allowed by a suitable structure like a salt bridge (as in the figure) or a semipermeable membrane.

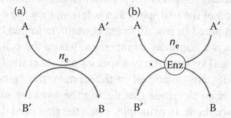

FIGURE A5.2 Formalism for the representation of a RedOx reaction: direct reaction (a) and enzyme-catalyzed reaction (b).

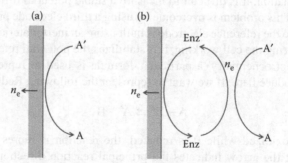

FIGURE A5.3 Formalism for the representation of a semi-RedOx reaction at an electrode (the anode in the figure case): direct reaction (a) and enzyme-catalyzed reaction (b).

modified as in Figure A5.3b, where the regeneration of the enzyme through electrons exchange with the electrode and with the RedOx species is evidenced.

A5.1 THE NERNST EQUATION

Let us consider a cell containing a solution of both R and O of known concentrations. The potential difference among the electrodes, when current flows through the circuit is due to the RedOx reaction taking place at the electrode surface. Let us write the electrode reactions as

$$R = O + n_e\, e^- \quad \text{(anode reaction)} \tag{A5.1a}$$

$$O + n_e\, e^- = R \quad \text{(cathode reaction)} \tag{A5.1b}$$

where n_e indicates the number of electrons that are exchanged by the single semi-reaction with the relative electrode. Since the current flow either generates electrical energy in the external circuit or is obtained at the expense of external electrical energy, has to balance the free energy change of the electrochemical cell due to the electrochemical reaction. If we assume that the reaction is completely reversible under a thermodynamic point of view this balance is exact and we can write

$$n_e N_a q \Delta\psi = -\Delta G \tag{A5.2}$$

where ΔG is a free energy per mole of substance, N_a is the Avogadro number, q the electron charge, and $\Delta\psi$ the potential difference among the electrodes. We can assume in practice that the semi-reactions are almost reversible when they are quite fast, so that no other phenomenon can enter to alter the balance (A5.2). When the electron exchange is slow, the assumption of thermodynamic reversibility is not acceptable. In this case, an empirical effectiveness factor α is inserted into Equation A5.2 to take into account nonreversible phenomena so that the energy balance becomes

$$\alpha n_e N_a q \Delta\psi = -\Delta G \tag{A5.3}$$

The factor α is smaller than 1 when the potential is applied by an external source, indicating that the external electrical energy is transformed in chemical energy with an efficiency smaller than 1, whereas it is greater than 1 when the system works like a battery, converting chemical energy into electrical energy in an external circuit. In this case, $1/\alpha$ represents the battery efficiency, that is the effective fraction of chemical energy that is transformed in electrical energy. Typical values of $1/\alpha$ in practical batteries comprises between 9.9 and 0.96 while, when the electrical energy is exploited to accumulate chemical energy in the cell, a wide range of values of α are observed in practice, depending on the RedOx couple that is under consideration and on the cell design, mainly on the electrodes material and shape.

Assuming a reversible reaction, we can say that the system is in thermodynamic equilibrium in every moment so that the difference of a state function along the transformation does not depend on the transformation itself but only on the initial and final state. Let us consider a single electrode semi-reaction, for example, the anode reaction (5.1a). Applying Equation 1.33 that gives the chemical potential of the reaction we can write

$$\mu_a = \mu_{0a} + RT \ln\left(\frac{\bar{c}_R}{\bar{c}_o}\right) \tag{A5.4}$$

where μ_{0a} is the chemical potential of the solution on the anode surface when the ratio of the surface concentrations of R and O, called $\bar{c}_R$ and $\bar{c}_O$, respectively are equal. Dividing by the charge of a mole transformed substance to pass from molar chemical potential to electrical potential we can write

$$\Delta\psi_a = \Delta\psi_{0a} - \frac{\kappa_B T}{q\, n_e} \ln\left(\frac{\bar{c}_o}{\bar{c}_R}\right) \tag{A5.5}$$

where κ_B is the Boltzmann constant and the electrical potentials are referred to the standard reference electrode. To evaluate standard potentials, the hydrogen reference electrode has been standardized, since it was the first reference electrode to be used by Nernst for determination of electrochemical potentials. Naturally, hydrogen electrodes are no more used in practice, replaced by much more stable and reliable solid state reference electrodes. Any electrode that is inert in the considered situation and has a stable potential difference with respect to a hydrogen electrode can be used as a reference electrode, adding to absolute potentials the difference between the potentials of the adopted electrode and of an hydrogen electrode. Potential differences, that are generally more important than absolute values, are naturally unaffected by the adopted reference.

Equation A5.5 is known as Nernst equation for the anode reaction. Similarly, for the cathode reaction it can be written as

$$\Delta \psi_c = \psi_{0c} - \frac{\kappa_B T}{q n_e} \ln \left(\frac{\overline{c}_R}{\overline{c}_o} \right) \tag{A5.6}$$

The potentials $\Delta \psi_{0a}$ and $\Delta \psi_{0c}$ are called formal anode and cathode potentials. Their expression can be derived by considering the cell at equilibrium, where no current flows, so that $\Delta \psi_c = 0$.

Considering the anode as example we have in this case

$$\psi_{0a} = \frac{\kappa_B T}{q n_e} \ln \left(\frac{\overline{c}_o}{\overline{c}_R} \right) = \frac{\kappa_B T}{q n_e} \ln k_{an} \tag{A5.7}$$

where we have used the mass action law for the anode semi-reaction (see Section 1.2.3) and we have indicated with k_{an} the anode electrons exchange rate. With a similar procedure, if we consider the cathode, we get

$$\psi_{0c} = \frac{\kappa_B T}{q n_e} \ln k_{cat} \tag{A5.8}$$

One important conclusion that we can draw is that the electrons exchange rates can be measured by the measure of the formal potentials, so that this is also an indication if a certain RedOx reaction can be considered reversible or not.

In general, it is not simple to relate the concentrations of the RedOx species on the electrodes surface with the concentrations in the bulk of the solution in the cell. This problem is extensively treated in Chapter 10 in lab on chip conditions, where diffusion is the only means of transport of molecules and the cell is designed for analytical application. If the cell is sufficiently small that the characteristic time for mass transport is of the order of the dynamic rate of the electrons transfer, that happens for example when strong convection happens in the solution. The surface concentration divided by the characteristic length of the thin layer around the electrode surface when the reaction happens can be identified with the concentration in the solution bulk.

In this case, it is possible to introduce a form of the Nernst equation for the whole electrochemical cell as

$$\Delta \psi = \psi_c - \psi_a = \psi_0 - \frac{\kappa_B T}{q n_e} \ln \left(\frac{c_R}{c_o} \right) \tag{A5.9}$$

where $\Delta \psi_0$ is called formal potential of the RedOx reaction, C_R and C_O are the concentrations of R and O, respectively, and

$$\psi_0 = \frac{\kappa_B T}{q n_e} \ln \left(\frac{k_{cat}}{k_{an}} \right) = \frac{\kappa_B T}{q n_e} \ln(k) \tag{A5.10}$$

where k is the global kinetic coefficient of the RedOx reaction.

TABLE A5.1
List of the Formal Potentials of Common Oxidation and Reduction Semi-Reactions

Semi-Reaction	$-\Delta\psi_{0o}$ (V)	Semi-Reaction	$\Delta\psi_{0R}$ (V)
$Li^+ + e^- \rightleftarrows Li$	3.045	$2H_3O^+ + 2e^- \rightleftarrows H_2 + 2H_2O$	0.000
$K^+ + e^- \rightleftarrows K$	2.924	$NO_3^- + H_2O + 2e^- \rightleftarrows NO_2^- + 2OH^-$	0.01
$Ca^{2+} + 2e^- \rightleftarrows Ca$	2.76	$S_4O_6^{2-} + 2e^- \rightleftarrows 2S_2O_3^{2-}$	0.08
$Na^+ + e^- \rightleftarrows Na$	2.7109	$S + 2H_3O^+ + 2e^- \rightleftarrows H_2S + 2H_2O$	0.14
$Mg^{2+} + 2e^- \rightleftarrows Mg$	2.375	$Sn^{4+} + 2e^- \rightleftarrows Sn^{2+}$ (in HCl 1F)	0.15
$H_3O^+ + e^- \rightleftarrows H_2O + H$	2.10	$Cu^{2+} + e^- \rightleftarrows Cu^+$	0.158
$Al^{3+} + 3e^- \rightleftarrows Al$	1.71	$Hg_2Cl_2 + 2e^- \rightleftarrows 2Hg + 2Cl^-$	0.2682
$Ti^{2+} + 2e^- \rightleftarrows Ti$	1.63	$Cu^{2+} + 2e^- \rightleftarrows Cu$	0.337
$ZnO_2^{2-} + 2H_2O + 2e^- \rightleftarrows Zn + 4OH^-$	1.22	$O_2 + 2H_2O + 4e^- \rightleftarrows 4OH^-$	0.401
$Mn^{2+} + 2e^- \rightleftarrows Mn$	1.03	$Cu^+ + e^- \rightleftarrows Cu$	0.521
$2H_2O + 2e^- \rightleftarrows H_2 + 2OH^-$	0.826	$I_2 + 2e^- \rightleftarrows 2I^-$	0.535
$Zn^{2+} + 2e^- \rightleftarrows Zn$	0.7628	$O_2 + 2H_3O^+ + 2e^- \rightleftarrows H_2O_2 + 2H_2O$	0.682
$Cr^{3+} + 3e^- \rightleftarrows Cr$	0.74	$Fe^{3+} + e^- \rightleftarrows Fe^{2+}$	0.771
$Te + 2H_3O^+ + 2e^- \rightleftarrows H_2Te + 2H_2O$	0.72	$Hg^{2+} + 2e^- \rightleftarrows 2Hg$	0.7961
$As + 3H_3O^+ + 3e^- \rightleftarrows AsH_3 + 3H_2O$	0.60	$Ag^+ + e^- \rightleftarrows Ag$	0.7996
$Cr^{2+} + 2e^- \rightleftarrows Cr$	0.557	$2NO_3^- + 4H_3O^+ + 2e^- \rightleftarrows N_2O_4 + 6H_2O$	0.80
$H_3PO_2 + H_3O^+ + e^- \rightleftarrows P + 3H_2O$	0.51	$NO_3^- + 3H_3O^+ + 2e^- \rightleftarrows HNO_2 + 4H_2O$	0.94
$Fe^{2+} + 2e^- \rightleftarrows Fe$	0.409	$NO_3^- + 4H_3O^+ + 3e^- \rightleftarrows NO + 6H_2O$	0.96
$Cr^{3+} + e^- \rightleftarrows Cr^{2+}$	0.41	$Br_2 + 2e^- \rightleftarrows 2Br^-$	1.065
$Cd^{2+} + 2e^- \rightleftarrows Cd$	0.4026	$Pt^{2+} + 2e^- \rightleftarrows Pt$	1.2
$Se + 2H_3O^+ + 2e^- \rightleftarrows H_2Se + 2H_2O$	0.40	$MnO_2 + 4H_3O^+ + 2e^- \rightleftarrows Mn^{2+} + 6H_2O$	1.21
$Tl^+ + e^- \rightleftarrows Tl$	0.3363	$O_2^- + 4H_3O^+ + 4e^- \rightleftarrows 6H_2O$	1.229
$Co^{2+} + 2e^- \rightleftarrows Co$	0.277	$Cr_2O_7^{2-} + 14H_3O^+ + 6e^- \rightleftarrows 2Cr^{3+} + 21H_2O$	1.33
$Ni^{2+} + 2e^- \rightleftarrows Ni$	0.230	$Cl_2 + 2e^- \rightleftarrows 2Cl^-$	1.356
$N_2 + 5H_3O^+ + 4e^- \rightleftarrows N_2H_3^+ + 5H_2O$	0.23	$ClO_3^- + 6H_3O^+ + 6e^- \rightleftarrows 6Cl^- + 9H_2O$	1.45
$Sn^{2+} + 2e^- \rightleftarrows Sn$	0.1364	$PbO_2 + 4H_3O^+ + 2e^- \rightleftarrows Pb^{2+} + 6H_2O$	1.455
$Pb^{2+} + 2e^- \rightleftarrows Pb$	0.1263	$MnO_4^- + 8H_3O^+ + 5e^- \rightleftarrows Mn^{2+} + 12H_2O$	1.50
		$2HClO + 2H_3O^+ + 2e^- \rightleftarrows Cl_2 + 4H_2O$	1.63
		$H_2O_2 + 2H_3O^+ + 2e^- \rightleftarrows 4H_2O$	1.776
		$Co^{3+} + e^- \rightleftarrows Co^{2+}$ (in HNO_3 3F)	1.842
		$F_2 + 2e^- \rightleftarrows 2F^-$	2.87

Note: The values are referred to the standard hydrogen electrode, and evaluated at 25°C.

Rigorously, the Nernst equation is valid only for completely reversible RedOx reactions, however, if a small degree of irreversibility is present, that is α is very near to one, the Nernst equation is frequently used after its phenomenological modification by the insertion of a coefficient in front of the potential.

A list of the formal potentials of common oxidation and reduction semi-reactions of inorganic species is reported in Table A5.1.

A5.2 REDOX POTENTIAL OF BIOMOLECULES

If biological macromolecules are considered, the RedOx reaction is driven by well-specified RedOx sites in the molecule. Considering proteins, strong RedOx sites are present in metal-binding proteins that has been the first RedOx proteins to be studied [4,5]. In this case, the RedOx sites are generally the metal-binding sites. A good example is the protein containing the nFe-mS group, where n and m are integer numbers. These are called iron–sulfur proteins and the RedOx properties of such molecules are driven by the Fe atoms that are bonded to the sulfur-containing site. Cytochrome is another well-known RedOx protein [6].

Many nonmetal proteins, however, show electrochemical activity due to the possibility of exchanging electrons with a suitable electrode through specific active sites [7–9].

Differently from the case of small inorganic molecules, the formal potential of a RedOx semi-reaction depends on the protein tertiary structure [10] that determines the accessibility of the RedOx site, and on the conditions in which the semi-reaction happens. Important factors are the species that are present besides the protein in the solution and the state of the electrode surface. Thus, even fixing the electrode type and the solution pH, the formal RedOx potentials for proteins generally are comprised within a range instead of having well-defined values, as shown in Table A5.2. Moreover, the formal potential for RedOx proteins is influenced also by part of the protein that are far from the RedOx site, mainly due to the fact that they influence the steric structure of the protein. This is demonstrated in many cases by the fact that substituting a lateral residue of the protein, that is not a part of the RedOx site, the formal potential can have relevant changes [6].

The electrochemistry of nucleic acids has been studied in detail both for its importance in biological reactions and for its analytical relevance [11]. Formal potentials of the nucleobases have been both experimentally measured and theoretically estimated with a good agreement with measured values [12]. To do this, the nucleobases are generally attached to a small support molecule instead of to the nucleic acid backbone to be able to study them individually. The methylated form of nucleobases, that is the nucleobase saturated with a methyl radical where it is connected to the backbone in a DNA, is the most used and structure formulas of methylated nucleobases are reported in Figure A5.4, while relative electrochemical data are reported in Table A5.3.

Carbohydrates are perhaps the biological molecule that more easily experience RedOx reactions due to their nature of fuel of living beings. The single carbohydrate unit CO_2/CH_2O has a redox potential of −470 mV at pH 7 and 25°C and it changes at −60 mV for each change of a unit in pH.

TABLE A5.2
Ranges for Formal Redox Potential for Selected RedOx Proteins

Redox Complex	Protein	$\Delta\psi_0$ Range (mV)	pH	Reference
4 Fe cluster	[7Fe–8S] Ferredoxins	−645 to −400	7	[4]
4 Fe cluster	[8Fe–8S] Ferredoxins	−500 to −390	7	[4]
3 Fe cluster	[7Fe–8S] Ferredoxins	−455 to −140	7	[4]
2 Fe cluster	[2Fe–4S] Ferredoxins	−435 to −230	7	[4]
4 Fe cluster	[4Fe–8S] Ferredoxins	−422 to −270	7	[4]
Heme binding site[a]	H10A24	−265 to −170[b]	8	[5]
Heme binding site	VAVH$_{25}$	−170[b]	8	[5]
Heme Binding Site[a]	MOP1	−170 to −110[b]	8	[5]
Heme binding site	H11A24	−166[b]	8	[5]
3 Fe cluster	[3Fe–4S] Ferredoxins	−142 to −121	7	[4]
Rubredoxins	—	−65 to 30	7	[4]
4 Fe cluster	HiP1P	81–500	7	[4]
Horse heart cytochrome c	—	262	7	[6]

[a] Indicates that the protein binds heme in two similar sites.

[b] Indicates that the half-way potential $\psi_{1/2}$ is measured, that can be approximated in the considered situation with the formal potential.

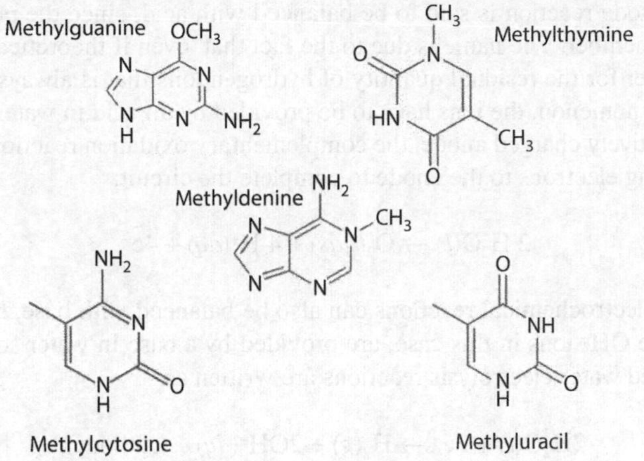

Methylguanine OCH₃   Methylthymine

Methyldenine NH₂

Methylcytosine   Methyluracil

FIGURE A5.4   Structure formulas of the methylated forms of the nucleobases.

TABLE A5.3

Formal Potential of the Methylated Forms of the Nucleobases in a Specific Isomer Form Indicated by the Number Preceding Their Name, all Data at 25°D and pH = 7

	Formal Potential (V)	
Nucleobase	Theoretical	Experimental
9-Methylguanine	1.37	1.58
9-Methyladenine	1.79	2.03
1-Methylcytosine	2.07	–
1-Methylthymine	1.86	–
1 Methyluracil	2.13	–

Source: Data from Psciuk B. T. et al., *Journal of Chemical Theory and Computation*, vol. 8, pp. 5107–5123, 2012.

In a reaction where a carbohydrate chain is oxidized each unit reacts almost independently so that the overall freed energy is approximately equivalent to the energy freed by each unit multiplied by the number of units.

A5.3   THE FARADAY EQUATION

Faraday's law is the fundamental law of electrolysis. An electrolytic phenomenon takes place in an electrochemical cell when the material undergoing a RedOx reaction at an electrode leaves the cell instead of remaining inside the cell and participating eventually to the opposite reaction at the other electrode.

A common example is water electrolysis. In pure water at the negatively charged cathode, a reduction reaction takes place, with electrons from the cathode being transferred to hydrogen cations to form hydrogen gas so as to give rise to the cathode semi-reaction:

$$2H^+(aq) + 2e^- \rightarrow H_2(gas) \tag{A5.11a}$$

This form of cathode reaction is said to be balanced with acid, since the positive hydrogen ion appears as the first member. The name is due to the fact that, even if theoretically water hydrolysis happens in pure water for the residual quantity of hydrogen ions that is always present, in order to obtain a sizeable phenomenon, the ions have to be provided by an acid in water solution, for example, HCl. At the positively charged anode, the complementary oxidation reaction occurs, generating oxygen gas and giving electrons to the anode to complete the circuit:

$$2\,H_2O(l) \rightarrow O_2(gas) + 4\,H^+(aq) + 4e^- \tag{A5.11b}$$

The same set of electrochemical reactions can also be balanced with base, that is, the ions driving the reactions, the OH^- ions in this case, are provided by a base in water solution, for example, NaOH. Base balanced water electrolysis reactions are written as

$$2H_2O(l) + 2e^- \rightarrow H_2(g) + 2OH^-(aq) \quad \text{(cathode)} \tag{A5.12a}$$

$$4OH^-\,(aq) \rightarrow O_2(g) + 2H_2O(l) + 4e^- \quad \text{(anode)} \tag{A5.12b}$$

Combining half-reaction pair yields the same overall decomposition of water into oxygen and hydrogen. Since both oxygen and hydrogen are produced in gaseous form they leave the electrolytic cell and no more participate in the electrochemical reactions.

The Faraday law of electrolysis relates the mass M of a substance that is freed at one electrode and the quantity Q of charge is absorbed at the electrode. The resulting equation can be directly derived from the observation that if N molecules react and each molecule has a molar mass m and releases or absorbs n_e electrons we can write

$$Q = n_e N q \tag{A5.13}$$

Multiplying both members by m/N_a, that is the molecular mass of the substance, after rearranging the terms we obtain

$$M = \frac{Q}{qN_A}\frac{m}{n_e} = \frac{Q}{F}\frac{m}{n_e} \tag{A5.14}$$

where $F = qN_A$ is the so-called Faraday constant. Due to the definition of transferred electrical charge, it can be expressed as the integral of the electrical current in the measurement interval so that the Faraday law can be also written as

$$M = \frac{m}{qn_e N_A}\int_0^t I(\tau)\,d\tau \tag{A5.15}$$

REFERENCES

1. Hamann C. H., Hamnett A., Vielstich W., *Electrochemistry*, Wiley-VCH; 2nd edition (April 9, 2007), ISBN-13: 978-3527310692.
2. Bard A. J., Faulkner L. R., *Electrochemical Methods: Fundamentals and Applications*, Wiley; 2nd edition (December 18, 2000), ISBN-13: 978-0471043720.
3. Wang J., *Analytical Electrochemistry*, Wiley-VCH; 3rd edition (April 28, 2006), ISBN-13: 978-047167879.
4. Bott A. V., Redox properties of electron transfer metalloproteins, *Current Separations*, vol. 18, pp. 47–54, 1999.

5. Moffet D. A., Foley J., Hecht M. H., Midpoint reduction potentials and heme binding stoichiometries of de novo proteins from designed combinatorial libraries, *Biophysical Chemistry*, vol. 105, pp. 231–239, 2003.

6. Rodkey F. K., Ball E. G., Oxidation–reduction potentials of the cytochrome c system, *Biological Chemistry*, vol. 182, pp. 17–20, 1950.

7. Chiku M., Nakamura J., Fujishima A., Einaga Y., Conformational change detection in nonmetal proteins by direct electrochemical oxidation using diamond electrodes, *Analytical Chemistry*, vol. 80, pp. 5783–5787, 2008.

8. Mazzei F., et al., Soft-landed protein voltammetry: A tool for redox protein characterization, *Analytical Chemistry*, vol. 80, pp. 5937–5944, 2008.

9. Hu N., Direct electrochemistry of redox proteins or enzymes at various film electrodes and their possible applications in monitoring some pollutants, *Pure and Applied Chemistry*, vol. 73, pp. 1979–1991, 2001.

10. Mao J., Hauser K., Gunner M. R., How cytochromes with different folds control heme redox potentials, *Biochemistry*, vol. 42, pp. 9829–9840, 2003.

11. Paleček E., František J., Electrochemistry of nucleic acids, in Perspectives in Bioanalysis, vol. 1, *Electrochemistry of Nucleic Acids and Proteins*, Paleček E., Scheller F., Wang J. editors, Elsevier Science, 1st edition (February 3, 2006), ISBN-13: 978–0444521507.

12. Psciuk B. T., Lord R. L., Munk B. H., Schlegel H. B., Theoretical determination of one-electron oxidation potentials for nucleic acid bases, *Journal of Chemical Theory and Computation*, vol. 8, pp. 5107–5123, 2012.

Appendix 6: Detection Requirements of Selected Clinical Blood Tests

One of the key diagnostic analyses in almost all human disorders is the blood test. A large number of chemical and biochemical substances provide important information when quantized in blood, which are used for medical diagnosis.

Blood tests are quite different in scope, requiring the assaying of ions and small molecules, proteins and other macromolecules such as carbohydrates, and cells of different types. A few assays require accurate quantification of substances that are present in relevant quantities, as albumin, while other assays require the quantification of very diluted substances, such as Troponin I and R.

Thus, considering the characteristics that are required in standard blood tests is very useful to have an idea of the requirements of lab on chip in terms of assay sensitivity.

Here, we cannot consider all the possible blood biochemical analysis that are used in the medical practice, but we will restrict ourselves only to the most frequent tests reported through a set of tables, the tested substance and a reference range of concentrations in healthy human blood. In interpreting these tables an important comment is necessary.

Standard levels of a huge number of substances in healthy human blood are defined by several medical bodies in the world, both related to public health administrations and to private companies like large hospitals. Different levels are often defined for a selected substance by different bodies and discussions exist on the clinical interpretation of individual values and of the correlation among different values.

It is completely beyond the scope of this book to open up such a discussion. Thus, the tables presented in this chapter do not aim to define reference levels usable for clinical purposes. They provide a reference for the design of lab on chip aimed to detect selected substances, so that very precise values are not required. This aim is also transparent from the adopted measurement units; we have used possible biochemical units, in line with units adopted in lab on chip design. Sometimes different units are adopted in the clinical practice that are defined in appropriate References [1,2].

The first set of substances that can be quantized in blood for diagnosis is related to base metabolism. They are ions such as sodium, potassium, chloride, bicarbonate, magnesium, and calcium, besides a set of small molecules such as blood urea nitrogen (BUN), creatinine, glucose LDL, and HDL cholesterol, as well as triglyceride. Levels of selected substances of this group in healthy blood are reported in Table A6.1 [1,2].

Another important set of substances that are frequently quantized in blood are blood proteins and hormones. A classification of the most common blood proteins has been reported in Section 3.6.2 in connection with the use of macroscopic electrophoresis to detect them from human plasma or serum. However, more diluted proteins can be important indicators in the diagnosis of several disorders, such as Troponin I and R for heart attacks [3,4] and the D-dimer for the diagnosis of deep-venous thrombosis [5,6].

Particular proteins like the Carbohydrate Antigen 19-9 (CA 19-9), the Carbohydrate Antigen 125 (CA125), and many others are used as tumor markers to monitor the effect of tumor therapy [7–9].

Several hormones are also quantified in blood either for diseases prevention or for therapy monitoring. Sex-related hormones are in addition detected and quantified for the control of the female reproductive cycle and for pregnancy detection and monitoring. Selected hormones quantified in human blood for clinical purposes are reported in Table A6.2 [7,9,10]. Hormones are present in the human serum, that is, blood after removal of cells. Besides hormones, enzymes are quite used in

TABLE A6.1

Reference Levels of Selected Ions and Metabolic Substances in Healthy Blood

Test	Low	High	Unit
Sodium	135	145	mmol/L
Potassium	3.5	5.0	mmol/L
Chloride	98	106	mmol/L
Calcium	2.2	2.6	mmol/L
Phosphorus	0.87	1.49	mmol/L
Iron (in serum)—male	11.6	32	μmol/L
Iron (in serum)—female	4.6	30.4	μmol/L
Copper	11	24	μmol/L
Zinc	9.2	20	μmol/L
Magnesium	0.6	0.85	μmol/L
Urea	2.5	6.4	mmol/L
Creatinine—male	62	115	μmol/L
Creatinine—female	53	97	μmol/L
Glucose	3.9	5.8	mmol/L

Source: Adapted from Burtis C. A., Bruns D. E., *Tietz Fundamentals of Clinical Chemistry*, Saunders; 6th edition (November 20, 2007), ISBN-13: 978-0721638652; McKenzie S. B., *Clinical Laboratory Hematology*, Prentice-Hall; 2nd edition (2010), ISBN-13: 978-0135137321.

Note: All values are referred to blood serum.

TABLE A6.2

Reference Levels for Selected Hormones in Healthy Blood

Hormone	Type	Patient Type	Lower	Upper	Unit
Free tyroxine (FT4)	Tyr.	Adult	10	18	pmol/L
Free triiodothyronine (FT3)	Tyr.	Adult	3.1	7.7	pmol/L
Thyroglobulin (Tg)	Tyr.	—	1.5	30	pmol/L
Testosterone	Sex	Male adult	8	35	nmol/L
Testosterone	Sex	Female adult	0.7	2.8	nmol/L
17-Hydroxyprogesterone	Sex	Male adult	0.18	9.1	μmol/L
17-Hydroxyprogesterone	Sex	Female adult in follicular phase	0.6	3.0	μmol/L
Estradiol	Sex	Adult male	50	200	pmol/L
Estradiol	Sex	Adult female: follicular and luteal phase	70	600	pmol/L
Estradiol	Sex	Adult female post-menopausal	0	130	pmol/L
Progesterone	Sex	Female adult in mid-lutean phase	17	92	nmol/L
Parathyroid hormone (PTH)	—	Adult	1.5	7.2	pmol/L
Adrenocorticotropic hormone (ACTH)	—	Adult	4.4	20	pmo/L

Source: Adapted from Burtis C. A., Bruns D. E., *Tietz Fundamentals of Clinical Chemistry*, Saunders; 6th edition (November 20, 2007), ISBN-13: 978-0721638652; Chernecky C. C., Berger B. J., *Laboratory Tests and Diagnostic Procedures*, Saunders; 6th edition (December 4, 2012), ISBN-13: 978-1455706945; Medline plus on-line encyclopedia, a service of U.S. National Library of Medicine (NLM) and National Institutes of Health (NIH), http://www.nlm.nih.gov/medlineplus/ency, last accessed on June 20, 2013.

Note: All values are referred to blood serum. Thyr. indicates that the considered hormone is used for assessment of thyroid functionality, Sex indicates that it is a hormone related to sexual activity.

TABLE A6.3
Reference Level for Selected Enzymes in Healthy Blood

Enzyme	Type	Patient Type	Lower	Upper	Unit
Alanine transaminase (ALT)	Liv.	Female adult	0.15	0.75	μkat/L
Alanine transaminase (ALT)	Liv.	Male adult	0.15	1.10	μkat/L
Aspartate transaminase (AST)	Liv.	Female adult	0.25	0.60	μkat/L
Aspartate transaminase (AST)	Liv.	Male adult	0.25	0.75	μkat/L
Lactate dehydrogenase (LDH)	—	Adult	1.8	3.4	μkat/L
Amylase	—	Adult	0.15	1.1	μkat/L
Creatine kinase (CK)	—	Male adult	0.42	1.5	μkat/L
Creatine kinase (CK)	—	Female adult	0.17	1.17	μkat/L

Source: Adapted from Burtis C. A., Bruns D. E., *Tietz Fundamentals of Clinical Chemistry*, Saunders; 6th edition (November 20, 2007), ISBN-13: 978-0721638652; Medline plus on-line encyclopedia, a service of U.S. National Library of Medicine (NLM) and National Institutes of Health (NIH), http://www.nlm.nih.gov/medlineplus/ency, last accessed on June 20, 2013.

Note: All values are referred to blood serum. Liv. indicates that the considered hormone is used for assessment of liver functionality. Hormone levels are expressed in units of enzyme activity (kat/L) (see Section 2.5).

diagnostic activity, for example, for the assessment of liver functionality. A list of selected blood enzymes with their reference concentrations is reported in Table A6.3 [1,10].

Antibodies are also frequently quantified in blood to detect the body's reaction to disorders, to detect and monitor immunity system diseases, to monitor the immunity system's reaction to the presence of selected pathogens, and to monitor allergic reactions. Generally, two types of immunoglobulin tests are performed: general tests in which the concentration of selected immunoglobulin types are measured without distinguishing antibodies with different specificity and tests in which antibodies that are specific to a selected antigen are specifically searched. Reference levels in healthy adult human blood for different types of antibodies are reported in Table A6.4 [1,10].

Finally, among proteins, lipoproteins are searched to measure the quantity of lipids that are present in blood and vitamins are searched for a variety of clinical reasons. Tables of reference levels for lipoproteins and vitamins are reported in Tables A6.5 and A6.6 [1,9,10].

Besides proteins, search for nucleic acids in blood is becoming increasingly important not only for its forensic use, where the DNA is used as the main way of recognizing the identity of a person from its biological traces [11,12], but also in medical diagnostics. The possibility of designing

TABLE A6.4
Reference Level for Different Types of Antibodies in Healthy Blood

Antibody Type	Lower	Upper	Unit
IgA	100	500	mg/dL
IgD	0.5	3.0	mg/dL
IgE	0.01	0.04	mg/dL
IgG	800	1800	mg/dL
IgM	54	220	mg/dL

Source: Adapted from Burtis C. A., Bruns D. E., *Tietz Fundamentals of Clinical Chemistry*, Saunders; 6th edition (November 20, 2007), ISBN-13: 978-0721638652; Medline plus on-line encyclopedia, a service of U.S. National Library of Medicine (NLM) and National Institutes of Health (NIH), http://www.nlm.nih.gov/medlineplus/ency, last accessed on June 20, 2013.

Note: All values are referred to blood serum and to an adult patient.

TABLE A6.5
Reference Level for Selected Lipoproteins in Healthy Blood

Lipoprotein	Patient Type	Lower	Upper	Unit
HDL cholesterol	Female adult	1.15	2.2	mmol/L
HDL cholesterol	Male adult	0.9	2.0	mmol/L
LDL cholesterol	—	2.2	3.2	mmol/L

Source: Adapted from Burtis C. A., Bruns D. E., *Tietz Fundamentals of Clinical Chemistry*, Saunders; 6th edition (November 20, 2007), ISBN-13: 978-0721638652; Chernecky C. C., Berger B. J., *Laboratory Tests and Diagnostic Procedures*, Saunders; 6th edition (December 4, 2012), ISBN-13: 978-1455706945; Medline plus on-line encyclopedia, a service of U.S. National Library of Medicine (NLM) and National Institutes of Health (NIH), http://www.nlm.nih.gov/medlineplus/ency, last accessed on June 20, 2013.

TABLE A6.6
Reference Level for Selected Vitamins in Healthy Blood

Vitamin	Lower	Upper	Unit
A	30	65	µg/dL
B_9 (serum)	3	16	ng/mL
B_{12}	140	800	ng/L
Homocysteine	45	210	µg/dL
C	0.4	1.5	mg/dL
D	8	80	ng/mL
E	1.2	—	mg/dL

Source: Adapted from Burtis C. A., Bruns D. E., *Tietz Fundamentals of Clinical Chemistry*, Saunders; 6th edition (November 20, 2007), ISBN-13: 978-0721638652, Chernecky C. C., Berger B. J., *Laboratory Tests and Diagnostic Procedures*, Saunders; 6th edition (December 4, 2012), ISBN-13: 978-1455706945; Medline plus on-line encyclopedia, a service of U.S. National Library of Medicine (NLM) and National Institutes of Health (NIH), http://www.nlm.nih.gov/medlineplus/ency, last accessed on June 20, 2013.
Note: All values are referred to blood serum and to an adult patient.

TABLE A6.7
Average Values of Blood Cells Count in Healthy Adults

Red Cells	4.50	5.30	10^6 Per Cube Millimeter
Platelets	130	400	10^3
White cells	4.8	10.8	10^3
Neutrophils	1.50	6.50	10^3
Lymphocytes	1.20	3.40	10^3
Monocytes	0.30	0.60	10^3
Eosinophils	0.10	0.80	10^3
Basophils	0.01	0.20	10^3

Source: Adapted from Rodgers G. P., Young N. S., *The Bethesda Handbook of Clinical Hematology*, Lippincott Williams & Wilkins; 3rd edition (May 20, 2013), ISBN-13: 978-1451182705; Rodak B. F., Carr J. H., *Clinical Hematology Atlas*, Saunders; 4th edition (April 17, 2012), ISBN-13: 978-1455708307; Medline plus on-line encyclopedia, a service of U.S. National Library of Medicine (NLM) and National Institutes of Health (NIH), http://www.nlm.nih.gov/medlineplus/ency, last accessed on June 20, 2013.

practical lab on chip for sequencing of parts of human DNA prelude to a possible revolution in the way important disorders are discovered in a very early stage or even before their manifestation [13,14]. In addition, the identification of the small nucleic acid molecules called miRNA (see Section 2.6.3.2) could be a key instrument for an early diagnosis of cancer [15–17].

Finally, a large number of blood tests are related to the abundance and functionality of blood cells. Not only are cell counts in blood important to determine the efficiency of processes like oxygen transport and blood coagulation and to measure the intensity of the ongoing immune system activity, but the functionality of cells is also monitored.

The hemoglobin content of red cells and the percentage of heme groups that bind oxygen inside blood cells are commonly measured through suitable analytical tests. Normal values for blood cell counts are reported in Table A6.7 [18,19].

REFERENCES

1. Burtis C. A., Bruns D. E., *Tietz Fundamentals of Clinical Chemistry*, Saunders; 6th edition (November 20, 2007), ISBN-13: 978-0721638652.
2. McKenzie S. B., *Clinical Laboratory Hematology*, Prentice-Hall; 2nd edition (2010), ISBN-13: 978-0135137321.
3. Babuin L. Jaffe A. S., Troponin: The biomarker of choice for the detection of cardiac injury, *Canadian Medical Association Journal*, vol. 173, pp. 1191–2002, 2005.
4. Ilva T. et al., Clinical significance of cardiac troponins I and T in acute heart failure, *European Journal of Heart Failure*, vol. 10, pp. 772–779, 2008.
5. Haemostasis and Thrombosis Task Force of the British Committee for Standards in Haematology, The Diagnosis of Deep Vein Thrombosis in Symptomatic Outpatients and the Potential for Clinical Assessment and D-Dimer Assays to Reduce the Need for Diagnostic Imaging, *British Journal of Haematology*, vol. 124, pp. 15–25, 2004.
6. Hayag J. E., Manchanda P. P., Predictive value of the rapid whole blood agglutination D-dimer assay (AGEN SimpliRED) in community outpatients with suspected deep venous thrombosis, *The Permanente Journal*, vol. 10, pp. 16–20, 2006.
7. Koepke J. A., Molecular marker test standardization, *Cancer*, vol. 69, 6 Suppl, pp. 1578–1581, 1992.
8. Bjerner J., et al. Reference intervals for carcinoembryonic antigen (CEA), CA125, MUC1, Alfa-Foeto-Protein (AFP), Neuron-Specific Enolase (NSE) and CA19.9 from the NORIP Study, *Scandinavian Journal of Clinical and Laboratory Investigation*, vol. 68, pp. 1–12, 2008.
9. Chernecky C. C., Berger B. J., *Laboratory Tests and Diagnostic Procedures*, Saunders; 6th edition (December 4, 2012), ISBN-13: 978-1455706945.
10. Medline plus on-line encyclopedia, a service of U.S. National Library of Medicine (NLM) and National Institutes of Health (NIH), http://www.nlm.nih.gov/medlineplus/ency, last accessed on June 20, 2013.
11. Butler J. M., *Fundamentals of Forensic DNA Typing*, Academic Press; 1st edition (September 3, 2009), ISBN-13: 978-0123749994.
12. Elkins K. M., *Forensic DNA Biology: A Laboratory Manual*, Academic Press; 1st edition (September 25, 2012), ISBN-13: 978-0123945853.
13. Hu P, Hegde M., Lennon P. A., editors, *Modern Clinical Molecular Techniques*, Springer; 2012 edition (May 14, 2012), ISBN-13: 978-1461421696.
14. Makowski G. editor, *Advances in Clinical Chemistry Series*, Academic Press; 1st edition (April 13, 2012), ISBN-13: 978-0123943842.
15. He L. et al., A microRNA polycistron as a potential human oncogene, *Nature*, vol. 435, pp. 828–833, 2005.
16. Lu J. et al., MicroRNA expression profiles classify human cancers, *Nature*, vol. 435, pp. 834–838, 2005.
17. Sassen S., Miska E. A., Caldas C., MicroRNA—Implications for Cancer, *Virchows Archiv*, vol. 452, pp. 1–10, 2008.
18. Rodgers G. P., Young N. S., *The Bethesda Handbook of Clinical Hematology*, Lippincott Williams & Wilkins; 3rd edition (May 20, 2013), ISBN-13: 978-1451182705.
19. Rodak B. F., Carr J. H., *Clinical Hematology Atlas*, Saunders; 4th edition (April 17, 2012), ISBN-13: 978-1455708307.

Index

A